Landmarks in Cardiac Surgery

Landmarks in Cardiac Surgery

By

Stephen Westaby

BSc, MS, FRCS

Oxford Heart Centre
John Radcliffe Hospital
Oxford, UK

with

Cecil Bosher

Toronto, Canada

ISIS
MEDICAL
MEDIA

Oxford

British Library Cataloguing in Publication Data.
A catalogue record for this title is available from
the British Library.

ISBN 1 899066 54 3

Westaby, S (Stephen)
Landmarks in cardiac surgery

Always refer to the manufacturer's Prescribing
Information before prescribing drugs cited in this book.

Typeset by
Selwood Systems Ltd., Midsomer Norton, UK

Reprinted in China

Distributed in the USA by
Books International, Inc., PO Box 605,
Hendon, VA 20172, USA

Distributed in the rest of the world by
Plymbridge Distributors Ltd., Estover Road,
Plymouth PL6 7PY, UK

Contents

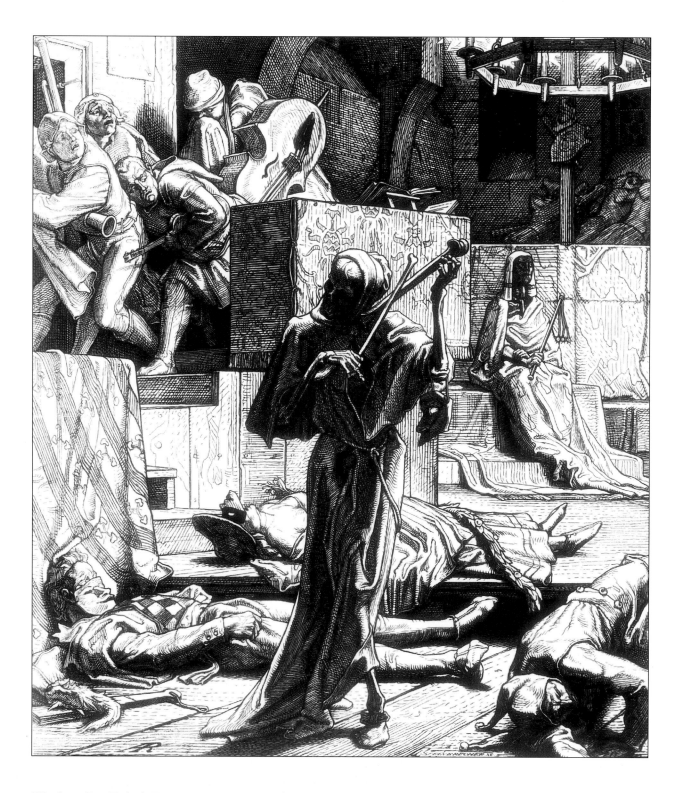

Woodcut: Der Tod als Erwurger; anon. after Alfred Rethel, 1851. (Courtesy of Wellcome Institute Library, London.)

Preface

One hundred years after the first successful heart operation by Rehn in Frankfurt (1897), few of us now involved in cardiac surgery appreciate the spectacular evolution of the speciality. The recent history is one of extraordinary characters with daring and resilience. Though remarkable, early progress was a hit-and-miss affair. Whereas the Ancient Egyptians (4000–2000 BC) attributed dyspnoea to the blockage of blood vessels and the Greeks (2000–1000 BC) described the clinical symptoms of heart failure, the great anatomist and physician William Harvey (1616) failed to recognize the connection with the circulation. This was left to Lower (1669) who described a syndrome attributable to 'impaired cardiac constriction'. Hope (1831) provided the concept of 'backward' cardiac congestion, but John Hunter missed the relationship between angina pectoris and coronary occlusion, despite extensive autopsy studies and his own crippling symptoms. When cardiac surgery began with the suture of stab wounds, medical treatment of heart disease remained primitive. As late as 1913, William Osler in his monumental work, *The Principles and Practice of Medicine*, summarized the whole of congenital heart disease in four pages. The state of the art at that time is evident from the following paragraph:

"The child should be warmly clad and guarded from all circumstances liable to cause bronchitis. In the attacks of urgent dyspnoea with lividity, blood should be let. Saline cathartics are also useful. Digitalis must be used with care; it is sometimes beneficial in the later stages."

Twenty-five years later, Robert Gross provided a surge of interest and growth in cardiac surgery when he performed ligation of a patent ductus arteriosus. Soon afterwards Gibbon's conception of a heart–lung machine to treat pulmonary embolism became a career-long quest. Perhaps the great stimulus towards the development of intra-cardiac surgery came during World War II through the fellowship of British and American surgeons in the European Theatre. Brock and Holmes-Sellors' pioneering closed operations were followed by Harkens' removal of intracardiac missiles and Bigelow's experiments with hypothermia. Cross-fertilization of ideas through joint clinical meetings between the allies stimulated determined young men to return home and find direct surgical solutions to intra-cardiac disease.

Developments in cardiac surgery during the 1950's were epic and fascinating to both physician and layman. Significant advances made international headlines and the true stories surrounding the operations were as compelling as the scientific advances. In those days the 'Grim Reaper' sat on every surgeon's shoulder. Charles Bailey, in a desperate attempt to perform successful mitral valvotomy, planned three operations in the same day at three different hospitals, each about to terminate his operating privileges through past failures. When the first two patients died he rushed to the third hospital in a taxi where he successfully dilated the mitral valve of a young woman. Within the week he took the patient 200 miles by train to a congress in Chicago and reported his resounding achievement. Tenacity was rewarded.

In the wake of Blalock's 'blue baby' operations his brilliant resident Cooley was sent from Johns Hopkins to the Brompton Hospital to train with Brock. There was a striking contrast between Brock — who was agitated and aggressive in the operating room — and the laconic and confident Texan. Cooley recalls being called to 'Pasty' Barrett's operating room in a moment of desperation. The left atrial appendage had torn during closed mitral valvotomy and there was blood everywhere. Barrett turned to Cooley and said, "Cooley, this operation should be awfully simple, but I've made it simply awful!". Cooley was less adept with the rigid bronchoscope. During a bit of a struggle an experienced technician invited Cooley to hold the instrument still whilst he thread the patient over it. Eventually humour prevailed over adversity.

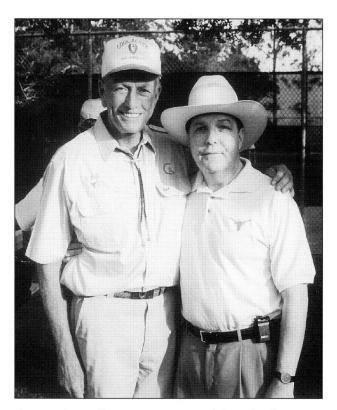

Progress in cardiac surgery emanated from the close
working relationship between surgeon and cardiologist.
Drs Denton Cooley and James Willerson (current editor
of Circulation*) of the Texas Heart Institute.*

Soon afterwards cardiac surgery was dominated by events in Minnesota. Three potential techniques held promise for direct vision intracardiac surgery. Systemic hypothermia with inflow occlusion provided only a short safe period for repair of simple defects. Lillehei's brilliant cross-circulation operations in Minneapolis were perhaps the most daring in the history of surgery but provided the potential for 200% mortality (never realized). Eventually the heart–lung machine prevailed in Kirklin's hands at the Mayo Clinic after Gibbon's single success was followed by demoralizing deaths in children.

Competition between surgeons was fierce; that between Lillehei and Kirklin was mutually productive, whilst Bailey and Harken's relationship was acrimonious. Eugene Braunwald, whose wife Nina was the pioneering lady cardiac surgeon, recalls the first live surgical teleconference transmitted nationwide from Philadelphia in the early 1960's. Charles Bailey flew in overnight from Hawaii and went directly to the operating room to perform coronary endarterectomy (a procedure he had not previously attempted). In front of an enormous audience the patient exsanguinated before cannulation for cardiopulmonary bypass. This tragedy gave the clear message that cardiac surgeons were not infallible.

By this time a huge industry supported cardiovascular surgery with technological advances in valve, pacemaker and heart–lung technology. With few exceptions, both the patient and surgeon have been well served by our commercial colleagues and both research and education rely on their support. The great societies and journals of cardiac surgery were established to disseminate knowledge and chronicle the new advances. Experienced editors such as John Kirklin, Tom Ferguson and Marko Turina have enormous influence through the quality and worldwide distribution of their publications.

Through the persistence of pioneers past and present, surgery now has a remedy for virtually every cardiac defect. The landmark advances are presented in this book, some with manuscripts in their original form. They provide a background to surgical treatment in most areas of the speciality and a detailed history of one of the great success stories of modern medicine. We are grateful to many of the pioneers who provided material for this book, and particularly to Charles Bailey and Dwight Harken who sent us important contributions in their last year of life. We hope that the book appeals to everyone involved in cardiology and cardiac surgery together with the student and general reader. Whilst developments continue, a career in cardiac surgery will never be the same again!

Stephen Westaby

Acknowledgements

I am grateful to those who made important contributions to this book; in particular to my assistant, Cecil Bosher, who assiduously persued the pioneers of cardiac surgery for their biographical details and to Dr Muir Grey for his constant encouragement. Without the generous support of James Deegan (Carbomedics), Roger Osborne (St Jude Medical) and Gordon Wright (Caledonian Medical) we could not have researched this compelling story.

Lastly, I am indebted to all who helped me down the long and difficult road to a career in cardiac surgery. Lord Brock left me his operating boots and with John Kirklin, I learned to wear them!

To my family,
particularly Gemma and Mark; two great characters who should have seen
more of their father.

Chapter 1: The foundations of cardiac surgery

THERE have been many landmarks in the evolution of cardiac surgery as a major speciality, but in the words of Sir Ernest Rutherford,

"Science grows step by step and every man depends on the work of his predecessors. Inevitably, the monuments of success have been built on the rubble of failure, rubble which nevertheless plays its part in the foundations of the subject."

Perhaps the difference between cardiac surgery and other fields of science or medicine is that the endpoint for failure is death. Claude Bernard wrote that, "The names of the prime movers of science disappear gradually in a general fusion, and the more science advances, the more impersonal and detached it becomes." Open heart surgery is now 40 years old and practised in most countries of the world. Current techniques already differ greatly from the time of its evolution in the early 1950s. Most of us involved in cardiac surgery have little knowledge or understanding of the epic discoveries and giant footsteps of the pioneer surgeons and their support teams.

Discovery of the circulation

PREHISTORIC humans recognized the importance of the heart. They hunted animals and learned that to achieve a quick kill, the spear should pierce the chest. The Cave of Pindal near Altamira in northern Spain contains magnificent polychrome frescoes of stone-age animals. Twenty thousand years ago, an Aurignacian man drew the outline of a mammoth and marked the heart within the chest with red ochre. Caves such as those in the cavern of Niaux in southern France contain fine drawings of bison, some with a spear embedded in the region of the heart.

The ancient Chinese had some awareness of the circulation of the blood. The *Neiching*, *Internal Classic* or *Canon of Medicine*, a text traditionally ascribed to the Yellow Emperor Huang Ti (2698–2598 BC), states that,

"The blood cannot but flow continuously like the current of a river, or the sun and moon in their orbits. It may be compared to a circle without beginning or end. The blood travels a distance of 3 inches during inhalation and another 3 inches during exhalation, making 6 inches with one respiration."

These statements appear to give insight into the nature of the pulmonary and systemic circulation, although it is clear they were not understood at that time. Another part of this classic describes the bloodstream as starting from the foot, and circulating to the kidneys, heart, lungs, liver and spleen and then from the spleen back to the kidneys. Early Chinese texts recorded the weights of organs including the heart, and various data involving the pulse. One Chinese work described the pulse or spirit as stored in the heart. Blood was said to be stored in the liver which contained the soul.

Ancient Egyptians were also conversant with the pulse and the heart. The Ebers Papyrus, dated 1550 BC, states,

"Begins the secret of the physicians. Knowledge of the going of the heart. Knowledge of the heart itself. There are vessels from it to every limb. On whatever part of the body a physician, a Sekhmet's priest, or a magician might put his finger—on the neck, on the hands, on the whole region of the heart, on both arms—he encounters the heart everywhere because its vessels are there for all the limbs; this means that it speaks through the vessels of the limbs."

The Edwin Smith Surgical Papyrus (c. 1600 BC) recognized the heart as the centre and pumping force for a system of distributing vessels. In the 16th century BC, the Brahdarankopanishad appeared in India. The composite term 'Hridaya' was used for heart, but segments of the word had different meanings. 'Hri' means that it imbibes air and other substances; 'da' means that it delivers up the air and substances; 'ya' means that it passes as nutrition to the body.

As in modern times, much was discovered during armed combat, when wounds of the heart and great vessels caused rapid death. It is also apparent that heart disease was recognized in the 26th century BC. The Yellow Emperor wrote,

> *"Long, slow pulse beats mark its good regulation; short, empty beats prove its disorderly condition. Quick pulse, with more than 6 heartbeats per one respiratory cycle, proves a sickness of the heart; a broadly slow pulse signifies a deterioration of the disease."*

The early Chinese and Egyptian texts had little influence on the evolution of Western medicine, probably through lack of availability and translation. The roots of European medicine stem from the Greeks, who clearly had information about the heart and vascular system as early as 600 BC. Alcmaeon of Corotonoa was aware of the difference between arteries and veins and recognized that the origins of sensation were in the brain and not the heart. In the Hippocratic era (400 BC), animal dissection was employed and the heart was found to be part of the vascular system. In the pseudo-Hippocratic *De Corde*, the heart was recognized as a muscle containing 'valves'. Aristotle (384–322 BC) described elements of the vascular system, including the heart and pericardium, though the heart valves were not mentioned. Although Aristotle had no concept of the circulation, he considered the body to be nourished by blood. His understanding was that blood emanated from the heart, supplied the rest of the body and was used up. Others noted the arteries to be empty after death (after combat and traumatic exsanguination) and inferred that arteries normally contained air. Although some of Aristotle's work was informative, many of his hypotheses were wide of the mark.

Erasistratus of Alexandria (310–250 BC) was the first to describe the atrioventricular valves and chordae tendonae (the semilunar valves had already been described in *De Corde*). His description of the distribution of arteries and veins was accurate enough to suggest that he dissected human bodies. Erasistratus described the method of closure and purpose of the heart valves. He suggested an anastomosis between arteries and veins, thereby anticipating the need for the capillary circulation. This was a remarkable insight, considering that the capillary was only described after William Harvey's work in the 17th century.

Herophilus of Chalcedon (300 BC) timed the pulse using a waterclock and commented on the systolic and diastolic phases. He described the four characters: frequency, rhythm, size and strength. The Roman physician Celsus (25 BC–50 AD) is accredited with the first account of heart disease in *De Medicina*. The first description of angina pectoris was by Seneca (4 BC), when he described his own symptoms. Rufus of Ephesus (98–117 AD), a notable surgeon of that time, first described attempts at haemostasis.

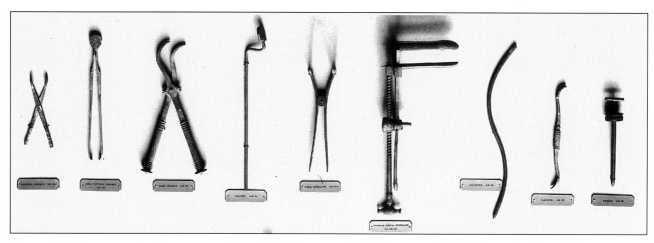

Figure 1.1. Roman surgical instruments from the 2nd century AD. (Courtesy of the Wellcome Institute Library, London.)

The works of Galen

GALEN (131–201 AD) worked in Rome as a surgeon to the gladiators. His experience, recorded in several million words, dominated medical teaching for 1500 years (Figure 1.2). As late as 1649, Riolan of Paris remarked that if anatomical dissections differed in nature from the observations of Galen, then the nature of anatomy itself must have changed. Galen's influence is particularly remarkable because he did not carry out dissection, vivisection or significant experiments. His findings were purely observational, but with careful and perceptive

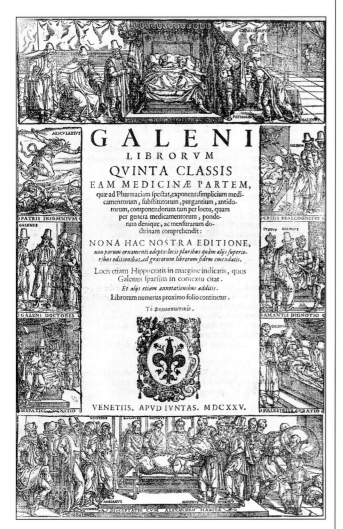

Figure 1.2. Title page of the latin edition of Galen's medical writings published in Venice in 1625. (Courtesy of The Library, History/Special Collections, University of California, San Francisco.)

interpretation. He recognized the motion of blood and the direction of bloodflow (mostly into the drains of the Colosseum!).

Galen's understanding of bloodflow through the heart and lungs is summarized by Fleming as follows,

"Blood on entering the right ventricle must pass a one-way valve opening inwards, so that only an insignificant portion can relapse into the vena cava whence it came. Some of the blood passes directly from right to left through the intraventricular septum. Much and apparently most of the blood moves into the arterial vein (our pulmonary artery) by passing a one-way valve opening outwards from the ventricle. On contraction of the thorax, the blood in the arterial vein, its retreat cut off from behind, can only go forward into the arterial system of the lungs."

The statement that blood passed through pores in the intraventricular system was accepted by others and passed down through many centuries. Galen's description of the general physiological workings of the vascular system including 'vital spirits', 'natural spirits' and 'animal spirits' (Figure 1.3), were incorrect, yet also remained part of fundamental medical thought. It is conceivable that Galen recognized an anastomosis between terminal arteries and veins and his concept of the function of cardiac valves was correct. He recognized the systolic and diastolic phases of the heart and wrote extensively on the nature of the pulse. He provided the first description of the pericardium as a protective structure and noted the complication of pericardial effusion. After Galen, significant advances in cardiology were surprisingly infrequent, until the anatomical drawings of artists in the 14th century. For a time, the spread of Islamic, Arabic and Eastern culture overshadowed the medicine and science of the Graeco-Roman civilization.

The Arabs made significant contributions to pharmacy, chemistry and mathematics. Ibn Al-nafis (1210–88) studied medicine in Cairo and Damascus and wrote at least 10 books on medical subjects. In one volume, entitled *The Perfect Man*, he offered a theory on the physiology of the pulmonary circulation. He suggested that blood returned from the body to the right side of the heart, where it was thinned. He was aware of Galen's description of bloodflow through the ventricular septum, but correctly refuted this because the openings did not exist anatomically. According to Al-nafis, blood flowed

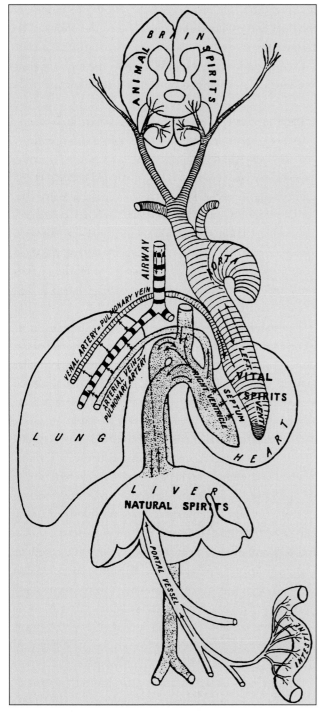

Figure 1.3. Diagram of Galen's description of the physiological working of the vascular system.

from the right ventricle to the lungs, then back to the left ventricle, where it was concocted with 'animal spirit' and distributed to other organs. He also recognized that the heart was nourished by its own blood vessels. Both concepts were revolutionary for the time, particularly as

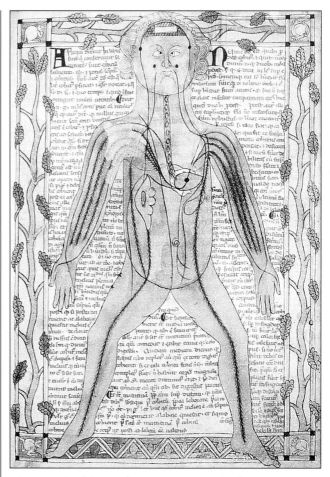

Figure 1.4. Thirteenth-century anatomical figure (English) illustrating the heart and blood vessels. (Courtesy of the Bodleian Library, Oxford, MS Ashmole 399, fol 19.)

Al-nafis (like Galen) was not an experimentalist and could not engage in dissection because of the prevailing Muslim law. His theories appear to be partly dependent on Galen's research and records, though Galen did not recognize the separate existence of the pulmonary circulation. Unfortunately, Al-nafis' strategic work was forgotten and discarded by his own students. Consequently, the pulmonary circulation was 'rediscovered' 200 years later by those unfamiliar with his work and insight.

The Renaissance period

THE RENAISSANCE bridged the gap between the Middle Ages and the Modern World, arbitrarily covering the period between 1450 and 1600. This was a time when art, architecture, sculpture and painting flourished with enormous vitality. The period was rich in culture, social and political life. Its beginnings were in the fall of Constantinople, which drove Arab scholars with their accumulated manuscripts and knowledge into Western Europe. The development of printing had a powerful influence on the spread of knowledge, and broad expansions in trade and commerce culminated in important geographical discoveries, including the Americas. Syphilis was widely disseminated and cardiological problems took on a new significance.

Many important anatomical works were produced by artists rather than physicians. Systematic drawings of the anatomical composition of the human body were made with great accuracy. Detailed knowledge of the heart and circulatory system evolved, although proof of circulation remained elusive.

Leonardo da Vinci (1452–1519) was a true Renaissance man. He was a superb painter and sculptor, an exceptional architect, a talented mechanical and hydraulic engineer and the founder of functional anatomy. His knowledge of architecture and engineering gave a mechanical perspective to his study of human anatomy. He regarded the human body as a God-created structure but governed by the laws of mechanics. Leonardo's remarkable understanding of functional concepts led him to design webbed gloves to enhance swimming, and wings and parachutes to promote flight.

Leonardo's anatomical work fell into two distinct periods: the first, between 1487 and 1493 in Florence and Milan, and the second, from 1506 to his death in France in 1519. The early period was preoccupied with the structure and function of the skull and eye, which he regarded as the 'window of the soul'. The later period concentrated on other organs, and in particular, the relationship between mechanics and human physiology. Leonardo is said to have dissected 30 cadavers and to have made almost 800 anatomical drawings. Two hundred of these remain in existence, all but a few housed in the private collection of Her Majesty the Queen at Windsor.

Leonardo's heart drawings (Figure 1.5) were overshadowed by the dogma of Galen. However, unlike his predecessors, Leonardo considered the heart to be a two-chambered organ dedicated to the 'warming of blood'. He described it as, "a vessel made of thick muscle, kept alive and nourished by arteries and veins, as

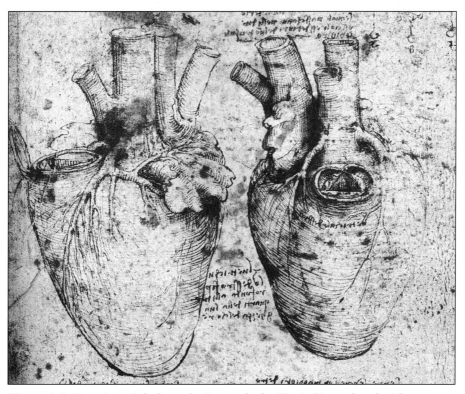

Figure 1.5. Drawing of the heart by Leonardo da Vinci. (Reproduced with permission of Her Majesty, Queen Elizabeth II.)

other muscles are." He wrote of the heart as having, "pre-eminent power over other muscles, a muscle that moves itself and does not stop if not forever." His drawings and descriptions of the heart clearly recognize both right and left ventricles and the atria, which he regarded as 'upper ventricles'. He described the atrial appendages as ears (auricula). The drawings accurately display the pericardial sac (capsula), the endocardium, the shape and structure of the atrioventricular valves and the moderator band (band of Leonardo). His structural and functional studies of the aortic valve and sinuses of Valsalva were amazing for the time. He was able to visualize the role of turbulence in closing the aortic valve and the pattern of bloodflow entering the thoracic aorta. He was also able to reproduce the mechanism of aortic valve closure systems in a primitive pulse duplicator. The experiments were performed on a glass model of the aortic root with a pig's aortic valve mounted at the base. Through this he pumped water and studied flow patterns, using markers such as finely shredded paper or grass seeds. The methods were described in his manuscripts, *Quadrati Anatomica*. Wax was poured into the aorta of a bull's heart to accurately reproduce the shape of the aortic valve and sinuses of Valsalva. One page of the manuscript contains drawings of the geometrical dimensions of the aortic valve, together with a design for construction of an artificial valve. Sketches of a cross-section of the left ventricular outflow tract and aortic root show vortices and the means whereby ejected blood causes valve closure. Both the drawings and text show that Leonardo had a clear understanding of the role of eddy currents within the sinuses of Valsalva:

> *"The effect of this revolution of the blood is to shut again the open valve, making by its primary reflected motion a perfect closure."*

Unfortunately, Leonardo could not completely disassociate himself from Galenic principles and persisted with the notion of communications through the ventricular septum by invisible pores. Despite detailed knowledge, he misunderstood the overall function of the heart. His concept that the left ventricular outflow tract had a sphincter-like function which assisted aortic valve closure was also misguided.

In later life, a papal decree barred Leonardo from performing autopsies, and probably prevented him from understanding the nature of the circulatory system 100 years before Harvey. Towards the end of his life, Leonardo reflected on his anatomical achievements and wrote the following to his pupils.

> *"But though possessed of an interest in the subject (anatomy), you may perhaps be deterred by natural repugnance of it. If it does not restrain you then, perhaps by the feat of passing the night hours in the company of corpses, quartered and flayed and horrible to behold. And if this does not deter you then perhaps you may lack the skill in drawing essential for such representations and even if you possess this skill it may not be combined with knowledge of perspective. While it is not combined, you may not possess the methods of geometrical demonstration, or the methods of estimating the forces and power of the muscles; or you perhaps may be found wanting of patients though you will not be diligent. Concerning which things whether or not they have all been found in me, the 120 folios I have composed will give their verdict, yes or no. In these I have not been hindered either by avarice or negligence, but only by want of time. Farewell."*

After Leonardo's death, his anatomical descriptions had little influence on medical science. Most of his drawings remained hidden for a century.

Leonardo apart, Andreas Vesalius (1514–64) arguably produced the most significant anatomical advances of the Renaissance period. He was the public prosecutor at the University of Padua and established a considerable reputation for his knowledge of morbid anatomy. In 1543, he produced the classic, *De Fabrica Humani Corporis*, which revolutionized anatomical knowledge and for the first time illustrated the many errors in the teaching of Galen. Consequently, Vesalius engendered considerable criticism and, disillusioned, he left the academic life of Padua to become Court Physician to Emperor Charles V. His most important contributions include accurate descriptions of the heart and coronary vessels, the venous system and aneurysms of the thoracic and abdominal aorta. In 1563, Vesalius made a pilgrimage to Jerusalem but died on the return trip. He was succeeded in Padua by the great Fallopius (of the tubes).

Fabricius of Aquapendente (1533–1619) was educated in Padua as a pupil of Fallopius, from whom he

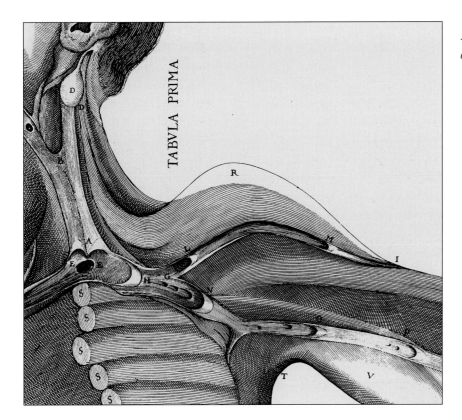

TABVLA PRIMA

Figure 1.6. Fabricius' dissection of the veins of the arm.

learned dissection. He graduated in 1559 (19 years before Harvey was born) and was appointed Professor of Surgery and Anatomy at the age of 32 (1565). He was required to dissect the whole human body in public, twice, between St Luke's day and the Feast of the Assumption. It was Fabricius who designed the famous oval anatomy theatre at Padua, built in 1594. This remains in existence, with its five steep and narrow galleries arranged almost vertically above the dissection table, enabling the students to look directly down upon the body.

Like most academics, Fabricius was far more interested in research than in teaching students, and frequently failed to appear for dissections or demonstrations. He was an energetic and enthusiastic researcher, intolerant of fools, and quick to take offence. Fabricius described the venous valves, which he called 'ostioles', but despite his accurate description he did not understand their function (Figures 1.6 and 1.7). Fabricius followed the Galenic view that blood from the alimentary system flowed from the liver to the periphery and that the venous valves prevented too rapid dissipation of the nutritious fluid.

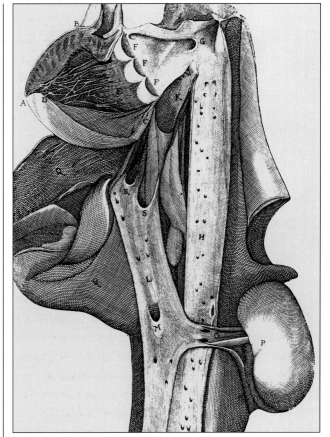

Figure 1.7. The heart and great vessels according to Fabricius.

Harvey and the circulation of the blood

WILLIAM HARVEY was born in Kent in the spring of 1578. His father, Thomas Harvey, was an intellectual Yeoman farmer who became Mayor of Folkestone and his mother was Joan Halke. William was sent to King's School, Canterbury and then to Gonville and Caius College, Cambridge, at the age of 16. In 1594, the college had recently opened a new anatomy school where Harvey began his lifelong studies. He also read the works of Plato and Aristotle. Harvey's choice of Padua for medical training was influenced by Dr John Caius, an enthusiastic anatomist and pupil of Vesalius.

Harvey was 22 when he attended the English College in Padua. In time, he became a councillor with a seat on the governing body. Harvey's most influential teachers were the great anatomist Fabricius and Galileo the astronomer. Demonstration of the venous valves by Fabricius probably played an important part in Harvey's understanding of the circulation. Harvey discussed the existence of the venous valves with his friend, the scientist Robert Boyle.

"When he (Fabricius) took notice that the valves of the veins of so many several parts of the body were so placed that they gave free passage of the blood towards the heart, but opposed its passage in the contrary way, no design seemed more probable than that the blood should be sent to the limbs by the arteries and return through the veins."

However, it was probably Harvey's grossly inaccurate calculation of cardiac output that finally convinced him that the Galenical concepts were unacceptable. It was obvious to him that most of the massive volume of blood pumped by the left ventricle must somehow be returned to the heart by the veins (Harvey's calculation of cardiac output was 23 lb and 4 oz (17 litres) in 30 minutes!).

On receiving his Doctorate in Medicine from Padua (April 1602), Harvey returned to England and took up medical practice in London. In 1604, he was married to Elizabeth Browne, the daughter of Lancelot Browne, a prominent London physician. In 1607, Harvey was elected Fellow of the Royal College of Physicians, in whose professional and political affairs he took an active interest for the rest of his life. In 1609, he was appointed

Physician to St Bartholomew's Hospital. The earliest evidence of his scientific research on the circulation comes from anatomical lecture notes written in 1616. These formed the basis for anatomical demonstrations as Lumleian lecturer at the College of Physicians. As well as his teaching of morphological anatomy, Harvey's lectures included extensive discussions on the function of various parts of the body. His philosophical basis was generally traditional, but with an increased under-standing of physiology, the Galenic doctrines were eventually discredited.

From Harvey's early notes it is clear that in Padua he had performed original investigations of the cardiac cycle, respiration, the functions of the brain and spleen, locomotion and embryology. Harvey's *Treties de Generatione Animalium* was an extension of Fabricius' work.

"I propose to follow of the ancients, Aristotle, and of the moderns, my former teacher at Padova, Fabricius of Aquapendente."

However, Harvey was both independent and critical of his teacher's work.

"He reliath on probability rather than experience and layeth aside the verdict of sense which is grounded upon dissections; he fleeth to petty reasonings borrowed from mechanicks which is very undeseeming in so famous an anatomist."

Harvey was also adrift in some of his observations. Whilst Fabricius taught that mammalian birth was accomplished by the power of the uterus assisted by the mother's abdominal muscles and diaphragm, Harvey claimed that the fetus propelled itself to freedom unassisted by the womb. Harvey cited clinical cases where he claimed to have witnessed infants born by their own efforts. Nevertheless, from the notes of 1616, it is clear that he had started original investigations of most anatomical systems and had planned a vast research programme that would lead to publication on a wide range of subjects. Unfortunately, only manuscripts on the heart and reproductive system survived. Many notes and documents were destroyed when his rooms at Whitehall were ransacked in 1642. Most of the rest were presumably lost in the Great Fire which destroyed his new library at the College of Physicians. Harvey was appointed Lumleian lecturer in 1615 and continued in this role for 41 years. The notes of his early lectures are preserved in the British Museum. They show that by 1616, Harvey had dissected more than 80 different species of animal and had developed preliminary concepts on the function of the heart and circulation.

Harvey demolished the Galenic description of communications between the chambers of the heart. It was thought that venous blood was conveyed from the liver directly into the left side of the heart and the arteries. In discounting this theory, Harvey resurrected the views of the Arab physician Ibn Al-nafis, Servetus and the Italian anatomist Colombo. They had each suggested that venous blood from the liver passed through the lungs before reaching the left heart and arteries. Harvey's claim that all venous blood passed through the pulmonary circulation (and not just a small volume from the liver) was new. Also, the concept that blood constantly circulated from the arteries to the veins

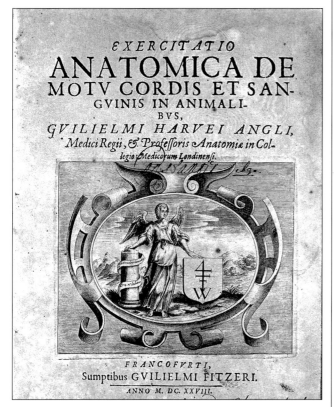

Figure 1.8. Title page of Harvey's classic text, Exercetatio Anatomica de Motu Cordis Etsanguinis in Animalibus *published in Latin in Frankfurt (1628). (Courtesy of Jeremy Norman & Co., Inc. San Francisco, CA, USA)*

contrasted with the traditional view that blood was consumed in the peripheral organs and constantly replenished. Harvey considered that heat was transmitted to the peripheral organs via the arteries and that the venous circulation returned cold blood to the heart, which regenerated heat. The key to Harvey's concept of the circulation was his experiments on cardiac output. His calculations suggested that the volume of blood ejected by the left ventricle per hour far exceeded the total blood volume. This entirely correct assumption proved that blood could not be constantly replenished from the outside (from food), consequently, the same blood ejected from the left ventricle must repeatedly return to the heart. Harvey proceeded to confirm this hypothesis by a brilliant series of comparative anatomical observations and incontrovertible experiments. He employed techniques such as vascular ligation and succeeded in determining the direction of bloodflow in both arteries and veins.

Harvey compared the heart with a fire-engine pump. He proposed that the right auricle initiated the cardiac cycle by heating the blood and setting it into motion. Nevertheless, the concept of the heart as a pump is conspicuously absent from Harvey's classic text, *Exercetatio Anatomica de Motu Cordis Etsanguinis in Animalibus*, published in Frankfurt in 1628 (Figure 1.8). This famous description of the discovery of the circulation was sufficient to ensure Harvey pride of place in the history of science and medicine. It is evident from this work that his ultimate realization came from careful observation of animal hearts in an agonal state. When the heartbeat slowed prior to death, the sequence of the heart's action was much easier to discern in slow motion. When choosing the questions to be answered by his experiments, Harvey was substantially influenced by Colombo's descriptions of the heartbeat (1559). Colombo emphasized that the arteries dilate as the heart contracts and vice versa. He also characterized the relaxed or diastolic phase of the heart during which the ventricles receive blood and contrasted this with the vigorous contractile phase as blood was ejected into the great arteries. Harvey established first that the heartbeat consisted of one active movement to which he gave the neutral designation 'erection'. This is followed by a completely passive relaxation. The word 'erection' stemmed from the observation that the apex of the heart appeared to uplift during systole. Harvey commented that during erection the heart strikes the chest and its flesh changes from soft to hard; at the same time the pulse of the arteries is perceived.

"Erection is slightly preceded by the obvious contraction of the auricles, during which they expel their blood and become whiter. Indeed the beat of the heart begins with the auricles and then proceeds to the apex of the ventricles so that the auricles arouse the somnolent heart."

Having determined the sequence of the cardiac cycle, Harvey applied himself to proving that erection represented the contraction of the ventricles. He considered a number of observations to support this hypothesis.

"When the beating heart is punctured, blood is forcibly expelled during erection; the heart becomes whiter during erection; the dissection of a beating heart shows that its walls become thicker during erection, which means that its cavities must become smaller."

Harvey also considered that the entire structure of the heart, with its valves, fibres and chordae tendonae, indicated that its essential action was to contract and expel its contents rather than to dilate and attract them. Harvey went on to note correctly that the arterial pulse followed ejection of blood by the heart and was not, in itself, an active movement. He observed that blood was expelled more vigorously from a cut artery during erection. He repeatedly compared the pulse in an artery to inflation of a glove, an analogy which he appears to have borrowed from Fallopius. The arteries now replaced the veins as the principal blood-distributing vessels and the vena cava became more concerned with transporting blood from the liver to the heart than from the liver to the peripheral veins. The heart, rather than the liver, became the principle circulatory organ, and Harvey recognized that the veins did not pulsate because valves interrupted the impulse caused by cardiac contraction. This latter observation is important as it shows that, in Harvey's view, the orientation of the venous valves was not merely upward in the body, as was previously thought, but inwards towards the heart. This probably caused him to conceive the nature of centripetal venous flow, having grasped the need for return of blood from the arteries to the heart.

In the first half of *de Motu Cordis*, Harvey presents his conclusions on the movements of the heart and arteries in a more comprehensive form, supported by vivisection and anatomical, pathological and embryological observations. The manuscript presents a devastating critique of Galen's doctrine on the motions of the heart and arteries, especially against the concept that these activities serve a ventilatory function. A contrary explanation to peripheral vascular connections was proposed in 1623 by Emilio Parigiano, who maintained that there must be a significant reflux of blood from the aorta back to the left ventricle during each cardiac cycle. He argued that,

"since the heart in systole expels the larger part of its blood into the aorta, and that in scarcely a moment of time, the aorta would always be so filled with blood that it could receive no more, while the heart would be emptied in a few beats."

Parigiano considered that both problems would be eliminated if there was constant reflux of blood back to the heart through the aortic valve. Harvey writes,

"When I had thus considered how large the amount of transmitted blood would be, and in how short a time the transmission would take place, I noticed that the juice of the ingested aliment could not supply this amount without our having the veins emptied and completely drained on the one hand, and the arteries disrupted by the excessive intrusion of blood on the other, unless the blood somehow permeates from the arteries back to the veins and returns to the right ventricle of the heart. I began to consider whether the blood might have a kind of motion, as it were, in a circle, and this I afterwards found to be true."

The second half of *de Motu Cordis* presents further evidence to confirm the circular movement of blood. Harvey notes that all the blood can be rapidly evacuated from an animal by cutting a large artery. Furthermore, if the vena cava of a live snake is pinched between the fingers, the beating heart rapidly empties itself of blood. In contrast, when the aorta is occluded, the heart soon becomes engorged with blood. Harvey's experiments with ligatures to obstruct the passage of blood from the veins are described (Figure 1.9). He notes that if an arm

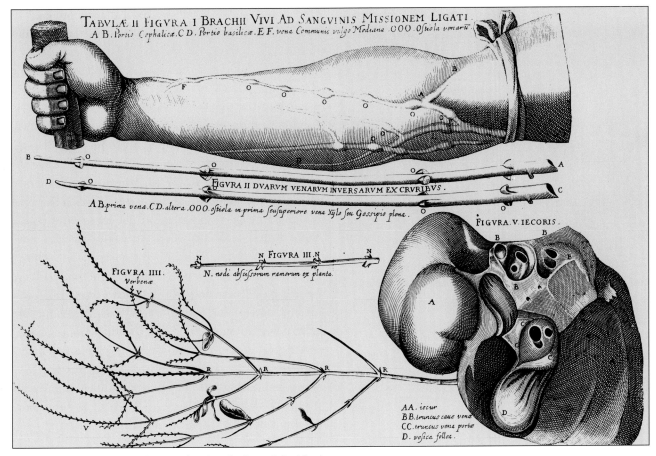

Figure 1.9. Harvey's studies on the circulation of the blood.

is ligated so tightly that the arterial pulse is interrupted, then it becomes pale and bloodless and the arteries above the ligature become swollen with blood. When the ligature is loosened sufficiently to restore the pulse, the arterial swelling above the ligature subsides and the arm becomes suffused with flowing blood. In contrast, the veins become swollen below a ligature, which means that blood must flow into them from the arteries at the periphery rather than from the central veins. Harvey notes that if a swollen, obstructed vein is opened for bloodletting, then within half an hour most of the blood within the body can be evacuated. This provides an index of the amount of blood that flows from the heart into the arteries and from the arteries into the veins.

Harvey stresses the cardiocentric orientation of the various valves and notes that a probe can be inserted inwards through them, but not outwards. He also shows that when an arm is ligated to make the veins swell, then a finger drawn along a vein with some pressure can push blood towards the thorax through the valve, but not

outwards. Furthermore, if a segment of vein is emptied by applying pressure with one finger, then the blood is squeezed into the valve with a second, it is apparent that the vein refills from the peripheral end when the first finger is removed. Harvey regarded these classical manoeuvres as confirmation that blood must circulate.

Inevitably, Harvey's hypothesis was treated with scepticism. Many physicians sought to incorporate the idea of the circulation within the traditional framework of anatomy, with the minimum of other changes. In 1618, Harvey was appointed Physician Extraordinary to James I, a position he retained after the accession of Charles I in 1625. The king took an interest in Harvey's scientific work and provided him with stags from the Royal Parks for some of his experiments (Figure 1.10). During the Civil War, Harvey accompanied the king on the Scottish campaigns of 1639, 1640 and 1641. He became a close friend of Charles I and remained with him at Oxford from the winter of 1642 until the surrender of loyalist forces to the Scots in 1646. Consequently,

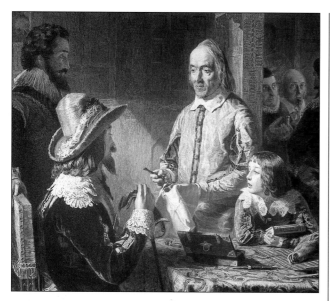

Figure 1.10. Harvey demonstrating an experiment on a deer to King Charles I and the boy prince. Engraving after the painting by Robert Hannah at the Royal College of Physicians, London. (Courtesy of Jeremy Norman & Co., Inc.)

Harvey was not popular with the Parliamentarians, and many of his manuscripts were probably destroyed at this time.

The description of the heart as a pump to drive the circulating blood marked a new era of scientific materialism in the West. Soon afterwards, the elusive communication between arteries and veins was discovered by Marcello Malpighi (1628–94). Malpighi was a great pioneer of microscopy and he described the histology of most organs in the mammalian body, including the newly discovered lymph glands. He also published many manuscripts on the anatomy of insects and plants and provided valuable insight into embryology. Malpighi described two separate systems of interconnecting vessels: the capillaries and the vesicles of air and blood networks in the lungs (Figure 1.11). He inflated excised lungs and noted that the pulmonary arterial system stands out like the branches of a tree. Injection of coloured fluid into the pulmonary artery confirmed its passage through to the veins, though he also noted oozing into the interstitial tissues and passage of fluid into the trachea. In a letter to his friend, Giovanni Borelli, Malpighi states that,

"Observation by means of the microscope will reveal more wonderful things than those viewed in regard to mere structure and connection; for while the heart is still beating, the contrary movement of the blood (in opposite directions in the different vessels) is observed in the vessels, so that the circulation of the blood is clearly exposed. This is more clearly recognized in the mesentery and in the other great veins contained in the abdomen. Thus by this impulse the blood is driven in very small streams through the arteries, like a flood into the several cells, one or other branch clearly passing through or ending there. Thus blood, much divided, cuts off its red colour, and carried round in a winding way is poured out on all sides till at length it may reach the walls, the angles, and the absorbing branches of the veins."

Malpighi goes on to describe ligation of the pulmonary hilum of a frog.

"This when dried will preserve the vessels turgid with blood. You will see this very well if you examine it by the microscope with one lens against the horizontal sun. Or you may institute another method of seeing these things.

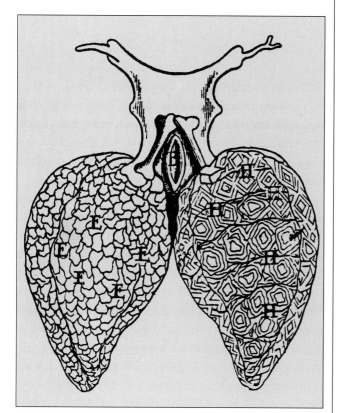

Figure 1.11. Lung of a frog showing capillaries by Malpighi.

Place the crystal plate illuminated below through a tube by a lighted candle. To it bring a microscope of two lenses and thus the vessels distributed in a ring-like fashion will be disclosed to you. By the same arrangement of the instruments and light, you will observe the movement of the blood through the vessels in question."

Malpighi also described the appearance of capillary circulation in the bladder wall (of frogs) swollen with urine. The motion of the blood is seen clearly through the transparent vessels joined together by anastomoses.

Malpighi's work was supported by that of the microscopist Anthony van Leeuwenhoek (1632–1723), who became one of the greatest scientific explorers of all

time. Leeuwenhoek was a draper by trade in the city of Delph. He devoted all his free time to the construction of single lens microscopes of remarkable precision and resolution. Through the use of his microscopes, he discovered protozoa, bacteria, sperm cells, red blood corpuscles, capillaries, crystal structures and hundreds of other biological and physical novelties (Figure 1.12). Many observations were extremely astute for a non-physician. He realized that as large arteries are thick walled, they could not be the site of nutrient diffusion into the tissues. Leeuwenhoek identified cells within blood and concluded remarkably that,

"The particles of blood from redness emanates deliver their juices through the capillary walls, whereby the blood, when returning in the veins, being deprived of those juices which are taken away, will appear blackish."

He observed blood clots in damaged vessels and was ingenious in determining the rate of bloodflow by observing the passage of cells and thrombi. With Leeuwenhoek's insight into the significance of the microcirculation and the cellular components of blood, an understanding of the importance of the heart and circulation was almost complete.

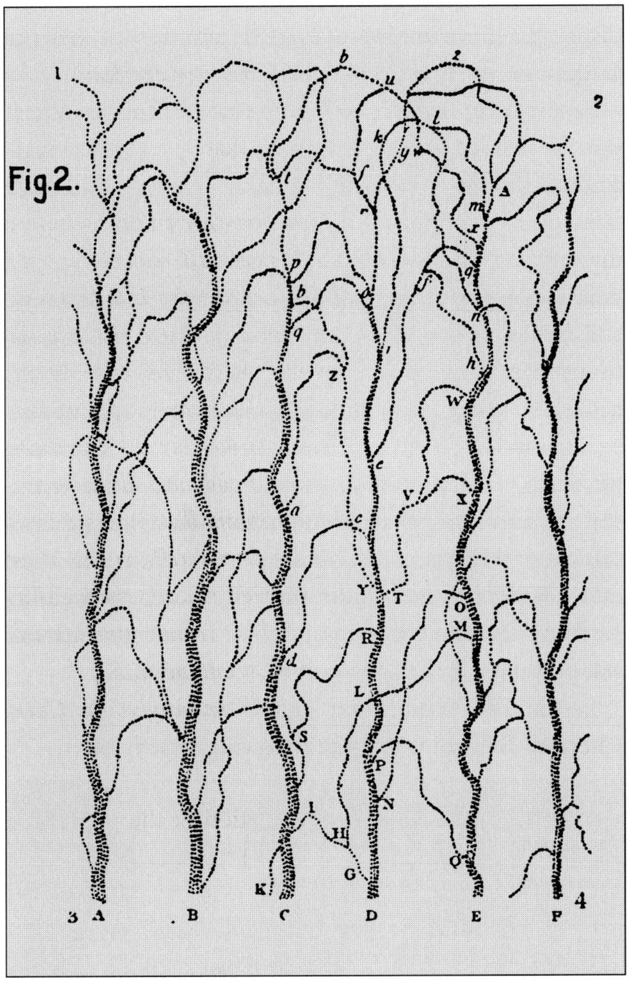

Wounds of the heart

THE ANCIENTS, including Hippocrates, considered all wounds of the heart to be fatal. Five hundred years after Hippocrates, Galen gained experience of every conceivable type of penetrating wound in the gladiatorial arenas of Pergamon and Rome, where he held appointments as Chief Surgeon. He drew attention to the rapidity of death if a ventricle was lacerated, and considered all cardiac wounds to be ultimately fatal. The first evidence to refute the inevitability of death from the wounded heart came from Bartholemy Cabrol of Montpellier. In his book of *Anatomical Observations*, published in 1604, he describes two autopsies of executed criminals, whose hearts contained the scars of previous penetrating trauma. Fallopius, the famous anatomist and pupil of Vesalius, proposed that "a cardiac wound could only be survived by a miracle. The heart could never heal as it was too hard, always in motion, and of an inflammatory heat."

Figure 1.12. Capillary network in a tail of an eel from Leeuwenhoek.

The 17th century physician, Paulus Zacchias, whose patients included the Popes Innocent X and Alexander VII, also subscribed to the 'invariably fatal' school. He recorded the incident of a mad priest who cut off his penis and testicles and then proceeded to stab himself with a needle many times in the left breast. He continued to live for 1 week and at postmortem it was evident that many wounds had penetrated the right ventricle. William Harvey also gave an account of scars in the hearts of animals that had survived arrow wounds.

During the 17th century, it became apparent that careful postmortem studies could shed light on symptoms and signs present before death. The potential importance of pathological findings was demonstrated by Theophile Bonet in his postmortem records, published under the title *Sepulchretum* in 1679. This work was a compilation of 3000 autopsy records, including a number of patients with haemopericardium. This led Bonet to observe that pressure from pericardial collections (pericardial tamponade) could stop the heart from beating. Giovanni Morgagni, Professor of Anatomy in Padua in the 18th century, criticized the deficiencies of *Sepulchretum* and spent 20 years carefully annotating his postmortem examinations in the light of symptoms during life. Published in 1761 as a collection of 70 letters, entitled *De Sedibus et Causis Morborum per Anatomen Indagatis* (The seats and causes of diseases investigated by anatomy), this text laid the foundations for modern pathology. Cardiac tamponade was described again and death attributed to pressure of blood within the pericardium.

The term 'Herztamponade' was coined by a German surgeon, Edmund Rose, in Berlin, more than 100 years later (1884). Rose's manuscript described the pathophysiology of cardiac tamponade and recorded 23 case histories of ruptured or wounded hearts, several of which did not cause death. In 1868, Georg Fischer of Hannover published a detailed analysis of 452 wounds involving the heart and pericardium. He recorded survival in 10% of cardiac wounds and 30% of wounds which involved only the pericardium. Realization that the pericardium could be drained surgically suggested for the first time that repair might prove possible for cardiac wounds.

The first occasion on which a surgeon deliberately operated on an injured heart was in October 1872. This followed a brawl in a public house in East London, after which a 31-year-old man could not find a needle he usually kept in the left side of his coat. The next day, he attended St Bartholomew's Hospital, but the needle was not found. Nine days later, pain and discomfort persisted, and on return to St Bartholomew's he was admitted. The surgeon, George Callendar, explored the area of discomfort and made an incision between the ribs. He eventually located the needle, which was embedded in the myocardium close to the apex. The needle was removed and the patient made an uneventful recovery.

Soon afterwards, the Danzig surgeon, Bloch, experimented by inserting sutures into the beating hearts of rabbits. From his experience he realized the feasibility of suture closure of wounds in the human heart. However, his promising career was ruined by an ambitious attempt at surgery for supposed tuberculosis in a young, female cousin. Bloch performed a thoracotomy with the intention of removing the diseased tissue, but the girl died on the operating table. When autopsy showed no evidence of tuberculosis, the distraught Bloch committed suicide and the possibility of surgery on the heart remained forbidden territory.

In the latter half of the 19th century, thoracic surgery was restricted to operations on the chest wall. Encroachment on the pleural cavity and the consequences of pneumothorax remained a physiological mystery and surgical disaster. However, it was recognized that in empyema thoracis the pleural cavity was adherent, and by the 1870s, physicians decided that it was a good thing to evacuate pus from the chest. This was initially achieved using tiny tubes, though lack of success eventually led to rib resection. In 1876, the Hamburg physician, Gottard Bulau, introduced the underwater-seal apparatus for patients who needed fluid drained from the chest. He inserted a drainage tube from the chest into a bottle of water under the bed, thereby preventing air from entering the pleural cavity. A strong reluctance still prevailed about approaching the heart itself.

In the 1897 edition of Paget's *Surgery of the Chest*, Christian Billroth wrote the following statement:

"Surgery of the heart has probably reached the limits set by nature to all surgery: no new method and no new discovery can overcome the natural difficulties that attend a wound of the heart. It is true that heart 'suture' has been vaguely proposed as a possible procedure, and has been done on animals, but I cannot find that it has ever been attempted in practice."

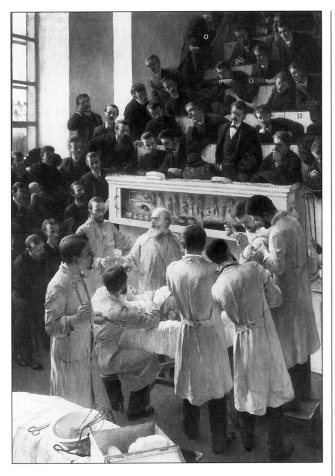

Figure 1.13. Billroth operating in the auditorium of the Allgemeine Krankenhaus, Vienna (1889) by Anton Seligmann. Although Billroth operated with sterile instruments, public spectators (including the Duke of Bavaria, who frequently attended Billroth's lectures for entertainment) were allowed to come extremely close to the operating conditions.(Courtesy of the Österreichische Galerie, Vienna.)

Billroth was widely influential, but unfortunately, this much-quoted remark was probably taken out of context and misquoted in innumerable publications since. In the 1864 edition of his *Surgical Textbook*, Billroth included the operation of pericardial incision and drainage for suppurative pericarditis, a procedure successfully performed by his former teacher, Bernhard Von Langenbeck, in 1850. Billroth states that he believed this operation to be the next best thing to frivolity and approaching what some surgeons might regard as a prostitution of the art of surgery. He relented, to a degree, by concluding that future generations might think differently. This part of his textbook was not

revised in subsequent editions and the remark was perpetuated through to the last edition.

Another much-quoted remark by Billroth in the early 1880s was that, "any surgeon who wishes to preserve the respect of his colleagues, would never attempt to suture the heart." This came shortly after Bloch's first experimental attempts at cardiac suture, and, of course, his demise. The remark was spoken by Billroth at a meeting of the Vienna Medical Society, around 1880. As the father of abdominal surgery, with a formidable list of operative 'firsts', his remarks made strong ammunition for those who regarded the heart as 'off-limits'. Nonetheless, drainage of pericardial effusions was by this time well established.

As early as 1653, Jean Riolan, the Galenistical Professor of Anatomy in Paris (who objected to Harvey's theory of circulation), had already advocated evacuation of fluid from the pericardium. "When copious humour collects and the heart is embarrassed, if hydrogues have no effect, is it not lawful to open the sternum with a trephine at a thumb's interval above the xiphoid cartilage?"

The first realistic attempt to deal with pericardial effusions was made by Francisco Romanero of Barcelona. Romanero incised the fifth intercostal space and probed the outside of the pericardium in order to identify a fluid collection. He then held the pericardium with forceps and incised it with curved scissors. With the fluid evacuated, he inserted a gauze drain for 3 days to draw

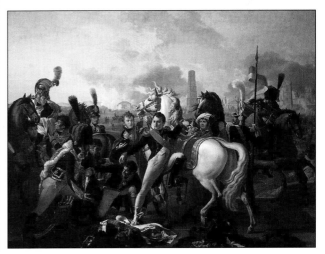

Figure 1.14. Napoleon wounded at Ratisbon by Claude Gautherot. The surgeon shown treating Napoleon is believed to be Dominique Jean Larrey. (Courtesy of the Versailles Museum.)

off any reaccumulation. Romanero undoubtedly had problems with pneumothorax, as he laid great stress on not allowing air to enter the pleural cavity. The Scandinavian, Skielderup, avoided the risk of pleural entry and laceration of the internal mammary artery by making a trephine hole in the sternum at the level of the fifth costal cartilage. His heroic, but painful attempts, in the pre-anaesthetic era were soon abandoned.

Napoleon's great surgeon, Baron Dominique Jean Larrey (Figure 1.14), who at the Battle of Limbourg advocated the use of ambulances to evacuate the wounded, and at the Battle of Borodino performed more than 200 amputations in 24 hours, is credited with operating for suppurative pericarditis (1810). The patient, Bernard Saint-Ogne, a 30-year-old foot soldier, stabbed himself in the left breast after being accused of a crime he did not commit. The left lung was injured and an increasingly painful empyema developed. Larrey's treatment initially consisted of embrocations of camphorated oil followed by scarification of the chest wall as counter-irritation. However, Saint-Ogne's condition deteriorated inexorably, with marked oedema of the legs. Diagnosing fluid in the pericardial cavity, Larrey decided to perform left thoracotomy between the fifth and sixth ribs. On incising the pericardium, a large volume of pus was evacuated in synchrony with the heartbeat. The patient improved initially, but the wound became infected and 10 days later, further signs of cardiac compression appeared. Larrey operated for a second time, but Saint-Ogne eventually died over 2 months after the initial wound.

In Larrey's book of *Surgical Experiences in Military Camps*, published in 1829, he describes six other cases of wounds of the heart and pericardium. One of these was a 24-year-old soldier with a bullet wound to the chest. In February 1824, before attempting surgery, Larrey tested his proposed approach on cadavers. He first performed débridement of the entry wound, removing all foreign material and dead and dying tissue. He then inserted a gum-elastic catheter into the pericardial cavity to drain the bloodstained fluid. The procedure was successful and the soldier recovered.

Billroth's own exposure to pericardial drainage consisted of the two patients operated on by his teacher, Bernhard Von Langenbeck, Professor of Surgery in Berlin. The first case resulted from a duel, during which a bullet caused severe derangement of the patient's chest

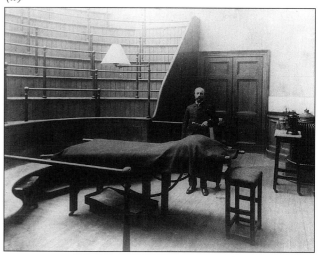

(a)

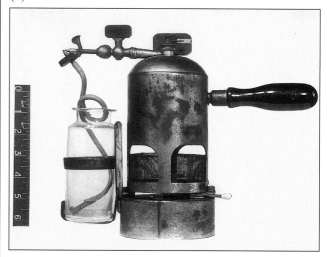

(b)

Figure 1.15. (a) *The old operating theatre of Guy's and St Thomas's Hospitals, London, the only operating theatre in England to remain intact since the 19th century. (Courtesy of St Thomas's Hospital, London.) (b) Lister's carbolic acid diffuser. (Courtesy of Wellcome Institute Library, London.)*

wall. Langenbeck incised the pericardium to evacuate pus and healing was uneventful. In the second patient, Langenbeck introduced a trocar and cannula into the pericardium to drain off purulent fluid. Despite Billroth's scepticism, developments in modern medicine, pathology and physiology in the second half of the 19th century created an environment in which surgery for heart disease became increasingly feasible.

The science of microbiology grew with the development of improved microscopes. An association between microorganisms and disease was noted in Henle's essay of 1840. He recognized that contagious diseases were caused by living things that had a parasitic relationship with the body. He proposed that cause and effect could be established by isolating the organism from a sick patient. The debate as to whether bacteria might be the cause or consequence of infection was settled in 1858 by the fermentation experiments of Louis Pasteur. In 1864, Joseph Lister used this information in his quest to eradicate surgical infection. He made efforts to exclude microorganisms from the surgical field by cleansing the hands and instruments with disinfectant and spraying the air above the operating table (Figure 1.15). He could then show that wounds would heal primarily without infection, which had generally been regarded as a necessary part of the repair process. Whereas surgeons had previously operated with bloodstained instruments and topcoats, Lister's principles of aseptic technique and the use of antiseptics spread rapidly through the West and greatly improved the prospects for surgical patients.

Anaesthetics and artificial respiration

PERHAPS the most significant step in the development of surgery as a science was the advent of anaesthetics. Since prehistoric times, alcohol made from fermented fruit juice or grain was used as a sedative to relieve pain. Herbs such as henbane, deadly nightshade, hemlock, poppy and mandragora were also used to produce pain-relieving powders and potions. A Chinese surgeon, Hua To, performed abdominal surgery using the coca-based sedative agent scopolamine. An 8th century manuscript from Monte Cassino describes a concoction for rendering patients unconscious through opium, juice of mandragora leaves, fresh poppy leaves and henbane juice. In the 12th century, ivy juice, mulberry juice and lettuce and sorrel seeds were added to this preparation. Distillation created a very strong alcoholic liquor. The resulting liquid was often soaked in a sponge which was allowed to dry out and then held over the face to induce unconsciousness. Revival was achieved by pouring vinegar into the nostrils.

During the Napoleonic Wars, anaesthetics other than alcohol were essentially unknown, but Larrey noticed

that during the bitterly cold winters, intense cold seemed to numb the limbs of those needing amputation. In 1839, Alfred Velpeau wrote, "The avoidance of pain during operations is a fantasy that should not be indulged in. Cutting instruments and pain are inextricably associated with each other in the mind of patients."

In 1776, Joseph Priestly, a gentleman farmer and chemist, discovered carbon dioxide and then nitrous oxide gas. In 1799, Humphrey Davy, a Cornish apothecary, investigated the properties of various gases on the human body, usually by self-application. Inhaled nitrous oxide produced a feeling of wellbeing, followed by persistent migraine, but the pain of a broken tooth disappeared. There was no practical application of this finding until December 1844, in Hertford, Connecticut, where a fairground entertainment included 'men who could not stop laughing'. This stemmed from the fact that humans who inhaled nitrous oxide burst into spontaneous uncontrollable laughter. One man fell off the platform, sustaining a fracture, but remained unaware of the pain. This attracted the attention of a dentist, Horace Wells, who tested the benefits on himself during a tooth extraction. Wells was greatly impressed and arranged a demonstration before other doctors and

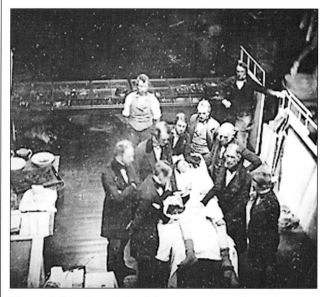

Figure 1.16. An original daguerrotype made at the second operation performed with the use of ether anaesthesia on 17 October, 1846. At the head of the table is William Morton, the surgeon is John Collins Warren and facing Warren is the orthopaedic surgeon, Henry Jacob Bigelow. (Courtesy of the Boston Medical Library.)

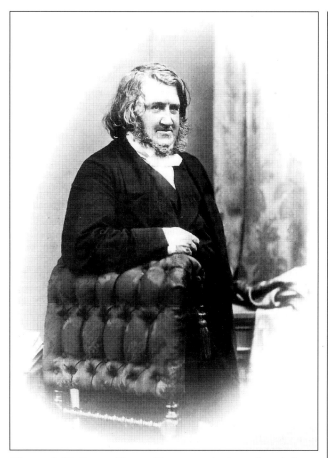

Figure 1.17. James Young Simpson, who introduced the use of chloroform as an anaesthetic in 1847. (Courtesy of Historical Collections, College of Physicians of Philadelphia.)

dentists. Unfortunately, the gas was badly prepared and the patient roared with pain.

Inevitably, experiments and antics with laughing gas produced hilarious results, but 2 years later, William Morton, another Boston dentist, found ether to be an effective anaesthetic. He devised a face mask onto which liquid ether was poured, causing the gas to be inhaled. On 16 October 1846, Morton administered an ether anaesthetic whilst his colleague, Warren, excised a tumour from the neck of Gilbert Abbot (Figure 1.16). Abbot remained unconscious during the procedure and the demonstration was extremely successful. Ether anaesthetic became popular in the US and was introduced into Europe, where Jobert de Lambelle was the first to use it successfully in Paris in December 1846.

In 1847, chloroform was employed by James Young Simpson, the Professor of Obstetrics at Edinburgh University (Figure 1.17). He first used the vapour early in November 1847 for a woman in labour. Within a month, he had recorded 50 applications in a wide variety of obstetric procedures. During 1853, whilst Queen Victoria was pregnant with her eighth child, Prince Albert discussed the use of chloroform with a Scottish doctor, John Snow. Snow explained that the technique was extremely simple and when the Queen went into labour 2 days later, Snow was summoned to the Palace. Inhaling a chloroform-soaked handkerchief, Prince Leopold was born, with the Queen largely unconscious and free from pain.

Chloroform soon became the most popular anaesthetic, particularly in Europe, where French and English ambulance teams used it to treat soldiers at the Siege of Sebastapol. An American physician, Oliver Wendall Holmes, coined the term anaesthetic from the Greek word 'no feeling'. However, chloroform resulted in a number of fatalities. A 15-year-old girl called Hannah Greener died in Newcastle whilst having a toenail removed in January 1848. The danger of 'chloroform syncope' became a popular subject for discussion in the medical journals, but also stimulated the evolution of techniques for cardiac resuscitation. Whereas ether was preferred by many on grounds of safety, chloroform worked more quickly, seemed more pleasant for the patient and was less irritating to the surgeon. Opinion was divided over the cause of deaths from chloroform syncope. Snow regarded heart failure from too high a concentration of the vapour as the likely explanation, whereas Simpson and Lister considered respiratory failure to be important.

On 3 July 1849, Charles Bleeck removed a breast from a 42-year-old woman using chloroform anaesthesia. This took only 4 minutes, but as the last incision was complete, the patient appeared to fall dead upon the floor. Bleeck could not feel a pulse and there was no respiratory effort. Cold water and ammonia were applied to no avail and Bleeck used mouth-to-mouth respiration. On the fourth inspiration, the woman gave a convulsive gasp and was revived. Undeterred, Bleeck went on to remove an enlarged lymph node from the woman's axilla, during which she complained of pain.

In the US, on 5 October 1850, Metcalf described a similar achievement at the New York Academy of Medicine. "I at once applied my lips to those of the patient, holding his mouth open with my right hand and closing his nose with the left, and inflated the lungs

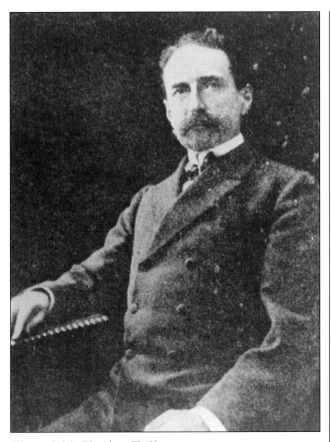

Figure 1.18. Theodore Tuffier.

slowly and gently, so as to imitate as much as possible a natural inspiration." After 15 to 20 breaths, the patient gave a feeble gasp and an artery in the surgical wound began to spurt blood. Metcalf went on to recommend that artificial resuscitation should be started immediately for chloroform syncope. In the 1870s, Moritz Schiff, Professor of Physiology in Florence, showed that deaths in dogs caused by ether could be overcome by artificial respiration. In contrast, chloroform fatalities usually occurred through heart failure, and resuscitation was ineffective unless the chest was opened and the heart massaged. "One makes rhythmic movements with the hand holding the whole heart." With remarkable insight, Schiff suggested that resuscitation was due to the massage filling the heart's own arteries and not to pure mechanical stimulation. He also drew attention to the value of compressing the abdominal aorta during cardiac massage, so as to ensure that the heart's output was supplied to the brain and coronary arteries.

Probably the first surgeon to attempt cardiac massage on a patient was Niehaus of Berne, whose patient, a 40-year-old man, died during chloroform administration for a goitre removal in 1880. Niehaus performed a left thoracotomy and began rhythmical compression of the heart, whilst the anaesthetist continued with artificial respiration. This attempt was unsuccessful and was not repeated for many years. The next attempt was made in 1898 by Theodore Tuffier (Figure 1.18) on a 24-year-old man who died suddenly, 5 days after drainage of an appendix abscess. Tuffier witnessed the demise, called for a knife and incised the left third interspace. Inserting his hand, he performed cardiac compression for between 1 and 2 minutes, during which the pulse and respiration returned temporarily, but could not be sustained. Autopsy showed death from pulmonary embolus.

The first successful cardiac massage was achieved by Christian Igelsrud of Tromso, Norway, at the turn of the century. Chloroform was used to anaesthetize a 43-year-old woman with carcinoma of the uterus, but at the end of the hysterectomy, the woman suffered cardiac arrest. After an unsuccessful attempt at artificial respiration, Igelsrud performed a left thoracotomy and massaged the heart between thumb and middle and index fingers. Using strong rhythmical massage for about 1 minute, the heart began to beat and the patient survived with complete recovery. Soon afterwards, in 1902, Sir William Arbuthnut Lane recorded a second success in a 65-year-old man undergoing abdominal surgery for colic. The heart stopped during ether anaesthesia and, inserting his hand into the abdominal incision, Lane felt and squeezed the motionless heart. Artificial respiration was continued for 12 minutes, after which the patient recovered uneventfully.

The first heart operations

EFFORTS to repair cardiac wounds continued. The Italian experimental surgeon, Simplicio Del Vecchio, incised dogs' hearts and successfully sutured them. He demonstrated his methods to a surgical congress in 1894 and showed a surviving dog that had been operated on 40 days before. Del Vecchio provided practical details of how a surgeon should conduct cardiac suture in a human patient. Practical application of cardiac suture came in September 1895, when the Norwegian surgeon, Axel Cappelen, operated on a 24-year-old man who had been stabbed through the fourth intercostal space on the left side. Cappelen opened the chest by removing the fourth rib and found a 1 inch wound of the left ventricle. Sutures were inserted into the wound and a lacerated coronary vessel was tied off. An injection of saline was given to improve the patient's condition, but he died 2 days later. Autopsy showed the wound to have closed satisfactorily, but death had occurred through coronary occlusion. In March 1896, Guido Farina of Rome operated on a 30-year-old man with a 7 mm stab wound of the right ventricle. This was easily closed with sutures, but the patient died 3 days later from bronchopneumonia. Again, the cardiac wound was already healing satisfactorily. Farina was refused permission to keep the heart following autopsy and did not publish his results. However, he later described the case to Sir John Bland Sutton, the famous London surgeon, who subsequently quoted Farina's work in a lecture on the treatment of injuries of the heart in 1908.

The first clinical success came in September 1896, when Ludwig Rehn of Frankfurt operated on a 22-year-old man stabbed in a drunken brawl. Rehn operated to relieve cardiac tamponade and closed a 1.5 cm wound of the right ventricle with three interrupted sutures. He then packed the pericardial cavity with iodoform gauze as a precaution against infection and secondary haemorrhage. Although pus accumulated in the pleural cavity, the man recovered and was known to be alive 10 years later.

For cardiac wounds, Paget advocated absolute rest of the body and mind, a light diet and, in some cases, morphine. If the patient became restless, excited or heavily oppressed and the external haemorrhage was not profuse, Paget advised venesection. If this was not successful, the pericardium could be tapped, or a small incision made in it to relieve cardiac tamponade. Paget also saw no future in chest drainage and believed Tuffier's successful resection of pulmonary tuberculosis in 1891 to have been a freak.

The first cardiac operation reported in the US took place on 14 September 1902 (Article 1.2, Appendix A). Luther Hill, of Montgomery, Alabama, was called to the home of a 13-year-old boy who had been stabbed five times in the chest. The boy was dyspnoeic, restless and in shock, with a barely palpable pulse and inaudible heart sounds. Recognizing cardiac tamponade, Hill proceeded to perform a thoracotomy by the light of oil lamps on the kitchen table. He reported the operation in some detail.

"The wound was about three-eighths of an inch in length and from it came a stream of blood at every systole. I removed the boy from his bed to a table, at 1 o'clock at night, 8 hours after the stabbing, and proceeded to cleanse the field of the operation and place the patient in as favourable a condition as my surroundings in the negro cabin would allow. Commencing an incision about five-eighths of an inch from the left border of the sternum, I carried it along the third rib for 4 inches. A second incision was started at the same distance from the sternum and carried along the sixth rib for 4 inches. A vertical incision along the anterior axerior line was made connecting them. The third, fourth and fifth ribs were cut through with the pleura. The musculo-osseous flap was raised with the cartilages of the ribs acting as the hinges. There was no blood in the pleural cavity, but the pericardium was enormously distended. I enlarged the opening in the pericardium to a distance of 2 inches, and evacuated about 10 ounces of blood. The pulse immediately improved and was commented upon by Dr LD Robinson, who so successfully and skilfully administered the chloroform. I had my brother, Dr RS Hill, to pass his hand into the pericardial cavity and bring the heart upwards and at the same time, steady it sufficiently for me to pass a cat gut suture through the centre of the wound in the heart and control the haemorrhage. I cleansed the pericardial sack with a saline solution and closed the opening in it with seven interrupted cat gut sutures. The pleural cavity was also cleansed with a saline solution and drained with iodoform gauze. On 17th September he commenced to improve, and his recovery has been uninterrupted."

Luther Hill had trained with Joseph Lister in England and christened his son Lister Hill. His son eventually became well known as Senator Hill of Alabama.

Evolution of cardiology

IN 1895, Wilhelm Konrad Roentgen, Professor of Physics at the University of Wurtzburg, discovered X-rays. This provided an enormous stimulus for many developments in medicine and surgery by opening up an entirely new field of diagnosis and study of disease. Roentgen was working with cathode-ray tubes, where a

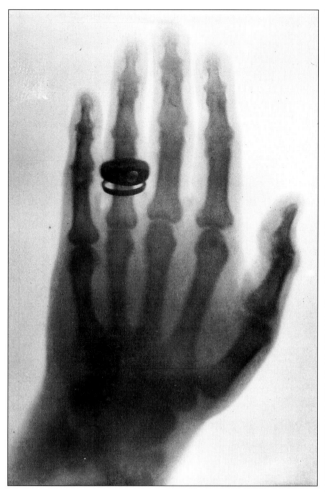

Figure 1.19. Roentgenogram of the hand of anatomist Rudolph von Kölliker made in the first and only public demonstration of X-rays by Roentgen in 1895. (Courtesy of Jeremy Norman & Co., Inc.)

beam of electrons is directed onto a fluorescent television screen to produce an image. On 8 November 1895, in his darkened laboratory, he passed a current of 20 A through the black paper-wrapped cathode tube. One end of the tube became fluorescent and a faint glow travelled 1 inch or so beyond the end. Unexpectedly, there was a greenish light about 1 yard away, and the glow appeared to emanate from a small screen coated with a fluorescent substance used to monitor cathode rays. Aware that cathode rays could not travel the distance in question, Roentgen postulated the production of a different type of ray. Holding a piece of paper between the cathode ray tube and screen did not cause the glow to disappear; nor did a book or various sheets of metal, apart from lead. Whilst holding a sheet of metal in front of the ray, Roentgen observed the shadowy outline of his hand with

the bones clearly showing through. In disbelief, he sought to confirm the ability to see through tissues by placing a wrapped photographic plate on the workbench and again energizing the cathode ray tube for several minutes. When the photographic plate was developed, the rays left a clear image of the bones of his hand and wrist. The first radiological negative of a human limb was that of his wife's hand, taken on 22 November 1895. A month later on 28 December, Roentgen announced the discovery of what he called X-rays because of the uncertain nature of the discharge (Figure 1.19). The discovery had an explosive effect on the medical world and, in 1901, Roentgen was awarded the first Nobel Prize for Physics. The first time X-rays were used for diagnosis was in 1896, when a drunken sailor was admitted to a London hospital with a stab wound in the back. He was paraplegic and X-rays of the spine showed the tip of a knife blade wedged between two vertebrae and encroaching on the spinal canal. Surgery to remove the blade resulted in resolution of the paraplegia. In 1903, Tuffier used X-rays to locate a bullet in the chest of a wounded soldier. The X-rays appeared to demonstrate the bullet in the region of the left atrium, and on 10 October Tuffier explored the pericardial cavity, located the bullet within fibrinous adhesions and removed it. The patient made an uneventful recovery.

The second half of the 19th century saw a tremendous amount of work on the heart and circulation, with the eventual evolution of medical specialization. The histological structure of normal and diseased hearts was actively investigated from the last part of the 19th century onwards. Wilhelm His described the bundle of conducting tissue between the atria and ventricles in 1893, and Stanley Kent identified accessory conduction pathways. Ludwig Aschoff characterized the myocardial changes of rheumatic fever, describing the perivascular cellular bodies known as Aschoff bodies. With his student, Tawara, he described the conduction system in mammalian hearts, with observations on the abnormalities in conduction in congenital heart disease. Tawara traced the communications between the bundle of His and the fibres previously described by Purkinje. Tawara also described the atrioventricular node in 1906, and the following year, Arthur Keith and Martin Flack located the sinoatrial node. In 1910, Thomas Lewis provided proof of the origin of the heartbeat from this site.

In 1889, Augustus Waller, a GP in Kensington, London, attempted to measure the electrical impulses created by the heart, but his equipment was insufficiently sensitive to give an accurate record. Willem Einthoven of Leiden adapted a string galvanometer for the purpose and connected this to electrodes on the chest wall. His apparatus was extremely cumbersome, with the subject sitting with his or her feet in a tub of salt solution. Nevertheless, he identified the P, Q, R and S waves in 1903, and published many basic clinical observations. Einthoven was also a Nobel Prize winner in 1924, and electrocardiography became a standard cardiological investigation, both in clinical and experimental studies.

Thomas Lewis, who had been acquainted with both Waller and Einthoven, used an ink-writing polygraph together with an electrocardiogram to study the normal mechanism of heartbeat and rhythm disorders. He attracted many students to London, particularly from the US, and contributed to the development of cardiology as a speciality. It was not until 1919 that James Herrick first described the electrocardiogram (ECG) after coronary thrombosis, and compared the clinical diagnosis with the electrocardiographic findings; autopsy confirmed the association. The ECG in angina was first noted by Bousfield in 1918, and in 1920, Harold Pardee described a survivor of acute myocardial infarction with ECG records.

William Osler, generally regarded as the greatest and most respected physician of his time, was one of the first to recognize the platelet as the third formed element of the blood and to recognize the importance of platelets in thrombus formation.

Creating an environment to support intracardiac surgery

THE DEVELOPMENT of angiocardiography began surprisingly soon after Roentgen's description of X-rays. Initial experiments involved injection of potential contrast media into animals and cadavers, but by 1918, water-soluble iodides and air contrast were in use in neurology.

The first intravenous pyelogram was reported in 1923 and indicated that the vascular system might easily be visualized. Experimental catheterization of the heart had been undertaken as early as 1855 by two Frenchmen, Auguste Chauveau and Etienne Marey. They sought to study the pressures inside the heart and discover whether all the chambers contracted together or not. They used tubes with two separate sausage-shaped recording balloons connected to a revolving drum with pen recorders. For the right heart the catheter was passed through an incision in the jugular vein and for the left side it was passed via a metal tube that passed into the carotid artery. The great French physiologist, Claude Bernard, also catheterized the heart and measured cardiac output by chemical and temperature measurements of the blood. He succeeded in passing catheters retrogradely through the aortic valve via the carotid artery. In 1905, Fritz Bleichroder, a physician from Berlin, passed a ureteric catheter through a vein in his own thigh into the inferior vena cava. He saw no future for the technique and did not publish his work until 1912. Later he used direct arterial catheterization for delivery of the agent Salvarsan in syphilis.

Along similar lines, the German urologist, Werner Forssmann, unaware of Bleichroder's work, also planned to use catheterization as a method for delivering drugs in an emergency on the operating table. Having achieved right atrial catheterization easily with a ureteric catheter in a cadaver, he engaged the aid of an assistant to catheterize himself. The assistant's nerve failed and Forssmann cut down on a vein in his own left elbow and threaded the ureteric catheter through a wide-bore needle into the vein. With a mirror arranged so that he could see the X-ray screen, he manipulated the catheter into the right heart, then walked upstairs to the X-ray department to confirm his achievement radiographically. Two years later, Forssmann obtained contrast X-rays of the heart in dogs and again attempted the technique unsuccessfully on himself. It was not until 1938 that George Robb and Israel Steinberg of New York used an iodized agent to demonstrate first the right heart and pulmonary circulation, then later the left heart chambers and aorta. This provided a tremendous impetus to cardiological investigation with a view to surgical treatment.

Adolph Fick began his basic physiological studies of bloodflow and haemodynamics in 1882, and heart muscle physiology evolved from previous studies of skeletal muscle. The relationships between fibre length and strength of contraction of skeletal muscle were known to Fick, and Otto Frank formulated the fundamental principles of cardiac contraction. Straub and Wiggers independently described the stress curve characteristics of the right ventricle in 1914, and Ernest Starling performed a series of experiments characterizing left ventricular volume and stroke output during variations of venous inflow and aortic resistance. Starling published a series of papers in 1914 describing how the mechanical energy of cardiac contraction depended on the length of the muscle fibres.

Another great discovery came from a medical student, McLean, in 1915. He discovered heparin whilst working on thromboplastins in the laboratory of Howell. Citrate had been used to render blood incoagulable since 1914, but only very small quantities could be tolerated in transfusion. Heparin permitted a great variety of new therapeutic interventions. Oral anticoagulants did not appear until the 1940s, after a disease of cattle was noted to produce excessive bruising and fatal bleeding. The cause was identified as a defect in the clotting mechanism caused by feeding cattle with spoiled sweet clover. Dicumarol was isolated and crystallized in the laboratory of Link in 1941 and applied clinically soon afterwards.

Despite significant advances in diagnostic cardiology, the problem of acute ventilatory disturbance persisted when the chest was opened. Nevertheless, some advances occurred after the discovery of anaesthesia in 1846. Trendelenburg, Langenbeck's assistant in Berlin in the 1860s, devised a curved metal tracheostomy tube and gauze mask to provide anaesthesia without inhalation of blood or secretions. He subsequently modified his device by incorporating an inflatable rubber cuff on the endotracheal aspect of the device. Next, the famous Glasgow surgeon, Sir William MacEwen, invented a flexible brass tube to be introduced into the upper airway of the unconscious patient, instead of tracheotomy. In 1885, a New York ear, nose and throat surgeon, Joseph O'Dwyer, devised a tube to be passed through the larynx in patients with diphtheritic obstruction. Two years later, George Edward Fell of Buffalo designed bellows for giving artificial respiration to patients with opium poisoning. The bellows system was combined with O'Dwyer's tube to become the Fell–O'Dwyer apparatus. This was used by Rudolph Matas for administering endotracheal anaesthesia in 1899. Bellows provided positive pressure to keep the lungs inflated with the chest open.

Invention of the laryngoscope, by Alfred Kirstein in

1895, meant that endotracheal tubes could be inserted under direct vision. Franz Kuhn introduced nasotracheal intubation with the use of cocaine as a local anaesthetic to prevent gagging and coughing. Kuhn also emphasized that the tube should be large enough to allow easy expiration as well as inspiration. It was then realized that surgery could be performed on the open thorax by insufflation anaesthesia, during which anaesthetic gas was introduced directly into the lungs; these were kept inflated and oxygenated. The method was not readily accepted, however, and the alternative of creating a negative pressure around the chest so that the lungs could not collapse with the chest open was introduced by Ferdinand Sauerbruch.

Sauerbruch was assistant to the Polish Professor of Surgery, Mikulicz, who, in turn, was a pupil of Billroth and an expert gastrointestinal surgeon who wished to operate on cancer of the oesophagus. When Sauerbruch joined Mikulicz in 1903, Mikulicz had already attempted rhythmic insufflation of the lungs by pumping air into them (with little success). Sauerbruch considered positive pressure anaesthesia to be actively harmful and proposed instead a negative pressure chamber, which allowed the chest to be opened widely with safety. Eventually, Mikulicz agreed to provide the negative pressure chamber and ordered a large one to be built for human operations. At the Congress of the German Society for Surgery in April 1904, Sauerbruch described his work and Mikulicz speculated on the revolution such a chamber would cause in thoracic surgery, perhaps by allowing surgery on the heart. A large glass chamber, equipped with telephone, was installed in June 1904. This was successful experimentally, but the suction apparatus failed during the first operation on a patient. Undaunted, the pair carried out more than a dozen technically successful operations on the lungs or oesophagus, though the temperature in the cabinet was unpleasantly high. Unfortunately, Mikulicz died from cancer of the stomach soon afterwards. Sauerbruch then lost his facilities until his appointment as Professor of Surgery in Zurich in 1910. There he continued his work with the negative pressure chamber, but was soon overtaken by positive pressure insufflation methods. The latter were further facilitated in 1909 by a notable paper from Samuel James Meltzer and John Auer of the Rockefeller Institute, New York. They described the use of muscle paralysis by curare to facilitate rhythmic pulmonary inflation. Their experimental findings were applied to human anaesthesia by Charles Elsburg in 1910, using an endotracheal tube directly inserted with the aid of a laryngoscope.

Competition between negative pressure chamber methods and inhalational positive pressure anaesthesia continued until after World War I, when two British anaesthetists, Magill and Rowbotham, improved endotracheal insufflation. They used positive pressure ventilation for many of Sir Harold Gillies' plastic surgery patients whose faces were badly burnt or wounded. Reconstructive surgery took many hours and face masks were obviously unsuitable. Many years later, Magill developed the simple method of intermittent endotracheal suction to remove secretions from the air passages.

Between the Great Wars

BETWEEN the wars, there were few forays into the realms of cardiac surgery, with the notable exceptions of Doyen's attempted mitral valvotomy in 1913, Tuffier's abortive aortic valvotomy the same year, and Elliot Cutler's mitral valvotomy of 1923. Notable achievements were nevertheless recorded in the surgery of pulmonary embolism. Best known in this field is Trendelenburg, Langenbeck's former assistant and founder of the German Surgical Society (1872). Reviewing the deaths of nine patients from pulmonary embolism in Leipzig Hospital, he observed that the majority survived for intervals of between 10 minutes and 1 hour after initial collapse. Reasoning that this gave time for surgical intervention, Trendelenburg produced experimental pulmonary embolism in the calf, and then intervened by thoracotomy. Working in the post-mortem room, he perfected his technique and applied it first on a 70-year-old man who had died on the operating table. The procedure was carried out through a window in the anterior chest wall, started along the second rib and extended vertically to the left of the sternum. The pericardium was incised and a rubber tube passed behind the aorta and pulmonary artery. Traction on this sling obstructed the bloodflow and allowed the pulmonary artery to be opened and the clot removed with forceps in less than 45 seconds. When his second patient died from secondary haemorrhage (internal mammary artery),

Trendelenburg, then aged 64, never attempted the procedure again.

The first successful pulmonary embolectomy was carried out by Martin Kirschener, a pupil of Trendelenburg, who operated on Johanna Kemphf on 18 March 1924. The pulmonary embolus followed a routine hernia operation and it was 4 days before the patient regained consciousness. By the 1930s, more than 300 attempts at pulmonary embolectomy had produced less than 10 survivors. To open the pleura was in itself hazardous and many survivors died from recurrent pulmonary embolus. The only surgeons to achieve success were Clarence Crafoord of Stockholm, Eric Nystrom of Uppsala and Arthur Mayer of Berlin, who modified Trendelenburg's technique with an extrapleural approach. This was easier said than done.

With the appearance of anticoagulant drugs, it was hoped that pulmonary embolectomy might become obsolete. In 1944, Alton Ochsner told the American Surgical Association,

"I hope we will not have any more papers on the removal of pulmonary emboli before this organization, an operation which should be of historic interest only. Certainly the way to prevent death from pulmonary embolism is to prevent the clot from becoming detached and getting into the pulmonary artery if thrombosis does occur."

Antibiotics

THE DEVELOPMENT of antibiotics occurred more by accident than by design, but changed the face of modern medicine and surgery. As recently as 60 years ago, any surgical wound infection was potentially fatal, with little else but arsenic, mercury or bismuth for treatment. Penicillin was discovered by chance in 1928, when Alexander Fleming, a Scottish bacteriologist working at St Mary's Hospital in London, was growing staphylococci on Petri dishes. These were left on a workbench whilst he and his staff left for a three week holiday. During this time, the dishes became contaminated with a mysterious mould, the spores of which must have entered through the laboratory window. When Fleming returned, he noticed that the colonies of bacteria in contact with the mould had been killed. Whatever the mould was, it had the property to eradicate a dangerous organism. Fleming cultured more of the mould, which he named *Penicillium notatum*. He put it in contact with other bacteria, including streptococci, pneumococci, gonococci, meningococci and the diphtheria bacillus, all of which were responsible for hundreds of thousands of deaths annually. In each case, the colonies of bacteria rapidly died in contact with the penicillin. Further experiments showed penicillin to be non-toxic to healthy animals, though attempts to isolate the active constituent of the mould were difficult. When mixed with blood in the test-tube, the antibiotic effect appeared to disappear. Frustrated by the inability to isolate the antibiotic substance, Fleming published only one short manuscript on the subject in 1929 and resumed other investigations. In the meantime, many patients continued to die from relatively simple traumatic or surgical infections.

In 1937, Howard Florey, a young Australian pathologist, was appointed head of the Dunn School of Pathology at Oxford and took on Ernst Chain, a Jewish biochemist who had escaped from Nazi Germany, to help him find a reliable antibiotic. Scouring the literature they found Fleming's report, obtained a small sample of penicillin and took the investigations further. Like Fleming, they had difficulty in separating the active substance from the mould, as less than one part in 2,000,000 was pure penicillin. Nevertheless, Norman Heatley, another biochemist in the team, succeeded in purifying it.

At the beginning of 1940 and World War II, research money was difficult to find, but with a simple experiment the team achieved dramatic success. In May 1940, they infected eight mice with a lethal dose of streptococci and four were then given penicillin. The following day, the treated mice were well whereas the others were dead. The significance of this finding was readily apparent to the Oxford team, who published a manuscript entitled *Penicillin as a Chemotherapeutic Agent* in *The Lancet* on 24 August 1940. The discovery was well timed for the treatment of war wounds and Florey, Chain and Heatley attempted to produce as much penicillin as they could by growing the mould in hospital bedpans. As man is about 3000 times larger than a mouse, it was obvious that a correspondingly larger dose of penicillin would be needed.

The first human test patient was Elva Ackers, who was dying from cancer and agreed to be treated with the first dose. After the injection, she suffered only minor shivering due to impurities, but no other side-effects. The first real patient was a 43-year-old policeman, Albert Alexander, who was dying from cellulitis resulting from a rose thorn scratch two months earlier. He was given 200 mg of penicillin (12 February 1941), followed at three-hourly intervals by a further 100 mg. Within 24 hours there was a dramatic improvement, with the temperature returning to normal. By 17 February, the treatment was stopped due to lack of further supplies. All the patient's urine had been collected during treatment and the remaining penicillin extracted and reinjected. Sadly, Alexander suffered a relapse for which insufficient penicillin was available and died on 15 March. The second patient was a 15-year-old boy, again, critically ill with septicaemia, but this time he was cured after 2 days of treatment. The third patient also survived.

The team worked around the clock to produce more supplies, but, unable to obtain funding from the Government or UK pharmaceutical companies, Florey and Heatley went to the US. The US government backed the penicillin project which was soon as well funded as the development of the atomic bomb. Heatley continued to work in the US with Andrew Moyer and penicillin was soon produced in quantities large enough to treat the wounded. In 1942, Fleming, who had taken no interest in the Oxford team's work, obtained some penicillin from Florey to treat a dying friend. This man recovered and an article appeared in *The Times* soon afterwards (followed by a letter) recounting Fleming's original discovery. This helped to generate the myth that Fleming alone was responsible for discovering the wonderdrug. British drug companies began to produce penicillin to treat allied servicemen in 1943, and in 1945, Fleming, Florey and Chain shared the Nobel Prize for their role in the discovery. Heatley was left in the cold.

Progress in closed cardiac surgery

BY THE END of the 1930s, experimental work that would prove to be the foundation of modern cardiac surgery was just beginning. Perhaps the first indication of future developments came in March 1937, when John Streider attempted to close a patent ductus arteriosus in a young woman with bacterial endocarditis. Only partial closure was achieved and she died on the fifth postoperative day from acute dilatation of the stomach; this probably resulted from interruption of the vagus nerve. Robert Gross then successfully closed a patent ductus in a 7-year-old girl on 26 August 1938. Between the two world wars there was a change in attitude towards surgery for penetrating wounds of the chest and heart. Before World War I there were about 380 operations recorded for cardiac wounds, with a mortality rate of 45–50%; World War I added about 60 more to the list. A British surgeon, Sir Charles Ballance, obtained the records of 58 of these, of which only 14 had died. Most operations had been performed by French surgeons, often with a substantial interval between wounding and surgery. This implied a self-selection process. For instance, a French soldier was wounded at Bapaume, on 27 August 1914, and taken prisoner by the Germans. Six months later, with increasing symptoms of dysrhythmia, the chest X-rays revealed a bullet in his heart. He was sent first to Switzerland and then back to Paris, where Henri Hartmann successfully excised the bullet from the wall of the right ventricle.

Bullet embolus was recognized in 1916, when Deneke removed a bullet that had entered the left ventricle, but impacted in the right axillary artery. There were six recorded operations on the heart by British military surgeons, with three successes. John Fraser, a Captain in the Royal Air Force Medical Corps, had observed two deaths from cardiac tamponade and realized that there was often enough time for surgical intervention. He decided to operate immediately on the next case where physical signs suggested a cardiac injury. His opportunity came in 1917 with a solider with multiple wounds of the face, arms and chest. When Fraser opened the chest, he found a perforation of the right atrium, which he repaired. With appropriate management of the other wounds, the soldier made an excellent recovery.

The second survivor came from Samson, who explored the chest but chose to leave the blood clot around the heart undisturbed, and simply sewed the wound together again. The third operation was performed by Berkley Moynihan (later to become Lord Moynihan). The 34-year-old patient had been wounded in France on 11 April 1917, but it was 3 May 1918 when Moynihan operated for chronic empyema and discovered the bullet embedded in the wall of the left ventricle. Moynihan inserted two sutures on either side of the site of entry, then cut down and removed the bullet. Recovery was uneventful and Moynihan went on to remove missiles from the pericardium on at least three other occasions. He noted that retained foreign bodies were often asymptomatic, but considered that, in general, they were a source of discomfort and anxiety and should be removed.

One of the unsuccessful cases was remarkable for the use of blood transfusion directly from a donor. A 21-year-old soldier was wounded in Salonica on 14 November 1917 and X-ray showed the bullet to be lodged in the wall of the left ventricle. He was evacuated to Malta where he came under the care of Ballance at Saint Elmo Hospital. Ballance operated on 16 February 1918 and found the bullet firmly embedded on the inner surface of the left ventricle, which he incised directly. The soldier lost a considerable amount of blood and was transfused directly from a donor until the donor's systolic pressure also fell below 90 mmHg (after about five minutes). Although the patient survived surgery, he eventually died from infection four weeks later. Ballance observed that, "It is a common experience that bullets frequently lodge in the tissue and induce neither local nor general infection until attempts at removal are made." This was also the view of Gerome Head of Chicago, who treated many World War I veterans with retained foreign bodies in the chest between 1926 and 1946. Surprisingly, these rarely caused problems.

In 1933, Albert Singleton, Professor of Surgery at the University of Texas, Galveston, wrote, "Aspiration of the pericardium is criticized as an unsafe procedure by many. We do not believe that aspiration of the pericardium is always unwise; on the contrary, with definite signs and symptoms of effusion and with reasonable care, one need not hesitate to puncture the pericardium." Singleton widely reviewed the literature on foreign bodies in the heart, concluding that their presence was not always fatal and removal might invite problems. In 1938, Bigger, of Richmond, Virginia, reported 17 patients with cardiac wounds. He advocated urgent surgery if a patient was dying, but suggested that conservative treatment should be considered for those who were stable. Conservative treatment consisted of pericardial aspiration, an unpopular manoeuvre even then due to the risk of puncturing a coronary artery. Shortly after this, Streider was faced with a 12-year-old Armenian schoolboy who had been stabbed accidentally in the precordium. It was

Streider's intention to operate on the boy, but recalling Bigger's experience, he decided to aspirate the pericardium first. Withdrawal of 100 ml of blood gave immediate and dramatic symptomatic improvement and the blood was directly returned to the circulation by intravenous injection. The boy was spared thoracotomy, but Streider concluded, "It would seem that not operating upon a patient with a stab wound is a very hazardous course to follow."

The beginning of World War II saw the development of penicillin and sulphonamides to combat infection and the beginnings of a blood-transfusion service. The American Military Manual, *Guide to Therapy for Medical Officers*, of March 1942 gave the following directions for management of cardiac wounds:

1. Aspirate the blood from the pericardium by the costo-xiphoid route, if possible.

2. Repeat if there is a recurrence.

3. If it again recurs, perform a cardiorrhaphy through an extrapleural exposure.

Reviewing the experience of the Second Auxiliary Surgical Group at forward hospitals in France, Paul Samson found cardiac tamponade to be unusual because of the large size of the pericardial lacerations. Cardiac wounds were frequently not diagnosed until surgical exploration of the chest, and in 10 of 16 lacerations of the myocardium, no repair was attempted and the patient survived. The pericardium was frequently sutured over a cardiac wound, or intercostal muscle grafts used to plug holes. Out of 75 patients, Samson's group had 30 deaths, including 27 of 57 penetrating myocardial injuries. Only three of 18 with pericardial wounds died.

Meanwhile, at the thoracic centre of the 160th General Hospital of the United States Army situated in England, Dwight Harken of Boston operated on 134 patients with retained missiles in the mediastinum without losing a single patient (Article 1.3, Appendix A). Thirteen of these foreign bodies were within cardiac chambers and 55 were pericardial. Harken sought specific indications for surgery and more foreign bodies were left alone than operated on. He sought to reduce the danger of infection or missile embolus and brought attention to the difficulties of locating a missile, even

with X-rays or fluoroscopy. Harken's achievements in removing foreign bodies from within the cardiac chambers whilst the heart supported the circulation were remarkable and laid the foundations for his outstanding future career in cardiac surgery. When Harken read a paper on his operations in 1947, Laurence Miscall of New York recounted that his unit in the north of England had also removed 39 foreign bodies from the heart or pericardium without mortality.

Two other significant cardiological events were reported in 1947. Based on the pioneering work on electrical defibrillation by William Kouwenhoven and Karl Wigger, Claude Beck performed the first successful defibrillation of a surgical patient by direct application of electrical paddles to the heart. It was 10 more years before Kouwenhoven and Paul Zoll independently developed alternating current machines, capable of performing transthoracic defibrillation. At St Anne's Military Hospital, Montreal, McKendry witnessed the demise of a 60-year-old obese patient with angina. The patient had developed signs of impending coronary occlusion and after a meal became distressed, received the last rites and stopped breathing. The attendants considered the patient dead, but whilst removing rings and dentures, McKendry noticed twitching of the muscles of the neck.

"For some inexplicable reason, this prompted the application of firm pressure with both hands over the lower part of the sternum, causing considerable depression of the front of the thoracic cage. This manoeuvre was carried out not less than 4 minutes after the heart had stopped. On release of the pressure, the patient took several jerky breaths."

Rhythmic pressure was continued until the patient recovered and subsequently left hospital alive. Again, it was not until 10 years later that real efforts were made to resuscitate the arrested heart without thoracotomy. In 1949, Callaghan of Toronto used an electrode catheter to electrically stimulate a dog's heart. Paul Zoll built on this information to construct a transthoracic pacemaker for patients in 1952.

At the end of World War II and the beginning of the 1950s, the stage was set for the great advances in cardiovascular surgery. Surgeons such as Harken and

Bigelow returned to the US with ideas and experience which would provide the stimulus for future developments. Closed cardiac operations had already caught the imagination of ambitious young men such as Walton Lillehei, John Kirklin, Denton Cooley, Donald Ross, Viking Björk, Brian Barrett-Boyes and many others who would mould cardiac surgery into a speciality. By this time, John Gibbon was already working towards development of the pump oxygenator which would eventually prove the key to direct vision intracardiac repair. Key areas of support such as safe anaesthesia, cardiac catheterization, electro-cardiography and defibrillation were now established, as were antibiotics and anticoagulants.

Development of the pacemaker

EFFORTS to restore life by mechanical or electrical means consumed the 18th and 19th century physicians and scientists. Harken, in his *History of Pacemaker Development*, notes that Harvey restarted an arrested pigeon's heart by a simple flick of the finger in 1600. Even before Benjamin Franklin's studies in 1747 showing the electrical nature of lightning, there were endless experimental demonstrations of reanimation by electricity of mammalian structures, such as frog legs, skeletal muscle, hearts and even human heads.

Franklin's experiment to harness lightning involved him standing dry under a shelter holding a dry silk string attached to a wet silk kite. The string was attached to either a grounding key or a Leiden jar and electrical discharge conducted to the ground. Franklin described his experiments to the American Philosophical Society, but when Richmond sought to replicate the experiment, he failed to observe the safety precautions and was electrocuted in an elegant demonstration of electrical fibrillation. Others provided similar information. In 1775, Nickolev Abilgaard of Amsterdam placed electrodes on the side of a hen's head and applied a discharge which caused it to fall dead. Application of electrodes over various parts of the hen's body failed to reanimate the bird, until placed across the chest. In this position, they presumably caused defibrillation, after which the hen staggered to her feet and walked.

In 1797, Alexander von Humboldt found a dead bird in his garden and placed a blade of zinc in the beak and a shaft of silver into the rectum. An electrical shock caused the bird to flap its wings and try to walk. When von Humboldt repeated the experiment on himself, he had an unpleasant surprise. Probably the first description of heart block was by Marcus Gerbezius in 1719, who described two cases of slow pulse and convulsive seizures. Similar accounts were provided by Morgagni (1769), Spens (1793) and Burnett (1824). Adams in 1827 and Stokes in 1854 independently described the syncope of heart block. Rudolph Albert Von Kolliker published important work on the 'action currents' of the heart in 1855. His experiments showed that with each beat of a frog's heart, a definite electric current was produced.

Physiological experiments with the electric torpedo fish in the late 17th century, and the contributions to the physics of electricity by Galvani, Volta and Matteuci, led to the beginnings of electrocardiography. In 1859, Michael Foster demonstrated that any part of a snail's heart separated from the rest could beat rhythmically, but at a different rate. He also showed that ganglia could be excised from the heart and it would still beat normally. Stannius established in 1852 that there was a descending order of automaticity in the frog heart, with the atria beating inherently faster than the ventricles. He demonstrated that the ventricles had the property of initiating their own rhythm. The work was continued by Walter Gaskell, a pupil of Foster, who confirmed the autonomous rhythm present in heart muscle. The myogenic theory of conduction states that the cardiac impulse is conducted by muscle tissue itself. Arising in the sinus venosus, the impulse passes to the atria and then the ventricles. In 1893, His defined the conduction pathways anatomically.

The first report of cardiac pacing came from the Third Congress of the Australian Medical Society in 1929. The anaesthetist Mark Lidwill, of the Royal Prince Alfred Hospital, Sydney, attempted to resuscitate a stillborn infant who failed to revive after chest compression and mouth-to-mouth ventilation. Lidwill passed a needle through the baby's chest and used an intermittent electric current applied through the needle to revive the child. The next, but little known, advance came from Albert Highman, a student at Harvard. Working under the physiologist Walter Cannon, Highman was fascinated by the fact that some hearts could beat indefinitely while those of identical appearance suddenly stopped. He explored the literature on resuscitation by mechanical or electrical stimuli and by 1924 had accumulated information from 80 cases with 13 successes. In 1930, he received a grant to develop an artificial pacemaker that could deliver a pacing current to the heart by way of an insulated needle. By March 1932, such a device had been used successfully in 43 patients. Surprisingly, Highman was unable to interest a manufacturer in the artificial pacemaker and faced considerable opposition, including that from the *Journal of the American Medical Association*. Consequently, he did not report his experiments.

The next pioneer was Zoll, who began the modern era of cardiac pacing in 1951 with a non-invasive pacemaker system used to resuscitate patients from ventricular standstill. In 1956, Zoll applied transthoracic electric shocks to reverse ventricular fibrillation in humans and soon afterwards developed the first cardiac monitors for clinical use. These formed the basis for cardiac monitoring in the coronary and intensive care units of the future. Like Harvey 350 years before, Zoll noticed that an arrested heart would respond to a simple flick of the finger by contracting and sometimes resuming its beat. He also realized that the closest access to the heart was via a lead in the oesophagus. Zoll was assisted in his work by the surgeon Howard Frank. Frank performed the first open intrathoracic myocardial electrode placement and later implanted the first miniaturized generator.

At the Beth Israel Hospital, Boston, Zoll and his colleagues used electrical stimulation to overcome heart block in patients suffering from Stokes–Adams attacks.

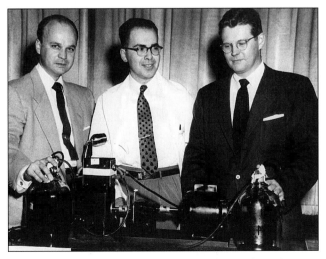

Figure 1.20. Lillehei, Cohen and Warden with pacing apparatus.

They placed electrodes on the skin of the chest directly over the heart and delivered periodic electric impulses with a frequency corresponding to the heart rate. Their ability to restore and maintain a normal heartbeat was offset by the fact that the electrodes irritated the skin and the patients found repeated electric shocks painful. Furthermore, the apparatus (a modification of the electrical stimulator used in physiological laboratories) was cumbersome and had to be kept connected to an electrical power source.

By this time, open cardiac surgery had begun at the University of Minnesota. Lillehei and colleagues (Figure 1.20) performed repair of intracardiac defects, firstly with cross-circulation and then with the pump oxygenator. At the time, there was little certainty about the site of the conduction pathways and heart block occasionally occurred after repair of ventricular septal defect or tetralogy of Fallot. Lillehei attempted to overcome this in the first seven patients with complete heart block using drugs such as adrenaline, atropine or sodium lactate. Although these efforts occasionally restored the heartbeat temporarily, none of the seven survived. In 1955, a new drug, isoprenaline, was available which proved to be more effective. A total of 60% of patients with complete heart block then survived the immediate postoperative period, although many died later from sudden recurrence of the condition.

At a pathology meeting in the summer of 1956, the heart of a child with ventricular septal defect and surgically induced heart block was discussed. The physiologist John Johnson was present and reminded the group that for years the Grass stimulator had been used to activate frog and animal hearts. He thought that a wire from the heart to an external stimulator should be tried. Vincent Gott brought Johnson's Grass stimulator to Lillehei's laboratory and studied different myocardial positions on which to connect the wire. The external stimulator was used to pace frogs with surgically created heart block. Gott was joined by William Weirich from California and they established that a cardiac rhythm could be restored by this method in other animals with heart block. With a wire inserted into the wall of the right ventricle and attached to an electrical pacemaker, a dog's heart could be stimulated with low voltages at the desired rate. The method was used to restore heartbeat following deliberate His bundle ablation and caused the blood pressure to return to normal levels.

On 30 January 1957, Lillehei called Gott and Weirich to the operating room to help him place a myocardial wire on a 3-year-old girl in whom heart block had complicated the repair of tetralogy of Fallot. The wire emerged to the external Grass stimulator. Cardiac pacing was performed successfully until the patient regained normal sinus rhythm and recovered uneventfully. Whereas the mortality of such patients following treatment with isoprenaline, atropine or body surface stimulation had been excessive, 17 of Lillehei's next 19 patients with heart block survived. Samuel Hunter, a resident at this time, described the early use of a pacemaker in a 12-year-old boy after repair of ventricular septal defect.

> "During the closing moments of the procedure we encountered a severe bradycardia of about 30 beats per minute. Dr William Weirich was summoned and appeared shortly with a device that resembled a large table radio. Two stainless steel Teflon coated wires connected to this device were immediately sutured to the right ventricle and subcutaneous tissue respectively by Dr Lillehei. The patient's rate immediately jumped from 30 to 85 beats per minute."

If temporary heart block occurred during the course of an operation, Lillehei electively left a pacing wire on the right ventricle which could be withdrawn later. Occasionally, heart block occurred late and for this reason the group developed a method to insert a pacing wire through the closed chest. After experimentally inducing heart block in dogs, they closed the chest and then passed a hollow needle through the fifth intercostal space. Through this needle, a wire was passed directly onto the wall of the right ventricle and could maintain a steady heartbeat and cardiac output. The studies were then repeated in cadavers and showed that a wire could be passed through the fourth or fifth intercostal space directly onto the wall of the right ventricle without penetrating the pleural cavity. This became the method for treating non-surgical patients with Stokes–Adams attacks.

The existing pacemakers were cumbersome and potentially dangerous. As electrical impulses of only 1 or 2 volts were required, Lillehei thought it possible to use a very small power source. Early in 1958, he enlisted the help of Earl Bakken, the electrical engineer responsible

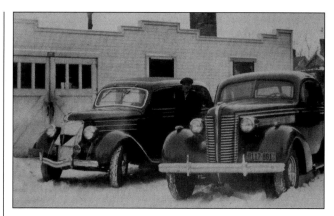

Figure 1.21. Medtronic's first office building and factory in northeast Minneapolis.

for maintenance of equipment in the Department of Surgery. At the time, Bakken was in partnership with his brother-in-law, Hermun Dsli, and together they operated an electrical equipment business in a garage in northeast Minneapolis. They repaired television sets and sold medical apparatus to physicians, often modifying equipment such as electrocardiographs to meet particular needs. Within a few weeks of the request, Bakken returned to the University Hospital with a small battery-powered pacemaker, which could be adjusted to give a desired heart rate and was easily carried by the patient in a small holster (Article 1.4, Appendix A). The device was made possible by new developments in electronics, including the transistor, improved mercury-cell batteries and other miniaturized components.

The new pacemaker was so successful that Bakken and Dsli had difficulty in keeping pace with the demand. They formed the Medtronic Company in 1958 and by 1960 Lillehei and co-workers had used the electronic pacemaker to correct complete heart block in 66 patients. Although the great majority regained sinus rhythm within a few weeks, one patient was kept on the device for 15 months.

Of 28 patients who recovered from heart block after surgery between 1956 and the end of 1961, 17 died later from recurrent heart block. This persuaded Lillehei that such patients should remain connected to a pacemaker indefinitely. Long-term pacing with a single wire also caused problems. Eventually, scar tissue formed around the area of stimulation and increased electrical resistance. This necessitated a progressive increase in voltage, and after several weeks the thoracic muscles began to twitch. In 1959, Hunter, by this time Assistant Professor of

Surgery and Director of Cardiac Research at St Joseph's Hospital, St Paul, worked with Norman Roth, Chief Engineer at Medtronic Incorporated, to develop a bipolar stainless steel electrode that required a much smaller electric current. The first such device was implanted by Hunter, on 4 April 1959, into a 72-year-old man suffering from complete heart block after myocardial infarction.

The first total implantation of a pacemaker was performed to avoid the infective complications associated with transcutaneous stimulation. The operation was performed by Åke Senning on 8 October 1959, using a unit developed by Elmquist. Senning recounts the circumstances of this occasion in a letter to Harken,

"What made me make the first clinical implantation was an energetic, beautiful woman who entered my lab on 6th October 1958 and told me I had to implant a pacemaker into her husband. He had been hospitalized with total AV block and frequent Stokes–Adams attacks for 6 months. Even though he had had an injection of digitoxin 10 days before, he still suffered 20–30 events a day. I told her we had not completed our experimental series and we did not have a pacemaker for human clinical implantation. She demanded, 'so make one'. That day she drove several times from Elmquist's electronic lab and back and finally convinced us. Elmquist coated two circuits in epoxy resin using shoeshine tins as a mould. On 8th October (1958), in the evening, when there were no extra people in the theatre, I implanted the first pacemaker, but it lasted only 8 hours. Presumably, I had damaged the output transistor or capacitance with the catheter and I did not have the other one, which was in the lab. I implanted the other one early the next morning. As the early pacemakers were short-lived, this patient now has his 24th pacemaker. He is well and has retired from an active and successful life. In the 1950s, we did not have any liability problems. The patient and relatives were happy if the patient survived."

Realizing the need for a fully implantable system for long-term pacing, Wilson Greatbatch of Buffalo, New York, designed a disc-shaped pacemaker small enough to be implanted unobtrusively beneath the skin. Greatbatch, an engineer, worked with William Chardack, and obtained the bipolar electrode from Hunter and Roth to use with the implantable pacemaker. The first

implant was in a 65-year-old man who suffered up to 20 Stokes–Adams attacks a day. He was cured of this problem, but died 1 month later from myocardial infarction. At autopsy, the tissues surrounding the bipolar electrode were found to be unchanged, with no sign of fibrosis. In 1960, Medtronic formed an agreement with Greatbatch to produce and market his implantable pacemaker. With wider application of cardiac pacing, the battery quality became a limiting factor. It became increasingly apparent that with zinc–mercury-powered batteries the pacemaker would have to be changed frequently. Greatbatch began to search for an alternative, looking into other chemical battery systems, rechargeable batteries, biological batteries and eventually nuclear batteries. Most of these alternatives proved unsuitable, and in 1970, the best option appeared to be a battery with a lithium anode, an iodine cathode and a solid state, self-healing crystalline electrolyte. Despite the fact that lithium batteries would last 5–10 times as long as the standard mercury battery, the lithium-powered pacemaker was rejected by Medtronic and others because lithium was potentially explosive. Greatbatch was nevertheless convinced that he had solved this problem and teamed up with a former Medtronic employee, Manuel Villafana, who had introduced the Medtronic pacemaker into South America. Villafana recognized the value of a long-lasting, lithium-powered pacemaker and left Medtronic to start Cardiac Pacemakers Incorporated (CPI). With the help of Lillehei's surgeon brother Richard, the lithium pacemaker was tested and commercialized. So successful was the project that Villafana sold CPI to Eli Lilly in 1975 for $126 million and went on to develop the St Jude and ATS heart valve companies.

Next to the development of the implantable pacemaker in 1960, the most significant advance was the endocardial pacing catheter which could be inserted through the cephalic or jugular vein into the right heart. The Canadians, Bigelow and Callaghan, worked with engineer Hops to achieve this goal experimentally in 1950. The first clinical implant of an endocardial electrode for temporary pacing was by Seymour Furman, of Montefiore Hospital, New York, in 1958. Initially, there were problems with constant movement and the difficulty of developing an unbreakable wire lead with an electrode that could remain in a stable position for a long time. Myocardial perforation also occurred initially. With satisfactory solutions, the system gained wide acceptance, because a transvenous lead could be implanted without a thoracotomy or general anaesthesia.

The next step was to develop a system that avoided competition between intrinsic heartbeats and the fixed-rate pulse generator. The first implantable units to respond to atrial activity were produced in 1965, and by the mid-1970s dual chamber pacing systems which stimulated first the atrium and then the ventricles were developed.

Biographies

William Osler (1849–1919)

AS THE most respected physician of his time, William Osler had an important influence on the practice of cardiology. Osler was born in Bond Head, near Toronto, the son of an Anglican clergyman. His mother lived past the age of 100 years. He enroled at Trinity College, Toronto, expecting to follow his father into the clergy, but influenced by the physician James Bovel, Osler switched to medicine and transferred to McGill University. He received his MD degree in 1872, then travelled to England and continental Europe. He spent a year in the Burdon/Sanderson Laboratory, where he became one of the first to recognize the platelet and its role in thrombus formation.

On his return to Canada he worked briefly as a general practitioner but was soon invited to join the medical faculty at McGill. He also worked in pathology at a smallpox hospital and performed nearly 1000 autopsies. During the next 10 years (1874–84) Osler rose to the rank of Professor and was recognized as an outstanding clinician and stimulating teacher. After a 4-year period as Professor of Clinical Medicine at the University of Pennsylvania, Osler was invited to become Chief of Medicine at the new Johns Hopkins Hospital and Medical School, where he remained until 1905 (Figure 1.22). In 1892, he published the first edition of his textbook *The Principles and Practice of Medicine*, which became the leading treatise on general medicine in the world for the next 40 years.

Many of Osler's clinical aphorisms were collected by his students during the Johns Hopkins years. Notable amongst these are "Medicine is learned at the bedside and not the classroom", "There is no disease more conducive to clinical humility than aneurysm of the aorta", "Angina pectoris may be precipitated by: muscular exertion, violent mental state, stomach upsets or cold weather", "Adhesions are the refuge of the diagnostically destitute", "The chief function of the consultant is to make a rectal examination that you have omitted", "A physician who treats himself has a fool for a patient". Osler was instrumental in establishing the Johns Hopkins as the foremost institution for medical education in the US. He applied the latest advances in medicine to the care of his patients, urging the board of the Johns Hopkins Hospital to acquire an X-ray machine within a few months of Roentgen's

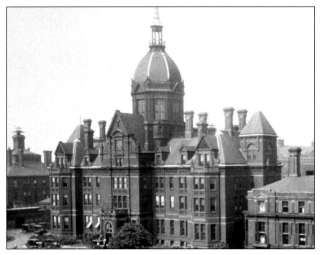

Figure 1.22. The Johns Hopkins Hospital and Johns Hopkins University School of Medicine designed by John Shaw Billings. Among its early faculty and staff were William Osler and William S. Halsted. (Courtesy of the Alan Mason Chesney Medical Archives of the Johns Hopkins Medical Institutions, Baltimore.)

first publication on its discovery. The term 'ward round' originated from the progression of bedside teaching by Osler and his surgical colleague, Halsted, around the circular building at the Johns Hopkins Hospital.

Osler emphasized the importance of travel and broad experience in the art of medicine,

"The all important matter is to get a breadth of view as early as possible, and this is difficult without travel. To walk the wards of Guy's or St Bartholomew's, to see the work at St Louis and the Salpetriere, to put in a few quiet months of study at one of the German University towns will store the young man's mind with priceless treasures. I assume that he has a mind. I am not heedless of the truth of the sharp taunt, 'How much the fool that hath been sent to Rome, exceeds the fool that hath been kept at home'."

In 1892, Osler married the widow of his friend Samuel Gross, the Philadelphian surgeon who helped recruit him to the University of Pennsylvania. In 1905, Osler left Baltimore to take up his new appointment as Regius Professor of Medicine at Oxford. He had considered that Oxford would offer a more relaxing atmosphere so that he could retire gradually but he was soon as busy as at the Johns Hopkins. He continued to practice medicine, carry out clinical teaching, publish further books and papers and was knighted in 1911. The Osler home was known as the 'Open Arms' to students, colleagues and friends before tragedy struck in 1917, when his son Edward was wounded in Flanders during World War I. Despite the attentions of Harvey Cushing (Figure 1.23), Edward died and Osler never recovered from the loss. Osler developed pneumonia and died in 1919.

A prolific writer, Osler had 1500 items in his bibliography, with one-third of the papers dedicated to cardiovascular disease, particularly infective endocarditis (Osler's nodes). He described hereditary haemorrhagic telangiectasia and characterized the aetiology and clinical course of polycythaemia vera. He recognized the value of historical knowledge in determining the direction for the future. "By the historical method alone, can many problems in medicine be approached profitably." "In science the credit goes to the man who convinces the world, not the man to whom the idea first occurs." This last comment is perhaps best exemplified in the giants of cardiac surgery.

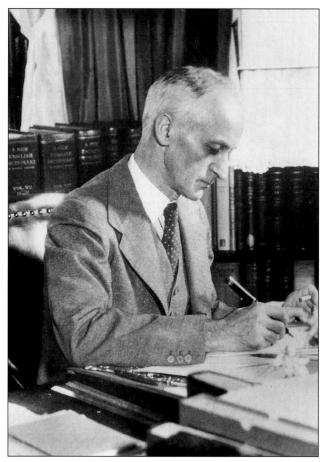

Figure 1.23. Harvey Cushing (c. 1930).

Rudolph Matas (1860–1957)

RUDOLPH MATAS was born at Bonnet Carre, New Orleans, the son of a Catalonian medical doctor. He entered the University of Louisiana at the age of 17 (MD, 1880) and interned at Charity Hospital,

> *"where the surgery of the blood vessels had become a proud historic tradition, my association with the great surgeons and teachers, who were especially concerned with the cure of aneurysm, and the anatomic experience that I had acquired early in my career as demonstrator of anatomy for over ten years (1885–95) in the dissecting rooms of the medical school, all combined to give me a special interest in vascular pathology..."*

As a student, Matas worked as medical clerk, microscopist and Spanish and French interpreter for the Chaillé Yellow Fever Commission in Havana, Cuba, in Brownsville, Texas and in

Mier, Mexico. He subsequently translated Carlos Finlay's thesis on the contagion of the female *Culex* mosquito. He commenced private practice in New Orleans (1881), where he was editor of the *New Orleans Medical and Surgical Journal* (1883–85) and president of the Medical and Surgical Society (1886). Matas organized the New Orleans Polyclinic (1888), which became the Tulane Medical School. He operated at Charity Hospital (1894–1928) and the Touro Infirmary (1904–35) and, as Professor of Surgery at the University of Louisiana (1894–1927), is said to have taught 3714 students. Among many distinctions, Matas was a founding fellow of the American College of Surgeons, honorary president of the Association Française de Chirurgie (1922), Chevalier de la Légion d'Honneur, honorary fellow of the Royal College of Surgeons (1927) and recipient of the first Carlos Finlay Award (1941).

Before Matas' treatment of Manuel Harris' multiple gunshot wound (Article 1.1, Appendix A), aneurysms were dealt with by proximal (Anel, 1710 and Hunter, 1785) or distal (Brasdor, 1798) ligation, wiring (Moore, 1864), compression, or

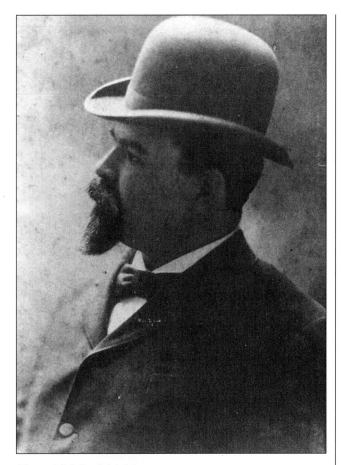

Figure 1.24. Rudolph Matas.

ORIGINAL ARTICLES.

TRAUMATIC ANEURISM OF THE LEFT BRACHIAL ARTERY.

Failure of direct and indirect pressure; ligation of the artery immediately above tumor; return of pulsation on the tenth day; ligation immediately below tumor; failure to arrest pulsation: incision and partial excision of sac; recovery.

BY RUDOLPH MATAS, M.D.,
VISITING SURGEON CHARITY HOSPITAL, ETC., NEW ORLEANS, LA.

NOTWITHSTANDING the fact that in these latter days the integrity of the brachial artery has ceased to be endangered by the practice of venesection, still, traumatic aneurisms of this vessel are sufficiently common and amenable to ordinary treatment to merit for the records of such cases no other than a commonplace interest. The exceptional features presented by this case, as indicated by the heading, are sufficiently instructive and interesting, it is hoped, to commend this report to the attention of the reader.

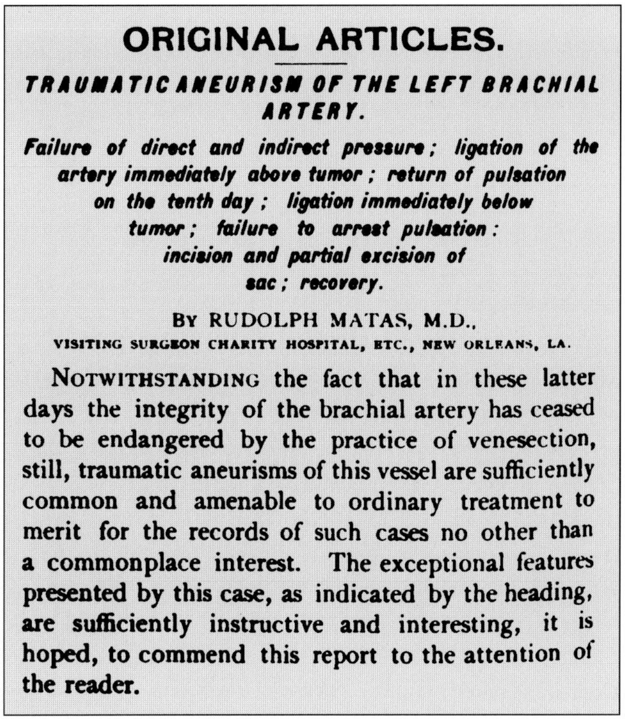

Figure 1.25. Matas' article of 1888 entitled 'Traumatic aneurism of the left brachial artery'. (*Reproduced with permission from* Medical News 1888; 53: 462–6.)

amputation followed frequently by infection, haemorrhage or gangrene. After little success with the prevailing Anel or Hunterian ligation, Matas wrote,

> *"It occurred to me then, that the easiest way out of this awkward dilemma was to seal the orifices of all the bleeding collaterals by suturing them as we would an intestinal wound, leaving the sac attached and undisturbed in the wound. This procedure was at once put into effect and the haemostasis was so perfect and satisfactory that it seemed to me strange that no one should have thought of so simple an expedient before."*

So radical did his endoaneurysmorraphy appear, that Matas was careful not to publish his report in New Orleans, but rather in Philadelphia. In addition, he did not repeat the operation until 1890 when he found Manuel Harris healthy and Souchon (his superior and the main antagonist to his break with the Anel tradition) dead. This was because he could not muster sufficient courage to battle against tradition which had imbued him, as it did almost every operator, with the fear of the dangers of atheroma and secondary haemorrhage in suturing injured arteries. The intrasaccular suture, attributed to Antyllus (300 AD) and since called the 'Matas operation', revolutionized aneurysmal surgery of peripheral arteries and is still employed today with only minor alterations.

By 1889, Matas had repaired an aneurysm of the femoral artery for the first time by the same procedure. In 1900, he began a series of over 600 operations on blood vessels, of which 260 were for aneurysms classified into obliterative, restorative or reconstructive types; by 1908 he reported 24 end-to-end arterial anastomoses and 120 lateral sutures of arteries. Matas performed his first complete ligation of the aorta in 1923, over a century after Astley Cooper's original procedure.

Pioneering in other surgical fields, Matas first described and used intravenous therapy for treatment of haemorrhage, shock and collapse (1888). He adopted spinal anaesthesia soon after Corning (1886); extended his friend William Halsted's use of cocaine in local anaesthesia and introduced direct intraneural anaesthesia with cocaine (1898). Matas developed the Matas–Smyth pump for artificial respiration (1901) and used the Fell–O'Dwyer apparatus for anaesthesia directly into the trachea (1902). He devised a test to determine collateral circulation before surgery of the great blood vessels. He was the first to describe and use nasogastric tube drainage and the gastroduodenal tube for siphonage in intestinal obstruction (1911) and first introduced films as a teaching technique in 1912.

Matas' surgical career continued until he was 78. It was not impeded by the loss of an eye (1908) which was infected by wiping his face with his operating gown after surgery of a gonorrhoeal tubo-ovarian abscess. He acquired enormous wealth and gave one million dollars and his medical library to the Tulane Medical School (1935). Matas was a key figure in the establishment of the field of vascular surgery.

Luther Leonidas Hill Jr (1862–1946)

LUTHER LEONIDAS HILL Jr was born on a farm near Montgomery, Alabama, son and grandson of Methodist ministers. A distinguished scholar of Latin and Greek, he had prepared himself to enter the ministry at Howard College, Marion, Alabama (1878) before deciding to study medicine at the University of the City of New York (MD, 1881). After he chose to specialize in surgery, he continued his studies at Jefferson Medical College, Philadelphia (MD, 1882 [2nd]) under Samuel Gross and at Wyeth's New York Polyclinic Medical School and Hospital (1883). Several months at King's College Hospital, London (1883–84) under Sir Joseph Lister made a great impression on Hill. "Lister's name," he wrote, "is imperishably embalmed in the memory of man wherever surgery is taught as a science, and practised as an art." He credited Lister with "the wondrous achievement of completely revolutionizing surgical treatment by the introduction of the methods of asepsis and antisepsis—the chart and compass of all surgical advancement."

Hill was appointed surgeon to the Second Regiment of Alabama State Troops (1888), Montgomery County physician to the Poor House and President of the Montgomery County Board of Health (1893). He was a member of the Board of Examining Surgeons (1896–99 and 1902–4), its president (1899) and visiting surgeon to the Laura Hill Hospital, Montgomery. This hospital, named after his mother, was owned and operated (1897–1932) by Hill and his brother, Robert Hill. Hill was appointed Surgeon-General to the Alabama National Guard (1911) and surgeon to the Mobile and Ohio Railroad (1915). He wrote many articles and a chapter, *Wounds of the heart* in the *Reference Handbook of the Medical Sciences* in print until 1923.

Senator Lister Hill, Luther Hill's son and Sir Joseph Lister's namesake, said that when Hill began his career in Montgomery in 1881, "my father had never seen an abdominal operation until he performed one himself, and though he was conversant with Billroth's statement, he went to work to study wounds of the heart and their possible suture." In an article preceding this one, *Wounds of the heart, with a report of seventeen cases of heart suture* (1900), Hill described Bloch's suture of animal heart wounds in the 1880s and Ludwig Rehn's first suture of the human heart (1896). In this earlier article, Hill also describes

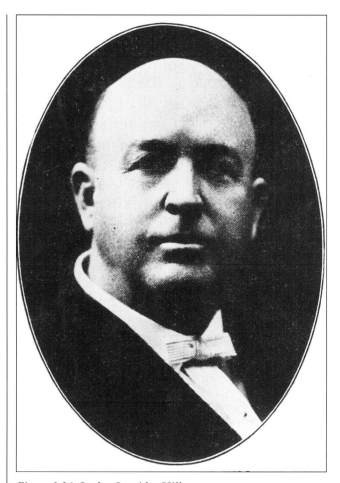

Figure 1.26. Luther Leonidas Hill.

his own first two cases: the removal of a 2.5 inch needle from the heart of an 8-year-old girl and the suturing of the heart of a stabbed 28-year-old coloured man who recovered briefly before traumatic pericarditis set in. Hill was encouraged by the remarks of John Roberts, who in 1881 suggested heart suture, and Del Vecchio, who in 1894 demonstrated its feasibility before the Eleventh International Medical Congress in Rome, by his experiments on dogs. Two years later, sutures of the human heart were attempted by Farina and Cappelen. Finally, the successful suturing of the heart by Rehn, Parrozzani, Parlavecchio and others, Hill concluded, had revolutionized the treatment and changed the probable outcome. Hill was not to be put off by Billroth's dictum in Paget's '*Surgery of the Chest*' (p. 14). Nor could the negative statistics on suturing the heart (collected by Fischer in 1868 and quoted by leading textbooks as late as 1900) dissuade Hill. Between his article of 1900 and this successful suture of 14 September 1902 (Article 1.2, Appendix A), Hill added 22 more attempts to his first list of 17 heart sutures, five of them European successes. Hill's own achievement, the first suture of the heart in North America, caused a sensation. 'Lived with Stabbed Heart' reported the headline of the article in the *New York Sun*, which described Hill's stitching of 13-year-old Henry Myrick's three-eighth-inch stab wound in the left ventricle with a single catgut suture on the kitchen table of a shack, lit by two kerosene lamps. Despite this success and Hill's plea to surgeons to "rescue the drowning heart", no further significant advances in repairing the heart were made in the US or Europe until Robert Gross closed the patent ductus arteriosus in 1938.

A REPORT OF A CASE OF SUCCESSFUL SUTURING OF THE HEART, AND TABLE OF THIRTY-SEVEN OTHER CASES OF SUTURING BY DIFFERENT OPERATORS WITH VARIOUS TERMINATIONS, AND THE CONCLUSIONS DRAWN.

BY L. L. HILL, M.D.,
MONTGOMERY ALA.,
SURGEON TO THE HILL INFIRMARY.

HENRY MYRICK, negro, thirteen years of age, of rather delicate appearance, was stabbed at five o'clock Sunday afternoon, September 14, 1902. About six hours after the injury Drs. Parker and Wilkerson were called, and, perceiving the nature of the case, advised that I should be sent for, and upon my arrival I urged an immediate operation. To this the parents readily consented, and I was

Figure 1.27. Hill's article of 1902 entitled 'A report of a case of successful suturing of the heart and table of thirty-seven other cases of suturing by different operators with various terminations and the conclusions drawn'. (Reproduced with permission from Medical Record 1902; 62: 846–8.)

J. Erik Jorpes (1894–1973)

J. ERIK JORPES, the son of a fisherman, was born in Finland on the island of Kökar in the Baltic Sea. His medical studies at the University of Helsinki were interrupted by the Finnish Civil War, when he worked in St Petersburg in a field hospital for Finnish refugees. For political reasons, he went to Sweden in 1919 to finish his medical education (MD, 1925). With the exception of a year at the Rockefeller Institute (1928–29), he remained at the Karolinska Institute as Associate Professor of Chemistry and Pharmacy (1929–47) and Professor of Physiological Chemistry (1947–63). He wrote the *History of Medicine* in retirement.

His thesis about nucleic acids in the pancreas developed into investigations of heparin and blood coagulation. He found heparin to be an acidic mucopolysaccharide able to block coagulation through—as then thought—interfering with thrombokinase. Decades later it was shown that heparin acts by potentiation of the activity of the protease inhibitor, antithrombin. Jorpes described the chemical composition of heparin and the importance of its sulphur content, proving its presence in high concentration in the so-called mast cells localized in blood vessel walls, capillaries and precapillaries. With Crafoord, he determined a dosage and mode of application of heparin, subsequently used over a period of 30 years. Jorpes' monograph, *Heparin*, a survey of the field to 1946, focused on the use of heparin in the treatment of venous thrombosis and other anticoagulant therapy, and contained a compilation of clinical literature showing that heparin promoted fibrinolysis. It gave clinical details on the use of indwelling needles suitable for injecting heparin.

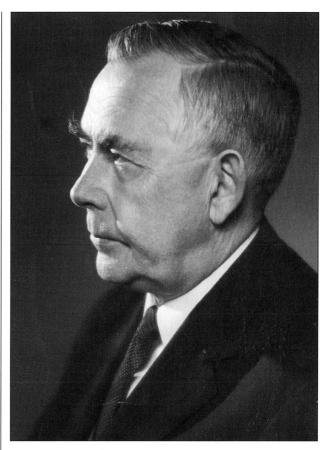

Figure 1.28. J. Erik Jorpes.

Jorpes purified heparin in cooperation with Swedish surgeons and industry, at the same time as Best, Murray, Jaques and Perrett in Canada, and introduced it as a specific and

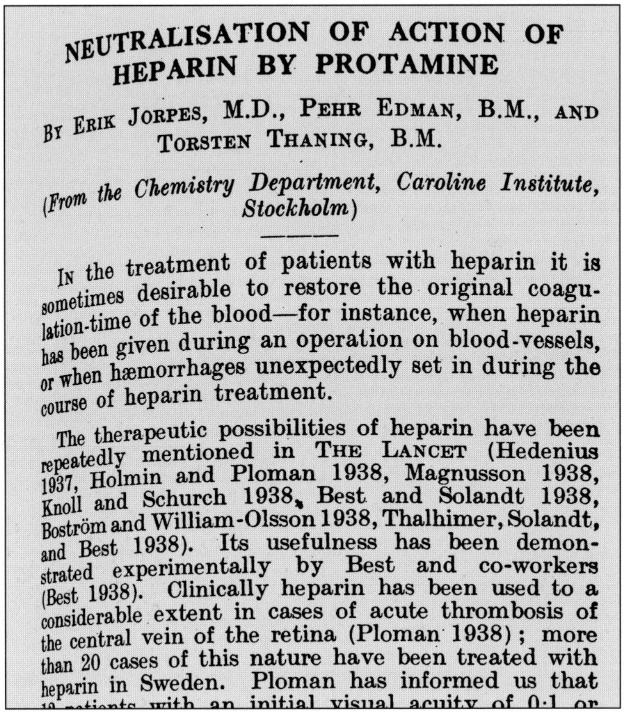

NEUTRALISATION OF ACTION OF HEPARIN BY PROTAMINE

By Erik Jorpes, M.D., Pehr Edman, B.M., and Torsten Thaning, B.M.

(From the Chemistry Department, Caroline Institute, Stockholm)

In the treatment of patients with heparin it is sometimes desirable to restore the original coagulation-time of the blood—for instance, when heparin has been given during an operation on blood-vessels, or when hæmorrhages unexpectedly set in during the course of heparin treatment.

The therapeutic possibilities of heparin have been repeatedly mentioned in The Lancet (Hedenius 1937, Holmin and Ploman 1938, Magnusson 1938, Knoll and Schurch 1938, Best and Solandt 1938, Boström and William-Olsson 1938, Thalhimer, Solandt, and Best 1938). Its usefulness has been demonstrated experimentally by Best and co-workers (Best 1938). Clinically heparin has been used to a considerable extent in cases of acute thrombosis of the central vein of the retina (Ploman 1938); more than 20 cases of this nature have been treated with heparin in Sweden. Ploman has informed us that

Figure 1.29. Jorpes' article of 1939 entitled 'Neutralisation of action of heparin by protamine'. (*Reproduced with permission from* Lancet 1939; 975–6.)

efficient remedy for thrombosis and, later, as an indispensable pre-requisite for extracorporeal circulation and haemodialysis. From heparin, he widened his investigations to purifying different coagulants, which improved the plight of haemophiliacs in Sweden. Later, he took up his earlier work on purification of secretin and cholecystokinin, which gradually expanded to include the purification of many other gastrointestinal peptide hormones used in the fields of physiology, neurophysiology and pharmacology.

His major contribution was to show that the effect of heparin could be abolished instantaneously, *in vitro* and *in vivo*, by addition of the strongly basic protein, protamine, which forms a complex with the acidic polysaccharide, heparin,

precluding its interaction with antithrombin. This discovery permitted a valuable time-limiting application of heparin, particularly useful in extracorporeal circulation.

Jorpes, a demanding and highly entertaining examiner, started the first training courses for nurses in clinical laboratory work, now a well-established branch of medical education in Sweden. He was a driving force in founding a National Medical Research Council in 1946 to improve economic security for Swedish scientists through state funds and career posts. Though he received extensive research funds, he used private and royalty monies from work on insulin and heparin to safeguard the working facilities of his institution and co-workers. He improved the technique of blood group testing and developed, together with Swedish industry, methods for improving the production of insulin.

Jorpes was central to Swedish medicine. He went to England early in 1946, hoping to encourage young men to go to Sweden to recreate a feeling of scientific unity, which he felt had been impaired by Sweden's neutrality in World War II. J.N. Howell spent the summer in Sweden as Jorpes' guest. He wrote,

"Together we worked at polishing the English of his heparin monograph, crossing out paragraphs, stapling on new ones, in his small office with the electrometric titration equipment in its cage at our backs. I had never before worked so closely with a man. He worked early and late, good-naturedly accepting criticism from a man half his age. I returned to England with a transplant of Jorpes' enthusiasm which survives until this day."

Jorpes had a complex personality, an enormous working drive attenuated by a sense of humour, a deep knowledge of botany, of classical literature and poetry which he quoted from liberally to illustrate his perspective. He loved the outer Stockholm archipelago with its bird life, fishing, light, low cliffs and free horizon.

André Frédéric Cournand (1895–1988)

ANDRÉ FRÉDÉRIC COURNAND was born in Paris, where he studied at the Sorbonne (BA (Licence), 1913) and the University of Paris (PCB (physics, chemistry and biology), 1914). After his thesis on acute disseminated sclerosis, *La Sclérose en Plaques Aigüe*, at the Faculté de Médecine de Paris (MD, 1930) and a year-long visit to the USA (1930–31), he

began a permanent collaboration with Dickinson Woodruff Richards. Cournand began as Chief Resident of the Tuberculosis Service at the Columbia University division of Bellevue Hospital and then became Professor of Medicine (1956) at the College of Physicians and Surgeons, Columbia University. Among many publications, Cournand wrote *Cardiac Catheterization in Congenital Heart Disease* (1949) and, with Lequime, *Chronic Heart Failure (L'insuffisance Cardiaque Chronique)* (1952). He received the Andreas

Retzius Silver Medal from the Swedish Society of Internal Medicine (1946), the Lasker Award (1949) and the Nobel Prize for medicine and physiology (1956) with Richards and Forssmann for their original work in catheterizing the heart.

For 40 years (1932–73), the two pulmonary physiologists, Cournand and Richards collaborated on a systematic and comprehensive examination of cardiopulmonary function in normal and diseased man, based on Henderson's concept of lungs, heart and circulation as a single apparatus for the transfer of respiratory gases between the outside atmosphere and working tissues. Richard Bing describes Richards as a great clinician, a quiet and reserved man, with a keen intellect and compassion for his fellow man, and Cournand as a meticulous worker, with a passion for accuracy.

Catheterization allowed them to measure the state of the blood as it entered the right heart, its respiratory gas content, pressure relations and rate of flow. There was no way to obtain samples of mixed venous blood until then, except by Grollman's lung–bag rebreathing technique with a balloon catheter in the pulmonary tree. This was inadequate, as Cournand pointed out while searching for a relationship between alveolar ventilation and perfusion,

"In patients with pulmonary disease, one could not predict the concentration of gas from the rebreathing method because of the different blood flow and gas distributions through different parts of the lung, normal and abnormal. We realized that we would have to get venous blood samples directly from the right heart in order to get accurate values of gas concentrations to compare with the arterial blood gas concentrations that we could get by sticking a brachial or radial artery. Using the difference between the two, we could directly apply the Fick principle."

They discussed using Forssmann's catheterization, first performed in 1929. Richards thought the possible danger of clot and embolus formation made it a dangerous procedure, but Cournand was reassured by a visit to his former teacher, Ameuille, in Paris, who catheterized the right atrium of 100 patients without complications. Cournand returned to New York in August 1936, armed with catheters, needles and instructions and began, with Richards, to catheterize the hearts of dogs, cadavers and a chimpanzee (1936–40). By 1942 they had performed nothing but a series of somewhat desultory trials in animals and an unsuccessful attempt in man.

When Homer Smith, renal physiologist at New York University College of Medicine who was interested in having a standard for Albert Starr's then invalidated ballistocardiograph, asked Cournand how to measure cardiac output, he replied, "I told him the best way of getting a good Fick cardiac output was

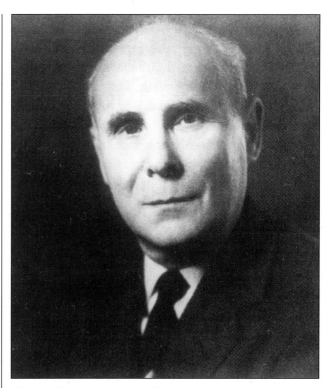

Figure 1.30. André Frédéric Cournand.

12029

Catheterization of the Right Auricle in Man.

ANDRE COURNAND* AND HILMERT A. RANGES.* (Introduced by Homer W. Smith.)

From the Departments of Medicine, College of Physicians and Surgeons, Columbia University, and of New York University College of Medicine, and the Third Medical Division (N.Y.U.), Bellevue Hospital, New York City.

Forssmann[1] first used catheterization of the right heart on himself, after exposure of a vein of the arm by a surgeon. Numerous other investigators since have used right heart catheterization for visualization of the right chamber of the heart and pulmonary vascular trees by means of contrast substance.[2–7] The introduction of the Robb and Steinberg method,[8] however, renders this method unnecessary for the latter purpose. Collection of right heart blood by catheterization of the right auricle for determining cardiac output in man[9] is mentioned by Grollman,[10] who discredits it because of the possible

*Supported by a grant from the Commonwealth Fund.
[1] Forssmann, W., *Klin. Wchschr.*, 1929, **8**, 2085.
[2] Forssmann, W., *Muench. Med. Wchschr.*, 1931, **78**, 489.
[3] Egas Moniz, Lopo de Carvalho, and Almeida Lima, *Presse med.*, 1931, **39**, 996.
[4] Heuser, C., *Rev. Asoc. med. argent.*, 1932, **46**, 1119.
[5] Conte, E., and Costa, A., *Radiology*, 1933, **21**, 461.
[6] Ravina, A., *Progres med.*, November 3, 1934, p. 1701.
[7] Ameuille, P., Ronneaux, G., Hinault, V., DeGrez, and Lemoine, J. M., *Bull. et mem. Soc. med. d. hop. de Paris*, 1936, **60**, 720.
[8] Robb, G. P., and Steinberg, I., *J. Clin. Invest.*, 1938, **17**, 507.
[9] Klein, O., *Muench. Med. Wchschr.*, 1930, **77**, 1311.
[10] Grollman, A., *The Cardiac Output of Man in Health and Disease*, Monograph, Williams and Wilkins Co., Baltimore, 1932.

Figure 1.31. Cournand's article of 1941 entitled 'Catheterization of the right auricle in man'. (Reproduced with permission from Proc. of Soc. of Exp. Biology (NY) 1941; 46: 975–6.)

by passing a catheter to the right atrium as had been done by Forssmann and others." Smith said, "If that's the best method, why not do it?" and arranged for Cournand and Hilmert Ranges to catheterize 250 hypertensive patients, demonstrating the innocuity of catheterization in a substantial series. Cournand and Richards showed that the catheter could be left in place for protracted periods without harm, that the tip could be advanced with safety into the right ventricle (1942) and thence into the pulmonary artery (1944). As the procedure was not only safe and painless, but involved no active cooperation by the subject, it was applicable to the study of patients with circulatory and pulmonary dysfunction. Alfred Blalock, Chairman of the Shock Committee, offered funds to the

Bellevue group to outline the effects of shock in 125 cases (1941–45). In 1942, Sir John McMichael corresponded with Cournand about techniques of right heart catheterization, although senior cardiologists warned that they would not defend him in court if he was charged with manslaughter. McMichael and Sir Edward Sharpey-Schafer successfully catheterized many patients in shock and myocardial failure.

Catheterization opened a whole new range of studies on heart and lung function in various diseases, which allowed comprehensive and exact descriptions of physiological conditions previously characterized only partially on the basis of bedside clinical observations.

Dwight Emary Harken (1910–1993)

DWIGHT EMARY HARKEN was born in Osceola, Iowa where his father was a physician. Harken studied at Harvard University (AB, 1931; MD, 1936) and served as house and resident surgeon on the Children's Service (1936–39) at Bellevue Hospital, New York City. In 1939, he won an appointment as junior clerk to A. Tudor Edwards, the first thoracic surgeon to make Brompton Hospital a mecca of thoracic surgery before the war. He received a New York Academy of Medicine Bowen Fellowship (1939–40) and became certified LMSSA (Licentiate in Medicine and Surgery of the Society of Apothecaries) (1939) to enable him to perform surgery in England. Harken was resident to the Fifth (Harvard) Surgical Service at Boston City Hospital (1940–42) until appointed director of the first thoracic unit of the European Theatre of Operations in the 160th General Hospital in Quonset Huts near Cirencester. After the war, he was Chief of Thoracic Surgery at Peter Bent Brigham Hospital, Boston (1948–70) where he designed, tested and implanted the first successful heart valve prosthesis, incorporated Barouh Berkovitz's direct current defibrillator to replace the alternating current and established, with nurse Edith Heideman, one of the first intensive care units. Among many honours, Harken received the Legion of Merit (1942–46), an honorary degree from Suffolk University (1964) and the Ray C. Fish Award. In addition, he received the 17th Texas Heart Institute Medal (1987) for the development of: heart valves; heart–lung machines; counter pulsation; the direct current defibrillator; correction of high health costs; awareness of dangers of smoking and the importance of animal research. He was awarded the Chadwick Medal (1991) from the Massachusetts Thoracic Society for pioneering contributions to thoracic surgery in the last half of this century. He was editor of *Medical*

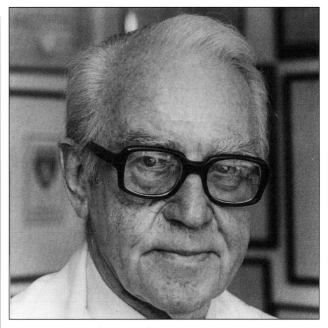

Figure 1.32. Dwight E. Harken.

Instrumentation and Emeritus Professor of Clinical Surgery at Harvard Medical School (late 1980s). Harken wrote,

"Before World War II, I had marvelled at the work of Drs. Whipple, Cutler, Churchill, Graham and Mr. Tudor Edwards of London, among others. I was confounded by their reluctance to touch, even retract, the heart. Some had flirted with intracardiac surgery, but heart surgery was mostly pericardiectomy for constrictive pericarditis....When I saw that largely mechanical heart with muscle power source and uniflow valves, I wondered about the reluctance of these master surgeons to touch it. It seemed incomprehensible that we surgeons, who are considerably mechanically oriented, should not attack this significantly mechanical organ."

During his two years at Boston City Hospital, he made his first sortie into experimental research at the Mallory Institute of Pathology. He investigated what was then a diagnosable and fatal disease of the heart, subacute bacterial endocarditis. He produced this condition experimentally on a safety pin, hooked to the margin of the mitral leaflet, visible by a cardioscope he had devised. "One might be able to cure the disease," he wrote, "if one could resect those early smaller vegetations that were limited to the edge of the mitral leaflet." Penicillin made his research obsolete, but his preoccupation with both foreign bodies and the mitral valve persisted.

With the outbreak of World War II, Harken's attention turned to shell fragments capable, in his opinion, of embolizing and damaging the heart. This was contrary to the current opinion enunciated by Ryerson Decker that free cavity, sharp needle-like bodies did not need immediate surgery. Cutler, heading the Allied Medical Command of the European Theatre of Operations, permitted Harken's removal of missiles, unlike Churchill, who, in the Mediterranean Theatre, considered the risks too great.

Harken, then aged 34, assisted by the cardiologist Paul Zoll, the surgeons Ashbel Williams, William Stanton and William Sandusky, the anaesthetist Charles Burstein and the artist Felix Weinstein, removed 134 missiles from the heart and great vessels of wounded soldiers, with no deaths: 13 from the myocardium, 17 from the pericardium, 13 from the heart chambers, 13 from the mediastinum and 78 from in, or about, the large thoracic blood vessels (Article 1.3, Appendix A). Penicillin, careful preparation of the patient for surgery, excellent anaesthesia, adequate replacement of blood loss with whole blood, postoperative rehabilitation based on breathing exercises and increased operative skill and experience improved the prognosis. However "'No deaths' was awesome," as Harken wrote, "and I knew no one would believe me so I went to Elliot Roosevelt in charge of the Signal Corp and he sent a camera crew to photograph these surgical procedures. His illustrator was a promising young man by the name of Walter

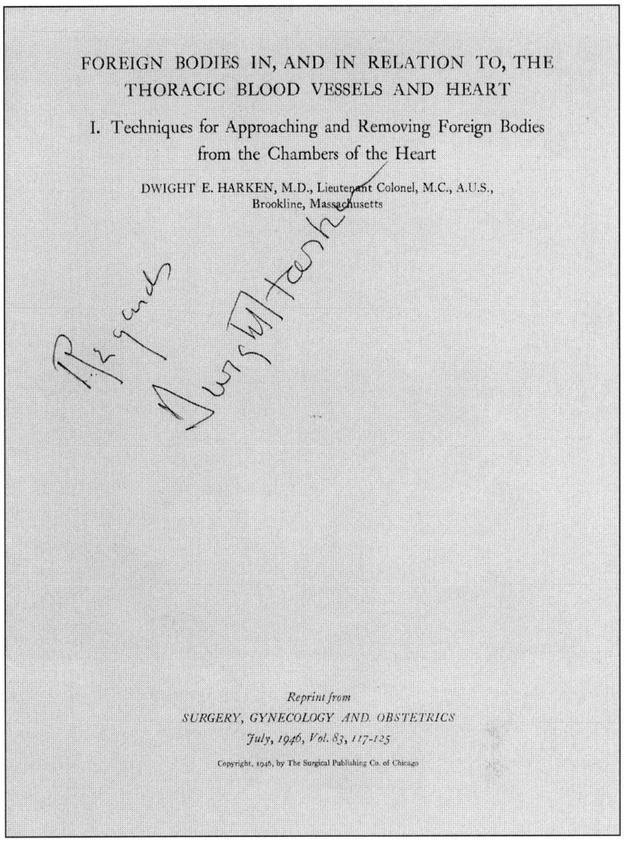
FOREIGN BODIES IN, AND IN RELATION TO, THE THORACIC BLOOD VESSELS AND HEART

I. Techniques for Approaching and Removing Foreign Bodies from the Chambers of the Heart

DWIGHT E. HARKEN, M.D., Lieutenant Colonel, M.C., A.U.S., Brookline, Massachusetts

Reprint from
SURGERY, GYNECOLOGY AND OBSTETRICS
July, 1946, Vol. 83, 117-125
Copyright, 1946, by The Surgical Publishing Co. of Chicago

Figure 1.33. A signed copy of Harken's article of 1946 entitled 'Foreign bodies in and in relation to the thoracic blood vessels and heart'. (*Reproduced with permission from* Surgery, Gynecology & Obstetrics 1946; 83: 117–25.)

Disney." The night before filming of the operation, Harken wrote to his wife, "If I kill this man, I shall be regarded as foolhardy rather than bold, and heart surgery could be set back by decades. If I succeed, heart surgery may well be on its way." This first safe intracardiac manipulation of bullets in the chambers of the heart marks the beginning of modern cardiac surgery.

Russell Claude, Baron Brock of Wimbledon (1903–1980)

RUSSELL CLAUDE, Baron Brock of Wimbledon, was born in London and studied at Christ's and Guy's Hospital medical schools (MRCS; LRCP, 1926) and London University (MB; BS, 1927; FRCS, 1928). A year in the US (1929–30) as a Rockefeller Fellow in Surgery and assistant to the thoracic surgeon, Evarts Graham, who performed the first one-stage removal of a lung for cancer, primed Brock's interest in thoracic surgery, "The impressions and inspiration I gained then as a young surgeon visiting Barnes Hospital and numerous other great surgical centers in your country were such a powerful influence that they had a permanent effect on my surgical thoughts and career." When Brock returned to London University (MS, 1932), he was appointed Surgical Registrar and tutor at Guy's, Research Fellow to the Association of Surgeons of Great Britain and Consultant Surgeon to the London County Council (1935) and Guy's and Brompton Hospitals (1936). He held these last two appointments until

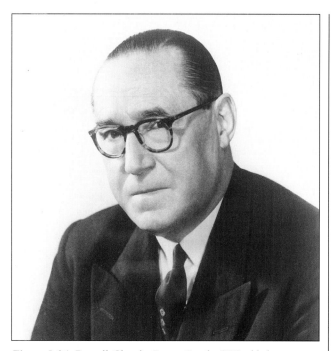

Figure 1.34. Russell Claude, Baron Brock of Wimbledon.

Sectional page 57

Proceedings of the Royal Society of Medicine

Vol. 44
995

Section of Surgery

President—Sir STANFORD CADE, K.B.E., C.B., F.R.C.S.

[*April 4, 1951*]

DISCUSSION ON THE SURGERY OF THE HEART AND GREAT VESSELS

Mr. R. C. Brock: *Intracardiac surgery.*—Heart disease may be caused by a lesion of the great vessels near the heart and may be relieved by an operation upon the great vessels. Alternatively, the heart itself may be malformed or diseased and relief may be accorded it by some indirect procedure such as a systemic-pulmonary anastomosis. The heart lesion may also be operated upon directly by some form of intracardiac surgery and I intend to confine my remarks almost entirely to this. I shall refer only briefly to the indirect operations for heart disease in so far as they introduce the subject of direct cardiac surgery. It is at once significant that 1 am able to discuss the intracardiac operations alone, because it would not have been possible three years ago. So far I have performed some 130 intracardiac operations; thus it would seem that we have here a thriving new branch of surgery.

I shall not refer to operations for injuries to the heart nor to the treatment of cardiac ischæmia nor to septal defects, but shall confine myself to the group of congenital lesions associated with pulmonary stenosis, and to mitral stenosis as representing acquired heart disease.

Figure 1.35. Brock's article of 1951 entitled 'Discussion on the surgery of the heart and great vessels'. (*Reproduced with permission from* Proc. of Royal Society of Medicine 1951; 44: 995–1005.)

by operating on the heart at a time when a large and influential body of British medical opinion believed that no form of heart surgery could be seriously contemplated. As Lord Brock said, the challenge of the early days of cardiac surgery was the actual recognition and acceptance of its very surgical nature. American advances, like Gross' ligation of the patent ductus and Harken's removal of foreign bodies from the heart, encouraged Brock to attempt direct operation of the stenotic valve. This cross-pollination is illustrated by Harken's conversation with Lord Brock at the 160th General Hospital in 1946,

"'I really don't see what useful purpose we can put this (intracardiac surgery) to after the war, Dwight,' he [Brock] said. 'We won't see such fragments in hearts then.' Harken emphatically disagreed. 'Russell, if you'd read the manuscript of your own marvellous Laurence O'Shaughnessy, you'd know he already had the idea of doing something very like what I'm doing! With this same technique, I could probably open up a congenital pulmonic valvular stenosis. If he hadn't died at Dunkirk, O'Shaughnessy would probably have come back and done it. I'll show you.'"

Lord Brock obediently examined Harken's copy of the unfinished manuscript of the Hunterian lecture O'Shaughnessy had been invited to deliver before war intervened. Included was a picture of an obstructed valve and a description of a projected operation to open the stenosis by inserting a cutting valvulotome by way of the ventricle. Brock read it carefully, remained sceptical but in 1948 himself performed mitral and pulmonary valvotomy and infundibular resection.

Lord Brock was said to give "the impression of perpetual disappointment at the unattainability of universal perfection."

1968. In the 1930s, he won the Royal College of Surgeons' Jacksonian Prize for his essay, *New Growths of the Lung*. As editor of *Guy's Hospital Reports* (1939–60) he made enormous contributions to the literature of pulmonary and cardiac surgery, although he considered only *The Anatomy of the Bronchial Tree* (1946); *The Life and Work of Astley Cooper* (1952); *Lung Abscess* (1952) and *The Anatomy of Congenital Pulmonary Stenosis* (1957) worthy of memory in Munk's *Roll*. Brock was knighted in 1954 and made a Life Peer in 1965. He gave the Bradshaw Lecture (1957) and the Hunterian Oration (1961) and became president of the Royal College of Surgeons (1963–66). When he retired from his National Health Services' appointments (1968), he became Director of the Department of Surgical Sciences of the Royal College and continued in private practice. Brock supported private medicine, hospital care and treatment complementary to the National Health Service, demonstrated by his chairmanship (1967–77) and presidency (1978) of the Private Patients' Plan, in succession to Lord Brain. Lord Brock lived through the development of hypothermia and the heart–lung machine and made significant preliminary contributions to heart transplantation. Just days before his death, he visited Papworth and Harefield hospitals to arrange gifts of equipment for their heart transplant programmes.

Lord Brock's career in thoracic surgery began before World War II, when his tentative approaches towards excision of the lung and studies of the anatomy of the bronchial tree gave him a widespread reputation. Nevertheless, he was mostly intrigued

Hanlon (personal communication, 1993) described Brock's visit to the Johns Hopkins on the Guy's exchange as,

"most impressive, and some of us who were later privileged to visit him in his last years carried away the warmest feelings for this mellowed master surgeon and investigator, a worthy clone of Astley Cooper. In contrast with the watch spring tension he

had manifested earlier in his precise, faultless operative essays in Baltimore, demonstrating his valvotomy for pure pulmonic stenosis, the elderly Lord Brock was a gracious guide to the House of Lords, masterfully elucidating its place in history."

Lord Brock was a great and unique character who played an important part in the progress of surgery.

Charles Philamore Bailey (1910–1993)

CHARLES PHILAMORE BAILEY was born in Wanamassa, New Jersey and studied at Rutgers University (1926–28), Hahnemann Medical and Homeopathic College (MD, 1932; LLD, 1953), and the University of Pennsylvania (MS, 1943; DSc, 1955). After internship at Fitkin Memorial Hospital, New Jersey (1932–33), he went into general practice (1933–37) and residency (1938–40) at Sea View Hospital, Stanton Island, New York. Bailey lectured at Hahnemann College (1940–48) where he became Professor and Head of Thoracic Surgery (1948–58) and wrote his textbook, *Surgery of the Heart* (1955), a compendium of all aspects of the burgeoning field of cardiac surgery. He taught at New York City College (1959–62) and St Barnabas Hospital in the Bronx for more than 10 years.

In the 1960s, Bailey was sued in four cases of medical malpractice in which all patients lived. Two of the cases involved awards of $25,000 to $50,000. Because no one in medicine or law could justify the lawsuits to him, Bailey decided to study law at Fordham Law School at night while performing heart surgery in the day. "In my abrupt fashion," he wrote, "I decided to go to law school so that I could understand what was happening and what to do about it." He became a licensed lawyer of New York State (DJ, 1973) but later considered medical malpractice insurance a better solution and became a full-time member of the Physicians Reliance Association in Marietta, Georgia (1993).

A vigorous and inventive surgeon, Bailey made many initial advances in heart surgery including the first combined mitral and aortic valvotomy (4 April 1952), the first excision of a postinfarctional aneurysm (15 April 1954) and the first coronary endarterectomy using the retrograde approach (29 October 1956).

The correction of atrial septal defects became the battleground upon which techniques of open heart surgery emerged and Bailey and Gross were the first to make significant

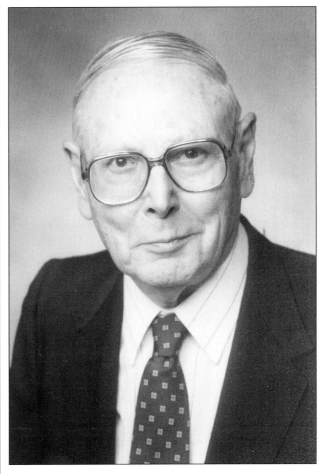

Figure 1.36. Charles Philamore Bailey.

clinical progress. Bailey described the patient preceding his first successful treatment of a septal defect by atrioseptopexy,

"A lady of 35 or so years came to me with a thoroughly diagnosed atrial septal defect. A theoretically 'corrective' approach had been made by a researcher in an animal laboratory, but no human had yet been so operated. Thorough explanations of the risks and possibilities were made, but the lady was in heart failure and desperate. So she was given

general anaesthesia, went into cardiac arrest, was resuscitated with difficulty, and the attempt at the operation was terminated. She died a few hours later. Her husband and 20-odd-year-old son approached me and requested that an autopsy be done, 'hopefully, so that a curative operation can be developed.' [Bailey's letter continues]

"Responding almost tearfully, I did the autopsy. There was the large central septal defect with a greatly dilated right atrial chamber. A deficiency of living tissue in one area and an excess of tissue in another! Right then, the concept of sewing the tip of the right atrial appendage to the margin of the septal defect— thus obliterating it—was born. It did not take much further cerebration to conceive of inserting the left index finger through the tip of the right atrial appendage to guide a suturing needle through the dilated right atrial wall, to pick up the margin of the septal defect, and to return the needle through the atrial wall. If an assistant then tied down the suture ends, one point on the defect margin would have become attached. By repeating the manoeuvre again and again the attachment of the right atrial wall or appendage to the margin of the septal defect could be applied for 360 degrees (about the margin of the defect). The large globular right atrium would have been 'dimpled in' and converted into a hollow doughnut-shaped chamber, still sufficiently large to transmit the returning blood from the two venae cavae to the tricuspid valve. By simply removing the finger and over-sewing the appendageal stump the septal defect would have been completely closed by a patch of living right atrial wall."

Two weeks later, on 11 January 1952, Bailey performed atrioseptopexy on the 4 cm septum secundum defect of a 38-year-old woman. Catheterization revealed complete abolition of the former large left-to-right shunt. Later that year he operated on five more patients: three were satisfactory, but two with advanced disease died. At first this technique only seemed suitable for correction of septum secundum defects, preferably centrally located, but it has been used in patients with

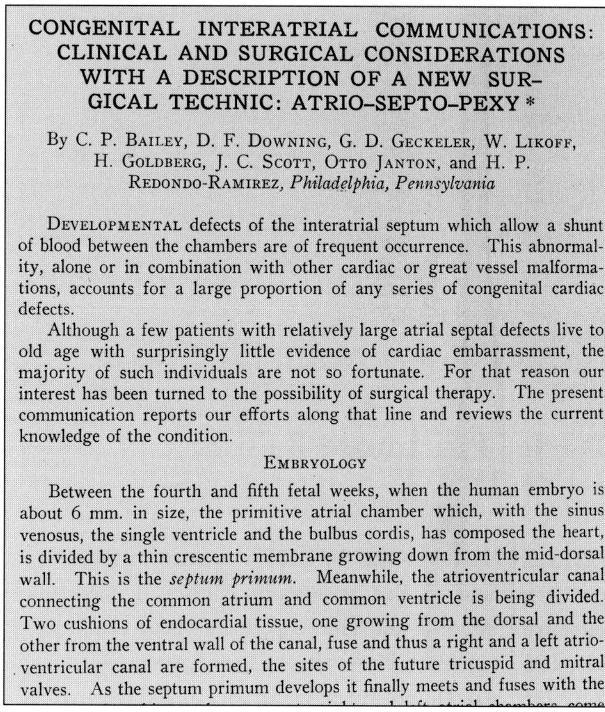

CONGENITAL INTERATRIAL COMMUNICATIONS: CLINICAL AND SURGICAL CONSIDERATIONS WITH A DESCRIPTION OF A NEW SURGICAL TECHNIC: ATRIO–SEPTO–PEXY *

By C. P. BAILEY, D. F. DOWNING, G. D. GECKELER, W. LIKOFF, H. GOLDBERG, J. C. SCOTT, OTTO JANTON, and H. P. REDONDO-RAMIREZ, *Philadelphia, Pennsylvania*

DEVELOPMENTAL defects of the interatrial septum which allow a shunt of blood between the chambers are of frequent occurrence. This abnormality, alone or in combination with other cardiac or great vessel malformations, accounts for a large proportion of any series of congenital cardiac defects.

Although a few patients with relatively large atrial septal defects live to old age with surprisingly little evidence of cardiac embarrassment, the majority of such individuals are not so fortunate. For that reason our interest has been turned to the possibility of surgical therapy. The present communication reports our efforts along that line and reviews the current knowledge of the condition.

EMBRYOLOGY

Between the fourth and fifth fetal weeks, when the human embryo is about 6 mm. in size, the primitive atrial chamber which, with the sinus venosus, the single ventricle and the bulbus cordis, has composed the heart, is divided by a thin crescentic membrane growing down from the mid-dorsal wall. This is the *septum primum*. Meanwhile, the atrioventricular canal connecting the common atrium and common ventricle is being divided. Two cushions of endocardial tissue, one growing from the dorsal and the other from the ventral wall of the canal, fuse and thus a right and a left atrioventricular canal are formed, the sites of the future tricuspid and mitral valves. As the septum primum develops it finally meets and fuses with the

Figure 1.37. Bailey's article of 1960 entitled 'Congenital interatrial communications: clinical and surgical considerations with a description of a new surgical technique atrio-septo-pexy'. (Reproduced with permission from Ann of Int Med 1960; 37: 888–920.)

eccentrically located defects and defects of the persistent ostium primum type associated with anomalous pulmonary venous drainage into the right atrium. Bailey's atrioseptopexy technique would have been widely used except that open-heart surgery soon became possible—and popular. Even now, this method is used in third world countries where open-heart surgery is not widely available. This was the first human atrial septal defect to be closed completely without prosthesis and the first example of true intracardiac suturing for relief of a cardiac defect considered by some to have been the zenith of blind tactile intracardiac surgery.

Clarence Walton Lillehei (1918–)

CLARENCE WALTON LILLEHEI was born in Minneapolis, Minnesota. After graduating from the University of Minnesota (BS, 1939) he completed a 3 year medical course in just 2 years (MS, 1941). During World War II, he was appointed Commanding Officer of the 33rd Field MASH Unit of the US Army Medical Corps, following troops fighting Rommel in North Africa. He returned to civilian life as a Lieutenant-Colonel decorated with the European Theatre Ribbon with five battle

stars, the Bronze Arrowhead Award for amphibious operations and the Bronze Star Medal for meritorious service at Anzio, Italy.

Lillehei fulfilled residency and doctoral studies at the University of Minnesota Medical School (1946–50) and on 1 July 1949 became a full-time clinical instructor. The day after he completed residency in February 1950, a growth on his left ear led to the removal of a tumour from his left parotid gland, which proved to be a lymphosarcoma. Lillehei underwent 12 hours of surgery, which involved left parotidectomy, radical neck dissection and mediastinal exploration by Wangensteen,

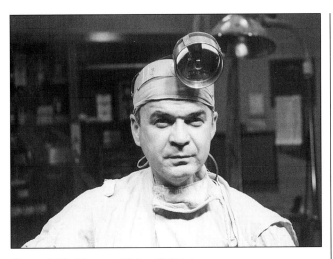

Figure 1.38. Clarence Walton Lillehei.

assisted by Varco and Lewis, followed by intensive radiation therapy to the surgical field. He became Associate Professor in the Department of Surgery (1951) (MSc (physiology); PhD (surgery, 1951). Between 1951 and 1967 at the University of Minnesota Hospital, 134 cardiothoracic surgeons trained under Lillehei, profiting from his incredible ingenuity and Wangensteen's insistence on research, among them Norman Shumway and Christiaan Barnard. Another 20 trained under Lillehei at the New York Hospital Cornell Medical Centre (1967–79) following his departure from the University of Minnesota.

In Maurice Visscher's physiology laboratory (October 1948–September 1949), Lillehei produced cardiovascular stress by surgically-created arteriovenous fistulas (aorta-inferior vena cava or femoral artery-vein) in dogs. When some of the animals developed endocarditis with typical vegetations on the mitral or aortic valves, a condition never thought to occur in the canine, the formation of valvular lesions in patients with congenital heart defects was explained. If congenital heart defects led inevitably to the development of bacterial endocarditis, then their correction became urgent, even when such defects appeared superficially benign. In the doctoral thesis *Role of Cardiovascular Stress in the Pathogenesis of Endocarditis and Glomerulonephritis* (1951), Lillehei reported these conclusions (arrived at in 1943) supported by clinical evidence from patent ductus arteriosus accrued by Shapiro and Keys at the University of Minnesota. For "outstanding research contributions to medical science" Lillehei received the Theobald Smith Award in Medical Sciences from the American Association for the Advancement of Science (1951). Lillehei, performed postmortem cardiotomies on infants and children with congenital heart disease and knew that through an incision in the outflow tract of the right ventricle, he could, with direct

vision, correct the anatomical defects with two or three well-placed stitches.

These investigations were followed by his initial major contribution, the phenomenal cross-circulation operations for intracardiac correction of congenital heart defects, beginning with a ventricular septal defect on 26 March 1954. Accused of performing an operation with a 200% risk—of the patient and the donor by the unorthodox cross-circulation—his paper proves that the method was not only safe but, in retrospect, the only one which was physiologically feasible. These operations established Lillehei as one of the greatest pioneers of cardiac surgery.

In the years that followed, Lillehei was one of the most productive innovators in heart surgery, developing a large number of techniques, concepts and devices. By 13 May 1955, DeWall and Lillehei had created their disposable bubble oxygenator. As early as 1957, Lillehei had replaced the aortic valve with a prosthetic plastic valve and had performed partial and total replacement of the aortic and mitral valves. This led to the concept that heart transplants were possible with donor hearts or a prosthetic organ. In 1960, Lillehei published his work on the pacemaker (Article 1.4, Appendix A) and in 1967, reported two assist devices to the American College of Cardiology; one, a rounded plastic sheet with a balloon lining to be implanted around the heart to assist in the rhythmic pumping of the blood and the other, a multilayered sandwich of plastic sheets and silicone rubber membranes, which could function as a miniature heart and lung. At the New York Hospital Cornell Medical Centre (1967–79) Lillehei performed his first heart transplant on 2 June 1968 ("I guess if the kids can do it so can the old man") and two more in

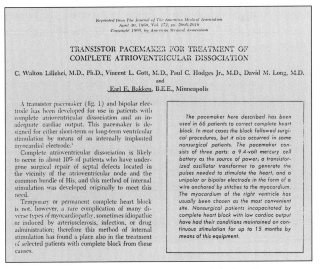

Figure 1.39. Lillehei's article of 1960 entitled 'Transistor pacemaker for treatment of complete atrioventricular dissociation'. (*Reproduced with permission from* JAMA 1960; 172: 76–80.)

January 1969. In February 1969, he performed the world's largest multiple organ transplantation, implanting one heart, kidneys and corneas into four recipients and the liver to another patient.

Lillehei threw an anchor beyond the perimeters of his time. He was the first to prove that complete correction of heretofore fatal congenital heart defects and extracorporeal circulation were not merely a hope, but an achievable reality.

William Bennett Kouwenhoven (1886–1975)

WILLIAM BENNETT KOUWENHOVEN was born in Brooklyn, New York and studied electrical engineering at the Brooklyn Polytechnical Institute (EE, 1906; ME, 1907), where the circuit analyst, Steinmetz, urged him to continue at the Karlsruhe Technische Hochschule in Baden (Diplôme Ingénieur, 1912; Doktor Ingénieur, 1913). At the Johns Hopkins, Kouwenhoven was Professor of Electrical Engineering (1930–38) and Dean of the School of Engineering (1938–54). On his retirement, he became Lecturer in Surgery (1956–75) at the Johns Hopkins School of Medicine under the aegis of Alfred Blalock, who summed up Kouwenhoven's achievements: "One, is that most important discoveries are simple in concept and design, and the second, is that an occasional person past three score and ten makes an important discovery, and it could not happen to a better fellow than Dr Kouwenhoven."

Kouwenhoven received the first honorary doctorate in medicine bestowed by Johns Hopkins (MD, 1969) for his lifetime study of defibrillation. When he received the Edison Medal from the American Institute of Electrical Engineers (1962), he explained the context of his work,

"In 1951, with the cooperation of the Department of Surgery at the Hopkins School of Medicine and with funds provided by the Edison Electric Institute, I began a further study of the possibility of developing a closed chest defibrillator ... From 1951 on, as our original team had disbanded, I had the cooperation of surgical trainees—a different one each year—and various staff members also collaborated in the work."

Among them were Vivien Thomas, Jerome Kay, G. Guy Knickerbocker, and Jude and Henry Bahnson.

The Johns Hopkins group, who had created Kouwenhoven's alternating current closed-chest defibrillator in the Hunterian Laboratory in early 1957, were stymied by the necessity of applying it within 3 minutes. Though Kouwenhoven knew of the early contribution of open chest massage by Carl Wiggers

and Claude Beck at Western Reserve University, he only slowly confirmed that this massage was equally effective on the closed chest. On the 6 May 1956 Kouwenhoven recorded that when electrodes were pressed on the chest there was a marked rise in the femoral arterial blood pressure. The hospital staff disagreed, saying that pressing on an animal's chest was like pressing on a balloon. When the pressure was relaxed the chest expanded and the pressure returned to normal and the rise was

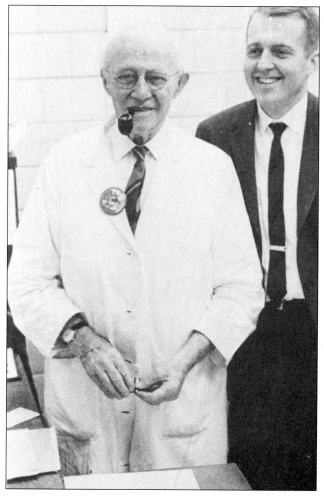

Figure 1.40. William B. Kouwenhoven.

not thought to be a sufficient indication of circulation. However, Kouwenhoven wrote,

"Mr Knickerbocker, who was working with me at that time, and I were not satisfied. We pressed on different areas of the chest and even applied blows to the chest wall. We found that the maximum rise in pressure occurred when we pressed vertically downward on the lower half of the sternum. We mounted strain gauges on the dogs' ventricles and found that the heart was definitely contracted by the pressure. Flowmeters were then installed, and evidence of blood circulation, was clear."[8]

The effectiveness of external rhythmic pressure on the heart was observed sporadically over a period of 30 years by many people. Its value was magnified by its simplicity, which made it possible for any person to perform it anywhere. It has saved thousands of patients from fatal cardiac arrest. Henry Beecher of Boston stated, "To our minds, this discovery ... ranks not too far behind that of the tourniquet in its lifesaving potentialities." Massage gave time for the application of the closed-chest defibrillator, making it a useful and effective device for depolarizing a fibrillating heart without opening the chest. Closed-chest massage, combined with mouth-to-mouth ventilation, was perfected by James Elam and Peter Safar of the Faculty of Anaesthesiology at Johns Hopkins (1954). Publications of the technique was urged by Blalock in 1960

**CARDIOPULMONARY RESUSCITATION
AN ACCOUNT OF FORTY-FIVE YEARS OF RESEARCH**

William B. Kouwenhoven and Orthello R. Langworthy

*Departments of Surgery and Psychiatry
The Johns Hopkins University School of Medicine and Hospital*

The electric public utilities, concerned about the rising electric shock accident rate among linemen and the public, sought to promote research directed toward understanding and partially alleviating this problem. This led to a research program starting in 1928 and continuing to the present time. The effort involved several men attacking the problem from different points of view. Often arduous work for a period of time led to a blind alley. Partial insight developed slowly and often somewhat fortuitously. Research grants from the National Institutes of Health as well as from the power companies and the Edison Electric Institute supported the effort. The results in terms of treatment exceeded all expectation and benefited not only the employees of the electric utilities, but also patients in hospitals. The cardiac defibrillator and the closed chest method of artificial circulation have made it possible to save many lives. The defibrillator is now standard equipment for hospitals. The closed chest method of cardiopulmonary resuscitation may keep the patient alive for at least an hour until a hospital is reached and the defibrillator used. These have become such standard methods in hospitals all over the world that younger physicians may take them for granted as having been always available. With the expansion of electric facilities new problems continue to present themselves. This report consists of a brief chronological review of previous studies.

Figure 1.41. Kouwenhoven's article of 1973 entitled 'Cardiopulmonary resuscitation: an account of forty-five years of research'. (*Reproduced with permission from* Johns Hopkins Med J 1973; 132: 186–93.)

because it was in danger of being claimed by visiting Russian clinicians as a Russian discovery; Gurvich and Yuniev's discussion of sustained circulation by external massage had appeared as early as 1947.

Chapter 2: Evolution of cardiopulmonary bypass and myocardial protection

BY 1950, closed cardiac surgery was well established in many clinics throughout the world. Nevertheless, the techniques were blind and limited to those that could be performed without entering the cardiac chambers. If cardiac surgery was to progress, there was a need for better operating conditions and direct visualization of internal cardiac anatomy and pathology.

The early experiments

VENOUS inflow occlusion had been recognized as an experimental method which gave access to internal cardiac structures as early as 1907. Rudolph Hacker achieved survival in a dog whose venous flow to the heart had been occluded for 10 minutes. In his paper, Hacker described a special clamp that he had devised for temporarily occluding venous inflow (usually for no more than 90 seconds) whilst he experimented with heart wounds and operations. In the same year, Sauerbruch and Rehn also described methods for inflow occlusion. Rehn's paper was concerned mainly with the treatment of heart wounds, but he also described experimental compression of the right atrium for 1.5 minutes during an operation performed by Magnus of Heidelberg. Sauerbruch illustrated the technique of occluding the inferior vena cava and right atrium between the middle and ring fingers, a simple method adopted later by surgeons for suturing heart wounds. Carrell and Tuffier independently used clamping of the whole pedicle of the heart for their experimental procedures. They discovered that a clamp could be left in place across the aorta and main vessels for 2–3 minutes without compromising survival. They also found that air remaining in the left heart could kill an animal if bubbles entered the coronary or cerebral circulation.

With reference to intracardiac surgery, Alexis Carrell

wrote in 1914, "It may even be regarded as extremely doubtful whether this class of operation may ever be applicable to human surgery." Two years before, in 1912, Ernest Starling had devised his isolated heart–lung preparation. This enabled him to study the behaviour of the heart in different circumstances, including variations in temperature of infused blood. In 1914, Jean François Heymans of the University of Ghent began his experimental work on the infusion of heated or cooled blood into the brain or heart of rabbits. He used a glass cannula connected to a fistula between the internal jugular vein and the common carotid artery. Despite Heymans' isolation from either libraries or scientific colleagues through the German occupation of Belgium, his many experiments laid the foundations for therapeutic temperature manipulation such as extra-corporeal cooling. Even at this time it was widely understood that the limitation to temporary arrest of the circulation was tissue hypoxia in sensitive organs, such as the brain.

Perfusion of isolated organs

THE GROUNDWORK for provision of an extracorporeal supply of oxygenated blood to isolated organs was already established 100 years before. Modern study of the circulation began with 18th century rationalism and the birth of the 'new science'. The aim of this scientific method was to eliminate religious mysticism and to discover the anatomical seat of the soul or 'essence of life'. The hypothesis was that removal of the seat of the soul would extinguish life. Classical experimentation to prove this hypothesis was the ablation of body parts until the animal died. The experiments then progressed to ablation of an individual function, for instance, asphyxiation of the animal by occluding the trachea, or interrupting the circulation to an organ by tying off arteries and veins. Le Gallois initially followed this format but became interested in reviving the animals. He realized the potential for extracorporeal circulation, as reported in his 1813 text, *Experiments on the Principles of Life,*

> *"But if the place of the heart could be supplied by injecting and if, with a regular continuance of this injection, there could be furnished a quantity of arterial blood, whether naturally or artificially formed, supposing such a function possible, then life might be indefinitely maintained in any portion."*

A decade later, James Kay performed such experiments by injecting venous blood through the lungs of a rabbit. In 1828, Kay described the restoration of contractility in isolated muscles by perfusing their arteries with oxygenated blood. In this report, he described resuscitation of a dog that exsanguinated through the carotid artery. The animal was restored with an infusion of blood into the abdominal aorta.

Workers such as Loebell, Brown-Séquard and Bidder infused defibrinated blood (oxygenated by simple stirring or shaking) by syringe perfusion into isolated muscle and kidneys. Electrical contractility and urine flow were investigated by these methods. A gravity reservoir perfusion apparatus was then developed by Ludwig and Schmidt in 1868. This enabled them to conduct studies of electrical excitability of muscle in relation to perfusion pressure and oxygen and carbon dioxide content of the blood. More complex systems were developed that allowed the return of venous blood to reservoirs by gravity, and illustrated the need for a blood pump.

The apparatus designed by Von Frey and Grubner consisted of a simple piston pump and an oxygenator, which covered the inside of a rotating cylinder with a thin film of blood. This apparatus was designed to make prolonged perfusion more efficient. It was described as the 'respiration apparatus' and was, in essence, the forerunner of the pump oxygenator. Jacobj developed a similar device in 1890, but he oxygenated the blood by allowing gas to flow through it. Both the rotating film

and bubble system caused considerable problems with haemolysis, and with the aim of solving this problem Jacobj used a set of animal lungs in his apparatus. By the end of the 19th century, long-term perfusion of isolated organs with oxygenated blood was feasible in the laboratory.

The debate as to whether constant or pulsatile bloodflow gave the best long-term results was studied independently by Hoffmann (1903) and Hooker (1910); at the time, pulsatility led to a greater degree of haemolysis. Hooker's apparatus was designed to give pulsatile rather than steady flow by using simple piston pumps. Dale and Schuster attempted to reduce haemolysis by removing the piston from mechanical contact with the bloodstream, and relied instead on the hydraulic pressure generated by an expanding rubber finger cot.

Although many problems persisted (including haemolysis and inadequate venous return), interest switched from perfusion of isolated organs to artificial support of the whole circulation. In 1930, the British pharmacologist, Gibbs, developed an artificial heart for cat experiments. His device consisted of a two-chamber pump complete with four valves, which was able to sustain the circulation for between 1 and 3 hours. Catheters connected the superior and inferior venae cavae to the device and re-routed the blood to the aorta. Gibbs' primary objective was to study the effects of drugs on the pulmonary circulation. Until the mid-1930s, extracorporeal circulation remained of interest only as a physiological laboratory research tool.

The first person to suggest that an extracorporeal circuit might have a place in cardiac surgery was the Russian, Bruchonenko, another pharmacologist with an interest in the effects of drugs on the heart. In the early 1920s, he had used a roller-type pump for blood transfusion work and in 1926, he and his colleague, Tchetchuline, designed an extracorporeal pump with a diaphragm and valves for canine experiments. He employed the excised lungs of a second dog as oxygenator. Venous blood was pumped from the experimental animal into the pulmonary vessels of the isolated lungs; the oxygenated blood was then withdrawn by a second pump back into the animal's arterial system. Using this circuit, the dog's heart stopped, but was kept alive by perfusion, sometimes for several hours. In 1928, when most other researchers regarded cardiac surgery as virtually impossible, Bruchonenko wrote,

> *"If this method were perfected, would it not be possible to use it in medicine, in particular when it is necessary to replace, if only temporarily, an inadequately functioning human heart? Without going much more deeply into the matter, we accept on the basis of our present work that in principle the application to man (in certain cases and perhaps even for the performance of certain operations on the temporarily arrested heart) of the method of extracorporeal circulation is capable of realization, but for this to come about an adequate technique must be worked out in detail. The whole solution to the problem of artificial circulation of the whole organism opens the way to the problem of operations on the heart (for example, on the valves)."*

Between 1935 and 1940, a modified version of the Bruchonenko machine was used by another Russian, Terebinskii, for animal experiments. He produced valvular lesions in the heart and then treated them successfully by surgery.

John Gibbon and the first heart–lung machine

IN FEBRUARY 1932, John Gibbon Jr was a Resident and Research Fellow with Edward Churchill in Philadelphia. He was given the task of nightwatching a young female patient suffering from massive pulmonary embolus. The following morning, when the patient was moribund, Churchill attempted pulmonary embolectomy, but the patient died. Gibbon then wrote, "During that long night's vigil, the idea occurred to me that the patient's life might have been saved if some of her cardiorespiratory functions might be temporarily taken over by an extracorporeal blood circuit." In discussion of this problem, Phemister suggested to Gibbon that the circulation could remain intact, independent of the heart or lungs, if a constant arterial transfusion from a series of donors could be performed. Realizing the difficulties of such a system, Gibbon set out to devise a mechanical pump oxygenator.

In 1934, Gibbon obtained a second surgical fellowship with Churchill, this time at the Massachusetts General Hospital, and began his research on a heart–lung machine. After 1936, he pursued this work at the University of Pennsylvania, where the physiologist Ravdin arranged laboratory space and assistance. During 1937, he developed a machine that would maintain gas exchange and bloodflow in experimental animals for 30–40 minutes during complete heart–lung bypass. At the conclusion of experiments, the normal function of the heart and lungs could be restored in only three of his animals, and they survived only briefly. Later in 1937, Gibbon moved back to Jefferson Medical College, Philadelphia and built a new heart–lung machine using two roller pumps designed by Michael DeBakey in 1934 (Figure 2.1). The new machine had sufficient capacity to replace the heart and lungs of experimental cats, but was too small to serve for dogs or humans.

The outbreak of World War II brought Gibbon's work to a halt temporarily, but on his return from war service (as Professor of Surgery at Jefferson) he resumed work on a larger and more efficient heart–lung machine. By then, Best and co-workers had produced heparin in clinically significant quantities and Gibbon immediately realized the importance of this substance for his research. He obtained a small quantity of heparin from the University of Toronto, and in 1939, he reported the survival of four animals after bypass at the American Association for Thoracic Surgery. However, most animals were still dying from severe haemolysis, air embolism, or the damaging effects of blood–foreign surface interaction.

In 1946, whilst on vacation, Gibbon met Thomas Watson, the Chairman of IBM, who agreed to support the project through both finance and technical assistance. This

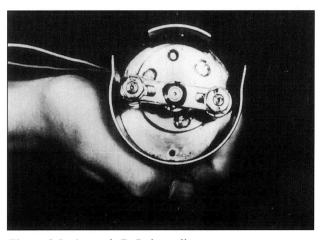

Figure 2.1. An early DeBakey roller pump.

association provided the vital breakthrough. With the engineers' help, a new heart–lung machine was designed to minimize haemolysis and prevent air bubbles from entering the circulation. The extracorporeal circuit was enclosed within a cabinet kept at body temperature and bloodflow was carefully controlled to maintain a constant blood volume. By 1947, Gibbon was able to perform complete heart–lung bypass in small dogs, and perform surgery inside their hearts. At first, 80% of the dogs died, but Gibbon gradually learned to avoid air embolism after cardiotomy. Within 2 years, the Philadelphia team were able to reduce the mortality rate to 10%.

Bigelow and hypothermia

THE FIRST interest in systemic hypothermia was expressed in 1940, when Temple Faye of Philadelphia attempted to cure or control brain tumours by cooling the patients with cold blankets and maintaining them in a moderately hypothermic state (31°C) for several days. He treated over 100 patients in this manner, at a time when there was a general fear of hypothermia. The procedure involved considerable risk and had a high mortality rate. Metabolic studies were also carried out at this time, with equivocal results. One German research programme (1943) was stimulated by the death of Luftwaffe pilots from hypothermia after ejecting into the North Sea. Experimental hypothermia in dogs had, paradoxically, shown an average increase in metabolism of about 200% and death from ventricular fibrillation at body temperatures below 20°C. Shivering was found to increase the basal metabolic rate by 400%.

The concept that metabolism and oxygen demand increased with cooling originated from the fact that shivering occurred whenever there was any significant decrease in body temperature. Most early experiments with cold baths probably did not achieve a significant fall in metabolic rate, with one documented exception published in 1797. James Curry of Liverpool used cold water baths as a remedy for fever, convulsions and insanity. He immersed two apparently normal men in a deep bath of sea water at 7°C and measured their temperature with a rectal thermometer, similar to the one designed by John Hunter. The thermometer, of questionable accuracy, recorded body temperatures as low as 25°C with survival.

Bill Bigelow's interest in hypothermia began as a resident at Toronto General Hospital (1941), when he encountered a young patient with frostbite that progressed to gangrene. Bigelow was surprised by the lack of information on frostbite, and consequently published his own review entitled, *The Modern Concept and Treatment of Frostbite*. This highlighted the fact that gangrene resulted from a secondary shutdown of the peripheral circulation and not from direct damage to tissue cells.

During World War II Bigelow served with the Canadian Army in England in preparation for the Normandy landings. As an army surgeon, he was interested in the treatment of vascular injuries, which usually resulted in amputation. Bigelow felt that therapeutic hypothermia might reduce the metabolism in an ischaemic limb and preserve the tissue's vascular repair system. He persuaded the British War Office to build a cooling cabinet for this purpose and also obtained heparin (first used at the Toronto General Hospital in 1935) and fine arterial sutures. He acquired some newly designed vitallium Blakemore–Lord tubes, which were designed to aid reconstruction of severed arteries. Bigelow landed in Normandy with the Sixth Casualty Clearing Station, but regardless of his careful preparation, he never encountered a wound for which major arterial repair was practicable.

After returning to Canada, Bigelow was seconded to the Johns Hopkins Hospital to train with Blalock, before returning to the Toronto General Hospital as a vascular surgeon. Blalock had described his subclavian artery–pulmonary artery shunt (1944) and was known as the 'blue-baby surgeon'. In 1941, Cournand and Richards developed right-heart catheterization, measured blood oxygen content and applied a mathematical formula (Fick's principle) to calculate cardiac output. Richard Bing, who established the Johns Hopkins' cardiac catheterization laboratory, modified this formula to measure bloodflow in congenital heart disease, taking into account shunting between chambers, or valve and muscular obstruction. The early success of Taussig, Blalock and Bing encouraged a continuous flow of cardiac cases to the Johns Hopkins for surgery.

Blalock's palliative surgery on wasted, poorly developed, cyanotic babies and children was inspired, but it was obvious to Bigelow that these infants were not cured by the operation. It was apparent that detailed

ANNALS OF SURGERY

VOL. 132   NOVEMBER, 1950   No. 5

HYPOTHERMIA

ITS POSSIBLE ROLE IN CARDIAC SURGERY:
AN INVESTIGATION OF FACTORS GOVERNING SURVIVAL IN DOGS
AT LOW BODY TEMPERATURES*

W. G. BIGELOW, M.D., W. K. LINDSAY, M.D.,
AND W. F. GREENWOOD, M.D.

TORONTO, CANADA

FROM THE DEPARTMENTS OF SURGERY, PATHOLOGICAL CHEMISTRY AND MEDICINE OF THE
UNIVERSITY OF TORONTO

THE USE OF HYPOTHERMIA as a form of anesthetic could conceivably extend the scope of surgery in many new directions. A state in which the body temperature is lowered and the oxygen requirements of tissues are reduced to a small fraction of normal would allow exclusion of organs from the circulation for prolonged periods. Such a technic might permit surgeons to operate upon the "bloodless heart" without recourse to extra corporal pumps, and perhaps allow transplantation of organs.

At the present time, pericardectomy as well as operations designed to revascularize[1, 2, 3] or repair[4] the myocardium are in the process of development; these involve the heart wall. Most so-called heart operations, however, are restricted to the anastomosis of vessels about the heart, the most notable in this category being the current operations for congenital heart disease[5, 6] and a shunt[7] for mitral stenosis. Intracardiac procedures upon human beings are heroic technics designed to open a stenosed mitral valve and close[11] or produce[12] a septal defect in an intact heart with little or no visual control. All these procedures represent advances in our knowledge, but the human heart until now has resisted serious inroads by the surgeon. The shunt operations produce a secondary, although less serious, defect and intracardiac operations under direct vision are still not possible.

A bloodless heart excluded from the circulation is necessary before much further progress can be made in the field of cardiac surgery. Methods to short circuit the heart by an extra corporal heart-lung pump have been under experimental study in different centers[13-16] for several years. We have used

* Financed in part by a Defence Board of Canada grant. Submitted for publication November, 1949.

840

Figure 2.2. Title page of Hypothermia. Its possible role in cardiac surgery. *A 1950 article by Bigelow, Lindsay and Greenwood. (Reproduced with permission from* The Annals of Surgery.*)*

intracardiac correction could only be achieved if circulation of blood through the heart could be stopped. Bigelow was aware that John Gibbon of Philadelphia was experimenting with a heart–lung pump, but in 1947, this was far from a clinical application. Bigelow decided that a simpler option would be to cool the whole body and reduce the oxygen requirements. It would then be possible to interrupt the circulation and open the heart. This concept simply transferred the idea of local limb hypothermia to whole body cooling.

When Bigelow started his experiments, it was still anticipated that the heart, brain and liver would require more oxygen during hypothermia. He began by using surface cooling of an anaesthetized dog down to –9°C in a temperature-controlled room, but this provided a difficult working environment (Figure 2.2). Cooling was then achieved by pumping cold saline solution through the coils of a cooling blanket. Again, with oxygenation maintained via an endotracheal tube and controlled respiration, cooling appeared to result in an increase in oxygen consumption and metabolic rate as the body temperature was lowered. Attempts to control shivering did not always prevent an increase in metabolism, as increased muscle tone and a fine tremor often remained. Only when more sophisticated anaesthetics managed to control shivering and eliminate muscle tone did the oxygen requirements fall in an almost linear relationship with temperature. This was a simple but important fundamental discovery.

Bigelow's experimental observations included the effects of low body temperature on blood pressure, cardiac output, heart rate, blood chemistry, oxygen delivery and the effects of cold on the microcirculation. It was noted that the lower limit of safe cooling in an adult animal was 20–23°C; newborn animals tolerated cooling to much lower body temperatures. Specific efforts were made to show that cold did not damage the brain. Once the basic physiological responses to hypothermia were established, it was time to consider hypothermia for a surgical approach on the heart.

The early dog experiments (1949) were based on the following premise.

1. If the heart stops for more than 3–4 minutes in an adult animal or human, permanent brain damage may result, presumably from lack of oxygen.
2. According to experimental data, cooling the body to 30°C reduces the oxygen requirements to 50% of normal, and cooling to 20°C reduces the requirements to 20%.
3. A body temperature of 20°C would allow safe interruption of the circulation for five times as long as at normothermia (up to 20 minutes), so the heart could be opened to allow direct vision repair.

The dog open heart operations were performed in the Banting Institute, Toronto. The anaesthetized and ventilated dog was cooled to 20°C using a cooling blanket and ice bags. With the chest open, the circulation could be interrupted by occluding the superior and inferior vena cava (inflow occlusion). The slowly beating heart then ejected blood and emptied. The right atrium was incised and retractors were used to provide a view within the right atrium and ventricle. After 15 minutes, the incisions were closed, the snares released and the dog rewarmed in a warm water bath to 37°C. Of the first 39 animals, only half survived. Nevertheless, the work was presented to the American Surgical Association in Colorado Springs in 1950, together with a film of the technique.

The presentation stimulated Henry Swan of Denver to pursue this line of research, and the following year, Boerema of Holland published independent experimental studies of hypothermia for cardiac surgery. For the next 2 years, Bigelow's team worked at increasing the safety of hypothermia. They studied cardiac irritability, management of acid-base balance, the problems of rewarming shock and improvements in the cooling technique. By 1952, they achieved 100% survival in 12 monkeys cooled to 18°C with cardiotomy for 20 minutes. At 30°C it was necessary to perform the cardiac repair in 8–10 minutes. The Toronto cardiologists began to identify children with relatively simple congenital anomalies (such as atrial septal defect or pulmonary stenosis) as the best prospective candidates for surgery.

The University of Minnesota

IN THE meantime, others were also working towards the goal of open cardiac surgery. At the University of Minnesota, the potential for intracardiac operations was of particular interest to the physician, Morse Shapiro. As Medical Officer in the US Army during World War I, he had been struck by the large number of men who had heart defects following rheumatic fever in childhood. His interest in cardiac diseases grew and extended to children with congenital heart defects. Shapiro and Keys studied a large number of patients with patent ductus arteriosus, noting that few survived beyond 35 years of age. About 40% developed subacute bacterial endocarditis, a disease that was fatal before the introduction of antibiotics. At the University Hospital, Owen Wangensteen ligated a ductus in 1939, only 1 year after the first successful operation by Robert Gross at the Children's Hospital in Boston. By 1943, Wangensteen had operated on 10 ductus patients with eight successes. Meanwhile, Shapiro's interest brought many children with rheumatic fever and rheumatic heart disease into the University of Minnesota

and exhausted its facilities. Shapiro persuaded Steffs, a senior member of the Variety Club in Minneapolis, and a motion-picture theatre owner, to take an interest. The Variety Club responded enthusiastically to Shapiro's appeal and raised $150,000 for the construction of a heart hospital on the campus of the University of Minnesota. As many of the Variety Club members were connected with the motion-picture industry, they decided to produce a short film on the urgent need for a heart hospital. Actor Ronald Reagan appealed to audiences to join in the battle against heart disease. Their fundraising campaign was given a boost in May 1945 by the first successful blue-baby operation by Blalock. When completed in March 1951 at a cost of more than $1.5 million, the Variety Club Heart Hospital was the first facility in the US to be devoted entirely to heart patients.

Late in 1945, when the appeal for the Heart Hospital was in full swing, Wangensteen and Maurice Visscher, the Head of Physiology, suggested to Clarence Dennis, Associate Professor of Surgery, that he undertake to develop a mechanical heart–lung apparatus that would permit complete bypass of the heart and lungs during surgical operations on the heart. Dennis was the son of a St Paul surgeon. He graduated from Johns Hopkins in 1935 and then returned to Minnesota for his residency in surgery under Wangensteen. In accordance with Wangensteen's requirement for residents to study physiology, Dennis spent the years 1938–39 working with Visscher in the Department of Physiology. Visscher was a well-known authority on the heart and circulation and held joint physiology seminars with Wangensteen for the residents.

Dennis began by studying the types of apparatus devised by others. He noted that an oxygenator must use the minimum amount of blood, do as little damage to the blood cells as possible and achieve a critical level of oxygenation without excessive foaming. Dennis first tried to pass blood through tubes of cellulose sausage casing in an oxygen atmosphere. The sausage casing was intended to serve as a dialysing membrane, which by separating the blood from direct contact with oxygen could prevent both foaming and bacteriological contamination. Unfortunately, the rate of oxygenation through the cellulose membrane was insufficient to be of clinical use. Dennis therefore resorted to direct injection of oxygen into blood which flowed through membranous tubes, but lost an excessive amount of blood through foaming. However, when the blood was filmed on the inner surface of a vertical rotating plexiglass cylinder containing oxygen, he discovered (as had Gibbon) that the blood did not foam and was oxygenated sufficiently to sustain experimental animals.

Dennis went on to build a modified Gibbon pump, consisting of a nest of vertically revolving stainless steel cylinders. These were mounted over a revolving funnel in which the blood, oxygenated on the walls of the cylinders, was collected. In place of DeBakey roller pumps, he used modified Dale–Schuster pumps, which caused less haemolysis. The assembled apparatus was both cumbersome and difficult to clean. Most dogs died, either during perfusion or shortly afterwards. Only nine of 46 dogs survived and half of their plasma protein was lost during 30 minutes on the machine. Platelet numbers fell to one-third and the white blood cell count was reduced by 50%. Dennis then discovered that the oxygenator was contaminated and that many animals were dying from septicaemia. The method of sterilization was changed, as was the design of the oxygenator. Viking Björk in Sweden then introduced an oxygenator with multiple screen discs rotating slowly in a shaft, over which a film of blood was injected. Oxygen was passed over the rotating discs and provided sufficient oxygenation for an adult human.

Many lessons were learned about how to avoid haemolysis. The Minnesota group redesigned their blood pumps to reduce turbulence and crushing of cells by sudden changes in pressure. They were also extremely careful to use healthy, dewormed dogs and gave them a preoperative preparation of penicillin and streptomycin. Despite such precautions, the experimental mortality remained formidable. On 5 April 1951, Dennis and colleagues used the new blood oxygenator for an open-heart operation on a 6-year-old girl with heart failure and pulmonary oedema from a large atrial septal defect. During the operation, Dennis was astonished by the amount of blood returning to the right ventricle via Thebesius' veins. So much blood was aspirated from the heart that they were forced, without having planned it, to return the aspirated blood to the oxygenator. Although the child died shortly afterwards, Dennis was encouraged by the performance of the blood oxygenator during the world's first operation with cardiopulmonary bypass.

In 1951, when the Minnesota and Philadelphia groups presented their findings to the American Surgical

Association, it was clear that many problems remained to be solved. The year before, in Toronto, Bill Bigelow and his colleagues had demonstrated that when the blood of a dog was cooled to 20°C, the animal's oxygen consumption fell to about 15% of normal, thereby allowing the heart to be isolated from the circulation for as long as 15 minutes and operated on with survival. Although many dogs died from ventricular fibrillation, Bigelow used electric shocks to defibrillate. He even used an artificial pacemaker, equipped to deliver repeated electrical impulses at a required heart rate for 15 minutes.

In Minnesota, Floyd John Lewis and Mansur Taufic began to experiment with hypothermia to lower the oxygen requirements of dogs, whilst they created and later corrected defects in the atrial septum. Using hypothermia, they produced atrial septal defects in 39 dogs, but only 27 survived the operation. As Bigelow had discovered in Toronto, the chief cause of death was hypothermia-induced ventricular fibrillation. They then operated on 26 of the surviving dogs to close the defect under hypothermia and direct vision. Seventeen dogs survived and, although the mortality was regarded as substantial, Lewis and Taufic were able to identify the cause in all but one. Most deaths occurred early in the series from coronary air embolism.

By the late summer of 1952, Lewis, Varco and Taufic felt sufficiently confident of their hypothermia technique to attempt an operation on a human. On 2 September 1952, they operated for an atrial septal defect on a sick and underdeveloped 5-year-old girl (Figure 2.3). When

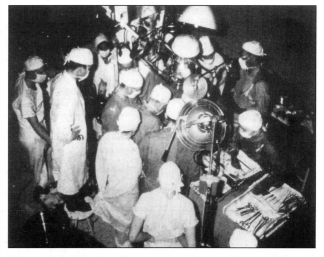

Figure 2.3. The first direct vision closure of an atrial septal defect in the University of Minnesota Hospital operating room on 2 September 1952.

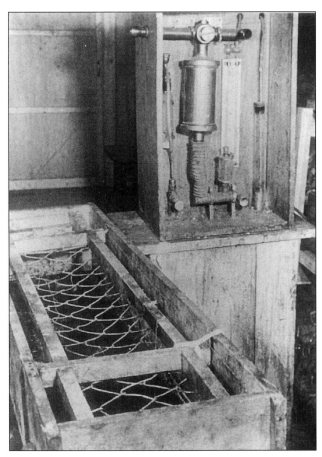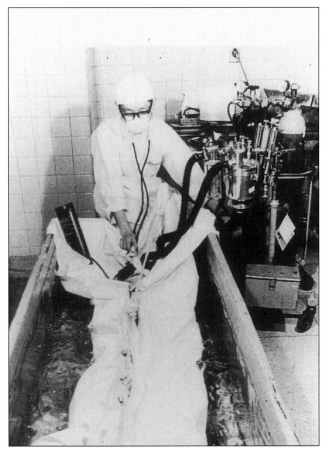

Figure 2.4. Water baths for immersion hypothermia and intracardiac repair. (Courtesy of Professor H. Koyanagi of Tokyo Women's Medical College, Japan.)

her body temperature had fallen to 28°C, they opened the chest and stopped the venous inflow to the heart for 5.5 minutes. During this time, they closed a secundum-type defect 2 cm in diameter. The child recovered uneventfully and went home 11 days after the operation. This was the first operation in history to be performed within the heart, under direct vision. Swan then reported successful correction of pulmonary stenosis and aortic stenosis in children using hypothermia. He frankly confessed, however,

> *"I have always been scared to death of it. My philosophy has been that I do not know what is going on; I have some very definite purposes for it, and I would like to induce it and get the job done and get the patient back up where I believe I can understand him a little better, as quickly as possible."*

But Swan's enthusiasm for the direct vision that hypothermia permitted was total,

> *"Finger vision is capable of limited success, and bears the same relation to real vision in surgery that it does in life—one can read Braille with moderate facility, but the chromatic values of the Mona Lisa escape one, and to shoot a winging mallard or to fly an airplane is impossible. That the blind but educated finger is capable of accomplishing much within the heart is to be fully admitted, and much admired; that it should be considered as the best method in the long run is absurd."*

Nevertheless, the method continued to impose limitations on the complexity of intracardiac repair. Only operations that could be achieved within 8–10 minutes were amenable to this technique (Figure 2.4).

One important characteristic of the successful hypothermia operations was the use of ether as the anaesthetic agent. By chance, both the Bigelow and Swan teams used ether. When more modern anaesthetics were employed, serious rewarming shock (metabolic acidosis) was encountered. Unpredictably, ether had dilated the peripheral capillary beds, providing better tissue perfusion and more efficient oxygen delivery.

C. Walton Lillehei

C. WALTON LILLEHEI was appointed Associate Professor of Surgery at the University of Minnesota in 1951 and was keen to pursue research in cardiac surgery experimentation. At the age of 33, Lillehei was one of the many young physicians who had returned from war service to begin a surgical residency. The day after completing his residency, he underwent radical surgery to the head, neck and chest for a lymphosarcoma that had appeared on his right ear. Undeterred by this, he spent the years 1948–49 working with Visscher in physiology. He discovered that when a large arteriovenous fistula was created in dogs, to cause volume overload of the heart, the animal invariably developed bacterial endocarditis and renal failure. Lillehei considered this to explain why bacterial endocarditis developed so frequently amongst patients with congenital heart defects. It seemed logical that the surgical correction of an intracardiac lesion should protect against endocarditis and prolong the patient's life.

Lillehei was assiduous in his pursuit of knowledge of cardiac pathology. He attended the autopsies of patients who had died from congenital heart defects and performed mock operations on the deformed hearts. He found that through an incision in the outflow tract of the right ventricle, the ventricular septal defect of tetralogy of Fallot could be closed with two or three well-placed sutures. He therefore assumed that if one could gain access to the interior of the heart and operate with direct vision, the surgery itself might be relatively simple. It was also clear that although shunt procedures could palliate tetralogy of Fallot in children, it did not correct the fundamental defect and the patient could not be expected to live a full life. Consequently, when Wangensteen asked what his research interest would be, Dr Lillehei replied, 'open heart surgery'. Wangensteen accepted this without question.

Lillehei was fully aware of the mechanical heart–lung devices developed by Gibbon, Dennis, Björk and others. He thought them complex, awkward to sterilize and consequently difficult to use repeatedly. He considered

that for open heart surgery to become routine, heart–lung bypass must be achieved by some simpler, more easily controlled method.

In 1952, the British surgeon Anthony Andreasen and his assistant Frank Watson were working in the laboratories of the Royal College of Surgeons at the Buxton Brown Farm (on the former estate of Charles Darwin) in Kent. Their aim was to determine the conditions under which dogs might survive occlusion of the venae cavae for the purpose of surgery on the interior of the heart. They noted that obstruction of both venae cavae at their entry into the heart resulted in death of the dog or severe brain damage after 5 minutes. No dogs survived 10 minutes of caval occlusion. In contrast, when the superior vena caval snare was situated above the entry of the azygos vein, the dogs would survive without brain damage for up to 40 minutes with both venae cavae occluded. In other words, flow through the azygos vein supplied sufficient cerebral bloodflow to prevent brain damage for periods as long as 40 minutes.

When Andreasen and Watson's work on azygos flow was published in 1952, Lillehei realized the significance of this finding for cardiac surgery. It appeared that the rate of bloodflow required to maintain life without damage to the brain (or other organs) was only about 8–9% of normal basal output. The requirements for bloodflow and oxygenation with the heart out of circuit during cardiac surgery may therefore be considerably less than had previously been supposed.

Meanwhile, Lillehei's senior colleague, Richard Varco, had taken over responsibility for the Blalock–Taussig shunt procedure and routinely opened the pericardium of cyanosed patients to check for the presence of pulmonary stenosis. Having noted that about 30% of tetralogy of Fallot patients had pulmonary valve stenosis, he decided to intervene by opening the valve and reducing the number of defects. With inflow occlusion (including the azygos vein), Varco found that the heart could be isolated for as long as 4 minutes with complete recovery. He applied this finding to patients and began to use very brief interruption of cardiac inflow in order to obtain direct visualization of the pulmonary valve.

In 1951, Morley Cohen (Figure 2.5) carried out more dog experiments and showed that with periods of caval occlusion, alternated with periods of recovery, tolerance could be increased up to 15 minutes. During this time, an atrial septal defect could be created and then closed.

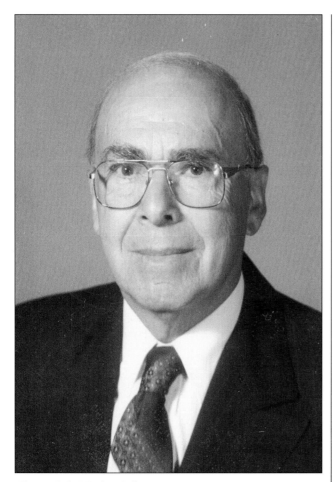

Figure 2.5. Morley Cohen.

jugular vein, circulate it through the left lower lobe, where it would become oxygenated, and supply it to the systemic arterial system through the right common carotid artery. The pumps maintained the circulation at a level corresponding to the azygos-flow principle, and the venae cavae were tied off by tightening the loops around them. A single pump was employed to drive both the pulmonary and systemic circuits; the priming volume of the circuit was small.

In physiological studies before, during and after heart bypass, Cohen and Herbert Warden measured changes in blood pressure, red cell count, plasma haemoglobin levels, kidney and liver function and respiratory exchange. They found that tissue oxygen saturation and elimination of carbon dioxide were efficient, and that only a slight acidosis had developed. Their success rate was strikingly better than results achieved using mechanical heart–lung machines. Lillehei suggested that difficulties with mechanical extracorporeal circulation were probably due to the much higher rates of perfusion that were necessary. With knowledge of Bigelow's work on hypothermia, Cohen and Lillehei thought that lowering body temperature would further reduce the tissue oxygen requirements. They suggested that moderate hypothermia might be used to prolong bypass operations if more time was required.

Further developments in supportive technology

ALTHOUGH the heart–lung machine was first used clinically in 1953, it was a further 4 years before cardiopulmonary bypass was in common use. During this time, hypothermia was the mainstay of open heart surgery. It was 1960 before it was considered safe to combine hypothermia with cardiopulmonary bypass. By using a heat exchanger to cool and rewarm the blood, it was possible to eliminate the somewhat tedious process of surface cooling. Some surgeons combined cardiopulmonary bypass with topical cardiac cooling with cold saline or ice chips in the pericardium. Packing the heart in ice effectively stopped its action, a technique known as 'ice-chip arrest'.

Cohen and Lillehei proposed that under conditions of reduced circulation, the capillary beds of the brain and heart become dilated, so as to receive a larger proportion of the limited supply. They also suggested that the tissues remove a much larger proportion of the available oxygen under these conditions. They confirmed this experimentally by showing that in dogs maintained on azygos flow, the oxygen level of venous blood was only about one-tenth of the normal level.

Cohen and Lillehei went on to perform cardiac bypass operations on a series of dogs, using just one lobe of the animal's lung as oxygenator. They first cannulated the right external jugular vein and the right common carotid artery. Next, they opened the chest, ligated the azygos vein and placed loops of tape around the venae cavae. They inserted a cannula into the branch of the pulmonary artery supplying the left lower lobe and another cannula into the pulmonary vein from the same lobe. The cannulae were then attached to a pump circuit, so that they would withdraw venous blood from the

In parallel with these advances, important supportive techniques were developing. In the early 1950s, blood oxygen measurements were seldom available and frank

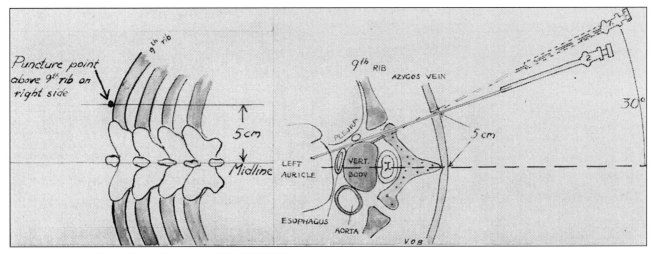

Figure 2.6. Left auricle catheterization by passing a 7 inch needle through the patient's back into the left atrium. (Reproduced with permission from Björk VO, Malmström G, Uggla LG. Left auricular pressure measurements in man. Annals of Surgery 1953; 138: 718–25.)

cyanosis was the working index of low oxygen saturation. Grey was alleged to be the best background colour to recognize cyanosis, and operating theatres were routinely painted grey. An ear oximeter was first employed to monitor arterial oxygen saturation in 1948. It soon became apparent that this could fall to 75% before the surgeon or anaesthetist was aware of a clinical problem.

Postoperatively, there were no recovery areas or intensive-care units. An oxygen tent on the ward served as the recovery area. Electrocardiogram (ECG) or electroencephalogram (EEG) transducers, arterial and venous pressure monitors and temperature recorders were not widely available. Even the concept of external cardiac massage did not exist. The only treatment for cardiac arrest in the 1950s was to open the chest, manually massage the heart, and apply defibrillator electrodes directly to shock it. As the patient was unconscious shortly after cardiac standstill, no anaesthetic was employed.

Right-heart catheterization was achieved in the mid-1940s by passing a long catheter through a vein in the groin or arm under X-ray control. Left-heart catheterization was pioneered by Björk in Stockholm, who designed a 7 inch needle to be passed through the patient's back into the left atrium (Figure 2.6). This required courage, skill and surgical standby in case of a complication. The 15 gauge needle accommodated a tiny

nylon catheter that was threaded through a side arm and down the lumen into the left ventricle. This system allowed simultaneous blood sampling and pressure measurements in the left atrium and ventricle. It provided new information about the mitral and aortic valves and greatly enhanced the accuracy of diagnosis and prognosis in cardiac disease. Some years later, the left side of the heart was entered by transvenous cannulation with a sharp-tipped, right heart catheter that could penetrate the intra-atrial wall and pass into the left atrium and ventricle.

The first donor cross-circulation experiments

DURING one of the discussions between Cohen and Warden, it occurred to them that all pregnant mammals provided a supply of oxygenated blood for their offspring *in utero*. They thought that an artificial placenta might be created by connecting the circulation of the patient to that of a suitable donor. The donor's lungs would then oxygenate the patient's blood (just as the maternal circulation oxygenates the blood of the fetus through the placenta), whilst the donor's heart would maintain the circulation.

Andreasen and Watson (1953) published their own results on controlled cross-circulation experiments in

CONTROLLED CROSS CIRCULATION FOR OPEN INTRACARDIAC
SURGERY

PHYSIOLOGIC STUDIES AND RESULTS OF CREATION AND CLOSURE OF VENTRICULAR
SEPTAL DEFECTS

HERBERT E. WARDEN, M.D.,* MORLEY COHEN, M.D.,** RAYMOND C. READ, M.D.,
AND C. WALTON LILLEHEI, M.D. (ALL BY INVITATION)
MINNEAPOLIS, MINN.

THE curative surgical attack on a number of intracardiac lesions has been stymied by the lack of a safe and satisfactory method for operating in a leisurely fashion under direct vision within the open chambers of the heart. Appreciating the historic lesson that the solution of many problems in medicine has ultimately been simple and, in most cases, obvious, once sufficient knowledge has been brought to bear upon the problem, we began work several years ago to look for a simple, safe, and efficient method for open intracardiac surgery.

The first step toward this goal was the definition of the tolerance of the canine heart and other organs to complete inflow stasis at normal temperatures.[4] The second major step was the demonstration by Andreasen and Watson[1] and Cohen and Lillehei[5] that dogs were able to survive long periods of complete vena caval occlusion without discernible injury if the flow through the azygos vein into the heart was unimpeded. Cohen then measured the azygos flow in terms of c.c./min./kg. of body weight. He found this azygos flow to be 8 to 14 c.c./min./kg. of body weight or slightly less than 10 per cent of the generally accepted basal cardiac output. Careful physiologic studies of these dogs uniformly surviving 30- to 60-minute periods on their azygos flow, indicated that under these conditions the dog's body became tremendously more efficient in its utilization of oxygen.

The significance of these studies in reference to cardiac by-pass was obvious, and the next step was to acquire a simple and efficient pump† capable of pumping blood in two circuits simultaneously and in exactly equal amounts.

Modification of the mode of oxygenation of blood was then approached. It was apparent to us that the intricacies of this process could be avoided if normal lung tissue could be employed for this purpose. Also, existing extracorporeal oxygenators inevitably removed platelets and fibrinogen so that postoperative clotting defects were likely. Likewise, in most mechanical oxy-

From The Department of Surgery, University of Minnesota Medical School, Minneapolis, Minn.

Supported by research funds of: Graduate School of Minnesota Medical School, Minneapolis, Minn., Minnesota Heart Association, Life Insurance Medical Research Fund, and the United States Public Health Service Research Grant (No. H-830).

Read at the Thirty-fourth Annual Meeting of The American Association for Thoracic Surgery at Montreal, Quebec, May 3 to 5, 1954.

*Heart Trainee, National Heart Institute.
**Life Insurance Medical Research Fellow.
†Available at Sigmamotor, Middleport, N. Y.

Figure 2.7. Title page of Controlled cross circulation for open intracardiac surgery. *A 1954 article by Warden, Cohen, Read and Lillehei. (Reproduced with permission from* Journal of Thoracic Surgery.*)*

dogs, in which they were able to support a recipient dog during heart–lung bypass for 30 minutes. They showed that cross-circulation must be controlled by a pump to prevent the donor animal bleeding excessively into the recipient. Warden and Cohen undertook similar experiments and used donor animals somewhat larger than the recipients. Using plastic cannulae that passed through a control pump, Warden connected the femoral artery of the donor to the right common carotid artery of the recipient, and the external jugular vein of the recipient to the femoral vein of the donor. The cannula inserted into the recipient's vein was passed down as far as the inferior vena cava, and had side holes so that it could receive venous blood from both the superior and inferior venae cavae. When the connections were completed, the cannulae filled with blood, the pump was turned on and set to circulate through the recipient at a rate of flow determined by the recipient's weight and the azygos flow principle. The dogs were perfused at the rate of azygos flow, twice azygos flow and three times azygos flow. This showed that blood pressure in the recipient corresponded to the rate of flow. At three times azygos flow, the blood pressure was about four-fifths normal systemic pressure. The degree of haemolysis was also proportional to the rate of flow (suggesting that lower perfusion rates were beneficial), but better levels of oxygenation were achieved with higher levels of flow.

There were no deaths among the donors and three deaths in recipient animals were found to be due to preventable causes. With further experimentation, Warden and his colleagues concluded that the optimum level of perfusion during full heart bypass was somewhere between 30–50% of resting cardiac output. Higher flow rates were unnecessary and actually harmful. In addition, when the heart was open, the faster the bloodflow, the more the coronary sinus venous return obscured the surgeon's vision.

Lillehei and the clinical donor cross-circulation operations

IN MARCH 1954, Lillehei and his group judged that the third option, that of donor cross-circulation, was sufficiently developed to be used for human patients. Because the method was new, with unknown risks to both the patient and donor, they resolved to operate only on children with severe symptoms who were likely to survive for only a short time without surgery. At that time, the concept of taking a healthy person to the operating room to provide a donor circulation, even temporarily, was considered unacceptable and even immoral by some critics. This was compounded by the general lack of success with the mechanical pump oxygenator and widespread doubt about the feasibility of open heart surgery in humans.

When the authorities at the University of Minnesota realized that Lillehei was about to embark on human cross-circulation, he was asked not to proceed. Nevertheless, when presented with a 1-year-old boy weighing 6.9 kg, who had spent most of his short life in hospital with heart failure, Lillehei decided to press on and informed Wangensteen of his intentions. With great foresight, Wangensteen had already left a note for

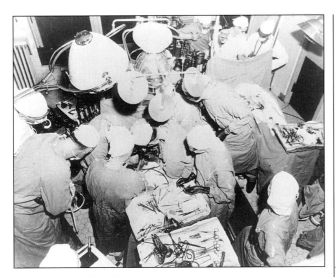

Figure 2.8. Lillehei's first donor cross-circulation operation.

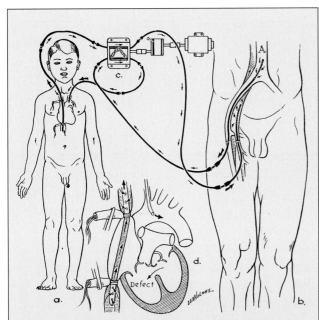

Fig. 1. Method of linking donor and patient for direct vision intracardiac surgery. a, Patient: showing sites of arterial and venous cannulations. b, Donor: showing sites of arterial (superficial femoral) and venous (saphena magna) cannulations. c, The pump assembly: Consisting of an electric motor, a speed changer, and the pumping unit. The pump consists of multiple cam operated metal fingers that massage the blood contained within the tubing. d, A magnified view of the patient's heart showing the plastic vena caval catheter which has been inserted through the internal jugular vein in the neck and positioned so that venous blood is withdrawn from both cavae during the interval of total cardiac by-pass. Note also the relative positions of the vena caval occluding tapes for securing inflow stasis during the intracardiac procedure. The arterial blood from the donor is circulated to the patient's body via the catheter inserted into either the right or left subclavian artery.

Figure 2.9. Lillehei's cross-circulation diagram.
(*Reproduced with permission from* Lillehei CW, Cohen M, Warden HE et al. The results of direct vision closure of ventricular septal defects in eight patients by means of controlled cross circulation. Surgery, Gynecology and Obstetrics 1955; October: 447–66.)

Lillehei instructing him to go ahead with the operation. On 26 March 1954, in operating room B of the University of Minnesota Medical Center, the first human-controlled cross-circulation procedure was performed, using the boy's father as donor (Figure 2.8). A long cannula was inserted through the infant's internal jugular vein to provide superior and inferior venae caval drainage with snares in place (Figure 2.9). Arterial return was via the left common carotid artery. The lightly anaesthetized father underwent cannulation of the femoral artery and great saphenous vein in the right groin. A sigma motor pump controlled the rate of flow between the donor and patient at an average of 40 ml/kg body weight/minute at normothermia. The ventricular septal defect was directly visualized through a right ventriculotomy. This allowed the hole to be closed by direct suture during 19 minutes of cross-circulation. Lillehei was assisted by Varco, whilst Warden and Cohen supervised the donor. The operation proceeded smoothly and the boy appeared to recover well, until he developed pneumonia and died 11 days after surgery. The autopsy showed severe pulmonary vascular disease which accounted for his episodic right-to-left shunt and cyanosis. Undaunted, Lillehei and colleagues operated on a second patient, on 20 April 1954, again using the child's father as the donor. This 4-year-old child survived, and by the end of August 1954, eight operations to close ventricular septal defects had been performed with only two deaths.

In the months that followed, a rapid succession of surgical firsts were achieved in Minneapolis for correction of defects previously deemed inoperable. There was no donor mortality in the 45 operations and no long-lasting adverse sequelae. Of the 45 patients, 28 survived surgery and were discharged from hospital. Only six of these patients died in the 30 year follow-up period. The others remained in good health and went on to live normal lives. Of the deaths, none were attributable to cross-circulation; most occurred in the postoperative period and were due either to surgical errors (inevitable at the time) or respiratory failure.

In April 1955, Lillehei reported his surgical experience of the correction of tetralogy of Fallot to the American Surgical Association. He had performed nine operations, with four deaths, but the beneficial effect on the five survivors was remarkable. During discussion of this paper, Alfred Blalock commented, "I never thought I would live to see the day when this type of operative procedure could be performed." He commended the Minnesota group for their imagination and courage. Perhaps surprisingly, in the light of Lillehei's success, Blalock predicted that the ultimate answer to the support of the patient's circulation would not be human cross-circulation, but the mechanical pump oxygenator, as described by Gibbon. Certainly, other cardiac surgeons were also afraid of a technique that could result in 200% mortality, and by that stage even Lillehei himself had gone on to develop a new pump oxygenator.

Clinical use of the pump oxygenator

GIBBON'S first operation with the pump oxygenator took place in 1952 on a 15-month-old baby, who was believed to have an atrial septal defect. However, at operation, no hole was found and the post-mortem disclosed a large patent ductus arteriosus. Two other attempts at intracardiac repair using the pump oxygenator were made in two 5.5-year-old girls, one with a multiply fenestrated atrial septum and the other with multiple intracardiac anomalies. Both were failures. Gibbon's moment of triumph came on 6 May 1953. An 18-year-old girl was connected to the machine for 45 minutes and was completely dependent on it for 26 minutes, whilst a secundum atrial septal defect was closed by direct suture. When Gibbon presented this success at a meeting, Dodrill stated that more than a year previously he had successfully operated on a mitral valve, under direct vision, using a left-sided bypass only (with the pulmonary circulation intact and the lungs as oxygenator).

The oxygenators of Gibbon and Dennis worked on the principle of creating a large interface between blood and oxygen. Their devices spread out the blood into a thin film that moved in an atmosphere of oxygen. However, a substantial blood–oxygen interface could also be created by bubbling oxygen through the blood, though this was previously associated with excessive foaming. Leyland Clarke and co-workers succeeded in preventing foaming by passing the blood through a tube containing small glass rods or beads coated with DC antifoam A, made by the Dow Corning Company of Michigan.

In the autumn of 1954, a young physician, Richard DeWall, asked to join Lillehei in his cardiac research programme. Lillehei needed someone to supervise the pumps during cross-circulation operations and invited DeWall to take over that job. He was originally appointed as a resident, but the Dean of the Graduate School instructed Wangensteen to refuse him admission because his medical school grades were too low. When DeWall was given the news, he elected to stay on as a laboratory attendant, and continued the same research as before, the only difference being that his wages were more substantial than those of a surgical resident.

Lillehei went on to develop a bubble oxygenator from first principles. The chief problem with bubble oxygenators had been that of debubbling and prevention of foaming. DeWall obtained plastic tubing coated with the DC antifoam previously employed for the commercial production of mayonnaise. The system could control foaming but did not remove all the bubbles. The possibility of air embolism persisted. DeWall realized that bubble-containing blood was lighter than bubble-free blood, so that when oxygenated blood was passed through a vertical settling tube, the bubble-free blood gravitated to the bottom, whilst the bubbles rose to the top. This system was inefficient because the hydrostatic forces that tend to move the lighter blood upwards were opposed by the downward movement of heavier blood through gravity. In order to overcome the viscosity resistance to separation of the bubble-containing blood, DeWall employed a spiral settling tube. The heavier blood could then flow beneath the bubble-containing blood and constantly push the lighter blood upwards. The hydrostatic force created by differences in density therefore acted across the short distance of the tube's diameter instead of along the full height of a straight, vertical settling tube. The helical system worked perfectly, giving rapid, dependable and complete elimination of bubbles.

During the winter of 1954–55, DeWall tested the bubble oxygenator thoroughly with experimental animals. He developed a waterbath heat exchange system to keep the blood at a constant temperature and to prevent hypothermia at the end of the procedure. On 13 May 1955, Lillehei used the DeWall oxygenator for a 3-year-old child suffering from ventricular septal defect and pulmonary hypertension. The child's venous blood flowed into the bottom of a vertical plastic tube, through which oxygen was bubbled via 18 intravenous needles inserted through an ordinary rubber stopper. As the blood flowed slowly upwards, the oxygen bubbles ascended through the rising column to the top of the mixing tube. From here, the blood entered a U-shaped debubbling chamber containing DC antifoam A. Most of the bubbles were separated in this chamber. Those remaining were removed as the oxygenated blood poured into the plastic helical coil, through which it flowed by gravity into a reservoir. At the bottom of the helical settling tube, oxygenated blood (now completely free of bubbles) passed into a reservoir and then through standard blood filters before entering the arterial system of the patient.

By 9 August 1955, Lillehei and his group had used the bubble oxygenator for seven paediatric operations with two deaths. All the patients woke up immediately after the operations without showing any signs of damage to the nervous system, liver or kidneys. The deaths were explained (at autopsy) by residual haemodynamic problems. Lillehei considered the bubble oxygenator a great success and cross-circulation was abandoned.

In contrast to the elaborate screen oxygenators with moving parts and complex controls, the DeWall–Lillehei bubble oxygenator was simple, cheap and easily assembled from lengths of polyvinyl plastic food hose (Figure 2.10). It could be sterilized completely by autoclaving and its size was adaptable. Consequently, donor blood required to prime the device could be kept to a minimum, particularly for small infants.

By May 1956, Lillehei and colleagues had performed 80 open heart operations with a bubble oxygenator. They carried out progressively more complex operations, not previously amenable to surgery, with hypothermia and short periods of inflow occlusion. From DeWall and Lillehei's early experience with the bubble oxygenator, considerable physiological and biochemical data were collected, analysed and compared with earlier animal studies. Their information confirmed the safety of perfusion with relatively low flow rates (the azygos flow concept). Tests performed by psychologists and neurologists before and after perfusion detected no significant cerebral damage. In the long-term follow-up of 106 patients operated on for tetralogy of Fallot, it was found that 32% had college or graduate degrees, including two in medicine, one in law and two PhDs. Putting humans on the bubble oxygenator was not expected to increase intelligence, but on these findings, the cerebral status was above the average compared with a random group from the general population.

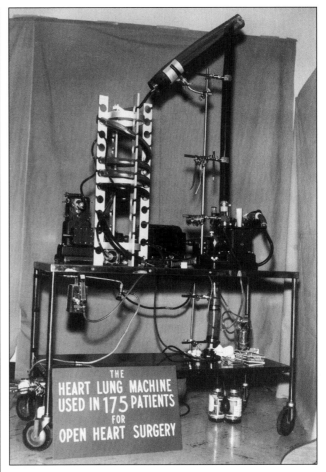

Figure 2.10. DeWall–Lillehei bubble oxygenator set up for exhibition (c. late 1955 or early 1956). (Courtesy of the University of Minnesota Archives.)

Although Gibbon abandoned his machine due to a general lack of success, the Gibbon-type pump oxygenator (originally built by IBM) was modified by Kirklin, Wood and colleagues at the Mayo Clinic and used with considerable success. Throughout 1955 and well into 1956 there were two hospitals in the world performing open heart surgery—the Mayo Clinic and University of Minnesota Medical Center—and these were only 90 miles apart. Visitors from all parts of the world travelled to both institutions to observe their methods. Though the surgery was superlative at both hospitals, there were substantial differences in equipment and approach. Denton Cooley, an early observer in June 1955, was later to write,

"The contrast between the two institutions and the two surgeons was striking. We observed Lillehei and a team composed mostly of house staff correct a ventricular septal defect using cross-circulation. During the visit we also

saw an oxygenator developed by Richard DeWall at the University of Minnesota. The next day we observed John Kirklin and his impressive team in Rochester that was made up of physiologists, biochemists, cardiologists and others as they performed operations using the Mayo–Gibbon apparatus. Such a device was beyond my organizational capacity and financial reach. Thus I was deeply disappointed on our return to Houston when Dr MacNamara stated that he would not permit me to operate on his patients unless I had a Mayo–Gibbon apparatus."

Although professional rivals, Kirklin and Lillehei remained lifelong friends, with great mutual respect.

In London and Stockholm, Dennis Melrose and Viking Björk worked independently on the rotating disc oxygenator. The Melrose machine was used clinically by Ian Aird and Bill Cleland at the Hammersmith Hospital (9 December 1953) to support the circulation (rather than to bypass the heart) during a closed aortic valvotomy. Towards the end of the 1950s, Melrose worked with Frank Gerbode at Stanford, California, and his rotating disc machine was compared with John Osborne's Stanford machine. This utilized a plastic screen oxygenator. There was no real difference in efficiency between the devices, but on the grounds of convenience and cost the Melrose machine was finally adopted, with one important modification. All parts with a blood interface were altered to facilitate sterilization in an autoclave and rendered disposable.

It soon became apparent that the keys to extracorporeal circulation were simplicity and biocompatibility, with minimal blood damage at the blood–foreign surface interface. Vincent Gott, during his residency with Lillehei, sought to incorporate the essential features of DeWall's device into an oxygenator that could be manufactured commercially (Figure 2.11). Gott flattened the helical tube to fit between two sheets of heat-sealed plastic. The oxygenated blood still descended in an inclined plane, which, though shorter than the helix, proved to be a dependable barrier to the transmission of bubbles. The great advantage of the plastic sheet oxygenator was that it could be manufactured easily and distributed in sealed, sterile containers to surgical operating rooms anywhere in the world.

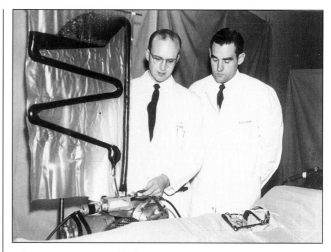

Figure 2.11. DeWall (left) with Gott (right) with the sheet bubble oxygenator (c. late 1956 to 1957). (Courtesy of the University of Minnesota Archives.)

In 1956, Kolff, (Figure 2.12) who had previously developed the renal dialysis apparatus, described a disposable membrane oxygenator for experimental use. This separated blood from gas and eliminated problems with bubbling. Klaus and Neville reported experimental studies with membrane oxygenation in 1958 and declared the system suitable for clinical perfusion. The main problem was to provide effective diffusion of gas across the membrane. With this achievement came the expectation that clinical results would exceed those with the bubble oxygenator. In practice, the early membrane oxygenators were only superior when perfusions lasted 6–8 hours. In these unusual circumstances, there were

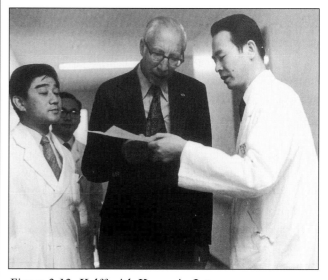

Figure 2.12. Kolff with Konno in Japan.

smaller reductions of platelets, fewer microemboli and less postoperative bleeding.

With widespread use of cardiopulmonary bypass, it became apparent that the pump oxygenator created a specific pathological entity soon to be known as the 'post-perfusion syndrome'. Extracorporeal circuits required priming before use, and in the early years, about 2 litres of cooled, heparinized blood was used for this. Complications often arose through incompatibility of the blood or biochemical disturbances due to citrate, known as the 'homologous blood syndrome'.

In an attempt to eliminate problems with the donor blood prime, Long and Lillehei experimented with low molecular weight dextran. They found that dextran prevented or minimized thrombosis and aggregation of red cells in the microvasculature. In 1961, they reported the use of this non-blood prime for all cardiac bypass procedures in the University of Minnesota, and the results presented dispelled anxiety about the effects of dilution and reduced haematocrit. Zuhdi and colleagues in Oklahoma City used 5% dextrose (in distilled water) and employed moderate hypothermia to reduce oxygen requirements, in order to compensate for haemodilution. Cooley adopted the dextrose prime, which conveyed a particular advantage when urgent preparation was needed as in emergency surgery, such as pulmonary embolectomy. By 1962, he had used the dextrose solution with a disposable plastic oxygenator at normothermia in 100 patients. He replaced blood lost at operation with compatible donor blood, and noted that postoperative bleeding was reduced, as was the incidence of cerebral, renal and pulmonary complications. Postoperative recovery appeared to be expedited through the use of the clear pump prime.

At this stage, the operative method for extracorporeal circulation was essentially the same, whatever type of pump oxygenator was used. Catheters were placed into the venae cavae, usually through the right atrial appendage. When bypass was commenced, caval snares were used to ensure complete venous return to the oxygenator. The oxygenated blood was then pumped back into the body through a catheter inserted into either the subclavian or common femoral artery. The aorta was clamped for periods of up to 30 minutes, during which time surgery could be undertaken on the intracardiac defects. Initially, operations with cardiopulmonary bypass suffered the same drawbacks as

did moderate hypothermia alone: the heart was still beating and coronary and bronchial bloodflow tended to obscure the operative field.

Hypothermia and the bubble oxygenator combined

UNTIL now, no-one had considered the possibility of combining hypothermia with the pump oxygenator in patients. A considerable amount of research in this area had already been undertaken by Frank Gollen of Nashville, Tennessee, who had worked on this combination before either method was widely adopted. Gollen employed the principle of extracorporeal cooling, first used by Heymans in his experiments during World War I. Gollen's oxygenator was of the bubble type and cooling took place in a heat exchanger that formed part of the apparatus. He demonstrated that the rate of bloodflow in dogs could be reduced to meet the diminished need for cardiac output as the temperature fell. By 1955, he had explored the influence of profound hypothermia to the point where cardiac action ceased (13°C), and with his extracorporeal circuit was able to rewarm the dogs with complete recovery. Gollen was the first to demonstrate that the combination of hypothermia and extracorporeal circulation overcame the difficulties of hypothermia alone (anoxia and irreversible ventricular fibrillation) and extracorporeal circulation alone (air embolism and an operating field obscured by coronary blood).

Will Sealy of Duke University, North Carolina was the first to employ these methods clinically. On 21 June 1956, he successfully repaired an atrial septal defect in a 7-year-old girl, though the combination of cooling and rewarming resulted in an operative duration of 7 hours 15 minutes. Sealy reasoned that extracorporeal circulation at normal temperatures and low flow rates allowed only a limited time inside the heart. At that time, the only machines giving rates of flow equivalent to normal cardiac output were both expensive to purchase and maintain, and difficult to clean and sterilize. He suggested that hypothermia could be used to lower oxygen requirements to a level that could be supplied by the simpler low flow pump and diffusion-type oxygenator.

In 1958, Sealy reported on 49 patients with a variety of defects repaired using the combined technique. The first 40 were cooled topically by packing in ice—a time-consuming procedure. For the other nine, Sealy incorporated a heat exchanger in the extracorporeal circuit, and the patients reached the same temperatures in 5–20 minutes. From the surgical standpoint, operating conditions were improved, as the aorta could be cross-clamped for longer periods. This provided a bloodless field and ventricular fibrillation was no longer a problem. On a number of occasions, Sealy electively arrested the patient's heart by ventricular fibrillation for up to 17 minutes.

Whereas Sealy reduced temperatures to between 29°C and 31°C, Charles Drew at the Westminster Hospital, London operated on two children after lowering their body temperatures to 15°C. Drew's ingenious method used the child's own lungs as the oxygenator and an extracorporeal heat exchanger to achieve profound hypothermia. He first exposed the left femoral artery and opened the chest. Catheters were inserted into both right and left atria for venous return. The femoral arterial cannula completed the left-sided circuit and about 20–25% of the left atrial flow was first drained into a reservoir via a heat exchanger and then returned to the femoral artery. This initiated the cooling process. When the temperature reached 25°C, ventricular fibrillation occurred and the heart could no longer act as a pump. Drew then established separate complete bypasses of both sides of the heart, with the lungs in circuit and inflated. The venous return to the right atrium was drained into a second reservoir and pumped into the lungs via a cannula in the main pulmonary artery. Likewise, all the pulmonary venous return into the left atrium was now routed through the heat exchanger, as cooling continued to below 15°C. This process took less than 30 minutes in infants; for adults the time was doubled. When a nasopharyngeal temperature of 12–15°C was achieved, the pump was turned off and respiration discontinued. The venae cavae were closed by snares and the heart was drained. The aorta was clamped to prevent air embolism and the cardiac repair performed. Complete circulatory arrest was maintained for 45 minutes and, on rewarming, the heart resumed sinus rhythm by spontaneous defibrillation.

By 1960, Drew had used this technique on more than 60 patients, aged from 3 months to 55 years, with results comparable to other methods of open heart surgery. Drew had remarkably few cerebral complications, but others who adopted the method reported temporary or permanent paralysis and psychological impairment. Although many of these events could be attributed to errors of technique, enthusiasm for profound hypothermia waned for some time.

Cardioplegia and myocardial protection

AS INTRACARDIAC repair extended to more complex lesions, a beating heart with coronary and bronchial venous return was a distinct disadvantage. Attention turned to methods to arrest the heart, although the greatest anxiety was how to start it again. As usual, clues to the solution of this problem were found in the literature. In 1878, Boehm of the Pharmacological Institute of the University of Dorpat studied resuscitation of cats whose hearts had been stopped by an overdose of chloroform, asphyxiation or the use of potassium salts. He successfully resuscitated hearts after potassium arrest. Five years later (1883), Sidney Ringer, of University College, London, showed that an excess of potassium salts in fluid, bathing an isolated heart, would stop it beating. In 1904, Martin, of Johns Hopkins University, performed extensive experiments on the isolated hearts of terrapins. He arrested the hearts for periods of up to 35 minutes by infusing potassium chloride solution. When the solution was washed out, the cardiac action resumed spontaneously.

Melrose, of the Hammersmith Hospital and Royal Postgraduate Medical School, translated the theory of cardioplegic arrest into practice. He performed experimental work on dogs and in isolated hearts at temperatures between 26°C and 35°C. Melrose was convinced that the heart could resume normal function after being stopped by an injection of potassium citrate. In 1955 (3 months after Melrose's preliminary communication in the *Lancet*), the Hammersmith Hospital carried out the first elective cardiac arrest on the operating table. With the patient on cardiopulmonary bypass, the aorta was cross-clamped and potassium citrate injected directly into the aortic root. This produced cardiac arrest in the flaccid, diastolic phase, and allowed the operation to be carried out in a dry, motionless heart. On release of the aortic cross-clamp, reperfusion of the coronary circulation washed out the potassium citrate and restored normal cardiac function in a very short time, much to the elation of the surgical team.

Once again, some surgeons who adopted this method in the US reported problems, and attributed them to potassium citrate arrest. Consequently, the method was not widely adopted. One year later, Conrad Lam (Henry Ford Hospital, Detroit) introduced acetylcholine as a method for elective cardiac arrest. This drug had been extensively investigated by physiologists and had been found to slow the heart markedly without actually producing cardiac standstill. Lam regarded continued action as an advantage, particularly when suturing close to the conducting tissue in ventricular septal defects. The surgeon could immediately see when conduction was disturbed by a suture near the His bundle. In 1956, Lam described operations in eight children with ventricular septal defects using the pump oxygenator and acetylcholine arrest. Two died on the operating table from ventricular fibrillation, leaving Lam uncertain as to whether the acetylcholine or the surgical procedure was responsible. Two others died in the immediate postoperative period from unrelated causes.

The problem of myocardial protection was then approached from a different direction. Lillehei investigated the possibility of direct coronary cannulation and perfusion, but this proved to be technically difficult, with the danger of direct injury to the coronary ostia or of coronary air embolism. However, Lillehei discovered the experimental work of Pratt (1898) and of Joseph Roberts (1943), who had independently demonstrated the ability of cardiac muscle to derive oxygen from retrograde bloodflow through the veins to the arteries. The Lillehei team then decided to perfuse the coronary system in a retrograde direction by cannulating the coronary sinus and using a pump to deliver 125 ml oxygenated blood per minute. This method was first used clinically during aortic valve replacement on 31 January 1956. The perfusion lasted for 11 minutes and the heart remained pink. The technique was particularly useful for operations on the aortic valve, as it helped to prevent coronary air embolism. Anterograde coronary perfusion with oxygenated blood was subsequently developed using improved atraumatic cannulae. Retrograde coronary sinus perfusion with blood cardioplegia was reinvented in the 1990s.

After 1960, cardioplegia was kept alive in Germany by Hölscher, Bretschneider and Kirsch. Bretschneider, working initially in Cologne and then in the Institute of Physiology at the University of Göttingen, published the principle of arresting the heart with sodium-poor, calcium-free, procaine-containing solutions, known as the 'Bretschneider solutions'. The rationale behind this formulation was that a sodium concentration equal to the intracellular sodium content would prevent the excitation potential and that lack of calcium ions would prevent activation of the contractile system. Finally, procaine would stabilize the cell membrane. Osmolality was maintained with mannitol. Søndergaard initiated the new wave of cardioplegia by adopting Bretschneider's solution for myocardial protection. Kirsch worked on the theory that a cardioplegic agent should contain no component that would stimulate and, from 1969, the Kirsch magnesium-aspartate-procaine bolus solution was in regular clinical use in Rodewald's unit in the University Clinic in Hamburg.

As Senior Registrar to Sir Russell Brock at the Brompton Hospital, Braimbridge was influenced by his early experiences with Frank Gerbode in Stanford. He recognized the importance of collaboration between the cardiac surgeon and the laboratory scientist. In the laboratories of the Royal College of Surgeons, he entered into discussion with the two cytochemists, Chayen and Bitensky, about why his patients were dying of low cardiac output from left ventricular failure after cardiac surgery, with seemingly normal myocardial histology at post-mortem. The cytochemists, who had established a method of identifying ischaemic muscle by adding adenosine triphosphate (ATP) and calcium and looking at the orientation of myosin with polarized light, asked Braimbridge to send biopsy specimens of the left ventricle, frozen to –70°C in hexane, so that they might examine the myosin fibrils. In air, myosin is disoriented and polarized light does not come through and, in normal muscle, the section looks dark. Looking at myosin with polarized light after the addition of ATP and calcium it becomes oriented, the polarized light is allowed through and the section immediately becomes brighter. Damaged or ischaemic muscle is already much brighter and more oriented in air, so that adding ATP and calcium makes less difference than in the undamaged muscle.

Where death from low cardiac output caused by

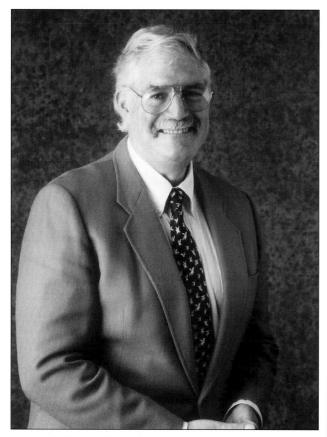

Figure 2.13 Gerald Buckberg.

THE VALUE OF HISTOCHEMISTRY IN THE ANALYSIS OF MYOCARDIAL DYSFUNCTION

THE very rapid advances in cardiac surgery during the past decade have tended to outstrip basic knowledge of the pathology of the myocardium. Thus, in many of those patients who were subjected to major cardiac surgery and who died apparently as a direct consequence of the operation, routine pathological investigations failed to reveal any abnormality which could account for the death. The lesion was likely, therefore, to be functional rather than morphological, and to involve a disturbance of the cellular biochemistry of the myofibres. It seems inadvisable to study this type of disturbance in postmortem tissue because the biochemistry is likely to be confused by autolytic changes. Yet, until recently, it was not possible to study such lesions in small biopsy specimens. This has now become possible because of the development of histochemistry, not as an " essentially morphological tool " as

12. Central Veterinary Laboratory, London. Report for 1963.

s3

Figure 2.14. The value of histochemistry in the analysis of myocardial dysfunction. *A 1964 article by Braimbridge* et al. *(Reproduced with permission from* Lancet.*)*

damage to the myosin was undetectable by routine histopathological methods, it could be detected by these histochemical procedures. Braimbridge and his collaborators validated their quantitative birefringence test by examining endomyocardial biopsies of the left ventricle from patients with aortic valve disease and either normal or abnormal left ventricular function. It was possible to identify patients with good or poor physiological left ventricular function by the degree of birefringence in response to ATP and calcium which, under polarized light, allowed them to measure contraction of the muscle fibres and estimate the amount of potential contractile reserve. By combining electron microscopy, cytochemistry and optical biophysics it became possible to identify those patients who had suffered ischaemic damage, to quantify this damage and to define whether its main effect had been on the epicardium or endocardium of the right or left ventricle.

Braimbridge found that results of cellular chemical assessment of preservation of the myocardium by biopsy during bypass correlated closely with clinical outcome in terms of low cardiac output and death. Quantitative birefringence tests applied to aortic valve replacements proved this relationship good, whether myocardial protection was intermittent perfusion with blood at 15°C or 30°C (in the 1960s), continuous coronary perfusion with a beating heart, or single or multiple infusion cardioplegia. It was not until the late 1980s that completely satisfactory biopsy and clinical outcomes were obtained with multiple infusion cardioplegia.

Vincent Gott researched high energy phosphate levels in the human heart during potassium citrate and selective hypothermic arrest as early as 1960 and Griepp, Stinson and Shumway described the protective influence of topical hypothermia in 1973. In the same year, Mark Braimbridge asked Sir Ernst Chain, Nobel prizewinner and Head of Biochemistry at Imperial College, how he could protect the myosin that was being damaged during aortic occlusion. Chain referred him to David Hearse. From their collaboration arose the Heart Research Unit in the Rayne Institute at St Thomas's Hospital, London in 1975. This institute is a broadly-based interdisciplinary unit formed to study myocardial cell damage, specifically its mechanisms and prevention. It has also sought to define basic guidelines for the

formulation and safe use of effective cardioplegic solutions. The St Thomas's Hospital cardioplegic solution has subsequently become one of the most characterized and widely used solutions of its type in the world.

For the past 20 years the clinical strategies and basis science of myocardial protection have been pioneered by Gerald Buckberg (Figure 2.13), Phillipe Menasche and others. The repertoire now includes anterograde and retrograde warm and cold blood cardioplegia which may convey advantages particularly during long ischaemic periods. As a result complex intra-cardiac anomalies can be considered accurately without risk of myocardial necrosis.

Buckberg's views of myocardial protection evolved as a consequence of extensive experimental and clinical studies beginning with multi-dose crystalloid cardioplegia in 1976. Cold blood cardioplegia was

The Development and Characterization of a Procedure for the Induction of Reversible Ischemic Arrest

DAVID J. HEARSE, PH.D., DAVID A. STEWART, M.SC.,
AND MARK V. BRAIMBRIDGE, B. CHIR., M.A.

SUMMARY An isolated perfused working rat heart model was used to investigate the extent to which various protective agents, used either singly or in combination, were able to increase the resistance of the heart to periods of transient ischemia. The aim of the studies was to develop a solution which, if infused into the coronary vessels just prior to the onset of ischemia, would rapidly induce arrest and would also counteract several of the deleterious cellular changes known to occur during myocardial ischemia. Agents which induce cardiac arrest, modify cellular ion loss, affect substrate utilization, energy production and energy stores, affect coronary vessel diameter and cell swelling, prevent dysrhythmias, and affect metabolic rate were investigated. The additive effects of these agents were evaluated. An aqueous solution was formulated which contained high concentrations of potassium and magnesium, in combination with adenosine triphosphate, creatine phosphate and procaine. This solution increased the recovery of the ischemic (37°C for 30 min) rat heart from 0% to 93%. The safe period of ischemia could be further increased by the use of hypothermia.

OPEN HEART SURGERY requires ideally a still and relaxed heart. Cardiac arrest (cardioplegia) in diastole can be induced by several procedures[1-10] which may or may not involve coronary perfusion. While few workers would question the metabolic and morphological advantages of maintaining coronary perfusion throughout the period of arrest, the simplicity and practical advantages of nonperfusion methods has resulted in the widespread use and advocation[7, 8] of ischemic arrest. However, the use of ischemic arrest has been criticized[11-13] because associated with its prolonged use is the onset of irreversible metabolic and ultrastructural damage. Two important questions have therefore arisen. First, what is the maximum duration of ischemia that can be tolerated by the myocardium before the onset of major irreversible damage? Second, is there any way in which this period can be extended or the onset of irreversible damage be reduced or delayed?

Immediately following the onset of ischemia a number of functional, metabolic, and morphological changes occur.[14] These changes are initially of a reversible nature and if blood flow is restored to the ischemic tissue during this phase of reversible damage there is a complete resumption of normal metabolism and function. If ischemia is maintained for longer periods of time, irreversible damage occurs, the restoration of blood flow no longer consistently reverses injury, and a permanent impairment of functional capacity occurs. The time taken for the onset of irreversible damage is determined by a number of factors such as the severity of ischemia, the nutritional and hormonal status of the tissue, the availability of energy supplies such as glycogen, adenosine triphosphate (ATP), and creatine phosphate (CP), the metabolic capacity for anaerobic energy production, the contractile state of the tissue, the age and temperature of the tissue, and the composition of the coronary blood in the tissue at the onset of ischemia.

The temperature of the myocardium and the composition of the extracellular fluid during ischemia provide an effective means of modifying the rate at which ischemic tissue deteriorates. The use of topical hypothermia and the consequent reduction of metabolic rate affords considerable protection to the ischemic myocardium.[4, 9, 15-18] Similarly,

From the Myocardial Metabolism Research Laboratories, The Rayne Institute, St. Thomas' Hospital, London SE1, United Kingdom.
Supported by grants from the Wellcome Trust and the British Heart Foundation.
Address for reprints: Dr. D. J. Hearse, Myocardial Metabolism Research Laboratories, The Rayne Institute, St. Thomas' Hospital, London SE1, U.K.
Received December 2, 1975; revision accepted January 13, 1976.

Figure 2.15. Title page of The development and characterization of a procedure for the induction of reversible ischemic arrest. A 1976 article by Hearse, Stewart and Braimbridge. (Reproduced with permission from Circulation.)

introduced in 1977, followed by warm blood cardioplegic reperfusion (1977), then warm induction in 1983. Retrograde cardioplegic delivery (Lillihei) was resurrected in 1989 with alternation between anterograde and retrograde warm blood cardioplegia. Buckberg (1994) now advocates the technique of simultaneous antegrade/retrograde perfusion and continuous cold, non-cardioplegic blood perfusion.

The original studies of cold blood cardioplegia showed complete recovery of myocardial function after up to 4 hours of aortic cross-clamping. The advantage of cold blood cardioplegia was the simultaneous provision of myocardial nourishment and perfusion hypothermia to lower myocardial oxygen demand and ischaemic damage. Warm blood cardioplegia was introduced (1977) to limit reperfusion damage. This approach was based on the fact that ischaemia increases the vulnerability to myocardial injury if unmodified blood is used as the initial reperfusate. This damage may be limited by a brief (3–5 minutes) period of warm blood cardioplegic reperfusion before aortic unclamping. Theorectically normothermia maximises the rate of metabolic repair by channelling aerobic ATP production to reparative processes.

Warm cardioplegic induction was introduced to limit further injury in the ischaemically damaged (energy and substrate depleted) heart. In this situation, cardioplegia is really the first phase of reperfusion. Experimental and clinical data showed that warm induction could actively resuscitate the ischaemic myocardium and improve its tolerance to cold ischaemic arrest during coronary surgery. The benefits of warm induction were amplified by enriching the cardioplegic solution with the amino acids glutamate and aspartate to replenish the key Krebs' cycle intermediates which are depleted during myocardial ischaemia. The strategy of multi-dose blood cardioplegia emerged from the need to counter non-coronary collateral flow. This rewarms the heart by replacing cardioplegic solution with blood at the temperature of the extracorporeal circuit. Systemic blood enters the heart through open mediastinal connections and is evident when blood fills the coronary arteries while the aorta is clamped.

With coronary surgery extending to increasingly severe and diffuse disease, the benefits conferred by cardioplegia are effective only if the solution is delivered to all parts of the myocardium. Maldistribution of anterograde flow is commonplace in patients with severe coronary disease. The problem was overcome by the introduction of retrograde cardioplegia. Transatrial coronary sinus cannulation techniques made this process feasible, simple and safe, though retrograde flow to the right ventricle via the coronary sinus is unreliable.

The damaging effects of cardiopulmonary bypass

"One of the most serious difficulties encountered in total body perfusion is the profound effect upon the lungs that may occur in certain patients. It is indeed discouraging to perform open cardiac corrective surgery, to have the patient remain in excellent condition throughout the procedure and for a day or two thereafter, finally succumbing to pulmonary insufficiency while the heart itself remains strong to the very end."

F.D. Dodrill, MD
Chicago, September 1957

THIS statement introduced the session on 'post-perfusion pulmonary dysfunction' at the first major international meeting devoted to the subject of cardiopulmonary bypass. In the 1980s, after 25 years of research and development in extracorporeal circulation, it was apparent that adverse effects continued to occur in every patient.

On the occasion of the 25th anniversary of open heart surgery at the Mayo Clinic, Dr John Kirklin stated:

"Some of the basic problems associated with the clinical use of pump oxygenators are as real and unsolved today as they were in 1953. They are not necessarily apparent since the knowledge and skills that have been developed by all concerned with cardiac surgery have reduced the risks of many kinds of heart surgery nearly to zero. But when we repair very complex kinds of heart disease, particularly in the very young, the very sick, and the very old, important risks are still imposed by the unsolved problems of cardiopulmonary bypass with pump oxygenators. These include the physico-chemical changes produced in the formed and unformed elements of the blood by exposure to non-biological surfaces which produce profound and widespread structural and functional abnormalities in the patients. Solutions to

these complex problems would not only be intellectually rewarding and save lives but would considerably increase the cost effectiveness of cardiac surgery.

We could, of course, set aside these problems, rejoice in our accomplishments and accept the idea that nature sets certain limits to everything including cardiac surgery. Billroth expressed such a view in 1897 when he said that cardiac surgery had reached the limits set by nature. Most in 1954 who urged aborting the pump oxygenator effort must have had a similar notion. Not the passage of time but the efforts of many people have proven the idea to be wrong at both points in time. I believe acceptance of such an idea today would also be wrong."

Cardiopulmonary bypass can never be truly physiological. The artificial environment created by plastics and metal results in many alterations in structure and function of the blood which traverses the extracorporeal circuit, and indirectly of the tissues of the body by virtue of these changes. Since the first bypass procedures in the 1950s, perfusion has been known to contribute to the mortality and morbidity of cardiac surgery. Collectively the manifestations of the damaging effects of cardiopulmonary bypass have been termed the 'post-perfusion syndrome'.

The classic manifestations of this condition were a generalized increase in pulmonary capillary permeability (sometimes with haemorrhagic pulmonary oedema despite low left atrial pressure), renal dysfunction, leucocytosis and fever, bleeding tendencies and vasoconstriction resulting in haemodynamic and metabolic problems. Traumatic red cell breakdown resulted in haemoglobinuria and anaemia. The overall consequence of this syndrome was multiple organ dysfunction which could be transient and inconsequential, as in most straightforward adult bypasses, or alternatively may necessitate prolonged respiratory or renal support, blood transfusion, or re-entry for diffuse abnormal bleeding. These problems were particularly seen in the very young, the very old or the seriously ill, especially when bypass was prolonged. Surgery for congenital heart disease in the first 3 months of life carried a substantial mortality from perfusion-related non-cardiac sequelae. It is notable that Lillehei's early results for correction of intracardiac defects in infancy using the child's mother as oxygenator achieved

a success rate that took almost 25 years to duplicate using cardiopulmonary bypass. Until recently it was safer to shunt a small infant with tetralogy of Fallot than to perform complete correction. There was no surgical reason for this — similar numbers of infants were ill in both groups; but many deaths after total correction were attributable not to cardiac failure but to pulmonary problems, bleeding disorders and other complications, which led people to believe that the limitation to successful surgery was the 'dose' of cardiopulmonary bypass.

Clinically, post-perfusion pulmonary dysfunction ranges from unnoticeable benign interstitial oedema to rare but lethal haemorrhagic pulmonary oedema which used to be the characteristic feature of perfusion-related damage. "Post-perfusion lung" is summarized as increased work of breathing, arterial hypoxaemia with increased alveolar arterial oxygen difference and fluid accumulation in the tracheobronchial tree. There is significant shunting due to both venous admixture and alveolar collapse. Total air flow resistance increases and there are measurable changes in pulmonary compliance. These changes in mechanical properties have been ascribed, in part, to a non-cardiogenic increase in extravascular lung water. Thus interstitial oedema may lead to alveolar collapse, or compressed or fluid-filled alveoli, all of which contribute to ventilation perfusion mismatch. Attempts were made to moderate the damaging effects by developing pulsitile perfusion systems. Though Taylor, Uttley and others demonstrated improvements in neurohormonal function and tissue perfusion, particularly of the kidney, pulsitile systems continued to be limited by the adverse consequences of blood–foreign surface interactions and were never widely adopted.

In the late 1970s, Craddock and colleagues at the University of Minnesota identified complement activation and intrapulmonary white cell sequestration as the cause of pulmonary dysfunction during haemodialysis. Uraemic patients were seen to develop leucopenia during treatment and infusion of autologous plasma incubated with dialyser cellophane caused sudden leucopenia and hypoxia in an animal model. Kirklin's group in Birmingham, Alabama, recognized this pathophysiological mechanism as the likely cause of problems after cardiopulmonary bypass. Eugene Blackstone put Stephen Westaby, James Kirklin and

Robert Stewart onto the project and soon the relationship between foreign material in the bypass circuit and complement activation was clearly established. As a result, the avid complement activator, nylon tricot was rapidly withdrawn from the Bentley bubble oxygenator. The group went on to study a large patient population and with Blackstone's superb analytical abilities showed a relationship between serum complement *anaphylatoxin* levels and morbidity. The anion–cation reaction of heparin neutralization by protamine was also found to activate complement, which accounted for the haemodynamic deterioration and sometimes catastrophic pulmonary oedema and collapse which follows this reaction clinically. The group went on to coin the term 'whole body inflammatory response' to describe the interaction of blood with the foreign materials of the bypass circuit. The work generated frantic activity in the industry to develop more biocompatible surfaces and materials.

Westaby returned to the Hammersmith Hospital and pursued the cellular and molecular basis of the post-perfusion syndrome. Identification of protease enzyme release (elastase) and generation of free radical species by the intrapulmonary neutrophils provided another piece to the jigsaw. The next step was to define methods to attenuate this reaction. Westaby met with Charles Wildevuur, a surgical scientist from Groningen, who had spent several years working in the same area. The only available antagonist to elastase was aprotinin (Trasylol). This agent had been used unsuccessfully in pancreatitis and was about to be withdrawn from the market. A trial of high dose intravenous aprotinin infusion in cardiopulmonary bypass was established at the Hammersmith Hospital and did show some attenuation of elastase release in aprotinin-treated patients. Of greater significance was the recognition that aprotinin patients had a dry operative field with less blood loss. It transpired that inhibition of the kallikrein and fibrinolytic system helped to preserve platelet function and haemostasis. This discovery generated an enormous amount of research into the mechanism of action of aprotinin and its applications in cardiac surgery.

Biographies

Viking Olov Björk (1918–)

VIKING OLOV BJÖRK was born in Sunnansjö, Dalecarlia, Sweden. An excellent private education necessitated by dyslexia and an interest in the circulation of the blood prepared him to study medicine at the University of Lund (MD, 1944). Through a British Council scholarship, he worked under A. Tudor Edwards on lung cancer at Brompton Hospital (1945). This resulted in the publication of *Bronchogenic Carcinoma*, the first of over 400 papers and monographs.

While Clarence Crafoord was in London in January 1946 describing his operation for coarctation of the aorta to the Royal College of Surgeons, he invited Björk to study his and Andersson's artificial heart at the Sabbatsberg Hospital. On his return to Sweden (October 1946) Björk started 18 months of experimental research into Andersson's perfusion machine with two milk machines as pumps. After an extensive series of *in vitro* oxygenation experiments with fresh heparinized blood, he attempted brain perfusion in 19 dogs. When all the dogs died, Crafoord left him to his own devices. Björk devised a blood filter and an artificial intima of silicon under the trade name UHB 300, prepared in collaboration with chemical engineers at the Uddeholm AB, Skoghall. He applied it to all parts of the perfusion machine, particularly the rough red rubber tubes, to delay clotting and save platelets. For 33 minutes (30 October 1947) his revamped machine supported the circulation of a 20 kg dog (Figure 2.17), which he transported from the hospital in the trunk of a Citröen belonging to his older brother, a dentist. At night, in his two-room flat, he and his wife were able to monitor the dog's progress by the thumping of his tail. His wife, a chemical engineer and his only surgical assistant surveyed the carpet in the morning and announced happily: "The urine is clear without blood so haemolysis is low and the kidneys are fine." Seven other dogs survived similar perfusion.

Björk's compressed air pump, and stainless steel disc oxygenator rotating at 120 rpm, demonstrated that a rapidly moving blood-stream could effectively oxygenate without excessive damage to the red cells. By adding twice as many discs, it could double the oxygenation at a time when Gibbon's oxygenator could only support cats. This was because the red

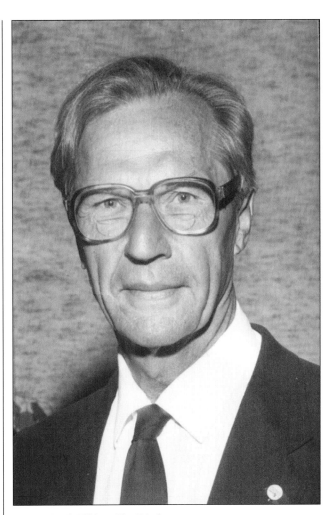

Figure 2.16. Viking Olov Björk.

cells, centrifuged to the wall of the cylinder, merely caused a thicker layer of plasma between the cells and oxygen. Björk's pump could not be found when the Smithsonian Museum wanted to exhibit it as the first oxygenator suitable for human use. Earle B. Kay of Cleveland and Fredrick Cross at the University of Minnesota adapted the Björk–Aga oxygenator to create the Kay–Cross model. This supported the first attempt at open heart surgery by Clarence Dennis on 5 April 1951. Gerbode in San Francisco and Melrose in London also used Björk's rotating disc oxygenator as a model for future developments.

> ## AN ARTIFICIAL HEART OR CARDIO-PULMONARY MACHINE
> ### PERFORMANCE IN ANIMALS
> #### VIKING OLOV BJÖRK
> ##### M.D.
>
> *From the Surgical Clinic of Sabbatsberg Hospital, Stockholm, Sweden*
>
> IN experimental and clinical work which he began in 1935 Crafoord found it possible to suspend the flow of blood to all organs but the brain for a considerable time without damaging them. Thus, in 33 patients undergoing operation for patent ductus arteriosus he double-clamped the aorta for 10–27 min.—in most cases more than 20 min.—just below the point where the left subclavian artery arises, without causing any subsequent disturbances in the patients' internal organs.
>
> In view of this experience Crafoord thought it possible to achieve a bloodless approach to the inside of the heart, arresting the circulation of blood but maintaining an adequate flow through the brain with a cardiopulmonary machine. In 1946 Crafoord and Andersson constructed an artificial heart, which I have studied in experiments on animals.[1] Thus in a dog I have clamped both superior and inferior venæ cavæ for 33 min., rendering the heart bloodless but maintaining the blood-flow to the brain alone with the cardiopulmonary machine. The dog survived with no sign of organic damage and became father to eleven puppies.
>
> Though all the other organs will tolerate an arrest of the circulation for half an hour, a few minutes' anoxia damages the brain. During a bloodless intracardiac
>
> 1. Björk, V. O., (1948) *Acta chir. scand.* suppl. 137.

Figure 2.17. An artificial heart or cardiopulmonary machine: performance in animals. *A 1948 article by Björk. (Reproduced with permission from* Lancet.)

A 7-month visit to American surgeons (1950) funded by the Swedish-American Foundation Zorn Scholarship, began a long and fruitful relationship with the United States. As associate Professor of Thoracic Surgery (1951–58) at the Karolinska Institute, Björk performed the first left heart catheterization (1952), which he considers his most original contribution to cardiac surgery. This despite the enormous success and application of the Björk Shiley Valve. As Chief of Thoracic Surgery (1958–66) at University Hospital, Uppsala, he established a cardiac programme and introduced an intensive care unit. Uppsala University conferred on him the title of Professor of Medicine (1962–66), making him only the 30th personal professor in the university's 500 year history. By appointment of the King of Sweden, Björk succeeded Crafoord as Professor of Cardiovascular and Thoracic Surgery at the Karolinska Institute (1966–83). Since 1966 Björk has served on the Nobel Prize (medicine) selection committee. He has been decorated knight, Order of St Charles and the North Star. In 1967 and 1982, the American Association for Thoracic Surgery and the American College of Cardiology, respectively, made him an honorary member. In 1983, incapable of retirement, Björk became Director of Research and Education at The Heart Institute of the Desert in affiliation with the University of Southern California in Los Angeles. He was chief editor (1984–90) of *Reflections on Cardiac Surgery*, a series of taped interviews with surgeons whose contributions changed the course of cardiac surgery. *The Scandinavian Journal of Thoracic and Cardiovascular Surgery* (1991), of which Björk was the first editor (1968–82), dedicated an issue to celebrate his 70th birthday with the citation, "Viking Björk has long held the position of eminence in Swedish thoracic surgery...Through his numerous and world-wide contacts with leading centres of thoracic surgery, he has guided his country to acknowledge international standards." Bjork's memoir, *50 Years of Thoracic Surgery* (1993), illustrates surgical landmarks in his own career and, through eyewitness accounts, the history of heart surgery in the 20th century. His biography, *One for the Heart* (1983), illustrates the life of a man who, according to his student Christian Olin, "is utterly responsible and hard working. He is so energetic that I sometimes wonder what drives him—maybe a nuclear plant hidden under his shirt."

Björk is certainly one of the foremost pioneers in cardiac surgery with multiple broad based contributions. The Björk Shiley Valve issue for which he cannot be held responsible must not detract from this.

Floyd John Lewis (1916–)

FLOYD JOHN LEWIS was born in Waseca, Minnesota. He studied at the University of Minnesota (MD, 1942; PhD, 1950), where he served on the Faculty of Surgery. Lewis subsequently became Chief of Thoracic Surgery at Anoka State Hospital, Minnesota and Professor of Surgery at Northwestern University Medical School (1957–76). Since retiring in 1977, he has written *Bicycling Santa Barbara* (1983) and *So Your Doctor Recommended Surgery* (1990). Lewis and Mansur Taufic were the first men to operate directly inside the open heart. On 2 September 1952, after months of laboratory experimentation and study of hypothermia (stimulated by Bigelow), Lewis and Taufic used moderate total-body hypothermia to 28°C with venous inflow occlusion to close a large interatrial septal defect (Article 2.1, Appendix A). Surface cooling of the 5-year-old girl, weighing less than 30 pounds, was achieved by refrigerated blankets; rewarming took place in a bath of water at 45°C. The intracardiac repair took only 5.5 minutes. Lewis and Taufic were assisted by Varco and Lillehei. Richard Varco had already

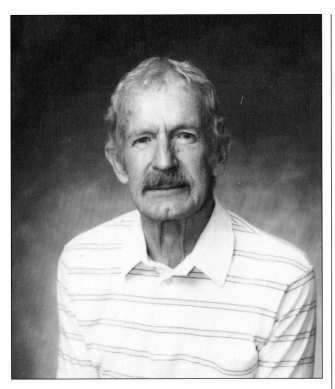

Figure 2.18. Floyd John Lewis.

CLOSURE OF ATRIAL SEPTAL DEFECTS WITH THE AID OF HYPOTHERMIA; EXPERIMENTAL ACCOMPLISHMENTS AND THE REPORT OF ONE SUCCESSFUL CASE

F. JOHN LEWIS, M.D., AND MANSUR TAUFIC, M.D., MINNEAPOLIS, MINN.

(From the Department of Surgery, University of Minnesota Medical School)

IN THE past the use of general or regional refrigeration in clinical medicine has been disappointing. Despite the fact that Fay,[13] a number of years ago, stimulated interest in the therapeutic potentialities of hypothermia when he reported on its use as a palliative method for treating patients with advanced cancer, little evidence developed to show that his method was better than the more simple treatments for incurable cancer, and it was never widely used. A little later, regional refrigeration, used as a preservative and anesthetic agent in treating gangrenous or severely wounded extremities, received consideration[9, 10] and many articles were published concerning the technique, but this method seems no longer to be of interest. Other anesthetic agents are better.

Despite these failures, it might still be expected that the production of greatly lowered body temperature would find use in medicine. The strikingly reduced metabolic rates associated with states of hibernation or artificially induced hypothermia[1, 3, 4] offer intriguing possibilities for the performance of operations requiring relatively prolonged vascular occlusion. A rewarding exploration of some of these possibilities has been undertaken by Bigelow,[2, 4] who has experimentally demonstrated the potentialities of hypothermia as an aid in cardiac surgery. He showed that during profound hypothermia in the dog, a longer cardiac inflow occlusion was possible than was tolerated without danger at normal body temperature. This maneuver made possible a cardiotomy in a dry field allowing examination of the interior of the heart for a number of minutes without the aid of complicated pumps or shunting procedures. With the body temperature reduced to 20° C., 51 per cent of his dogs, including 11 which had a cardiotomy during the operation, survived a fifteen-minute period of total cardiac inflow occlusion.

Boerema[6] also has used body cooling in dogs for the performance of intra-cardiac operations. In a number of animals the circulation was interrupted for ten to twenty minutes and in four dogs portions of the atrial septum were removed.

It has been our purpose to continue in this direction, using hypothermia experimentally as an aid for the production and correction of intracardiac defects under direct vision. We have tried to make the technique simple and safe enough so that its use for the closure of similar defects in human beings

This work was supported, in part, by a grant-in-aid from the Graduate School of the University of Minnesota and by a grant from the Minnesota Heart Association.
Received for publication. Sept. 15, 1952.

Figure 2.19. Closure of atrial septal defects with the aid of hypothermia. *A 1953 article by Lewis and Taufic. (Reproduced with permission from* Surgery.)

demonstrated the feasibility of normothermic inflow occlusion when operating for pulmonic stenosis. Lillehei, seeing the open heart for the first time on this occasion, considered the potential of open heart surgery so staggering that he left the operating room for the laboratory to plan a research programme. It was Bigelow who, by detailed physiological studies, arrived at the concept of hypothermia. He wrote "Our dismay at not performing the first successful human operation was offset by the pleasure of learning that the theory was correct and that the technique was effective."

Success, together with relative simplicity, led to the popularity of hypothermia. With inflow stasis, for less than 10 minutes repairs of atrial defects (of the *secundum* type) and correction of isolated congenital pulmonary or aortic valve stenosis were possible. By February 1954, Lewis had used hypothermia to correct atrial septal defects in 11 patients with two deaths. The first death had been caused by haemorrhage because the defect was more complicated than Lewis anticipated; the second came from heart block, 3 days after the

operation. Ventricular fibrillation in three other patients following surgery was overcome by electric shock and massage of the heart, by an apparatus built at Minnesota for surgical use. Failure was uniform when hypothermia was applied to more complex lesions, such as atrioventricular canal, infundibular pulmonary stenosis or ventricular septal defect. The basic problem was rewarming a cold, non-beating heart.

Whilst the medical world debated the risks involved in hypothermia and open heart surgery. Lewis appreciated its limited simplicity: "Hypothermia allowed open repair in a bloodless field without complex equipment, without a special team of assistants, without heparinization of the patient, and without special blood donors."

Ian Aird (1905–1962)

IAN AIRD was educated at George Watson's College, Edinburgh where he received the Annandale Gold Medal and Wightman Prize in clinical medicine (MB; ChB, 1928; FRCS (Ed), 1930). While he was clinical tutor in the wards of Graham at the Royal Infirmary (1931–35), he won a Rockefeller travelling fellowship (1934) to study under Evarts Graham at Barnes Hospital, St Louis, Missouri and at the University of Washington. On returning to Scotland in 1935, Aird was appointed to the staff of the Royal Edinburgh Hospital for Sick Children (ChM, 1935), and in 1939 he became temporary assistant surgeon at the Royal Infirmary, Edinburgh. During World War II, Aird served as lieutenant-colonel in the Royal Army Medical Corps (1939–43), mostly in North Africa, and was twice mentioned in dispatches. When he was released because of ill health, he became Assistant Surgeon to the Royal Infirmary and the Professorial Surgical Unit of the Edinburgh municipal hospitals (1943), where, with characteristic energy, he contributed to the neurovascular unit and built up a museum of surgery. Aird was an examiner for the Royal College of Surgeons of England and Edinburgh and the universities of London, Birmingham and Malaya. He provided a professional link between the English-speaking countries and particularly admired the openness and energy of Americans. He likened them to his fellow Scots, whom he said had "a keen eye to see the main chance." He was pleased to be made an

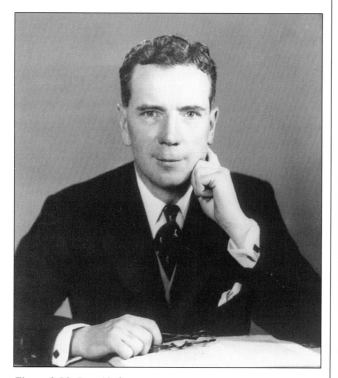

Figure 2.19. Ian Aird.

ASSISTED CIRCULATION BY PUMP-OXYGENATOR DURING OPERATIVE DILATATION OF THE AORTIC VALVE IN MAN

BY

IAN AIRD, Ch.M., F.R.C.S.
Professor of Surgery

D. G. MELROSE, B.M.
Assistant Lecturer in Surgery

W. P. CLELAND, F.R.C.S.
Lecturer in Thoracic Surgery

AND

R. B. LYNN, M.D., F.R.C.S.
Assistant Lecturer in Surgery

Postgraduate Medical School of London, Hammersmith Hospital

Interest in the clinical application of the various forms of pump-oxygenator (extracorporeal circulation or artificial heart–lung machine) is growing so rapidly, and the use of this type of apparatus in man has so seldom been followed by recovery, that it is customary for isolated examples of its use to be reported (Dennis *et al.*, 1951; Dogliotti, 1952; Gibbon, 1953; Dodrill *et al.*, 1953; Helmsworth *et al.*, 1953).

Three authors, Dogliotti (1952) in Turin, Gibbon (1953) in Philadelphia, and Dodrill *et al.* (1953) in Detroit, report survivors, and Helmsworth *et al.* (1952) have used an oxygenator for vein-to-vein perfusion in a case of fibrosis of the lung. The pump-oxygenator employed in the case here reported was that designed and developed by Melrose in the department of surgery of the Postgraduate Medical School. Melrose (1953a) has described the machine and Melrose *et al.* (1953b) have reported the animal experiments performed in the Buckston Browne Laboratories of the Royal College of Surgeons, which seemed to prove that the machine might be used with safety in man. The machine consists essentially of a rotating oxygenator and two rotary pumps. Its chief advantages are a high degree of efficiency in oxygenation (100 ml. of oxygen per litre of blood) and a low initial charge of blood.

The circumstances in which the machine might be used with profit in a clinical way have also been discussed (Aird, 1953), and the opinion was then expressed that the use of such a machine to by-pass heart and lung totally and to provide safely a dry heart for surgery was an aim not then immediately obtainable. We

Figure 2.20. Assisted circulation by pump-oxygenator during operative dilatation of the aortic valve in man. A 1954 article by Aird, Melrose, Cleland and Lynn. (Reproduced with permission from The British Journal of Medicine.*)*

honorary member of the American College of Surgeons in 1957 when the James IV Association of Surgeons, of which he was the first president, was inaugurated.

In 1946, at the age of 41, Aird succeeded E. Grey-Turner to the Chair of Surgery at the Royal Postgraduate Medical School with special certification of FRCS *ad eundem*. Under his direction, the Department of Surgery rose to occupy a unique position in British medicine by the vigour and freshness of its programmes and the calibre of its faculty. Aird's teaching affected every school of surgery in England and abroad. His *magnum opus*, *A Companion in Surgical Studies* (1949), was one of the most outstanding textbooks of its time. He expressed himself completely in words; no illustration appeared in the first edition and only two diagrams were permitted in the second. Aird's *The Making of a Surgeon* (1961) contains avuncular advice for the aspiring surgeon like "knife before wife," as he observed the deleterious effect of surgical training on marriage.

Though he seldom worked in the laboratory himself, his ideas and practical support sparked a team of investigators whose efforts produced the two major innovations of modern surgery—organ grafting and open heart surgery. In addition, the group produced some of the earliest work in extracorporeal circulation, organ and tissue transplantation, peripheral vascular disease, studies of the relation of blood groups to incidence of cancer of the stomach and peptic ulceration, and studies in body mineral metabolism.

Under Aird's guidance at the Royal Postgraduate Medical School, Melrose modified and improved the Björk pump creating a piece of precision engineering using a rotating plastic cylinder packed with 76 discs, reducing the amount of blood needed to prime it. It was first used in a patient on 9 December 1953, when Cleland of the Hammersmith Hospital dilated a stenosed aortic valve by open operation through the left ventricle. Melrose wrote,

> "As a measure of the man, it is noteworthy that in the first clinical trials of this machine Aird took on himself full clinical responsibility, and as soon as success was ensured, relinquished it, leaving the rewards to others. He took immense pleasure in this, striving always to direct the limelight away from himself towards his staff."

His separation of Nigerian-born Siamese twins in 1953 somewhat obfuscated his more serious contributions and thrust him before the public, causing him a fair amount of distress. According to Burman, who assisted at that operation,

> "Aird lived every moment as though it were his last. He drove himself with a passion and fury that caused grave concern to his friends. He was a whirlwind of a man, larger than life with day merging into day with no interval of rest and no visible flagging of his energy."

He appeared completely extroverted, full of zest, a little ruthless and very worldly, and it was tragic when he was found dead in bed from barbiturate poisoning, while suffering from depression, at Hammersmith at the age of 57. Irreverently his room became the hospital bar—the 'Waterhole' much frequented by cardiac surgeons of the future.

John Heysham Gibbon Jr (1903–1973)

JOHN HEYSHAM GIBBON JR a fifth-generation physician and third-generation surgeon, studied at Princeton (AB, 1923) and Jefferson Medical College (MD, 1927). He interned at Pennsylvania Hospital (1927–29) and had a year's fellowship to study under Edward Churchill at Harvard Medical School (1930–31), where on 31 October 1930, Gibbon cared for one of Churchill's patients who was dying of massive pulmonary embolism. He wrote,

> "During the 17 hours by this patient's side, the thought constantly recurred that the patient's hazardous condition could be improved if some of the blue blood in the patient's distended veins could be continuously withdrawn into an apparatus where the blood could pick up oxygen and discharge carbon dioxide and then pump this blood back into the patient's arteries."

In 1931, Gibbon went to the University of Pennsylvania with his wife, Mary Hopkinson Gibbon, who had been Churchill's research assistant, to continue working on a heart–lung machine in association with Landis: "It was this man," he wrote, "who gave me unwavering encouragement in what had by now become a principal ambition, to build an extracorporeal-blood circuit capable of temporarily taking over the cardiorespiratory functions." Churchill, though sceptical of Gibbon's ideas, granted him and his wife another year's funding in 1934 to build a heart–lung circuit at the Harvard Surgical Research Laboratories. On 10 May 1935, Gibbon demonstrated that his perfusion apparatus could maintain blood pressure and respiration for up to 3 hours in an animal, followed by spontaneous re-establishment of normal circulation and respiration. In 1949, six engineers from the Endicott Laboratories of International Business Machines (IBM) built Gibbon's Model I heart–lung machine. This incorporated a larger revolving vertical oxygenator with the

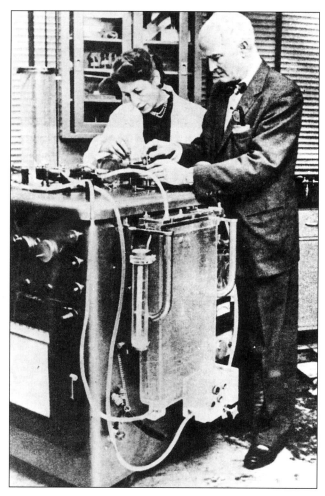

Figure 2.21. John Heysham Gibbon and his wife Mary Hopkinson with the heart–lung machine.

APPLICATION OF A MECHANICAL HEART AND LUNG APPARATUS TO CARDIAC SURGERY

JOHN H. GIBBON, Jr., M.D.
Philadelphia, Pennsylvania

IT IS A PLEASURE to be here and to talk about a subject in which I have been interested for many years. The ultimate objective of my work in this field has been to be able to operate inside the heart under direct vision. From the beginning, I have not only been interested in the substitution of a mechanical device for the heart, but also for the lung. We have always considered congenital abnormalities of the heart the most suitable lesions for operative repair. Many of these abnormalities are septal defects. In the presence of a septal defect, shunting the flow of blood around one side of the heart with a pump, will not provide a bloodless field for operative closure of the defect. An apparatus which embodies a mechanical lung, as well as pumps, enables you to shunt blood around both the heart and lungs, thus allowing operations to be performed under direct vision in a bloodless field within the opened heart. Furthermore, an apparatus which embodies a mechanical lung enables you to provide partial support to either a failing heart or failing lung where a major operative procedure is not contemplated. Such an apparatus can also be used as an adjunct during the course of a major operative procedure. This partial support of the cardiorespiratory functions consists in removing venous blood from some peripheral vein continuously, oxygenating the blood and getting rid of the carbon dioxide in it and then injecting the blood continuously in a central direction in a peripheral artery. Of course, such partial circulation, or cardiorespiratory support, requires the use of a mechanical lung in the circuit.

I shall not describe in detail the entire apparatus. I shall merely discuss six aspects of the problem which I consider of fundamental importance. Four of these concern the apparatus itself, and two concern problems which arise on opening the heart and operating within it under direct vision.

The first feature of a mechanical heart-lung apparatus is a suitable pumping mechanism to move the venous blood from the subject, through the apparatus, and back into an artery of the subject. There is no real problem about a pumping apparatus. There are many ways of moving blood through tubing without producing significant amounts of hemolysis. We have used for many years a roller type of pump which does not contain any internal valves. Such pumps are extremely simple. Because of the absence of valves, the blood circuit is easy to clean and there are no stagnate regions where fibrin might be apt to form. There are many other advantages in this type of pump such as the simple and rapid control of the rate of blood flow. The pumps cause no significant hemolysis. In human patients in which we have used the apparatus, hemolysis has always been well below 100 mg. of free hemoglobin per 100 ml. of plasma. In animal experiments, hemolysis is similarly minimal.

The second main feature of a mechanical heart-lung apparatus is the mechanical lung itself. This presents far more difficulties than pumping blood. I am sure that the most efficient apparatus for performing the functions of the lung has not yet been devised. Our present mechanical lung, however, provides a reasonably satisfactory working solution to this problem. The mechanical lung performs the gas exchange required for respiratory function by filming blood on both sides of screens which have a somewhat larger mesh than ordinary fly screens. These screens are made of stainless steel wire and are suspended vertically and parallel in a plastic chamber. As the blood flows over these screens, it takes up oxygen and gives off carbon dioxide. It should be remembered that it is equally important to remove carbon dioxide from the blood as it is to add oxygen. It is easy to observe that sufficient oxygen is being picked up in the apparatus, as the blue blood entering the oxygenator becomes red as it leaves. This can be determined more accurately, of course, by intermittent sampling or by continuous reading with a Wood cuvette and oximeter. On the other hand, there is no way of estimating the carbon dioxide tension by observing the color of

Presented in the Symposium on Recent Advances in Cardiovascular Physiology and Surgery, University of Minnesota, Minneapolis, September 16, 1953.
Dr. Gibbon is Professor of Surgery and Director of Surgical Research, The Jefferson Medical College, Philadelphia, Pennsylvania.

MARCH, 1954   171

Figure 2.22. Application of mechanical heart and lung apparatus to cardiac surgery. *A 1954 article by Gibbon. (Reproduced with permission from* Minnesota Medicine.*)*

entire blood circuit enclosed in a cabinet, maintained at body temperature with an oxygenating capacity sufficient to replace cardiorespiratory function in dogs.

The great turning point came when, in Gibbon's laboratory, Thomas Stokes and John Flick discovered that lining the surface of the revolving cylinder with a closely adherent, fine wire screen increased contact between red cells and oxygen by 700–1000%. In December 1949, Gibbon instructed IBM to replace the revolving cylinder with a parallel series of six flat, stainless steel screens which exposed both surfaces of blood film to oxygen. Model II was delivered to Jefferson Medical College Hospital on 19 June 1951 and was cannibalized to create Model III in 1954.

In February 1952, the first repair of a defect in an open heart supported by Model II failed because the defect, assumed to be in the atrial septum, was found at autopsy to be a huge patent ductus arteriosus. However, on 6 May 1953, 18 years after Gibbon's bypass of the heart and lungs of a cat, his Model II heart–lung machine allowed open and bloodless repair of the heart of Cecilia Bavolek, an event which formed the basis of

modern cardiac surgery. The operative note was handwritten by Robert K. Finley Jr,

"With patient under pentothal and oxygen endoanaesthesia, Dr Gibbon opened the chest through the 4th interspaces bilaterally. The right atrium was large and by invaginating the appendage, a large interauricular defect could be felt. The patient was then placed on the oxygenating apparatus (26 minutes on total substitution of heart and lungs), the right auricle opened and the defect sutured closed with 50 silk (dekanate)...The patient tolerated the procedure well."

That night Gibbon telephoned Alfred Blalock at Johns Hopkins and Clarence Crafoord at the Karolinska Institute to tell them the news. In July 1953, he operated on two 5-year-old girls. When both died, Gibbon declared a moratorium on bypass surgery until more work could be done on the coagulation problems. He never returned to cardiac surgery.

Shown is the last paper from Gibbon's research laboratory (Article 2.2, Appendix A). Had Clarence Dennis not asked him to describe his one successful operation to the Symposium on Recent Advances in Cardiovascular Physiology and Surgery at the University of Minnesota on 16 September 1953, it would not have been recorded. Gibbon thought the apparatus could not be accepted on the basis of one positive outcome, but Dennis insisted that success in even one case warranted publication. Gibbon attributed his failure to human error, confirmed by John Kirklin's successful application of a modified version of Model II. Kirklin wrote, "In the deepest recesses of my heart, I felt that those four patients died in part because of his [Gibbon's] lack of appreciation of some of the technical aspects of cardiac surgery."

Gibbon, like his father, became Samuel D. Gross Professor of Surgery and chairman of the department at Jefferson Medical College (1956–67). He became interested in cancer of the lung and oesophagus, and devoted his remaining years of professional practice to thoracic surgery.

Denis Graham Melrose (1921–)

DENIS GRAHAM MELROSE was born in Capetown, South Africa and was educated in England at Sedbergh School. He studied medicine at University College, Oxford and University College, London (MA; BM; BCh, Oxon, 1945; Hon MRCP, London, 1964; Hon FRCS, 1969). After 6 months each at the Royal Postgraduate Medical School, Hammersmith and the Edgeware General Hospital in London, he joined the Navy and was posted to HMS Tamar, Hong Kong, as ear, nose and throat specialist to the British Pacific Fleet (1947–48). On his return to England, he rejoined the Department of Surgery at the Royal Postgraduate Medical School to begin what was to become his life's work: to make surgery of the heart possible. He became Emeritus Professor of Surgical Science there.

Progress was at first painfully slow. Many had tried to keep isolated organs alive by mechanical pumps and artificial lungs, but had failed. It was therefore difficult to remain optimistic that similar methods would have a better fate when used to perfuse the whole body. But this proved the right approach and by 1953 Melrose was able to publish a description of suitable equipment and its successful use in man.

With the courageous support of the surgeons Cleland and Bentall, and the superlative cardiology of Shillingford (who rarely referred a patient for surgery), Goodwin and Oakley, the cardiac department at Hammersmith came to have substantial influence in the development of cardiac surgery in Europe and throughout the world.

Melrose described operating conditions in the early 1950s, which precipitated the need for 'elective cardiac arrest', in 1955:

> "Consider a group of people practising in animals the management of an open heart operation. Remember the clumsy perfusion equipment, primitive anaesthesia; little or no measuring equipment, a host of mysteries gradually overcome, and then the first attempt at clinical application. Suddenly the rules established are completely without validity, drowned in a torrent of blood streaming into the opened heart from a patent ductus, a large bronchial anastomosis or an incompetent aortic valve above the septal defect."

Clearly conditions were not ideal, especially in complicated congenital defects.

In 1955, 3 months after Melrose's preliminary communication in the *Lancet* (Article 2.3, Appendix A), the Hammersmith Hospital carried out the first elective cardiac arrest in a patient on cardiopulmonary bypass, with the aorta cross-clamped and

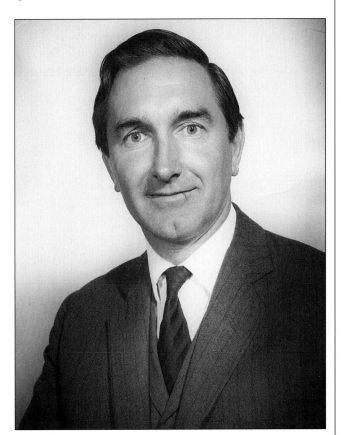

Figure 2.23. Denis Graham Melrose.

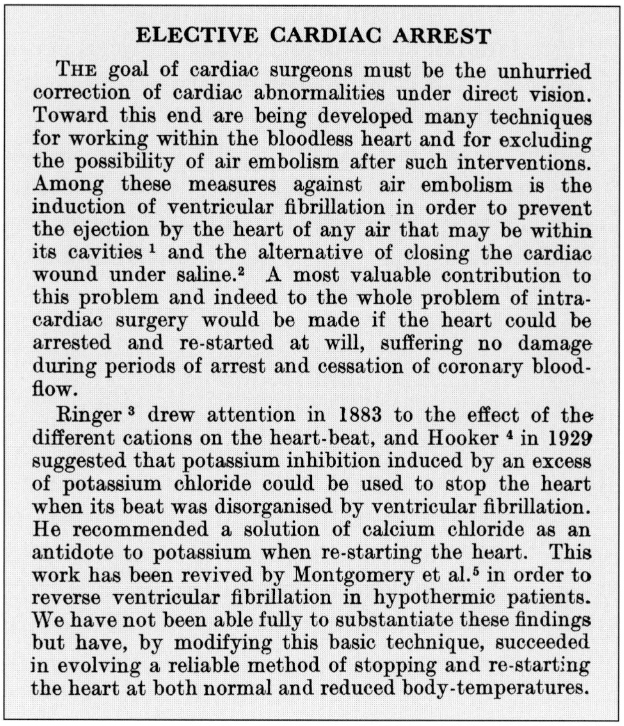

ELECTIVE CARDIAC ARREST

THE goal of cardiac surgeons must be the unhurried correction of cardiac abnormalities under direct vision. Toward this end are being developed many techniques for working within the bloodless heart and for excluding the possibility of air embolism after such interventions. Among these measures against air embolism is the induction of ventricular fibrillation in order to prevent the ejection by the heart of any air that may be within its cavities [1] and the alternative of closing the cardiac wound under saline.[2] A most valuable contribution to this problem and indeed to the whole problem of intracardiac surgery would be made if the heart could be arrested and re-started at will, suffering no damage during periods of arrest and cessation of coronary blood-flow.

Ringer [3] drew attention in 1883 to the effect of the different cations on the heart-beat, and Hooker [4] in 1929 suggested that potassium inhibition induced by an excess of potassium chloride could be used to stop the heart when its beat was disorganised by ventricular fibrillation. He recommended a solution of calcium chloride as an antidote to potassium when re-starting the heart. This work has been revived by Montgomery et al.[5] in order to reverse ventricular fibrillation in hypothermic patients. We have not been able fully to substantiate these findings but have, by modifying this basic technique, succeeded in evolving a reliable method of stopping and re-starting the heart at both normal and reduced body-temperatures.

Figure 2.24. Elective cardiac arrest. *A 1955 article by Melrose. (Reproduced with permission from* Lancet.*)*

potassium citrate injected directly in the aortic root. This produced cardiac arrest in the flaccid diastolic phase and allowed the operation to be carried out in a dry, motionless heart. To deliberately cause cardiac arrest was enormously controversial and provided an ethical dilemma similar to cardiac transplantation. The coroner, present in the operating room for this first use of elective cardiac arrest, gave the team his blessing as did the leaders of the Anglican, Catholic and Presbyterian churches.

At the Cleveland Clinic, Effler, who had built a Melrose-type oxygenator with Kolff, was the first to use potassium citrate solution clinically in the United States. Through a telephone conversation with Kolff, Melrose (in London) advised Effler (in Cleveland) to limit himself to 15 minutes in the heart. Their first repair of a septal defect using 'cardioplegia,' a convenient word for elective cardiac arrest, (17 February 1956) was successful. After 73 such 'stopped-heart' operations in the next 15 months, Effler reported that the safety and benefits of elective cardiac arrest justified its international adoption.

By the end of the 1960s, however, doubts arose about the safety of potassium citrate-induced cardiac arrest. An influential paper by MacFarland from the National Heart Institute (USA) described the discovery of unusual areas of necrosis in the hearts of two patients who had died. This led to an examination of the solution used to stop the heart and it was noticed that in the glass containers in which it had been stored, 'flaking' had occurred forming a precipitate. Making up the solution freshly from crystals of potassium citrate at the time of operation did not prevent an incidence of similar lesions and it was felt that the technique should be abandoned. The National Heart Institute replaced it with intermittent aortic occlusion or coronary perfusion and the rest of America went with them. Most of the world followed, but small pockets of resistance remained to rework the original experiments and, in the fullness of time, to reintroduce heart-stopping techniques dependent on the manipulation of potassium and calcium ions. The method produces the best conditions for safe cardiac surgery and it is unlikely to be challenged again.

Melrose's final assessment was that it was not only the adverse reports which led to the abandonment of cardioplegia, but also the fact that extracorporeal circulation was felt emotionally by cardiac surgeons to be the best method of keeping the patient, and, by inference, the myocardium alive during open heart surgery. An arrested heart, Melrose concluded, was conceptually repugnant to the surgeons of the early 1960s.

Charles Edwin Drew (1916–)

CHARLES EDWIN DREW was born and obtained his qualifications in England (MVO, VRD; MB; BS (Lond); MRCS (Eng); LRCP (Lond), 1941; FRCS (Eng), 1946). He was subsequently Chief Assistant and Surgical Registrar at the Westminster Hospital, civil consultant in thoracic surgery to the royal Navy, honorary consultant in thoracic surgery at St George's Hospital, London and the King Edward VII Hospital, Midhurst, and honorary consultant to the Army. Drew was a fellow of the Royal Society of Medicine and member of the Society of Thoracic Surgeons. He was first assistant to Sir Clement Price Thomas, who performed a pneumonectomy for cancer on King George VI. A few years later Sir Clement, a smoker himself, also developed lung cancer, but was successfully operated on by Charles Drew and survived to the age of 80. Drew wrote *Clinical Use of Hyperbaric Oxygen Bed* (1969) and *Heart Transplantation* (1970).

Drew and Anderson combined profound hypothermia, using a heat exchanger with two extracorporeal circuits to bypass the left and right ventricles when they fibrillated as the temperature

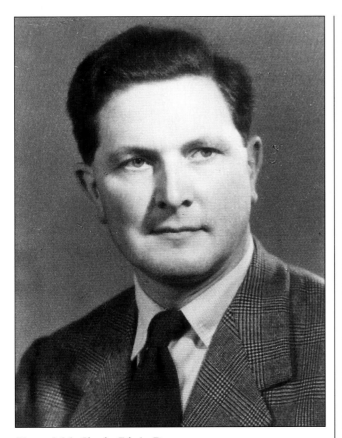

Figure 2.25. Charles Edwin Drew.

PROFOUND HYPOTHERMIA IN CARDIAC SURGERY

REPORT OF THREE CASES

C. E. DREW
M.V.O., F.R.C.S.
ASSISTANT SURGEON, WESTMINSTER HOSPITAL, LONDON, S.W.1; THORACIC SURGEON, ST. GEORGE'S HOSPITAL, S.W.1

IAN M. ANDERSON
M.D. Glasg., F.R.C.P.
PHYSICIAN, CHILDREN'S DEPARTMENT, WESTMINSTER HOSPITAL; PHYSICIAN, QUEEN ELIZABETH HOSPITAL FOR CHILDREN, LONDON, E.2

THE technique of inducing profound hypothermia described in the preceding paper was carried out in animals with normal hearts. It depended on the ability to direct part (eventually most) of the systemic and pulmonary venous streams from the atria into reservoirs, from which the blood was pumped respectively into the aorta and the pulmonary artery.

In the presence of a septal defect—especially a large one at atrial level—this might present some difficulty, particularly in the early stages of the cooling process. On the other hand it had been observed that, later on, the oxygen saturation of systemic venous blood became so high that mixing of pulmonary and systemic blood would no longer be so important. Whether the technique would in fact prove satisfactory in such cases was a question which would be difficult to answer in the laboratory.

With this in mind, we chose as our first patient a child with a large atrial septal defect, whose condition would be considered inoperable by other techniques.

Figure 2.26. Profound hypothermia in cardiac surgery. *A 1959 article by Drew and Anderson. (Reproduced with permission from* Lancet.)

lowered. One circuit perfused the patient's lungs to oxygenate the blood during cooling and rewarming, and the other maintained systemic and coronary perfusion. At 15°C, the aorta and cavae were occluded, providing the surgeon with a still, bloodless field and 1 hour in which to complete the operation before cerebral or detectable myocardial damage occurred. On 11 April 1959, the *Lancet* carried two articles by Charles Drew. The first described his experimental methods for biventricular bypass with core cooling using a heat exchanger. In this method, the lungs remained as the oxygenator as the pharyngeal temperature was taken down to 8°C. A relatively small number of experiments were sufficient to show that profound hypothermia could be induced in a dog followed by safe, circulatory arrest for 30 minutes. This allowed an operating time of about 1 hour. On rewarming, complete recovery was achieved. In the second article, Drew described three children in whom cooling to 15°C was undertaken with a circulatory arrest time of up to 45 minutes (Article 2.4, Appendix A).

The principles devised by Drew were sound and are still applicable, although his protocol has been abandoned. Drew predicted that profound cooling with an extracorporeal circuit whilst maintaining the lungs as oxygenator would prove a more attractive proposition than the use of the pump oxygenator. This was a logical expectation given the increasing awareness of the damaging effects of bubble oxygenators. His prediction was never realized, although profound hypothermic circulatory arrest became standard for the repair of complex congenital cardiac defects in infants and for problematic thoracic aneurysms. More complex types of atrial septal defect, ventricular septal defect and Fallot's tetralogy also became correctable. Profound hypothermia did not gain general acceptance for routine use because of the continual improvement of the regular heart–lung machine and dangers of deep hypothermia. Working at the Westminster Hospital in London, Drew persisted with his methods almost until retirement in the 1970s.

William Evans Neville (1919–)

WILLIAM EVANS NEVILLE was born in Fairbury, Nebraska. He studied at Creighton University, Nebraska and the University of Nebraska College of Medicine (MD, 1943). He interned at Santa Rosa Hospital, Texas. After residency under George Crile Jr and Thomas Evans Jones at the Cleveland Clinic, Neville 'migrated across town' to the Cleveland City Hospital, where he and George Clowes made the first attempt at direct surgery of the aortic valve supported by a heart–lung machine (1954). Their patient, a man of 55 years, suffering from severe aortic stenosis, mitral stenosis and hemiparesis from a cerebral infarction, died an hour after closing the chest. Beginning in 1958, Clowes and Neville, using their large, cumbersome membrane oxygenator and a recirculation pump with a small priming volume, performed about 250 open heart operations (1958). In 1962, Neville began the open heart programme at Hines Veterans Administration Hospital, University of Illinois, which he directed until 1989. He wrote a monograph on extracorporeal circulation in *Current Problems in Surgery* (1967), as well as *The Care of the Surgical Cardiopulmonary Patient* (1983) and *Intensive Care of the Surgical Cardiopulmonary Patient* (1983). Neville, remembers operating on patients with 'some sort of congenital heart

defect' before cardiologists had equipment to make diagnoses and soldiers being given anyone's blood when bleeding from wounds during World War II. He is currently writing a book on the circuitous route taken to arrive at current methods of cardiac surgery and continues his professional duties as Emeritus Professor at the University of Illinois.

The Neville tracheal prosthesis evolved from surgery of the trachea at the Veterans Administration Hospital in Illinois, a 2500-bed hospital with 300 beds allocated to pulmonary disease. Having successfully implanted silicone bifurcated grafts in animals with good long-term results, Neville went on to implant them in man.

Several articles in the early 1960s demonstrated the advantage of a clear prime for the pump oxygenator during cardiopulmonary bypass (Figure 2.28). Neville had a particular interest in the damaging effects of cardiopulmonary bypass, but highlights the work of Zuhdi, Long, Cooley and Roe who

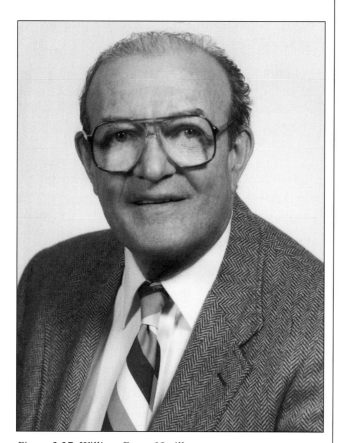

Figure 2.27. William Evans Neville.

Total Prime of the Disc Oxygenator with Ringer's and Ringer's Lactate Solution for Cardiopulmonary Bypass
Clinical and Experimental Observations*
WILLIAM E. NEVILLE, M.D., F.C.C.P., L. PENFIELD FABER, M.D.
AND HOWARD PEACOCK, B.T.
Hines, Illinois

MANY OF THE UNDESIRABLE SEQUEL-lae attendant to open heart surgery is due to the donor blood.[4,7,9] For this reason, the substitution of another ingredient for priming the pump oxygenator has been the goal of most cardiac surgeons. The original work of Neptune[6] suggested the feasibility and practicability of priming the bubble oxygenator with normal saline for cardiopulmonary bypass. Since then Zuhdi and associates[10] have promulgated 5 per cent dextrose in water for perfusion with the Lillehei-De Wall unit, and Long et al.[5] have had success with the same oxygenator using low molecular weight dextran. Recently Cooley and colleagues[8] have advocated 5 per cent D/W for filling the plastic disposable bubble oxygenator** prior to open heart surgery and Roe[9] has used a balanced electrolyte solution for extracorporeal perfusion. The distinct advantage of a low priming volume is proferred with these techniques.

The purpose of this paper is to present our experimental and clinical experience with Ringer's solution and Ringer's lactate to prime the disc oxygenator (Kay-Cross) with the Gebauer heat exchanger. Hemodilution ranged from 140 ml./kg. to 53 ml./kg. body weight in the dog and in man the extracorporeal prime was 35 to 52 ml./kg. In addition the biochemical alterations in two patients perfused with 5 per cent glucose in water will be briefly discussed.

Our results conclusively demonstrate that this method of cardiopulmonary bypass is feasible when one is aware that metabolic acidosis can occur during prolonged perfusion. Even though high flow rates can be achieved with this technique, the oxygen capacity of the blood is reduced, thus exposing the tissues to hypoxia. However, by determining the pH, buffer base, bicarbonate and pCO₂ at frequent intervals during the perfusion, irremedial metabolic acidosis can be prevented with the addition of sodium bicarbonate into the oxygenator. At the end of cardiopulmonary bypass, the hematocrit can be restored to near control by the slow return of the blood in the oxygenator to the organism.

METHODS AND MATERIALS
Experimental

Mongrel dogs weighing from 10 to 18 kg. were anesthetized with intravenous pentobarbital sodium (Nembutal) without prior medication. The Mark 8 Bird respirator was used for pulmonary insufflation through an endotracheal tube and the right chest was opened in the fourth interspace. Concomitantly the femoral vessels were exposed bilaterally and cannulated for measurement of arterial and venous blood pressure and the arterial inflow from the pump oxygenator. Catheters were inserted into the superior and inferior vena cavae through the right auricle for gravity drainage into the oxygenator.

The buffer base, standard bicarbonate pCO₂, base excess and pH were determined in the arterial blood before and after

*From the VA Hospital.
**Mini-prime bubble oxygenator, Travenol Laboratories, Morton Grove, Illinois.

320

Figure 2.28. Total prime of the disc oxygenator with Ringer's and Ringer's lactate solution in cardiopulmonary bypass: clinical and experimental observations. *A 1964 article by Neville, Faber and Peacock. (Reproduced with permission from* Diseases of the Chest.)

independently reported similar observations with different solutions. Neville emphasizes that in order to avoid metabolic disturbances haemodilution should not exceed 60 ml/kg body weight. Extraneous blood need only be added to the system if bleeding occurs or if the flow rate becomes too low during prolonged bypass as the Ringer's solution diffuses into the tissues. The following year, Kirklin and colleagues produced important data on renal performance during cardiopulmonary bypass with and without haemodilution. They demonstrated significantly greater volumes of urine flow with lower osmolality during and immediately after cardiopulmonary bypass when haemodilution was used. Glomerular filtration rate, effective renal plasma flow and postoperative urine electrolyte excretion were essentially similar with or without

haemodilution, but the authors concluded that increased production of urine in haemodilution patients might well protect renal tubular integrity.

In 1973, Rabelo and colleagues from São Paulo, Brazil, investigated the nature of the pump primer on post-perfusion pulmonary changes. Using lung biopsy specimens before and after bypass, electron microscopy showed a predominance of abnormalities in patients where blood was used to prime the extracorporeal circuit. The alterations which included leucocyte migration into the septa and alveoli, desquamation of alveolar epithelial cells and vacuolization of type 2 pneumocytes were not found to the same extent in patients primed with clear fluid.

Sir Brian Barratt-Boyes (1924–)

SIR BRIAN BARRATT-BOYES was born in Wellington, New Zealand and studied at the University of Otago Medical School (MB; ChB, 1946). After 7 years of postgraduate work in general and orthopaedic surgery and pathology (FRACS, 1952), he spent 2 years at the Mayo Clinic as a fellow in cardiothoracic surgery (1953–55) under John Kirklin and a year at the Royal Infirmary, Bristol through a Nuffield Fellowship (1956). He was appointed Senior Thoracic Surgeon (1957–65) (ChM, 1962) and, since 1965, has been Surgeon-in-Charge of the cardiothoracic surgical unit at Green Lane Hospital, Auckland. Since 1966, Sir Brian has been surgeon to the Mercy Hospital, Auckland and Honorary Professor and Consultant in Surgery at the University of Auckland. He was named Companion (1970) and Knight of the British Empire (1971). Sir Brian was awarded the R.T. Hall Prize of the Cardiac Society of Australia and New Zealand (1966) for his original work on homograft valve replacement beginning with his placement of an aortic homograft valve on 23 August 1962, a month after Donald Ross's in London, and the René Leriche Prize, by the Société Internationale de Chirurgie (1987). In 1981, Sir Brian and John Kirklin published *Cardiac Surgery,* a comprehensive textbook, widely regarded as the definitive work in the specialty, reflecting a lifetime's experience from two pioneers.

When Viking Björk asked why Sir Brian became a doctor, he replied:

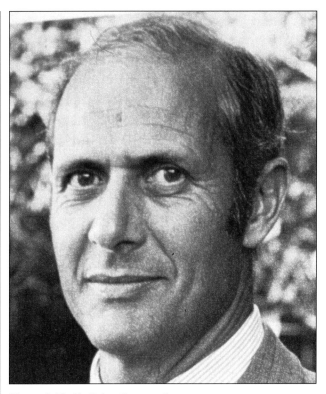

Figure 2.29. Sir Brian Barratt-Boyes.

"I was one of those fortunate people, i.e. it was specifically the only thing that I wanted to do from the time I was a small child. I really have no idea why that was. There were only two other things that interested me and which I toyed with perhaps a little, one was music. I used to spend a lot of time playing the

piano...I sold my piano when I first went over to the States, in order to get enough money to travel with my wife and then two children...The other profession I did toy with was going into the Church...but I always wanted to be a doctor...He had a terrible bout of tuberculous laryngitis. Those of you who remember those early days know what a killer tuberculosis could be. It was a dreadful situation. That affected me a great deal and it wasn't too unexpected I suppose, that I went into what was then thoracic surgery."

Sir Brian spearheaded the development of cardiovascular surgery in the Asian Pacific region. He demonstrated the advantages of primary intracardiac repair in infancy for many types of congenital heart disease. The first such operation, using profound hypothermia–circulatory arrest in infants, was undertaken at Green Lane Hospital early in 1968. Earlier work reported by the Japanese differed in that their operations were performed on a very limited group of older infants. Sir Brian wrote:

> "The introduction of the technique in our unit was a direct result of a visit to Auckland by two Japanese surgeons who came to us to learn the technique of aortic homograft valve replacement! We learned from them about their experience with profound hypothermia. Subsequently, one of them returned as a senior resident for 1 year, and it was during that period that we initiated our program and developed it."

In 1969, Atsumi Mori from Kyoto told the Green Lane staff about profound hypothermia and minimal support by cardiopulmonary bypass, which allowed radical corrective surgery in very small infants with gross cardiac deformities under direct vision.

The 1970 article in *Chest* (Article 2.5, Appendix A) was published at a time when the damaging effects of cardiopulmonary bypass accounted for considerable morbidity and mortality in the surgery of congenital heart disease. Infants, particularly those less than 3 months of age, tolerated prolonged cardiopulmonary bypass with a bubble oxygenator badly, and frequently died from multisystem failure after a completely satisfactory cardiac repair. Core cooling required a relatively short period of perfusion and minimized the duration of blood—foreign surface interaction. Heat exchange with the pump oxygenator was supplemented by surface cooling and rewarming. Profound hypothermia also conveyed a myocardial protective effect before the advent of cardioplegia. The

Intracardiac Surgery in Neonates and Infants Using Deep Hypothermia with Surface Cooling and Limited Cardiopulmonary Bypass

By Brian G. Barratt-Boyes, M.B., Ch.M., M. Simpson, M.B., Ch.B., and John M. Neutze, M.D.

SUMMARY

In an attempt to achieve safe intracardiac surgery in severely ill babies with congenital heart defects, a technique of deep hypothermia with surface cooling and limited bypass has been used. Under halothane anesthesia, these infants were cooled to a nasopharyngeal temperature of 26 C on a circulating water blanket and the temperature was lowered further to 22 C by a short period of total body perfusion. After a period of circulatory arrest which averaged 48 minutes at 22 C, during which the intracardiac repair was carried out, rewarming to 32 C was achieved by 20 minutes of total body perfusion and final rewarming to 36 C by surface means.

Thirty-three of 37 infants under 10 kg in weight, with correctable lesions, survived this procedure, including 25 aged 8 days to 12 months. Conditions corrected were transposition (13), tetralogy of Fallot (9), total anomalous pulmonary venous connection (6), ventricular septal defect (6), and atrioventricular canal (3). The technique gave ideal operating conditions and is believed to have wide application in the neonatal and infant group.

Additional Indexing Words:
Circulatory arrest   Bypass rewarming   Ventricular septal defect
Cyanotic heart disease   Transposition of great vessels   Tetralogy of Fallot
Pulmonary circulation   Total anomalous pulmonary venous connection

INTRACARDIAC surgery for congenital heart disease in neonates and infants by conventional cardiopulmonary bypass techniques has carried a high mortality and morbidity, particularly for complex prolonged procedures. This has been due in part to metabolic disturbances and pulmonary complications which are difficult to manage in this age group. In addition, with total body perfusion caval cannulation, which can be technically difficult, is usually required. Moreover, this technique tends to be associated with the presence of some intracardiac blood and with incomplete myocardial relaxation,

both of which hinder rapid accurate repair of complex defects within these tiny hearts.

These disadvantages can be avoided by a technique of deep hypothermia and circulatory arrest, which is designed to limit the duration of total body perfusion to an absolute minimum, does not require caval cannulation, and provides a completely bloodless, relaxed heart.

Technique

The infant is placed supine on a cooling blanket and is anesthetized with equal parts of nitrous oxide and oxygen, halothane (0.5% to 1%), and intravenous d-tubocurarine (1 mg/kg). Plastic bags of crushed ice are positioned to cover the trunk, the upper parts of the limbs, and the crown of the head, avoiding contact with peripheral parts. At 26 C nasopharyngeal, the ice

From the Cardio-thoracic Surgical Unit, Green Lane Hospital, Auckland, New Zealand.

Supplement 1 to Circulation, Vols. XLIII and XLIV, May 1971

Figure 2.30. Intracardiac surgery in neonates and infants using deep hypothermia with surface cooling and limited cardiopulmonary bypass. *A 1971 article by Barratt-Boyes, Simpson and Neutze. (Reproduced with permission from* Chest.*)*

demonstration that these repairs were possible with deep hypothermia and total circulatory arrest stimulated a major push forward in this area. Large clinical series by Dillard, Subramanian, Castaneda and others followed, demonstrating the feasibility of this method.

Philip R. Craddock (1943–1983)

PHILIP R. CRADDOCK was born in Sydney, Australia. After graduating from Sydney University Medical School (MD, 1965), he became a Fellow of the Royal Australian College of Physicians (FRACP, 1974), the American College of Physicians (1981) and Associate Professor in the haematology section of the Department of Medicine at the University of Minnesota (1973–81). Craddock received a number of National Institute of Health grants and the Research Career Development Award

for work entitled *Granulocytes, Complement and Vascular Endothelium*. He won international recognition in the field of immunological mechanisms in the adult respiratory distress syndrome. His appointment as Professor and Chief of the Haematology/Oncology Division of the Department of Medicine at the University of Kentucky (1981–83), where he set up a bone marrow unit, was cut short by his premature death by suicide, precipitated, in the view of his physician and neurosurgeon, by a brain tumour.

As early as 1968, observations were made that a profound

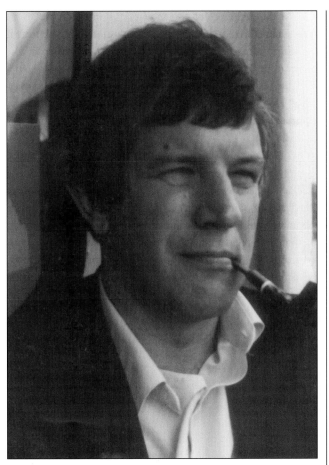

Figure 2.31. Philip R. Craddock

acute transient granulocytopenia occurred during the initial phase of haemodialysis when cellophane membrane dialysers were used. In 1977, Craddock first demonstrated that this granulocytopenia was caused by complement activation and, furthermore, that the responsible complement breakdown fragment C5a caused pulmonary leucostasis. Demonstration of the plugging of pulmonary capillaries by aggregated granulocytes allowed a better understanding of this phenomenon, which adversely affected pulmonary function. Craddock extended his work to include the role of complement–granulocyte interactions in other important pathogenic processes, such as adult respiratory distress syndrome and myocardial infarction, and the mechanism of inhibition of C5a-induced granulocyte aggregation.

A report by Craddock and co-workers (Figure 2.32), though

The New England
Journal of Medicine

©Copyright, 1977, by the Massachusetts Medical Society

Volume 296   APRIL 7, 1977   Number 14

COMPLEMENT AND LEUKOCYTE-MEDIATED PULMONARY DYSFUNCTION IN HEMODIALYSIS

PHILIP R. CRADDOCK, M.B., B.S., F.R.A.C.P., JORG FEHR, M.D., KENNETH L. BRIGHAM, M.D., RICHARD S. KRONENBERG, M.D., AND HARRY S. JACOB, M.D.

Abstract During hemodialysis, cardiopulmonary decompensation may appear in uremic patients, possibly caused by plugging of pulmonary vessels by leukocytes. In 34 patients we noted leukopenia (20 per cent of initial levels) during hemodialysis that in 15 was associated with impaired pulmonary function. When we infused autologous plasma, incubated with dialyzer cellophane, into rabbits and sheep, sudden leukopenia and hypoxia occurred, with doubling of pulmonary-artery pressures and quintupling of pulmonary-lymph effluent. Histologic examination showed severe pulmonary-vessel leukostasis and interstitial edema. The syndrome was prevented by preinactivation of complement but was reproduced by infusions of plasma in which complement was activated by zymosan. Thus, acute pulmonary dysfunction from complement-mediated leukostasis may play a major part in the acute cardiopulmonary complications of cellophane-membrane hemodialysis. (N Engl J Med 296:769-774, 1977)

TRANSIENT leukopenia, selectively involving granulocytes and monocytes, occurs in all patients during the first two hours of hemodialysis with cellophane-membrane apparatus.[1,2] We recently reported that such leukopenia results from pulmonary sequestration of leukocytes, somehow provoked by low-molecular-weight (7000 to 20,000 daltons) complement component (or components), which, in turn, were shown to be activated by dialyzer cellophane.[3,4] Thus, immunoelectrophoretic analysis of plasma from dialyzed patients revealed conversion of both C3 and factor B during the first hour of each dialysis, and simple incubation of human plasma with cellophane from a dialyzer caused identical complement activation. Moreover, infusions of cellophane-exposed, autologous plasma into rabbits confirmed the role of complement in causing sudden decrements in circulating granulocytes and monocytes and provided histologic evidence of associated pulmonary-vessel engorgement with these cells.

Patients, particularly those with antecedent cardiopulmonary dysfunction, are also prone to acute cardiopulmonary decompensation during induction of hemodialysis; dyspnea, congestive cardiac failure, cardiac arrhythmias, angina pectoris and frank myocardial infarction have been documented.[5] Such complications are generally attributed to inadequate volume replacement, or to excessively rapid induction of blood flow into the dialyzer.[5] We performed the present studies in patients, rabbits and sheep to evaluate instead the possibility that the acute cardiopulmonary complications of hemodialysis resulted from complement-mediated, pulmonary-vessel leukostasis, respiratory dysfunction and associated arterial hypoxemia.

METHODS

Patient Studies

We studied patients 18 to 65 years of age with diverse congenital and acquired renal diseases, undergoing routine hemodialysis with single-use, disposable, parallel-plate cuprophane equipment (Gambro Lundia, Gambro Incorporated, Northbrook, Illinois). Dialyzer circuits were primed with isotonic saline (200 to 300 ml). Circulatory access was achieved with Quinton–Scribner[6] or Buselmeier[7] shunts, or arteriovenous fistulas,[8] and heparin anticoagulation induced within the dialyzer circuit.[9] Automated blood cell counts (Coulter Model S, Coulter Electronics, Hialeah, Florida) and 200-cell leukocyte differential counts were performed upon blood drawn from the arterial line, proximal to the dialyzer and the site of heparin infusion. Arterial gas and pH determinations were made upon samples drawn from the same site into cold, heparinized plastic syringes; such assays accurately reflect levels in femoral-artery blood.[10] Arterial oxygen (Pa_{O_2}) and carbon dioxide (Pa_{CO_2}) tensions and pH were assayed with a pH/blood gas analyzer (Model 213, Instrument Laboratories, Lexington, Massachusetts) and oxygen saturation, hemoglobin concentration and carboxyhemoglobin in a co-oximeter (Model 182, Instrument Laboratories). Alveolo-arterial oxygen-tension differences were calculated from simultaneous values for arterial and carbon dioxide tensions with the standard formulas.[11]

From the Hematology and Pulmonary sections, Department of Medicine, University of Minnesota, Minneapolis, and the Pulmonary Section, Department of Medicine, Vanderbilt University, Nashville, TN (address reprint requests to Dr. Craddock at the Department of Medicine, Box 480, Mayo Memorial Bldg., University of Minnesota, Minneapolis, MN 55455).

Supported by grants (CA 15627, HL 18210, HL 13714, AM 15730 and HL 19725) from the U.S. Public Health Service and by grants from the Minnesota Medical Foundation, the University of Minnesota Graduate School and the Parker B. Francis Foundation (Dr. Brigham is an established investigator of the American Heart Association).

Figure 2.32. Complement and leukocyte-mediated pulmonary dysfunction in hemodialysis. *A 1977 article by Craddock* et al. *(Reproduced with permission from* New England Journal of Medicine.*)*

not directly related to cardiac surgery, provided an important clue to the aetiology of the damaging effects of cardiopulmonary bypass. Recognition of complement activation and pulmonary white cell sequestration during haemodialysis provided vital evidence that the same sequence of events might follow the interaction of blood with the foreign surfaces of the pump oxygenator. This study again highlights the importance of laboratory investigation in elucidating complex pathophysiological processes. It appeared in the literature at a time when Kirklin and Blackstone were taking a further look at the morbidity of cardiopulmonary bypass in infants at the University of Alabama at Birmingham.

James Karl Kirklin (1947–)

JAMES KARL KIRKLIN was born in Rochester, Minnesota and attended Ohio State University (1965–69) and Harvard Medical School (MD, 1973). His internship, residency (1974–77) and chief residency in cardiothoracic surgery (1978) were fulfilled at Massachusetts General Hospital. He was Chief Resident in Cardiothoracic Surgery at the Children's Hospital, Boston (1979) and Cardiothoracic Resident at the University of Alabama School of Medicine (1979–81). Kirklin has been Director of Cardiac Transplantation since 1986 and Professor of Surgery since 1987 at the University of Alabama School of Medicine.

James' father, John Kirklin, had a long-standing interest in the damaging effects of cardiopulmonary bypass, particularly relating to morbidity and mortality in infancy. In 1989, he wrote "We know today as we did then that Dick Varco was in part correct. And today, in my opinion, the damaging effects of cardiopulmonary bypass, generated particularly by the oxygenator continue to be the limiting factor in our ability to have nearly a 100% survivorship after open heart operation." The discovery of complement activation and pulmonary white cell sequestration during renal dialysis presented an important clue to the aetiology of the 'post-perfusion syndrome'. This was characterized by pulmonary dysfunction, abnormal bleeding and renal failure in patients who had otherwise undergone an uncomplicated operation. Kirklin's chief resident, Bob Stewart (now at the Cleveland Clinic) worked with Dennis Chenoweth of the Scripps Institute and demonstrated complement activation during cardiopulmonary bypass.

In 1981, James Kirklin was Chief Resident in Cardiac Surgery at the University of Alabama. Stephen Westaby was a cardiac surgical research fellow (from the Royal Postgraduate Medical School in London). Together they worked both in the laboratory and in the clinical setting on the relationship between complement anaphylatoxin release and clinical events. With Eugene Blackstone's formidable analytic methods it was possible to correlate complement activation with morbidity, a process which led to the concept of 'whole body inflammatory reaction', initiated by contact of blood with foreign surfaces

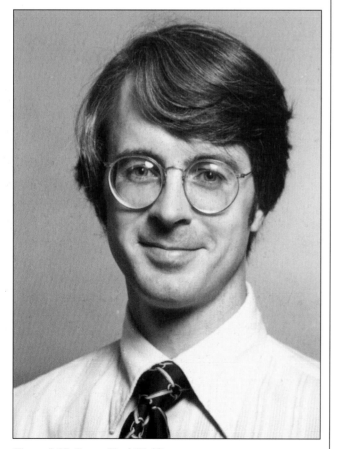

Figure 2.33. James Karl Kirklin.

J Thorac Cardiovasc Surg 86:845-857, 1983

Complement and the damaging effects of cardiopulmonary bypass

Postoperative cardiac, pulmonary, renal and coagulation dysfunction, along with C3a levels, were studied prospectively in 116 consecutive patients undergoing open cardiac operations and 12 patients undergoing closed operations in the same time period. The level of C3a 3 hours after open operation was high (median value 882 ng · ml⁻¹ plasma) and was related to the C3a level before cardiopulmonary bypass (CPB) (p = 0.03), the level at the end of CPB (p < 0.0001), elapsed time of CPB (p = 0.07), and older age at operation (p < 0.0001). It was inversely related to the cardiac output as reflected by the strength of the pedal pulses (p = 0.006). In contrast, C3a levels did not rise in patients undergoing closed operations. The probability of postoperative cardiac dysfunction after open operations (present in 27 of 116 patients) was predicted by C3a levels 3 hours after operation (p = 0.02), the CPB time (p = 0.02), and younger age (p < 0.0001). The same risk factors pertained for postoperative pulmonary dysfunction (present in 41 of the 116 patients); renal dysfunction (present in 24 of the 116 patients) except that CPB time was not a risk factor here; abnormal bleeding (present in 21 of the 116 patients); and important overall morbidity (present in 26 of 116 patients). As regards important overall morbidity, the C3a level effect became evident at about 1,900 ng · ml⁻¹ (a level reached by 9% of patients); the effect of increasing time of CPB became evident at about 90 minutes of CPB time; and the effect of young age became evident as age decreased from 10 to 4 years. This study demonstrates the damaging effects of CPB, relates them in part to complement activation by the foreign surfaces encountered by the blood, and supports the hypothesis that the mechanisms of the damaging effects include a whole-body inflammatory reaction.

James K. Kirklin, M.D. (by invitation), Stephen Westaby, F.R.C.S.* (by invitation), Eugene H. Blackstone, M.D. (by invitation), John W. Kirklin, M.D., Dennis E. Chenoweth, M.D. (by invitation), and Albert D. Pacifico, M.D., *Birmingham, Ala., and San Diego, Calif.*

Cardiopulmonary bypass (CPB) with maintenance of the circulation by a pump oxygenator has become an established modality for support of the patient during cardiac operations. However, whether or not damage to the patient results from its use and, if so, the mechanisms underlying the damage, remain contentious.

Changes in plasma proteins, including those of the coagulation system, have been shown to result from the contact of blood with foreign surfaces, including blood-gas interfaces, during CPB.[1-4] Complement levels fall,[5] and the complement degradation products C3a and C5a are elaborated during CPB.[6] C3a and C5a have physiological effects similar to those observed in many patients after CPB, including vasoconstriction and increased capillary permeability.[7,8] Previous work from this institution has evolved the hypothesis that a whole-body inflammatory reaction of variable magnitude develops as a result of CPB and that a transient damaging effect results.[9]

This clinical study was undertaken to investigate further the possibility that CPB has a damaging effect and that certain phenomena, including complement activation on the foreign surfaces of the pump oxygenator, may be related to its magnitude.

From the Department of Surgery, School of Medicine and Medical Center, University of Alabama in Birmingham; the Alabama Congenital Heart Disease Diagnosis and Treatment Center; and the Department of Pathology, University of California School of Medicine, San Diego, Calif.

Supported in part by Research Grant No. HL27440, National Heart, Lung and Blood Institute, U.S. Public Health Service.

Read at the Sixty-third Annual Meeting of The American Association for Thoracic Surgery, Atlanta, Ga., April 25-27, 1983.

Address for reprints: James K. Kirklin, M.D., Department of Surgery, University of Alabama School of Medicine and Medical Center, Birmingham, Ala. 35294.

*Current address: Royal Postgraduate Medical School, Hammersmith Hospital, London, England.

845

Figure 2.34. Complement and damaging effects of cardiopulmonary bypass. *A 1983 article by Kirklin et al. (Reproduced with permission from* Journal of Thoracic and Cardiovascular Surgery.*)*

(Article 2.6, Appendix A). The work had important clinical relevance as some materials in the circuit, such as nylon, were found to promote anaphylatoxin release strongly whereas others were inert. As a result, nylon tricot was removed from bubble oxygenators and more biocompatible materials and circuits were developed. The importance of complement activation during interaction between heparin and protamine was also identified.

Stephen Westaby (1948–)

STEPHEN WESTABY grew up in a steel town in Northern England and decided to be a cardiac surgeon at the age of 7 when his parents acquired a television set. This coincided with the development of direct vision intracardiac surgery (1955) which featured prominently in the media both in fact and fiction. From the local grammar school Westaby gained a place at Charing Cross Hospital Medical School (University of London) in 1966. He obtained degrees in Biochemistry (BSc., 1969), Medicine and Surgery (MB.BS., 1972) and captained the Medical School's cricket and rugby teams.

From the beginning, Westaby watched the once weekly heart operation from the operating theatre viewing gallery. The early rotating disc oxygenator was used and most patients died either in the operating room or afterwards from the 'post perfusion syndrome'. In 1972, he won a scholarship to the Albert Einstein Medical College in New York city where his time was divided between cardiac surgery and trauma in the emergency rooms of hospitals in the Bronx and Harlem. On returning to England he was awarded the Medical School prize for the most promising graduate and given internships in the academic departments of medicine and surgery. Still determined to be a cardiac surgeon, his next position was Resident Surgical Officer at the Brompton Hospital (1974) with Mattias Paneth and Christopher Lincoln (two of the best surgical technicians in Britain at that time). He was Oswald Tubbs' last resident and inherited Lord Brock's operating boots recently discarded in an operating theatre cupboard. Cardiac surgery was still difficult in those days and most nights were spent in the intensive care unit increasing the dose of inotropes. With no previous surgical experience, his first median sternotomy (a re-operation) opened the right ventricle.

Training in general surgery was in Cambridge with Roy Calne during the evolution of liver transplantation and discovery of Cyclosporin. Calne, a sporting enthusiast encouraged Westaby to play rugby every Saturday afternoon and this led to a fractured mandible between the written papers and oral examination for the Fellowship of the Royal College of Surgeons. This was generally regarded as a good thing since he could not talk himself out of a pass mark (FRCS, 1977). Whilst waiting for the facio-maxillary surgeon in the Accident Department, a young Cambridge student was admitted with exsanguinating traumatic rupture of the thoracic aorta. With no one else willing to intervene, Westaby wearing rugby kit and covered in mud performed an emergency room thoracotomy whilst spitting his own blood into the sink nearby.

After transferring to cardiac surgery at the Hammersmith Hospital in the latter days of Hugh Bentall and Dennis Melrose, Westaby took a research fellowship at the University of Alabama with John Kirklin (1981). At the time Nicholas Kouchoukos, Robert Karp and Albert Pacifico were all at UAB and the analytical genius, Eugene Blackstone supervised the research projects. James Kirklin and Robert Stewart of the Cleveland Clinic were chief residents and worked with Westaby on Complement activation and the 'damaging effects of cardiopulmonary bypass'. The term 'Whole Body Inflammatory Response' through blood foreign surface interaction was adopted at that time. This was the most stimulating environment in cardiac surgery of that era with inexhaustible clinical and scientific material. Visits to DeBakey, Crawford, and Cooley in Houston and Shumway at Stanford added further perspective and consolidated Westaby's affinity for the American approach.

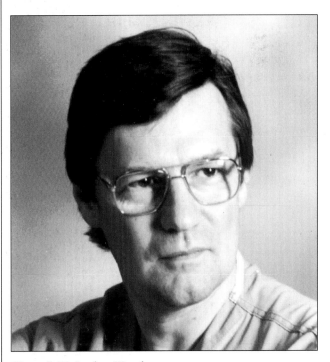

Figure 2.35. Stephen Westaby.

On return to the Hammersmith he pursued the pathophysiology of the 'Whole Body Inflammatory Response' with work on protease enzymes, oxygen free radicals and cytokine release during cardiopulmonary bypass. This work led to a Masters degree and numerous scientific papers (M.S., 1985). Knowledge that the interaction of blood with foreign surfaces activated the Complement and Kallikrein cascades (as well as coagulation and fibrinolysis) stimulated the quest for inhibitors to intervene against the 'Post Perfusion Syndrome'. For 25 years, heparin had been the only agent given during cardiopulmonary bypass. When it was found that intrapulmonary white cell sequestration caused release of the protease enzyme elastase, Westaby suggested that the protease inhibitor aprotinin might be used to prevent increased capillary permeability. At a meeting convened by the Beyer Company (Luxembourg 1982), Westaby met with Charles Wildevuur to discuss the possibility of aprotinin infusion. Their initial objective was to assess the inhibitory action of aprotinin on the Fibrinolytic and Kallikrein systems. The project was established at the Hammersmith Hospital with the technical help of Van Oeveren and Jansen from Groningen (Netherlands) and clinical assistance of Bidstrup (Cardiac Surgeon), and Royston from the Department of anaesthetics. The trial showed that aprotinin inhibited both Kallikrein and plasmin but had little effect on elastase release. However, the most interesting finding was that the surgical field appeared abnormally dry in patients who received aprotinin, so much so that it was readily apparent which patients had received the drug or placebo. This serendipitous finding stimulated enormous interest in the role of aprotinin and led some workers to advocate its use for all patients undergoing cardiopulmonary bypass. The Wildevuur group identified inhibition of fibrinolysis as the primary effect with a protective effect on platelet membrane receptors and adhesive function.

As Senior Registrar at the Hammersmith, Great Ormond Street (Hospital for Sick Children) and Harefield Hospitals, Westaby spent virtually every day in the operating room and operated day or night at every opportunity. As a thoracic surgeon at Harefield he designed the silicone rubber 'Tracheo-Bronchial Stent' for treatment of inoperable major airways obstruction. Harefield covered many district general hospitals for thoracic trauma and extensive operating experience in this area led to two early books entitled, *'Wound Care'* and *'Trauma, Pathogenesis and Treatment'*.

In 1986 at the age of 37, Westaby was appointed Chief of Cardiac Surgery for the new regional unit in Oxford. This presented a unique opportunity for a new direction in cardiac surgery since there were no senior colleagues. At the time Alf Gunning's facilities had been eroded to eight beds on a general surgical ward and there were no dedicated intensive care

Effects of Aprotinin on Hemostatic Mechanisms during Cardiopulmonary Bypass

Willem van Oeveren, M.Sc., Nicolaas J. G. Jansen, M.D., Ben P. Bidstrup, M.D., Dave Royston, M.D., Steven Westaby, M.D., Heinz Neuhof, M.D., Ph.D., and Charles R. H. Wildevuur, M.D., Ph.D.

ABSTRACT Cardiopulmonary bypass (CPB) is associated with activation of humoral systems, which results in the release of proteases. These proteases may affect platelets and stimulate granulocytes. In the present study, the protease inhibitor aprotinin was given in high doses to 11 patients to achieve plasma concentrations of more than 150 kallikrein inactivator units per milliliter during CPB. At such concentrations, kallikrein and plasmin are effectively inhibited. This treatment resulted in platelet preservation during CPB. Platelet numbers were virtually unaffected, and thromboxane release was prevented in the aprotinin-treated group in contrast to the control group. Postoperatively, hemostasis was significantly better preserved after aprotinin treatment (blood loss of 357 ml in the treated group versus 674 ml in the untreated group; $p < 0.01$). Since tissue-plasminogen activator activity was similar in both groups, the improved hemostasis most likely should be attributed to platelet preservation. Furthermore, aprotinin lessened neutrophilic elastase release, which might contribute to decreased pulmonary dysfunction in patients at risk.

The damaging effects of cardiopulmonary bypass (CPB) continue to contribute to the morbidity and mortality of cardiac procedures, particularly in patients at risk. The so-called postperfusion syndrome, comprising fever of noninfective origin, pulmonary and renal dysfunction, leukocytosis, and abnormal bleeding, has recently been interpreted as a "whole-body inflammatory response" possibly initiated by contact of blood with the nonbiological materials of the extracorporeal circuit [1]. The patible polymers of the extracorporeal circuit [2]. Particularly through the activation of the fibrinolytic and complement systems, the generalized inflammatory reaction may also affect platelets and leukocytes, and this result might contribute in a major way to postbypass complications such as impaired hemostasis and pulmonary dysfunction. To identify the importance of the fibrinolytic and complement systems in this regard, patients undergoing CPB were treated with aprotinin, which in high doses inhibits plasmin. The effect of aprotinin was determined by differences in platelet and leukocyte numbers and their release products in treated and nontreated patients. The clinical relevance of platelet preservation was indicated by the hemostatic capacity, expressed as postbypass blood loss and blood requirements.

Material and Methods

Informed consent was obtained from 22 otherwise healthy patients undergoing elective coronary artery bypass grafting. Eleven patients were randomly assigned to aprotinin treatment during CPB; the other 11 served as controls. Aprotinin (Trasylol) was supplied by Bayer AG (West Germany) in bottles containing 50 ml of saline solution without any additives or preservatives, each milliliter containing 10,000 kallikrein inactivator units (KIU).

The study protocol was approved by the ethical committee. The following dosage regimen was used in the treatment group. At the start of anesthesia, an infusion of $2 \cdot 10^6$ KIU (200 ml) was given over a 20- to 30-minute period. Thereafter a continuous infusion of $0.5 \cdot 10^6$ KIU (50 ml) per hour was administered until the end of the operation after the last blood sample had been collected.

Figure 2.36. Effects of aprotinin on hemostatic mechanisms during cardiopulmonory bypass. *A 1987 article by Westaby* et al.

facilities. Most patients were sent to London for surgery. With a small group of dedicated nursing staff, Westaby operated all day every day and no further patients were referred elsewhere. Five months later, after resources for eighteen months had been spent, the cardiac beds and operating theatre were closed and Westaby left to operate in Saudi Arabia. When the 'political smoke' cleared six weeks later he took over a second operating room and made plans for the Oxford Heart Centre.

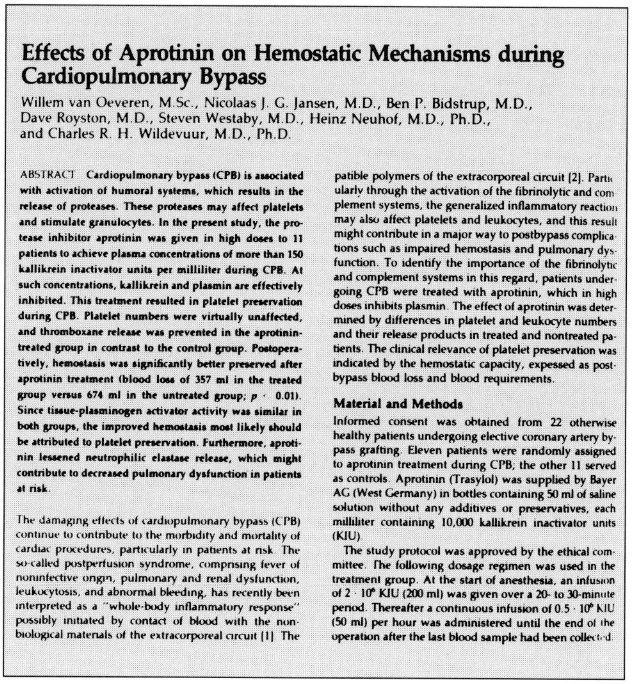

When lack of intensive care beds became an important limiting factor (1992), Westaby withdrew cardiac surgery from the intensive care unit and established a small cardiac recovery area within the operating suite. Anaesthetic and perfusion techniques were modified to allow six patients per day to pass through three recovery beds. 'Fast Track Surgery' began in this unit where patients operated in the morning returned to the surgical floor in the afternoon. Rapid recovery prompted early discharge from hospital on the fifth or sixth post operative day. The 'Fast Track' approach reduced the cost of a coronary bypass to £4,000. With progressive economic constraints in Europe and the United States the 'Cardiac Surgery Without Intensive Care' approach caused great interest and attracted many overseas visitors. The activity rate grew rapidly with a comprehensive paediatric programme and an expanding thoracic aortic practice. Within ten years of Westaby's arrival at Oxford the surgical volume expanded from 100 to 1800 patients per year.

1994 provided a new challenge when Westaby met Robert

Jarvik who showed him the prototype of the Jarvik 2000 axial flow impeller pump. Oxford had been frustrated by the difficulties of having patients accepted onto a transplant list and particularly by seeing children die whilst waiting. Westaby persuaded Jarvik to establish a research programme in Oxford and contribute to the development of a centre for mechanical circulatory support. By this time Frazier and others had demonstrated the potential for myocardial recovery after prolonged mechanical left ventricular unloading. Progress in the lab with the Jarvik 2000 and the excellent results of bridge to transplantation with the pneumatic Thermo Cardio Systems LVAD in the United States led to permanent TCI electric LVAD implants in Oxford for patients not eligible for transplantation. To overcome the risk of driveline infections during long term use Jarvik and the Oxford team developed an electric system which included a carbon button screwed to the outer table of the skull based on artificial hearing technology. The current aspiration is that a combination of prolonged left ventricular offloading perhaps with surgical ventricular remodelling at the time of LVAD explant will provide a preferable alternative to transplantation particularly for children.

Westaby has produced 6 books (including 'Stentless Bioprosthesis' and 'Surgery of Acquired Aortic Valve Disease' with Armand Pinwica and 'Atlas of Surgery for Ischaemic Heart Disease' with Brian Buxton and Bud Frazier) together with more than 150 scientific papers.

Chapter 3: The palliation and correction of congenital heart defects

IN 1672, Stensen described the anatomical features of what is now termed tetralogy of Fallot. By the 18th century, many congenital malformations had been described, mostly as isolated events. For instance, William Hunter (1784) described the combination of ventricular septal defect with pulmonary stenosis. In 1861, Henri Louis Roger described the characteristic murmur and thrill (*bruit de Roger*) of ventricular septal defect. In 1866, Thomas Peacock adopted a systematic classification of congenital defects in his textbook. Soon afterwards, in 1888, a more comprehensive account of cyanotic congenital heart disease appeared, by Etienne Louis Fallot. He described the tetralogy of ventricular septal defect, pulmonary outflow tract or valvular obstruction, aortic override on the ventricular septal defect, together with right ventricular hypertrophy. Although Fallot's description of the tetralogy was by no means unique, his account illustrated the mechanism of cyanosis by right-to-left shunting. In 1897, Victor Eisenmenger described ventricular septal defect with cyanosis but without right ventricular outflow obstruction. The term 'Eisenmenger's syndrome' was adopted to describe several different kinds of venoarterial shunt in the presence of pulmonary hypertension.

Measurement of pulmonary arterial and intracardiac pressures was achieved by Auguste Chauveau, a veterinarian, and Etienne-Jules Marey. They modified instruments initially designed by Ludwig and employed air-filled manometers, introduced via the jugular veins of a horse, to record right-sided cardiac pressures. They introduced a second tube through the carotid artery into the left ventricle and recorded systolic pressures in both ventricles.

Maude Abbot (Figure 3.1) made a comprehensive study of congenital anomalies of the heart whilst curator of the McGill University Museum. In 1908, she published a monograph concerning 412 specimens, and in 1936 she published the comprehensive *Atlas of Congenital Heart Disease*, with critical analysis of more than 1000 cases. She was responsible for a unique understanding of congenital cardiac defects that eventually stimulated the development of surgery in this area. Helen Taussig, the cardiologist, was a friend of Abbot. In 1932, she assumed responsibility for a cardiac clinic in Baltimore and worked closely with cyanotic children. In 1935, she recorded the clinical features of the hypoplastic right ventricle and noticed that when the ductus arteriosus closed soon after birth in cyanotic infants, they quickly died. Acyanotic children with congenital abnormalities often developed cyanosis after duct closure. These were the observations which would later stimulate development of the systemic pulmonary arterial (Blalock–Taussig) shunt, to increase pulmonary bloodflow and oxygen saturation in patients with

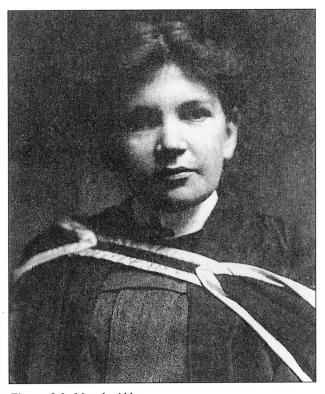

Figure 3.1. Maude Abbot.

cyanotic congenital heart disease. The first direct attack on congenital pulmonary stenosis was made by Doyen in a 20-year-old woman with heart failure. He devised a special tenotome, which was introduced through the right ventricle and blindly cut into the obstruction. The procedure was doomed to fail because of unfavourable anatomy, which included a large ventricular septal defect.

Early attempts at diagnosis and palliation

JOHN MUNRO, Professor of Surgery at Tuft's Medical School and visiting surgeon at Boston City Hospital, described ligating a persistent ductus in the cadaver of a newborn child in *Annals of Surgery* (1907). No patient was referred to him, though he tried to inspire the paediatric specialists with his views. When Elliott Cutler examined a 22-year-old woman on the verge of heart failure from patent ductus at the University of Minnesota in 1935, Wangensteen tried to persuade him to ligate the ductus; Cutler agreed, but the patient refused. Then, Ashton Graybiel, a physician at Massachusetts Memorial Hospital in Boston, persuaded John Streider, a thoracic surgeon, to develop a suitable operation. Like Munro, Streider had previously dissected cadavers.

In March 1937, an extremely sick 22-year-old woman presented in Boston with *Streptococcus viridans* bacterial endocarditis on a patent ductus arteriosus. At the time, it was generally understood that congenital cardiac anomalies were more susceptible to bacterial endocarditis than normal hearts. Streider reasoned that if the ductus could be closed, the infection might resolve. Certainly, in pre-penicillin times, recovery was unlikely and medical management had little to offer. Endotracheal intubation and positive pressure ventilation had only recently been described in the UK by the anaesthetists McGill and Rowbotham, and the principles of surgery with an open chest were barely established. Streider nevertheless decided to attempt surgical duct closure, and partially achieved this with a series of plicating sutures. The patient died on the 5th postoperative day from acute dilatation of the stomach. Eighteen months later, Robert Edward Gross successfully ligated a ductus in a 7-year-old girl. There was no infection on this occasion and the procedure was both uneventful and successful. As a result, elective closure of the patent ductus arteriosus was

widely adopted to prevent both bacterial infection and pulmonary hypertension. Oswald Tubbs of St Bartholomews and the Brompton Hospitals in London was the first to cure infective endocarditis on a ductus by surgical ligation.

Figure 3.2 shows the first cardiac operation in Japan in 1951. Professor Shigeru Sakakibara performed ligation of ductus arteriosus on the daughter of a Taiwanese millionaire at Tokyo Womens Medical College (Figure 3.3). Sakakibara was assisted by his elder brother, Tohru, to whom the patient had been referred. Recalling the operation Sakakibara said "we took 2000 years for just 3 cm to the heart".

At this time, diagnostic techniques were restricted. Forssmann had achieved cardiac self-catheterization using a ureteric catheter through an arm vein in 1929, but it was not until 1938 that George Robb and Israel Steinberg of New York City developed a practical method to visualize the heart and great vessels in

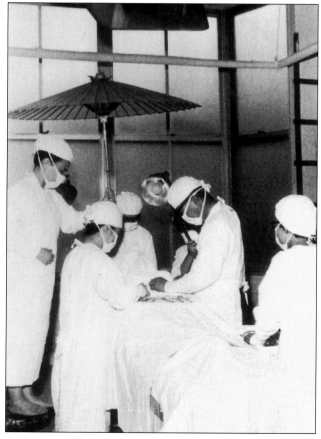

Figure 3.2. The first Japanese cardiac operation carried out in 1951 at Tokyo Womens Medical College. The operating room ceiling was in poor repair at the time. (Courtesy of Professor H. Koyanagi.)

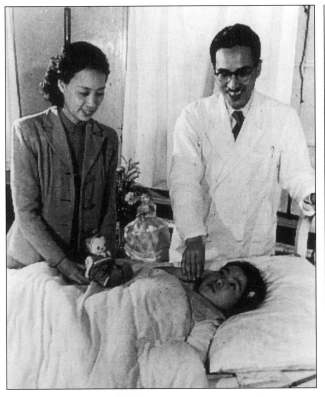

Figure 3.3. Professor Shigeru Sakakibara and the patient at the Tokyo Women's Medical College.

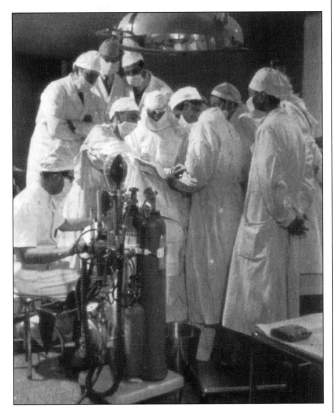

Figure 3.4. Ake Senning and Clarence Crafoord operating in 1949 at the Karolinska Institute.

humans. Their technique involved the injection of between 20 and 40 ml of iodine-based contrast into the patient's arm, with radiography 3–5 seconds later. The method exposed the human heart to radiological examination, and in 1941, André Cournand and Hilmert Riches catheterized the right heart to obtain samples for blood gas analysis.

As early as March 1938, Gross and Hufnagel planned to excise aortic coarctation and reconnect the cut ends by end-to-end anastomosis using a new aortic clamp and continuous mattress suture. Clarence Crafoord, who had visited Gross and Hufnagel in the Harvard Research Laboratory, beat Gross to the first reported correction of aortic coarctation. In Sweden, on 19 October 1944, assisted by Gustav Nylin, he excised a coarctation of the aorta and joined the cut ends together. The first patient was a 12-year-old boy and the second, 12 days later, was a 27-year-old farmer.

Gross, who had spent about 7 years working out a technique and was close to clinical implementation, maintained, although he seldom articulated it, that Crafoord learned the end-to-end anastomosis technique in his laboratory. Crafoord's manuscript was received by *Journal of Thoracic Surgery* on 1 June 1945 and sent to Gross for peer review (Figure 3.5). Reading it precipitated Gross's own first correction in a 5-year-old boy on 28 June 1945, when he was joined by Hufnagel. After he excised the coarctation, rejoined the aorta and

---

CONGENITAL COARCTATION OF THE AORTA AND ITS
SURGICAL TREATMENT

CLARENCE CRAFOORD, M.D.,* AND G. NYLIN, M.D.†
STOCKHOLM, SWEDEN

IN EXPERIMENTAL studies on dogs in 1935-1936, one of us (C. C.) demonstrated that the flow of blood to all the organs could remain suspended for as long as twenty to twenty-five minutes without there being any subsequent signs of organic damage, provided an adequate flow to the brain was secured. This circulation to the brain was maintained by creating anastomoses between the carotid and jugular vessels on one side in the animal under operation with the corresponding vessels in a dog of the same size lying beside it. On the strength of this observation Crafoord, in certain patients with a patent ductus arteriosus, took the risk of placing clamp forceps on the aorta above and below the point of entry of the duct into this artery and of keeping them attached during the time necessary to divide the duct and suture the aorta. In one of the patients this part of the operation took no less than twenty-seven minutes to perform. In spite of this long period during which the aorta was shut off just below the point where the subclavian artery arises, no noticeable disturbances were subsequently observed in the patient's internal organs.

While performing this type of operation on other patients with a patent ductus arteriosus, Crafoord began to wonder whether it might not also be possible to treat congenital coarctation of the aortic isthmus by surgical means.

Figure 3.5. Title page of Congenital coarctation of the aorta and its surgical treatment. *A 1945 article by Crafoord and Nylin. (Reproduced with permission from* Journal of Thoracic Surgery.)

removed the aortic clamps, the heart stopped beating. Despite cardiac resuscitation the child died. Attributing the failure to too rapid release of the aortic cross-clamps, he tried again on 6 July 1945. This time, he took a full 10 minutes to withdraw the clamps from a 12-year-old girl with a coarctation completely obstructing the upper thoracic aorta; 19 days later she was discharged from the hospital in excellent health. This was the first correction of coarctation in the United States.

At this time there were no arterial substitutes, and for the eventuality that the resected ends could not be easily approximated, Alfred Blalock and Edward Park, at the Johns Hopkins, developed the method of coarctation bypass (1944). This operation, in which the divided left subclavian artery was turned down and anastomosed to the distal end of the aorta, below the coarctation, was first performed clinically by Claggett at the Mayo Clinic (1947). The patient was a 34-year-old man with a coarctation close to the origin of the left subclavian artery. Claggett considered excision with end-to-end anastomosis as unlikely to succeed. He therefore ligated the coarctation, dissected the dilated left subclavian artery, and anastomosed it end-to-end with the small descending thoracic aorta. Other surgeons, such as Gordon Murray, adopted this method electively for coarctation bypass and noted that the blood supply to the left arm was rarely compromised. The development of transient or permanent paralysis of the backlegs in 4 out of 10 of Blalock's experimental animals caused him to delay performing this operation until after Crafoord and Gross' successes in 1945. They reported that extensive collateral circulation in cases of coarctation allowed cross-clamping, resection of the coarctation and end-to-end anastomosis with impunity.

Following perfection of arterial anastomosis for which he was awarded the Nobel Prize in 1912, Alexis Carrel demonstrated that either an artery or a vein, from the same or another animal, could substitute for a damaged artery with routine success. In 1948, Gross and Hufnagel similarly used segments of aorta from cadavers to bridge otherwise unresectable lengths of hypoplastic aorta. Gross first employed homograft aortic replacement on 24 May 1948 for coarctation in a 7-year-old boy who made an uneventful recovery. Fear of paralysis was lessened when John Alexander and Francis Byron ligated the thoracic aorta with a thoracic aneurysm and probable coarctation with no paralysis

(1944). End-to-end aortic anastomosis was performed by Shumacher during the first successful aortic aneurysm resection with restoration of arterial continuity in 1947. Shumacher's patient was an 8-year-old boy with a thoracic aortic coarctation and an aneurysm of 4 cm.

By 1950 Gross had performed 130 corrections of coarctation with 12 deaths. He used an aortic homograft in 16 cases, but calcification in one graft after 1 year diminished his enthusiasm. During the next few years surgical correction of aortic coarctation was performed in many centres throughout the world with excellent results. This was a critically important period in aortic surgery, as surgeons began to realize their ability to clamp and suture the aorta without adverse effects. In the 1950s there was an explosion in the knowledge and clinical application of surgery of the arteries. A number of young American surgeons performed immediate repair of injured arteries with remarkable success during the Korean war, and markedly reduced the incidence of leg amputation.

Blalock and Taussig

IN PARALLEL with the operations for coarctation of the aorta, were the first attempts to palliate cyanotic congenital heart disease. In 1943, after a surgical conference at the Johns Hopkins Hospital, Taussig asked Blalock whether he had any thoughts about surgical correction of pulmonary stenosis in children. Blalock described his experimental work involving mobilization of the left subclavian artery for coarctation repair. From this it was apparent that anastomosis of the subclavian artery to the pulmonary artery might provide the means for additional pulmonary bloodflow to relieve cyanosis. At the same time, Blalock had a young patient with tetralogy of Fallot who was deteriorating. On feeding, the child became deeply cyanosed and often lost consciousness.

On 29 November 1944, at the Halstead Clinic, Blalock performed the first subclavian to pulmonary artery anastomosis (Figure 3.6). William Longmire (Chief Resident at the time) was first assistant and Denton Cooley, a 24-year-old junior resident, administered fluids. Blalock's experienced technician, Vivien Thomas (Figure 3.7), who had pioneered the procedure in the laboratory, stood by while Merel

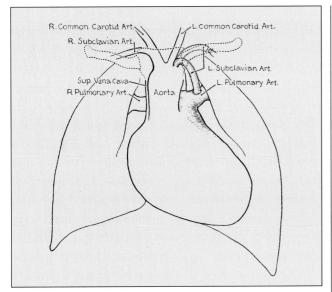

Figure 3.6. Blalock's subclavian to pulmonary artery anastomosis.(Reproduced with permission from Blalock A, Taussig HB. The surgical treatment of malformations of the heart in which there is pulmonary stenosis or pulmonary atresia. Journal of the American Medical Association 1948; 128: 189–202.)

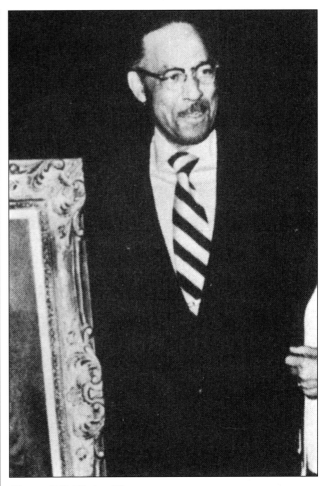

Figure 3.7. Vivien Thomas.

Harmel administered the anaesthetic of ether and oxygen. Taussig watched the operation from the head of the table, as Blalock used bulldog clamps to occlude the pulmonary artery. The anastomosis was performed with some difficulty, using china beaded silk and fine needles (Blalock was not a gifted technician). On removal of the clamps, the child's colour immediately improved. The postoperative course was stormy, but the child survived with excellent symptomatic relief.

Blalock gave Taussig credit for her participation in the first clinical report, though Taussig went as far as to suggest that she had devised the procedure. She published several articles on follow-up studies without acknowledging Blalock. In a letter to Willis Potts which addressed this controversy, Blalock wrote,

> *"I must say that if I make a statement to you that you could improve the condition of patients with aortic stenosis should you be able to find a means to allow more blood to reach the body, I would be far from solving the practical problem."*

Blalock and Taussig remained at loggerheads and Cooley was appointed house officer to the Cardiac Service with

a specific brief to liaise between surgery and cardiology. He was soon promoted to first assistant.

Following the first few 'blue baby' operations, Blalock and Taussig were invited to tour Europe to demonstrate the procedure. Blalock was accompanied by Henry Bahnson, a junior resident, as Cooley was in Italy on war service. Russell Brock invited Blalock to operate at Guy's Hospital, where the shunt procedure was performed successfully on 10 children with tetralogy of Fallot. Taussig and Blalock presented their experience in the Great Hall of the British Medical Association. At the conclusion of Blalock's lecture, the hall remained dark after the projection of slides, when suddenly a long searchlight beam traversed the length of the hall. The spotlight fell on a Guy's nursing sister, dressed in blue uniform and holding a small but vivacious, blonde, curly haired 2-year-old girl with tetralogy, now pink after surgery at Guy's 1 week before. The effect was theatrical and dramatic and provoked tumultuous applause from the audience. The tour probably changed the course of cardiac surgery in Europe and was soon to be reinforced by the cardiotomy procedures of Dwight Harken for war wounds in 1946 and the mitral valvotomy of Charles Bailey in 1947.

As a modification of the shunt procedure, Potts performed direct anastomosis between the descending aorta and left pulmonary artery using a partial occluding clamp (Figure 3.8). His first operation was on 13 September 1946 on a 21-month-old girl. Within 2 weeks, Potts had operated again on an 11-year-old girl who died the following day and an 8-year-old girl who survived and did well. Nevertheless, the Blalock and Potts shunts gradually gave way to direct closed interventions for pulmonary outflow and valvular obstruction.

Brock and Holmes-Sellors

BROCK performed detailed studies of hearts with right ventricular outflow obstruction in the postmortem room. Observing the occasional pinhole orifice of the pulmonary valve with secondary muscular hypertrophy, he considered a direct surgical attack on the obstruction as the procedure of choice. Brock designed a valvulotome for this purpose and initially elected for retrograde insertion via the left pulmonary artery. When attempts to pass a cardioscope from this direction failed (which

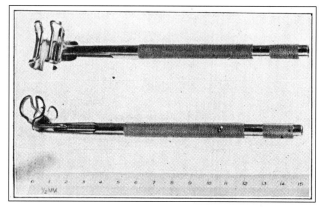

Figure 3.8. Potts' occluding clamp used for anastomosis of the aorta to a pulminary artery. (Reproduced with permission from Potts WJ, Smith S, Gibson S. Anastomosis of the aorta to a pulmonary artery: certain types of congenital heart disease. Journal of the American Medical Association 1946; 132: 627–31.)

contributed to the death of a 17-year-old patient after a Blalock anastomosis), he resorted to a transventricular approach. At the first operation, on 16 February 1948, he was able to pass a curved valvulotome effortlessly into the pulmonary artery of an 18-year-old girl. Further operations were performed on two other patients and both were technical successes. Brock published in the *British Medical Journal* during the summer of 1948 (Figure 3.9), and 2 weeks later a separate manuscript from Thomas Holmes-Sellors of the Middlesex Hospital appeared in the *Lancet*. It is likely that Holmes-Sellors performed the first successful pulmonary valvotomy. His 20-year-old male patient had advanced tuberculosis of both lungs and the typical features of tetralogy of Fallot. Holmes-Sellors originally planned to perform a shunt on the left side but encountered dense tuberculous adhesions. He therefore opened the pericardium and passed a long tenotomy knife through the right ventricular wall until it engaged the stenosed pulmonary valve. Making cuts in two directions, the pulmonary stenosis was relieved and the patient survived for 9 years before dying from tuberculosis.

Before cardiac catheterization and angiography, it was difficult to distinguish between the membrane type of pulmonary valve stenosis (with or without secondary hypertrophy) and the infundibular narrowing of tetralogy of Fallot. For infundibular stenosis, Brock designed a blunt-nosed punch which could be passed through an incision in the right ventricle to core out the obstructing muscle. He used this instrument successfully in 1949 and introduced it to the United States on an exchange visit to Johns Hopkins.

Just as Blalock had profoundly impressed the surgeons of Europe, Brock's impact in Baltimore was no less dramatic. He arrived at Johns Hopkins whilst Blalock and his staff were presenting patients to a clinical staff meeting of the Medical School. Brock appeared in the rear of the auditorium wearing a grey top coat, Homburg hat and carrying his own suitcase. Blalock introduced him to the audience and invited him to examine the patient under consideration. Brock put down his suitcase and, without removing hat or coat, stepped on the stage, took a stethoscope from his pocket, examined the child and his X-ray and stated, "Coarctation of the aorta, surgical correction advised." It was on this visit that Brock invited Cooley to be visiting chief resident at the Brompton Hospital.

BRITISH MEDICAL JOURNAL

LONDON SATURDAY JUNE 12 1948

PULMONARY VALVULOTOMY FOR THE RELIEF OF CONGENITAL PULMONARY STENOSIS

REPORT OF THREE CASES

BY

R. C. BROCK, M.S., F.R.C.S.

Surgeon to Guy's Hospital

The surgery of the heart may be said to have begun in 1896 when Rehn (1897) first successfully sutured a wound of the heart. Until a short time before this a semi-mystical, mediaeval attitude prevailed in relation to the heart, which was generally thought to be untouchable surgically. Thus even as late as 1883 Billroth declared that the surgeon who attempted to suture a wound of the heart would lose the respect of his colleagues. Rehn's epoch-making operation demonstrated conclusively that the heart of man was, in some measure at any rate, tolerant of interference. Surgeons were quick to profit by this lesson, so that within ten years Rehn was able to collect reports from the literature of 124 cases of a wound of the heart treated by suture.

The early promise of the development of direct cardiac

The most sustained effort to solve the problem of relief of valvular stenosis by direct attack on the valves was made by Cutler and his associates (Cutler and Beck, 1929); they used a tenotome in their first three cases and a cardio-valvulotome in four others. Their first patient survived four and a half years and was thought to have been improved; six other patients died soon after operation, as also did single cases reported by Allen and Graham (1922) and Pribram (1926).

These early efforts were succeeded by a long period of inaction, and in the minds of many these operations of a quarter of a century ago seem to have proved that direct surgical attack on the diseased valves of the heart is too dangerous to be practicable.

Figure 3.9. Title page of Pulmonary valvulotomy for the relief of congenital pulmonary stenosis, *the 1948 article by Lord Brock. (Reproduced with permission from* British Medical Journal.)

A different approach to right ventricular outflow tract obstruction had been considered by Tuffier and Carrell 40 years previously. They stitched a venous patch on the outside of the pulmonary outflow of a dog and, with a pair of scissors inserted beneath the patch, they divided the valve ring so that the pulmonary valve fell open. This produced an additional 1 cm circumference in the outflow tract. In 1950, Hufnagel in Boston carried out similar experiments in dogs, this time using patches of aorta, superior vena cava, or the animals' own pericardium. The only difference in technique was that Hufnagel used a stainless steel suture to 'cheesewire' through the outflow tract. This was inserted before suturing the patch over the area for section. This technique was translated into clinical practice by John Kirklin in 1952. Operating on a 17-year-old girl, he passed a stainless steel wire through the anterior wall of the right ventricle, negotiated the infundibular obstruction and brought it out again through the wall below the pulmonary valve. He then oversewed the wire on the outside of the heart by plicating the muscle and sewing the edges together. Under the tunnel so created, he used the wire to cut through the obstructed infundibulum and achieved both haemodynamic and symptomatic improvement.

In 1955, Davidson reported the first central aortopulmonary shunt by direct suture, and in 1962, Waterston performed the ascending aorta to right pulmonary artery anastomosis, an important alternative to the Blalock–Taussig and Potts operations. Klinner

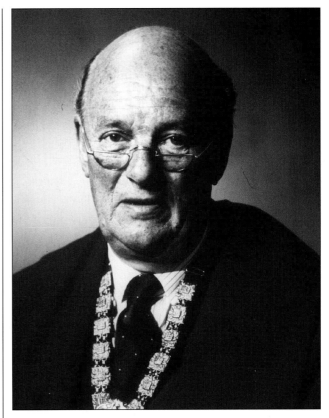

Figure 3.10. Holmes-Sellors.

(1962) was the first to use a prosthetic conduit between the subclavian and pulmonary arteries. Whereas relief of intracardiac obstruction became a reality with closed methods, the possibility for blind closure of atrial or ventricular defects proved more difficult.

Correction of atrial septal defects by closed methods

PRIOR to direct vision intracardiac repair, many innovative techniques were suggested for closure of atrial septal defects. Cohen produced atrial septal defects in dogs and repaired them by suturing the inverted right atrial appendage onto the defect. A wire snare was first passed into the right atrium and the appendage was inverted against the septal defect through the snare. One suture was placed at each quadrant of the defect and mattress sutures positioned on the outside of the atrium, in preparation for reconstitution of the free wall. With the inverted appendage attached to the septal defect, the snare was used to amputate this from within and the mattress sutures tied to close the defect. Although this method worked experimentally, no attempt was made to use it on patients.

Murray (1948) carried out anterior–posterior suturing of the atrium along the line of the septum, using external landmarks for guidance. However, while anterior–posterior plication could reduce the size of the defect, it was doubtful whether it ever completely closed the hole. A restudy of one patient by Keith and Forsythe showed a considerable residual left–right shunt. Henry Swan (1950) reported the method of double invagination of both atrial appendages against the septal defect. He used plastic buttons and approximating sutures of silk in an attempt to promote adherence of the inverted and opposed appendages to each other around the edges of the septum. The method was first applied in a patient in October 1949 and then in five others. With large septal defects, however, the appendages did not adhere to the septum and failed to close the hole.

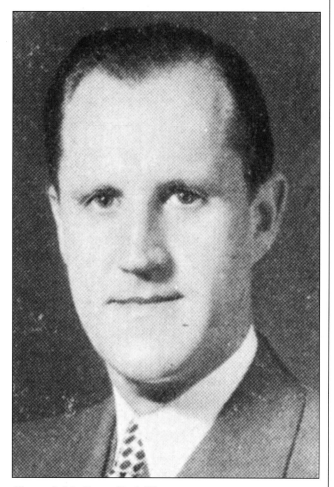

Figure 3.11. Forest Dodrill

In 1949, Forest Dodrill (Figure 3.11) designed a method whereby metal rings on an ice-tong type of mechanism approximated left and right atrial walls against the interatrial septum. The excluded part of the atrial free wall was then opened to expose the septal defect, which was sutured directly. Dodrill also suggested that very large interatrial septal defects might be covered or bridged by suturing the left atrial free wall to the periphery of the opening. This method was attempted clinically, but with limited success. Hufnagel and Guillespie (1951) devised an ingenious method to close experimentally produced septal defects in dogs using male and female plastic buttons. These could be screwed together from the outside to occlude the defect mechanically. The method was never used in a human patient, probably because the technique would not leave a large enough atrium after the operation.

Other experimental methods were never adopted clinically. Kiriluk used an invaginated plug of epicardial fat surrounded by pericardium to close experimental defects. Donald reported the use of polyvinyl sponge covered by a pericardial sac to close a defect. Although these methods were recognized as unsuitable for patients, the surgeons considered that they might prove useful after closure of persistent ostium primum-type defects, when the defect was reduced in size but not completely obliterated.

In January 1952, Bailey performed what is believed to be the first complete closure of an atrial septal defect. His operation, referred to as 'atrioseptopexy', was performed on a 38-year-old woman with a 4 cm secundum-type defect. The procedure again consisted of invaginating a portion of the redundant, dilated right atrial wall against the defect. The invaginated atrial wall was then sutured to the periphery of the hole using multiple interlocking mattress sutures. This was accomplished by inserting an ungloved left index finger through an incision in the tip of the right atrial appendage. Atrioseptopexy was adopted clinically and applied to primum-type defects as well as the fossa ovalis variety.

Gross (1953) described an ingenious method of repair using a 'latex well' sutured to the right atrial wall (Figure 3.12). When the wall was incised, the patient's venous pressure caused the blood to rise by 10–12 cm within the well, and local heparinization was thought sufficient to prevent thrombosis. The atrium was explored with a finger to locate the septal defect and directly suture the

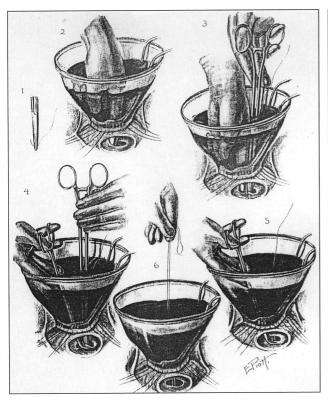

Figure 3.12. Gross' atrial repair technique employing a latex well.(Reproduced with permission from Gross RE, Watkins E, Pommeranz AA, Goldsmith EI. A method for surgical closure of interauricular septal defects. Surgery, Gynecology and Obstetrics 1953; 96: 1–23.)

edges together. In patients with larger defects, it was even possible to use a patch of polythene sheeting to bridge the defect. Gross also used atrioseptopexy, considering that the well technique excluded the use of redundant atrial wall to close the hole. At this time, Shumacher modified atrioseptopexy by enlarging the right atrium with a pouch of pericardium. The increased expanse of atrial wall facilitated suture to the edges of the septal defect. Pericardium soon proved unsatisfactory and nylon fabric was used in its place.

In the early 1950s, Søndergaard developed a method whereby a heavy silk suture was passed through the upper portion of the interventricular septum, from the anterior aspect of the heart to the posterior. The suture emerged posteriorly on the interatrial groove. The groove was then deepened by dissection and the suture passed along it, turning anteriorly just to the left of the superior vena cava. When the circumferential suture was tied down, the region of the septum was obliterated by a

pursestring action. This greatly reduced the size of the interatrial communication and shunt. Husfeldt subsequently reported four complete closures out of 10 cases, with four others symptomatically improved. Björk and Crafoord modified the method by checking the degree of closure with a finger within the right atrium.

The first attempts at open heart surgery

ON 29 AUGUST 1952, Cookson, Neptune and Bailey used surface-induced hypothermia at 34°C, together with temporary vena caval occlusion to close an ostium primum defect in a 32-year-old woman. This defect had been digitally explored at a previous operation, and the technique of atrioseptopexy considered inappropriate. Although the hole was closed, the patient suffered coronary air embolism and fatal ventricular fibrillation. On 2 September 1952, Lewis and Taufic successfully performed closure of an atrial septal defect using hypothermia, inflow occlusion and direct vision in a 5-year-old child. Swan followed this lead with three survivors out of four patients.

On 6 May 1953, 3 weeks after Swan's first successful case, Gibbon used his heart–lung apparatus to perform closure of an atrial septal defect in an 18-year-old girl. Bailey's textbook *Surgery of the Heart*, published in 1955, contained the following statement:

"Numerous proposed methods and actual surgical attempts give one some idea of the creative thought and energy which has been expended in trying to provide a suitable method for correcting atrial septal defects. However, it would seem to be time for clarification of our ideas and the requirements which the situation demands. First, at the present time, the use of various lung machines in human cases, in the leading clinics throughout the world, usually in an attempt at repair of atrial septal defects (with complete vena caval obstruction), has been attended by only a few operative survivals in some 40 or 50 attempts. While this method offers brilliant prospects, ultimately, it would seem to the author that its general applicability for cardiac surgery lies further in the future than we like to hope. Furthermore, it is doubtful that it will even then be as

safe or as significantly more satisfactory than our present-day closed cardiac surgical methods for the correction of a good many conditions, including interatrial septal defects. In other words, it is felt that the inherent danger of air embolism occurring during the surgery of intra-atrial septal defects when open techniques are used, and the difficulties encountered in re-establishing adequate cardiac function after completely stopping the heart for this purpose, will cause the majority of surgeons to continue to prefer the closed techniques for this purpose, even after the heart–lung apparatus becomes fully perfected. Practically all of the foregoing remarks are equally applicable against the use of hypothermia with complete vena caval obstruction as adjuncts in the correction of interatrial septal defects. In addition, one must then contend with the present effects of cold upon myocardial irritability and contractility."

Bailey went on to say that any surgical technique adopted for closure of an atrial septal defect should be simple, and not involve elaborate equipment or manoeuvres that require an experienced or specially trained surgical team. Bailey thought that the number of patients with atrial septal defects worldwide did not justify the development of specialized operating teams. He considered that his operation of atrioseptopexy was both suitable and desirable for practically every type of atrial septal defect, with the exception of complete atrioventricular canal defects. Bailey considered the operation inappropriate for infants below the age of 1 year, and in persistent ostium primum defects where there was no true inferior rim to the defect. He recognized that direct closure in these patients would cause distortion of the aortic valve and severe aortic insufficiency. The bundle of His was also in danger.

By 1954, Lewis and co-workers had performed surgical correction of atrial septal defects in 11 patients by the hypothermia and inflow occlusion method. Two patients died during the operation; in a third, the heart fibrillated during cooling and the surgery was abandoned after defibrillation. Other deaths occurred from bleeding and heart block.

Surgery for ventricular septal defect

ON 13 MARCH 1953, Bailey attempted direct suture of a ventricular septal defect using hypothermia and vena caval occlusion. The defect may have been completely closed, but it was soon clear that it had reopened. Bailey attributed this failure to the sutures having cut out of the soft muscular septum. He considered that the continuous and vigorous systolic impulse of the left ventricle essentially precluded direct closure of ventricular septal defects. The Hufnagel type of button prosthesis was then considered, but again, lack of a defined upper edge to the defect seemed disadvantageous. It was also apparent that the circular button might impinge on the aortic cusps. Bailey proposed that Hufnagel's buttons might be modified to provide a circular element for the right ventricular outflow side, and an elongated transverse band for the left ventricular aspect. A transversely elongated button was considered unlikely to encroach on the aortic valve cusps.

Bailey himself found an ingenious method to plug a small-to-medium-sized defect. The operation was first performed on 6 February 1951. An autogenous pericardial tube was inserted through the free wall of the left ventricle, into the septal defect and out of the free wall of the right ventricle. The pericardial tube was thought to swell to fill the hole. Between 7 and 14 days after operation, the oedema would disappear and the pericardial tube would shrink; at this time it was firmly welded to the septal edge, rendering the seal permanent. Bailey realized that if the right ventricular outflow tract was narrow, or the aorta had an extreme overriding position, serious left or right ventricular outflow tract obstruction might be produced. Several patients were operated on in this way; but, without direct vision, opportunities for successful surgery were limited.

Pulmonary artery banding

A simpler approach was to balance the circulation by reducing the large left-to-right shunt. On 29 March 1950, Bailey performed a pulmonary valvotomy on a 17-year-old girl with tetralogy of Fallot. The cyanosis disappeared immediately, but she promptly developed gross left–right shunting. This led to cardiac hypertrophy and chronic congestive heart failure, manifested by hepatomegaly, right-sided pleural effusion, ascites and peripheral oedema. On 21 June 1950, almost 3 months later, an attempt was made to reduce the left–right shunt by applying a Satinsky clamp to occlude two-thirds of the lumen of the pulmonary artery. The excluded portion of the arterial wall was excised and the free edges oversewn to permanently reduce the arterial lumen. Bailey noted that partial occlusion of the pulmonary artery caused the systemic blood pressure to rise by 20 mmHg; on removal of the clamp the pressure fell again. This first pulmonary artery banding was initially successful, but the patient died from hepatitis 3 weeks later. Nevertheless, it was recognized that the right ventricle could sustain the burden of increased afterload for an indefinite period.

Ventricular septal defect was the first congenital anomaly to be corrected routinely by open methods before the development of the pump oxygenator. In 1954, Lillehei, Varco and Warden began to repair ventricular septal defects at the University of Minnesota, using normothermic low-flow pump controlled cross-circulation between adult and infant, with the adult donor used as the oxygenator. The performance of the Lillehei team was extraordinary, both in surgical skill and daring. Right ventriculotomies were performed on the beating heart without aortic cross-clamping. The ventricular septal defects were identified and closed by direct suture in a field partially obscured by blood. Remarkably, heart block was avoided in most patients, a situation which led Lillehei to state,

"These observations would seem to deny the classical concept that the conduction system of the human or canine heart (atrioventricular node and bundle of His) is concentrated in a small localized discrete locus which is thereby very vulnerable to mechanical injury."

Only two of the first 10 patients died and both were less than 12 months of age. Lillehei appreciated the importance of the conducting system, as heart block at this time was invariably fatal. This stimulated him to work on the development of the pacemaker. The location of the conduction tissue in hearts with ventricular septal defect was described by Truex and amplified by Maurice Lev. Lev's extensive studies formed the basis on which guidelines to avoid surgical heart block were formulated in many congenital anomalies.

The very first operation to employ a pump oxygenator (Dennis and Varco, 1952) unexpectedly encountered an atrioventricular canal defect. The surgeons anticipated closure of a fossa ovalis defect, but the patient died and autopsy showed the true diagnosis to be partial atrioventricular canal. Remarkably, in 1954, Kirklin successfully repaired a partial atrioventricular canal defect using the atrial well technique of Gross. The following year, the same team at the Mayo Clinic began to repair atrioventricular canal defects by open cardiotomy using the pump oxygenator. Although Abbot in her *Atlas of Cardiac Defects* (1936) had recognized the difference between an ostium primum atrial septal defect and a complete atrioventricular canal, Rogers and Edwards (1948) pointed out that they were morphologically similar. The terms 'partial' and 'complete atrioventricular canal' were introduced by Wakai and Edwards (1956), and soon afterwards, Lev described the position of atrioventricular node and conducting bundles for these conditions.

In 1956, Kirklin reported 20 patients with ventricular septal defect who had undergone direct vision intracardiac repair with the mechanical pump oxygenator and normothermic perfusion rates of 70 ml/kg/minute. Only four of these patients died. Soon afterwards in 1957, Lillehei demonstrated the feasibility of the transatrial approach to ventricular septal defect using cardiopulmonary bypass.

Atrioventricular canal defects

LILLEHEI was the first to achieve successful repair of complete atrioventricular canal defect using parenteral cross-circulation in 1954. The atrial rim of the septal defect was sutured directly to the crest of the ventricular septum. Remarkably, the patient avoided complete heart block, a condition associated with high hospital mortality at that time. In the early repairs, residual left atrioventricular valve regurgitation and left ventricular outflow tract obstruction also caused substantial morbidity. Many of the early operations employed a separate patch for the ventricular and atrial septal defects. In 1962, Maloney described the use of a single patch from which the valve tissue could be suspended. A similar method was also used by Gerbode the same year. Dubost and Blondeau showed that the cleft anterior mitral leaflet need not be repaired to obtain left atrioventricular valve competence in partial canal defects. These improvements in technique, together with Lev's description of the location of the bundle of His, provided the basis for safer repair of atrioventricular valve defects. In 1966, Rastelli and Kirklin, at the Mayo Clinic, further characterized the distribution of valve leaflet tissue with definitions that were accepted for many years. The basic defect in these malformations was recognized to be absence of the atrioventricular septum due to an embryological endocardial cushion defect. Dwight McGoon emphasized the importance of committing leaflet tissue preferentially to the left atrioventricular valve orifice, and more recently, Carpentier suggested that the left atrioventricular valve functions best when repaired as a three-leaflet structure.

Transposition of the great arteries

EVEN BEFORE the advent of open cardiac surgery, complicated problems such as transposition of the great arteries were palliated surgically. Blalock's initial approach to transposition began with animal experiments. It was impossible to create transposition experimentally, but working with Rollins Hanlon, Blalock anastomosed the pulmonary veins to the superior vena cava in one set of dogs and the pulmonary veins to the right atrium in another. The plan was to next transpose the great vessels and see whether the previous operation brought sufficient oxygenated blood to the aorta in its new position. The anastomosis between the pulmonary veins and superior vena cava remained patent in more than three-quarters of their dogs and Blalock considered this type of anastomosis to be feasible for human patients. He therefore conceived the operation of redirecting venous return whilst leaving the transposed arteries alone.

In 1950, Blalock and Hanlon reported on a variety of procedures for palliation of transposition in 33 children aged between 8 days and 8 years. In each case, the preoperative diagnosis had been made non-invasively by Taussig. In the first nine children, they performed an extracardiac anastomosis, such as pulmonary veins to vena cava or pulmonary artery to vena cava. Some of these children also had their subclavian artery anastomosed end-to-end to the right pulmonary artery. This last procedure proved universally fatal. In another group of children, Blalock made use of the observation that children with septal defects had a better prognosis than those with some other form of compensatory anomaly, such as patent ductus. In 12 children, he created an atrial septal defect, but only three survived and without great symptomatic improvement. In a third group of 12 children, an anastomosis was made between the subclavian and pulmonary arteries as well as an artificial atrial septal defect. Eight of these children survived and Blalock considered them to be symptomatically improved.

In another remarkable series of operations, William Mustard of Toronto used a monkey lung as a biological oxygenator to facilitate surgery on babies with transposition. The first operation took place on 17 January 1952 on a 3-month-old girl, and by November of the same year, Mustard had operated on seven babies. Attacking the transposed vessels directly, he divided the pulmonary artery about half an inch beyond the valve and then cut the aorta obliquely, leaving the right coronary artery on the proximal stump, but taking the left coronary artery so that it was moved with the aorta. This was possible, as the left coronary artery was conveniently close to the original pulmonary artery. After dividing the aorta, Mustard perfused the left coronary artery with oxygenated blood pending reanastomosis. None of the infants lived for more then a few hours. On 10 November 1952, Bailey performed a switchover anastomosis in a 7-month-old boy, who also died postoperatively.

Lillehei realized that the obstacle to anatomical correction of transposition was the origin of the coronary arteries, so he decided to switch the veins instead. Beginning in March 1952, he anastomosed the right pulmonary veins to the right atrium in four babies, and two survived. Because of the venous imbalance created by this procedure, he decided to perform a second anastomosis between the inferior vena cava and the left atrium. However, the first anastomosis between the right pulmonary veins and right atrium often proved fatal before the second anastomosis could be undertaken. To counteract this, Lillehei inserted a temporary shunt between the superior vena cava and the left atrium, which could be opened as soon as the first anastomosis was complete. In 1955, he reported a series of 32 infants, seven of whom survived between 15 and 36 months after operation. By this time, Lillehei had already achieved intracardiac closure of ventricular septal defects using his cross-circulation technique.

In 1954, Björk used arterial grafts obtained from stillborn births to join the aorta to the pulmonary artery.

He then divided the two arteries and stitched the cut ends, so that all the blood flowed through the grafts in the correct direction. Björk considered this method to be suitable only when the pulmonary artery pressure was elevated. In 1955, Earle Kay and Frederick Cross of Cleveland joined the right pulmonary artery to the aorta, then the pulmonary conus to the arch of the aorta just beyond the innominate artery. They finally bridged the gap between the left pulmonary artery and aorta with a homologous arterial graft. On completion of the anastomoses, the result resembled normal anatomy except that the coronary arteries still came off the pulmonary arteries. Kay and Cross considered transposing the coronaries, but decided against it and all three infants died.

In transposition of the great arteries the idea that transposing the systemic and pulmonary venous return

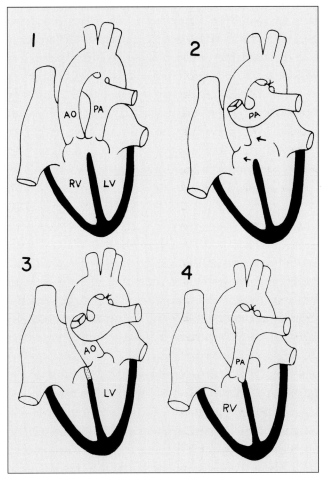

Figure 3.13. Senning's transposition of the great arteries. (Reproduced with permission from Senning Å. Surgical correction of transposition of the great vessels. Surgery 1959; 45; 966–80.)

to the heart would restore the normal arrangement of the two circulatory systems gained widespread clinical acceptance. In 1955, Senning attempted an arterial switch procedure in which the aorta and pulmonary artery were transected just above the aortic and pulmonary valves respectively, and transposed, moving both the coronary arteries *en bloc* with the aorta (Figure 3.13). This correction of supracardiac total anomalous venous return was unsuccessful and was abandoned.

Thomas Baffes, working with Potts in Chicago, persisted with the venous option and essentially adopted the Lillehei operation. Instead of direct anastomoses, however, he used aortic homografts to join the inferior vena cava to the left atrium and the right pulmonary vein to the right atrium. The amount of blood carried in these channels was essentially balanced and his first patient, a girl of 3.5 years, survived surgery and began to walk for the first time in her life. Within a year he had operated on 38 patients with 19 survivors, all of whom were symptomatically improved. Remarkably, all of these operations were performed without cardiopulmonary bypass. Although Baffes contemplated a second stage to join the superior vena cava and left pulmonary veins, this was never performed clinically. Baffes' original procedure remained the treatment of choice for transposition over the next 10 years.

The first operations to employ extracorporeal circulation were by Kay and Cross in 1956, who changed from their arterial operation to venous transposition within the atria. Unfortunately, none of their patients survived. On 20 March 1957, Alvin Merendino, at the University of Washington School of Medicine, used extracorporeal circulation and elective cardiac arrest to completely excise the interatrial septum and insert a plastic baffle to reroute the venous return of a 6-year-old girl. The object was to direct bloodflow entering via the pulmonary veins into the right atrium, and similarly the flow from the vena cava and coronary sinus into the left atrium. The prolonged first operation failed when the girl's heart went into irreversible ventricular fibrillation. A second 6-year-old girl died from cerebral embolus, but the procedure created interest and a potential solution for transposition at atrial level.

Senning (1957) reconstructed the atrial walls in such a way that flaps of autogenous tissue created venous and arterial pathways (the Senning repair). This allowed redirection of caval blood to the pulmonary artery and pulmonary venous drainage to the aorta. Kirklin adopted this ingenious technique at the Mayo Clinic and by 1961 had operated (using extracorporeal circulation and profound hypothermia) on 11 infants, with four survivors. In 1961, Christiaan Barnard also succeeded with the Merendino operation on a 16-year-old boy.

The next great advance came from Toronto, when Mustard was forced to re-operate on an 18-month-old girl who had previously undergone a Blalock–Hanlon septectomy. On 16 May 1963, using cardiopulmonary bypass, Mustard first repaired a small ventricular septal defect and then excised the entire interatrial septum. Using autogenous pericardium, he then fashioned a flap-like baffle that divided the atria into separate, functionally correct chambers. The girl made an uncomplicated recovery, was no longer cyanosed and developed normally. In 1966, Mustard presented four patients, all with full arterial oxygen saturation and normal venous pressures. The Mustard and Senning procedures subsequently remained the treatment of choice in transposition until the development of the arterial switch operation by Jatene and then Yacoub. This operation provided complete correction of the problem during the first few months of life.

Right ventricular outflow obstruction

AFTER Blalock's description of the subclavian–pulmonary artery anastomosis, other methods for systemic to pulmonary artery anastomosis were introduced by Potts, Smith and Gibson (1964) and Waterston (1962). Holmes-Sellors and Brock both described direct relief of pulmonary stenosis by closed methods in 1948. Although Russell Brock's account of the operation which bears his name appeared 2 weeks before Holmes-Sellors' (*Lancet*, 26 June 1948), Holmes-Sellors first performed the procedure at Middlesex Hospital on 4 December 1947.

Brock was convinced through post-mortem examinations that the valve in tetralogy of Fallot could be opened surgically. Brock conceived the idea of a retrograde approach to the valve during the course of pneumonectomy. He intended to look at the valve by a cardioscope inserted through the left pulmonary artery. Encouraged by his observations he decided to proceed

and in May 1947, the cardioscope was used in a 17-year-old man. However, the valve appeared normal and a shunt was performed instead. The patient died as did the next one, whose pulmonary artery was so small that the cardioscope could not be introduced. A third patient died from irreversible cardiac arrest as the scope was introduced. Brock then decided to introduce the cardioscope through the anterior wall of the right ventricle but, in fact, on 16 February 1948, he found it easier to perform a transventricular valvotomy with a curved valvulotome of his own construction. The operation became known as the Brock procedure. Both Holmes-Sellors and Brock recognized the importance of a direct attack upon narrowed valves both in congenital and acquired cardiac disease. Although their hospitals were only 3 miles apart it appears that neither was aware of the other's efforts. Brock went on almost immediately to design a punch for excision of infundibular muscle in tetralogy and this was used successfully in four patients in 1949. Brock's clinical experience demonstrated that even a severely underdeveloped pulmonary outflow tract could be restored to full growth by a successful direct operation.

The Brock–Holmes-Sellors technique was adopted by other pioneers including Blalock, Potts, Kirklin and Lillehei. The right ventricular approach was used almost universally via left anterolateral thoracotomy until 1952, when Shumacher called attention to the 'complete sternal splitting incision' (median sternotomy) which provided excellent exposure and required less dislocation of the heart.

In 1951, Charles Hufnagel of Georgetown University developed an experimental technique whereby a wire was passed into the pulmonary artery, manipulated through the pulmonary valve into the ventricular cavity and brought out through the right ventricular free wall. The pulmonary trunk and right ventricular outflow were then covered with a homograft patch, sutured into place. The wire was then used to cut through the free wall of the pulmonary artery, valve and right ventricular outflow tract. As the wire was withdrawn, the last sutures on the outflow patch were tied with little or no blood loss and the lumen of the outflow tract greatly increased in size. John Kirklin employed this method at the Mayo Clinic in 1953 when a transventricular valvotomy failed to improve the condition of a young female patient. Using the wire in the manner of a Gigli saw, the right ventricular outflow tract was incised and opened. In

October 1952, Dodrill successfully treated a patient with congenital pulmonary stenosis by an open procedure using a pump bypass circuit without oxygenator to bypass the right ventricle.

In 1957, Björk described a direct open operation on the pulmonary valve using normothermic venous inflow occlusion, considering that the operation itself could be performed safely in 2 minutes. Nevertheless, most surgeons preferred to follow Swan's approach and employ hypothermia to increase the safe inflow occlusion time. Soon afterwards the heart–lung machine came into general use and greatly facilitated intracardiac operations of increased duration.

The first open repair of tetralogy of Fallot was achieved by Lillehei and Varco, at the University of Minnesota (1954), using controlled cross-circulation. In the following year, at the Mayo Clinic, Kirklin performed the first successful repair using the pump oxygenator. Lillehei, Warden and colleagues then introduced patch enlargement of the right ventricular infundibulum and Kirklin employed transannular patching (1959) for the hypoplastic valve ring and main pulmonary artery. Kirklin also used a right ventricle to pulmonary artery conduit for tetralogy of Fallot with pulmonary atresia (1965); Donald Ross subsequently used a valved homograft for this purpose (1966). Whereas correction of tetralogy in older children was achieved with relatively low operative mortality, primary repair in infancy carried substantial risk, predominantly due to the damaging effects of cardiopulmonary bypass. This stimulated the use of a two-stage approach: firstly, a Blalock shunt; then open, total correction at a later stage. It was Barratt-Boyes, at Green Lane Hospital, New Zealand, who first pursued the policy of routine primary repair in infancy with satisfactory results (1969).

Pulmonary valve stenosis with intact ventricular septum was initially treated by closed valvotomy, notably by Holmes-Sellors, Brock and then Blalock, who reported 19 patients with two hospital deaths using the Brock method (1950). Swan first performed an open pulmonary valvotomy in 1952, using moderate hypothermia by surface cooling. Inflow occlusion was used to provide a bloodless approach to the valve via pulmonary arteriotomy. Kirklin's early experience at the Mayo Clinic soon led to an appreciation of the importance of right ventricular outflow obstruction through secondary hypertrophy. This could only be relieved adequately by

open operation with cardiopulmonary bypass.

Pulmonary atresia with intact ventricular septum was a still more difficult problem. John Hunter is accredited with the first description of this condition in 1783. The premature infant died on the 13th day of life and Hunter described the right ventricle as having "scarcely any cavity with a tricuspid valve" which was "especially small". The size of the right ventricular cavity was soon recognized to be an important limiting factor. In 1955, Greswold, working with Edwards, proposed pulmonary valvotomy for infants whose right ventricle was of adequate size. The same group advised an initial aortopulmonary shunt for those in whom the right ventricle was too small. Successful total correction was achieved at the University of Minnesota, the Mayo Clinic and Henry Ford Hospital, Detroit, all in 1961.

Tricuspid atresia

TRICUSPID atresia was described with both concordant ventriculoarterial connections, and in association with transposition of the great arteries by Kuhne in 1860. The clinical features were described by Bellet in 1933 and by Taussig in 1936. Cyanotic children were palliated by Blalock, Potts or Waterson shunts and in 1958, the superior vena caval–right pulmonary artery anastomosis was applied specifically to tricuspid atresia by Glenn (Figures 3.14 and 3.15). This followed comprehensive, independent, experimental work by Cowlon (1951), Glenn (1958) and Robicesk (1956), who clearly showed that systemic venous pressure was adequate to drive blood through the pulmonary circulation in patients without pulmonary hypertension. The potential for complete cavopulmonary anastomosis was demonstrated experimentally by Isaac Starr and colleagues (1943), who showed that destruction of a dog's right ventricle could be survived without systemic venous hypertension. In 1954, Warden, DeWall and Varco showed the feasibility of bypassing the right ventricle by right atrial to pulmonary artery anastomosis. Hurwitt and associates first attempted clinical correction of tricuspid atresia by right atrial to pulmonary artery anastomosis in 1955, but the patient died.

It was not until 1968 that complete separation of the right and left circulations was achieved in tricuspid atresia by François Fontan. He performed cavopulmonary

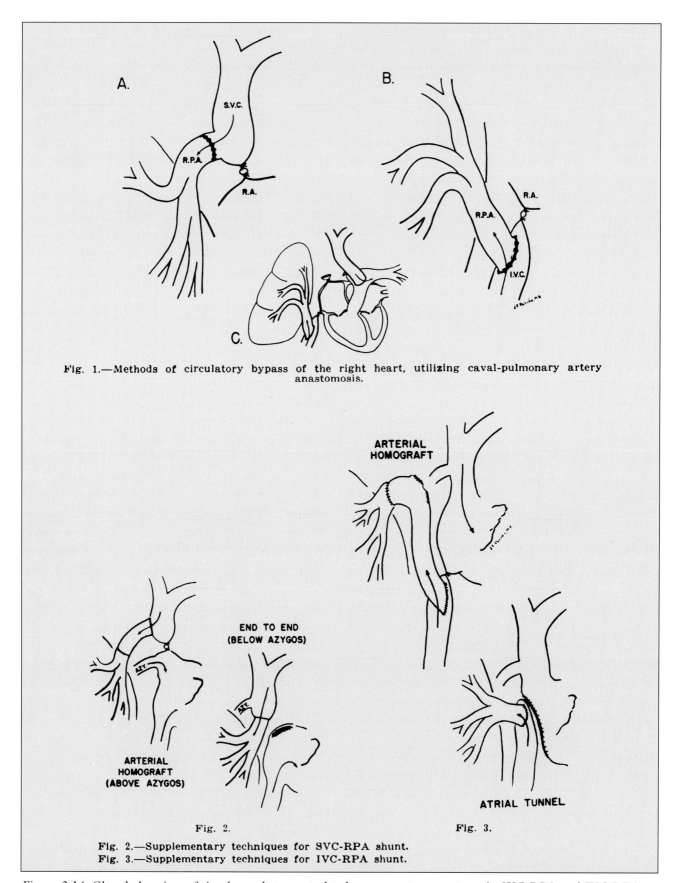

Fig. 1.—Methods of circulatory bypass of the right heart, utilizing caval-pulmonary artery anastomosis.

Fig. 2.

Fig. 2.—Supplementary techniques for SVC-RPA shunt.
Fig. 3.—Supplementary techniques for IVC-RPA shunt.

Figure 3.14. Glenn's drawings of circulatory bypass: caval-pulmonary artery anastomosis, SVC-RPA and IVC-RPA.

connection through direct anastomosis between the right atrial appendage and the divided main pulmonary artery. In his second and third patients, Fontan inserted a valved aortic homograft between the right atrium and pulmonary artery. All three patients received an aortic homograft valve in the inferior vena caval orifice, together with closure of the patent foramen ovale or atrial septal defect. The proximal end of the main pulmonary artery was oversewn. The Fontan operation has since been modified on numerous occasions.

Kreutzer (1973) dislocated the patient's main pulmonary artery with the valve intact and anastomosed the pulmonary root to the right atrial appendage. Björk described direct anastomosis between the right atrial appendage and right ventricular outflow tract for patients with an outflow chamber and normal pulmonary valve (1979). These methods did not require a Glenn anastomosis.

The bidirectional Glenn anastomosis has recently been resurrected as an excellent first-stage procedure for those who will eventually require their circulation to be based on a single ventricle. Total cavopulmonary anastomosis can then be achieved at a second stage by disconnecting the main pulmonary artery and anastomosing the right atrium to the right pulmonary artery, as described by De Leval.

Congenital aortic stenosis

THE PROBLEM of congenital aortic stenosis has been recognized by cardiac morphologists for many years. In 1910, Alexis Carrell attempted experimentally to place a conduit between the left ventricular apex and aorta to relieve this problem. In 1955, Marquis and associates used dilators introduced through the apex of the left ventricle to treat infants with congenital aortic stenosis. The first valvotomies performed by Swan and Lewis in 1956 under discrete vision employed inflow occlusion and moderate hypothermia through surface cooling. The same year, Kirklin used cardiopulmonary bypass (unpublished), though his method was first reported by Frank Spencer and colleagues in 1958. Discrete subvalvular aortic stenosis was discussed in *Guy's Hospital Reports* by Chevers in 1842. Diagnosis during life, together with characterization of the subvalvular lesion (as opposed to valvar aortic stenosis), was described by Brock, who employed transventricular puncture to measure differential pressures in the left ventricle. Brock then used closed transventricular dilatation, with only moderate success. Spencer published the first substantial report and described excision of the discrete subvalvular ring under direct vision using cardiopulmonary bypass

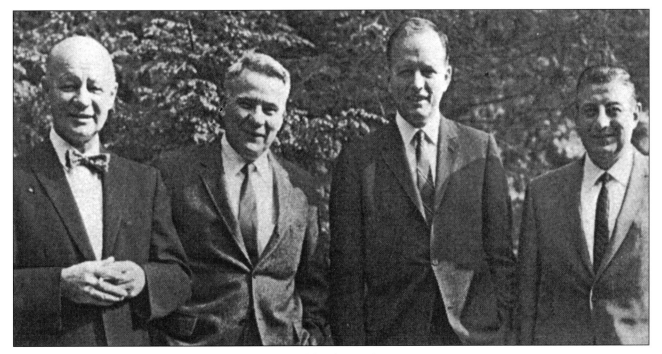

Figure 3.15. Photo of Glenn, Mustard, Cooley and Rashkind in 1968.

(1960). The long fibrous tunnel form of subaortic stenosis was also described by Spencer in 1960. Treatment of the 'funnel-type' defect was achieved by aortoventriculoplasty, an operation described independently by both Rastan and Konno (Figures 3.16 and 3.17) in 1975. The apical left ventriculo-aortic valved conduit was described by Cooley in the same year and adopted for otherwise inoperable left ventricular outflow obstruction.

Supravalvular aortic stenosis was recognized by Mancarelli in 1930, but the condition could not be differentiated from aortic valve stenosis until the development of retrograde arterial catheterization. In 1961, the Green Lane Hospital group, described the association of supravalvar aortic stenosis with "elfin faces and mental retardation". Multiple peripheral pulmonary artery stenoses were also documented in this condition, as was severe infantile hypocalcaemia, described by Black and Bonham Carter (1963). Patch graft enlargement of the non-coronary sinus of Valsalva was used by Kirklin at the Mayo Clinic in 1956 to correct the supravalvar stenosis.

For infants and children with aortic regurgitation due to ventricular septal defects, George Trusler at the Children's Hospital Toronto described valve repair by resuspension of the prolapsing cusp. (Figure 3.18.)

Truncus arteriosus

TRUNCUS arteriosus was recognized by Wilson in 1798 and described accurately by Buchanan in an autopsy of a 6-month-old infant in 1864. The condition continued to be confused with single arterial trunk in either aortic or pulmonary atresia, until Lev proposed the morphological criteria in 1942. In 1949, Collett and Edwards reviewed previously reported cases and established a classification. Van Praagh presented an alternative classification in 1965. At first, surgery was restricted to banding of the main or branch pulmonary arteries. Intracardiac repair, with separation of the systemic and pulmonary circulations, was achieved at the University of Michigan (1962), and this first patient was reported alive 11 years later. In 1966, Ross used an aortic

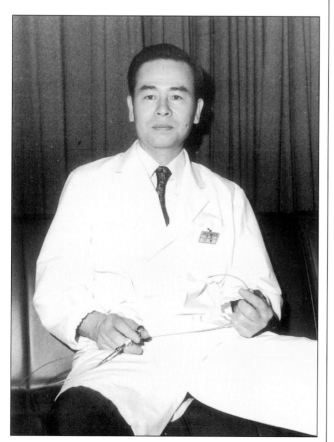

Figure 3.16 Konno holding his cardiac biotome.

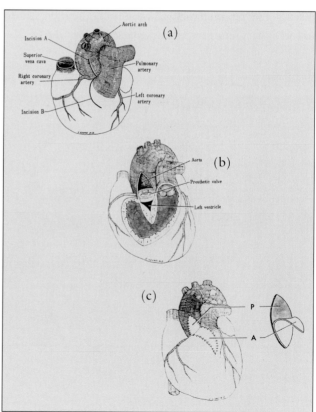

Figure 3.17 Konno's valve replacement operation in congenital aortic stenosis.

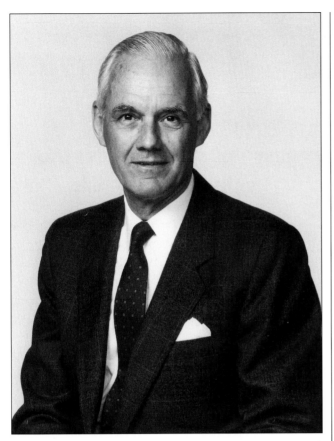

Figure 3.18. George Trusler of Toronto Children's Hospital.

homograft conduit to reconstruct tetralogy of Fallot with pulmonary atresia. The following year, Rastelli and McGoon adopted the homograft conduit for truncus arteriosus repair. Apparently, Barratt-Boyes had attempted the same method unsuccessfully several months before. Others, such as Binet in France and Barratt-Boyes, utilized heterograft (porcine) valves sewn into Dacron tubes (1971).

Total anomalous pulmonary venous drainage

TOTAL anomalous pulmonary venous drainage was recognized by Wilson in 1798. The first attempted surgical correction was by Muller, at the University of California Medical Centre, Los Angeles, in 1951. Without cardiopulmonary bypass, he anastomosed the common pulmonary venous sinus to the left atrial appendage. The first successful open repair was achieved using surface cooling, moderate hypothermia and temporary venous inflow occlusion, by Lewis and Varco (University of Minnesota, 1956). The same year, Kirklin performed three successful operations using the pump oxygenator, and also described a remarkable early repair using the atrial well technique.

Conclusion

SURGICAL correction of congenital heart disease has now reached an advanced level of sophistication thanks to major contributions from Brom, Buckley, Castanada, Danielsen, Ebert, Stark, Pacifico, Lincoln, Subramanian, Arciniegas and others. Second generation pioneers such as Norwood, Turley, Doty, Laks, Quaegebeur, Mee and Bove continue to refine operative techniques and reduce mortality. Outcome in many complex anomalies has been improved by the detailed anatomical studies of cardiac morphologists such as Lev, Van Praagh, Anderson, Becker, Allwork and Bharati. It remains to be seen whether detailed intrauterine ultrasound will allow prenatal intervention or termination of more complex anomalies in the future.

Biographies

Robert Edward Gross (1905–1988)

ROBERT EDWARD GROSS was born in Baltimore, Maryland, USA, seventh of eight children. Mechanically-gifted, he dismantled the engine of the family car at the age of 12. When his father found the pieces strewn around the garage floor, he ordered his son to put the engine together before morning, which he did. Later, Gross kept a tool chest in his operating room, painted gold by his nurses and residents, which he used between operations to fix an overhead light, an autoclave or squeaking door. Gross was offered a scholarship in chemistry to the University of Wisconsin after a BA (1927) from Carleton College, Minnesota. However, Harvey Cushing's biography of Sir William Osler, given to him as a Christmas present in his senior year, so impressed him that he applied to study under Cushing, then Professor of Surgery at Harvard Medical School.

During his 4 years of medical training, Gross worked as a volunteer in the old surgical research laboratory and always maintained that thorough training in pathology and the experimental laboratory were indispensable to academic surgical training. One month in his senior year under William Ladd at Boston Children's Hospital, persuaded him to specialize in paediatric surgery. After graduation (MD, 1931), he trained in pathology under S. Burt Wolbach and in surgery under Elliott Cutler (1931–33), followed by a year as surgical house officer to Ladd. Gross studied pathology for another 2 years under Wolbach (1933–35) and was Surgical House Officer (1935–37) to Cutler. After a Peters Travelling Fellowship (March–August 1937) to visit European clinics and work in the surgical laboratories of the University of Edinburgh, he became Ladd's chief resident. He went on to become the second Ladd Professor of Children's Surgery at Harvard Medical School, Surgeon-in-Chief of Cardiovascular Surgery at Boston Children's Hospital (1947–65) and finally, Chief of Cardiovascular Surgery at Boston Children's Hospital (1967–72). Gross received two Lasker awards for medical research (1954 and 1959) and Harvard University granted him an honourary degree (1984) and established the Robert E. Gross Chair in Surgery in 1984.

When Gross ligated the patent ductus arteriosus in 1938 the condition made up 17 of every hundred cases of congenital heart disease. While still a resident, he worked out the procedure

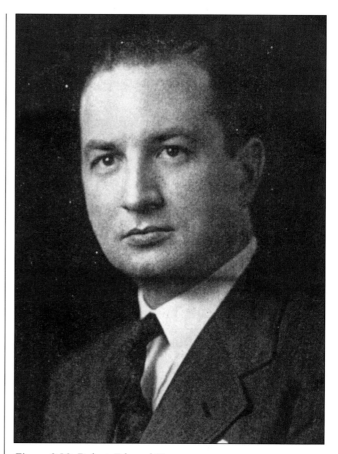

Figure 3.19. Robert Edward Gross.

in the autopsy room with a single, heavy, braided silk ligature. John Perry Hubbard, in charge of paediatric cardiology and one of the few cardiologists who believed in surgical correction of congenital defects, referred Lorraine Sweeney to him (Article 3.1, Appendix A). Nadas and Bing wrote:

"At that time, Green and Emerson ran the congenital heart clinic at Children's Hospital every Thursday afternoon. Neither of their names appeared on Gross's original publication. How the head of the rheumatic fever clinic (Hubbard) had access to a patient with patent ductus arteriosus remains a mystery, but it certainly happened and is another example of Gross's firm determination, skill and good luck."

SURGICAL LIGATION OF A PATENT
DUCTUS ARTERIOSUS

REPORT OF FIRST SUCCESSFUL CASE

ROBERT E. GROSS, M.D.

AND

JOHN P. HUBBARD, M.D.

BOSTON

The continued patency of a ductus arteriosus for more than the first few years of life has long been known to be a potential source of danger to a patient for two reasons: First, the additional work of the left ventricle in maintaining the peripheral blood pressure in the presence of a large arteriovenous communication may lead eventually to cardiac decompensation of severe degree. Second, the presence of a patent ductus arteriosus makes the possessor peculiarly subject to fatal bacterial endarteritis. While it is true that some persons have been known to live to old age with a patent ductus of Botalli, statistics have shown that the majority die relatively young because of complications arising from this congenital abnormality. Dr. Maude Abbott[1] presented a series of ninety-two cases which came to autopsy in which it was shown that the patient had had a patent ductus arteriosus without any other cardiovascular abnormality. Of these patients, approximately one fourth died of bacterial endarteritis of the pulmonary artery and an additional one half died of slow or rapid cardiac decompensation. The average age of death of patients in this series was 24 years.

Figure 3.20. Surgical ligation of patent ductus arteriosus: report of first successsful case. *A 1939 article by Gross and Hubbard. (Reproduced with permission from* Journal of American Medical Association.)

On 26 August 1938, Gross, then 33, ligated the patent ductus of the 7-year-old girl, in spite of Ladd's precise instructions as he left for his holidays: "Don't try to operate on that little girl's patent ductus. She will die." She recovered without complications. Legend has it that Gross and his group of young associates celebrated the success by attending one of the Longwood tennis matches and met Ladd, who asked Gross, "Anything new, Bob?" The laconic chief resident replied "Nothing much." When he and the patient reminisced about the surgery, in his retirement home in Vermont, Gross laughed and said, "You know, Lorraine, if you hadn't made it, I might have ended up here in Vermont as a farmer."

This first surgical correction of a congenital heart defect led to more clinical and laboratory evaluation. Modifications, like Willis Potts' ductus clamp, made the operation safer. In 1944, Gross went on to describe division and suture of the ductus. The first successful cure of bacterial endocarditis by ligation of the infected ductus was achieved a short time later, on 5 December 1939, by Oswald Tubbs, in London. Arthur Touroff, from

Mount Sinai Hospital, performed a similar operation in the USA on 27 January 1940. By 1947 Gross, Crafoord and Wangensteen had performed a total of 172 sections of ductus arteriosus with no fatalities and it was considered so safe that all children with patent ductus were to be operated on whether they showed signs of strain or not. Gross and his associates performed this operation on nearly 1600 patients. Marquis summed up this landmark of cardiac surgery:

"The foresight of this calculated risk established the feasibility of the surgical treatment of congenital heart disease at a time when accuracy of diagnosis depended on the correct interpretation of clinical features and the experience of thoracic surgery was limited. This achievement fired the imagination and heralded a new era. The ductus had pointed the way, had emphasised the importance of natural history in timing, and revealed the potential of surgical treatment."

Gross' *Abdominal Surgery of Infancy and Childhood*, with Ladd (1941), *Surgery of Infancy and Childhood* (1953) and *Atlas of Children's Surgery* (1970) have appeared in numerous editions and have been translated into many languages. Over 200 papers by Gross contain the largest reported experience of certain operations with the lowest incidence of complications. Gross worked out an extraordinarily innovative approach to intra cardiac structures with his atrial well technique (Article 3.4, Appendix A). With a clear understanding of the physiology of intracardiac pressures, Gross used careful animal experimentation to demonstrate that it was possible to open

A METHOD FOR SURGICAL CLOSURE OF
INTERAURICULAR SEPTAL DEFECTS

ROBERT E. GROSS, M.D., F.A.C.S., ELTON WATKINS, JR., M.D.,
ALFRED A. POMERANZ, M.D., and EDWARD I. GOLDSMITH, M.D.,
Boston, Massachusetts

OPENINGS in the interauricular septum allow shunting of blood from the left to the right atrium, thereby increasing the flow through the right side of the heart and through the pulmonary circulation. Although the condition is frequently encountered as the sole cardiac abnormality, its influence on longevity is poorly documented. In the average run of cases, there seems to be little doubt that a septal defect reduces life expectancy. While there is no direct correlation between the size of a septal opening and the duration of life, in general the smaller defects are known to be compatible with a long and active existence, while the larger openings are very apt to bring about right-sided heart failure or fatality in childhood or early adult years. If possible, it is highly desirable to find some surgical means whereby the larger defects can be closed and cardiac invalidism or fatality thereby be prevented. With careful clinical evaluation and with the use of modern ancillary diagnostic methods, it should be possible to select those humans who have atrial defects of considerable size and who might logically be expected to be in considerable danger from the abnormality. Such patients would constitute a group who should be greatly benefited by an adequate corrective procedure.

Described is a method devised for the closure of interauricular septal defects. Investigations in the Laboratory for Surgical Research have permitted development and perfection of the technique; experiences gained from surgical undertakings in humans indicate that the method is of practical value for treatment of interauricular septal defects in man.

Figure 3.21. A method for surgical closure of interauricular septal defects. *A 1953 article by Gross, Watkins, Pomeranz and Goldsmith. (Reproduced with permission from* Surgery, Gynecology and Obstetrics.)

the right atrium whilst the heart supported the circulation. A great deal was learnt from these experiments, such as the need for blood transfusion as the atrial well filled with blood. The fact that there was no difficulty in achieving leak-proof attachment of the rubber well to the atrial wall was a tribute to Gross' surgical skill. The case reports give superb insight into the difficulties, excitement and triumphs of cardiac surgery of that era. The article also provides important documentation of other methods used for the closure of atrial septal defects at the time, all of which were destined for extinction when safe and reproducible extracorporeal circulation became a reality.

By 1953, Gross had moved beyond this unique procedure and had begun building his own pump oxygenator with stainless steel parts made by his machinist, Fred Savage, in the basement of the Children's Hospital. When the machine was finally ready for testing on dogs (by this time in its third re-design), Gross sat on the floor and ran the pump oxygenator while Elton Watkins and a medical student inserted the cannulas and opened the heart. Over the next few years, Gross' heart–lung machine supported 2000 patients during open-heart surgery.

Alfred Blalock (1899–1965)

ALFRED BLALOCK was born in Culloden, Georgia. When his internship at Johns Hopkins (MD, 1922) did not lead to chief residency, he accepted a surgical residency at Vanderbilt University (1925–41) where his research led to a new understanding of the pathophysiology of shock. Other research focused on the production of chylothorax by ligation of the superior vena cava, measurement of thoracic duct pressure in concretio cordis, the effects of adrenalectomy and thymectomy for myasthenia gravis.

The early advances in cardiac surgery began with pericardial disease. Then came repair of vascular anomalies (patent ductus and coarctation of the aorta) adjacent to the heart. There soon followed the rapid and dramatic advances in the correction of other congenital defects and of acquired valvular disorders. In each of these areas, Blalock was a pioneer, and in the surgical approach to the treatment of the congenital intracardiac anomalies, he may be properly considered to have been 'the pioneer'.

On the strength of his insights into shock, Blalock returned to Johns Hopkins as Chief Surgeon and Professor of Surgery (1941–65). On the strength of the Blalock–Taussig procedure for the palliation of tetralogy of Fallot, Blalock and Johns Hopkins became the centre of cardiac surgery in the mid-1940s.

In Blalock's obituary, Lord Brock wrote:

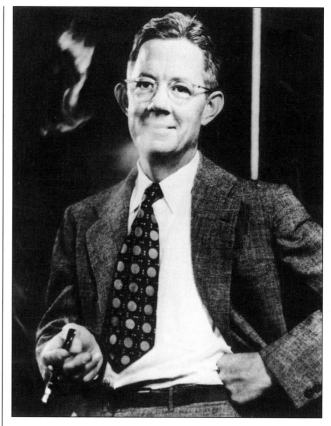

Figure 3.22. Alfred Blalock.

"*The conception and execution of this operation was brilliant in several ways. It was a triumph of technique to achieve this manoeuvre in very ill and often very small children. It was brilliant in conception as a method of relieving the severe disability, and it decided once and for all the argument as to the cause of the cyanosis by demonstrating that it must essentially be due to a deficient pulmonary blood flow, since the cyanosis was relieved by the increase of blood flow to the lungs. Last and perhaps most important of all, it showed that cyanotic congenital heart disease, previously incurable and always fatal, could be cured by surgery. This inspired and stimulated the enormous advances in cardiac surgery which followed with almost breathless rapidity within a very short time.*"

While at Vanderbilt in 1938, Blalock, with Sanford Leeds, had become interested in producing pulmonary hypertension by anastomosing a systemic artery to a pulmonary artery. At Johns Hopkins in 1942, Blalock presented this anastomosis to Edward Park and his paediatric staff as a solution for coarctation of the aorta. Helen Taussig who was present, asked Blalock if he could not devise a ductus for increasing bloodflow to the lungs of patients with pulmonic stenosis in tetralogy of Fallot. Blalock's ductus of the left subclavian artery to left pulmonary artery, devised in Vanderbilt days, eventually provided the palliation needed for patients with cyanotic congenital heart disease (Article 3.2, Appendix A). By 1950 about 1000 children between the ages of 2 and 5 had been operated on with a loss of every sixth patient.

Blalock's unassuming personality was as captivating as his epoch-making surgical accomplishments. Dubost in Paris remembered him during his European tour in 1947.

> *"Blalock impressed me so much that then and there I decided to forget about stomachs, colons and the rest, to devote my career exclusively to what was to become an entirely new surgical specialty."*

Björk remarked that Blalock was the most loved professor he had ever known. Ravitch, Longmire, Sabiston, Thomas and others have written eloquently of the idiosyncrasies of the fabulous Blalock: of the whisky still in his research laboratory; of his eight cold cokes a day; of his frustration at not being able to give away a colleague's (Samuel Crowe, MD) grand piano which he eventually wheeled to the bottom of his driveway, covered in gasoline and burned; of his charisma as a speaker, enunciating lucid surgical analyses in "a voice with a southern drawl so long drawn that it was said that when he arrived in Baltimore the far end was still in Nashville!"; of his unerring judgement in hiring residents such as Denton Cooley who, in his opinion "operated circles around him"; of maintaining a research programme run by a technician (Vivien Thomas) who was considered the best surgeon of the first half of this century. Bahnson (Chief Resident 1950–51) wrote,

> *"He was unusually personable, had a real interest in others, and a desire to help them. I rarely heard from him adverse comments about anyone, although he did allow that he would deserve a star in heaven for being able to work with Taussig."*

THE SURGICAL TREATMENT OF MAL-FORMATIONS OF THE HEART

IN WHICH THERE IS PULMONARY STENOSIS OR PULMONARY ATRESIA

ALFRED BLALOCK, M.D.
AND
HELEN B. TAUSSIG, M.D.
BALTIMORE

Heretofore there has been no satisfactory treatment for pulmonary stenosis and pulmonary atresia. A "blue" baby with a malformed heart was considered beyond the reach of surgical aid. During the past three months we have operated on 3 children with severe degrees of pulmonary stenosis and each of the patients appears to be greatly benefited. In the second and third cases, in which there was deep persistent cyanosis, the cyanosis has greatly diminished or has disappeared and the general condition of the patients is proportionally improved. The results are sufficiently encouraging to warrant an early report.

Figure 3.23. The surgical treatment of malformations of the heart in which there is pulmonary stenosis or pulmonary atresia. *A 1945 article by Blalock and Taussig. (Reproduced with permission from* Journal of American Medical Association.*)*

According to Denton Cooley,

> *"He had great confidence in his staff and gave all of us awesome responsibilities and opportunities. Equally striking was his legendary generosity in giving primary credit to his faculty while minimizing his own contributions. He subtly created a strong but unspoken attitude that any one of us was capable of doing some of the best work in the country. If he was not, he simply was not working hard enough. I consider this enormous impact of Blalock 'The Professor' on his residents as one of his most outstanding contributions."*

Helen Brooke Taussig (1898–1986)

HELEN BROOKE TAUSSIG was born in Cambridge, Massachussetts and studied at Radcliffe College (1917–19) and the University of California at Berkeley (BA, 1921). Refused admittance to Harvard Medical School, she registered at Boston University (1922) where Alexander Begg, Professor of Anatomy and Dean of the Medical School, gave her a beef heart, advising that it would do "no harm to be interested in one of the larger organs of the body." He encouraged her to go

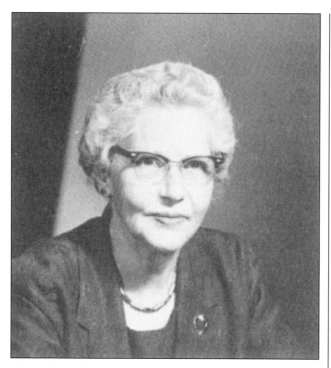

Figure 3.24. Helen Brooke Taussig.

on to Johns Hopkins (MD, 1927). After internship (1928–30), Edward Parks put her in charge of the Harriet Lane Children's Heart Clinic (1930–64), which became her base of operations for the next 50 years. Installing a fluoroscope, Parks ordered her to take an electrocardiogram and fluoroscope of every patient. Gordon Murray visited Taussig at this period:

> *"...the equipment was placed in a tiny cubicle in which was scarcely space, even with the best organization, for the small X-ray machine, a small child under observation and Dr Taussig. With careful manipulation, one additional observer could be squeezed in behind the door and the door closed to keep out the light. In these restricted quarters Dr Taussig did her examinations of these sufferers."*

Richard Bing wrote of Taussig:

> *"She really understood the anatomy of congenital cardiac malformations. Her hearing was seriously impaired from an early age, thus auscultation was not her forte. Under the fluoroscope, however, she could see the anatomy very clearly and could correlate it with her profound knowledge of pathology.... Seeing many cyanotic children, she gradually defined the clinical, radiologic, and electrocardiographic profile for tetralogy of Fallot, the most common subgroup of blue babies. She noticed that among this group, those who had continuous murmurs were significantly less blue than the others. From this observation came the original idea of attempting to create an*

> *artificial ductus to increase pulmonary flow in children with tetralogy of Fallot. One of Taussig's most striking characteristics was her straight, uncluttered even unsophisticated thinking."*

Earlier theories lacked her precision, as Lord Brock pointed out, "Until then it had been assumed that arteriovenous mixing was probably the more important factor."

When Taussig journeyed to Boston to ask Gross to consider reversing his ligation, he was in the full flush of his successful closure of the patent ductus and told her he was not interested in creating a ductus for a cyanotic child. "It was extremely fortunate for me," Taussig wrote "when Dr Alfred Blalock was appointed Professor of Surgery as he was known as a vascular surgeon." On an occasion when Blalock was ligating a patent ductus she said, "The truly great day will be when you build a ductus for the child dying of anoxemia and not when you tie off a ductus for a child with a little too much blood going to his lungs." Two years to the day, Blalock did his first anastomosis. He accepted the challenge first to test the theory and then to perfect the operation (Article 3.2, Appendix A). Harry Minetree, in describing the operation included many of the participants:

> *"On November 29, 1944, students and professors crowded into the double-deck observation gallery above the eighth-floor operating room in Halsted Clinic. Because there was a danger of losing the child before the operation began, Dr Merel Harmel decided not to use a strong anaesthetic and put her slowly to sleep with a diluted mixture of ether and oxygen. Dr William Longmire, the Chief Resident, was first assistant. Charlotte Mitchell was the scrub nurse. After inserting an arterial needle for blood-oxygen tests, Vivien Thomas, who in the dog lab had proved himself a master at vascular suturing, stood by in the event that his advice might be needed. Dr Denton Cooley administered fluids. The tiny, pliable ribs were retracted and the pleural cavity, containing the child's atrophied lungs and small, twisted heart, was opened...the heart and lungs seemed infinitely more complex in miniature. With the assistance of Thomas, Dr Blalock found the subclavian artery, clamped it at its origin and began dissecting away the tissue that clung to it. The instruments were too large and awkward... Using bulldog clamps fitted with rubber tubing so as not to crush the vessels, Blalock, with Thomas' help, carefully prepared a site for attaching the subclavian to the pulmonary artery. A small traverse incision was made between two clamps on the pulmonary artery then, using china beaded silk on fine needles, Dr Blalock completed the juncture that rerouted the baby's blood. She immediately went from waxen blue to pink. Dr Helen Taussig had watched the operation from the head of the table..."*

Taussig wrote *Congenital Malformations of the Heart* (1947), providing in depth clinical diagnosis of congenital heart disease in living patients. She kept up with children under her care through generations, which gave her an unrivalled view of the natural and surgically modified history of congenital cardiac defects. She maintained professional concern about thalidomide and acute rheumatic fever long after retirement in 1963. Taussig was still working on congenitally-defective bird hearts sent to her by friends in retirement when she was fatally injured while backing out of her driveway.

Willis J. Potts (1895–1968)

WILLIS J. POTTS was born in Sheboygan, Wisconsin. In World War I, he served in the USA and France; during World War II, he served as a colonel in the southwest Pacific with the 25th Evacuation Hospital. Potts studied at Rush Medical College, University of Chicago (MD, 1924) and interned at the Presbyterian Hospital. He was Clinical Associate Professor of Surgery at Rush, and quite unknown in paediatric surgery before he returned from World War II, when "some astute person", recounts Ravitch, "engineered his appointment as Surgeon-in-Chief at Children's Memorial Hospital [Chicago]." Eventually, he became Professor of Surgery at Northwestern University (1946–60). Ravitch describes Potts as "Tall, lanky, sandy-haired, with a marvellous wit and an elegant use of language, able to jest at himself, he was a great contributor to all fields of paediatric surgery."

An early visitor to Blalock's operation for tetralogy of Fallot, Potts attributed his courage to attempt the modification of the Blalock–Taussig procedure to Blalock and Taussig's careful description of the alternative operation. Three dangers were pointed out: paralysis in a dog whose aorta was occluded for 40 minutes; the sometimes friable nature of the aortic wall; and the difficulty in obtaining an accurate approximation of the intimal surfaces of the aorta and the pulmonary artery. Potts resolved the problems of the friability and paralysis with a specially designed clamp. This was conceived while Potts was watching a plastic surgeon using an instrument to stretch skin in order to cut grafts. This clamp "which partially occluded the aorta, and furnished a lip to which the pulmonary artery could be sewn" was designed by Potts and Smith and built by Bruno Richter, an instrument maker. Inaccuracy was resolved by Potts's insistence on the incision for the anastomosis being exactly 4/16 of an inch, measured with a calliper.

Potts, Sidney Smith and Stanley Gibson at Northwestern University Medical School reported the survival and improvement of two children (Figure 3.26):

"The first aortic–pulmonary anastomosis was performed in 1946 on a child who was deeply cyanotic with a red blood cell count of 10,300,000 per cubic centimetre, completely helpless

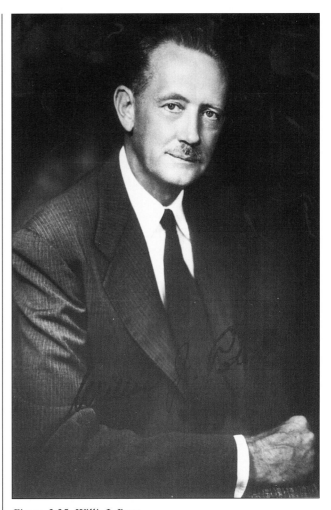

Figure 3.25. Willis J. Potts.

and subject to many attacks of syncope daily. Now, in 1958, she is 13 years old, healthy and active, in junior high school. Her heart is only slightly enlarged. She is too active to suit her mother. Last summer she pedalled 15 miles on a bicycle in one day. Why can't all results be as good?"

From 1946 to 1956 early mortality was approximately 8% in 600 patients, although later statistics showed some children reverted to cyanosis 10 years later. Björk wrote in 1950,

ANASTOMOSIS OF THE AORTA TO A PULMONARY ARTERY

Certain Types in Congenital Heart Disease

WILLIS J. POTTS, M.D.
SIDNEY SMITH, M.D.
and
STANLEY GIBSON, M.D.
Chicago

In 1945 Blalock and Taussig[1] introduced a new surgical procedure for the relief of anoxemia due to pulmonary stenosis or pulmonary atresia. By anastomosing the subclavian or innominate artery to either the right or the left pulmonary artery they have been able to increase the flow of blood to the lungs. Their work is an outstanding contribution to the relief of children whose outlook without aid is hopeless. Sacrifice of the subclavian artery for the anastomosis of its proximal end to the side of a pulmonary artery is associated with little danger to the circulation of the arm. Use of the innominate artery for such an anastomosis entails the hazard of an inadequate supply of blood to the brain.

Figure 3.26. Anastomosis of the aorta to a pulmonary artery: certain types in congenital heart disease. *A 1946 article by Potts, Smith and Gibbs. (Reproduced with permission from* Journal of American Medical Association.)

"The further to the west I travelled in the USA the more popular was Potts's aortico-pulmonary side-to-side anastomosis. In Chicago, Potts had performed 225 such operations. The youngest survivor with improvement was only 10 days old and the aorta had a diameter of only 5 mm which was why his special clamp with the narrow jaws was essential for the side occlusion of the aorta."

Potts was overwhelmed by the rapid advances in open heart surgery which, within weeks, appeared to obliterate his labours. At the First International Symposium on Cardiac Surgery in 1955, his scholarly dissertation on the Potts procedure was followed by Lillehei's film of correction of ventricular septal defects and tetralogy of Fallot by direct vision in the open heart with the patient's circulation maintained by a parent. In spite of his chagrin, Potts' spirit of fair play and intellectual honesty, combined with his wonderful sense of humour came to the fore. He ran down the aisle of the international symposium, calling out, "Does anyone here remember an old operation called the Potts' procedure for blue babies? What about my clamp?" Potts' chapter on palliative procedures, subclavian-pulmonary and aortic-pulmonary anastomoses and infundibulectomy in *The Surgeon and the Child* concludes:

"In self-defence, in defence of Smith, Blalock, Taussig and Brock, I am sure I may say we are not grieving as the incomplete operations for tetralogy of Fallot are being laid aside for an operation which will cure and be relatively safe. As future surgeons pass the markers of these operations all we ask is that they say a few kind words."

Donald Walter Gordon Murray (1894–1976)

DONALD WALTER GORDON MURRAY was born near Stratford, Ontario, Canada. His medical studies at the University of Toronto (MD, 1921) were interrupted by service as a gunner in France (1915–18) in World War I. He was said to have been blown up, presumed dead and buried until his burial site, recaptured from the Germans, was disinterred and he was discovered alive. Murray studied anatomy and surgery in London, England (1922–27), where he was resident at the West End Hospital (1922); house surgeon at Hampstead General (1923) and All Saints Hospitals (1924); demonstrator in anatomy at the University of London (1925–26); house surgeon at St Mary's Hospital; and demonstrator of anatomy and minor surgery at the University of London and the London Hospital (FRCS, 1926).

Murray returned to the USA and was house surgeon at both the New York Hospital (1927) and Hospital for Ruptured and Crippled Children (1928) in New York City. While Murray was working at Cornell University, Starr, Chief of Surgery at the Toronto Hospital, asked him to return to the University of Toronto as surgeon and lecturer (1928). His experiences with heparin were the subject of his Hunterian Lecture to the Royal College of Surgeons (1939), and an international lecture tour in the UK, Scandinavia, France and the USA.

In 1948 he was appointed Head of the Third Division of General Surgery at the Toronto Hospital. When he retired from the University of Toronto in 1953, he continued as consultant surgeon to the Toronto Hospital and Director of the Gardiner Medical Research Institute until 1963. He wrote three autobiographical works, *Medicine in the Making* (1960), *Quest in Medicine* (1963) and *Surgery in the Making* (1965). He was named Companion of the Order of Canada at 73, at which time he proposed an unorthodox method of regeneration of transected spinal cord for quadriplegia and paraplegia which was never proven correct.

Murray's contributions to surgery were enormous, imaginative and varied. Nineteen years after heparin was isolated (1916) by McLean and purified by Best, Charles and Scott in Toronto (1932) and Jorpes and Crafoord in Sweden, Murray was the first to use it clinically in 1935. He showed that heparin prevented thrombosis in veins at the site of arterial anastomoses, in venous grafts in the arterial tree, in the portal system and anywhere an experimental embolus had been removed. Patency in reconstructed vessels permitted by heparin and his rare technical skill, allowed Murray to make great advances in experimental vascular surgery in the 1930s, decades before such techniques had become clinically routine. Using heparin, he also performed haemodialysis with two artificial kidney machines which he made independently of Kolff, in 1946 and 1952–53.

In 1938, he demonstrated that cardiogenic shock, following myocardial infarction, was caused by a local area of inert muscle that could be resected. Throughout the moratorium on clinical surgery of the mitral valve between 1928 and the successes of 1948, his experimental work continued. He described replacing a cusp of the mitral valve with a homograft and two successful corrections of mitral stenosis in the discussion of Bailey's paper, *The Surgical Treatment of Mitral Stenosis*. Murray's ingenuity, including fascia lata for valve replacement and closure of atrial septal defects, were not recognized in Canada. As Murray said, "the nature of the medical climate was such that, as on so many other occasions, the luxuriant growth and expansion of the field occurred in the United States." His report on the attempted closure of three ventricular septal defects and one atrial septal defect using fascial strips in 1948 represented the first surgical intervention in this area (Figure 3.27). The last case, performed in August 1948, resulted in clinical improvement but a

> **CLOSURE OF DEFECTS IN CARDIAC SEPTA***
> GORDON MURRAY, M.D., F.R.C.S. (CAN.), F.R.C.S. (ENG).
> TORONTO, CANADA
>
> THE HIGH INCIDENCE of defects in cardiac septa in 350 congenital hearts examined, about 50% being diagnosed as patent inverventricular or interauricular septa, stimulated my interest in the subject.
> Only those defects in the septum which appear to be single lesions are included in this consideration. The perforated septum in tetralogy of Fallot, tricuspid atresia or patent ductus arteriosus and so on are not included and only those are considered when the septum is thought to be the predominant congenital defect and the one causing symptoms.
> It is obvious that a small interventricular or interauricular septal defect, in the absence of infection, is of little or no significance. Cases are recorded where soldiers have gone through commando training and through the recent war with known congenital interventricular septal defects with no change in size of heart and no ill effects.
> On the other hand, if the septal defect in either auricle or ventricle is large, it is possible that it may be the source of symptoms, and may be accompanied by cyanosis. The symptoms and the cyanosis may depend on several factors, but perhaps the size of the opening is one of the most important, which opinion is supported by Toussig[1] in her recent excellent book on Congenital Heart Disease.

Figure 3.27. Closure of defects in cardiac septa. *A 1948 article by Gordon Murray. (Reproduced with permission from* The Annals of Surgery.)

follow-up report by Keith and Forsyth showed that only a slight diminution in the shunt had occurred. Murray's procedure was nevertheless the direct forerunner of Søndergaard's circumclusion operation and Gross' atrial well technique.

Murray participated in each stage of the evolution of coronary artery surgery with the exception of the denervation procedures. He placed arterial grafts in the coronary circulation (1954), aware that they could not be proven viable until science produced angiography. In 1956, Murray's insertion of a fresh and viable homograft in the descending thoracic aorta of a patient with aortic regurgitation, stimulated further use of homograft valves and eventually orthotopic replacement. Heimbecker reported the valve to be functional 20 years later.

C. Rollins Hanlon (1915–)

C. ROLLINS HANLON was born in Baltimore and studied at Johns Hopkins (MD, 1938). He was resident to Mont Reid at the Cincinnati General Hospital. Hanlon served in the neurosurgical service of Howard C. Naffziger in San Francisco and with the United States Fleet in the Pacific (1944–46) during World War II, before his appointment as Chief Surgical Resident to Blalock (1947–48) at the Johns Hopkins. He became Professor and Chairman of the Department of Surgery

at St Louis University School of Medicine (1950–69). In the 1960s, he conducted systematic pharmacological, histological and physiological studies of cardiac function in surgically denervated and autotransplanted hearts in dogs and anthropoids. This was done in conjunction with Cooper and Willman in preparation for cardiac transplantation. As an 'academic' surgeon, Hanlon made an immense contribution to the American Surgical Association as secretary (1969). He was Director of the American College of Surgeons (1969–88) and President of the Society of University Surgeons (1959), the

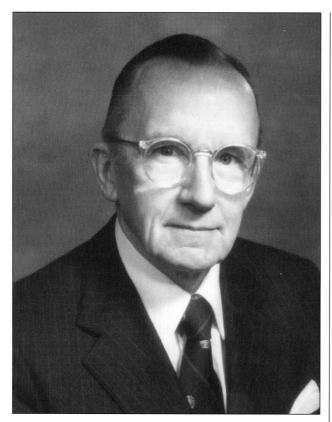

Figure 3.28. C. Rollins Hanlon (courtesy of Fabian Bachrach).

THE SURGICAL TREATMENT OF COMPLETE TRANSPOSITION
OF THE AORTA AND THE PULMONARY ARTERY

ALFRED BLALOCK, M.D., F.A.C.S., and C. ROLLINS HANLON, M.D.,
Baltimore, Maryland

COMPLETE transposition of the aorta and pulmonary artery is a relatively common congenital anomaly. In complete transposition of the great vessels the aorta arises from the ventricle receiving systemic venous blood and the pulmonary artery arises from the ventricle receiving oxygenated blood. Blood that is pumped by the left ventricle through the pulmonary artery to the lungs returns by the pulmonary veins and left auricle to its point of origin in the left ventricle. Blood that is propelled by the right ventricle through the aorta to the body is returned by the systemic veins and the right auricle to its starting point in the right ventricle. In other words, there is transposition of the great arteries without transposition of the great veins. The systemic and pulmonary circulations are thus basically separate; a condition obviously incompatible with long survival. However, there is generally some degree of communication between the two circulations by way of septal defects or other abnormalities. These abnormal communications allow some oxygenated blood to be shunted into the systemic circulation, and some venous blood is similarly transferred to the pulmonary circulation.

Because of these compensating abnormalities certain individuals with transposition may survive for a long time. The usual life expectancy, however, is quite short. In 123 collected cases (4) the average duration of life was 19 months. If 6 patients who lived 10 years or longer are excluded, the average duration of life for the remaining 117 patients was only 5½ months.

We have discussed elsewhere (4) the relation between longevity and the presence of specific abnormalities associated with complete transposition. As might be expected, the duration of life depends on the degree of mixing between the two circulations. A ventricular septal defect is associated with the greatest life expectancy in these patients, presumably because it results in the best interchange of blood between the two circulations. Patency of the auricular septum is the next most favorable isolated defect and the combination of an auricular and a ventricular defect gives an even better prognosis. Various other abnormalities may provide a means of mixing between the systemic and pulmonary circulations in cases of transposition. Among these are patent ductus arteriosus, and partial transposition of the great veins.

Figure 3.29. The surgical treatment of complete transposition of the aorta and the pulmonary artery. *A 1950 article by Blalock and Hanlon. (Reproduced with permission from Surgery, Gynecology and Obstetrics.)*

American Surgical Association (1981), the American College of Surgeons (1987) and executive consultant to the College of Surgeons. As Emeritus Professor of Surgery at the Northwestern University School of Medicine, he currently teaches ethics and human values.

As a medical student, Hanlon volunteered to work under Taussig, who meticulously dissected macerated stillborn foetuses at any hour of the day or night in the Pathology Department. In fact, Hanlon married Margaret Hammond, a young paediatric cardiologist working with Taussig. During their honeymoon in Rome, Hammond performed diagnostic cardiac catheterizations on young cyanotic patients who were then operated on by Hanlon and Professor Pietro Valdoni.

The technique of closed atrial septostomy, performed while the heart supported the circulation, provided better oxygen saturation of the arterial blood by improved interatrial mixing of the systemic and pulmonary venous returns. Before Hanlon's work, Blalock's technician Vivien Thomas created atrial mixing in 27 dogs by anastomosing the right pulmonary vein to an oval opening in the atrium. He used a specially-curved clamp, which made it possible to cut out most of the atrial septum without interrupting the circulation. Suture of the right atrial wall to the anterior wall of the pulmonary veins followed. After the autopsies on the first series of dogs Blalock

wrote on the manuscripts that this atrial septostomy was devised by Thomas. As Clarence Weldon noted, this "ought to surprise no one, for in 1946 and 1947, he [Thomas] was possibly the most skilled and experienced cardiac surgeon in the world."

When Hanlon began operating in Blalock's Hunterian Laboratory at the Johns Hopkins in 1947, he created a shunt from the pulmonary vein through an enlarged orifice of the azygos vein into the superior vena cava. This gave a smoother surface for bloodflow than Thomas' anastomosis to the right atrium. Hanlon wrote:

"The perception that the ventral walls of the pulmonary veins blend into a fusion with the dorsal wall of the right atrium to constitute a lamellar interatrial septum would be clear to any surgeon who had divided the azygos vein and used the stump to retract the vena cava and right atrium for deep exposure of the pulmonary vasculature in a difficult pneumonectomy. I had, at times, divided the pulmonary venous outflow by suturing a portion of what was essentially the left atrium at its fusion with the right atrium."

The Blalock–Hanlon pulmonary vein to superior vena cava anastomoses had a patency of 80%, whereas Thomas' pulmonary vein to right atrium anastomoses resulted in a patency of less than 20%.

Blalock was not happy with this palliative measure and was

aware that an arterial switch operation was necessary. Although the artificial atrial septal defect procedures for transposition actually compounded the basic anatomical problem by adding another anomaly, Hanlon maintained that surgical palliation allowed many patients to live on until definitive correction was available.

The Blalock–Hanlon technique was the first to permit survival of infants with transposed great arteries incompatible with life. It provided an impetus for continuing investigation of surgical methods to establish an efficient and durable circulation in this problem. Ochsner and Cooley modified the creation of an atrial septal defect with encouraging results (1961). The technique was superseded by reopening of the foramen ovale with a balloon catheter devised by William Rashkind in 1966. The advent of cardiopulmonary bypass then provided safer and simpler techniques for excising the entire intra-atrial septum or performing definitive repair by the venous inflow methods of Senning and Mustard.

Tyge Søndergaard (1914–1990)

TYGE SØNDERGAARD was born in Køge on the island of Zealand in Denmark, about 50 miles south of Copenhagen. He studied at the University of Copenhagen (MD, 1941) and received his surgical training in Denmark and the USA. In 1952, he established the Department of Thoracic and Cardiovascular Surgery at the Municipal Hospital in Århus, where kidney transplantations were also performed. In 1960, his work and ideas stimulated the establishment of the Institute of Experimental Clinical Research at Århus. In 1963, Søndergaard was the first surgeon to use cold chemical cardioplegia in open heart surgery. He received honourary degrees from the University of Wrocław in Poland and the University of Berne in Switzerland, where he worked for a few weeks each year in the 60s and 70s. Søndergaard was regarded as a hard worker and an excellent and demanding teacher and colleague. He retired in 1984.

Søndergaard's international reputation was based on his closure of atrial septal defects of the secundum type and relief of valvular pulmonary stenosis without extracorporeal circulation. His method of circumclusion of an atrial septal defect entailed creating a cleavage plain between the two atria. By means of a probe, a suture was passed from in front of the pulmonary veins, the long end carried up behind the superior vena cava then posterior to the inferior vena cava and the aorta, into the septum and tied in the ventricular myocardium to the left of the inferior vena cava. When this suture was tied down, the double atrial chamber became partially divided in two by a pursestring-like action.

Although it seemed improbable that a complete separation of the two atria could be accomplished by this method, a great reduction in the size of the communication and hence of the shunt, could be achieved. In dogs with experimentally produced atrial septal defects, a semicircular suture was employed successfully by Søndergaard (1952), but in patients, the defect was not always closed. Søndergaard's first operation on 11 November 1952 succeeded, though the patient died of whooping cough 8 months later. Autopsy showed that the atrial defect had been reduced to one-third its original size. In 1954, Søndergaard reported three successful cases.

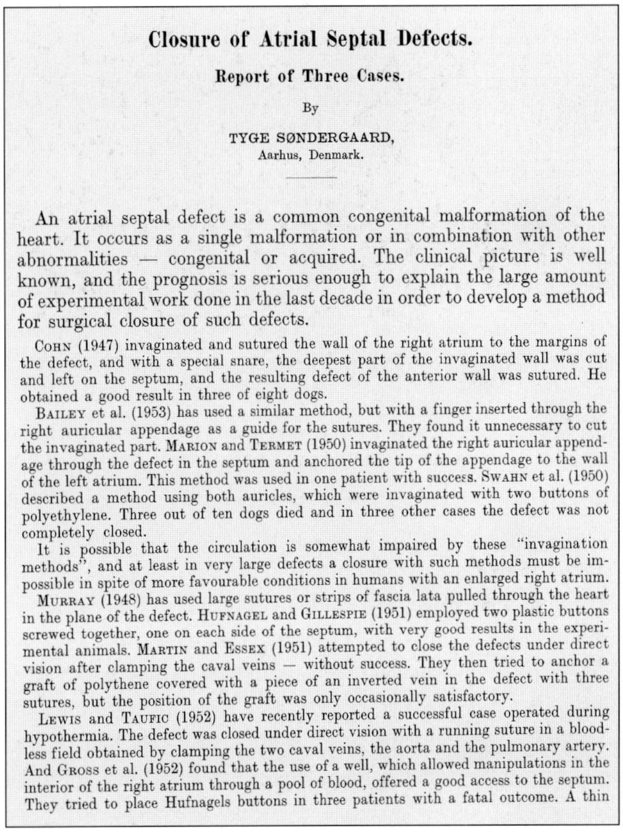

Closure of Atrial Septal Defects.

Report of Three Cases.

By

TYGE SØNDERGAARD,
Aarhus, Denmark.

An atrial septal defect is a common congenital malformation of the heart. It occurs as a single malformation or in combination with other abnormalities — congenital or acquired. The clinical picture is well known, and the prognosis is serious enough to explain the large amount of experimental work done in the last decade in order to develop a method for surgical closure of such defects.

COHN (1947) invaginated and sutured the wall of the right atrium to the margins of the defect, and with a special snare, the deepest part of the invaginated wall was cut and left on the septum, and the resulting defect of the anterior wall was sutured. He obtained a good result in three of eight dogs.

BAILEY et al. (1953) has used a similar method, but with a finger inserted through the right auricular appendage as a guide for the sutures. They found it unnecessary to cut the invaginated part. MARION and TERMET (1950) invaginated the right auricular appendage through the defect in the septum and anchored the tip of the appendage to the wall of the left atrium. This method was used in one patient with success. SWAHN et al. (1950) described a method using both auricles, which were invaginated with two buttons of polyethylene. Three out of ten dogs died and in three other cases the defect was not completely closed.

It is possible that the circulation is somewhat impaired by these "invagination methods", and at least in very large defects a closure with such methods must be impossible in spite of more favourable conditions in humans with an enlarged right atrium.

MURRAY (1948) has used large sutures or strips of fascia lata pulled through the heart in the plane of the defect. HUFNAGEL and GILLESPIE (1951) employed two plastic buttons screwed together, one on each side of the septum, with very good results in the experimental animals. MARTIN and ESSEX (1951) attempted to close the defects under direct vision after clamping the caval veins — without success. They then tried to anchor a graft of polythene covered with a piece of an inverted vein in the defect with three sutures, but the position of the graft was only occasionally satisfactory.

LEWIS and TAUFIC (1952) have recently reported a successful case operated during hypothermia. The defect was closed under direct vision with a running suture in a bloodless field obtained by clamping the two caval veins, the aorta and the pulmonary artery. And GROSS et al. (1952) found that the use of a well, which allowed manipulations in the interior of the right atrium through a pool of blood, offered a good access to the septum. They tried to place Hufnagels buttons in three patients with a fatal outcome. A thin

Figure 3.30. Closure of atrial septal defects: report of three cases. *A 1948 article by Søndergaard. (Reproduced with permission from* Annals of Surgery.*)*

The suture encircling the atrial septum was difficult to place correctly because it was done blind. In 1955, at the suggestion of Crafoord, Søndergaard placed his finger in the right atrium to direct the placement of the suture. Husfeldt reported four great improvements and four complete closures in 10 cases. Crafoord and Björk, who adopted and modified the procedure, emphasized that the suture should pass entirely subendocardially in the septal rim so that no part lay within the cavity of the atria to promote thrombus formation; also that a guiding finger should be placed within the right atrial chamber.

The advantages of circumclusion, emphasized by Søndergaard, were that the established septum was located in the normal septal plane and consisted of normal atrial septal tissue; that neither the right nor the left atrium were altered in shape or in function and there was no possibility of blocking the inflow veins. The technique was the same in multiple defects. No sutures or other foreign bodies were left exposed inside the heart; no needle was used and the blunt probe eliminated the danger of piercing the aortic wall — a mishap

reported a couple of times in the literature. There was no need for hypothermia or any other elaborate procedure, just ordinary anaesthesia as in any other thoracic case. A standard right thoracotomy was used. The probe was slid parallel to the bundle of His and not at a right angle as in direct suture or in atrioseptopexy. Mortality, Søndergaard concluded, had been zero in experiments and clinical cases. All the patients catheterized postoperatively had a complete closure of the defect, and the pressures had returned to normal in 2 weeks!

Others took up the operation for the short time before open heart surgery became a reality. Søndergaard's operation, with Bailey's atrioseptopexy and Gross' atrial well, were widely used as they could be performed on a normothermic patient. In the USA, circumclusion was modified by a number of surgeons, particularly Lam.

John Webster Kirklin (1917–)

JOHN WEBSTER KIRKLIN was born in Muncie, Indiana. Although his father was a pioneer radiologist, Kirklin recalls that he was mostly interested in managing the college football team. During his junior year at the University of Minnesota (BA *summa cum laude*, 1938), he decided to study medicine at Harvard University (MD, 1942). During Kirklin's first year, Robert Gross received universal acclaim for being the first person to successfully close a patent ductus arteriosus. For Kirklin, Gross was a powerful stimulus towards cardiac surgery.

Under a wartime plan, Kirklin interned at the University Hospital of Pennsylvania (1942–43), the Mayo Clinic (1943–44) and in neurosurgery at O'Reilly General Hospital, Missouri. Afterwards he spent 2.5 years as an army neurosurgeon, receiving war casualties from the Pacific and European fronts. Discharged from the army in 1946, he completed a general surgical residency at the Mayo Clinic (1946–48). Although Kirklin considered a career in neurosurgery, he fortuitously spent another 6 months as assistant resident to Gross at the Children's Hospital, Boston. Gross " looked like a surgeon sent up from central casting — handsome, quiet and very stimulating".

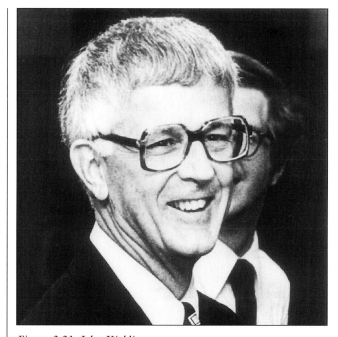

Figure 3.31. John Kirklin.

"My fellow residents and I filled pages of notebooks with drawings and plans of how we would close ventricular septal defects and repair the tetralogy of Fallot once science gave us a method to get inside the heart."

"Gross," Kirklin said, "was such a magnetic personality and his

work was so fascinating to me that I went back to the idea of being a cardiac surgeon."

Kirklin and his team at the Mayo Clinic were successful in their pioneering efforts to 'get inside the heart' (Article 3.12, Appendix A). In 1954, he applied Gross' atrial well technique to the repair of atrial septal defects (Figure 3.33). Later that year, he used the well technique for repair of partial atrioventricular canal defects. Several hundred such procedures were performed by the Mayo Clinic team in the early 1950s.

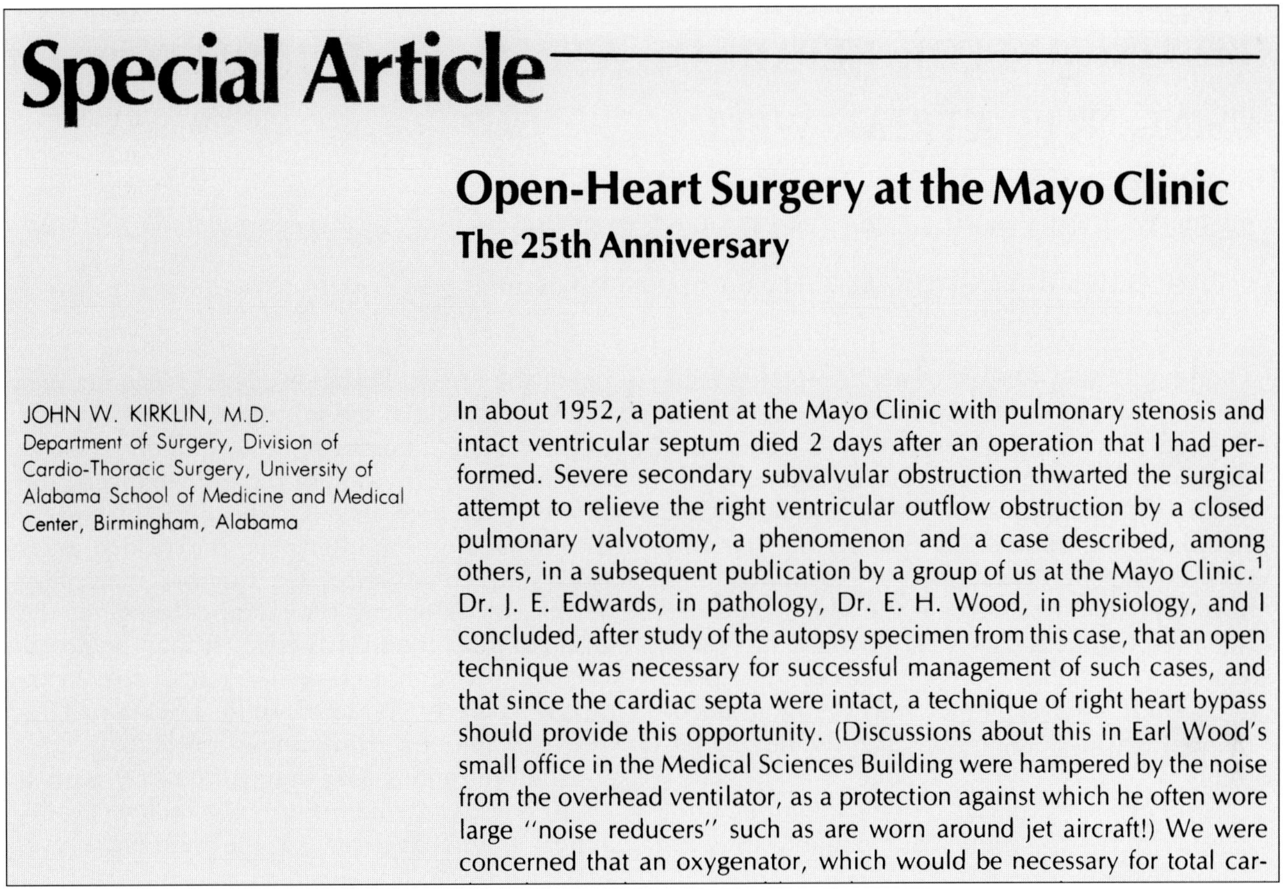

Special Article

Open-Heart Surgery at the Mayo Clinic
The 25th Anniversary

JOHN W. KIRKLIN, M.D.
Department of Surgery, Division of
Cardio-Thoracic Surgery, University of
Alabama School of Medicine and Medical
Center, Birmingham, Alabama

In about 1952, a patient at the Mayo Clinic with pulmonary stenosis and intact ventricular septum died 2 days after an operation that I had performed. Severe secondary subvalvular obstruction thwarted the surgical attempt to relieve the right ventricular outflow obstruction by a closed pulmonary valvotomy, a phenomenon and a case described, among others, in a subsequent publication by a group of us at the Mayo Clinic.[1] Dr. J. E. Edwards, in pathology, Dr. E. H. Wood, in physiology, and I concluded, after study of the autopsy specimen from this case, that an open technique was necessary for successful management of such cases, and that since the cardiac septa were intact, a technique of right heart bypass should provide this opportunity. (Discussions about this in Earl Wood's small office in the Medical Sciences Building were hampered by the noise from the overhead ventilator, as a protection against which he often wore large "noise reducers" such as are worn around jet aircraft!) We were concerned that an oxygenator, which would be necessary for total car-

Figure 3.32. Open-heart surgery at the Mayo Clinic: the 25th anniversary. *A 1980 article by Kirklin. (Reproduced with permission from* Mayo Clinic Proceedings.)

In 1955, Kirklin and his team began to use a modified form of Gibbon's pump oxygenator, to repair atrioventricular canal defects under direct vision (Figure 3.34). Kirklin wondered if the artificial oxygenator would be as dangerous as Richard Varco declared it to be in *Time* magazine in 1955 (because of its damaging effects on the blood). He was pressured from inside and outside the Mayo Clinic to abort his efforts in favour of Lillehei's controlled cross-circulation method. Nevertheless, between March and October 1955, Kirklin and his colleagues produced a successful series of intracardiac operations using the Mayo–Gibbon machine. This work established cardiopulmonary bypass as a safe and reproducible platform for progress in open-heart surgery.

In 1955, Kirklin and his colleagues undertook the second open intracardiac repair of tetralogy of Fallot, less than a year after Lillehei and Varco performed the first operation using cross-circulation at the University of Minnesota. When the first five patients died, Kirklin stopped operating while he and the team worked to overcome technical difficulties. They resumed surgery later that year and reduced the mortality rate to one in five.

Kirklin became Professor and Chairman of the Department of Surgery at the Mayo Clinic (1960–66) and then Surgeon-in-Chief and Chairman of the Department of Surgery at the University of Alabama, (1966–82). His opinion on the teaching of surgeons was expressed at this time:

"The resident must learn to think about alternatives to his plans, and about the times when he must improvise in a light-footed way to meet some unexpected development. The most critical and important part of the cardiovascular resident's learning is in the operating room, and this is where we try to be certain that he learns well and completely the thousand and one little details of operative cardiac surgery. This means endless hours of scrubbing with them, of searching for their wasted motions and helping them to get rid of them, of increasing their perception of tissue planes and insisting that they use them in their dissection, that they keep the operation moving forward, and so on, and so on, and so on..."

He received honorary degrees from the Universities of Munich, (1961); Hamline (1966); Alabama (1978); Bordeaux (1982);

TECHNIQUE FOR REPAIR OF ATRIAL SEPTAL DEFECT USING THE ATRIAL WELL

JOHN W. KIRKLIN, M.D., F.A.C.S., F. HENRY ELLIS, JR., M.D., F.A.C.S., and

BRIAN G. BARRATT-BOYES, M.D., Rochester, Minnesota

TECHNIQUES FOR REPAIR of atrial septal defects must entail a low operative mortality, and must allow opportunity for complete and permanent repair of the type of defect encountered. The atrial well technique of Gross has met these criteria in our experience. Seventy-one patients with atrial septal defect and left-to-right shunts have been operated upon at the Mayo Clinic by this method, with 3 deaths, giving a mortality rate of 4 per cent. Complete closure has been obtained in all except a few early cases, as documented by physiologic studies in the first 33 patients (2).

Although apparently complex and difficult of execution, the technique can be made easily re-neath the breast. Posteriorly, the incision curves below the angle of the scapula to follow the line of the vertebral border of the scapula for a short distance. After division of the muscle layers, the thorax is entered through the fifth interspace. The incision in the interspace is extended anteriorly, after ligation of the internal mammary vessels, by detaching the costal cartilage of the fifth rib from the sternal edge. It may be necessary, on occasion, to sever the fourth costal cartilage similarly. Wide exposure is obtained by the insertion of a self-retaining retractor.

After retracting the lung posteriorly with a moist pack, the pericardium is incised vertically, parallel and anterior to the phrenic nerve.

Figure 3.33. Technique for repair of atrial septal defect using the atrial well. *A 1956 article by Kirklin, Ellis Jr and Barratt-Boyes. (Reproduced with permission from* Surgery, Gynecology and Obstetrics.)

Universidad de la Republica, Uruguay (1982); and Indiana (1983). Kirklin outlined his philosophy on academic surgery as:

"Academic surgery is variously defined, but to me it is the practice of surgery in an environment and with an attitude that results in excellent patient care but also in the generation of new knowledge and in the organization and presentation of available knowledge so that it will be useful to others now and in the future. It is a fusion of clinical surgery, research, teaching, and administration. Those who have experienced only one of these interlinked phases cannot understand the whole."

With Robert Karp, Kirklin wrote *Tetralogy of Fallot from the Surgical Point of View* (1970), *Cardiac Surgery and the Conduction System* (1983). With Sir Brian Barratt-Boyes, he produced *Cardiac Surgery* (1990), the definitive and enduring textbook in the field. He was editor of the *Journal of Thoracic and Cardiovascular Surgery* and author of more than 500 scientific papers.

In the 1980s, Kirklin reflected on the improvements in the treatment of tetralogy of Fallot over the years:

"During 1955 our mortality rate was high for the repair of tetralogy of Fallot in children. We were discouraged by our inability to make most of these patients live. Mortality in these 'blue babies' was 50% or higher in 1955; within 5 years it had fallen to 15%. By 1970 it was around 8%. In 1980, it approached 0% overall and is never higher than 4% at the Birmingham Medical Center."

Kirklin concurred with Barratt-Boyes and Castaneda regarding the safety and advantage of early one-stage repair of tetralogy of Fallot. In 1987, he said

"I think congenital heart disease will all be treated surgically in the first few years of life and there will not be, except in areas where there are residual patients because of slower development, any surgery of congenital heart disease in older patients. I think it will be a different world."

One of Kirklin's many major contributions was the use of his operating rooms and intensive care unit as laboratories to make systematic measurements and deductions on which to base

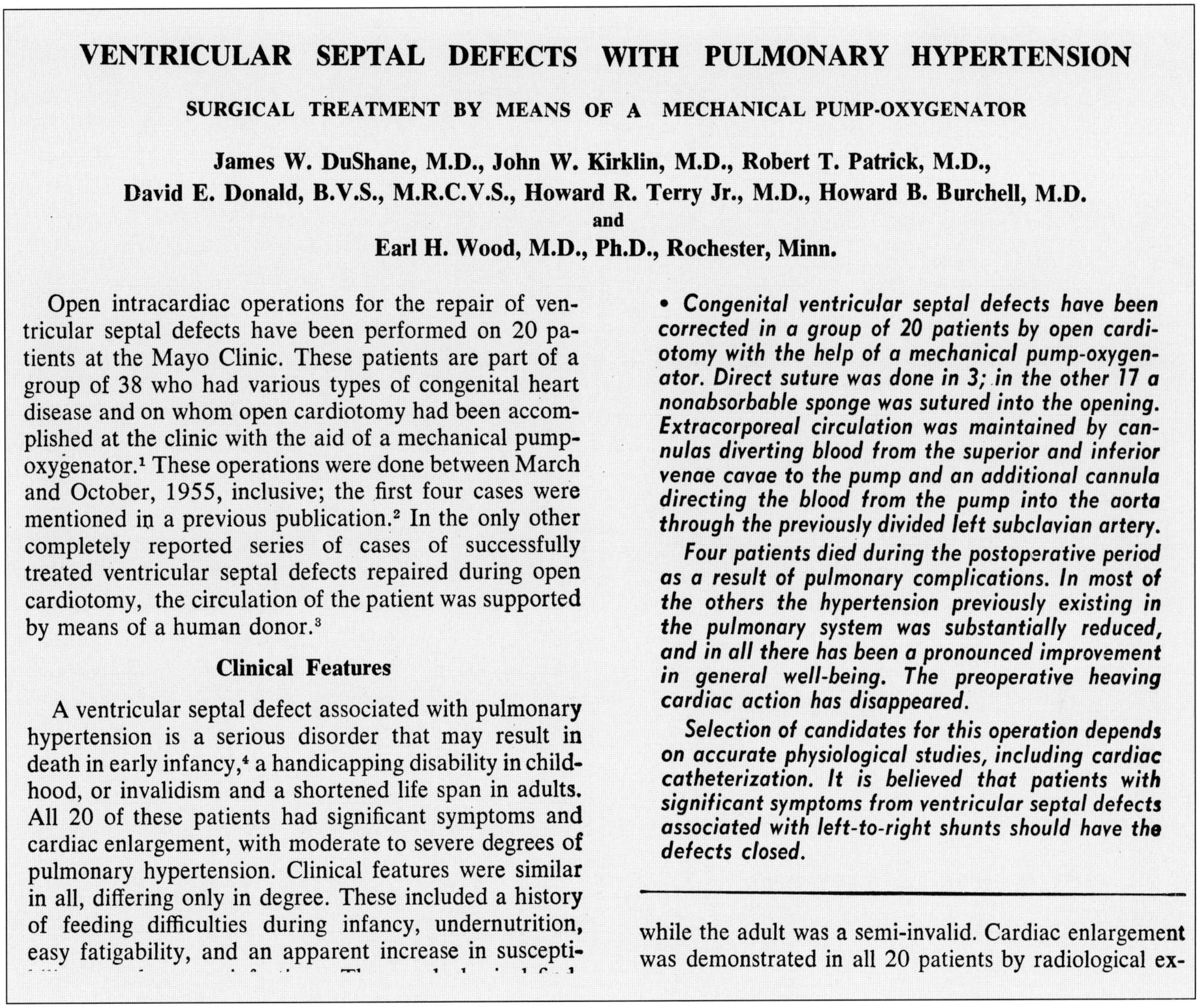

VENTRICULAR SEPTAL DEFECTS WITH PULMONARY HYPERTENSION

SURGICAL TREATMENT BY MEANS OF A MECHANICAL PUMP-OXYGENATOR

James W. DuShane, M.D., John W. Kirklin, M.D., Robert T. Patrick, M.D.,
David E. Donald, B.V.S., M.R.C.V.S., Howard R. Terry Jr., M.D., Howard B. Burchell, M.D.
and
Earl H. Wood, M.D., Ph.D., Rochester, Minn.

Open intracardiac operations for the repair of ventricular septal defects have been performed on 20 patients at the Mayo Clinic. These patients are part of a group of 38 who had various types of congenital heart disease and on whom open cardiotomy had been accomplished at the clinic with the aid of a mechanical pump-oxygenator.[1] These operations were done between March and October, 1955, inclusive; the first four cases were mentioned in a previous publication.[2] In the only other completely reported series of cases of successfully treated ventricular septal defects repaired during open cardiotomy, the circulation of the patient was supported by means of a human donor.[3]

Clinical Features

A ventricular septal defect associated with pulmonary hypertension is a serious disorder that may result in death in early infancy,[4] a handicapping disability in childhood, or invalidism and a shortened life span in adults. All 20 of these patients had significant symptoms and cardiac enlargement, with moderate to severe degrees of pulmonary hypertension. Clinical features were similar in all, differing only in degree. These included a history of feeding difficulties during infancy, undernutrition, easy fatigability, and an apparent increase in suscepti-

• Congenital ventricular septal defects have been corrected in a group of 20 patients by open cardiotomy with the help of a mechanical pump-oxygenator. Direct suture was done in 3; in the other 17 a nonabsorbable sponge was sutured into the opening. Extracorporeal circulation was maintained by cannulas diverting blood from the superior and inferior venae cavae to the pump and an additional cannula directing the blood from the pump into the aorta through the previously divided left subclavian artery.

Four patients died during the postoperative period as a result of pulmonary complications. In most of the others the hypertension previously existing in the pulmonary system was substantially reduced, and in all there has been a pronounced improvement in general well-being. The preoperative heaving cardiac action has disappeared.

Selection of candidates for this operation depends on accurate physiological studies, including cardiac catheterization. It is believed that patients with significant symptoms from ventricular septal defects associated with left-to-right shunts should have the defects closed.

while the adult was a semi-invalid. Cardiac enlargement was demonstrated in all 20 patients by radiological ex-

Figure 3.34. Ventricular septal defects with pulmonary hypertension: surgical treatment by means of a mechanical pump-oxygenator. *A 1955 article by Kirklin et al. (Reproduced with permission from* Journal of American Medical Association.)

formulae and nomograms to assist decision-making (Figure 3.36). These were used to indicate when, for a given cardiac lesion, the operation should be performed, and by which technique. "It is in the intensive care unit," he wrote, "that we reap the enormous and irreplaceable human rewards for all of our study and research." Kirklin believed that cardiac surgery should be scientific and reproducible, using international scientific language, research methods and proper statistical analysis when reporting results:

"When the rules and logic are correct, they are really better than human decisions, if only because they are reproducible in any setting. Now, getting the correct rules and logic is really difficult, but it can be done. If we are going to get along a little bit better, and to take the risks of operation say from 8 percent

to 4 percent, or 4 percent to 1 percent, or from 3 percent to 0.5 percent, we have to put in a great deal of new knowledge and a lot of new effort. So our job is to see if we can make those improvements like closed-loop interventions, automated history taking, automated decisions."

Kirklin possessed a unique ability to simplify and apply new surgical techniques by harvesting, distilling and presenting multifaceted experimental and clinical data in usable form. He was assisted in this for many years by the analytical genius, Eugene Blackstone, who supervised the residents' and fellows' research efforts (including those of the author). Kirklin's superb technical performance in large numbers of patients consistently produced excellent results and permitted him to make substantial contributions at each phase in the evolution of

SURGICAL TREATMENT FOR THE TETRALOGY OF FALLOT BY OPEN INTRACARDIAC REPAIR

John W. Kirklin, M.D., F. Henry Ellis, Jr., M.D., Dwight C. McGoon, M.D. (by invitation), James W. DuShane, M.D. (by invitation), and H. J. C. Swan, M.B., Ph.D. (by invitation), Rochester, Minn.

THE PROGRESSING invalidism usually imposed by the combination of malformations known as the "tetralogy of Fallot" has long stimulated search for effective treatment. Wide acclaim properly greeted the discovery of Blalock and Taussig[1] that an anastomosis between a systemic and pulmonary artery resulted in amelioration of cyanosis and polycythemia and improved exercise tolerance in the patient with tetralogy of Fallot. The beneficial effect of increased pulmonary blood flow was again demonstrated in the results obtained by Potts[2] utilizing anastomosis of the aorta and pulmonary artery. Brock[3] logically argued that pulmonary flow could be increased by directing the surgical endeavor toward relief of the pulmonary stenosis. He showed that good palliation could be achieved in many patients by pulmonary valvotomy and infundibular resection done by a closed technique. Many surgeons dreamed of complete repair of the tetralogy of Fallot, but it was first accomplished by Lillehei and associates in 1954 using whole body perfusion established by the technique of controlled cross-circulation.[4]

Figure 3.35. Surgical treatment for the tetralogy of Fallot by open intracardiac repair. *A 1959 article by Kirklin* et al. *(Reproduced with permission from* Journal of Thoracic Surgery.*)*

cardiac surgery. In a reflective mood towards the end of his operating career he said:

> "But after many years of cardiac surgery, and many tests and challenges from different operations, from patients, from colleagues, from difficult scientific and operational problems, and even more after too many deaths through the years that could not then be prevented, we tend gradually to become a little weary and in some small sense infinitely sad because of life's inevitabilities."

Now in his late seventies, John Kirklin is widely regarded as the foremost surgical scientist. Many of the world's leading cardiac surgeons were residents or research fellows at Mayo or U.A.B and have much to thank him for.

Author's note: With Kirklin, Pacifico, Kouchoukos and Karp all in the same unit, 1981 was a remarkable year at the University of Alabama, Birmingham. The residents' morning rounds began at 5 a.m. and Kirklin was called at 6 a.m. with a progress report on the patients. Surgery began after breakfast at 7 a.m. and usually lasted until the early evening. Morbidity and

Routine Primary Repair vs Two-stage Repair of Tetralogy of Fallot

JOHN W. KIRKLIN, M.D., EUGENE H. BLACKSTONE, M.D., ALBERT D. PACIFICO, M.D., ROBERT N. BROWN, B.S., AND LIONEL M. BARGERON, JR., M.D.

SUMMARY   Fifteen of 194 patients (7.7%) with tetralogy of Fallot operated upon since January 1, 1972 under a protocol of routine primary repair despite young age died in-hospital. Most deaths were from low cardiac output. Young age and smallness of size increased the risk of operation. No deaths occurred among patients older than 4 years. High hematocrit was also a risk factor. Transannular patching has an independent effect in increasing risk. The post-repair ratio of peak pressure in the right ventricle to that in the left did not exert an independent effect. To project current risks of a two-stage approach, we determined that five of 158 patients (3.2%) died in-hospital after secondary intracardiac repair after a previous Blalock-Taussig or Waterston anastomosis between 1967–1978. Using these data and those we have published on the risk of shunting, we project that except in very small babies, the risks of hospital death of a two-stage approach are not less than those of primary repair done without a transannular patch, except when body surface area is less than about 0.35 m². When a transannular patch is used in the primary repair, the two-stage approach is projected to be safer when the child has a body surface area of about 0.48 m² or smaller.

Figure 3.36. Routine primary repair vs. two-stage repair of tetralogy of Fallot. *A 1979 article by Kirklin* et al. *(Reproduced with permission from* Circulation.*)*

mortality were unacceptable particularly if through human error. Then there were evening rounds. There were full departmental academic meetings on Wednesday evening and Saturday morning beginning at 8 a.m. Topic presentations or journal reviews had to be flawless. On Sunday morning at 7 a.m., Kirklin and Blackstone held academic business meetings to review progress in the various research projects and finalize manuscripts. Kirklin usually went riding on Sunday afternoon. Blackstone went to church. The pace was unrelenting, particularly for the residents. When they complained of sleep deprivation through long nights in the ITU, Kirklin replaced them with clinical nurse practitioners. For the fellows, laboratory research alternated with operating theatre sessions. Follow-up for clinical reports was exhaustive with telephone calls to the coroner's office, prisons and overseas embassies (even Iran) if a patient could not be located. One fellow spent 2 years following 5000 coronary bypass patients to produce a single manuscript. This was the University of Alabama work ethic. Some thrived, others capitulated. Most of us came away with at least one prized paper and an attitude and plans for the future. The system produced good cardiac surgeons with the versatility to perform both paediatric and adult operations on a broad spectrum of clinical material.

William Wallace Lumpkin Glenn (1914–)

WILLIAM WALLACE LUMPKIN GLENN was born in Asheville, North Carolina. He studied at the University of South Carolina (BS, 1934), Jefferson Medical College (MD, 1938) and trained at the University of Pennsylvania and Massachusetts General Hospitals. He has been at Yale University School of Medicine since 1948, where he has been Professor of Cardiothoracic Surgery since 1962 (MA [Hon.] 1962) and is now Charles W. Ohse Professor Emeritus. Although best known for his circulatory bypass of the right side of the heart, he is also recognized, with Mauro, for intraoperative cardiac defibrillation devices which eventually yielded to totally implantable equipment.

Cyanotic children were first palliated by Blalock, Potts or Waterston shunts and in 1958, the superior vena cava/right pulmonary artery anastomosis was applied specifically to tricuspid atresia by Glenn (Article 3.5, Appendix A). The first experimental studies in the USA were carried out by Shumacker in Indiana, followed by the first partial and complete right heart bypass operations in cases so unsuitable that they were all unsuccessful. In 1956, the Russian, Meshalkin, had performed the first successful cavo-pulmonary anastomosis, though by virtue of prolific experimental and clinical work, Glenn's name is attached to the procedure. In 1957, Glenn at Yale and Sanger in North Carolina started experimental work on pulmonary artery vena caval anastomosis, after Glenn and Patiño in 1954 described increasing pulmonary blood flow by anastomosing the superior vena cava to the right pulmonary artery. Glenn's first clinical operation was performed on 25 February 1958. Glenn wrote to Stephen Westaby:

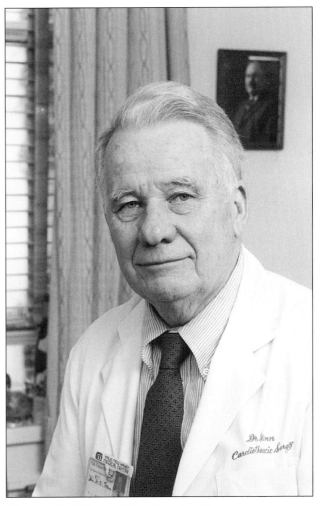

Figure 3.37. William Wallace Lumpkin Glenn.

"More than 40 years after a venous bypass of the right ventricle was proposed for treating patients with uncorrectable congenital malformations of the right side of the heart. Still there continues to be evaluation of operations that test the hypothesis that venous pressure alone is sufficient to propel the venous return through the pulmonary circuit. Investigation has proceeded along two courses, one that includes the pumping

CIRCULATORY BYPASS OF THE RIGHT SIDE OF THE HEART*

IV. Shunt between Superior Vena Cava and Distal Right Pulmonary Artery — Report of Clinical Application

WILLIAM W. L. GLENN, M.D.†

NEW HAVEN, CONNECTICUT

IN the first publication of this series of papers attention was called to the need of a method for the direct delivery of venous blood into the pulmonary arterial circulation.[1] The congenital anomalies of the heart that might be remedied from this operation are characterized by malfunction of the right atrium or right ventricle or both. More specifically, the cardiac conditions that would benefit from circulatory bypass of the right side of the heart include stenosis or atresia of the tricuspid and pulmonary outflow tracts, Ebstein's anomaly, single ventricle, bilocular heart and transposition of the great vessels with an associated pulmonary valvular stenosis. Also, in certain cases of pulmonary hypertension in which the changes in the pulmonary arterioles have not become irreversible, the direct delivery of systemic venous blood into the pulmonary arterial circulation may be beneficial at some time after temporary ligation of the right pulmonary artery. Finally, bypass of the right side of the heart may be indicated when there is obstruction of the cavae where they join the heart, or when there is an abnormal insertion of either cava into the left atrium. Other literature pertinent to this problem has been reviewed previously.[1-3]

*From the Department of Surgery, Yale University School of Medicine.

Supported in part by grants from the Victoria Foundation for Cardiovascular Research at Yale and United States Public Health Service (H851-C-7).

†Associate professor of surgery, Yale University School of Medicine.

Figure 3.38. Circulatory bypass of the right side of the heart. IV. Shunt between superior vena cava and distal right pulmonary artery — report of clinical application. *A 1958 article by Glenn (Reproduced with permission from* New England Journal of Medicine.)

force of the right atrium in the circuit and the other that excludes it. In the second circumstance, blood from either or both venae cavae being shunted instead directly into the pulmonary artery. Uncertain results with a right atrium–pulmonary artery shunt in laboratory animals and early failure of this in patients caused this course to be sidelined temporarily in the mid-1950s.

On the basis of extensive research with cavopulmonary artery shunts in dogs, superior vena cava–right pulmonary artery anastomosis was recommended for clinical trial. Diversion of inferior vena caval flow to the pulmonary artery was not recommended at that time, as pooling of venous blood below the diaphragm caused life-threatening hypovolemia in the immediate postoperative period. Long-term, ascites and congestive hepatomegaly resulted. The popularity of the SVC–RPA operation began to wane when it was apparent that after 5 to 8 years there was a gradual decline in oxygenation ascribed to a decrease in venous return to the shunted lung. Ways of increasing oxygenation consisted of shunting arterial blood to either lung, embolizing widened arteriovenous connections in the lower lobe of the shunted lung and ligating venous collaterals to the inferior vena cava. These caused a modest improvement in arterial oxygen saturation. To enable

perfusion of both lungs, the SVC–RPA operation was modified by the use of end-to-side anastomosis. This bidirectional shunt was first used in experiments in the 50s and 60s and was also applied to patients in the 60s.

In 1971, a major improvement in arterial oxygen saturation was gained when the right atrium to pulmonary artery shunt was revived. In general, the clinical results were excellent in selected cases. However, late-onset atrial dysrhythmias and the anatomical configuration of the atriopulmonary shunt have restricted its efficiency as a right heart bypass. Although the venous *vis a tergo generated during atrial systole should increase pulmonary bloodflow, this did not necessarily occur because of energy dissipation in the right atrium, greater resistance in the pulmonary vascular circuit relative to peripheral venous pressure.*

To take advantage of the full force of the vis a tergo *a tubular connection was made between the inferior and the superior vena cava intra-atrially. The SVC was transected above the right atrium and its central end anastomosed to the inferior side of the RPA. The peripheral end of the transected SVC was anastomosed to the superior side of the RPA to complete the bicaval connection to the pulmonary artery. In an effort to avoid an intracardiac procedure that may induce dysrhythmia,* an extracardiac shunt was introduced between the IVC and the PA using a tubular dacron graft. The initial clinical results of the total cavopulmonary artery operations have been favorable, and for high-risk patients have been improved by temporary venting (fenestration) of the bypass channel.

Is it realistic to expect the venous hemodynamics in homo sapiens erectus to be normal following bypass of the right heart? In evolution, the right heart becomes a more clearly defined muscular structure as we ascend in the vertebrate kingdom. This reflects the need for additional support of the vis a tergo for propelling the venous return through the pulmonary circuit. That such support is necessary for the maintenance of optimal circulatory dynamics is indicated by the increase in peripheral venous pressure and accumulation of extra vascular fluid postoperatively. That support is not necessary for survival is shown by the large number of patients who have benefited from right heart bypass operations. The first patient in our series (case report is reprinted herein), received a SVC–RPA shunt to treat single ventricle with pulmonary stenosis at the age of 7 and later had a supplementary atriopulmonary shunt. He is now 42 years old, physically active, married and employed full time, and is asymptomatic on digitalis and a diuretic. It is indeed encouraging that serious complications have not been prominent in many other long-term survivors of the total venous bypass operations."

Åke Senning (1915–)

ÅKE SENNING was born in Rativik, Sweden. He studied at Uppsala and Stockholm medical schools and became Associate Professor of Experimental Surgery at the University Thoracic Clinic, Karolinska Hospital, Stockholm (1956) and Professor of Surgery and Director of the University Surgical Clinic, Zurich (1961–85).

When Senning joined Crafoord at Sabbatsberg Hospital in 1948 he took over Crafoord's experimental laboratory. He immediately abandoned Björk's disc oxygenator because, as he told Björk, he could not duplicate his results. Together with Astradsson, an engineer from the AGA company, Senning constructed another pump-oxygenator, combining oxygen bubbles and wide rollers in a trough. In 1951, it was used successfully on dogs who survived 40 minutes of total cardiopulmonary bypass with right ventricular cardiotomy. In the same year, extracorporeal circulation was combined with hypothermia (26–28°C) to allow lower pump flows, thus diminishing blood trauma and the risk of perfusion complications. To avoid air embolism during cardiotomy, the heart was 'arrested' with electrically induced ventricular fibrillation, a technique which originated with Senning in 1952. Senning used cooling and rewarming with left ventricular bypass as his standard perfusion technique. The oxygenator was used only during intracardiac manipulations and when the right ventricle was unable to maintain sufficient pulmonary circulation. Left ventricular bypass was continued until normal body temperature was reached and the heart could be weaned from the pump.

On 8 October 1958, Senning inserted the first totally implantable pacemaker (developed by the engineer Elmquist of

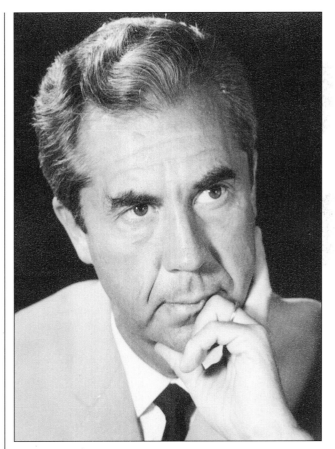

Figure 3.39. Åke Senning.

the Elema Company) in a patient with complete atrioventricular block. The aim was to avoid infection of transcutaneous electrodes which occurred along percutaneous pacemaker leads. That same month he also operated on a patient with stenosis of the left anterior descending circumflex and right coronary arteries. Endarterectomy of the left coronary was performed, and the arteriotomies were repaired with saphenous vein patches. Senning used autologous fascia lata to repair and reconstruct aortic valves in humans (1958).

He studied external counterpulsation with Clarence Dennis and Wesolowski and developed circulatory assist techniques using left heart bypass (1963). The Senning intra-atrial baffle repair of transposition was a surgical 'tour de force' and one of his most important contributions.

William Thornton Mustard (1914–1987)

WILLIAM THORNTON MUSTARD was born at Clinton, Ontario and studied at the University of Toronto (MD, 1937). He was awarded the MBE in 1941 following his military experience. During World War II, he bridged a lacerated artery with glass tubing — the first prosthetic material to conduct blood in human arteries. Although Mustard himself had only one success with this technique, the United States Army Medical Corp profited from his initiative by attempting to salvage limbs during the Korean War. Mustard, who had written a thesis on orthopaedic scoliosis (MS, 1947), became the Director of General, Orthopaedic and Cardiac Surgery at the Hospital for Sick Children (1947–76). His surgical advances include: the first total replacement blood transfusion in infancy; the iliopsoas muscle transfer for paralysed hip muscles (devised during an epidemic of poliomyelitis in Ontario); and a technique for overcoming prolonged spasm of major arteries. With Welch, Mustard edited the *Textbook of Paediatric Surgery* (1962) and wrote *Techniques in the Treatment of Congenital Heart Disease* (1965). In 1976, he received the Order of Canada.

Since the start of his career, Mustard was interested in correcting transposition of the great arteries (TGA). He attempted arterial repair of TGA in a 3-month-old girl on 17 January 1952 and in seven more babies in November of that year. A heart–lung machine, with monkey lungs as the biological oxygenator, was used. The procedure involved dividing the pulmonary artery about half an inch beyond the valve and then cutting the aorta obliquely. The right coronary artery was left on the proximal stump, but the left coronary artery was kept with the aorta. After dividing the aorta, Mustard perfused the left coronary artery with oxygenated blood pending reanastomosis. None of the babies lived more than a few hours.

In 1957 Mustard gave up general and orthopaedic surgery to devote himself entirely to finding a correction for TGA. He found Senning's operation difficult with a high mortality and believed a simpler repair possible. According to his resident, Firor, Mustard was so impressed by the progress of patients in whom a caval vein had been accidentally diverted into the left atrium during earlier closure of an atrial septal defect, that he

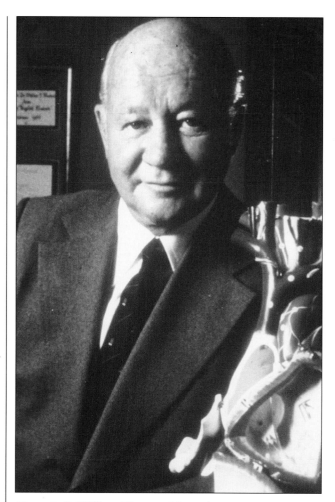

Figure 3.40. William Thornton Mustard.

decided to do it intentionally. He tried partitioning the atrial chambers with a pericardial patch, which worked well in dogs.

The Mustard operation was first attempted clinically on 16 May 1963 (Figure 3.41). After repairing a small ventricular septal defect using cardiopulmonary bypass in an 18-month-old girl who had previously undergone a Blalock– Hanlon septectomy, he excised the entire interatrial septum. Using autogenous pericardium, Mustard made a flap-like baffle that divided the atria into separate, functionally correct chambers. On the 16th birthday of Maria Surnoski, one of Mustard's early successes, he recalled his career's finest hour, when, after a horrifying moment during which he thought he had done the operation upside down, (red blood coursed through the

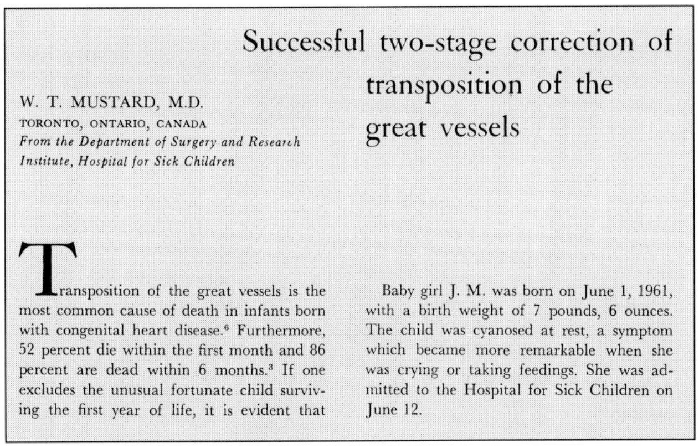

Successful two-stage correction of transposition of the great vessels

W. T. MUSTARD, M.D.
TORONTO, ONTARIO, CANADA
From the Department of Surgery and Research Institute, Hospital for Sick Children

Transposition of the great vessels is the most common cause of death in infants born with congenital heart disease.[6] Furthermore, 52 percent die within the first month and 86 percent are dead within 6 months.[3] If one excludes the unusual fortunate child surviving the first year of life, it is evident that

Baby girl J. M. was born on June 1, 1961, with a birth weight of 7 pounds, 6 ounces. The child was cyanosed at rest, a symptom which became more remarkable when she was crying or taking feedings. She was admitted to the Hospital for Sick Children on June 12.

Figure 3.41. Successful two-stage correction of transposition of the great vessels. A 1964 article by Mustard. (Reproduced with permission from Surgery.)

inferior vena cava) he realized it had worked perfectly. In 1982, Mustard's patient had borne her second child, was active and well although taking digitalis for moderate right ventricular enlargement. By the end of 1987, at the Hospital for Sick Children alone, 506 children had undergone the Mustard operation.

Technical modifications to avoid the complications of venous obstruction and arrhythmias were devised. Late right ventricular failure and tricuspid incompetence raised doubts about long-term prospects and stimulated the search for alternative methods. The Mustard operation prompted widespread interest in the management of TGA and although current results, particularly with neonates, suggest that arterial repair may displace the Mustard operation, it remains a milestone in the history of TGA.

Mustard was a mercurial and ebullient man. At a meeting in Houston, Texas, where Lord Brock was the guest speaker, Mustard, who had a passion for diving and spent most of his time in the pool at conferences, recognized the dark-suited man, climbed out, and said, "Hello, Sir. I did enjoy your lecture today." "Thank you, Dr Mustard," said Lord Brock, "It is tomorrow morning." On another occasion, after a particularly tense operation, when his residents had begun to close the chest, Mustard eased the pressure on the operating room staff by dropping to his knees and crawling out of the theatre on all fours. Outside, in the corridor, John Law, the administrator of the hospital, was escorting two VIPs on a tour of the building as the surgeon crawled toward them. "May I present our Chief of Cardiovascular Surgery," said the dignified Mr Law. The surgeon waved a paw and said, "If you live a dog's life you might as well behave like one," and kept on crawling, leaving John Law to explain as best he could.

Donald Nixon Ross (1922–)

DONALD NIXON ROSS was born in South Africa and studied at the University of Capetown (BSc; MB; ChB, 1946; FRCS, 1949). He was appointed senior registrar (1952), resident fellow (1953) and senior thoracic registrar (1954) at the Royal Infirmary, Bristol. He trained under Lord Brock at Guy's Hospital, where he became Consultant Thoracic Surgeon (1958).

In 1959, Ross and Brock described six methods of cardiac excision and replacement, including a method in which the native heart was separated from the venae cavae and pulmonary veins by sectioning the walls of the atria, thus forming both right and left atrial cuffs. This was the first method to combine the multiple pulmonary venous and venae caval anastomoses into two atrial anastomoses.

During a long and distinguished career at the National Heart Hospital, as Consultant (1963), Senior Surgeon (1967) and Director of the Department of Surgery (1970), Ross pioneered many surgical techniques in adults and children. He was responsible for describing the sinus venosus congenital defect. He performed the first cardiac transplant in the UK on 3 May 1968, the same day Denton Cooley performed his first transplant at St Luke's Hospital, Houston.

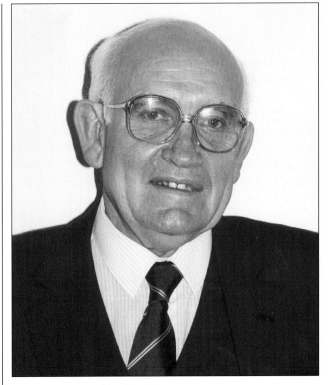

Figure 3.42. Donald Nixon Ross.

1446   DECEMBER 31, 1966   ORIGINAL ARTICLES   THE LANCET

CORRECTION OF PULMONARY ATRESIA WITH A HOMOGRAFT AORTIC VALVE

D. N. Ross
M.B., B.Sc. Cape Town, F.R.C.S.
CONSULTANT THORACIC SURGEON

JANE SOMERVILLE
M.D. Lond., M.R.C.P.
SENIOR LECTURER, INSTITUTE OF CARDIOLOGY

NATIONAL HEART HOSPITAL, LONDON W.1

IN any large series of patients with Fallot's tetralogy, a few will be found with a complete obstruction of the right ventricle at the pulmonary valve or infundibular level. Lillehei et al. (1955) first described the management of such a case by reimplanting the distal pulmonary artery into the right ventricle, and subsequently the practice has been to reconstruct the outflow tract with plastic material (Lillehei et al. 1964, Sabiston et al. 1964). Although these procedures relieve the obstruction of the right-ventricular outflow tract, significant pulmonary regurgitation inevitably results and imposes a serious volume load on the already hypertrophied right ventricle. In order to correct this, Lillehei has attempted to insert a monocusp valve and others have tried various pericardial reconstructions (Rastelli et al. 1965).

In view of the maintained function of the homograft aortic valve in the descending aorta (Murray 1956) and in the subcoronary position (Ross 1962, 1966), it was decided to use an aortic-valve homograft as a substitute for the absent pulmonary valve.

Case-report

This was an 8-year-old boy. Cyanosis was first noted at the age of 3 months and was constantly present after 1 year. Because of severe intolerance of effort he had to be

Electrocardiogram.—P pulmonale, right axis-deviation. R wave in V_1 32 mm. T inversion V_1–V_3.

Cardiac catheterisation.—The findings were as follows:

	Oxygen Saturation (%)	Pressure (mm. Hg)
Femoral artery ..	74	100/40
Superior vena cava	57	
Right atrium ..	57	a=4, v=0
Right ventricle ..	60	100/0

Angiocardiogram showed complete pulmonary-valve atresia. Pulmonary arteries filled from a possible ductus, and collaterals from a large right aortic arch.

Operation

Exploration by D. N. R. on Feb. 14, 1966, through a midsternal incision confirmed the presence of a large aorta, 3 cm. in diameter, and a main pulmonary artery 7 mm. across.

An attempt to find a way through the outflow tract was made by probing, and no connection was found between the right ventricle and main pulmonary artery. After hypothermic bypass was instituted, the right-ventricle outflow tract was opened through a vertical incision, and a blind-ended outflow was seen just beyond the hypertrophied infundibulum. A complete septum was present where the pulmonary valve should have been. A large ventricular septal defect, 2·5 × 1·5 cm., was closed with a 'Teflon' patch and multiple circumferential sutures.

The outflow tract was reconstructed by inserting a small homograft aortic valve with a segment of aorta above, and the anterior cusp of the mitral valve below, which acted as a gusset. A patch of pericardium was inserted between the anterior mitral cusp and a remaining defect in the ventriculotomy.

Postoperative systolic pressures in the main pulmonary artery and right ventricle were 60 mm. Hg when the aortic pressure was 75 mm. Hg.

Postoperative Course

After operation the patient developed features of pulmonary œdema, which was treated with tracheostomy and intermittent positive-pressure respiration as well as anti-failure medication.

Figure 3.43 Correction of pulmonary atresia with a homograft aortic valve. *A 1966 article by Ross and Somerville. (Reproduced with permission from* Lancet.)

Ross progressed from placing aortic valve homografts in the orthotopic position, in 1962, to using aortic homografts in right ventricular outflow reconstruction for the correction of pulmonary atresia in 1966 (Article 3.7, Appendix A). For Ross, this was one of the most important and wide-ranging developments in complex congenital heart disease. The striking feature of this type of reconstruction was that although the homograft aortic wall calcified early, especially in children, the conduit did not stenose and cusps remained functional for many years. This right ventricular outflow tract reconstruction with valve conduit has been called the 'Rastelli operation' (1969), although Ross described it before Rastelli. Kirklin used a right ventricle to pulmonary artery conduit for tetralogy of Fallot with pulmonary atresia in 1965.

Replacement of the pulmonary root with an aortic or pulmonary homograft was preferable to the use of dacron conduits containing a stent mounted pig valve.

Ross is best known for the formidable pulmonary autograft procedure for aortic valve replacement, which is now the treatment of choice for infants and children requiring aortic valve or aortic root replacement. Ross believed the acme of his biosurgical achievements came in 1967, when he autotransplanted the patient's pulmonary valve to the aortic position and, less well known but equally important, to the mitral position. He wrote:

"When one considers that the autogenous living pulmonary valve is immediately transferred to the aortic area, inserted freehand without delay or any form of chemical treatment, that is, conforming to our ideal criteria, you will not be surprised that these autografts function as you might expect when living cells are placed in their natural environment and with perfect design characteristics. In other words, they persist and function perfectly and do not show signs of degeneration. Although Shumway's team had reported some experimental moves in this

direction, this was the first clinical experience offering the prospect of a truly permanent living valve replacement. The problem of tissue failure adds weight to the safety of the autograft. Different sterilization and stage methods have not eliminated the problem of tissue failure as far as we are concerned. This feature has been the main stimulus responsible for our development of the pulmonary autograft operation, which we consider to offer a permanent valve uniquely suited to children and young adults."

Ross demonstrated that the autogenous pulmonary valve excised from its own position and transplanted into the aorta grows naturally with the child, with an almost indefinite life span. Because of the technical difficulties, including potential damage to the left anterior descending coronary and its principal septal branch, together with the prolonged duration of the procedure, the Ross operation was initially adopted by relatively few surgeons. With improved methods for myocardial protection, the 'Ross operation' is now performed with increasing frequency. Encouraged by the impressive function of the autogenous pulmonary valve in the aortic position, Ross advocated use of the pulmonary homograft, for aortic valve replacement.

For many years Ross worked closely with the formidable paediatric cardiologist Jane Somerville at the National Heart Hospital. Somerville was most particular about whom she allowed to operate on her children and liked to 'orchestrate' the procedure whenever possible. With an enormous experience of surgical follow-up Somerville is now the foremost authority on congenital heart disease in adolescence and adult life.

Ross was Yacoub's teacher and the pre-eminent cardiac surgeon in Britain during the last 25 years. Many believe he should have been honoured with a knighthood.

Gian Carlo Rastelli (1933–1970)

GIAN CARLO RASTELLI was born in Pescara, Italy. He attended the Classical Lyceum of Romagna and studied at the University of Parma (MD, 1957), where he won the Lepetit Prize for the best thesis. He fulfilled internship and residency at the University of Parma Hospital (1958–61). Rastelli entered the Mayo Graduate School of Medicine as a North Atlantic Treaty Organization (NATO) scholar in 1961 and became a research assistant (1962–64) and research associate (1964–68). During this time he received the Allen Welkind Award for outstanding research in cardiovascular surgery in 1965 and the Mayo Clinic Staff Memorial Award in 1968. Two exhibits concerned with advancements in cardiovascular surgery, of which he was a co-author, received awards from the American Medical Association: the Billings Gold Medal in 1968 and the Hektoen Gold Medal for originality of investigation in 1969. In May 1968, he was appointed a Mayo Foundation Scholar in cardiovascular surgical research; then in December of the same year, Head of Cardiovascular Surgical Research and finally, Head of the Cardiovascular Surgery programme at St Mary's Hospital, Rochester.

Rastelli was diagnosed as having Hodgkin's disease in the late 1960s and elected to return to the laboratory to continue his investigative work. It was during this period that he developed his classification of atrio-ventricular canal defects (Article 3.8, Appendix A) and the method for correction of transposition of the great arteries with ventricular septal defect and pulmonary stenosis, called the 'Rastelli operation'. He worked fervently right up to his death, after which the

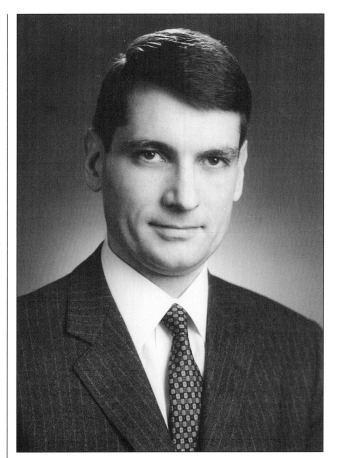

Figure 3.44. Gian Carlo Rastelli.

University of Parma named a new cardiovascular centre in his honour.

Surgical repair of the complete form of persistent common atrioventricular canal

G. C. Rastelli, M.D., Patrick A. Ongley, M.D., John W. Kirklin, M.D., and Dwight C. McGoon, M.D., Rochester, Minn.

Repair of the complete form of persistent common atrioventricular (A-V) canal with its severe anatomic derangement is still a formidable task for the cardiovascular surgeon. With the exception of Gerbode and Sabar's[1] report of only one surgical death in 13 cases, the surgical mortality has been 63, 75, and 67 per cent in reported series.[2-4] The technique of repair is far from standardized, and the reports of long-term follow-up have been too scarce to allow appraisal of late results. The whole experience of repair of this lesion at the Mayo Clinic is reviewed herein.* The technical problems of repair are analyzed in the light of new anatomic observations on pathologic ma-

terial, and a more appropriate repair, used in recent operations, is described.

Material

A total of 38 patients were operated upon between December, 1955, and September, 1967.* There were 21 females and 17 males; the median age was 6 years (range, 10 months to 51 years). Most of the patients had severe symptoms, including heart failure. Clinically mild cyanosis was present in 5 patients; severe cyanosis was present in 2 who had associated pulmonary stenosis. The average preoperative cardiothoracic ratio was 0.62 (range, 0.48 to 0.78). The electrocardiogram showed a negative mean frontal plane QRS axis between –45 degrees

Figure 3.45. Surgical repair of the complete form of persistent common atrioventricular canal. *A 1968 article by Rastelli* et al. *(Reproduced with permission from* Journal of Thoracic and Cardiovascular Surgery.)

Early experiences with complete forms of atrioventricular canal gave poor results before the Rastelli classification was published in 1966 by Rastelli and Kirklin. On the basis of the improved pathological description, surgical success with the more complicated forms of complete atrioventricular canal was achieved by the late 1960s.

The association of severe pulmonic stenosis with ventricular septal defect proved a formidable challenge to the intra-atrial method of physiological repair of TGA devised by Mustard and Senning. In 1969, Rastelli conceived of intraventricular rerouting of left ventricular output through the ventricular septal defect to the aorta, together with a new right ventricular outflow through the ventriculotomy via an extracardiac conduit to the pulmonary artery. By the early 1970s, repair could be accomplished with a high degree of success, even when conducted on infants. This procedure opened possibilities for the total correction of various congenital anomalies, including persistent truncus arteriosus, and pulmonary atresia with ventricular septal defect.

Dwight Charles McGoon (1925–)

DWIGHT CHARLES McGOON was born in Marengo, Iowa. He studied at Johns Hopkins (MD, 1948), where he and

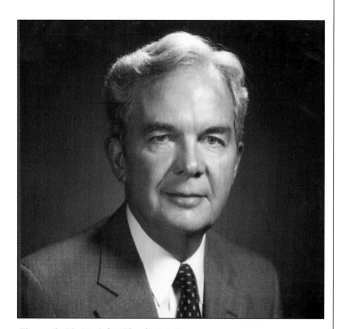

Figure 3.46. Dwight Charles McGoon.

Complete repair of truncus arteriosus defects

Robert B. Wallace, M.D. (by invitation), G. C. Rastelli, M.D. (by invitation), Patrick A. Ongley, M.B., Ch.B. (by invitation), Jack L. Titus, M.D. (by invitation), and Dwight C. McGoon, M.D., Rochester, Minn.

Previous attempts at complete repair of a truncus arteriosus have been unsuccessful.[1, 2] Recently, 3 patients have undergone successful repair of this anomaly with the use of a homograft of the ascending aorta and aortic valve to construct a pulmonary trunk.

Case reports

CASE 1. A 5½-year-old boy was first seen at the Mayo Clinic in April, 1962, at 14 months of age because of recurrent respiratory infections, cyanosis, exertional dyspnea, and failure to gain in height and weight. A cardiac murmur had been noted since birth. Cardiac catheterization and angiocardiography demonstrated a truncus arteriosus defect, apparently type 1. Digitalis was prescribed and he was dismissed.

The patient was readmitted in September, 1967. During the interim he had had frequent respiratory infections and his exercise tolerance had decreased considerably. He did not appear cyanotic at rest but mild cyanosis developed with exercise. The heart was overactive. A loud single second sound was audible at the second left intercostal space, an ejection murmur (Grade 3 on the basis of 1 to 6) along the upper left sternal border, and a separate continuous murmur, Grade 3, in the same area. A decrescendo

diastolic murmur was audible along the left sternal border. The electrocardiogram showed a normal sinus rhythm, a QRS axis of +70 degrees in the frontal plane, and hypertrophy of both right and left ventricles. The roentgenogram of the thorax showed evidence of an enlarged heart (cardiothoracic index of 0.67), a left aortic arch, and a mild increase in pulmonary vascular markings.

A second cardiac catheterization was performed (Table I). The oxygen saturation of the arterial blood was 89 per cent. The systolic gradients between the truncus arteriosus and the distal right and left pulmonary arteries were 42 and 53 mm. Hg, respectively. The ratio of pulmonary to systemic blood flow was 1.8 and the ratio of pulmonary to systemic vascular resistance was 0.38. There was a left-to-right shunt of 52 per cent and a right-to-left shunt of 31 per cent. Selective angiocardiograms from the right ventricle and a thoracic aortogram demonstrated a ventricular septal defect and a truncus arteriosus, apparently of type 1, with a short pulmonary trunk originating from the dorsal aspect of the truncus and immediately dividing into a right and a left pulmonary artery (Fig. 1). The truncus valve appeared to have four cusps and the aortogram showed it to have minimal incompetence directed toward the right ventricle.

Figure 3.47. Complete repair of truncus arteriosus defects. *A 1969 article by McGoon* et al. *(Reproduced with permission from* Surgery, Gynecology and Obstetrics.)

Jerome Harold Kay were co-chief residents to Alfred Blalock (1953–54). After 2 years in the medical corps of the US Air Force and as surgical consultant to the Surgeon General for the European Theatre of Operations, McGoon was the first Hopkins resident in surgery to join the Mayo Clinic (1956) and John Kirklin's progressive cardiac surgery programme. He was appointed to the staff of the Mayo Clinic as Head of the Section of General Surgery and became Professor of Surgery in the Mayo School of Medicine (1957). Ravitch described him as

"quiet, modest, a masterful technician achieving results in the 'standard' operations of cardiac surgery ranking with the

world's best, presenting in some areas of complicated congenital anomalies a dazzling and almost unique experience which has led to his being termed 'Mr Surgery-of-the-Impossible' in congenital heart disease and a quiet perfectionist in speech, manuscript and operation."

He has been the editor of the *Journal of Thoracic and Cardiovascular Surgery* (1977), a prolific and learned contributor to the literature of cardiac surgery and one of the editors of *Classics of Cardiology*, with Callahan and Key.

In 1968, McGoon, Rastelli and Wallace recorded the first successful repair of truncus arteriosus.

Robert B. Wallace (1931–)

ROBERT B. WALLACE was born in Washington, DC and studied at Columbia University and Columbia University School of Medicine, New York City (BA, 1953; MD, 1957). He served internship (1957–58) and residency in surgery (1958–62) at St Vincent's Hospital. After residency in thoracic surgery at Baylor University (1962–63), he became a Fellow and First Assistant in Cardiovascular Surgery (1963–64) and Consultant in Surgery (1964–69) at the Mayo Clinic. Wallace was instructor and Associate Professor of Surgery at the Mayo Graduate School of Medicine (1969–73), Professor of Surgery, Mayo Medical School (1973–79) and Chairman, Department of Surgery, Mayo Clinic (1968–79). He has been Professor of Surgery at Georgetown University School of Medicine, Washington, DC since 1980 and in 1994–95, was President of the American Association for Thoracic Surgery. Wallace described the first successful repair of truncus arteriosus in the *Journal of Thoracic and Cardiovascular Surgery* in 1969.

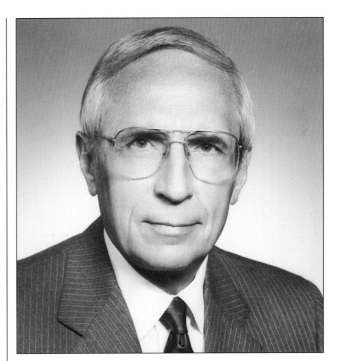

Figure 3.48. Robert B. Wallace.

François Maurice Fontan (1929–)

FRANÇOIS MAURICE FONTAN was born at Nay in the region of the Pyrénées Atlantique. He has been Assistant Surgeon (1960–63) and Surgeon to the Bordeaux Hospitals and Professor of Surgery at the University of Bordeaux since 1963. Fontan is a member of the French Society of Cardiology, French Society of Thoracic Surgery and French College of Vascular Diseases. In 1959, he wrote *Anoxic Cardiac Arrest in Extracorporeal Circulation*.

As early as 1943, Starr and co-workers destroyed

approximately 75% of right ventricular musculature by cautery without producing an increase in peripheral venous pressure. This confirmed that extensive right ventricular damage was not incompatible with life.

Complete bypass of the right ventricle was first performed by Fontan and Baudet for patients with tricuspid atresia. Glenn's work with cavopulmonary anastomosis and partial right heart bypass was the conceptual stimulus for Fontan's operation. By applying existing knowledge to properly selected patients they dramatically improved the prognosis of children with tricuspid atresia (TA) and other forms of univentricular heart. The

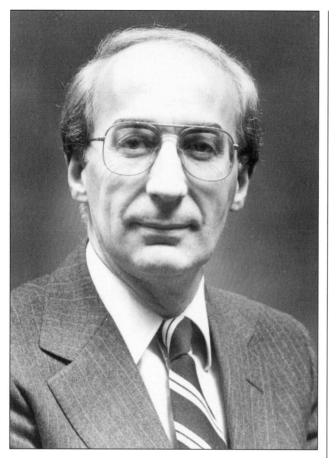

Figure 3.49. François Maurice Fontan.

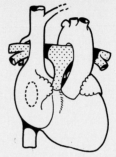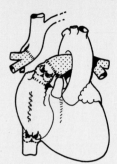

Surgical repair of tricuspid atresia

F. FONTAN and E. BAUDET

Centre de Cardiologie, Université de Bordeaux II, Hôpital du Tondu, Bordeaux, France

Surgical repair of tricuspid atresia has been carried out in three patients; two of these operations have been successful. A new surgical procedure has been used which transmits the whole vena caval blood to the lungs, while only oxygenated blood returns to the left heart. The right atrium is, in this way, 'ventriclized', to direct the inferior vena caval blood to the left lung, the right pulmonary artery receiving the superior vena caval blood through a cava-pulmonary anastomosis. This technique depends on the size of the pulmonary arteries, which must be large enough and at sufficiently low pressure to allow a cava-pulmonary anastomosis. The indications for this procedure apply only to children sufficiently well developed. Younger children or those whose pulmonary arteries are too small should be treated by palliative surgical procedures.

Only palliative operations (systemic vein to pulmonary artery anastomosis; systemic artery to pulmonary artery anastomosis) have been performed in tricuspid atresia. Although these procedures are valuable, they result in only a partial clinical improvement, because they do not suppress the mixture of venous and oxygenated blood.

We have initiated a corrective procedure for tricuspid atresia, which completely suppresses blood mixing. The entire vena caval return undergoes arterialization in the lungs and only oxygenated blood comes back to the left heart. This procedure is not an anatomical correction, which would require the creation of a right ventricle, but a procedure of physiological pulmonary blood flow restoration, with suppression of right and

FIG. 1. *Case 2. Tricuspid atresia type II B. Drawing illustrates steps in surgical repair: (1) end-to-side anastomosis of distal end of right pulmonary artery to superior vena cava; (2) end-to-end anastomosis of right atrial appendage to proximal end of right pulmonary artery by means of an aortic valve homograft; (3) closure of atrial septal defect; (4) insertion of a pulmonary valve homograft into inferior vena cava; and (5) ligation of main pulmonary artery.*

Figure 3.50. Surgical repair of tricuspid atresia. A 1971 article by Fontan and Baudet. (Reproduced with permission from Thorax.)

Fontan operation has become increasingly useful for other forms of complex congenital heart disease not amenable to complete intracardiac repair and when pulmonary stenosis has protected the pulmonary vasculature from injury.

In 1968, complete separation of the right and left circulations was achieved by Fontan by performing cavopulmonary connection through direct anastomosis between the right atrial appendage and the proximal end of the divided pulmonary artery. In Fontan's second and third patients he used a valved aortic homograft conduit between the right atrium and right pulmonary artery. All three patients received an aortic homograft valve in the inferior vena caval orifice together with closure of the patent foramen ovale or atrial septal defect operation and division of the main pulmonary artery. The Fontan operation has been modified on numerous occasions. Kreutzer, in 1973 dislocated the patient's main pulmonary artery with the valve intact and anastomosed the pulmonary root to the right atrial appendage. Björk described direct anastomosis between the right atrial appendage and right ventricular outflow tract for patients with an outflow chamber and normal pulmonary valve (1979).

The concept of an operation for tricuspid atresia that eliminated shunting, both congenitally and surgically acquired, still stands as one of the major breakthroughs in congenital heart surgery (Article 3.9, Appendix A). Before 1971, shunts (systemic artery or superior vena cava to pulmonary artery) were used for the majority of patients with TA with restricted pulmonary bloodflow. Alternatively, a Brock procedure (enlargement of ventricular septal defect) was occasionally used, also to increase left-to-right shunting. Compared with the more common cyanotic disorders, shunts carried a higher operative mortality in TA patients; Taussig and Bauersfeld reported an 8-month postoperative mortality of 26% after the Blalock–Taussig shunt. Sommers and Johnson reported that two thirds of all patients with TA died before 1 year of age owing to congestive failure and anoxia, whether or not operation had been performed.

A distinguished French gentleman, Fontan has made many important contributions in cardiac surgery and has received many international honours. He continues to operate in his retirement and produces excellent wine from his vineyards.

Aldo R. Castaneda (1930–)

ALDO R. CASTANEDA was born in Genoa, Italy where his parents landed en route from Guatemala to Germany. He spent his childhood and adolescence in Munich under the Nazi regime. Castaneda came from a distinguished medical family in Guatemala, where both his father and uncle were professors at the medical school. He returned home to enrol in the medical school at the University of Guatemala (MD, 1957).

While a medical student, Castaneda met Louis Diamond, Senior Physician at the Children's Hospital, when Diamond visited Guatemala. Young Castaneda acted as an interpreter to Diamond, who, being much impressed by him, was anxious to help him obtain the best possible training in surgery — his chosen career. He arranged for Castaneda to go to Boston and be interviewed by Gross for a job in his surgical training programme. Castaneda went to Boston, saw Gross, but nothing came of it.

Castaneda pursued postdoctoral training at the Hospital General de Guatemala (1957–58) and entered the surgical

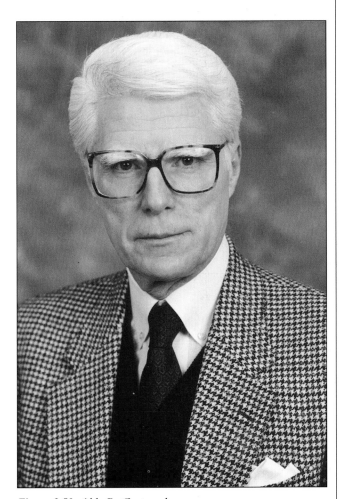

Figure 3.51. Aldo R. Castaneda.

Open-heart surgery during the first three months of life

Twenty-eight of 70 infants (40 per cent) with critical congenital heart disease required corrective surgery within the first 3 months of life. They were operated upon by means of deep hypothermia with surface cooling and limited cardiopulmonary bypass. These infants weighed between 2 and 5 kilograms. Twenty-six (93 per cent) of these patients had correctable lesions: ventricular septal defect (VSD), 9 infants; tetralogy of Fallot, 6 infants; d-transposition of the great arteries (d-TGA) with intact ventricular septum, 4 patients; d-TGA with VSD, 2 infants; total anomalous pulmonary venous connection (TAPVC), 4 children, and aortic stenosis, 1 patient. Twenty-two (85 per cent) of these patients survived. Two other infants died because the lesions were noncorrectable: a 1-day-old infant with rhabdomyoma and a 30-day-old infant with both Type II truncus arteriosus and complete endocardial cushion defect. The technique of deep hypothermia with surface cooling and limited cardiopulmonary bypass proved very useful in these tiny infants, because it provides optimal operative conditions. The bloodless and motionless operating field and the absence of intracardiac cannulas and suction lines permit delicate technical maneuvers inside the very small heart.

Aldo R. Castaneda, M.D., John Lamberti, M.D. (by invitation), Robert M. Sade, M.D. (by invitation), Roberta G. Williams, M.D. (by invitation), and Alexander S. Nadas, M.D. (by invitation), *Boston, Mass.*

Figure 3.52. Open-heart surgery during the first three months of life. *A 1974 article by Castaneda* et al. *(Reproduced with permission from* Journal of Thoracic and Cardiovascular Surgery.*)*

training programme at the University of Minnesota (1958–63). He specialized in surgery (PhD, 1963) and physiology (MS, 1964) and finally became Professor of Surgery (1963–72) there. Castaneda, whose surgical brilliance was recognized early, was strongly influenced by Wangensteen and Lillehei as well as Varco, whose right-hand man he eventually became. While at the University of Minnesota he carried out extensive laboratory work on the effect of cardiopulmonary bypass on formed blood elements and the use of cardiopulmonary bypass for combined heart–lung autotransplantation in primates. He then applied his laboratory work to the correction of complicated cardiac lesions in the first few months of life, using deep hypothermia and circulatory arrest (Figure 3.52).

In September 1972, Castaneda succeeded Gross as Chief of Cardiovascular Surgery at Boston Children's Hospital and in 1975, became the third William E. Ladd Professor of Surgery at Harvard Medical School and Cardiovascular Surgeon-in-Chief at the Children's Hospital. Gross, who retired in June 1972, was pleased by the selection of a practical, no-nonsense operating surgeon with an interest in the laboratory as his successor.

Castaneda wrote about his continued concern for early repair of congenital heart defects:

"In general, we have pursued, during the last two decades, the philosophy of earliest possible repair of complex congenital heart defects. We have made much progress. For example, anatomic repair of transposition of the great arteries with the arterial

switch operation was initiated at our institution by preference within the first 2 weeks of life with a mortality of 1%. Also, the risk of other complex congenital lesions, including truncus arteriosus corrected in neonates, is similar to our TGA results. We are accumulating solid hemodynamic evidence that early repair is advantageous for the heart and the lungs, after the

arterial switch operation. We will have to wait for another few years before some longer term information becomes available. Although there were some initial concerns by many colleagues in paediatric cardiac surgery, I think that the notion of early repair has now gained much support and is being practised worldwide."

Adib Dominges Jatene (1921–)

ADIB DOMINGES JATENE was born in 1921 in Xapuri, Brazil. He studied at the School of Medicine at the University of São Paulo (MD, 1953) and pursued postgraduate studies under Zerbini at the Hospital de Clinicas. He started a thoracic surgery group in Uberaba, Minas Gerais, Brazil and built the first heart–lung machine in that region. Jatene was Professor of Topographic Anatomy at the Medical School of Triangulo Mineiro (1955–57).

While at the Hospital de Clinicas and the Dante Pazzanese Institute of Cardiology (1958–61), Jatene built the university hospital's first heart–lung machine in an experimental laboratory which he developed into a large bioengineering department. In 1961, he left the Hospital de Clinicas to work exclusively for the Dante Pazzanese Institute of Cardiology (1961–83), where he was Head of the Experimental Research Laboratory, Head of the Department of Surgery and Medical and General Director, successively. Jatene also organized another bioengineering facility where he developed valvular prostheses, a pacemaker and a bubble oxygenator. The Jatene–Macchi disposable oxygenator is still used in Brazil as well as internationally.

In 1983 Jatene succeeded Zerbini as Professor of Thoracic Surgery at the School of Medicine and as Director of the Heart Institute at the University of São Paulo. Jatene has been Surgeon-in-Chief at the Children's Hospital since 1981. He has also been Brazil's Minister of Health since February 1992. He is the author or co-author of more than 700 scientific papers, a member of 50 scientific societies throughout the world and recipient of 168 titles from more than 10 countries.

The 'Jatene operation' (Article 3.10, Appendix A) varied from previous arterial switch procedures in that the aorta and pulmonary artery were divided distally from the aortic and pulmonary valves, avoiding coronary artery and valve distortion. The coronary arteries were removed with a button of aortic wall, facilitating the anastomosis to the neoaorta. The ventricular septal defect was closed with a Dacron patch through a right ventriculotomy.

At the 1976 meeting of the American Association for Thoracic Surgery, Jatene presented two successful cases and, in

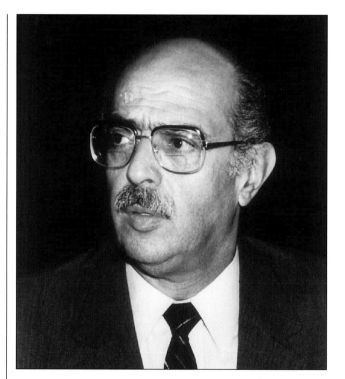

Figure 3.53. Adib Dominges Jatene.

Anatomic correction of transposition of the great vessels

We present a new approach for anatomic correction of transposition of the great arteries. The two coronary arteries, with a piece of the aortic wall attached, are transposed to the posterior artery. The two aortic openings are closed with a patch. The aorta and pulmonary artery are transected, contraposed, and then anastomosed. The interventricular septal defect is closed with a patch, through a right ventriculotomy approach, because the right ventricle is no longer part of the systemic circulation. Two patients, aged 3 months and 40 days and weighing 4,200 and 3,700 grams, respectively, were operated upon with deep hypothermia and total circulatory arrest. There was good recovery from the operation, with normal cardiocirculatory conditions. Renal failure developed in the first patient, and she died on the third postoperative day. During this time the cardiocirculatory conditions were good. The second patient made an uneventful recovery. Hemodynamic studies 20 days after the operation showed complete correction of the malformation. Five and one-half months after the operation, he weighs 7,500 grams, and his development is very good. We believe that this operation will be reproducible by most cardiovascular surgeons and will be an alternative to the Mustard procedure, especially for those patients with interventricular septal defect and pulmonary hypertension.

Adib D. Jatene, M.D. (by invitation), V. F. Fontes, M.D. (by invitation), P. P. Paulista, M.D. (by invitation), L. C. B. Souza, M.D. (by invitation), F. Neger, M.D. (by invitation), M. Galantier, M.D. (by invitation), and J. E. M. R. Sousa, M.D. (by invitation), *São Paulo, Brazil*
Sponsored by E. J. Zerbini, M.D., *São Paulo, Brazil*

Figure 3.54. Anatomic correction of transportation of the great vessels. *A 1976 article by Jatene* et al . *(Reproduced with permission from* Journal of Thoracic Cardiovascular Surgery.)

his comment, included five more patients, all of whom died. After the early experience of Jatene and others, attention was turned to modifications. Although Jatene's repair initially used no graft material in the aortic or pulmonary anastomosis, conduits and graft material were introduced to prevent tension or obstruction. Lecompte and associates (1981) placed the aorta behind the dissected pulmonary artery reducing tension and eliminating the need for a prosthetic graft. Modifications of Jatene's repair have been devised so that all but a few coronary patterns can be successfully repaired. In 1987, John Kirklin said,

"There is a very small place for the Senning or Mustard operation. I think that it will not be long that surgeons will not know how to do those operations because the arterial switch seems quite clearly to be a better operation, can be done in the first few weeks of life, no repeated hospitalizations and delayed surgery. I think it is one of the major changes in pediatric cardiac surgery in recent years."

Magdi Yacoub (1935–)

MAGDI YACOUB was born in Cairo, Egypt, the son of a village doctor. He studied medicine at the University of Cairo followed by postgraduate work in the UK (FRCS [Eng.]; FRCS [Ed.]; FRCS [Glas.]; MRCS [Eng.]; LRCP [Lond.]). He was Assistant Professor of Cardiothoracic Surgery at the University of Chicago. Since 1969 he has been Consultant Cardiothoracic Surgeon at the Harefield Hospital and to the National Heart Hospital, London. He is now Professor of Cardiac Surgery at the National Heart and Lung Institute at the Brompton Hospital (since 1986).

As a result of Sir Magdi's pioneering techniques in heart–lung transplants, Harefield Hospital has become Britain's leading transplant centre. It is renown internationally, not only for the 200 or more heart transplants performed there each year, but also for its pioneering work in paediatric cardiac surgery (Figure 3.56).

Sir Magdi started performing transplants in 1974 and was responsible for Britain's first combined heart–lung graft at Harefield in December 1983. He conducted the world's first 'domino' transplant, in which a patient with lung disease received a new compatible heart and lungs while donating his own healthy heart to another patient. Sir Magdi remains passionately opposed to artificial hearts. He remains unconvinced of their long-term ability to make up the shortfall of available human organs. He believes that,

"Transplant patients who receive human organs can, by and large, enjoy a very good quality of life —70% are well enough to travel extensively, have children and lead normal lives. I think it will be very hard to match that standard with artificial hearts."

Anatomical correction of complete transposition of the great arteries and ventricular septal defect in infancy

M H YACOUB, R RADLEY-SMITH, C J HILTON

British Medical Journal, 1976, 1, 1112-1114

Summary

Two patients, aged 8 weeks and 5 years, with D transposition of great arteries and large ventricular septal defect were treated by transection of both aorta and pulmonary arteries and reattaching them to the appropriate ventricles. This included the origins of the coronary arteries. The ventricular septal defect was closed through a transverse ventriculotomy using a Dacron patch. The younger child was operated on as an emergency because of cyanosis and severe heart failure resistant to intensive medical treatment. The older child had had previous banding of the pulmonary artery at the age of 1 year. In both patients pulmonary artery pressure dropped to below half systemic pressure immediately after the operation. Postoperative progress was satisfactory with relief of cyanosis and heart failure. Early anatomical correction of transposition of the great arteries and ventricular septal defect is feasible and should play an important part in the management of these patients.

months with progressive cyanosis and tachypnoea. In spite of full medical treatment (digitalis and diuretics) his respiratory rate was 80/minute, his liver was palpable three fingers below the costal margin, and he required tube feeding. The chest radiograph showed increasing cardiomegaly with plethoric lung fields (fig 1). On 29 October 1975 his condition deteriorated further and it was decided that operation should be performed as soon as possible. This was performed the next day. At that time he weighed 4350 g.

Surface-induced profound hypothermia combined with cardio-pulmonary bypass and circulatory arrest was used. The ascending aorta, aortic arch, and main pulmonary artery were mobilised. The ligamentum arteriosum was divided. The anteriorly placed ascending aorta was transected 3 mm above the top of the sinuses of Valsalva. The pulmonary artery, which was about twice the size of the aorta, was transected at the same level. The coronary ostia with a cuff of aortic wall about 1 mm wide were detached from the aorta and anastomosed to the corresponding sinuses of Valsalva of the pulmonary valve using 7/0 sutures. The proximal end of the pulmonary artery was then anastomosed to the distal end of the ascending aorta using 6/0 sutures. To match the size of the aorta to the large pulmonary artery the former was incised longitudinally on its posterior surface before starting the anastomosis. The defects in the aortic sinuses, produced by detachment of the coronary ostia, were then repaired using two patches of autogenous tissue (pericardium for one defect and free pulmonary arterial wall for the other). The proximal end of the aorta was then joined to the distal end of the pulmonary artery using a 10-mm Dacron graft.

Figure 3.55. Anatomical correction of complete transposition of the great arteries and ventricular septal defect in infancy. *A 1976 article by Magdi Yacoub* et al. *(Reproduced with permission from* British Medical Journal.)

A pupil of Donald Ross, Yacoub is also a great protagonist of homograft and autograft techniques with a dislike for mechanical valves. He is a pioneer of aortic root repair and the switch operation for transposition; techniques which adequately reflect his enormous technical ability. This together with an incomprehensibly frenetic work rate—seeing outpatients in the early hours of the morning—have made Yacoub a legend in cardiac surgery.

Chapter 4: Development of surgery for valvular heart disease

THE 10-YEAR period around the turn of the 19th century could be regarded as a time of discovery in cardiac surgery. In 1897, Herbert Milton, of the Kasr El Aini Hospital in Cairo, sent an article to the *Lancet* in which he described his sternum-splitting incision for access to the chest. This was a landmark in itself. Milton remarked that, "Heart surgery is still quite in its infancy, but it requires not a great stretch of fancy to imagine the possibility of plastic operations of its valvular lesions." Milton's article had little impact at the time, but the following year, Daniel Samways suggested that the obstructed valve in rheumatic mitral stenosis might be amenable to surgical enlargement. His first article in the *British Medical Journal* explained that the characteristic alteration in the left atrium in mitral stenosis was hypertrophy and not dilatation. He considered (contrary to popular belief) that the atrium responded well to the extra work of valve stenosis and only in the late stages did the atrium dilate. In a second article in the *Lancet*, he concluded with the prophecy, "I anticipate that with the progress of cardiac surgery, some of the severest cases of mitral stenosis will be relieved by slightly notching the mitral orifice." Samways already considered that regurgitation due to overenthusiastic valvotomy might itself prove troublesome.

Sir Lauder Brunton and mitral stenosis

THESE comments were disregarded until 1902, when a note in the *Lancet* by Sir Lauder Brunton resulted in correspondence that dispelled the possibility of cardiac surgery in Britain for many years to come. Brunton was an eminent physician at St Bartholomew's Hospital, London, a Fellow of the Royal Society and had a lifelong interest in the effects of drugs on the heart. Whilst a house physician in Edinburgh (1867), he described the beneficial effect of amyl nitrate in relieving the pain of angina, a treatment that remains the mainstay of symptomatic relief today. In his *Preliminary Note on the Possibility of Treating Mitral Stenosis by Surgical Methods* in the *Lancet*, he drew attention to the hopelessness of medical treatment for the incapacitating symptoms of severe rheumatic heart disease. His work in the post-mortem room showed that the adherent cusps of the mitral valve could be separated quite easily by blunt dissection. Brunton, therefore, proposed surgical intervention and suggested that a suitable instrument might be passed blindly through the wall of the left ventricle and "by sense of touch" into the mitral valve orifice. He considered the transventricular route to be preferable to atrial perforation for practical reasons. Whilst participating in a commission to investigate the effects of chloroform on the heart (1889), Brunton had noted that wounds of the ventricle bleed less than those of the atria. Furthermore, he had experimented on animal hearts for 35 years and had found that they withstood considerable manipulation. Consequently, he spoke from experience and had a genuine desire to obtain symptomatic relief for the many seriously debilitated young patients who filled his clinics and wards. He commented, "The wish unconsciously arises that one could divide the constriction as easily during life as one can after death."

Brunton's manuscript prompted an unpredicted, vitriolic attack on his integrity and judgement. The following week, a leading article in the *Lancet* viewed his suggestion with 'disapprobation'. The authors criticized him for recommending so momentous an undertaking on the basis of postmortem room experiments, and considered that the invitation to others to pursue the work could not absolve him from the responsibility for what he had started. The *Lancet* thought that the difficulties of the operation had been underestimated and that the technique itself "would prove fatal to its adoption". Brunton made an indignant reply, saying that he had no intention of abandoning the idea and reiterated the need for surgeons to find a solution.

Only two physicians supported Brunton's proposal. Samways drew attention to his earlier articles and Arbuthnot Lane reported that the idea of surgical relief had also been suggested to him by Lorriston Shaw. In fact, Lane himself had discovered through work on cadavers how to approach the valve through the left ventricle. Lane boldly stated that he was "quite prepared to act as soon as Dr Shaw succeeded in finding a case likely to derive benefit." Shaw responded negatively by claiming that he had "decided quite definitely that there was no benefit to be gained by operation", which he felt to be an unjustified form of treatment. He stated, "It is possible to do many things that are useless and things that are harmful." Nevertheless, he did agree that the operation was technically feasible and suggested that Brunton should persist in persuading his medical colleagues of the usefulness of the procedure. The cardiologist, Theodore Fisher, terminated the discussion by claiming that myocardial fibrosis was the most important factor in rheumatic heart disease, so that even if the patient survived operation, he or she would not accrue symptomatic benefit. This belief pervaded medical thought until surgeons were able to prove otherwise.

The eminent British cardiologist, Sir James McKenzie, supported the myocardial fibrosis theory in his textbook *Diseases of the Heart*. McKenzie wrote, "In chronic valvular affectations, the symptoms only arise where exhaustion of the heart muscles sets in." With regard to mitral stenosis specifically, he stated,

"It is important to bear in mind the progressive nature of the lesion, for it accounts for the varying changes in the symptoms. It should also be borne in mind that a cicatrizing process may be going on in the muscle, causing contraction of the chordae tendineae, impairing at other places the functional activity of the heart muscle. The manner in which heart failure is brought about in many cases is somewhat complicated."

McKenzie obviously recognized that both muscle and valves could be primarily affected. Discussing the cardiac changes of rheumatic fever, he wrote, "The myocardium rarely escapes and the changes in it are of great importance both for the acute condition and for the subsequent integrity of the heart muscle." With regard to the mitral valve, he stated,

"With the increased narrowing of the orifice, the heart becomes much more distressed and finally, dilatation of the heart may set in. But even without the progressive narrowing, dilatation may appear early and then it may be inferred with certainty that the rheumatic process has permanently injured the heart muscle."

These conclusions provided sufficient justification for those who were antagonistic towards surgical intervention. At the same time in the United States, the proposal by John Cummings Monroe of Boston, for ligation of the patent ductus, met with a similar response. Monroe had also demonstrated the feasibility of duct ligation in cadavers of newborn children. At that time, accurate diagnosis during life was difficult and in many cases, impossible. Clearly, the medical profession was neither mentally nor physically prepared for cardiac surgery.

Early experimental work on the heart valves

EXPERIMENTAL studies on the heart valves were initially undertaken without consideration of their application to human surgery. In 1872, the German ophthalmologist, Otto Becker, sought to reproduce the retinal changes exhibited by patients with aortic regurgitation. He did this by passing a glass rod down through the left common carotid artery and making a hole in the aortic valve. With this method, he confirmed that the retinal changes were secondary to the cardiac problem and not inherent within the eye itself. Soon afterwards, in 1876, Edwin Klebs, a pupil of Rudolph Virchow, used a small knife at the end of a rod-like handle to produce lesions of the aortic and tricuspid valves. Julius Cohnheim, Professor of Pathology at Breslau, and another pupil of Virchow, wanted to confirm that the work done by the healthy heart increased in proportion to the demands made upon it. He created aortic regurgitation in rabbits and dogs, and pulmonary stenosis, by passing a strong thread around the pulmonary artery to form a constriction. Cohnheim noted that the constriction had no effect until a certain point was reached. He surmised that the natural disease must also produce a critical degree of narrowing of the valve orifice before symptoms appear.

The pioneers

THE SUCCESSFUL suturing of a cardiac wound in 1896 by Rehn led to speculation about the further possibilities for cardiac surgery. The work of Klebs and Cohnheim was later developed by the eminent neurosurgeon, Harvey Cushing, of Johns Hopkins Hospital, Baltimore. Cushing also had an interest in the heart, and in 1905, together with his colleague, McCallum, he devised a valvulotome, which was introduced through either a ventricle or an atrium to create valvular incompetence. Stenosis was mimicked by passing a ligature on a curved needle around the valve orifice. The animals were anaesthetized by direct inflation of the lungs through a tracheostomy. Although Cushing and McCallum speculated on the benefits of surgery of the mitral valve in humans, both considered that the main value of the work was in teaching students the clinical signs of valve pathology. Their work was continued by Bernheim, who operated to relieve experimentally created stenoses.

Interest in cardiac surgery was then perpetuated by two surgical giants, Alexis Carrel and Theodore Tuffier, who worked closely together. Between 1902 and 1905, Carrell perfected his technique for vascular anastomosis and methods for organ transplantation. In 1910, he published work on the experimental surgery of the thoracic aorta and heart. This manuscript stressed a simple and easily duplicated approach to surgical techniques. Using insufflation anaesthesia, he used a preserved homograft to anastomose the left ventricle to the descending aorta, thus bypassing the aortic valve and arch. Tuffier sought to apply some of their experimental principles and the opportunity arose with a 26-year-old patient with severe calcific aortic stenosis.

On 13 July 1912, Tuffier, supported by his friend Carrel in the operating theatre, exposed the patient's heart and considered making an incision in the aorta to palpate the valve directly. However, he stopped, probably through anxiety, and conferred with Carrel. They decided to attempt to invaginate the aortic wall a short distance above the valve using the index finger. With this blunt closed method, he reached the diseased valve and attempted to dilate the narrow ring. Afterwards, Tuffier remarked on the "extremely lively vibrations" he felt. Carrel and Tuffier considered the man to have been improved by the procedure and presented their experience at the Fifth Congress of the International Surgical Society.

The next and more ambitious procedure took place in France a few months later. Eugenie Louis Doyen was a flamboyant and skilled surgeon. He had been instrumental in popularizing gastroenterostomy for peptic ulcer. When the opportunity to operate on the heart presented itself, Doyen was keen to proceed. The patient, a 20-year-old woman, was severely ill with right ventricular outflow tract obstruction. Doyen thought it possible to section the orifice of the pulmonary valve and devised a special tenotome. At operation, he introduced the tenotome through the anterior wall of the right ventricle and blindly cut the obstruction (a forerunner of the Brock procedure). However, cyanosis persisted, there was little haemodynamic improvement and the girl died a few hours later. From the description at post-mortem, it was apparent that the infundibular stenosis was severe and the tenotome had caused little surgical relief. In his report, Doyen stated that he had studied the problems of mitral stenosis and had worked out a precise technique for its surgical treatment. What he had in mind and whether it would have succeeded remains unknown, since he died 3 years later, at the age of 57.

Efforts to visualize the diseased heart

WITH THE French otherwise occupied during World War I, interest in cardiac surgery shifted to the US. In St Louis, Missouri in 1922, Evarts Graham and Duff Allan decided that accurate intervention for diseased valves required direct vision. They invented a cardioscope with a lens at the tip which would come into direct contact with the intended structure. The knife with which they proposed to cut the stenosed valve was carried alongside the tube of the cardioscope and had a sharp blade set at right angles to the lens. The instrument was initially introduced through the left ventricular apex, but later changed to the left atrial appendage. The mortality rate for experimental animals was low, though the view of the valves was restricted. In August 1923, they sought to use the cardioscope clinically on a 31-year-old female patient with mitral stenosis. Unfortunately, the patient died before the cardioscope was even introduced and they were unable to solicit another patient.

Meanwhile, in Cushing's laboratory at Harvard, Rhea and Walker devised a sophisticated instrument on the lines of a cystoscope. This had an electric bulb and small knife at the tip with which to divide the fused commissures of the mitral valve. Cutler and his two associates, Samuel Levine and Claude Beck, inherited this equipment, but abandoned the cardioscope because of poor vision in flowing blood (cardioscopy was reinvented in the 1950's). Cutler was nevertheless determined to find a surgical solution to the problem of mitral stenosis and reasoned that mitral incompetence was of less importance. Accordingly, he aimed to resect part of the valve in mitral stenosis and deliberately produce a moderate degree of regurgitation. Cutler began to experiment on dogs, cats and goats using a tenotome type of knife, similar to that of Klebs and Cushing.

Elliot Cutler's operation

LEVINE recognized that the medical treatment of mitral stenosis would never achieve symptomatic relief from attacks of cardiac failure and pulmonary oedema. After

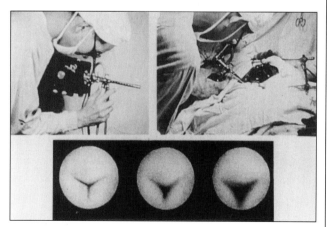

Figure 4.1. Aortic valvotomy for aortic stenosis with the cardioscope originally developed in the Heart Institute of Japan in 1953. (Courtesy of Professors Hitoshi Koyanagi and Masahiro Endo, The Heart Institute of Japan, Tokyo Women's Medical College.)

several years of study, Cutler operated for the first time at the Peter Bent Brigham Hospital in Boston (1923). The patient was a bedridden 12-year-old girl, terribly short of breath and with alarming haemoptysis (Figure 4.2). The child was expected to die soon and the parents were keen for Cutler to proceed. The operation lasted 1½ hours and utilized a modification of Milton's sternotomy, known as the Duval–Barasty approach. The sternum was split down the middle and the cut continued to 2 inches above the umbilicus. This gave excellent exposure to the heart and enabled the pleura to be dissected away from the pericardium without opening the pleural space. Cutler inserted a valvulotome into the apex of the left ventricle and attempted to cut both cusps of the stenotic valve. The patient survived surgery, but improvement was questionable. Signs of mitral stenosis persisted and her activity remained restricted. Nevertheless, she lived for another 4½ years and the haemoptysis ceased. Post-mortem examination showed that the mitral orifice had been partly enlarged by the incision.

Because of their initial success, more patients were referred and Cutler operated twice more during the next few months. The patients died 10 and 20 hours afterwards and examination of the heart suggested the valvulotome to be insufficient for the task. Cutler designed a further device consisting of a circular tube with a blunt point and cutting mechanism. This instrument was introduced through the left ventricle and passed through the valve into the atrium. By operating a spring-loaded handle, the valvulotome acted as a punch. The point was brought to a closed position on the body of the tube, thus cutting out a section of valve. Two patients were operated on with the new instrument, but survived for only 7 and 3 days, respectively. In the second patient, Cutler was unable to reach the valve, and this caused him to abandon further attempts. In retrospect, Cutler proposed that all four fatalities were inevitable, due to advanced disease, myocardial fibrosis, preoperative fever or adherent pericardium.

In the UK, Strickland Goodall, a cardiologist and physiologist at the Middlesex Hospital, worked on cadavers with rheumatic mitral stenosis. With the assistance of his colleague, Lambert Rogers, Goodall performed many operations using a double-edged knife to slit the fused cusps. They saw clearly that mitral stenosis could be relieved surgically and debated the relative merits of the transventricular and atrial routes.

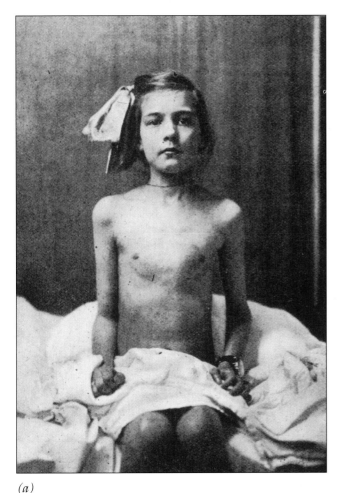
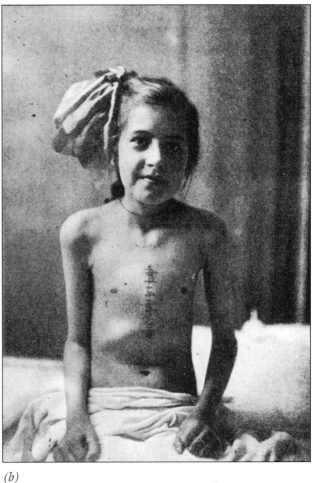

(a)   *(b)*

Figure 4.2. Cutler's 12-year-old patient (a) before and (b) after his first operation for mitral stenosis in 1923. (Reproduced from Cutler EC, Levine SA. Cardiotomy and valvulotomy for mitral stenosis: experimental observations and clinical notes concerning an operated case with recovery. Boston Medical Journal 1923; 188: 1023–7.)

They also explored the possibility of bypassing the valve with a pericardial tube from the left atrium to left ventricle. Because of the negative climate in the UK, their work was published in journals in New Zealand and the United States.

Sir Henry Souttar

IT WAS at the London Hospital on 6 May 1925 that the first great advance in surgery of the mitral valve was achieved. Sir Henry Souttar, a general surgeon, performed a pioneering alternative to the cutting procedure of Cutler, when he introduced a finger into the left atrial appendage and split the fused commissures of a rheumatic mitral valve with finger pressure alone.

The patient, Lily Hine from Bethnal Green, was one of six children of a tuberculous labourer and had suffered three attacks of rheumatic fever. At the age of 10, she was admitted to the London Hospital under Lord Dawson of Penn, with Sydenham's chorea and rheumatic carditis. In 1925, at the age of 19, she was again admitted with mitral stenosis, haemoptysis, orthopnoea and heart failure. Against current opinion, the physicians encouraged Souttar to attempt the operation.

The anaesthetic of ether vapour was given by intratracheal insufflation. Positive pressure was increased as necessary to keep the left lung expanded with the pleural cavity open. Souttar entered the chest by the fourth intercostal space and divided the ribs above to produce a rectangular flap. The left atrial appendage was clamped and incised between stay sutures. On removal of the clamp, Souttar's index finger was easily inserted into the valve orifice. He intended to use an instrument on the valve, but when his finger separated the leaflets and produced mitral regurgitation, he decided not to proceed further. As he withdrew the finger, the lower stay suture tore out and he was faced with a "voluminous gush of blood". Souttar managed to grip the appendage and squeeze it against the atrium before a clamp was applied and the defect sutured. The operation was completed in 1 hour without further incident. The patient improved symptomatically, but suffered a further attack of rheumatic fever the following year. In 1930, she was admitted for the last time with severe heart failure and atrial fibrillation. She suffered multiple cerebral emboli and died.

Although Cutler's work earned him a non-committal editorial note in the *British Medical Journal*, Souttar's paper only resulted in four letters. These were all complimentary and included one from Samways, who could not resist the temptation of drawing attention to his correspondence in the *Lancet* a quarter of a century before. Even though Souttar's operation had been successful, he was never asked to operate again (cardiologists reverted to their unshakeable belief that the state of the myocardium, and not the valves, was the important problem in rheumatic heart disease). Mitral valvotomy was not attempted again in the UK for more than 20 years.

Further attempts at mitral valvotomy

NEWS of Cutler's and Souttar's efforts reached Germany, and on 14 November 1925, Bruno Pribram of Berlin operated on what appeared to be a clear-cut case of mitral stenosis. The patient, a 38-year-old woman, was deteriorating inexorably despite medical treatment. He used a valvulotome and succeeded in excising a portion of the valve. The immediate response was satisfactory, but the patient died on the 5th postoperative day from pneumonia. At postmortem it was apparent that severe aortic stenosis had been obscured by the signs and symptoms of mitral stenosis. The patient also had bacterial endocarditis with fresh vegetation on the aortic valve.

This first era of surgery for mitral stenosis ended after two final, abortive attempts by Cutler. By this time he had abandoned the cardioscope because of poor vision, and during both attempts with the valvulotome he had difficulty in locating the mitral orifice. In their manuscript of 1929, Cutler and Claude Beck analysed their experience and reviewed all mitral valvotomies that year. The authors favoured median sternotomy, which gave easy access to the apex of the left ventricle and avoided opening the pleura. They considered that the left atrial approach provided easier entry into the mitral valve orifice and caused less dysrhythmia. Apart from this, little useful information was derived from the 12 operations. The only survivors had been Tuffier's and Souttar's patients, who had finger dilatation of their valves.

Soon afterwards, experimental work by William Wilson at the University of Edinburgh suggested that the heart could not easily withstand the sudden change from mitral stenosis to regurgitation. Wilson created mitral stenosis in dogs by using strips of rolled pericardium across the orifice. After a suitable interval, he operated to relieve the obstruction, using an operating cardioscope capable of performing a number of bites without losing the excised tissue. Wilson's experiments were never translated into clinical practice and further intervention for valvular heart disease was to await the conclusion of World War II. In 1954 Claude Beck wrote,

> *"I have been asked the question, "Why did Cutler stop the operation for mitral stenosis?". There were several reasons. The valves we examined were calcified and rigid, and it looked as though a piece of valve should be cut away in order to relieve the stenosis. It is probable that the pathology of mitral stenosis has been changed by the use of sulphonamides and antibiotics, for we did not then see soft, pliable valves that could be opened by finger dilatation. Furthermore, I cannot recall any words of encouragement for Cutler after he operated on his seventh and last patient with mitral stenosis."*

Gordon Murray and mitral regurgitation

THROUGHOUT the moratorium on valve surgery between 1928 and 1948 experimental work continued. In 1936, Gordon Murray addressed the problem of mitral regurgitation after valvotomy. He believed that the only way to relieve mitral stenosis was to cut out a piece of valve; however, he sought to counteract the inevitable regurgitation that resulted. He resected the postero–lateral cusp of the mitral valve in dogs and inserted a sling made of an inverted segment of external jugular vein across the valve opening. This was thrust in blindly from outside and sutured to the left ventricular wall under slight tension. The procedure was well tolerated and several animals survived for many years without signs of deterioration. Murray constantly modified and improved his techniques and eventually used them clinically, beginning in 1945. His first patient was a North American Indian. The cephalic vein was excised from the arm, turned inside out and a strip of palmaris longus tendon from the forearm inserted within its lumen to provide strength. Two of these lengths were inserted through an incision in the left ventricle and guided into place by a finger invaginating the left atrium. The valve was suspended from the ventricular aspect of the mitral orifice so that blood could flow through the atrium and fill the ventricle. When the ventricle contracted, the strips were forced back against the orifice to minimize regurgitation. Murray operated on 10 patients, aged 23–47 years, and seven were known to have a satisfactory outcome. This work was not published until 1950, however, by which time the significance was lost through more successful and well-publicized methods for closed mitral valvotomy.

Post-war cardiac surgery: Brock, Smithy, Bailey and Harken

UNTIL the conclusion of World War II, rheumatic and degenerative aortic valve disease remained inaccessible to surgical treatment. Patients with aortic stenosis always presented late, with a severely deformed, calcified valve not amenable to blind commissurotomy. Added to this were attacks of dysrhythmia from an irritable hypertrophied ventricle, and coronary embolus from air or calcific deposits. Blind efforts were also likely to create or aggravate aortic regurgitation. There were no realistic operations on the aortic valve between Tuffier's efforts in 1912 and 1946. In that year, Brock worked on a simpler

and safer route to the aortic valve than through the left ventricle. In the post-mortem room of Guy's Hospital he found that an instrument passed through the innominate artery or one of its branches would pass directly down the aorta into the valve. On 27 March 1947, more than a year before his first operation for mitral stenosis, Brock passed a cardioscope retrogradely through the subclavian artery of a 40-year-old man via a small incision in the neck. This gave him a view of exuberant calcific masses on the aortic valve and no orifice could be seen. Realizing the risks of a blind attempt through the cardioscope, he withdrew. During the next 2 years, Brock made further clinical attempts by the retrograde approach, but the results were so bad that the method was abandoned. Souttar (1925) had suggested the possibility of access to the aortic valve by a finger inserted through the left atrium and hooked through the mitral valve. Brock attempted this approach in 1950, but caused severe mitral regurgitation through papillary muscle injury. The patient died 48 hours later. His efforts then focused on the transventricular route.

In 1947, Horace Smithy in the United States reported some experimental operations in dogs, for which he used a thin, barbed valvulotome. He inserted this retrogradely through the aorta to divide one or more of the valve cusps. Smithy believed that moderate aortic regurgitation would be acceptable, but more than one-third of his dogs died, either during surgery or later from haemorrhage. Smithy worked on the aortic valve with a degree of urgency and the knowledge that his own severe aortic stenosis might benefit from surgery. Realizing the risks of blind aortic valve procedures, Smithy turned his attention to mitral valvulectomy. The object was to excise a segment of scarred valve leaflet from the margin of the constricted orifice and to accept the inevitable mitral regurgitation. He repeated Cutler's experiments and opted for the transventricular approach, as access through the atrium was more difficult and haemorrhage harder to control. However, in eight consecutive operations he used both the atrial and ventricular approach four times.

The first patient was a 21-year-old woman with endstage rheumatic mitral stenosis and chronic congestive heart failure. She travelled several hundred miles by plane to see Smithy in Charleston, South Carolina. On arrival, she was exhausted and dyspnoeic at rest. On 30 January 1948, Smithy approached the mitral valve through the apex of the left ventricle and punched out a segment of anterior leaflet about 0.8 cm long. The procedure was uncomplicated, though the piece of valve was lost on its way to the pathology laboratory. The patient survived surgery, but eventually died 10 months later. Autopsy showed a false aneurysm at the apex to the left ventricle where the valvulotome had been introduced. Smithy's second operation (1 March 1948) was unsuccessful, because the valvulotome was unable to cut into the solidly calcified valve. The 25-year-old man died 10 hours afterwards. The next patient was operated on 1 week later and also died postoperatively from pneumonia. Nevertheless, Smithy's next four patients all survived, including one 36-year-old woman who underwent two separate procedures. Her first operation was unsuccessful via the atrial approach, when the valve could not be entered. Nineteen days later, the transventricular approach was attempted and proved successful. Some of Smithy's patients were dramatically improved, but his own aortic stenosis overtook him and he died on 28 October 1948, at the age of 36. With the exception of Gordon Murray, no-one had achieved similar success. It is unfortunate that Smithy's obituary in the *Journal of the American Medical Association* (25 December 1948) contained the non-committal phrase "is said to have performed the first successful heart valve operation".

Charles Bailey was the next to achieve success, which he attributed to his extensive animal studies as well as an understanding of ladies girdles! As a boy, he sold these door-to-door after school and during summer holidays. He saw the girdle as a skirt-like structure with numerous garters arising from its lower margin, attaching front and back to the tops of two stockings (Figure 4.3). The mitral valve similarly has multiple strings (chordae tendineae) which attach front and back to the two papillary muscles arising from the subapical interior of the left ventricle. The added impetus to correct the stenosed mitral valve came from seeing the terrible consequences of this condition in his father, who died at a young age when Bailey was just 12 years old.

Bailey understood the pathology of mitral stenosis and realized that it was possible to restore fairly normal mobility to fused mitral leaflets, without producing regurgitation. He considered the left atrial approach to be safer and knew that sudden mitral regurgitation was poorly tolerated. Also, if a cutting instrument was used it

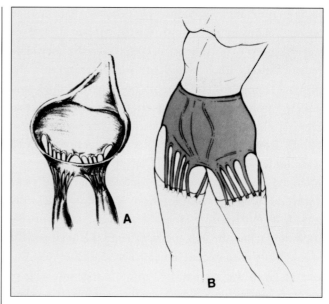

Figure 4.3. Bailey attributed his understanding of the mitral valve to his earlier experience of selling ladies girdles door-to-door as a boy. This cartoon is believed to have been drawn for Bailey by Walt Disney, working as a medical artist at the time.

was necessary to palpate the valve and carefully guide the instrument. Bailey's determination was eventually rewarded, though his first four clinical attempts were failures. The first patient (November 1945) died from atrial bleeding before the valve was reached. The second patient (June 1946) died 48 hours postoperatively. Autopsy showed that the valve commissures were barely separated and that thrombus had narrowed the orifice further.

Twenty-one months later at the Memorial Hospital in Wilmington, Delaware, Bailey used a commissurotomy knife fixed to the palmar surface of the index finger and almost succeeded in a 38-year-old man (Figure 4.4). The initial result was satisfactory, but because of thrombosis in the previous patient, anticoagulant therapy was started; this resulted in bleeding. Again, autopsy showed that the commissural splitting had been inadequate. Three of five hospitals in Philadelphia had by then cancelled his operating privileges. He reflected on his state of mind:

"Finally however, you have to face the 'moment of truth', and the poignancy is so great that I can't really express it. You know that almost all the world is against it; you

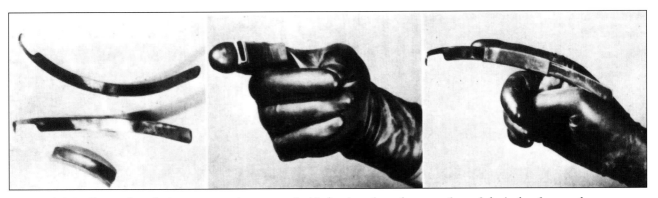

Figure 4.4. Bailey preferred to use a commissurotomy knife fixed to the palmar surface of the index finger when operating on the mitral valve. (Reproduced with permission from Bailey CP. The surgical treatment of mitral stenosis (mitral commissurotomy). Diseases of the Chest 1949; 15: 377–397.)

know that you have a great personal stake and might even lose your medical license or at least your hospital privileges if you persist. In fact, the thought crosses your mind that maybe you really are crazy. And yet you feel that it has to be done and that it has to be right. At the time I did the last of those five operations, the finally successful one, I was sure that I was, at the very least, in danger of losing all of my hospital operating privileges."

He then scheduled, on the same day, one case at the Philadelphia General Hospital where he still had morning privileges and another at Episcopal Hospital where he had afternoon privileges. If one attempt failed, the other would be underway before he could be stopped.

On the appointed day Bailey, at 38, developed measles and had to postpone both operations. One month later, on 10 June 1948, at Philadelphia General Hospital, the fourth patient, an elderly man with advanced disease and pulmonary complications, died before Bailey reached his mitral valve. As arranged, he and his team drove directly to Episcopal Hospital where Claire Ward, the fifth patient, advised by her family physician not to be operated on, survived Bailey's 80 minute operation for mitral commissurotomy performed with a knife along his finger to cut the lateral commissure. Soon afterwards she travelled 1000 miles by rail to the American College of Chest Surgeons Conference in Chicago, where Bailey triumphantly presented the case. She died some 38 years later of respiratory complications following a severe episode of Herpes simplex.

Bailey's great rival at this time was Dwight Harken.

Before the war, Harken had carried out a variety of experimental intracardiac operations. He put some of his experience into practice whilst working in the UK at the Thoracic Centre of the 160th General Hospital of the United States Army. Harken successfully removed 134 bullets or metallic fragments from the mediastinum without losing a single patient. Thirteen of these were within cardiac chambers and gave Harken confidence for his future civilian practice. Using a modified Cutler valvulotome, Harken operated on his first patient, a man of 26, on 22 March 1947. The instrument was passed through the left superior pulmonary vein and segments of valve were excised. During the manipulations, the patient deteriorated and died 24 hours later from pulmonary oedema. Harken then moved away from leaflet resection towards excision of tissue from the fused commisures, in an attempt to restore mobility. He was prepared to accept mitral regurgitation, which he termed 'selective insufficiency'. On 16 June 1948, he operated on a man of 27, using the transatrial approach. This patient survived and claimed dramatic symptomatic improvement. Objectively, there was little change in cardiac function. Six of Harken's next ten patients died, which so devastated him that he left the operating theatre and went home to bed, insisting that he would never do another heart operation. His cardiologist and collaborator, Laurence Ellis, dissuaded him from his decision: "You have never killed anybody. I have never sent you a patient who wasn't dying." Harken resumed his series and lost only one of the next 15 patients. Harken went on to use finger or instrumental dilatation.

In the UK, Brock followed the example of Souttar and used his index finger to split the stenosed valve. His first operation, on a 24-year-old woman (16 September 1948), was successful, and in six of his first eight patients (reported in 1950), Brock achieved separation of the valve cusps adequately with the finger alone. Only twice did he resort to the use of a finger knife. Two patients, the second and third, died from cerebral embolism and bleeding, respectively. The encouraging finding from Brock's experience was that mobilization of the fused commissures (without leaflet resection) could largely avoid the problem of mitral regurgitation. In fact, when regurgitation existed before leaflet mobilization, this was often less pronounced afterwards.

The operations of Smithy on 30 January 1948, Bailey on 10 June 1948, Harken on 16 June 1948 and Lord Brock on 16 September 1948 made 1948 the *annus mirabilis* of mitral valve repair. Their success was anticipated by Cutler some 20 years earlier. Unfortunately, Cutler did not live long enough to witness this advance. He died in 1947 at the age of 59.

Left atrial bypass in mitral stenosis

WHILST these surgeons attempted a direct attack on the stenosed valve, alternative methods were explored. As symptomatic deterioration in mitral stenosis results from left atrial hypertension and pulmonary oedema, might it not be possible to reduce left atrial pressure and palliate symptoms by decompression? In 1916, Renée Lutenbecker observed that patients with mitral stenosis and an atrial septal defect did not suffer from pulmonary oedema. This led Alexander Jarotzky to suggest deliberate creation of an atrial septal defect, a procedure which was undertaken experimentally in dogs (1925). No further efforts were made until after World War II, when Blalock and Hanlon revived the bypass concept. Both Bailey and Harken performed this operation despite their direct attacks on the valve; Harken's two patients derived only short-lived benefit and their symptoms returned.

Richard Sweet and Edward Bland, at Massachusetts General Hospital, Boston, favoured an extracardiac approach by linking the pulmonary and systemic circulations. They observed that in patients with severe mitral stenosis, the brachial veins (which drained through the azygos system into the venae cavae) became enormously dilated, thus providing a limited outlet for the congested pulmonary vessels. On 23 March 1948, Sweet performed a decompression operation on a 17-year-old girl, who had almost died from pulmonary oedema, by the anastomosis of a branch of the right inferior pulmonary vein to the azygos vein. This seemed to improve the symptoms and five more operations were performed with limited success.

In France, D'Allains used a similar operation on 10 patients, beginning on 29 January 1949. There were three postoperative deaths and seven relative successes. However, with improvements in mitral valvotomy guided by the finger, together with a variety of more sophisticated valvulotomes (such as those of Tubbs and Brock), closed mitral valvotomy flourished. Perhaps the most significant was the instrument devised by Charles Dubost, who reported its use to the French Society for Cardiology in December 1953. The new instrument had two parallel blades and was guided through the atrium and into the valve orifice by a finger. Once in place, the two blades were carefully separated, thereby splitting the fused commissures. This provided an excellent anatomical split, usually with no regurgitation. Left atrial bypass, which effectively lowered cardiac output, was then abandoned. The practice of closed mitral valvotomy spread to centres all over the world and in a short time, hundreds of operations had been performed. With increasing experience, the mortality rate fell, and it was apparent that surgery should be undertaken earlier, before endstage symptoms or gross valvular calcification.

Surgery for aortic stenosis

MORE INGENIOUS methods were required for relief of aortic valve disease. It was known that to punch out a piece of aortic valve resulted in sudden and potentially fatal aortic regurgitation. Bailey tried various methods to alleviate aortic regurgitation in the laboratory. He first tried an equivalent of Murray's method for mitral regurgitation. After excising a piece of aortic valve to relieve the stenosis, he treated the aortic regurgitation by slinging a length of the dog's external jugular vein, turned inside out, across the native valve to act as an artificial valve. He positioned the vein by pushing a hollow cork borer through the aorta from one side to the other and passing the vein through its lumen. This method was ineffective, but Bailey followed it by using direct grafts of small sections of aorta or pulmonary artery bearing their respective valve cusps. In 1950, it was difficult to control haemorrhage from the aorta and it was considered too risky to apply this method in patients. Another possibility was to bypass the aortic valve. For this Bailey adopted the technique of an apico-aortic conduit of homograft material containing a valve. A long segment of resected homograft aorta was first divided and reconstituted so that the valve came to lie in the middle of the bypass. Although sound in principle, there were more failures than successes. He therefore returned to simply punching out a piece of valve and, on 9 March 1950, operated on a 26-year-old woman. Through a stab incision in the left ventricle, he first passed a knife but was unable to reach the valve. He removed this and introduced a dilating instrument, which went through the valve orifice but became stuck. Attempts to remove the dilator caused immediate heart failure and death.

Bailey was undeterred and believed that if he could divide the cusps along their lines of fusion, he might be successful. He devised an instrument with an umbrella-like tip, which could be expanded by a screw at the end of the handle. On 6 April, less than a month after his previous attempt, he used this device to enter the valve via the right common carotid artery. After crossing the valve, he pulled the instrument back forcibly. The patient survived but with severe aortic regurgitation. Bailey then resorted to using the instrument via the transventricular route, and over the next 2 years operated on 11 more patients. One-third of these died, but survivors were improved symptomatically. With refinements of the device to an expandable tri-radiate instrument that could adjust automatically to the distorted valve orifice, he improved his results. On 8 April 1952, he performed the first combined mitral and aortic valvotomy. Bailey considered that for accurate aortic surgery without direct vision, it was necessary to palpate the deformed valve as with transventricular mitral valvotomy. Attempts to perform transaortic palpation using a pursestring suture often resulted in excessive bleeding. He then resorted to using a sleeve of pericardium anastomosed to the aortic wall over a Potts clamp. A finger was introduced into the pouch of pericardium and when the clamp was removed,

it was invaginated into the aorta to palpate the valve and guide the dilator.

The first operation of this type was performed on 3 March 1953 and Bailey subsequently recorded 11 of these operations with three deaths. Harken adopted a similar method, but used a small cylinder of plastic material sutured around the aortic incision. Nevertheless, closed techniques were soon destined to become obsolete, with the use of hypothermia and inflow occlusion, and then cardiopulmonary bypass.

George Clowes and William Neville were the first to attempt direct vision surgery of the aortic valve in 1954. Their 55-year-old male patient with severe aortic stenosis also had moderate mitral stenosis and a hemiparesis from previous cerebral infarction. Using a heart–lung machine, aortic valvotomy was performed under direct vision, but the patient died 1 hour after closure of the chest. It was hypothermia that provided the means for the first successful open aortic valvotomy on 17 November 1955, when Swann operated on a 29-year-old man with severe calcific aortic stenosis. Using inflow occlusion, an incision was made directly into the aorta and the fused commissures mobilized.

This operation was soon followed by that of Brock (26 January 1956) using hypothermia, and by Lillehei (31 January 1956) using an improved pump oxygenator and retrograde perfusion of the coronary sinus. Lillehei's patient was a 37-year-old female with calcific aortic stenosis. Besides mobilizing the fused commissures, he performed decalcification of the cusps which helped restore valve mobility and improved the anatomical result. The patient made an uneventful recovery. Continuous retrograde perfusion of the coronary sinus with blood allowed an oxygen supply to the myocardium and served to eliminate the hazard of coronary air embolism.

The problem of mitral regurgitation

IN PRACTICE, correction of valve regurgitation proved considerably more difficult than valve stenosis. At the Jefferson Medical College, Philadelphia (1949), John Templeton and John Gibbon performed experimental reconstruction of the tricuspid valve and compared grafts of autogenous vein or pericardium. They resected a portion of the tricuspid valve in a dog, then repaired the leaflet with autogenous material sutured into the defect. The pericardium produced the better result in a few long-term survivors. Shrinkage of both grafts occurred at a later stage. This work was known to Bailey, who considered that graft durability could be improved by maintaining native vascularization. The pericardium was mobilized and part of it folded into a tube with the smooth surface on the outside. With a finger in the left atrial appendage, the tube could be passed through the heart from front to back beneath the mitral orifice. The front end was anchored by the pedicle containing the blood supply and the rear end by sutures when appropriate tension had been obtained. When he achieved this, the pericardium showed no tendency to contract.

Bailey used this method clinically and in 1950, reported on seven patents, two of whom had also undergone commissurotomy for valve stenosis. He considered six of these operations to be successful in controlling regurgitation. Andrew Logan in Edinburgh used a similar technique for 11 patients with incapacitating and deteriorating symptoms. The first patient was a woman of 37, who presented with haemoptysis and whose operation took place on 1 October 1951. A sheet of pericardium was mobilized on a pedicle and a free corner sutured to the eye of a 7 inch silver probe. Logan opened the left atrial appendage and confirmed the presence of mitral regurgitation. He passed the probe through the anterior wall of the left ventricle, guided it across the underside of the mitral valve orifice with his finger, and brought it out through the back of the heart. The sheet of pericardium was pulled through after the probe and the tension adjusted by palpation. The object was to fill the valve orifice when the ventricle contracted, but not to provide significant obstruction as the ventricle filled. Remarkably, the first patient made an uninterrupted recovery and 10 months later had no further haemoptysis or shortness of breath. The remaining 10 patients all survived and nine claimed symptomatic improvement.

Bailey recognized that the valve deformity in rheumatic mitral regurgitation usually produced a pear-shaped gap towards the posterior aspect of the valve. He therefore suggested a pericardial baffle for this aspect of the valve alone. The strip of pericardium was passed through the wall of the left ventricle, below the level of the valve annulus. Guided by a finger in the atrium, the strip was taken out of the heart and the long end passed through a hole in the short end to produce a loop. Tightening of the loop approximated the edges of the leaflets at the broad end of the pear-shaped deformity, thus reducing the propensity for regurgitation. In a series of 72 patients, there were 20 hospital deaths and Bailey considered the procedure inherently too dangerous. However, William Jamison refined the method with his own instrument and the use of nylon sutures to fix the pericardial strips across the valve. He operated on 25 patients with only four deaths.

Harken, who by this time had a somewhat acrimonious relationship with Bailey, adopted a different form of closed annuloplasty by using nylon sutures to plicate the valve annulus. With interrupted sutures anchored outside the heart with buttons, he produced an elongated ellipse to approximate the deformed leaflets. Harken's method was also used successfully by Earl Kay and Frederick Cross. In 1955, they reported four clinical cases, one of which died from suspected pulmonary embolus. Harken next tried to create an artificial valve leaflet by inserting a moveable plastic baffle across the mitral orifice. The first baffles were ball shaped and were inserted into the left ventricle via the left atrial appendage. A suture was inserted through the wall of the ventricle below the valve annulus, then through a hole in the middle of the ball and out of the ventricular wall. Suspended in this way, the ball moved into the valve orifice during systole but tended to cause inflow obstruction in diastole. Clearly, it was extremely difficult to place the baffles accurately and a single size was not appropriate for all patients. In an attempt to overcome these difficulties and lessen the risk of obstructing the valve orifice, Harken produced a spindle-shaped baffle in a variety of sizes. These were used on 17 patients and reported in 1954.

It was soon apparent that blind intracardiac manoeuvres to reduce regurgitation were futile and doomed to failure. Surgeons then decided to intervene with the second component of mitral regurgitation, that of the dilated valve annulus. Robert Glover and Julio Davila, of the Philadelphia team, argued that with the onset of left ventricular failure, the mitral annulus dilated, producing a relative deficiency in valve leaflet size. They attempted to place a constricting ligature around the atrioventricular ring in an attempt to break the vicious cycle. In May 1956, the surgeons reported annuloplasty in 27 patients aged between 7 and 52 years, all with rheumatic heart disease in an advanced state of congestive cardiac failure. Their pursestring consisted of umbilical tape with a sleeve of pericardium stitched over its midportion, designed to lie in the transverse sinus. A finger inside the heart guided the needle and assessed the degree of regurgitation as the circumferential suture was pulled tight. About half of the patients were significantly improved. Another Philadelphia surgeon, Henry Nichols, used a plication technique with pericardium to take a tuck in the valve annulus and lessen the gap at the incompetent (usually the posterior) pole of the valve. In 1958, he reported on 93 patients with a 27% mortality. All patients over the age of 50 died.

In effect, surgery for mitral regurgitation remained ineffective until the development of the pump oxygenator. Even then, with no reliable repair available it was unacceptable to operate before endstage mitral regurgitation. By the time the patients were symptomatic and deteriorating, heart failure had damaged other organs and increased the risk of operation. Many were regarded as too ill for major surgery with hypothermia or extracorporeal circulation. Most surgeons had to bide their time until the pump oxygenator was improved and satisfactory techniques of valve repair or replacement were worked out.

The evolution of cardiac valve prostheses

IT WAS THE particularly difficult problem of aortic regurgitation which led to artificial valve development. Hufnagel began experiments with ball valves in 1946. By this time it was known that the descending thoracic aorta could be safely cross-clamped for coarctation repair. Hufnagel thought that it might be possible to place a valve in the descending aorta for patients with aortic regurgitation. By 1952, his ball and cage valve was sufficiently advanced for clinical use, and when inserted into the descending aorta, it effectively reduced aortic regurgitation by 70%. Hufnagel's valve consisted of a chamber made of a single piece of methyl methacrylate with fixation rings of nylon at both ends (Figure 4.5, page 167). The valve was implanted through a left thoracotomy after mobilisation of the descending

thoracic aorta from a number of intercostal branches. The aorta was then transected and the prosthesis invaginated into the cut ends. It was attached to the aortic wall by the multiple point nylon fixation rings. The first clinical implantation was undertaken on 11 September 1952. Most of the patients were extremely ill and in 12 of 80 operated on by Hufnagel himself, the procedure was abandoned in the anaesthetic room when the blood pressure fell precipitously. Hospital mortality was approximately 20% occurring mostly through ventricular fibrillation. However, many of the survivors were dramatically improved with an impressive decrease in cardiac size. This first effort demonstrated above all that foreign material could be implanted within the blood stream without disastrous effects.

The dynamics of bloodflow through the valve and its method for implantation were complex for the time, and a tremendous amount of work was necessary in both the construction and fixation methods. About 10% of the early patients suffered from thrombosis and embolism, but with improvements in technique the problems were largely eliminated. Initially, the metal ball clicked in the cage and could be heard opening and closing from across the room. This led to the metal ball being replaced by a silicone-covered ball. Hufnagel suggested that if direct aortic cross-clamping proved problematic, then a temporary bypass could be inserted between the subclavian artery and distal aorta or femoral artery. As an alternative method, the valve could be placed in a permanent bypass tube followed by resection of the intervening length of aorta.

Hufnagel's efforts clearly heralded the era of the cardiac valve prosthesis. Meanwhile, others attempted to insert various types of valve in the orthotopic situation. (Figure 4.6) In 1952, Bailey began to experiment with balls or plastic-flap valves, which were suspended in the aorta by one or two tails and designed to fall back into the regurgitant orifice during diastole. In addition, he described a constriction ring of nylon fabric tied around the outside of the aorta, and tightened using finger control. Neither of Bailey's methods were satisfactory, though the constriction procedure was partially effective if the aortic cusps were not severely deformed. Murray considered bypassing the regurgitant valve with an aortic xenograft taken from a donor animal. This was somewhat similar to Bailey's bypass for aortic stenosis. At the same time, Murray also experimented with bypass of the mitral

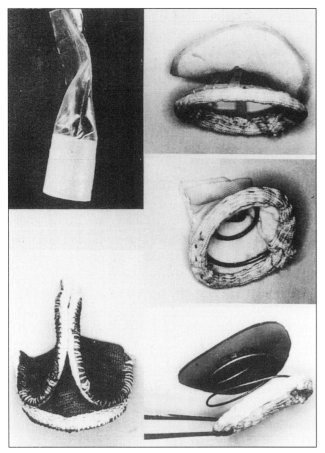 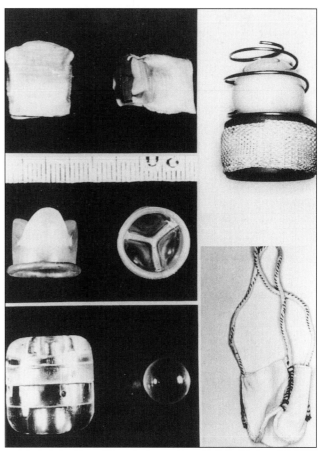

Figure 4.6. Valve prosthesis developed in the Heart Institute of Japan in the 1950s. (Courtesy of Professors Hitoshi Koyanagi and Masahiro Endo, The Heart Institute of Japan, Tokyo Women's Medical College.)

valve from the left atrial appendage to the left ventricle. In both instances, he had difficulty in suturing the graft to the muscular wall of the left ventricle. Murray then experimented with aortic homografts. When the dog's own aortic valve was competent and functioning normally, the transplanted valve in the descending aorta stayed open. If the animal's own valve was damaged to produce regurgitation, the transplanted valve functioned effectively, in some cases for 9 months.

The first aortic homograft operation

ENCOURAGED by these results, Murray operated on a 22-year-old man in October 1955. The donor valve was taken from a cadaver and preserved in physiological saline solution at 4°C for 36 hours. It was then inserted into the patient's descending thoracic aorta at the level of the sixth thoracic vertebra. The cross-clamp time was 37

minutes, after which the valve functioned well. The man was a heavy manual worker and when seen 6 years later he was asymptomatic. Three more patients with severe regurgitation were operated on with the same method and all were clinically improved.

By this time, the pump oxygenator was in use and on 23 May 1956, Lillehei operated on a 52-year-old female with mixed rheumatic aortic stenosis and regurgitation. He first performed a valvotomy and then used mattress sutures to reconstruct the valve from an incompetent tricuspid configuration to a bicuspid valve that closed effectively. Lillehei repeated the plication procedure using retrograde coronary sinus perfusion for myocardial protection and to eliminate air. He also used polyvinyl sponge or plastic to compensate for valve cusp deficiency. These early operations by Hufnagel, Murray and Lillehei had great significance, as they showed that both natural and prosthetic valves could be tolerated by the body. This was also the beginning of the competition between tissue and mechanical valve prostheses. In the late 1950s, cardiopulmonary bypass provided direct access to all four cardiac chambers, but many problems remained before a satisfactory artificial valve could be produced. All foreign materials used inside the heart tended to promote clot formation and embolism. It was also difficult to obtain secure fixation between the prosthesis and native tissues.

By 1959, Hufnagel had developed a single valve cusp substitute for use in patients with aortic regurgitation. The cusp was made of Dacron cloth impregnated with silicone rubber to prevent tissue ingrowth (which might impair flexibility). The device was moulded to directly mimic an aortic cusp, with pins at the edge which simply passed through the aortic wall and bent like staples. By 1961, Hufnagel had repaired more than 150 regurgitant aortic valves with this device, using cardiopulmonary bypass and topical cardiac cooling. The cusps were inserted either singly or in groups of three, united at the commissures. However, this initial experience persuaded Hufnagel that for patients with severe aortic regurgitation, complete replacement of the aortic valve was necessary.

McGoon devised an aortic prosthesis from a tube of closely knitted Teflon, which was cut and flattened to approximate shape before insertion. He attempted to preserve as much of the native valve as was functional. If part of a cusp was destroyed, but the remnant was flexible, he incorporated it into the repair by trimming the base of the prosthesis accordingly. In this way, the length of original tubing could be transformed into a bicuspid or tricuspid valve that was stitched to the aortic annulus or to functional remnants of flexible cusps as appropriate. Sutures of knitted Teflon tape were used to anchor the prosthesis at the commissures. Seven patients were operated on with this device in 1960, though three died within the first 24 hours.

The first mitral valve replacement

THE COMPLEXITY of the mitral valve with its subvalvar apparatus presented greater difficulties. Nina Braunwald and Andrew Morrow produced a mitral prosthesis made of polyurethane, reinforced with Dacron fabric (Figure 4.7, page 167). Besides two leaflets, it had tails that were passed through the ventricular wall and secured to act as imitation chordae. With dog experiments using cardiopulmonary bypass, they continually modified and improved the valve design. Eventually, when four animals survived for between 8 and 40 hours, they decided to translate their experience to the clinical situation.

The first complete excision and replacement of the mitral valve took place on 10 March 1960, in a 16-year-old girl with severe mitral regurgitation. Using cardiopulmonary bypass, the mitral valve was excised from the annulus and the papillary muscles and chordae transected. In their place, Morrow sutured the new valve and anchored the leaflets with the tails. Though the patient survived the operation, the valve failed to function adequately and the girl died 60 hours later. A second patient, a 44-year-old woman, had the operation the following day and this time made an uneventful but protracted recovery and was well 8 weeks later.

Experience demonstrated that accurate positioning of the artificial subvalvar apparatus was both critical and difficult. Because of this, Henry Ellis experimented with a single-hinged plastic cusp for replacement of the whole mitral valve. The prosthesis, made of mylar coated with polyurethane, was inserted in such a way that the suture lines and knots at the annulus were covered to leave a smooth surface. Of 42 dogs, 33 survived surgery and one lived for 10 months. Although the surviving dogs were treated with anticoagulants, this did not prevent the frequent occurrence of massive thrombosis or, in some cases, fracture of the valve hinge, resulting in sudden death. From autopsies on some long-term survivors, it was clear that there was firm healing between the ring of the prosthesis and the mitral annulus. Ellis also demonstrated that relatively normal haemodynamics could be achieved with this prosthesis.

The first aortic valve replacement

IN MAY 1960, Harken reported on the first patients in whom he had inserted a ball and cage valve within the aortic annulus. His prosthesis consisted of a stainless steel cage, containing a lucite ball and a sewing ring backed with Teflon (Figure 4.8, page 167). This was anchored to the native valve annulus by interrupted silk sutures, after removing the pathological valve. Harken used cardiopulmonary bypass at 26°C, together with topical cooling. Most of the patients were in endstage left ventricular failure. The first operation (10 March 1960) on a patient from Jacksonville, Florida, was a success and the second valve was implanted on 6 June 1960 in a patient from Massachusetts. This second valve lasted for 22 years and was functioning well when the patient developed sub-acute bacterial endocarditis following genito-urinary surgery without antibiotic prophylaxis. Harken's five other patients died, causing him to wait for a year before carrying out the procedure again. (The original design for the aortic position was subsequently modified for use as a mitral prosthesis [1963].)

Meanwhile, Albert Starr and his engineering colleague Miles Lowell Edwards, of the University of Oregon, designed and manufactured their own ball and cage valve. This was cast in one piece of stainless steel, carefully shaped, and given a high quality finish by electropolishing (Figure 4.9 page 167). The sewing ring made of knitted Teflon was attached to the cage by Teflon spreader rings and braided Teflon cloth. The ball was of medical grade, heat-cured silastic, and the valve responded well to accelerated fatigue tests. Edwards, a retired pump engineer, conceived the idea from an 1858 wine bottle stopper patent.

In 1960, no-one had lived for more than 3 months after mitral valve replacement. Starr's first patient was a woman of 33, who had previously undergone Ivalon sponge repair of the posterior mitral leaflet in an attempt to relieve severe mitral regurgitation. This was unsuccessful and on 25 August 1960, her mitral valve was replaced with the ball and cage prosthesis. On cardiopulmonary bypass with cooling to 32°C, the left atrium was open and the mitral valve excised, leaving a margin of valve leaflet on the annulus. Through this, 16–20 interrupted sutures were inserted to anchor the prosthesis. Unfortunately, the operation was complicated by massive air embolism and the patient sustained irreversible brain damage. She died 10 hours later.

The next procedure took place on 21 September in a 52-year-old man with combined rheumatic mitral stenosis and regurgitation. The surgery proceeded uneventfully and he recovered. Anticoagulants were commenced 7 days after surgery, although Starr was not convinced of their necessity. Many dogs had survived for prolonged period without anticoagulant drugs. This second patient, a truck despatcher, survived for 10 years then died following a fall from a ladder whilst painting

his house. The valve functioned impeccably until the accident. Only two other valves of this type were implanted. The lucite cage design was soon replaced by a stainless steel cage, which in turn was abandoned in favour of stellite 21 cast by the lost wax technique. This resulting aortic model 1260 has been available since 1968 to the present time (Figure 4.10, page 168). Model 1260 is a modification of the previous model 1200 but with the sewing ring cloth extended to the orifice, leaving no exposed metal on the inflow. The orifice ring has raised studs which project above the cloth so that the ball sits on the metal surface rather than on the orifice cloth which has been subject to wear. The struts of the cage were then covered in cloth consisting of two layers: polypropylene over teflon. The sewing ring cloth was of composite yarn. The object of strut coverage was to encourage epithelialization and reduce the potential for thromboembolism. Since the mid-1970s, the Starr valve sewing ring has been made of teflon and polypropylene yarns twisted together before knitting.

The mitral valve equivalent, model 6120 (1966), has a basic design that has been in clinical use for three decades. Early models used a metal ball which was rather noisy. This was hollow and formed from cast stellite hemispheres that were electron beam welded. The Starr valve was further modified in 1972 to incorporate a double cage with a metal lining on the inner aspect and polypropylene cloth on the outer aspects of the struts. The orifice cloth was changed to siliconized multi-filament dacron in a lock stitch to prevent runs. The sewing ring became a composite knit with a cloth lattice for neo-intimal growth. Ball and cloth contact were eliminated to minimise wear. Both aortic and mitral versions were available, the object being to prevent embolisation of worn cloth from the struts. Some of these valves were used without anticoagulation but had prohibitive thromboembolic rates. Both models were discontinued in 1980 in favour of uncovered struts and a silicone ball.

The first double valve replacement

WITH INCREASING experience, the ball and cage valve grew in popularity and on 1 November 1961, Robert Cartwright of Pittsburg carried out the first combined aortic and mitral replacement. Cartwright had experimented in the laboratory with the intention of gaining access to the aortic valve through the left atrium. Clinically, he achieved this by first removing the anterior leaflet of the mitral valve to gain access to the left ventricle and thereby to the aortic valve, which was excised and replaced with a Starr–Edwards prosthesis. He then excised the remainder of the mitral valve and inserted a second prosthesis. The patient was on cardiopulmonary bypass at 25°C for 55 minutes, during which the aorta was cross-clamped to prevent air embolism. Saline iced slush was packed around the heart to produce hypothermic arrest, and at the end of the procedure the operative field was filled with carbon dioxide to displace air. The patient survived and was greatly improved until a paraprosthetic leak caused sudden deterioration and death. Starr himself reported multiple valve replacement in 13 patients in 1964. Eleven underwent aortic and mitral replacement and two had triple valve replacement. Eight of the patients survived and six left hospital greatly improved.

Although the ball and cage valve was a great advance, not all surgeons were attracted to the idea of implanting a mechanical device within the circulation. Murray's first patients with aortic homograft implantation in the descending thoracic aorta were doing well 6 years later, and at Baylor, Beall, Cooley and DeBakey had used this technique successfully on four patients. Murray's group in Toronto persisted with the notion of aortic homograft substitution in the orthotopic position. In 1961, Murray's colleague, Heimbecker, performed the first orthotopic aortic homograft replacement using a valve obtained aseptically from a cadaver and preserved in a saline–penicillin mixture at 4°C. Using cardiopulmonary bypass and continuous coronary perfusion, the graft was sutured into the subcoronary position with a combination of continuous sutures reinforced by mattress sutures at the commissures. These were tied outside the aortic wall over pledgets. The first patient died 24 hours later from coronary thrombosis and acute myocardial infarction and Heimbecker did not attempt a further aortic replacement for 3 years. The following year, he attempted two aortic homograft replacements of the mitral valve, but both patients died within four weeks with the manuscript in preparation.

Other synthetic valves

AFTER the Hufnagel, Harken, Rowe and Starr valves, a fifth synthetic trileaflet valve was introduced by Muller and Littlefield for the aortic position. This consisted of three single cusps in an attempt to mimic the native aortic valve (Figure 4.11, page 168). It was implanted in about 75 patients at the National Institute of Health by Andrew Morrow. Initial results were encouraging with symptomatic improvement in all patients. However, with time the cusps stiffened producing prosthetic valve stenosis and virtually all had to be replaced within 8 years of implantation. Braunwald and Morrow published late evaluation of this flexible teflon prosthesis in the *Journal of Thoracic and Cardiovascular Surgery* in 1964. At about the same time, Earle produced a teflon mitral valve prosthesis with chordae tendineae which was also used clinically for complete mitral valve replacement. The leaflets of teflon fabric were coated with polyurethane but the valve proved unsatisfactory and was soon abandoned.

Aortic homografts

MEANWHILE at the Radcliffe Infirmary in Oxford, Alfred Gunning† (Figure 4.12) and Carlos Duran worked to establish a reliable method for aortic homograft valve harvest and preparation. Their intention was to use homografts in the orthotopic position, as first performed by the Toronto group in 1961.

Knowledge of this work allowed Ross to perform the first landmark subcoronary homograft implantation on 24 June 1962 (Figure 4.13, page 168). He described the circumstances surrounding the operation:

† Author's note: Alfred Gunning is an extraordinary character. Born in South Africa he was trained as an Ear, Nose and Throat surgeon. In Professor Alison's Department of Surgery in Oxford, Gunning worked as a general surgeon but took responsibility for developing thoracic, then cardiac surgery and was essentially self taught. An enthusiast, he functioned as a generalist interposing valve operations with herniae or gall bladders. He often took a lunch time break to play squash at neighbouring Green College with Tony Fisher, his anaesthetist. Forced to retire at 67, Gunning returned to work in South Africa until the age of 75. He is still a first class squash player.

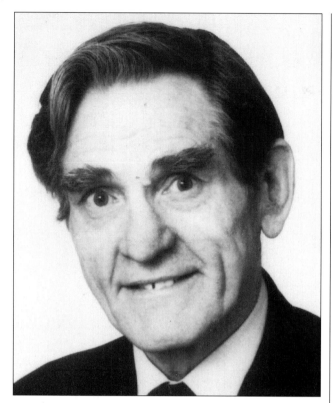

Figure 4.12. Alfred Gunning.

"*Such was our state of unpreparedness that in June 1962, an aortic valve that I was decalcifying disappeared down the sucker tubing at a time when Starr valves were only a distant rumour. We had no alternative but to reconstitute one of our freeze-dried aortic homograft valves and sew it in with a single suture layer — a technique which fortunately had already been suggested to us by our colleagues Gunning and Duran of Oxford. You can imagine our delight when the first valve was not rejected and continued to function in that patient for 4 years. We forgot about the newly available mechanical valves — a state of amnesia which I must confess persists to this day. The homograft valve became an established surgical technique although eventually with only a few persistent and courageous exponents of the method, largely in the Antipodes.*"

This success was followed on 23 August 1962 by that of Barratt-Boyes at Green Lane Hospital, New Zealand. Soon afterwards Mattias Paneth (Figure 4.14), assisted by Mark O'Brien, at the Brompton Hospital implanted a homograft which had been preserved in formalin for 6

months. Others such as Kirklin, Angell and Shumway adopted and pioneered homograft aortic replacement at a time when most surgeons preferred the simplicity of Starr valve insertion with a single row of sutures through a generous sewing ring. Mechanical prostheses offered the prospect of indefinite durability whilst crude homograft preservation techniques caused early clinical failure. Also the supply of suitable homografts was limited and a valve of appropriate size was not always available when needed. The homograft operation was more demanding at a time when myocardial preservation was primitive and there was less appreciation of the homograft's haemodynamic superiority.

To simplify homograft implantation, Weldon from the Johns Hopkins Hospital, published laboratory experience with aortic homografts mounted on a frame. Angell adopted stent mounted homografts for aortic, mitral and tricuspid replacement in the late 1960s. In the short-term, these valves were easy to implant and proved acceptable in all but the smallest aortic annulus. Stent mounting significantly decreased the incidence of early

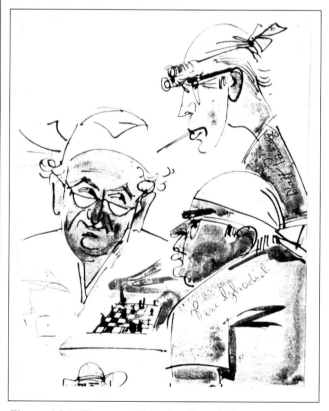

Figure 4.14. Cartoon of Mattias Paneth (surgeon), Ian English (anesthetist) and Pese Ghadiali (perfusion technologist) operating at the Brompton Hospital in the 1960s.

post-operative aortic regurgitation in comparison with the 20–30% incidence with freehand sewn aortic homografts. However, medium term follow up showed limited durability of the stent mounted homograft tissue. The stent caused accelerated tissue failure four to five years in advance of the freehand sewn homograft which usually functioned for 12–15 years.

Access to human cadaveric material remained limited and led to the search for other substitutes. In Zurich, Senning removed fascia lata from the thigh and fashioned this into a trileaflet valve sutured freehand in the subcoronary position. Marion Ionescu (Figure 4.15) in Leeds mounted both autogenous fascia lata and heterologous pericardium on a frame with a sewing ring to facilitate implantation and suspension of the commissures. Autologous fascia lata was soon found to be disappointing, with a 22% failure rate during the first 14 months after implantation. Various innovative methods were then used to stent mount aortic homografts or insert them into dacron sleeves (Top Hat valve) for the mitral position. In 1969, Donlap reported 10 such patients who had haemodynamic results equivalent or better than those with the Starr–Edwards mitral valve replacement or valve repair. Comparing the stent mounted homograft with the Starr–Edwards valve, Yacoub showed haemodynamic improvement to be superior with the tissue prosthesis. The orifice area of the aortic homograft in the mitral position was better than the Starr–Edwards valve, though mild to moderate mitral regurgitation was common on exercise. The theoretical disadvantage of the comparatively small valve area of an aortic homograft compared with the normal mitral valve was addressed by Angell and Shumway. They showed that the orifice area of a large adult aortic valve always exceeded that of the native mitral orifice in symptomatic mitral stenosis.

The pulmonary autograft (Ross) operation

LOWER, Shumway and Stofer began to investigate the potential for autogenous pulmonary valve aortic replacement in 1960 when they experimentally implanted pulmonary valve cusps in the descending thoracic aorta. In 1967, Ross first performed the pulmonary autograft operation for aortic valve

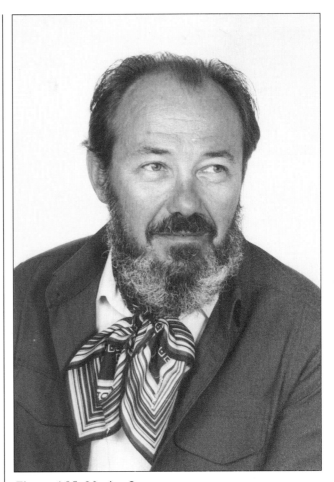

Figure 4.15. Marion Ionescu.

replacement in patients. The pulmonary outflow tract was reconstituted initially with an aortic homograft but then with a pulmonary homograft whose rate of degeneration and calcification was slower in the low pressure area. Initially the autogenous pulmonary valve was used as a subcoronary implant and later as a full aortic root substitute. Ross anticipated that the autologous pulmonary valve would remain viable within the blood stream and maintain the potential for growth in children. Experience over 25 years has shown this to be true, with real growth as opposed to distension. Whilst Ross persisted with the method, others were reluctant to perform a complex double root operation for isolated aortic disease which otherwise carried very low mortality with a stented valve. One of the principal risks of the Ross procedure was damage to the first septal branch of the left anterior descending coronary whilst mobilising the pulmonary root; on many occasions this proved fatal. Homografts were in short supply, myocardial protection was poorly developed and cardiopulmonary bypass still damaging in long operations. Attention therefore turned to the pig who many considered to closely resemble the human. The diversity of early valve substitutes prompted Gerbode to comment: "Once a valve has been rendered inert through preservation, it matters little whether it was human or animal." Ross disagreed and maintained a career-long dislike for porcine and mechanical valves.

Development of porcine bioprostheses

BACK IN OXFORD, Duran and Gunning transferred their attention to preservation of heterograft valves. On 23 September 1964, they performed the first human stent mounted porcine valve implant. Their experimental work with insertion of freeze-dried pig aortic valves in the descending thoracic aorta of dogs was published the following year but did not mention this clinical case. In 1965, Binet, Duran (now in Paris), Carpentier and Langlois presented their early experience of preserved frame mounted heterografts and acknowledged Gunning's contribution. Their report described five patients with porcine valves preserved in mercurochrome,

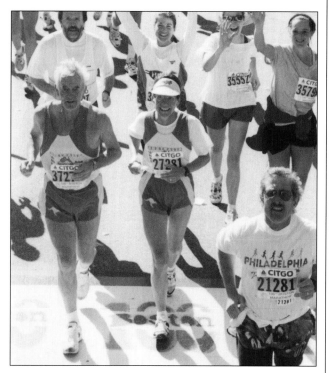

Figure 4.16. Mark O'Brien (left) running the Philadelphia marathon in his seventies.

all of whom survived without anticoagulants. In 1966, O'Brien (Figure 4.16), now in Melbourne, reported his experience with formalin preserved pig and calf aortic heterografts in nine patients. Long term results were poor because of the primitive preservation methods.

In 1966, Ionescu and Wooler developed a stent for mounting aortic xenografts (Figure 4.17, page 168). The titanium support had three legs and was covered inside and outside with dacron velour. A dacron felt ring covered with velour cloth served as the sewing ring. The porcine aortic valve was sutured within the frame and was kept with the aortic sinuses packed with cotton wool, soaked with formaldehyde to ensure cusp coarptation and shape. This titanium framed valve was marketed in both the UK and the United States and was the precursor of the Ionescu–Shiley pericardial valve. Carpentier next produced his round rigid stent of teflon coated stainless steel to which two rings of teflon cloth were attached so that the valve could be implanted with two suture lines. These suture lines were designed to enable complete covering of all peripheral portions of the frame with host tissue to minimise thromboembolism. The central portion was covered by the porcine xenograft, prepared in a mercurial salt solution. Human valve implants followed animal experiments in 1967 and this stent became the model used in the Carpentier–Edwards valve.

Carpentier's metal frame was intended to overcome the problems associated with freehand suturing of unmounted aortic homografts and xenografts. The round rigid stent was constructed from teflon coated stainless steel to which rings of teflon cloth were attached to facilitate implantation. A similar graft support ring was designed by Shumway and Angell and manufactured by Cutter Laboratories (Figure 4.18, page 168). The first human implant of a valve with this stent was on 22 May 1967. In the following 5 years, 426 patients from infants to octogenarians underwent mitral valve replacement with fresh aortic homografts mounted on this device. However, in a relatively short time it was evident that stent mounting caused excessive stress on the biological tissue with accelerated degeneration and calcification. Accelerated valve failure consequently caused the practice of homograft mounting to disappear.

At the same time, Warren Hancock, employed at Edwards Laboratories until 1967, designed a porcine valve with a machined stellite stent and aortic cusps fixed in formalin. Hancock's valve was implanted in animal experiments by Lester Sauvage (June 1968), after which Robert Litwak began implanting the valves clinically. Later models incorporated a polypropylene stent, which allowed flexibility and motion at the commissures and reduced stress on the tissues. The first of these valves was implanted at the National Institute of Health, Washington DC. A stellite stiffener ring was added later to act as a radio-opaque marker.

Carpentier, DuBost and colleagues then described stent mounted heterograft replacements of the mitral and tricuspid valves (1968). In the UK, Ionescu and Wooler used beta propriolactone sterilized freeze-dried heterografts for aortic and mitral replacement, followed by formalin fixed, stent mounted valves. Although the initial results with formalin fixation were satisfactory, the medium term durability was poor.

The preservation problem was soon resolved by Carpentier, who employed glutaraldehyde fixation in 1968. Following the efforts of Carpentier, Hancock and Angell, gluteraldehyde fixed stented porcine valves became readily available commercially, did not require anticoagulants and were soon in great demand. Though Binet had reported his experience with stentless pig aortic roots in 1965, ease of implantation of stented porcine xenografts rapidly superseded freehand stentless techniques. In discussion of Angell's paper on 'Five Year Study of Viable Aortic Valve Homografts' at the 52nd Annual Meeting of the American Association for Thoracic Surgery (1972), Carpentier made the following comments:

"My only criticism of the homograft is the practical problem of getting enough specimens of different sizes. Because of this difficulty the technique cannot be routinely used. As a result we are still concentrating our efforts on heterografts. If the durability of the homograft depends upon the viability of the tissue, the durability of the heterograft depends on the stability of the tissue, with absence of collagen denaturation and immunological reaction. This is achieved by an appropriate chemical treatment which decreases the antigenicity of the tissue by elimination of the antigenic components and prevents the denaturation of collagen by means of glutaraldehyde. The valve substitute so obtained is a 'bioprosthesis' rather than a graft. Its durability is based on the unfailing stability of the tissue and not upon regeneration by the host cells."

In this same discussion, Cooley (not a pig valve enthusiast) recalled the case of a 12-year-old boy with rapid degeneration of a xenograft.

"About 6 months earlier this patient had had a porcine graft placed in the aortic annulus in a city in Louisiana. The poor, bewildered mother knowing that her son had received a pork graft, asked me what type of valve we would now use. I told her we would use a Björk valve. She said, 'What kind of an animal is a Björk?'"

The stent mounted porcine xenograft is a hybrid of biological and mechanical structures, hence the term bioprosthesis. Central unobstructed flow characteristics are retained to an extent but the stent is partly obstructive and produces turbulent flow. Much less judgement and skill were needed on the part of the surgeon to insert the bioprosthesis and ensure competence. Haemodynamic characteristics of these valves lay somewhere between the homograft and the first generation mechanical valves. Long-term function of stented porcine xenografts soon proved to be less favourable than that of freehand homografts with improved preservation methods. Degeneration, calcification and cusp rupture occurred earlier in porcine xenografts, especially in children or young adults. The difference in durability could be partly accounted for by the stent, which led to suboptimal valve geometry and maldistribution of stress on the leaflets. A similar rate of valve failure was found in stent mounted aortic homografts.

Ross, with his strong preference for human tissue, used stent mounted homografts for the mitral position and confirmed that a normal cardiac output could be achieved without a significant increase in left atrial pressure. The valves had low thrombogenicity, central flow and relatively low profile when compared to the Starr valve, which tended to obstruct the left ventricular outflow tract. Durability of the stent mounted mitral homograft was soon found to be unsatisfactory and by 1973, Ross reported unacceptable rates of valve failure over 5 years. The results were even worse when Ross briefly tried pulmonary homografts mounted on a frame or dacron tube in the mitral position. Nine of 11 failed within 1 year of surgery, confirming the suspicion that rigid frame mounted valves in the mitral position were subject to unusually high stress. Yacoub's preferred operation was to select the largest available aortic homograft (25 to 30 mm in diameter) and to fix it inside a 35 mm dacron tube with a teflon collar at the inflow portion. The distal end of the tube was fixed to the mitral annulus whilst the collar suspended the proximal end of the tube to the left atrial floor above the annulus. This valve had a very low thromboembolic rate (actuarial freedom from thromboembolism 98% at 5 years and 97.5% at 9 years). Unfortunately, freedom from valve degeneration was only 48% at 10 years and reoperation was hazardous. Ross then attempted to replace the mitral valve with a mitral homograft in nine patients. The operation was complex and whilst early post-operative haemodynamics were satisfactory, seven patients sustained ruptured chordae tendineae within a few months of implantation The mitral homograft has never regained widespread acceptance in the high pressure mitral position but was used for tricuspid valve replacement by Pomar (Barcelona) and Westaby (Oxford) in the 1990's.

The idea of substituting a porcine cusp from another pig valve in order to eliminate the partially obstructive right coronary cusp muscle shelf gave rise to the modified orifice Hancock valve. Removal of the right coronary cusp with replacement by the non-coronary cusp of a larger valve resulted in a 1 mm increase in orifice area. The first clinical implant of a modified orifice bioprosthesis was performed in October 1976 at The Peter Bent Brigham Hospital, Boston. The flexible stent concept was reported by Reis in the *Journal of Thoracic and Cardiovascular Surgery* in 1971.

Further developments in mechanical valve technology

IN 1962, Christiian Barnard and the engineer, Carl Goosens, developed the Barnard lenticular mitral valve and the biconical aortic valve (Figure 4.19, page 168). Both were implanted by Barnard at the Groteschur Hospital. The original components were stainless steel and silicone rubber. The silicone was later changed to polypropylene and the valve was adopted and implanted by the Mayo Clinic. Barnard reported successful aortic valve replacement with the prosthesis (*Lancet* 1963) but it was soon superseded by other valves with better flow characteristics. Barnard also performed the first tricuspid replacement for Ebstein's anomaly with the Lenticular valve.

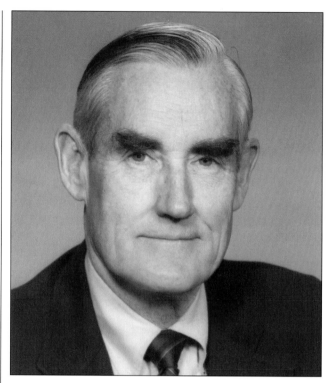

Figure 4.20. Vincent Gott.

In 1963, Vincent Gott (Figure 4.20) and William Daggett produced a butterfly valve which evolved through a number of early designs with several different materials (Figure 4.21, page 169). In animal studies, the most satisfactory was polyvinyl fluoride as most other polymers tested (including silicone coated plastic rings) induced thrombosis within a matter of hours. The commercially produced model had a lexan ring coated with colloidal graphite which appeared relatively non-thrombogenic. The moving poppet was silastic vulcanized dacron and the sewing cuff was made from rigid teflon. The Gott–Daggett valve was described in the *Journal of Thoracic and Cardiovascular Surgery* in 1964 but produced stasis distal to and between the leaflets and turbulence over the free edges of the leaflets. Both structural and embolic problems resulted in the valve being withdrawn at an early stage.

There followed a series of mechanical prosthetic valve designs from the United States, the majority of which were abandoned within a relatively short period. In 1963, a sutureless valve was designed by Harry Cromie of the Surgitool Company, Pittsburg and featured a row of horizontally orientated pins to secure a stainless steel cage containing a poppet. The valve was subsequently modified to incorporate two plates with vertically orientated pins. In 1964, a silicone rubber cuff was attached to the upper plate and the poppet was barium sulphate impregnated to convey radiolucency. The valve was further modified in 1965 by substituting dacron fabric for the silicone rubber cuff and covering the inflow surface of the valve with teflon. In 1968, dacron cloth was used to cover the entire base of the valve leaving only the orifice and cage bare. It was described by McGovern as a sutureless artificial heart valve in *Circulation* and the *Journal of Thoracic and Cardiovascular Surgery* in 1963 and remained in use by McGovern's group until 1991.

The Smeloff–Cutter valve was developed from its forerunner the Smeloff–Cutter–Davey–Kaufman valve in 1964. This was a full orifice, double cage ball valve with an open apex. The housing was machined from titanium and the struts were shorter than other cage ball valves, projecting less into the left ventricle (Figure 4.22, page 169). The silicone rubber ball allowed a small amount of regurgitation theoretically to wash the ball. The prosthesis was manufactured by Cutter Laboratories in Berkeley, California and the first clinical implant performed at Sutter Hospital in Sacramento, California. The valve name was eventually changed to the Sutter valve when sold to another laboratory. It was used clinically and the results reported in *Circulation* by McHenry in 1967.

The Braunwald–Cutter cloth-covered valve was released in 1965 by Cutter Laboratories (Figure 4.23, page 169). Braunwald first modified a standard Starr–Edwards mitral valve by covering the struts with porous polypropylene and the exposed metal orifice with netted dacron in order to reduce thromboembolic events. This resulted in high pressure gradients, particularly in smaller size valves, and prompted a redesign. With Cutter Laboratories, Braunwald produced an open apex, totally cloth covered ball valve with the housing machined from titanium. Between 1968 and 1974 about 5000 valves were implanted with excellent clinical results.

Origin of disc valves

IN 1965, Frederick Cross and Richard Jones developed a valve with a lens-shaped disc of silicone rubber in a low-profile cage with a woven teflon fixation flange (Figure 4.24, page 169). The free-floating disc was reinforced with a thin titanium ring. This allowed the lens weight and thickness to be reduced and prevented disc distortion and escape when subject to high closing pressure. The weight of the disc was further reduced by incorporating an air pocket within the body of the lens. Animal studies were undertaken in 1964 and the first human implant of the valve took place in January 1965. The clinical series was reported by Cross in *Annals of Thoracic Surgery* (1965).

Three prosthetic valves were developed by the Lillehei team at the University of Minnesota. The first, a toroidal disc design, was described in 1966 as the Lillehei–Nakib valve. This was constructed entirely from titanium with a low profile housing and a lightweight free-floating discoid poppet with a central orifice. *In vitro* hydrodynamic measurements in a pulse duplicator confirmed the superior flow characteristics of the toroidal design (with both central and peripheral flow) compared with the Starr ball valve and the Kay–Shiley disc valve, both of which had peripheral flow only. Five hundred toroidal prostheses were implanted worldwide between 1967 and 1970 without a single long-term structural failure. Panus occlusion and thrombosis occurred in 2% of the patients but thromboembolism and endocarditis were rare. The Lillehei–Kaster pivoting disc valve introduced a free-floating pyrolytic carbon disc that opened to 80° in an orifice ring machined from a single block of titanium (Figure 4.25, page 169). The valve first described in 1967 offered greatly improved central flow with rapid disc closure, relatively low profile and for the first time a rotatable teflon sewing cuff. This prosthesis with projected life time durability gained widespread clinical acceptance. Sixty-five thousand prostheses were implanted in humans between 1971 and 1990. There has been no reported incident of a valve failure due to degeneration and only three instances of disc escape with two survivors. Event-free survival rates at 13 years were 70% for aortic prostheses and 68% for mitral prostheses.

The original design concept for the Kalke–Lillehei bileaflet prosthesis began in 1965 when Kalke suggested a design based on the one-way dam in the irrigation system of India. Although the initial prototypes were crude, the bileaflet design concept produced the best hydrodynamic performance of any implantable device on the pulse duplicator. Subsequent *in vitro* and animal implantation studies resulted in refinements to the 1968 model. This prosthesis had a low profile with leaflets opening to 60°. The housing was of titanium and as the leaflets opened, they moved apart to create a central orifice, thereby eliminating stagnation and improving central lamina flow. Each leaflet had two short cylindrical cams that rotated within a semi-open ovoid recess in the orifice ring. A series of titanium valves were handcrafted by Cromie of the Surgitool Company and one of these became the first and only clinical implantation of this forerunner to the St Jude prosthesis.

Hufnagel produced a discoid valve in 1967, making the disc out of polypropylene because of its extremely low biological reactivity (Figure 4.26, page 169). This modification allowed the poppet to weigh approximately one-fifth of the ball in his cage ball valve. Perhaps the most significant feature of this prosthesis was the coating of hepcone. This combination of silicone rubber and heparin had the theoretical aim of slow release of heparin as prophylaxis against thromboembolism. Even the sewing ring cuff was coated, apart from a 5 mm strip in contact with the native annulus. The valve was implanted clinically between 1968 and 1970.

By the mid-1960s most eminent cardiac surgeons had devised their own valve prosthesis in association with either Edwards, Cutter or Surgitool. Cooley and DeBakey were no exception. In 1967, DeBakey, together with Cromie and Jack Bokros of Gulf Central Atomic Incorporated developed a pair of prosthetic heart valves whose occluders and orifice rings were coated with pyrolytic carbon (Figure 4.27 page 170). The cages were of titanium and the sewing ring a double layer of dacron velour. The ball and cage aortic valve was developed in 1967 and the low profile disc and cage mitral prosthesis soon afterwards. The inner surface of the aortic ball was covered with radio opaque tungsten. The DeBakey–Surgitool valve was inserted into 623 patients between 1968 and 1978 and compared favourably with similar valve designs. Aortic valve replacement with this valve was reported in the *Journal of Thoracic and Cardiovascular Surgery* in 1976. By this time the constituents of cardiac valves were both durable and minimally thrombogenic but there was room for improvement in the haemodynamic aspects.

Second generation mechanical valves

VALVE DESIGN continued to improve in the late

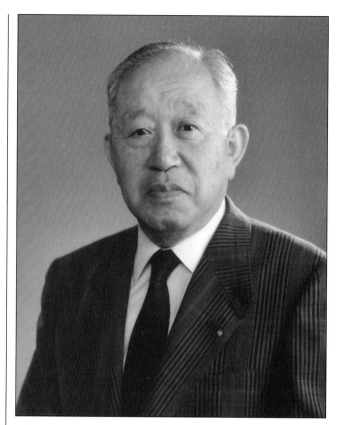

Figure 4.28. Juro Wada.

1960s and in Japan, Juro Wada (Figure 4.28) of the Sapporo Medical College developed the concept of a pivoting disc occluder (Figure 4.29, page 170). This was manufactured by Cutter Laboratories in Berkeley, California, using titanium for the housing, a teflon cloth sewing ring and hard teflon for the disc. The wafer-thin valve profile compared with bulky ball valves and disc poppet valves of intermediate height, made this valve immediately attractive. The Wada prosthesis was implanted clinically by Cooley, Rowe, Björk and others. The first total artificial heart implanted by Liotta and Cooley in 1969 employed four Wada–Cutter valves, which functioned successfully during the 64-hour life of the device.

Björk visited Wada in Japan and decided to use Wada's tilting disc valve. He found that the gradients were substantially lower (about half) than in the Kay–Shiley valve. Eventually, fibrin formation in the hinge caused malfunction of the occluding mechanism and localized wear of the hinges caused embolisation of the disc. Björk was of the opinion that disc valves provided lower gradients but that a hinge mechanism should be avoided. Don Shiley was Chief Engineer at Edwards Laboratories

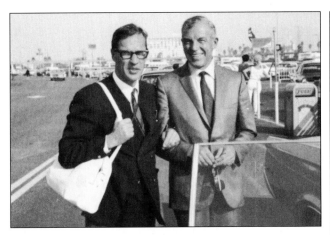

Figure 4.29. Viking Björk with Don Shiley in the mid 1960s.

when he first met Björk at the American Association of Thoracic Surgery Meeting. By 1964 Shiley had started his own heart valve company in the garage of his Southern Californian home and by 1966 he released the Kay–Shiley mitral valve in conjunction with Jerome Kay of St Vincent's Hospital in Los Angeles. The valves were constructed by Shiley and the suture rings were sewn in the family's bedroom. Björk implanted a number of Kay–Shiley valves at the Karolinska Institute and was the first to use it in the aortic position. Shiley visited Björk in Stockholm in May 1968 to see the valve used in the aortic position first hand. Björk showed him the data on patients who returned to post-operative investigation by transeptal heart catheters at rest and on exercise. After a series of 88 patients it was clear that the Kay–Shiley valve (and all central occlusive valves) had too high an outflow gradient. Despite this, the patients could tolerate tachycardia during exercise without a decrease in blood pressure (a persistent problem with ball valves). Björk was familiar with the Wada tilting disc valve which had only half the gradient and convinced Shiley that this was the way forward for a new mechanical prosthesis. Shiley returned to the United States and immediately began working on a tilting disc valve. Within a short time he manufactured two each of five sizes of disc valve and sent them to Stockholm. The first Björk–Shiley valve was implanted on 16 January 1969. On the evening of the first operation, Björk discussed with Shiley the necessity to rotate the valve after it had been sutured into place. They found that if the valve was soaked in a heparin/penicillin solution and revolved in its valve holder ten times in each direction, it was possible to turn

it after implantation into the patient. Björk used the same valve upside down for the mitral position. Modifications occurred rapidly with the opening angle reduced to 50° for the mitral position and the sewing ring improved. Within a short time, 100 aortic and 50 mitral valves had been implanted and Björk presented his data worldwide. The disc of the first model was made of delrin and some of these valves are still functional 20 years later. The disc was then changed to pyrolytic carbon for increased durability and provided with a radio-opaque marker. The inlet strut of the convexo-concave disc model was an integral part of the orifice ring but the outlet strut was welded. The disc opened to 60° with a greater and lesser orifice for flow. Turbulence through the lesser orifice of a disc valve is now known to encourage fibrin deposition and thrombus formation. In 1971, the delrin disc was exchanged for the so-called conical pyrolyte carbon disc when it was recognised that delrin could retain water and swell. In 1975, the conical disc valve was replaced by a spherical disc with a radio-opaque marker. Radiological screening could then verify disc excursion easily and recognise abnormal movement. In a series of 1657 patients who underwent aortic valve replacement with an early model, the 15 year actuarial survival was 54%; 25% of late deaths were valve related: 8.3% from anticoagulation related bleeding and 5.4% from thromboembolic complications. An early attempt by Björk to omit anticoagulation for 32 aortic replacement patients for 12 months resulted in 15.6 thromboembolic complications per 100 patient years. Subsequently, anticoagulation was started in every case. Similar attempts to eliminate anticoagulation at the Brompton Hospital proved disastrous and remained unpublished. For the mitral position 15 year actuarial survival was 51%; valve related death was dominated by thrombosis in 10%, embolism in 3% and anticoagulation related fatal bleeding in 4%.

The convexo–concave disc valve was introduced in 1976 (Figure 4.30, page 170). The disc configuration was changed, principally to improve the flow through the lesser orifice and thereby diminish thromboembolic complications. When open, the hydrodynamic force caused the disc to slide out of the orifice by 2 mm and eliminate the low flow area caused by the disc edge touching the valve ring (as occurred in the earlier models with a flat disc). The clinical results of the convexo–concave valve models with a 60° or 70° opening

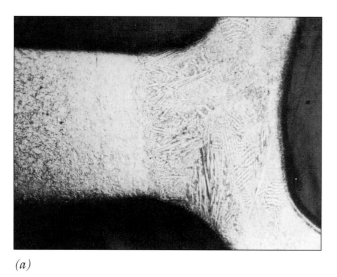

(a)

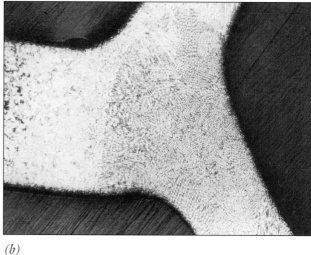

(b)

Figure 4.31. Examples of (a) good and (b) bad welding. (Reproduced with permission from Björk VO. Metallurgic and design development in response to mechanical dysfunction of Björk–Shiley heart valves. Scand J Thor Cardiovasc Surg 19: 1–12.)

showed a reduction in thromboembolic complications of 50% over the earlier models with flat discs.

The Björk–Shiley strut fractures

AT THE OUTSET, both the inflow and outflow struts of the Björk–Shiley valve were welded into the valve ring (Figure 4.31). Of the 1100 patients with a flat disc valve, only one suffered inflow strut fracture. The inflow strut was then made an integral part of the valve ring after which no fractures occurred. In 1978, came the first report of an outlet strut fracture with disc escape and rapid death of the patient. The opening angle of the valve was then increased from 60° to 70° in an attempt to moderate the opening forces on the outlet strut. The 70° opening angle also reduced vortex formation behind the smaller hole and diminished the gradient, making the valve more suitable in the small aortic root.

In March 1982, Björk himself had two fatal outlet strut fractures in large (31 and 33 mm) 70° mitral valves and immediately stopped using larger size convexo-concave valves (Figure 4.32). Between the first strut fracture (1978) and 1982, a new valve ring known as the monostrut valve was developed with an opening angle of 70° (Figure 4.33, page 170). The principal change was

in the valve housing, with both struts incorporated as an integral part of the ring and no welding. Björk advised against further production or sale of the welded convexo–concave model soon after the first reports of strut fracture. Clearly the welded outflow strut was an area of weakness, particularly for large size mitral prostheses. This eventually caused hundreds of

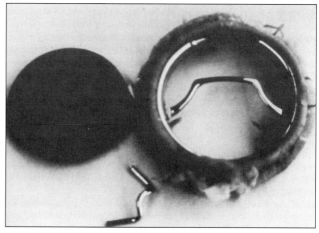

Figure 4.32. Outlet strut fracture of Björk–Shiley convexo-concave valve. (Reproduced with permission from Teijeira FJ, Mikhail AA. Cardiac valve replacement with mechanical prostheses: current status and trends. In Hwang NHC et al. Advances in Cardiovascular Engineering (Vol. 235), p.217. New York, Plenum Press, 1992.)

MECHANICAL FAILURE OF THE
BJÖRK-SHILEY VALVE

DAN LINDBLOM, M.D.,
VIKING O. BJÖRK, M.D.,
and
BJARNE K. H. SEMB, M.D.,
Stockholm, Sweden

From the Department of Thoracic Surgery, Karolinska
Hospital, Stockholm, Sweden.

Reprinted from
THE JOURNAL OF THORACIC AND
CARDIOVASCULAR SURGERY,
St. Louis

Vol. 92, No. 5, pp. 894-907, Nov., 1986
(Copyright © 1986, by The C.V. Mosby Company)
(Printed in the U.S.A.)

Figure 4.34. Mechanical failure of the Björk–Shiley valve. *A 1986 article by Lindblom, Björk and Semb. (Reproduced with permission from* Journal of Thoracic and Cardiovascular surgery.*)*

premature deaths through early mechanical failure (Figure 4.34). Despite protests by Björk and the Shiley engineers the valve was kept on the European market by the Shiley Company until 1986.

By 14 June 1987 there were 213 outlet strut fractures reported from 83,000 prostheses implanted. Of these, 76% occurred in mitral valves sized 29–33 mm, but fractures also occurred in aortic prostheses 21–27 mm in size. Risk of strut fracture ranged from 0.21 events per 100 patient years for small (21–27 mm) valves to 0.318 events per 100 patient years for large (29–33 mm) valves manufactured between 1 February 1981 and 30 June 1982. *In vitro* analysis showed that excessive stress on the outlet strut occurred during closure of the prosthesis. In October 1985, 29 mm, 31 mm and 33 mm convexo–concave Björk–Shiley valves manufactured between February 1981 and June 1982 were recalled and in November 1986, all unimplanted convexo–concave valves were removed from the market through risk of outlet strut fracture. The high risk 70° convexo–concave disc valve was never sold in the United States. Large valves processed between 1 February 1981 and 30 June 1982 had the highest risk of fracture (average 0.32%/year). Large valves processed after 30 June 1982 had a relatively low risk (0.08%/year). The 29–31 mm, 70° convexo–concave valve had an actuarial

incidence of mechanical failure of 12.5% over a 7 year follow-up period and prophylactic replacement of this selected group of valves is still considered advisable.

Investigation by the Food and Drug Administration (FDA) revealed many irregularities in the internal handling of the affair, though Björk himself was blameless. When the FDA prevented further sales in the United States, stocks were disposed of in Europe and other parts of the world. The ensuing patient deaths, anxiety in those with an 'at risk' prosthesis and monumental legal fees and compensation eventually led to the disintegration of the Shiley Company. The situation was compounded by premature failure of the Ionescu–Shiley stent mounted pericardial valve, resulting in thousands of valve reoperations within a few years of implantation. The Texas Heart Institute alone inserted more than 2000 Ionescu valves and faced the formidable task of wholesale rereplacement.

Björk went on to use the mono strut valve in over 2000 patients at the Karolinska Institute, with very satisfactory results. Nevertheless, the Björk–Shiley outflow strut fracture episode had a profound effect on the cardiovascular industry worldwide. Much tighter regulatory rules were introduced, particularly in the United States, where the FDA now prevent surgeons from using many useful drugs and devices which are freely available in Europe.

The St Jude valve

IN MARCH 1976, Manuel Villafaña (Figure 4.35), a former Medtronic employee and founder of Cardiac Pacemakers Incorporated (the lithium powered pacemaker), met with Victor Parsonnet, who suggested that the time had come for a better heart valve. Almost simultaneously Villafaña was approached by the Minneapolis surgeon, Demetre Nicoloff, and the engineer, Christopher Possis, with a crude bileaflet heart valve design. When their project was rejected by the Board of Directors of Cardiac Pacemakers Incorporated, Villafaña decided to pursue the idea further and formed another company, St Jude Medical Incorporated, to develop the valve. St Jude is the Patron Saint of Lost Causes and Villafaña had named his son Jude after surviving serious medical problems in infancy. Soon afterwards Cardiac Pacemakers Incorporated was

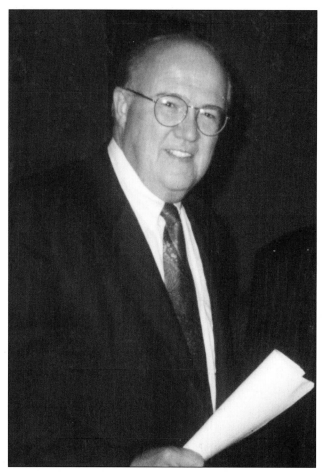

Figure 4.35. Manuel Villafaña.

acquired by Eli Lilly and Villafaña concentrated on the new valve design. The bileaflet concept had been proposed by Lillehei, Wada and Gott independently but the introduction of pyrolytic carbon as a thrombo-resistant surface came from Jack Bokros at General Atomic (subsequently CarboMedics Incorporated). The valve design incorporated four pivots and two leaflets at a time when there was a serious question mark over the durability of such fittings. Pyrolytic carbon is highly durable but expensive. Consequently the two semi-circular leaflets were constructed from tungsten and coated with pyrolytic carbon (Figure 4.36, page 170). This also rendered them radioopaque. The leaflets opened to 85°, allowing near lamina flow, and the butterfly shaped pivot was recessed in the orifice ring. This was also made of solid pyrolytic carbon with a dacron sewing ring.

The valve was first implanted clinically in October 1977 and demonstrated excellent haemodynamics with low thrombogenicity. Durability and freedom from primary valve failure have been outstanding and low levels of anticoagulation (INR 2.0–2.5) appear satisfactory for the aortic position. The principal competitor to the St Jude valve became the Medtronic Hall tilting disc valve (Figure 4.37) with its one piece machined housing and improved pivot design. This prosthesis also proved safe and durable with low thrombogenicity and excellent haemodynamics. Further bileaflet designs were also adopted including the DuroMedics valve, designed and developed by Hemex Scientific Incorporated in the early 1980s (first human implant in 1982). This valve was removed from the market in 1988 after 12 unexplained cases of leaflet escape.

After supplying pyrolytic carbon to other valve companies, CarboMedics introduced their own bileaflet pyrolytic carbon valve in 1986, comprising a solid pyrolytic carbon valve ring without struts, pivot guards or orifice projections (Figure 4.38, page 170). Their design also incorporated pivot recess washing, enhanced radiographic visualization and rotatability. The sewing ring was carbon coated to discourage panus ingrowth.

More recently, Villafaña left St Jude Medical Incorporated to establish the ATS (Advancing the Standard) Heart Valve Company with a design similar to that of St Jude but with a number of potential improvements, including convex self-washing pivots, absence of pivot guards and rotatability. Excellent

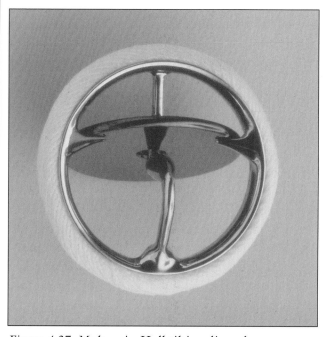

Figure 4.37. Medtronic–Hall tilting disc valve.

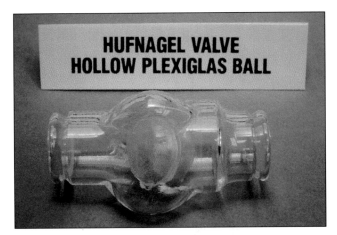

Figure 4.5. Hufnagel's ball and cage valve.

We wish to thank Baxter (Edwards division) for access to their library of historical valve photographs.

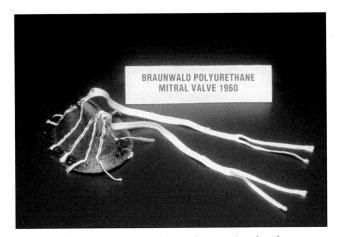

Figure 4.7. Braunwald's polyurethane mitral valve.

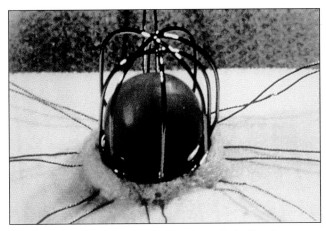

Figure 4.8. Harken's double-caged aortic ball valve.

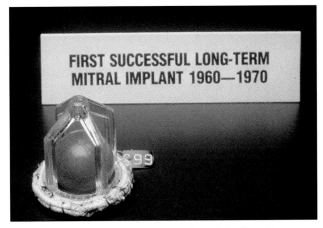

Figure 4.9. The original Starr–Edwards ball and cage valve.

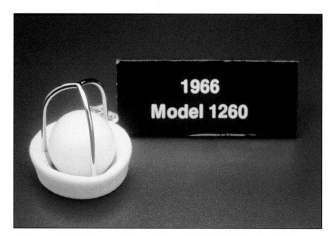

Figure 4.10. Starr–Edwards model 1260 silastic ball valve.

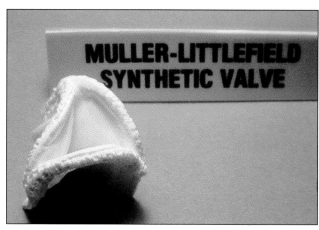

Figure 4.11. Muller–Littlefield synthetic trileaflet valve.

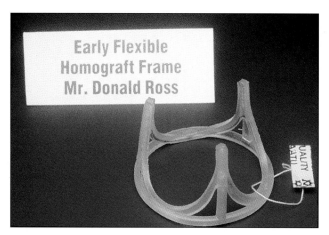

Figure 4.13. Ross flexible homograft support.

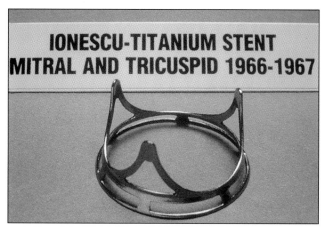

Figure 4.17. Ionescu–Wooler heterograft rigid titanium support.

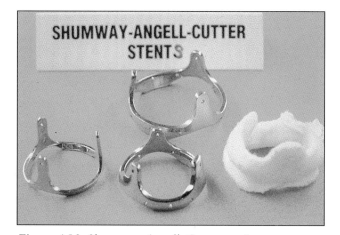

Figure 4.18. Shumway–Angell–Cutter graft supports.

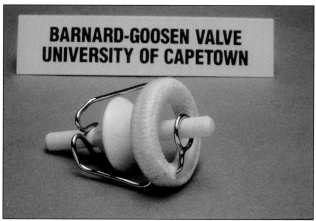

Figure 4.19. Barnard–Goosens biconical aortic valve.

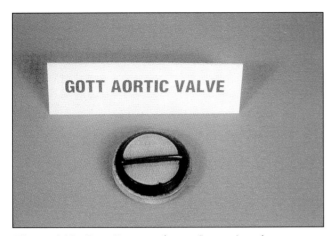

Figure 4.21. Gott–Daggatt butterfly aortic valve.

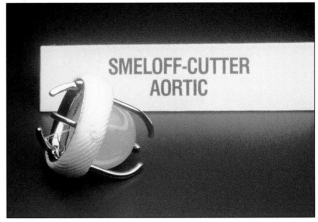

Figure 4.22. Smeloff–Cutter double-caged valve.

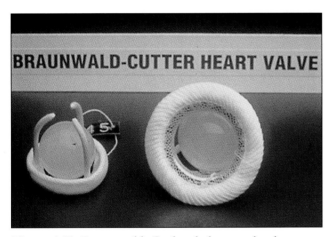

Figure 4.23. Braunwald–Cutler cloth-covered valve.

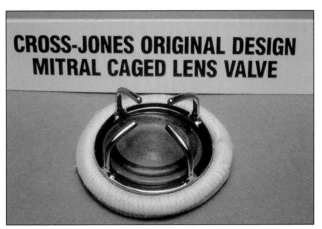

Figure 4.24. Cross–Jones lenticular disc valve.

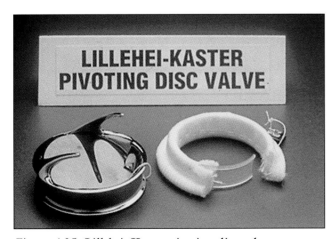

Figure 4.25. Lillehei–Kaster pivoting disc valve.

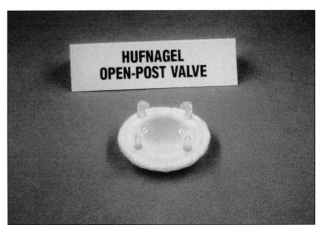

Figure 4.26. Hufnagel's discord valve.

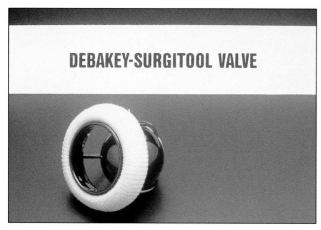

Figure 4.27. *The DeBakey–Surgitool ball and cage aortic valve.*

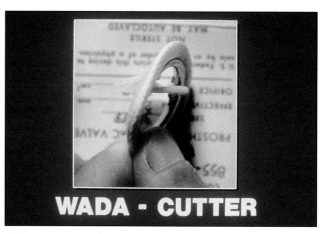

Figure 4.29. *Wada–Cutter hingeless disc valve.*

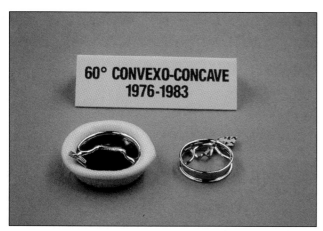

Figure 4.30. *Björk–Shiley tilting disc valve with convexo-concave disc valve (60°).*

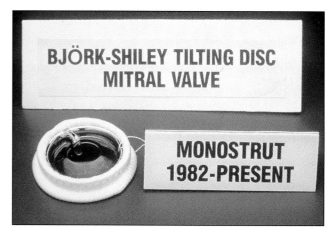

Figure 4.33. *Björk–Shiley monostrut tilting disc valve.*

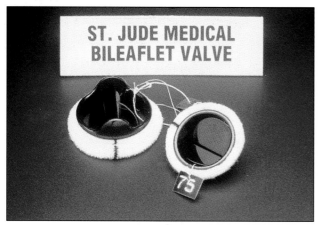

Figure 4.36. *St Jude Medical bileaflet valve constructed from tungsten and coated with pyrolytic carbon.*

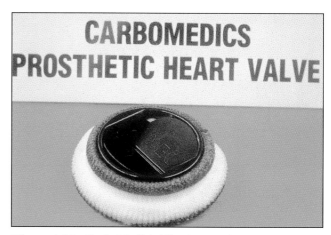

Figure 4.38. *CarboMedic's bileaflet pyrolytic carbon valve.*

haemodynamics translated into very low thrombogenicity for both valves.

Resurrection of the stentless valve

STUDIES taking into consideration the concept of patient orientated treatment failure and patient related variables, have suggested superior results in adult patients who receive bioprostheses in contrast to mechanical valves in the aortic position. Most patients who require mitral valve replacement, as distinct from repair, require continued anticoagulation whether a biological or mechanical prosthesis is inserted. Consequently, the advantage of the bioprosthesis is lost and it is illogical to use a valve subject to degeneration in these circumstances. For the aortic position the benign mode of bioprosthetic valve failure in conjunction with a low incidence thromboembolic events or anticoagulation related bleeding, has been seen to compensate for the risk of bioprosthetic reoperation. In contrast to mechanical prostheses, the patient with a true biological valve substitute, such as the pulmonary autograft (Ross operation) or aortic homograft inserted by the freehand technique, is able to live an unrestricted life without anticoagulants, threat of embolism or sudden death. Whilst the autogenous pulmonary valve remains vital and grows in children with an indefinite life span, structural failure of the aortic homograft occurs through calcification or cusp rupture, though later than in the stented xenograft.

Whilst preservation methods in bioprostheses account for some differences in durability, accelerated fatigue tests show that the stent of a bioprosthesis is a major factor governing stress on the biological component. Clearly the best stent for a glutaraldehyde fixed porcine xenograft is the native aortic root, where the structure of the sinuses is such that mechanical stress is dissipated during leaflet closure at high aortic pressure. This may account for the difference in durability between freehand sewn aortic valve homografts and stented aortic homografts used for valve replacement in humans. The average time for aortic homograft failure exceeds 12 years when handsewn but is approximately 8 years when stent mounted. The average time for failure of the stented porcine xenograft in the aortic position (though varying with age at implantation) is also 8 years.

Though the durability of stented porcine xenografts proves sufficient to prevent re-operation for the majority of the over 70s, haemodynamic function and freedom from structural valve failure remains less satisfactory than for mechanical valves or homografts. Given that the aortic wall and sinuses provide the best stent for valve leaflets, it is logical to expect that elimination of an artificial stent will reduce stress and improve durability. Absence of a stent and sewing ring provides reduced transvalvar pressure gradients and the native aortic root and sinuses dissipate mechanical stress during leaflet closure at high pressure.

Stentless aortic bioprostheses

In 1988, Tirone David (Figure 4.39) re-explored the use of stentless glutaraldehyde fixed aortic xenografts both experimentally and in humans. Haemodynamic evaluation showed very small resting gradients and minimal aortic regurgitation in these early implants. David went on to develop a low pressure fixed stentless

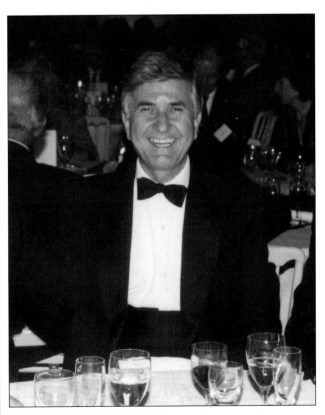

Figure 4.39. Tirone David, honoured guest at the European Society Meeting in Paris (1995).

but cloth covered valve, initially manufactured by Johnson and Johnson Cardiovascular Products but later acquired by St Jude Medical Incorporated. This stentless bioprosthesis known as the Toronto SPV (stentless porcine valve) has been used extensively by David and others with excellent medium-term results. The stentless valve allows a larger valve to be inserted into an individual annulus through elimination of the stent and sewing ring. The flow characteristics are inherently superior to the stented xenograft and there is a suggestion that improved haemodynamics and reduced leaflet stress will translate into prolonged durability for the porcine xenograft. Progressing along these lines, Medtronic introduced the stentless Freestyle valve in the form of a porcine aortic root with dacron covering of the inflow portion. This glutaraldehyde treated root was fixed with a zero transvalvar pressure drop to preserve the natural collagen crimp and integrity of the cusp structure. Added to this was an advanced anti-calcification treatment with alpha amino-oleic acid. These stentless porcine xenografts provide an alternative to aortic homografts, which remain in limited supply despite cryopreservation.

O'Brien and Angell reintroduced a trileaflet composite valve without a muscle bar, first used in 1966. At that time, formaldehyde had been used as a fixative and resulted in early leaflet failure. In 1991, the valve was manufactured again using the modern glutaraldehyde preservation techniques by Cryolife Incorporated. This stentless valve is unusual in that it can be implanted with a single suture line. The stentless concept was then applied to the mitral position. The use of mitral homografts was re-explored by Carpentier and Accar, who designed more secure implant techniques for the subvalvular apparatus and Frater constructed a stentless mitral bioprosthesis from pericardium.

Increasing experience with the Toronto SPV (David and Pepper) and the Freestyle valve (Westaby, Huysmans and others) demonstrated greatly improved haemodynamics when compared to stented bioprostheses. In particular, resolution of left ventricular hypertrophy occurred at a similar rate to that with aortic homografts. This new direction in valve surgery was stimulated by the International meeting on 'Stentless Bioprostheses' convened by Piwnica (Figure 4.40) (Paris) in 1994.

It is 500 years since Leonardo da Vinci described the flow characteristics through the aortic valve using a glass model of the aortic sinuses. With his prototype of the pulse duplicator and particles of carbon in the hydraulic fluid, Leonardo identified the mechanism of closure of the native aortic valve and would never have considered stent mounting. At the outset of valve replacement surgery, Ross, Barratt-Boyes and others in tandem with Leonardo and the Almighty considered the aortic homograft to be of perfect design to ensure central non-obstructive flow. After almost half a century of stent mounted tissue valves, we have reached the same conclusion.

Mechanical versus tissue valves

FOR THE PAST 20 years mechanical and tissue valves have continued to improve, though debate over their relative merits continues. Most modern mechanical

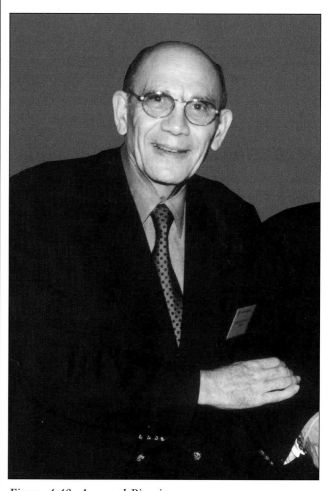

Figure 4.40. Armand Piwnica.

prostheses have an indefinite life span with little risk of structural failure. Their haemodynamic characteristics are acceptable but the need for anticoagulation with warfarin remains. This is a distinct disadvantage since the predominant valve related morbidity is firstly through bleeding and then thromboembolism. There is increasing evidence that event-free survival is better with a tissue prosthesis despite the need for reoperation. With improved cardiopulmonary bypass and myocardial protection, elective reoperation carries a low risk of mortality.

Biological tissue mounted on a stent suffers accelerated degeneration and for the last few years of their projected life span many stented bioprostheses have rigid, obstructive leaflets. Attempts to reduce this problem included elimination of the porcine muscle bar in the Hancock valve, flexible valve stents, anti-mineralisation treatments and zero pressure leaflet fixation as advocated by Grant Christie and Sir Brian Barratt-Boyes. Eric Jamieson (Vancouver) spent many years characterising the durability of bioprostheses through careful documentation of large, clinical series. Stent mounting leads to suboptimal valve geometry and maldistribution of stress on the leaflets. Degeneration, calcification and cusp rupture occur early in children or young adults.

Throughout their careers, Ross, Kirklin, Yacoub, Barratt-Boyes and O'Brien have been great protagonists of the freehand sewn aortic homograft. The principal problem with this approach was the availability of human tissue.

Ross' persistence with the autograft operation has produced persuasive long-term results, showing that the pulmonary valve is ideal for aortic replacement in infancy, childhood and the teenage years. With increasing availability of pulmonary homografts for reconstruction of the right ventricular outflow tract, protagonists such as Elkins (Oklahoma City), Oury (Missoula, Montana) and Petterson (Copenhagen) advocated the Ross procedure for any patient with a life expectancy greater than 20 years. Quaegebeur, Mee, Westaby and others have used this technique for infants with congenital aortic stenosis. As long as normal leaflet coaptation is established at the time of operation, the viable autograft remains competent and grows with the developing child or teenager. The biological problems of homograft degeneration are transferred to the low pressure pulmonary position, where optimal valve function is less important and failure occurs slowly. Consequently, the pulmonary autograft fits the criteria for the ideal aortic valve substitute, including indefinite durability, central non-obstructive flow, zero risk of thromboembolism or haemolysis and no requirement for anticoagulation. Nonetheless, by 1995 fewer than 100 surgeons worldwide had performed the procedure.

Valve replacement versus repair

THE PROBLEMS associated with mechanical and porcine bioprostheses stimulated efforts to repair rather than replace diseased valves. Valve repair techniques were attempted before the evolution of valve prostheses but the era of modern mitral repair began in Leeds in the early 60s where Geoffrey Wooler pursued surgical methods to correct mitral incompetence. Reed (1965) modified Wooler's annuloplasty to add a degree of haemodynamic predictability, but it was not until the development of the annuloplasty rings by Carpentier, then Duran, that widespread adoption of repair techniques occurred. Carpentier worked with Chauvoud to annotate the numerous mitral valve lesions amenable to surgical correction. Stimulated by Lev's comment, "Mitral valve diseases are like women, the more you study them, the less you understand them", Carpentier and Chauvoud described 10 acquired and 14 congenital valve lesions. Surgical strategy then concentrated on both the individual abnormalities and function of the valve as a whole. In rheumatic disease with commissural fusion and restricted leaflet motion, Carpentier extended standard mitral valvotomy by resecting secondary chordae and fenestrating marginal chordae to increase leaflet motion. For posterior leaflet prolapse with ruptured or elongated chordae, the technique of quadrangular resection was developed. For anterior leaflet prolapse, Carpentier developed chordal shortening , transposition of chordae from the mural leaflet and chordal replacement. The Carpentier Annuloplasty Ring was used to restore the size and shape of the native annulus and to prevent further dilatation. During the 1970s, these progressive techniques were limited to relatively few centres. Carpentier's achievements in the field were recognized at the 63rd Meeting of the American Association for Thoracic

Surgery (1983), where he presented the landmark guest lecture *Cardiac valve surgery — the French correction.* Both Carpentier and Duran gained enormous experience with valve repair on patients from North Africa and Saudi Arabia, who could not be safely anticoagulated. Duran considered that 80–90% of mitral valves with degenerative diseases could be repaired, as could 40–60% of rheumatic valves.

The benefits of mitral repair became increasingly apparent when both operative and long-term survival were found to exceed that of valve replacement. David, Duran, Gams and others showed that retaining the subvalvular apparatus during mitral replacement played an important part in preserving the mechanics of left ventricular function. Resection of the mitral subvalvar apparatus causes a significant decrease in ejection fraction. Consequently, most surgeons make every effort to repair rather than replace the mitral valve and to preserve annulo chordal continuity if replacement is required.

Valve replacement in the low pressure right heart carries a substantial thrombotic risk. Consequently, tricuspid repair is also preferable to replacement in most patients. Bailey first proposed closed tricuspid commissurotomy for rheumatic disease in the 1950s. Kay then proposed the simple but enduring technique of bicuspidalization for tricuspid regurgitation. Perhaps the most popular operation for tricuspid valve insufficiency was that of DeVega (1972) who described semi-circular annuloplasty to reduce the circumference of the tricuspid annulus without interfering with the conduction system. Carpentier and Duran then introduced annuloplasty rings in the tricuspid position. For drug addicts with infective endocarditis, Arbulu and associates showed that tricuspid valve excision could be well tolerated in the short term.

Reparative techniques for the aortic valve were less successful. Cabrol described a technique for aortic annuloplasty in 1966. Decalcification of the valve in aortic stenosis proved unsatisfactory. In Saudi Arabia, Fagih and Duran separately established principles for cusp repair or extension using pericardium in young patients with aortic regurgitation.

Biographies

Elliott Carr Cutler (1888–1947)

ELLIOTT CARR CUTLER was born in Bangor, Maine, USA and studied medicine at Harvard University (BA, 1909; MD, 1913). He interned under Harvey Cushing at Peter Bent Brigham (1913–15) and did further research in pathology at the Frank B. Mallory Laboratory and Heidelberg University (1913). During World War I, Cutler supervised the Harvard American Ambulance Unit (1915) and the Fifth General Hospital in Paris (1917–18) and was awarded the DSM. He was Resident Surgeon at Peter Bent Brigham (1919–21), Director of Surgical Research at Harvard Medical School (1921–24), Professor and Chairman of Surgery at Western Reserve University Medical School and surgeon at Lakeside Hospital, Cleveland (1924–32). He subsequently succeeded Cushing as the Moseley Professor of Surgery at Harvard and Surgeon-in-Chief at Peter Bent Brigham (1932–47) and Boston Children's Hospital (1937–47). It was in the late summer of 1932 that Cushing, returning from a summer abroad, found his books and papers in boxes outside his office and Cutler installed within.

During World War II, Cutler was in England as American Chief Surgical Consultant in the European Theatre with the first wave of the US medical units. His reputation preceded him in medical circles and he took the initiative in organizing interallied conferences on war medicine held at the Royal Society of Medicine. He advanced Anglo-American surgical relationships and encouraged the interchange of trainees. Cutler was made an Honorary Fellow of the Royal College of Surgeons in 1943 and President of the American Surgical Society (1946–47), but died before he fulfilled his term. Ravitch describes Cutler as a magnetic individual and teacher; Harken knew him as a forthright man, of high standards and integrity, who thought of himself as the complete surgeon-general, thoracic-, neuro-, and probably was as near to being one as was humanly possible that late in the evolution of surgery, a veritable Roger Bacon of surgery, "the last man to know everything." With Zollinger, Cutler produced the best-selling *Atlas of Surgical Operations* (1930), which is perennially reprinted. Cutler contributed to the understanding of postoperative atelectasis and introduced total thyroidectomy to relieve heart failure. His name is associated with advances in the

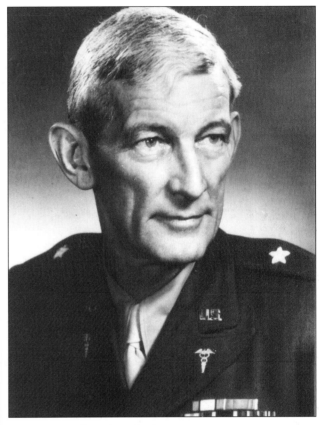

Figure 4.42. Elliott Carr Cutler.

surgery of the central and autonomic nervous systems and the gall bladder. He also encouraged prosthetic implants. His residents included Hufnagel, Gross, Beck, Zollinger, Swan and Hume.

Cushing, who eloquently declared that "The mitral valve may become the gateway to the last great Northwest of surgery," was the first to successfully produce valvular lesions in hearts of dogs with subsequent recovery while at Johns Hopkins. While studying immunology under Simon Flexner at the Rockefeller Institute (1916–17), he decided that the mitral valve was amenable to surgical correction and that mitral regurgitation would be better tolerated than stenosis. Cutler and Levine spent 2 years at Harvard in the Surgical Research Laboratories (1917–19) learning to handle open pneumothorax and endotracheal anaesthesia, in preparation for operating within the human thorax. Not only were the physical problems overwhelming, but the ambient medical opinion was completely opposed to Cutler's efforts. Cutler confessed in 1931 that "The trials, tribulations, and great mental anguish of the responsibility assumed at that time are still very bright in my mind." Sir James Mackenzie's reply to Levine's account of Cutler's effort to open a stenosed mitral valve, "Dear Sam, what a foolish thing to try to do. Have you forgotten that the myocardium is all-important?", illustrated the widely-held view that the cause of mitral stenosis was a weakened heart muscle not a diseased valve.

In May 1923, Cutler's valvulotomy through the wall of the left ventricle with a slender tenotome knife in an effort to resect each cusp of the stenotic mitral valve succeeded, miraculously, in this one case (Article 4.1, Appendix A). The patient died 4 years later and postmortem examination showed that the mitral orifice had been enlarged by the incision. After the tenotome knife was used unsuccessfully in two more cases, a cardiovalvulotome was devised by his associate, Claude Beck. This actually excised a piece from the stenosed valve and removed the piece from the blood stream. It was used unsuccessfully in two further cases.

In 1929, Cutler and Back reviewed the 12 cases of stenotic valves (10 mitral, one pulmonic and one aortic) treated between 1913 and 1928 and observed that besides Cutler's single case by tenotome only patients undergoing Souttar's and Tuffier's finger dilation survived. Cutler and Beck, although insisting that these mortality figures should not deter further investigation in a new field, were not stirred to attempt digital splitting or doubt the correctness of cutting the cusps of the stenotic valve. It was John Powers, a surgical resident under Cutler, who produced mild mitral stenosis in dogs and demonstrated that partial resection of a valve cusp led to death from fulminant mitral regurgitation. From experimental work, they soon learned that when he cut the anterior leaflet death occurred in minutes, but when he cut the posterior leaflet death

Original Articles.

CARDIOTOMY AND VALVULOTOMY FOR MITRAL STENOSIS. EXPERIMENTAL OBSERVATIONS AND CLINICAL NOTES CONCERNING AN OPERATED CASE WITH RECOVERY.

BY ELLIOTT C. CUTLER, M.D., BOSTON,
AND
S. A. LEVINE, M.D., BOSTON.

[From the Surgical Clinic of the Peter Bent Brigham Hospital and the Laboratory of Surgical Research of the Harvard Medical School.]

DURING the recent decennial celebration of the former and present members of the nursing and professional staff of the Peter Bent Brigham Hospital, we presented (May 24, 1923) a case of mitral stenosis upon which we had operated four days previously in an attempt to alleviate the condition by diminishing the degree of stenosis of the valve.

Figure 4.43. Cardiotomy and valvulotomy for mitral stenosis. Experimental observations and clinical notes concerning an operated case with recovery. *A 1923 article by Cutler and Levine. (Reproduced with permission from* Boston Medical and Surgical Journal.*)*

was delayed for as long as 24 hours. Beck admitted in 1954 that the creation of the cardiovalvulotome probably delayed the surgery of mitral stenosis by some 20 years. Cutler gave his valvular surgical instruments to Harken and abandoned cardiac surgery in the 1920s. No surgeon attempted this procedure again until 1948, when Smithy, Bailey, Harken and Brock prevailed.

Sir Henry Sessions Souttar (1875–1964)

SIR HENRY SESSIONS SOUTTAR was born in Birkenhead, Oxfordshire and educated at Oxford High School and Queen's College, Oxford University. He took a double first in mathematics and studied engineering and medicine (BA, 1901). In 1903, he became a clinical student at the London Hospital and after qualifying (BM, BCh, 1906; FRCS, 1909), held most house appointments, including resident accoucheur. He became surgical registrar and demonstrator in anatomy (1910), assistant surgeon on the staff of The West

London Hospital (MCh, 1912) and was appointed, 3 years later, to the staff of The London Hospital (1915). In 1916, Souttar became senior surgeon at the Red Cross Hospital at Netley where he developed many ideas for rehabilitating wounded men. He was Vice President of the Council of the Royal College of Surgeons, a Bradshaw lecturer and Hunterian orator. In addition, he was chairman of the Central Medical War Committee and of the Medical Planning Commission and President of the British Medical Association in 1945. Souttar received the CBE in 1919 and was knighted in 1949. The cardiologist Maurice Campbell wrote:

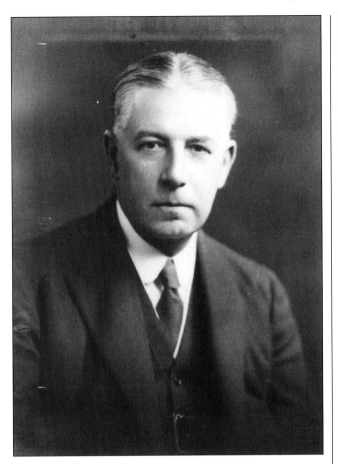

Figure 4.44. Sir Henry Sessions Souttar.

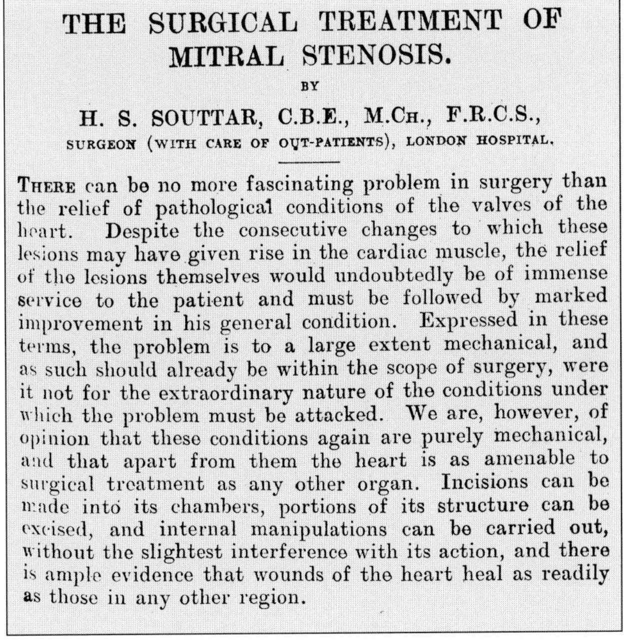

"Few can have been chairman of so many important bodies. His friendliness and his large impressive figure with his bull-dog face and his hearty laugh no doubt helped, but his colleagues must have trusted his good judgement and commonsense."

Souttar wrote *Injuries of the Peripheral Nerves* (1920) and *Art of Surgery* (1928), this last reaching its 4th edition in 1942. In *A Surgeon in Belgium*, Souttar described his experiences in World War II as Surgeon-in-Chief of a field ambulance at the Siege of Antwerp and war surgeon in Furnes on the Flanders coast, for which he received the Order of the Crown of Belgium. When radium was first discovered, Souttar, having encountered Marie Curie during the war in Belgium, rushed to Paris to meet the Curies. He wrote a great deal on the subject, including *Radium and its Surgical Applications, and Radium and Cancer*. As chairman of the Radium Technical Committee set up by the joint Royal Colleges, he played a leading part in the development of radium therapy.

He had an engineering workshop over his Harley Street house and a fine mahogany breakfront bookcase in his operating theatre at The London Hospital for his instruments: his hollow atraumatic intestinal needle, special tubes for

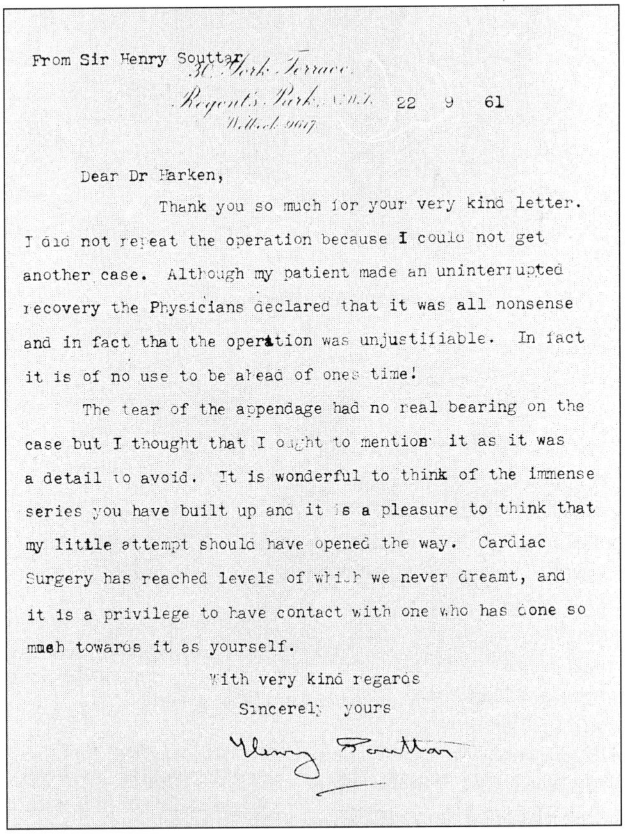

THE SURGICAL TREATMENT OF MITRAL STENOSIS.

BY

H. S. SOUTTAR, C.B.E., M.Ch., F.R.C.S.,
SURGEON (WITH CARE OF OUT-PATIENTS), LONDON HOSPITAL.

THERE can be no more fascinating problem in surgery than the relief of pathological conditions of the valves of the heart. Despite the consecutive changes to which these lesions may have given rise in the cardiac muscle, the relief of the lesions themselves would undoubtedly be of immense service to the patient and must be followed by marked improvement in his general condition. Expressed in these terms, the problem is to a large extent mechanical, and as such should already be within the scope of surgery, were it not for the extraordinary nature of the conditions under which the problem must be attacked. We are, however, of opinion that these conditions again are purely mechanical, and that apart from them the heart is as amenable to surgical treatment as any other organ. Incisions can be made into its chambers, portions of its structure can be excised, and internal manipulations can be carried out, without the slightest interference with its action, and there is ample evidence that wounds of the heart heal as readily as those in any other region.

Figure 4.45. A 1925 article by Souttar entitled 'The surgical treatment of mitral stenosis'. (Reproduced with permission from British Medical Journal.*)*

From Sir Henry Souttar
                                          22 9 61

Dear Dr Harken,

Thank you so much for your very kind letter. I did not repeat the operation because I could not get another case. Although my patient made an uninterrupted recovery the Physicians declared that it was all nonsense and in fact that the operation was unjustifiable. In fact it is of no use to be ahead of ones time!

The tear of the appendage had no real bearing on the case but I thought that I ought to mention it as it was a detail to avoid. It is wonderful to think of the immense series you have built up and it is a pleasure to think that my little attempt should have opened the way. Cardiac surgery has reached levels of which we never dreamt, and it is a privilege to have contact with one who has done so much towards it as yourself.

With very kind regards
Sincerely yours

Figure 4.46. Sir Henry Souttar's reply to Harken (1961).

intubation, the steam cautery, the craniotome, an introducer for radon seeds and the famous spiral oesophagoscope for inserting through the growth of an inoperable oesophageal cancer. In spite of the prevailing view of the cardiologist, Sir James MacKenzie, who was reputed to have said "The only heart disease I know of is that of the muscle, and no operation will correct it," Souttar was convinced of the mechanical aspect of mitral stenosis.

On 6 May 1925, *after the death of MacKenzie*, Souttar used his finger to dilate the mitral valve of a 19-year-old patient, Lily Hines, instead of the small knife he had prepared for incision of the anterior mitral leaflet (Article 4.2, Appendix A). He wrote, "The information given by the finger is exceedingly clear, and personally I felt an appreciation for the mechanical reality of stenosis and regurgitation which I never before possessed." Lily

Hines lived in fair health for 5 years when she suddenly developed a cerebral embolus, presumably from a clot in the atrium, and died shortly after. The physician, failed to recognize that her apparent lack of improvement was caused by preponderant mitral regurgitation, and would not send him another case, Souttar never operated on the mitral valve again. Souttar wrote to Brian Blades, "It was an article of faith with physicians that the valves were of no importance and that the only thing that mattered was the condition of the cardiac muscle." He made the following reply to Harken who wrote to enquire as to why Souttar had not repeated the operation (see Figure 4.46).

Instead of ushering in a new era, this first successful operation on the mitral valve in the UK marked the beginning of a 22-year-long hiatus.

Conrad Ramsey Lam (1905–)

CONRAD RAMSEY LAM was born in Ogelsby in the scrublands of West Texas, the first of 10 children, and studied at Simmons College and at Yale University (MD, 1932). He fulfilled internship and chief residency under Roy McClure at The Henry Ford Hospital, where his enthusiasm, inexhaustible work habits and surgical skill earned him a staff appointment (1938). As the youngest member of staff, he was responsible for burns and thoracic problems and eventually became Surgeon-in-Charge of the Department of Thoracic Surgery (1946–70). As a result, thoracic surgery moved from a world of thoracoplasty and phrenic nerve crush to the high-tech world of open heart surgery. For his relentless pursuit of new achievements in the laboratory, Lam was honoured as one of the 'Ten Pioneers of Cardiac Surgery' in 1980 by Shiley Laboratories.

Lam pioneered techniques for surgery of congenital and acquired heart lesions before direct vision was possible. He used newly purified heparin as early as 1939. With Gahagan, he conducted physiologic studies on the mechanism and treatment of intracardiac air embolism. He also performed 30 successive transarterial pulmonary valvotomies under normothermic inflow occlusion. Once the heart–lung machine was available, Lam was the first in Michigan to use it for correction of pulmonic stenosis and insertion of homograft valves and grafts.

Lam introduced acetylcholine for elective cardiac arrest one year after Melrose. "We thought," he remarked, "we originated the idea of induced or elective cardiac arrest, but to our surprise, this became known later as the 'Melrose technic'." Acetylcholine slowed the heart markedly without actually

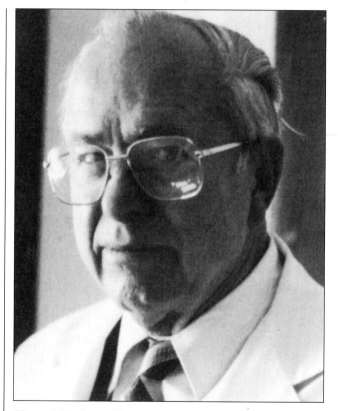

Figure 4.47. Conrad Lam.

producing cardiac standstill. Lam considered this an advantage, particularly when suturing close to the conducting tissue in ventricular septal defects, as the surgeon could see immediately whether conduction was interrupted. Lam recorded operating on eight children for ventricular septal defects with the aid of a pump oxygenator and acetylcholine arrest in 1956. Two died on the operating table from ventricular fibrillation, but Lam was uncertain whether the arrest or the surgical procedure was responsible. Two others died in the immediate postoperative period from unrelated causes.

Early homograft valve replacement, conceived of in laboratory experiments by Lam and associates, was successful in dogs. In Lam and Munnell's first animals, aortic valves were transplanted into the descending thoracic aorta, but the valve cusps shrivelled within a few days and showed no evidence of functioning. The same outcome was experienced by Hufnagel when he attempted to implant aortic homografts in the descending aorta while the aortic flow was maintained via a bypass tube. Hufnagel wrote:

"Many of these grafts showed failure of the valve cusps to function. Since it is necessary to leave some muscle attached at the base of the graft, suturing was hazardous, and secondary haemorrhage was frequent."

Munnell, Lam's co-worker, suggested that if the animal's own aortic valve was incapacitated, then the homograft might function for a longer period of time. This idea was taken up in the second experimental series in dogs. After the homograft was inserted into the descending thoracic aorta, a left

SURGERY

GYNECOLOGY AND OBSTETRICS

VOLUME 94   FEBRUARY, 1952   NUMBER 2

AN EXPERIMENTAL STUDY OF
AORTIC VALVE HOMOGRAFTS

CONRAD R. LAM, M.D., F.A.C.S., HARTLEY H. ARAM, M.D., and
EDWARD R. MUNNELL, M.D., Detroit, Michigan

Figure 4.48. An experimental study of aortic valve homografts. *A 1952 article by Lam, Aram and Munnell. (Reproduced with permission from* Gynecology and Obstetrics.*)*

ventricular stab wound was made and the non-coronary cusp of the aortic valve deliberately incised. This produced immediate aortic regurgitation and heart failure, but with increased pulse pressure on the homograft, it began to function. This was the first successful placement of a homograft valve in a dog. As Ross said, "To set the record straight, the use of a homograft was first tried in the descending aorta of dogs in 1952 in Detroit."

Andrew Logan (1906–)

ANDREW LOGAN was born in Scotland and studied at the University of St Andrew's (MA, 1926; MB; ChB, 1929; FRCS [Edin.], 1932; FRCP; FRCS [Eng.], 1934). He was Reader in Thoracic Surgery at the University of Edinburgh (1964) and Surgeon-in-Charge of the Department of Thoracic Surgery at The Royal Infirmary. With the cardiologist, Marquis, Logan's paper (Figure 4.49), which appeared in the *British Heart Journal* in 1955 before cardiopulmonary bypass was available in the UK, is a classic description of an early attempt to apply Bailey's transventricular approach to congenital as opposed to acquired aortic stenosis. In 1955, dilators were introduced through the apex of the left ventricle to treat infants with congenital valve aortic stenosis. Angiocardiography was employed in a proportion of patients in an attempt to exclude subaortic stenosis in surgical candidates. Predictably the results of blind valvotomy were extremely variable; the procedure usually led to aortic regurgitation but did provide symptomatic relief from severe stenosis.

It was clear from these early attempts that direct vision was essential for accurate repair of the aortic valve. Whilst this was first achieved through moderate hypothermia and inflow stasis, by April 1955, Kirklin and colleagues at the Mayo Clinic

CONGENITAL AORTIC STENOSIS AND ITS SURGICAL
TREATMENT

BY

R. M. MARQUIS AND ANDREW LOGAN

*From the Department of Cardiology of the Royal Infirmary and the Department of Surgery of the University,
Edinburgh*

Received November 20, 1954

The purpose of this paper is to assess the place and timing of surgery in the treatment of aortic stenosis of congenital origin. The diagnosis of aortic stenosis is readily made at the bedside and the clinical features are well known (Levine, 1945; Kiloh, 1950; Campbell and Kauntze, 1953). Its congenital origin is more difficult to substantiate. In the hope of excluding cases of acquired stenosis, we consider here only those patients in whom heart disease was recognized in infancy, or, at latest, on their first routine school medical examination at about five years of age, or in whom the site of stenosis was sub-aortic. Twenty-eight such patients form the basis of this review (Table I): their ages ranged from birth to 25 years. The length of follow-up extended in some instances to ten years and, excluding two infants, averaged nearly four years. Aortic incompetence was also present in six patients and the adult type of coarctation of the aorta in three others. Five patients died as a result of the lesion during the period of follow-up; two in infancy, two before puberty, and one in his middle teens. In six others the stenosis was considered sufficiently severe to justify aortic valvotomy.

Figure 4.49. Congenital aortic stenosis and its surgical treatment. *A 1955 article by Marquis and Logan. (Reproduced with permission from* British Heart Journal.*)*

approached the aortic valve using cardiopulmonary bypass. Kirklin also used the Melrose technique of potassium citrate arrest of the myocardium. Of the 33 patients with valvular aortic stenosis operated on at the Mayo Clinic between 1955 and 1960, there were only two hospital deaths; the outcome in 90% of patients was fair or good. With the direct vision approach no patient developed severe aortic regurgitation.

Oswald Sydney Tubbs (1908–93)

OSWALD SYDNEY TUBBS studied medicine at Cambridge University (MA; MB; BCh, 1932; FRCS [Eng.], 1935; MRCS [Eng.]; LRCP [Lond.]). Tubbs held the posts of Consultant Cardiothoracic Surgeon at St Bartholomew's and the Brompton Hospital (1932). He was President of the Society of Thoracic Surgeons of Great Britain (1932).

His first ligation of an infected patent ductus on 5 December 1939 in London was an important landmark in the history of congenital heart surgery. In his Hunterian Lecture at the Royal College of Surgeons in April 1943, Tubbs reported nine operations on infected ductus arteriosus with six survivors.

To those struggling with a finger against unyielding fibrotic and calcified mitral valves, the advent of the Dubost dilator and later the Tubbs dilator, was a great relief. The tendency of the mitral valve to yield at the commissures and not split through the leaflets themselves gave rise to the idea of using mechanically-expandable dilators. This also solved the problem of strictures that resisted the finger. Charles Dubost of Paris was the first to use an expanding dilator, which he described to the French Society of Cardiology in December 1953. It had two parallel blades and was guided through the atrium into the mitral valve orifice by a finger. When in place, the two blades were carefully separated. In his successful cases, Dubost achieved a good anatomical result with no evidence of mitral regurgitation. In 1954, Tubbs, developed a screw which adjusted Brock's old aortic dilator from 3.3 cm to 4.5 cm. He described the origins of the "Tubbs dilator" in a letter of June 1989 to Naef:

"When the Brown's Club (a club of British chest surgeons) visited Andrew Logan in Edinburgh (1954) I saw him do a combined aortic and mitral valvotomy by passing a (Brock) dilator through a small incision at the apex of the left ventricle. I was impressed but it seemed to me that the dilator should be adjustable according to the circumstances. I asked the Genito-Urinary Manufacturing Company to make such an instrument, which they did, and I was delighted because there was so little disturbance to the heart function. I thought the dilator was made solely for me, but they advertised it in their catalogue and it sold in enormous numbers throughout the world..."

Tubbs said, "This is my contribution to cardiac surgery, this little screw. All it does is limit the opening of a Logan dilator. Never in the field of cardiac surgery has a surgeon become so famous for so little."

Ten years later, closed mitral valvotomy was a well-established procedure, with a low mortality rate and good

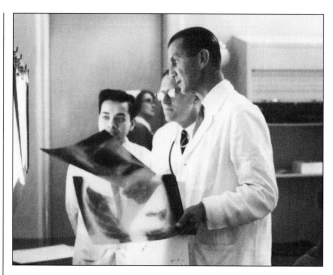

Figure 4.50. Oswald Sydney Tubbs.

short- and long-term results. By then it was appreciated that direct vision was necessary for the management of mitral regurgitation, and not blind baffles and pericardial tube grafts. The aortic valve was a more formidable problem and only resolved by direct vision and a reliable valve prosthesis.

O. S. TUBBS (London), *Transventricular mitral valvotomy* (film)

Following the description of successful mitral valvotomy by BAILEY, BROCK and HARKEN in 1950 the standard operation for the relief of mitral stenosis had been performed with the right index finger passed into the left atrium through the appendage.

In 1953 DUBOST designed an expanding dilator which he passed through the atrial appendage into the mitral orifice, and, with the end of the instrument in this position, he forcibly compressed the handle, thus separating the expanding members which caused the commissures to rupture.

Recognising the advantages of using an expanding dilator but dissatisfied with the inability to confirm the position of the instrument by palpation, LOGAN of Edinburgh in July 1954 passed his right index finger into the left atrium and then guided a Brock aortic dilator into the mitral orifice through a small incision in the left ventricle: before opening the instrument the position of the expanding members was readily confirmed from above by palpation with the right index finger. The Brock aortic dilator has a maximum expansion of 3.3 cms., and this is usually insufficient to cause rupture of both commissures. Consequently, in order to relieve the stenosis as fully as desirable I arranged for the manufacture of a dilator which has a maximum expansion of 4.5 cms. This was later modified by placing a screw on the handle which allows the maximum separation of the expanding members to be adjusted to any distance up to 4.5 cms. For severely scarred and calcified valves the maximum expansion should be set at 3,8 cms. or even less: for a good quality valve in an average sized patient I set the maximum expansion to 4.2 cms.: I rarely exceed this.

Figure 4.51. A 1962 article by Tubbs entitled 'Transventricular mitral valvotomy'. *(Reproduced from* Ned Tijdschr Geneeskd.*)*

Geoffrey Hubert Wooler (1911–)

GEOFFREY HUBERT WOOLER studied at Cambridge University and the London Hospital (MRCS [Eng.]; LRCP [Lond.], 1937; MA; MB; *BChir*, 1938; FRCS[Eng.], 1941; MD, 1947). He has been Consultant Cardio–Thoracic Surgeon at United Leeds Hospitals, Surgical First Assistant at The London Hospital, Lieutenant-Colonel in the Royal Army Medical Corps, Surgical Specialist (mentioned in despatches) and is now Honorary Thoracic Surgeon at the Leeds General Infirmary. He was co-editor of *Modern Trends in Cardiac Surgery* (1968) and author of many papers on the oesophagus, heart and lungs. He received an honorary degree from Szeged University, Hungary (1983) and became an honorary fellow of the Hungarian Surgical Society. Wooler is an English gentleman who spends his retirement years collecting materials for the war-injured in Croatia.

With the help of private benefactors and the Nuffield Foundation, in 1956, the University Hospital at Leeds bought their first heart–lung machine, leading to a new epoch in direct surgery of the mitral valve. Wooler began operating experimentally on healthy dogs because it was not possible to work out repair of the diseased valve in humans. After 6 months, with more dogs surviving, he moved the equipment into the Leeds General Infirmary where the cardiologists were happy to hand over a great number of cases, (many with liver and kidney disease and in the last stages of cardiac failure). Lord Brock said that he was surprised Wooler accepted such cases for surgery!

The Leeds group's first successful repair of the mitral valve was in February 1957 and Wooler persevered in spite of about 50% mortality in the early days. At this time there was no prosthesis available so the existing valve, whether mitral or aortic, had to be repaired or at least improved in function. Improvement was frequently achieved, but patients died a few days later from deficiencies in post-operative care. Initially, Wooler had no mechanical ventilator and in one case, he stayed in the hospital for 5 days and nights taking turns to hand ventilate the patient with the bag on the anaesthetic machine.

Wooler developed an annuloplasty to correct mitral incompetence due to a dilated valve ring (Figure 4.53). He started by inserting single deep stitches through the annulus across both commissures, which was satisfactory provided there was moderate dilatation of the ring. Wooler recounts using ring pessaries to reinforce an enormously dilated mitral annulus in two patients, where simple suturing had previously broken down, the tissues and annulus being too thin. When this did not work, the pessaries were removed and a double layer repair performed; the first being deep mattress sutures reinforced with teflon patches and the second layer being a continuous suture which buried the mattress sutures, plicated the atrial wall and

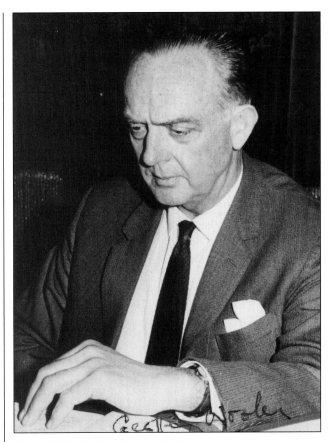

Figure 4.52. Geoffrey Hubert Wooler.

EXPERIENCES WITH THE REPAIR OF THE MITRAL VALVE IN MITRAL INCOMPETENCE

BY

G. H. WOOLER, P. G. F. NIXON, V. A. GRIMSHAW, AND D. A. WATSON

From the General Infirmary, Leeds

(RECEIVED FOR PUBLICATION NOVEMBER 20, 1961)

The mitral valve comprises four structures: annulus fibrosus, cusp tissue, chordae tendineae, and papillary muscles. The annulus fibrosus is strong at the base of the aortic cusp, where it forms part of the aortic valve ring, and weak at the base of the mural cusp. From every part of the annulus cusp tissue hangs vertically downwards into the cavity of the left ventricle in the form of a short sleeve (Fig. 1). Medially and laterally the tissue is elongated, and thickened by the insertion of chordae tendineae, to form the major aortic and mural leaflets. Anteriorly and posteriorly cusp tissue exists in the form of a delicate junctional band that may contain minor leaflets (Chieche, Lees, and Thompson, 1956). In health there are no commissures (Fig. 2). In mitral stenosis division of the junctional band may cause severe regurgitation. Chordae tendineae arise from papillary muscles and fan out as they insert into the edges and ventricular surfaces of the major cusps. It is important to realize that each papillary muscle distributes chordae to both cusps in such a way that contraction of the muscle tends to approximate the cusps (Fig. 3).

When the valve is closed the atrial surfaces of the major cusps have a wide area of contact, and eversion is prevented by chordae and papillary muscles.

the vicious circle described so well by Burchell and Edwards (1953). The annulus at the base of the aortic cusp is strong and firmly anchored to the aortic valve ring (Fig. 4) and so dilatation of the annulus enlarges the weak lateral annulus at the base of the mural cusp, which becomes correspondingly stretched and displaced downwards. Stretching may be so extreme as to split the cusp, and downward displacement causes the illusion of the aortic cusp prolapsing into the atrium. This downward displacement has been well described by Grant (1953). Building up the mural cusp with plastic sponge may make the valve competent, but we feel that such a repair is less efficient than one that shortens and elevates the cusp.

The following observations were made at operation in 38 cases. Adhesion between major cusps was present in five cases, but in only one was the long diameter of the orifice reduced to less than 2.5 cm. Gross dilatation of the annulus without apparent disease of the cusps, chordae or papillary muscles was present in eight patients. One of these was a man, 6 ft. in height and 14 stones in weight, who had heart failure four years before surgical treatment. At operation the clenched fist could be passed through the mitral valve. Repair appears to have been successful, for he has returned to work and presents little

Figure 4.53. Experiences with the repair of the mitral valve in mitral incompetence. *A 1962 article by Wooler, Nixon, Grimshaw and Watson. (Reproduced with permission from Thorax.)*

closed the atrial appendage. This extensive repair in a greatly enlarged left atrium produced a funnel-shaped appearance leading to the mitral orifice. The valves, perhaps a little too narrow, were still competent. After these two cases, Wooler always performed a double layer annuloplasty, but did not always plicate the atrial wall or close the appendage. Of the 12 early efforts to correct mitral incompetence in patients, Wooler and his colleagues had only three postoperative deaths. Thirty years later, mitral valve repair, in preference to replacement, remains the mainstay of surgery for mitral regurgitation. Most of Wooler's patients would not have survived the deterioration in left ventricular function that follows excision of the mitral subvalvar apparatus.

Albert Starr (1926–)

ALBERT STARR was born in New York City and studied at Columbia College of Physicians and Surgeons (MD, 1949). He interned at Johns Hopkins, served residency in thoracic surgery at Columbia Presbyterian Medical Center, New York City and became instructor in surgery at the University of Oregon, Portland in 1957. He was Professor and Chairman of the Division of Thoracic Surgery at the University of Oregon when he developed his ball-valve prosthesis. Starr wrote:

"In 1958, Lowell Edwards presented himself in my office with a proposal to develop an implantable artificial heart. I learned that he was a retired engineer, with considerable financial resources.... His visit was fortuitous because just about that time I had become interested in valvular prostheses. The few Bahnson leaflets that we had inserted seemed unsatisfactory. Edwards agreed to begin the project by working on one valve at a time....The obvious direction then was toward the ball-valve prosthesis. I drew out for Edwards the general configuration of the Hufnagel valve. He then drew out for me how he thought that particular valve could be adapted for intracardiac use, using an open cage. The first animal to have this implant survived for more than a year, but all subsequent animals died of thrombosis. The big breakthrough came at the end of 1958 when we developed the Silastic shield for the ball valve, which allowed an 80% long-term survival. I remember very well the day I thought of the idea of a Silastic shield. It was a beautiful spring afternoon...I was bounding up the steps of the Basic Science Building with my mind wandering aimlessly when it suddenly struck me that a Silastic shield over the area where thrombus formed on the valve would give us a chance to have long-term survivors..."

Starr and Edwards progressed through Teflon, lucite and silicone poppets in their ball-valve designs, and finally settled upon a Teflon-rimmed stainless steel cage enclosing a silicone rubber ball.

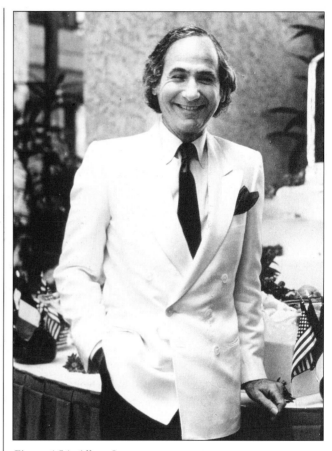

Figure 4.54. Albert Starr.

In May 1960, Starr and Edwards had their first long-term animal survivor and this was followed by successful use in patients. The first operation was done in September 1960, on a young girl in her mid-20s. Instead of presenting the first operation as a case report, Starr waited for medium-term follow up after eight operations (Article 4.3, Appendix A). This report in October 1961, was the first documentation of mitral prosthetic valve replacement with long-term survival of six out of eight patients. The presentation was the pièce de résistance of the 1961 American Surgical Association meeting.

Previous attempts at mitral valve replacement were associated

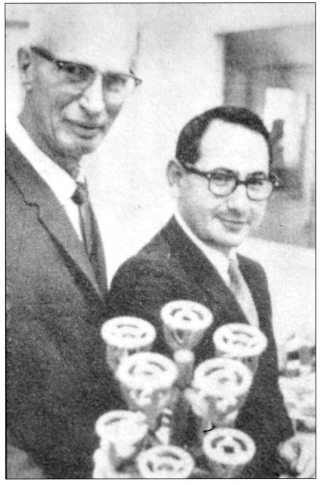

Figure 4.55. Albert Starr (right) with M. Lowell Edwards (left).

> ## Mitral Replacement: °
> ### Clinical Experience with a Ball-Valve Prosthesis
>
> ALBERT STARR, M.D., M. LOWELL EDWARDS, B.S.
>
> *From the Department of Surgery and Division of Thoracic Surgery,
> University of Oregon Medical School, Portland, Oregon*
>
> THE MORBID ANATOMY of rheumatic mitral disease is such that in many instances nothing short of excision and replacement will allow adequate relief of the hemodynamic abnormality. Experience with eight such patients in whom mitral replacement has been performed with a ball-valve prosthesis forms the basis of this report.
>
> Considerable work has been performed by other investigators in the development of a total mitral prosthesis for the dog and experience with human mitral replacement series have evolved. Firm and lasting fixation has been achieved by the use of interrupted sutures placed through the mitral annulus and through a knitted Teflon cloth ring to which the prosthesis is attached as shown in Figure 2. Satisfactory hydraulic function in the dog was demonstrated by left atrial pressure tracings immediately following implantation (Fig. 3) and by postoperative cardiac catheterization, angiocardiography, and cine-angiocardiography performed from two to 12 months follow-

Figure 4.56. Clinical experience with a ball-valve prosthesis. *A 1963 article by Starr and Edwards. (Reproduced with permission from* Annals of Surgery.*)*

such as ease of insertion, mechanical reliability, tolerance by the blood and tissues, acceptable noise level, simplicity of design and reasonable cost.

The Starr–Edwards valve transformed the treatment of heart valve disease. By mid-1961, the valve was employed in four countries and in at least five centres in the United States. By 1991, the valve had had a substantial impact on the lives of more than 175,000 patients and remains in wide use today. Progressive changes have been made to several aspects of the prothesis, including the configuration of the cage, the cloth covering the ring and the cage, and the materials used for the ball. In 1991, Starr commented that although the mitral prosthesis went through a series of rapid changes from 1960 to 1965, the performance of model 6120 could not be surpassed. This was also the case for the aortic prosthesis, the last modification of which was model 1260 in 1968.

Besides his enormous contribution to valve surgery Starr has made innumerable advances in other aspects of cardiac surgery including congenital heart disease. He is a fine teacher and has published several excellent books.

with thrombosis, infection, septicaemia or cardiac failure. Starr recognized that the major problem of thrombosis, which interfered with leaflet function was less likely to occur with a ball valve. The valve proved more than adequate in reducing thromboembolism and achieving other desired characteristics,

Alain Frédéric Carpentier (1933–)

ALAIN FRÉDÉRIC CARPENTIER was born in Toulouse, France and studied at the Faculté de Médecine at Nancy and Paris and the Faculté de Médecine, Paris-Orsay (Docteur d'Étatés Sciences, Docteur en médecine). He interned in the Paris Hospitals in 1961, became Chief Clinical Assistant (1966) and Associate Professor of Cardiac Surgery at the University of Paris VI (1972). He received the Bronze Medal from the Centre National de la Recherche Scientifique (1967) and became a member of the Association Française de Chirurgie and L'Académie de Médecine (1968). Carpentier was appointed Surgeon to the Paris Hospitals (1972), Professor of Cardiac Surgery (1978), Director of the Laboratory for Studies in Cardiac Prosthetics (1978) at the University of Paris VI and Chief of Cardiovascular Surgery at Broussais Hospital (1983). He became an honourary member of the American College of Surgeons in 1988.

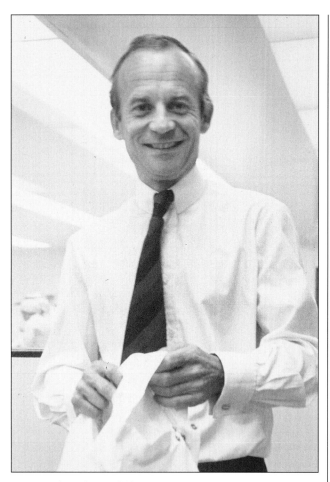

Figure 4.57. Alain Frédéric Carpentier.

Alain Carpentier has been one of the most prolific and consistent contributors to the development of cardiovascular surgery. Whilst best known for his contributions to bioprosthetic valve development and mitral valve repair, he has made enormous contributions to surgery for congenital heart defects and to cardiac support through cardiomyoplasty, transplantation and artificial hearts.

As a young resident in thoracic surgery in 1964, Carpentier was asked by Jean Paul Binet, Chief of Service, to collect homograft valves from cadavers. Studies of the anatomy of valves in various animal species (calves, pigs and sheep) showed that valves from pigs were closest to those of humans. In comparison with aortic homografts, porcine xenografts were easily obtained in unlimited numbers and under sterile conditions from selected animals. Carpentier performed the first human implantation of an aortic xenograft in collaboration with Binet in 1965, followed by 12 other implants of formalin-preserved valves (Article 4.4, Appendix A). All of the valves had to be replaced within 5 years through formalin-related tissue degeneration.

It became obvious that the future of tissue valves would

Biological factors affecting long-term results of valvular heterografts

Alain Carpentier, M.D. (by invitation), Guy Lemaigre, M.D. (by invitation), Ladislas Robert, M.D. (by invitation), Sophie Carpentier, M.S. (by invitation), and Charles Dubost, M.D. (by invitation), Paris, France
Sponsored by Frank Gerbode, M.D., San Francisco, Calif.

The use of biological tissue in surgery springs from a natural tendency of man to consider with affection all natural material and with suspicion any artificial substitute. This more sentimental than scientific attitude is, however, still justified at the present time in cardiac surgery because of the real advantages of valvular graft replacement, such as excellent hemodynamic function, absence of hemolysis, thrombosis, and embolism, and avoidance of postoperative anticoagulant therapy.

phasized to show this method of valvular replacement in its true aspect.

Having been the subject of a great deal of study in this laboratory[10, 11, 14] as well as in others,[16, 21, 30] the technical problems seem to be solved whereas the biological problems still remain relatively unknown, although they play a great part in the long-term results of such grafts.

Thus, despite continuous investigations, several questions still remained unanswered, such as: What is the host reaction to dif-

Figure 4.58. Carpentier's 1969 article 'Biological factors affecting long-term results of valvular heterografts. *(Reproduced with permission from* Journal of Thoracic and Cardiovascular Surgery.)

depend upon the development of reliable preservation methods capable of preventing an acute inflammatory reaction and rejection of the tissue. Finding his background in chemistry insufficient, Carpentier, at the age of 35 devoted 2 days a week to prepare for a doctorate in chemistry at the University of Paris. He began to investigate tissue cross-linking factors and found that glutaraldehyde was able to virtually eliminate the inflammatory reaction. During 1968, he used glutaraldehyde as an agent to attenuate antigenicity in xenograft valves. Glutaraldehyde preservation remains the mainstay in the manufacturing and processing of biological cardiac valves.

In 1966, Carpentier began mounting valves on a stent, which permitted the use of heterograft valves in the mitral position. The first implantation of a stented mitral xenograft took place in 1967, in collaboration with Charles Dubost. (Article 4.4, Appendix A). The stent-mounted valve was much easier to implant than the aortic homograft and this simplicity proved attractive to surgeons at a time when myocardial protection was less than perfect. More recently, he has developed new biochemical techniques aimed at preventing calcification of tissue valves. He coined the term 'bioprosthesis' in 1970.

Between 1970 and 1980 Carpentier became the champion of mitral valve repair operations, culminating in his honoured guest address at the 63rd Annual Meeting of the American Association for Thoracic Surgery (1983) entitled "Cardiac Valve Surgery 'The French Correction.'" His valve reconstruction techniques were also applied to congenital heart disease notably for repair of complete atrioventricular canal defects. He performed the first clinical cardiomyoplasty in 1985 and the first implantation of a heterotopic biventricular artificial heart in 1986. Carpentier has made important contributions in thoracic aortic surgery, notably in the treatment of acute Type A dissection and the development of the thrombo-exclusion technique for Type B dissection. The Carpentier–Edwards porcine xenograft is the tissue valve against which all others are compared; few have proven as durable and successful. Only now, with the resurrection of stentless porcine valves combined with zero pressure leaflet fixation and anti-mineralisation treatments, are improvements likely to be seen.

Chapter 5: Surgery for coronary artery disease

THE RELATIONSHIP between coronary atheroma and the symptom angina was not easily defined. Coronary artery disease was often found at post-mortem in patients who had never complained of angina. The Irish physician, Dominic Corrigan, maintained that angina was due to disease in the aorta itself, since many patients with syphilis, died during an anginal attack but had no coronary occlusive disease. In 1772 William Heberden published his description of angina pectoris in the literary magazine *Critical Review* (II, 203–204). A 51-year-old male reader recognised his own symptoms and wrote to Heberden, "I have never troubled myself much about the cause of it, but attributed it to an obstruction of the circulation or a species of rheumatism". In the event of sudden death he gave permission for an autopsy to establish the cause. Less than three weeks later his premonition was fulfilled and Herberden engaged the experienced anatomist John Hunter to open the body. Allegedly nothing was found to account for the death and Heberden concluded that angina was not due to an organic illness.

Hunter's first resident student, Edward Jenner attended the necropsy and was troubled by the negative outcome. Years later after Jenner had ascribed the anginal symptom to coronary obstruction he wrote that "almost certainly the coronary arteries were not examined". Hunter's extensive necropsy records certainly held clues to the association. In one case of cerebral embolus from a left ventricular thrombus Hunter noted (1770) "when I cut into the right ventricle I found the coronary artery as it goes between the auricle and ventricle, ossified". On 13th March 1775, Mr Rook, a 54-year-old man with angina pectoris died "in a sudden and violent transport of anger". The eminent physician John Fothergill suspected angina and heart failure and asked Hunter to perform the autopsy. Hunter found calcific aortic and mitral stenosis and that the coronary arteries "from their origin to many of their ramifications upon the heart were

become one piece of bone". Although Hunter's notes indicate that Rook "felt frequent pain in the arms" still "there was nothing very remarkable in his case worth taking notice of". Hunter's own anginal symptoms began in 1773 with an attack of severe epigastric pain accompanied by pallor ("the appearance of a dead man"). The pain lasted for 45 minutes and he was "perfectly recovered in two hours". In 1777 with worsening angina he was advised to go to Bath for spa therapy. Here Jenner made the correct diagnosis, recognised the relationship between angina and coronary disease but did not inform Hunter because he did not want to disturb his friend. In 1783 Hunter described three cases of congenital heart disease, one of which was tetralogy of Fallot and in 1793, the year of his death, he identified bacterial endocarditis in a six-year-old boy. Despite unstable and nocturnal angina from 1789 onwards, Hunter failed to make the important pathological association. Hunter's autopsy confirmed Jenner's prediction that coronary atheroma would be found but Hunter's wish that his heart should be preserved was disregarded.

The first physician to establish the diagnosis of coronary thrombosis in a living patient was Adam Hammer of St Louis (1876). He correctly reasoned that the onset and rapid progression of anginal pain could be attributed to interruption of the coronary supply and that myocardial ischaemia occurred through thrombotic occlusion of "at least one of the coronary arteries". In Hammer's own words,

"I mentioned my convictions to my colleague at the bedside. He, however, had a nonplussed expression and burst out, 'I have never heard of such a diagnosis in my life' and I answered, 'Nor I also'".

Nevertheless, a carefully conducted post-mortem proved Hammer to be correct.

The range of symptoms and cardiac events attributable to coronary artery disease were defined by James Herrick, of Chicago, in 1912. Differentiation between a prolonged anginal attack and acute myocardial infarction was difficult, until electrocardiography came into general use in the 1920s and 1930s. After that, it was possible to recognize the electrical changes of myocardial ischaemia and distinguish them from the permanent changes of infarction.

Having identified the association between angina pectoris and coronary artery disease, the next step was to define an appropriate method of treatment.

T. Lauder Brunton and amyl nitrate

"Few things are more distressing to a physician than to stand beside the suffering patient, who is anxiously looking to him for that relief of pain which he feels utterly unable to afford. Perhaps there is no class of case in which such occurrences as this take place frequently as in some kinds of cardiac disease in which angina pectoris forms at once the most prominent and most painful and distressing symptom."

THESE WERE the words of T. Lauder Brunton from his manuscript, *On the use of nitrate of amyl in angina pectoris*, published in the *Lancet* in 1867. Brunton was the first physician to achieve effective relief of angina by inhalation of amyl nitrate. This treatment provided the mainstay of anginal therapy in the early 1900s, but was of limited value. Consequently, early consideration was given to the possibility of surgical intervention. Three different approaches were considered. The first efforts to relieve angina were by blocking the nervous innervation of the heart. Second, it seemed logical to reduce the metabolic requirements of the myocardium by reducing workload. Finally, it seemed logical to increase the blood supply to ischaemic areas.

Charles Emile Francois-Frank first suggested thoracocervical sympathectomy for angina in 1899. His reasoning was indirect, in that sympathectomy was used for the treatment of thyrotoxicosis and some of Francois-Frank's thyrotoxic patients also had aortitis and angina. It was probably Charles Mayo (one of the Mayo brothers who, together with their father, founded the Mayo

Clinic) who first performed cervical sympathectomy for angina in a US Army major (1913). In 1916, the Bucharest surgeon, Thomas Jonnesco, who devoted most of his career to the surgery of the sympathetic nervous system, operated on a 20-year-old man with angina due to syphilitic aortitis. Jonnesco removed the last two cervical ganglia and the first two thoracic ganglia on the left side, and wanted to follow with right-sided sympathectomy. However, the patient was so much improved that he declined the second operation. When seen 4 years later, he was completely asymptomatic and able to do heavy work.

An alternative method was proposed by the physicians Gastineau Earle and Strickland Goodall. They suggested that the sensory roots should be cut from the cardiac plexus at the point where they entered the spinal cord (posterior rhizotomy). In 1913, they persuaded Sampson Handley, their surgical colleague at the Middlesex Hospital, to attempt the operation experimentally. Although he was able to section the second, third and fourth thoracic nerve roots on a cadaver, they collectively decided that injection of alcohol or novocaine into the nerve roots would be simpler and just as effective.

The concept of posterior nerve root section was resurrected 10 years later, when Danielopolu (Director of the Second Medical Clinic at the University of Bucharest) criticized the Jonnesco-type sympathectomy on the grounds that it produced an irreversible deterioration in cardiac function. He therefore directed his surgical colleague, Hristide, to cut the posterior roots of the upper thoracic spinal nerves which divided only sensory fibres. Danielopolu later declared cervicothoracic sympathectomy to be disastrous, from the therapeutic point of view, and concluded that removal of the stellate ganglion for angina was incompatible with life. In the 1920s, many forms of sympathectomy were undertaken and alcohol was injected into the upper thoracic sympathetic ganglia or nerve roots. About two-thirds of patients were relieved of their anginal pain, though the natural history of coronary artery disease progressed inexorably.

Elliot Cutler and thyroidectomy

EFFORTS to reduce cardiac workload were made by lowering the metabolic rate. This reduced oxygen requirements in those areas of limited myocardial perfusion. The concept of creating thyroid underactivity as a treatment for angina came in stages. Thyroidectomy was commonplace in the early part of the century, and occasionally, patients with congestive cardiac failure were seen to improve after remission from thyrotoxicosis. In 1927, Elliott Cutler in Boston saw a 61-year-old woman with severe heart failure, who was thought to be suffering from latent hyperthyroidism. At operation, the thyroid gland appeared normal, but the surgeon pressed on with the thyroidectomy regardless. Despite normal thyroid histology, the patient was greatly improved from the cardiac standpoint. On 15 June 1932, Cutler carried out the first subtotal thyroidectomy with the specific objective of relieving angina. This patient was symptomatically improved, as were several others. Total thyroidectomy was then undertaken to induce myxoedema, which in turn moderated the cardiovascular response to adrenaline. Eventually, the operation was reduced to simple ligation of the superior and inferior thyroid arteries in order to preserve the recurrent laryngeal nerves and parathyroid glands.

Thyroidectomy was said to provide symptomatic relief in 80% of patients, although they were often transformed physiologically and psychologically into a vegetative existence. Within a decade, thyroidectomy fell into disrepute, partly because surgeons such as Singer (who performed section of the posterior nerve roots) and Rainey (who advised surgical division of the upper thoracic pre-ganglionic fibres) were achieving satisfactory results without the disadvantage of myxoedema. Some physicians, such as Sir James McKenzie, also felt that the anginal syndrome should be preserved to prevent unduly severe exertion and ventricular fibrillation.

Early attempts to increase myocardial blood supply

AN INCREASED understanding of the pathophysiology of angina spawned efforts to increase myocardial blood supply. The initial attempts were indirect. In 1932, Claude Beck, Professor of Neurosurgery at the Western Reserve School of Medicine, Cleveland, sought to increase myocardial bloodflow by creating collateral circulation within the pericardium. Beck's colleague,

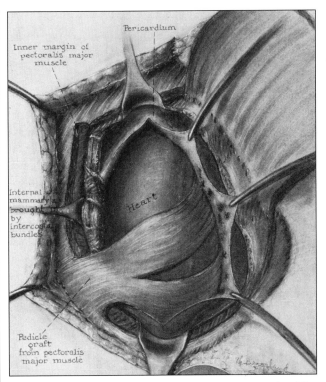

Figure 5.1. Diagram from Beck's 1935 article 'The development of a new blood supply to the heart by operation' *showing pedicle grafts carried posteriorly to the circumflex bed and sutured to the parietal pericardium. (Reproduced with permission from* Annals of Surgery; *102: 801–13.)*

Alan Moritz, drew attention to a report from Thorel (1903), where at post-mortem a patient was found to have longstanding complete obstruction of both main coronary arteries. There were diffuse vascular adhesions around the heart and Thorel suggested that these must have supplied the myocardium with blood. Beck suggested that it might be possible to imitate this situation by creating adhesions between epicardium and pericardium. After a great deal of experimental work, he operated on his first patient, a 48-year-old man, on 13 February 1935. He roughened the inside of the pericardial sac with a burr and denuded the epicardium. Between the two raw surfaces he grafted part of the pectoralis major muscle on its vascular pedicle (Figure 5.1). Within a year, the patient was asymptomatic. Beck then used pericardial fat and omentum as a source of vascularity and showed that after promoting adhesions, experimental animals could survive almost complete occlusion of the native coronaries.

In Britain, Laurence O'Shaughnessy used a pedicle of

greater omentum to wrap the thoracic oesophagus after oesophagogastrectomy. This rapidly enhanced vascularity in the area of the anastomosis. In April 1933, he began to apply omental grafts to the epicardium and vascular anastomoses were soon formed with the epicardial blood vessels. O' Shaughnessy then sought to test his method in greyhounds, who are prone to heart failure. The dogs on which he performed coronary occlusion followed by omental grafts recovered and were able to return to the track. In 1936, he used the technique on a 64-year-old man at Lewisham Hospital. The patient survived, but in later operations, O'Shaughnessy avoided suturing the myocardium by a applying omentum to the pericardium and using adhesive paste between the epicardium and graft. In 1938, he reported symptomatic relief for all patients who had survived 6 months or more. Regrettably, O'Shaughnessy's work was truncated in World War II, when he was killed at Dunkirk at the age of 40.

Other tissues, such as skin, jejunum and stomach, were used experimentally as grafts during the 1950s, but the only satisfactory alternative to omentum appeared to be lung. This was used by the German surgeon, Lezius, in 1937. He created a pericardial window, painted acriflavine onto the epicardium and then sutured the lung to this area. In animals, he succeeded in demonstrating anastomoses between coronary and lung vessels radiographically. This relatively simple approach was used on patients by several enthusiasts in the 1950s, but the results were never impressive.

Another even simpler method to create adhesions was to stimulate chemical pericarditis. Thomson and Raisbeck, of New York, used sterile talc and instilled 2% novocaine on to the epicardium to prevent the irritant powder from producing ventricular fibrillation. Thomson used this technique extensively and 14 years later reported that most of his patients had been relieved of their symptoms. The operation only lasted about 20 minutes, although four of the first 16 patients died in the post-operative period. Other irritants included carborundum sand, powdered beef bone or asbestos, kaolin, iron filings, iodine, ether, alcohol, formaldehyde, cotton, human skin and water glass. In 1955, Harken used 95% carbolic acid to remove the epicardium and followed this by instilling powdered talc. Although many patients claimed to have fewer and less severe anginal attacks, experimental work gave no objective evidence of improved circulation to the myocardium. The alleged symptomatic improvement also occurred much too soon to be attributable to newly vascularized adhesions. Carbolic probably destroyed all the nerve endings.

Revascularization through the coronary sinus

IN 1935, Louis Grosse and Lester Blom, at the Mount Sinai Hospital, New York, observed that the severity of anginal pain was reduced if the patient developed right heart failure. They argued that the congested myocardium had a sluggish bloodflow from which more oxygen could be extracted. They then demonstrated that complete ligation of the coronary sinus (in dogs) could prevent death when a major coronary artery was occluded. After some time, the congestion disappeared due to collateral channels, but by that time intercoronary arteriolar connections had opened up. Mercier Fauteux, a Canadian working in Boston, attacked the problem from two different directions: first by removing the sympathetic nerves from around the coronary vessels (pericoronary neurectomy), and then by ligating the veins. He later switched to ligation of the great cardiac vein, which drains into the coronary sinus. Fauteux operated on humans in 1940 and by 1946, had a series of 16 patients, all with previous acute myocardial infarction confirmed by ECG. Eleven had been severely disabled by angina beforehand, but reported substantial clinical improvement. By 1941, Beck stopped using muscle grafts and resorted to venous ligation. He described the Beck I operation in 1945. This comprised abrasion of the pericardium and epicardium, application of an inflammatory agent and partial occlusion of the coronary sinus. Mediastinal fat or pericardium were grafted to the surface of the myocardium.

If bloodflow and oxygenation could be achieved by retrograde flow through the coronary sinus, it seemed logical that arterial blood should prove more satisfactory than venous blood. In 1943, Joseph Roberts (University of Texas Medical School, Galveston) showed, by dye studies on dogs' hearts, that it was possible for Thebesius' veins to carry blood retrograde from the left ventricular cavity into the myocardium. This occurred when the pressure in the ventricle exceeded that in the coronary arteries. Of greater significance were experiments that showed that ischaemic myocardium could be revascularized by joining a large artery to the coronary sinus or veins. When the brachiocephalic, subclavian or innominate artery was anastomosed to the coronary sinus via a glass cannula, the coronary veins became distended and pulsatile. The myocardium then continued to contract when the coronary arteries were ligated.

Beck followed this lead with his own experiments and on 27 January 1948, performed the first Beck II operation on a human patient. He excised a length of brachial artery and used this to join the descending aorta to the coronary sinus. The coronary sinus itself was ligated at its junction with the right atrium. This was a difficult operation and Beck soon changed to a two-stage procedure, whereby the graft was inserted first, and between 2 and 6 weeks later, the coronary sinus was partially ligated. The Beck II operation produced impressive, longstanding intercoronary connections, even though the graft tended to thrombose after a few weeks. However, the operative mortality was 15–20% and this soon brought the procedure into disrepute.

Vineberg and the internal mammary artery

IN 1939, the Italian physician, Fieschi, suggested that bilateral ligation of the internal mammary arteries below their pericardiophrenic branches might increase myocardial bloodflow. These branches normally give rise to small pericardial vessels, which in turn anastomose with other small arteries from the aorta. Fieschi persuaded his colleagues Zoja and Cesa-Bianchi to undertake this procedure on a patient with myocardial infarction. Bilateral ligation was performed under local anaesthetic through an incision in the second intercostal space. Two years later, the patient remained well. The procedure was undertaken by other Italians, including Battezzati, who reported 11 cases in 1955. The operation had the merit of being simple, with no operative mortality. It could be performed safely during recuperation from an acute myocardial infarction and was said to produce worthwhile results. Other investigators failed to demonstrate a significant increase in cardiac bloodflow. When patients with angina were divided into two groups, one in which ligation was carried out and the other in which only the skin was incised (no ligation), the results showed patients in both groups to benefit equally. Such was the power of suggestion! The internal mammary artery was nevertheless destined to play an important part in the future of myocardial revascularization.

Arthur Vineberg began his experimental work at McGill University in 1946. He mobilized the left internal mammary artery, ligated the vessel distally and implanted the bleeding end into a tunnel in the left ventricular muscle close to the left anterior descending coronary artery. Remarkably, no haematoma formed and he could later show that the artery formed anastomotic channels with neighbouring vessels. Why should this work? If a bleeding artery were to be implanted in any other muscle, it would simply result in a large haematoma. It appears that the myocardium has a potential sponge-like quality. In early embryonic life, the sponge is soft and loose, deriving its oxygen from blood squeezed in and out of it. This is the method by which the hearts of many lower vertebrate animals, such as fish, obtain their nutrition. With further development of the human embryo, the sponge tightens and the coronary vessels and capillaries condense out of the spongy network. However, when intercoronary connections are opened under the stress of ischaemia or a surgical procedure, there is a tendency to revert towards the sponge stage. This is the theoretical basis on which Vineberg based his procedure and in 1950, he operated on the first human patient. Three years later, he reported that the patient "from a condition of complete disability could walk 10 miles through the bush". Vineberg also used pads of pericardial fat, grafted to the surface of the left ventricle, and in 1963, he employed a mesenteric graft. The greater omentum was detached completely from the gut and wrapped around the heart after denuding the epicardium.

In 1964, Vineberg reported 140 operations with a 33% mortality, though for the decade 1954–63 the mortality was less than 2%. Of 109 surviving patients (1964), 91 had either no angina or slight pain on effort. In general, clinical improvement was good, with a high percentage of patients able to return to work. Later, with the introduction of coronary arteriography by Sones, of the Cleveland Clinic, the Vineberg procedure was shown to produce worthwhile anastomoses with the native coronary circulation in 70–80% of internal mammary implants.

On 4 October 1955, Sidney Smith, of Florida, using a modification of the Vineberg procedure, harvested the long saphenous vein from the leg, anastomosed this proximally to the aorta and pulled the substance of the vein graft through the myocardium from base to apex. The 43-year-old patient was asymptomatic 18 months later. Smith then abandoned the saphenous vein and used a perforated nylon prosthesis instead.

Favaloro and Sones at the Cleveland Clinic

JUST before Favaloro's arrival at the Cleveland Clinic in 1962, two important events occurred. First, on 5 January 1962, Effler successfully operated on a severe obstruction at the left main coronary artery using the patch graft technique described by Senning. The first patch operations were performed using a pericardial graft to enlarge the lumen of the left main coronary artery. With increasing experience, longer patch reconstructions were performed. Sones' post-operative angiograms showed that there was a direct relationship between the length of repair and post-operative thrombosis; the longer the repair the greater the failure. Secondly, on 12 January 1962, Sones examined a patient operated on by Vineberg in Canada (1946). Using selective cannulation of the left internal mammary artery he showed that collateral circulation from the systemic artery implanted in to the myocardium was sufficient to diminish the myocardial perfusion deficit in the territory of an occluded left anterior descending coronary. As a result of these events Effler and the Cleveland Clinic were motivated towards a surgical solution to coronary artery disease.

At the Clinic Favaloro had difficulties with the authorities and could only be accepted as an observer without payment. Nevertheless, Effler cut through the red tape and put Favaloro to work in his unit. At the time the Department of Thoracic Surgery consisted of Effler and his partner, Harry Groves with a senior and junior resident. Most of the routine work was lung or oesophageal surgery. Only 3 or 4 open cardiac procedures were performed each week.

Favaloro was put to work in the intensive care unit and helped clean, siliconize and assemble the enormous heart–lung machine and Kay–Cross oxygenator. From the beginning Favaloro spent time with Sones and Shirey, who had by then performed hundreds of coronary angiograms with a degree of precision exclusive

to the Cleveland Clinic. While the basic concepts of myocardial revascularization evolved, a lasting friendship developed between Sones and Favaloro. After a few months with Sones, it became clear to Favaloro that coronary patients fell in two groups: first, those with diffuse disease that involved most of the coronary branches and second, those with localized obstructions occurring mainly at the proximal segments of the coronary arteries but with good distal run-off.

Favaloro passed the Educational Council Foreign Medical Graduate Examination and eventually became Chief Resident at the Cleveland Clinic in 1964. When median sternotomy became the standard approach for most heart operations, Favaloro had the idea that both internal mammary arteries might be implanted by the Vineberg method. He discussed the idea with Sones several times, but it was suggested that necrosis might occur if the sternum was deprived of that blood supply. Reviewing the anatomy he wrote, "I thought it logical to think this a senseless warning." Finally, in 1966, and by that time a staff member in the Department of Thoracic and Cardiovascular Surgery, he dissected both mammaries and implanted them in the left ventricle. The right was implanted parallel to the left anterior descending coronary and the left on the lateral wall in a tunnel beneath the branches of the circumflex coronary. He went on to perform 38 consecutive bilateral implants without mortality or significant morbidity, possibly because the patients were selected very carefully.

The assistants at these operations soon grew tired of manually retracting the sternal edges, so Favaloro designed his self-retaining retractor (Figure 5.2). Late restudies of Favaloro's modification of the Vineberg procedure showed many patients existing on a well-perfused coronary collateral system with both implants patent. A parallel series of patch graft operations on the left main stem carried substantial mortality (11 deaths in 14 patients), so much so that the kidney transplant team asked if they could cross match these patients as prospective donors before surgery.

Evolution of coronary angiography

WITHOUT direct visualization of the diseased coronary arteries, effective myocardial revascularization remained

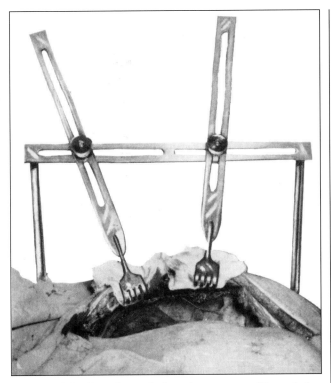

Figure 5.2. Favaloro designed a new self-retaining retractor to list the left side of the sternum, giving good exposure of the left mammary artery. (Reproduced with permission from Favaloro's 1967 article 'Bilateral internal mammary artery implants'. Cleveland Clinic Quarterly; 34: 61–66.)

only a remote possibility. However, by the end of the 1950s, the development of microvascular techniques (for surgical reconstruction of blocked vessels) stimulated efforts towards a reproducible method for coronary angiography. The first deliberate experimental attempt to X-ray the coronary arteries was in 1933, when Peter Rousthoi, of Stockholm, injected contrast medium directly into the aorta or via the carotid artery. Interest waned until 1945, when Stig Radner, of Lund, Sweden, injected contrast into the ascending aorta of patients via a puncture hole in the sternum. Opacification of the coronary arteries was only moderate and serious complications in two of five patients caused him to abandon the method. In 1948, Jorge Meneses Hoyos and Carlos Gomez del Campo, of Mexico City, produced images of the thoracic aorta, its brachiocephalic branches and the coronary arteries. They used intra-aortic injection of 30 ml contrast medium through a needle inserted via the second intercostal space to the left of the sternum.

Retrograde transarterial catheterization of the heart began in the 1940s, but was initially abandoned because of arterial spasm. In 1946, Pedro Farinas, of Havana, catheterized the aorta via the femoral artery and obtained good contrast pictures of the abdominal aorta and iliac arteries. Retrograde arterial catheterization was not widely adopted until Sven Seldinger, of Stockholm, published his technique for percutaneous catheterization in 1953. Seldinger punctured the brachial or femoral artery with a hollow needle, then inserted a flexible guidewire through the needle and into the aorta. The catheter was threaded over the guidewire, which was withdrawn to allow the catheter to be manipulated safely to its destination. The advantage of this method was that catheters the size of a needle could be used to gain access to the cardiac chambers.

In 1952, the Italians, Lucio de Guglielmo and Mariano Guttadauro, working in Stockholm, passed a catheter through the radial artery into the ascending aorta. They then injected contrast, which they claimed would provide 100% imaging of the coronary arteries. At that time it was thought necessary to slow, or even stop, bloodflow in the arteries whilst contrast was injected. Temporary cardiac arrest was induced by injection of acetyl choline and methods sought to block the aorta above the coronary arteries. An occlusive inflatable balloon catheter was used in an early attempt to obtain satisfactory opacifications of the coronaries.

In 1962, Sones and Shirey, of the Cleveland Clinic, achieved (by accident) direct and reproducible catheterization of the coronary arteries. Using the brachial arterial approach under X-ray control, they manipulated a catheter into the coronary ostia and injected between 2 and 5 ml of contrast whilst watching the image intensifier. A permanent record was taken on cinefilm at 60 frames per second. By demonstrating the site of coronary occlusion, this method added a new dimension to coronary artery surgery and opened the way for direct arterial revascularization. To quote Floyd Loop, "Collectively, all of the cardiological advances in this century pale in comparison with this priceless achievement." In the early 1960s, selective coronary angiography was carried out and if a major branch of the left coronary was occluded, a left internal mammary artery was implanted into the muscle of this territory. If a major branch of the right coronary was diseased, a right internal mammary artery implant was undertaken. If both vessels were occluded, bilateral Vineberg procedures were performed. When atheroma was localized to the coronary ostia, these were attacked directly through the aorta. If the patient had widespread coronary disease deemed unsuitable for internal mammary implants, thoracic sympathectomy was employed. However, as a leading article in the *British Medical Journal* in 1967 concluded, "No operation has yet been shown to increase the patient's expectation of life". Inevitably, the results of this type of surgery were difficult to assess, as the natural history of coronary disease varied greatly. One patient might suffer acute myocardial infarction and die suddenly, with no previous history of angina. Another patient might have stable angina for many years, or suffer an acute myocardial infarction and be alive, well and active 20 years later.

Direct myocardial revascularization

IT WAS ONLY a matter of time before the suggestion arose to operate directly on the coronary arteries to achieve normal flow. Alexis Carrell (1910) had performed experimental vascular grafts between the descending aorta and left main coronary artery. He suggested that an operation of this nature might find a place in the treatment of angina when the ostia of the coronary arteries were calcified; at this stage, the cause was usually syphilis. Direct vascular surgery remained primitive until 1945, when Gross and Crafoord independently described resection of coarctation of the aorta with end-to-end anastomosis. In 1953, Gordon Murray reported (at a congress in Lisbon) that he had resected the diseased part of the left anterior descending coronary artery in five patients and had replaced it with a vascular graft. This was done after experimental work on dogs, but without the benefit of coronary angiography. He used the internal mammary, the axillary or the carotid artery as the graft. In Russia, Vladimir Demikhov worked along similar lines, by joining the left internal mammary artery of dogs to their left anterior descending coronary a few millimeters beyond the origin. In 1955, he developed the operation further in experiments on human cadavers and live baboons. He then devised a three-way plastic tube to connect the internal mammary artery to two coronary branches

beyond their obstruction. As usual, reports of Demikhov's pioneering work did not reach the West until after the initial clinical and experimental successes of Murray and Lillehei.

In 1956, Lillehei gave an account of two experimental procedures for coronary disease. On human cadavers he performed endarterectomy and on dogs he repeated Murray's type of anastomosis, using a plastic prosthetic tube to join the subclavian artery to the circumflex branch of the left coronary. The latter method was largely unsuccessful, due to thrombosis within the prosthetic graft. He therefore proceeded to attempt direct anastomosis between the left internal carotid or internal mammary artery to the circumflex coronary. Many of these grafts remained patient, but at the time Lillehei did not translate the work into clinical practice.

Angelo May, working with Charles Bailey in Philadelphia, experimented with endarterectomy on human cadaver hearts. He passed a special instrument beyond the atheroma and pulled back to cut and remove the blockage. When he attempted to reproduce the procedure in dogs (by stripping off part of the vessel lining), all the animals developed thrombosis at the site of intervention. Soon afterwards, Bailey carried out the first human coronary endarterectomy (29 October 1956), by incising the coronary artery itself at a point beyond the blockage and passing a curette retrogradely through the vessel. The 51-year-old patient was given heparin to prevent thrombosis and made a satisfactory recovery. Encouraged by this, Bailey performed seven similar operations, with survival and symptomatic improvement in each case. Remarkably, these initial operations were undertaken without cardiopulmonary bypass. Because of the obvious technical limitations, Bailey subsequently changed to a direct approach through the aorta and coronary ostium using the Gibbon pump oxygenator. Without the benefit of coronary angiography, these procedures were largely based on the pathological principles outlined by Monroe Schlesinger, of Beth Israel Hospital, Boston. In 1940, Schlesinger worked with cadaver hearts to characterize the zones of coronary occlusion by comparing radiographs with dissection. He found that most zones of coronary occlusion were less than 5 mm long and occurred within 3 mm of the ostia of the main coronary arteries. Bailey suggested that endarterectomy should be restricted to well localized short segments of coronary

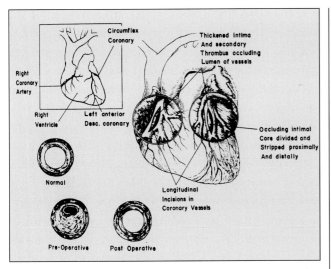

Figure 5.3. Exposure of the right main coronary and left anterior descending coronary arterieswith longitudinal incisions in to the vessels. (Reproduced with permission from Longmire WP et al. Direct-vision coronary endarterectomy for angina pectoris. The New England Journal of Medicine 1958; 259: 993–99.)

artery. In practice, this occurs in less than 20% of coronary artery patients.

Coronary endarterectomy (Figures 5.2 and 5.3) or segmental excision with saphenous vein or internal mammary artery grafts were performed in the late 1950s before cardiopulmonary bypass came into widespread use. Longmire recalls the first direct anastomosis between the left internal mammary artery and the right coronary in 1958 (Figures 5.4 and 5.5):

> "At the time we were doing the coronary thromboendarterectomy procedure and we also performed a couple of the earliest internal mammary to coronary anastomoses. We were forced into it when the coronary artery we were endarterectomising disintegrated and in desperation we anastomosed the left internal mammary artery to the distal end of the right coronary artery and later decided it was a good operation."

From Bailey's early work, it was apparent that when the endarterectomy passed across the mouth of a branch, the sheared-off atheroma detached from the main channel and tended to retract, form a clot and occlude. A death from this cause stimulated Senning to open the coronaries more extensively, peel out the diseased areas

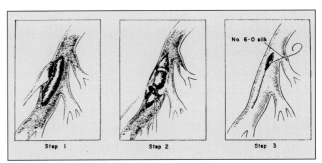

Figure 5.4. Stripping of the intimal core. (Reproduced with permission from Longmire WP et al. Direct-vision coronary endarterectomy for angina pectoris. The New England Journal of Medicine 1958; 259: 993–99.)

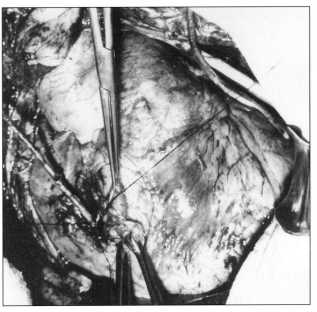

Figure 5.5. Longmire's direct anastomosis of a skeletonised right internal mammary artery to the right coronary artery.

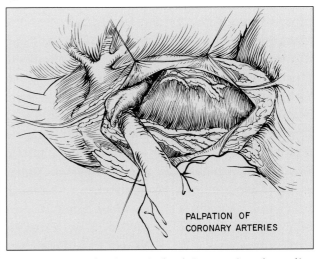

Figure 5.6. Palpation of the left anterior descending coronary to determine the site of atheromatous obstruction.

under direct vision and avoid the important side branches. The arteriotomy was then enlarged using a vein patch along the length of the incision. For this procedure, Senning used cardiopulmonary bypass at 23°C and closed the incisions with saphenous vein taken from the ankle.

For a short time, Bailey considered that emergency thromboendarterectomy might be used for treatment of acute myocardial infarction. He proposed that with cardiopulmonary bypass, the patient might undergo removal of the thrombus and endarterectomy of the atheromatous narrowing. He also reasoned that pre-operative angiography was unnecessary, since the affected artery could be readily identified from the site of myocardial infarction. In 1963, George Nardi and Robert Shaw, of Harvard Medical School, reported four patients in whom they attempted this procedure. All died and the operation was never widely adopted.

Sabiston first employed aortocoronary saphenous vein bypass in 1962, during a re-operation. He made an end-to-end vein to right coronary artery anastomosis. Unfortunately, the patient died 3 days later of cerebral complications. Probably the first successful saphenous vein bypass graft was by Edward Garrett (1964), whilst he was working with DeBakey. He performed the bypass graft in order to wean a patient from cardiopulmonary bypass, and the long-term result of the procedure was not reported until 10 years later.

It was the work of René Favaloro, at the Cleveland Clinic, and Dudley Johnson in Milwaukee, beginning in 1967, that launched the widespread application of coronary artery surgery.

The possibility of studying the pathological anatomy of coronary arteries by cine-arteriography was the springboard for Favaloro's coronary bypass procedures. The idea of working directly on the coronary arteries in patients with severe localized proximal obstructions, but with good distal run-off encouraged Favaloro to attempt bypass of the obstruction. At first pericardial- and venous-patch graft repairs in segmental localized obstructions were used. A single longitudinal incision was performed through the obstruction and the lumen of the artery enlarged by patch closure. Although occasionally successful in patients with a sharply localized obstruction of the right coronary artery, its application to the left coronary artery was seldom successful, with an operative mortality of 65%. In patients who needed long segmental reconstructions (2–4 cm) the patch graft was

a tedious task and the irregular surface left inside the artery produced turbulence and thrombosis.

Early experience with saphenous femoropopliteal bypasses and renal artery reconstruction, led Favaloro to think that if saphenous grafts worked in the distal circulation why not in the coronary arteries close to the ascending aorta, with high flow and high pressure! (Article 5.5, Appendix A). In May 1967, his colleague, David Fergusson, referred a 51-year-old woman who had had typical angina pectoris for 3 years. Selective cine-coronary angiography showed that the right coronary artery was totally occluded in the proximal third. The left coronary artery did not have significant occlusive disease and through collateral filling the distal portion of the right coronary artery appeared normal. Sones and Favaloro decided to begin with this patient with a completely occluded right coronary since failure of the reconstruction was unlikely to result in fatality. On May 7, Favaloro resected the occluded portion of the artery and performed a saphenous vein interposition graft. Angiography eight days later showed excellent flow in the resected vessel. Recatheterized 10 years later, the graft and right coronary artery were patent. However , after a few operations using only interposed saphenous grafts, the technique showed certain limitations and he turned to the concept of aorto-coronary saphenous vein bypass grafts.

A bypass from the anterolateral wall of the aorta to the distal end of a resected segment using end-to-end anastomosis was attempted in 15 patients before this was changed to an end-to-side anastomosis with the coronary distal to the blockage. This was simpler and soon became the enduring technique.

After this initial success several substantial advances took place in 1968. Aorto coronary bypass with saphenous vein was applied to the left coronary. The first operation was performed on a patient with obstruction of the left main stem but minimal distal disease in the left anterior descending or circumflex branches. A single vein graft to the proximal segment of the left anterior descending coronary showed excellent perfusion of the entire left coronary tree on post operative angiography. Left main coronary obstruction could then be treated and coronary bypass was combined with left ventricular aneurysmectomy and valve replacement.

By the end of 1968, Favaloro had accumulated a series of 171 patients who had undergone direct myocardial revascularization. After that first full year, they knew that saphenous vein bypass grafts had a future. The concept of coronary artery bypass surgery developed by Favaloro was expanded from a single saphenous vein bypass of the right coronary artery to procedures involving the left coronary artery, to double and triple bypass procedures and mammary artery bypass procedures.

Although, as Mason Sones said, twentieth century cardiology could be divided into the pre-Favaloro and the post-Favaloro era, at the time it was difficult for Favaloro to persuade his colleagues. Nevertheless, he persisted in spite of their lack of confidence and disbelief expressed at different national meetings and at visits to hospitals. One of the main reasons for scepticism was that previous myocardial revascularization attempts had been performed in that "twilight zone" — where there was no objective demonstration that the surgeons' approach had changed the ischaemic myocardium. In 1968, Favaloro already knew that this was an operation that could be performed efficiently with a well-defined technique, a very low mortality rate, and with excellent postoperative results. During the early days, some doctors simply did not believe the operative mortality — always below 5% — and their scepticism led them to doubt the truth of the statistics.

Direct anastomosis of the internal mammary artery to an obstructed coronary artery was described by Kolessov in 1967 and by George E. Green in 1968. Green worked on experimental microvascular suture anastomosis and demonstrated the potential for direct mammary artery to coronary artery anastomosis under the operating microscope. He recognized that suture of the internal mammary artery directly to a coronary arteriotomy should offer substantially more benefit than intramyocardial implantation. Green spent many hours examining hearts at the New York City Mortuary to convince himself and others that the distal segments of diseased coronary arteries were usually free from atheroma and greater than 1 mm in diameter. He practised mammary artery anastomosis to canine coronary arteries and demonstrated that these could sustain cardiac function. In February 1968, David Tice, Director of Surgery at the New York Veterans Administration Hospital, encouraged Green to proceed with a human bypass graft. The successful early operations were presented as footnotes to the experimental data published in *Annals of Thoracic Surgery* (May 1968).

Soon afterwards, it became clear that this new form of revascularization offered substantial benefits over previous therapeutic modalities, particularly for intractable angina. When bypass grafting was performed in cases of angina that were unresponsive to medical management, symptoms were relieved in most cases. Widespread adoption of coronary revascularization came from 1968 onwards, with improvements in cardiopulmonary bypass and cardioplegic arrest. These facilitated the coronary anastomosis and provided the stimulus for a dramatic increase in the number and complexity of procedures.

Within a short time, following the experimental contributions of Cox and others, Favaloro proceeded to apply coronary bypass to acute myocardial infarction. On the first occasion a patient awaiting elective coronary surgery at the Bolton Square Hotel across the street from the clinic was reported to be suffering from severe, persistent central chest pain. The coronary angiogram had previously shown subtotal occlusion of the proximal left anterior descending coronary. Favaloro rushed to see the patient who was sweating, dyspnoic and hypertensive. The electrocardiogram confirmed extensive anterolateral myocardial injury. Favaloro rapidly discussed the patient with Mason Sones and decided to proceed with emergency revascularization. This was performed uneventfully and the patient recovered function in the ischaemic segment. The postoperative left ventriculogram demonstrated only a small area of impaired wall motion and normal left ventricular end-diastolic pressure. The graft was patent.

Within a year Favaloro and Sones had reported 18 impending myocardial infarctions and 11 acute infarctions treated by coronary bypass in the *American Journal of Cardiology*. They concluded that when surgery is performed within six hours of acute myocardial infarction most of the heart muscle can be preserved. The first double bypass to the right and left anterior descending coronaries was undertaken in December 1968, though a double inter position operation had been performed in March that year. These advances are summarized in the *Journal of Thoracic and Cardiovascular Surgery* as presented. Others soon adopted Favaloro's methods. In particular, Dudley Johnson of Milwaukee showed that grafts could be placed in distal segments of the coronary tree.

In 1970 endarterectomy was combined with coronary bypass either by the simple mechanical methods described by Groves, or by carbon dioxide gas endarterectomy as described by Soya. In the same year Favaloro began to use direct internal mammary to coronary artery anastomoses as developed by George Green of New York. By June 1970, 1086 bypasses had been performed with an overall mortality of 4.2 percent. Coronary anastomoses were performed with interrupted sutures, a method which has persisted at the Cleveland Clinic since that time.

Favaloro was invited to attend the 6th World Congress of Cardiology in London during 1970 and Donald Ross invited him to perform coronary surgery at the National Heart Hospital. During the first operation, after opening the right coronary and placing the first stitch, the scrub nurse accidentally pulled the vein off and tore the vessel. At least she did not drop the vein!

It was during the Congress in London that a large delegation from Argentina asked Favaloro to return home. Consequently in October 1970 Favaloro wrote a letter of resignation to Effler and pointed out that his work could be continued by the outstanding residents, Loop and Cheanvechai. Favaloro's decision to leave the Cleveland Clinic caused great sadness particularly to Mason Sones. Favaloro told his colleagues that he would leave at the beginning of July 1971 but he accepted an invitation to lecture in Boston in June and flew straight home to Argentina.

It transpired that Favaloro's first saphenous vein bypass operation was proceeded by that of Garrett in November 1964. Garrett was trying to perform a patch repair of a localised obstruction in the left anterior descending coronary and resorted to a vein graft for complications. Garrett eventually published this case in 1973 by which time thousands of operations had been performed in Cleveland and other centres in the United States. When Donald Effler left the Cleveland Clinic, Floyd Loop became Chief of Cardiac Surgery and with others (notably Delos Cosgrove and Bruce Lytle) created one of the largest cardiac surgical centres in the world, and certainly the best known for research and development in coronary artery surgery.

Surgery of left ventricular aneurysm

BAILEY was the first surgeon to excise a post-infarction left ventricular aneurysm. The 56-year-old man was operated on 15 months after sustaining a large anterolateral myocardial infarction (15 April 1954). Bailey approached the pericardium through a left sixth interspace thoracotomy and dissected away the pericardial adhesions from "a smooth ovid bulge" involving the entire anterior wall of the left ventricle. Without cardiopulmonary bypass, he applied a large sideclamp to the aneurysm, which resulted in immediate improvement in cardiac ejection. He then applied a continuous suture beneath the clamp, followed by a series of interrupted mattress sutures. Then, tentatively removing the clamp, the aneurysm was slowly cut away and the raw edges closed over with a third layer of sutures. The patient survived and remained in good health 3 years later.

In 1957, Bailey reported on nine patients after left ventricular aneurysmectomy; eight survived and were much improved. The single failure was due to thromboembolism and stroke, through dislodging clots in the aneurysm wall. Bailey learned to avoid damage to the mitral subvalvar apparatus by inserting a finger into the left ventricle. He also emphasized that it was unnecessary to attempt to remove all scar tissue and important to restore the left ventricle to as near normal size and shape as possible. Bailey's closed technique for ventricular aneurysm excision was soon superseded by the operation on cardiopulmonary bypass. On 17 January 1958, Cooley, at Baylor, Houston, used cardiopulmonary bypass to excise an aneurysm in a 50-year-old male. This patient had sustained a myocardial infarction 3 months previously and his aneurysm was full of blood clot. For this patient there was a risk of massive embolus. The open technique allowed the thrombus to be removed, after which the aneurysm was excised and the ventricle repaired with a clear view of the internal structures. Lillehei followed with the same operation soon afterwards.

The advent of coronary angiography provided a powerful stimulus towards revascularization by direct arterial anastomosis.

The early clinical trials

ALTHOUGH it is now known that 85% of patients with severe or unstable angina are relieved of symptoms, early and widespread acceptance of coronary bypass was delayed by clinical trials in stable angina that compared surgery with improving medical treatment. The trials were also designed to permit surgery in any individual who developed problematic angina, a situation that led to crossover in 25–40% of patients in the medical arms of most major trials. Another confounding factor was the rapid improvement in all aspects of management of coronary disease. Revascularization techniques improved dramatically after the late 1960s, with the development of cold potassium cardioplegia, oxygenated blood cardioplegia, retrograde cardioplegia, multiple dose cardioplegia, use of the internal mammary artery and intra-aortic balloon pumping for cardiac support. Medical treatment improved with the introduction of beta-receptor and calcium-channel blockers, documentation of the efficacy of nitrates and recognition of the importance of thrombotic occlusion and thrombolysis in ischaemic heart disease.

The best known cooperative studies (conducted in the 1970s and early 1980s) were the Veterans' Administration (VA) Cooperative Study, the Coronary Artery Surgery Study (CASS) and the European Coronary Surgery Study. All were multicentre efforts to examine the efficacy of coronary artery bypass grafting versus medical treatment, in stable clinical situations.

The Veterans' Administration Cooperative Study

THE VA Cooperative Study screened more than 5000 patients between January 1970 and December 1974. Of these, 686 were entered into the final phase of the study. Ninety patients had severe left main coronary disease and 596 had multiple vessel disease. Patients were randomly assigned to medical or surgical management. The majority of all surgical patients received saphenous vein grafts and operative mortality was 5.6%. When patients were stratified according to the number of vessels grafted, operative mortality at 30 days was 0% for single vessel disease, 6.1% for two vessels and 7.3% for three vessels. Graft angiography in 84% of patients showed 69% of grafts to be patient at 10–15 months.

One of the most important findings of the VA Cooperative Study was that chronic stable angina in association with high-grade, left main coronary artery disease is a definite indication for coronary artery bypass

grafting and that survival is clearly improved for this group of patients. In the 596 patients with coronary artery lesions in vessels other than the left main coronary artery, no clear short-term (36 months) or long-term (7 or 11 years) survival advantage was documented. At 36 months, 87% of the medical group and 88% of the surgical group were alive; at 7 years, 70% of the medical group and 77% of the surgical group were alive. Nevertheless, a statistically significant difference in survival was found for patients in two high-risk subgroups: patients with three-vessel coronary artery disease and impaired left ventricular function; and those with prior myocardial infarction, hypertension or resting ST depression on the ECG. Only 52% of patients with three-vessel disease and impaired ventricular function were alive at 7 years when treated medically, compared to 76% in those treated surgically; at 11 years, survival was 37% and 50%, respectively. Survival at 7 years in those with two of the three clinical risk factors (hypertension, previous myocardial infarction and resting ST depression) was better if treated surgically than medically. Patients who fulfilled criteria for both high-risk subgroups had the largest benefit from surgery (76% versus 36% survival at 7 years, and 54% versus 24% at 11 years).

The CASS study

CASS was a multicentre, North American investigation which enroled patients from August 1975 to May 1979. It assessed the effects of coronary surgery on mortality and selected non-fatal endpoints. The register included 24,959 patients who underwent coronary angiography during the enrolment period. Of this group, 33% were recruited from study centres that did not participate in the final randomized study, or they were studied in a pilot trial only; 16,626 patients were screened for entry into the randomized trial. Subsequently, subjects were excluded from randomization if they had normal, minimal, or non-operable disease by angiography; class III or class IV angina; left main coronary artery disease; prior coronary bypass grafting; congestive heart failure; or were older than 65.

After all exclusions, only 780 patients were randomized to medical or surgical therapy. Not surprisingly, mortality in both groups was low. Annual mortality rates in the surgical arm were 0.7%, 1.0% and 1.55% for patients with single-, double- and triple-vessel disease, respectively.

Mortality in the medical group was remarkably low, at 2.4%, 1.2% and 2.1% for single-, double- and triple-vessel disease, indicating the rather benign nature of this type of coronary disease. No statistical difference was noted at 5 years between medical and surgical survival, although 5% of the medical group underwent coronary artery bypass grafting for amelioration of progressive symptoms. These patients remained in the medical group for data analysis. Of the 160 patients with ejection fractions of less than 0.5 and three-vessel disease, survival was better (although not statistically) in the surgical arm at 7 years. Those with triple-vessel disease and ejection fractions higher than 0.34, but lower than 0.50, also had an improved 7-year survival with surgery when compared with medical treatment (84% versus 70%).

Non-randomized patients from the CASS trial with either class I or class II angina (who refused randomization) and those patients with class III or class IV angina, who were excluded from the study by design, were also analysed. This showed that medical treatment of patients with class III or class IV angina, three-vessel disease and normal left ventricular function produced only a 74% 5-year survival, compared with 92% for surgical treatment. Comparison of those patients with class III and class IV angina, three-vessel disease and abnormal left ventricular function revealed a 5-year survival rate of 82% with surgery, but only 52% for those treated medically. In contrast, patients with class I or class II angina and normal left ventricular function had a 5-year survival in excess of 92% with medical or surgical treatment. These later results confirmed the superiority of surgical treatment for patients with severe angina, amidst considerable scepticism based on the earlier analyses.

Another purpose of the CASS study was to examine quality of life under the two different treatments. Patients treated surgically had significantly less chest pain, fewer activity limitations and required less therapy with nitrates or betablockers. At 5 years, surgically treated patients had significantly longer treadmill times, less exercise-induced angina and less ST segment elevation than medically treated patients. In the US, these improvements in physiological findings were not reflected by an increase in employment or recreational status. This led to the policy that patients who were moderately symptomatic after infarction, or had chronic, stable angina, should be managed medically first. If symptoms worsened, or the patient became dissatisfied

with his or her lifestyle, coronary artery bypass grafting was recommended. At the same time, quality of life and work status studies in the UK demonstrated considerably better rehabilitation statistics. Westaby, at the Royal Postgraduate Medical School, reported a greater than 70% return to work and increase in physical activity in chronically disabled patients with angina, including those performing heavy manual work.

The European Coronary Surgery Study

THE THIRD major randomized trial was the European Coronary Surgery Study. This multicentre prospective randomized trial studied 768 men under the age of 65 with mild to moderate angina, 50% or greater stenosis of at least two major coronary arteries and normal left ventricular function. Results showed that coronary artery bypass grafting improved survival overall, but especially in patients with severe three-vessel disease or proximal left anterior descending lesions. Surprisingly, the subgroup with left main coronary artery disease did not have a statistically significant increase in survival after surgery when compared with medical treatment. However, the numbers with left main disease were small. Symptoms (including anginal attacks, use of beta-adrenergic blockers and nitrates, and poor exercise performance) were significantly ameliorated in the surgical group at 5 years. Operative mortality was 3.6%. For patients with three-vessel disease, the 5-year survival was 94% in the surgical group and 90% in the medically treated group. When an important left anterior descending stenosis was present, a 5-year survival of 92.7% was achieved with surgery, whereas only 82% of medically treated patients were alive. Both findings were statistically significant. For patients with left ventricular dysfunction and ischaemic ST segment depression of greater than 1.5 mm, surgery improved survival to 91.7% at 5 years, compared to 79% without surgery.

In summary, the European study documented significantly improved survival in patients with proximal left anterior descending stenosis, associated with disease in one or two other vessels, and also in those with an ECG showing ST segment depression of greater than 1.5 mm at rest.

Patients with myocardial infarction and cardiogenic shock were an especially difficult group to treat, and consequently attracted the early interest of both medical and surgical teams. With the introduction of intra-aortic balloon counterpulsation, many of these patients could be stabilized. Inability to wean the intra-aortic balloon pump was a situation in which early angiography and coronary bypass surgery improved survival. By 1973, the Massachusetts General Hospital was able to report improved 1-year survival, from 20% with balloon pumping alone to 37% with intra-aortic balloon support plus early coronary bypass grafting.

Based on these major and sometimes contradictory landmark studies, controversies surrounding indications for coronary artery surgery were inevitable. Each study had problems when compensating for important improvements in treatment and crossover from medical to surgical groups. Differences in the types of patient enroled, particularly the relatively benign class of patient, made comparisons between the studies difficult. Nevertheless, broad clinical indications for coronary artery surgery were agreed upon and summarized by Cohen. These were: class III angina that was unresponsive to medical therapy, unstable angina, left main coronary stenosis and symptomatic patients with triple-vessel disease. Relative indications were high-risk subgroups, post-myocardial infarction (with positive stress test at low workload) and those in cardiogenic shock.

Later, single centre studies of high-risk patients confirmed clear superiority of surgery over medical treatment. For those with triple-vessel disease and impaired left ventricular function, the difference in survival for medical versus surgical treatment was 53% versus 89%. Coronary bypass became the most frequently performed operation in the US and heralded widespread expansion in cardiac surgical facilities to cope with the commonest cause of death in adult males. The Cleveland clinic maintained its dominance in the field through the efforts of Loop, Cosgrove, Lytle and others who performed thousands of primary and re-operative procedures. Long-term follow-up of their patients has formed the basis for numerous publications to define the risks and benefits of coronary surgery.

Evolution of coronary angioplasty

THE NOTION OF dilating narrowed blood vessels using a balloon catheter began with Dotter, who was the first to apply the concept to lesions of the peripheral arteries. The idea arose when he inadvertently passed an angiography catheter retrogradely through an occluded iliac artery into the abdominal aorta. This stimulated the idea of purposely enlarging stenotic arterial segments by catheter techniques. In 1964, Dotter and Judkins reported the first successful transluminal dilatation of a popliteal artery stenosis. A co-axial catheter system was used, which involved placing a small guide catheter across the stenosis followed by dilating catheters of various sizes to enlarge the narrowed area. The 'Dotter technique' was never widely accepted and initial attempts to design a balloon catheter failed through lack of appropriate materials. However, in 1974, Andreas Grüntzig, in Zurich, produced a polyvinyl chloride balloon catheter and used it to dilate peripheral arterial stenoses, with good results. Encouraged by his initial success, he modified the system for use in the coronary arteries and experimented with this on dogs in the autopsy room. Grüntzig and Miller then inserted the small balloon catheter intraoperatively in patients undergoing coronary artery surgery, and demonstrated that human coronary narrowings could be enlarged in the same way. By 1977, the catheter system had been refined sufficiently to allow percutaneous use in humans, and on 16 September, the first percutaneous coronary artery dilatation was performed in Zurich. In 1978, Grüntzig published the results of the first five patients. Clearly, the prospect of dilating coronary atheroma by a percutaneous catheter method had widespread appeal for both the interventional cardiologist and the patient who might avoid surgery. Coronary angioplasty was adopted widely, particularly for the treatment of isolated single- and then double-vessel coronary stenoses. Improvements in balloon technology and the developments of atherectomy (laser and mechanical) and intracoronary stents has greatly increased the scope of catheter techniques. As a result, coronary artery bypass surgery is now reserved for cases of increasing difficulty and an ever increasing number of patients requiring re-operation.

The resurrection of less invasive coronary bypass

THERE IS SELDOM logic in the sequence of scientific or surgical development, and significant advances are often recycled. Whilst improved operating conditions with cardioplegic arrest provided the stimulus for an explosion in surgical myocardial revascularization, recent years have witnessed a swing back to the so-called 'less invasive' techniques. Coronary bypass is undertaken without opening a cardiac chamber, and consequently it is not necessary to divert blood from within the heart. With continued ventilation of the lungs and unimpaired blood flow there is no need for a pump oxygenator. The only technical requirement for coronary bypass is a bloodless anastomotic field, which can be achieved by temporary coronary occlusion whilst the circulation is supported through uninterrupted cardiac action.

When emerging technology stifled attempts to operate on the beating heart a few surgeons persisted. Ankeney (1972) described 143 patients in whom cardiopulmonary bypass was not used. Buffolo, from Saö Paulo, Brazil, reported coronary bypass by simple interruption of coronary flow (1985) and in the same year, Benetti, from Buenos Aires, described 700 operations. Benetti's experience, which now includes more than 2000 cases, was stimulated by limited resources. In Argentina, non-pump coronary surgery allowed a substantially greater throughput of patients than would otherwise have been possible. Post-operative angiography showed no difference in graft patency between bypass and non-bypass patients when the saphenous vein or the internal mammary artery were used.

Others followed the lead of Benetti and Buffolo in a range of selective, emergency and re-operative coronary operations. Pfister, of the Washington Hospital Center, reported 220 operations without cardio-pulmonary bypass, comparing the outcome with 220 conventional operations matched for number of grafts, left ventricular function and date of operation. He concluded that for selected patients with disease of the left anterior descending and right coronary arteries, coronary bypass could be performed successfully without extracorporeal circulation. Also, that left ventricular function was better preserved that after cold cardioplegic arrest.

The superior preservation of left ventricular function in non-pump patients despite periods of unprotected regional ischaemia is persuasive. Akins, from the Massachusetts General Hospital, performed a comparative study of coronary operations with and without cardiopulmonary bypass. He found that post-operative septal wall motion was abnormal in all cardiopulmonary bypass patients with aortic cross clamping (global ischaemia). Those operated without had either no change or an improvement in septal motion after revascularization. Benetti also investigated myocardial injury by performing intra-operative left ventricular biopsies and showed superior preservation of the mitochondria in non-bypass patients. Collectively, the data from these groups suggested that non-pump coronary operations were safe, avoided the damaging effects of cardiopulmonary bypass and were advantageous, particularly for those with impaired ventricular function or a wish to avoid blood transfusion. Increasing experience of non-pump coronary bypass through a median sternotomy then led to the concept of minimally invasive coronary bypass. Benetti, Calafiore, Subramanian and others then achieved direct anastomosis between the left internal mammary artery and the left anterior descending coronary through a 10 cm incision in the 4th left intercostal space. Fonger demonstrated the feasibility of the subxiphoid approach for anastomosis of the gastro-epiploic artery to the posterior descending branch of the right coronary. These procedures, whilst of limited use in routine coronary surgery, are useful for re-operations and in high risk patients where sternotomy and cardiopulmonary bypass are deleterious. Videoscopic harvest of the internal mammary artery, new types of instrument and chest wall retractors together with pharmacological slowing of cardiac action have been introduced to facilitate this new approach.

Transmyocardial laser revascularization

THE 1990s brought increased expectations from patients and a demand for treatment from those previously regarded as inoperable. With an increasingly elderly population, the number of patients with severe diffuse coronary disease or occluded vein grafts (but preserved left ventricular function) expanded rapidly. Transmyocardial laser revascularization (TMR) was introduced to treat patients with medically and surgically refractory angina and has been applied to cardiac transplant patients with severe diffuse graft atherosclerosis where conventional revascularization in untenable. The procedure involves firing a laser through the epicardial surface of the myocardium to drill channels and connect intra-myocardial sinusoids with the left ventricular cavity. Initial work by Frazier and Cooley at the Texas Heart Institute, and Cohn at Brigham and Women's Hospital, Boston, provided anecdotal reports of dramatic relief of markedly debilitating angina. A multicentre trial sponsored by the Food and Drug Administration then demonstrated reproducible relief of angina, though experimental observations suggest that most laser channels occlude early and little myocardial blood flow originates from the left ventricle. Clinical improvement may reflect enhancement of coronary collateral circulation and the future role of the method remains to be defined.

THE ORIGINS OF DYSRHYTHMIA SURGERY

THE MECHANISM and order of cardiac electrical activity was determined at the beginning of the 20th Century through the penetrating observations of Gaskell (1883), Woller (1887), Kent (1893), His (1893), Einthoven (1903), Tarawa (1905), Keith (1906), Flack (1907), MacKenzie (1908) and Lewis (1925). Their pioneering work was undertaken before the emergence of catheters, electrodes, monitoring devices or stimulators. Interest in electrophysiology was brought to the United States by the trainees of Sir Thomas Lewis, in particular Paul White and Frank Wilson, who provided a broader dimension to electrocardiography with correlation between electrophysiological and clinical events.

The Wolff–Parkinson–White Syndrome

WHITE returned to the Massachusetts General Hospital from England in 1914 and introduced electrocardiography. He first noted the electrocardiographic combination of a short PR interval and prolonged QRS complex (delta wave) in 1917, but the patient was asymptomatic. Fourteen years later, White identified the same pattern in a 35-year-old callisthenics instructor, who presented with paroxysmal atrial tachycardia. The patient was under the care of

Louis Wolff, who subsequently collected six other patients with similar electrocardiographic abnormalities. During a return trip to Europe, White showed the electrocardiograms to various experts, including Lewis who suggested that the abnormality occurred through bundle branch block with atrioventricular nodal rhythm. John Parkinson, however, recognized the abnormality and provided other patients similar to those from the Massachusetts General Hospital. Wolff then published 11 cases in the *American Heart Journal* (August 1930) under the title *Bundle branch block with short PR interval in healthy young people prone to paroxysmal tachycardia*. Parkinson and White were co-authors with Wolff for the seminal manuscript, though the three physicians did not meet until 1954.

Similar findings were described by Wilson in 1959 and by Holzmann and Scherf in 1932, and subsequently many patients were diagnosed as having electrocardiographic evidence of pre-excitation. Most experienced a benign course, though Kimball, in 1947, reported eight dysrhythmic deaths in patients with the Wolff–Parkinson–White (WPW) syndrome. At this time, there was no evidence to suggest that anatomic pathways of pre-excitation existed, though Stanley Kent had suggested this possibility. Kent's observations were disregarded, as were those of Holzmann and Scherf, who postulated the presence of atrioventricular muscular bridges as accessory pathways in 1932. In 1933, Charles Wolferth and Francis Wood studied the abnormal electrocardiograms of ten patients similar to those in the Wolff–Parkinson–White paper. Wolferth recognized the fact that the electrocardiogram (ECG) in the Wolff–Parkinson–White paper could not be attributed to bundle branch block and must be due to the early arrival of an impulse from the atrium. Reviewing Kent's writings, Wolferth and Wood proposed the presence of a true "Kent's bundle" — an accessory atrioventricular pathway. When they encountered a patient who died suddenly with this ECG anomaly, Wood cut sections through the atrioventricular groove and found three potential tracks along the right cardiac margin. In his manuscript of 1943, Wood proposed the mechanism of accessory pathway conduction, and noted that the proof of the hypothesis must rest with direct evidence that the tracks were capable of transmitting the excitatory impulses. Subsequently, it was the collaborative work of Bionic from Duke University and More of the University of Pennsylvania, that would prove the existence of conductivity in anatomically demonstrable accessory tracks.

Surgery for dysrhythmia

SURGERY FOR DYSRHYTHMIA evolved through the collaboration of John Boineau and Andrew Wallace with their surgical colleague, Will Sealy, of Duke University. Wallace became interested in cardiac conduction during his residency with Harvey Estes, who worked on vector electrocardiography. Wallace then worked with Stanley Sarnoff at the National Institutes of Health and employed epicardial surface electrodes to study propagation of the atrioventricular impulse. By stimulating the stellate ganglion and vagus nerve, a considerable amount of information was obtained about re-entry around the atrioventricular node. Wallace returned to Duke University in 1962, and deprived of facilities, was invited to collaborate with Sealy in the thoracic surgical laboratory. Sealy's interest in dysrhythmia stemmed from the work on his original concept of combining extracorporeal circulation with hypothermia in order to permit lower perfusion flow rates and prolong the safe period of cardiopulmonary bypass. Extending the work to deep hypothermia, Sealy encountered the problem of ventricular fibrillation at temperatures below 28°C and became interested in the effects of hypothermia on cardiac conduction and arrhythmogenesis. Sealy asked Wallace to teach clinical electrophysiology in exchange for laboratory facilities and together they collaborated on several experimental electrophysiology papers. Their main thrust was to correlate the ECG with different pathologic conditions using Hofmann electrodes.

Wallace's group performed intra-operative electrophysiological mapping on Sealy's patients with atrial septal defects, tetralogy of Fallot and left ventricular hypertrophy. They measured His bundle recordings, including patients undergoing His ablation for supraventricular tachycardia. Boineau joined the group from a cardiology fellowship at Georgetown University under Proctor Harvey. Together they used intramural electrodes and probes to map patients undergoing congenital cardiac repairs. In 1963, Boineau travelled to Amsterdam to study mapping in myocardial infarction

with Dirk Durrer. Durrer was a pioneer in electrophysiology and identified an accessory pathway in a 21-year-old woman with Type B WPW syndrome, who was scheduled to undergo closure of an atrial septal defect. Durrer recognized that the type of epicardial excitation pattern present in this patient was completely different from that in hearts with normal conduction. Durrer and Roos located an accessory conduction pathway which ran from the lower lateral part of the right atrium towards the adjoining part of the right ventricle. This tract corresponded to others identified by anatomic studies in hearts of patients who died from the WPW syndrome and in whom a muscle bundle was identified.

Durrer and Roos also studied four additional patients with WPW syndrome using intracardiac catheters introduced into the right atrium and ventricle. These showed that a 'Kent pathway' could conduct either anterograde or retrograde (ventriculo-atrial) and that a premature stimulus could render the His bundle refractory. This suggested that any conduction during this period must travel via an accessory atrioventricular connection. With what he had learned from Durrer, Boineau collaborated with Wallace and Sealy at Duke University to map a number of patients suffering from ischaemia and infarction. Boineau also participated with Sealy in experimental excision of the sinus node of dogs in an attempt to define the mechanics of a new intrinsic pacemaker. In this environment, Sealy's interest grew in the potential for surgical intervention in dysrhythmia.

In August 1966, at The Mayo Clinic a patient presented for surgery with the combination of asymptomatic atrial septal defect and disabling arrhythmia from a co-existing WPW syndrome. The patient came under the care of Burchell and McGoon, who were familiar with the work of Durrer and Roos. McGoon planned to close the atrial septal defect and simultaneously use epicardial excitation to identify the pathway with a view to surgical ablation. At operation, the right ventricle was mapped below the atrioventricular groove and the point of earliest excitation localized to the basal acute margin, just caudal to the right atrium. McGoon injected procaine into this site to confirm ablation of the impulse and then made a transverse cut, 1 cm in length, inside the right atrium to interrupt the pathway. Unfortunately, after closing the chest the ECG showed a return of the WPW syndrome. Nevertheless, this operation demonstrated the feasibility of surgical ablation and McGoon suggested a more extensive epicaridal incision, with complete atrioventricular separation in the region of the accessory pathway. Shortly afterwards, Dreifus and colleagues at the University of Georgia ligated the His bundle in a patient with symptomatic WPW syndrome instead of attempting to identify the accessory pathway.

Sealy and the fisherman

IN MARCH 1968, a 32-year-old fisherman, Norman Salter, from North Carolina, presented to Duke University for treatment of an intractable tachycardia. Salter had an intermittent but symptomatic tachycardia from the age of 4 years and eventually developed progressive cardiomegaly and heart failure. On admission, his heart rate was 150–180 bpm for more than 70% of the time and when the rhythm slowed, the ECG showed the classic appearance of the WPW syndrome. Dreifus' approach had been discussed at the 1967 Meeting of the American Heart Association and Sealy's team considered the creation of heart block in Salter's case. After reading Wood's description of an accessory pathway, Sealy decided to attempt identification and interruption of this directly.

The operation took place on 2 May 1968. The electronic mapping equipment was already in place from previous studies in the observation deck above Operating Room 1 of the University Hospital. Boineau rehearsed the mapping procedure in the laboratory for 2 weeks before the procedure on Salter. Sealy, assisted by his Chief Resident, Hattler, exposed the heart through a median sternotomy and attached reference electrodes to the right ventricle. Boineau and Wallace performed the mapping with the technicians, Bob Clark and Jackie Kassell, who had developed most of the electrophysiology equipment at Duke. Before commencing cardiopulmonary bypass, approximately 60 points were measured on the epicardial surface of both left and right ventricles. There was no timing device on the recorder and Clark measured intervals by hand on paper emerging at 500 mm/sec all over the observation room. The area of earliest activation (100–110 msec) was localized to an area 1 cm along the acute margin of the right ventricle at the atrioventricular groove. Bypass was

then established using a disk oxygenator and roller pump. A right atriotomy was made just above the atrioventricular groove and on each side of the electronically determined site, the right coronary artery was dissected free of the epicardial fat and retracted inferiorly. Influenced by McGoon's experience, Sealy adopted a more aggressive approach to the Kent's bundle. He made a 5 cm incision extending from the base of the right atrial appendage to the right border of the right atrium, completely transecting the right ventricular muscle at the site of pre-excitation. This caused the delta wave to disappear and established a normal PR interval and QRS complex in sinus rhythm. Salter recovered uneventfully and Sealy had provided definite proof that the WPW syndrome resulted from an anomalous pathway of pre-excitation. The operation was reported in *Circulation* (December 1968), with Frederick Cobb (who had recognized WPW syndrome in Salter) as first author.

Evolution of surgery for re-entry tachycardia

THE EARLY intracardiac dissections for WPW syndrome were performed with epicardial mapping and ventricular fibrillation. Unfortunately, the second patient with a very unstable arrhythmia pattern could not be satisfactorily mapped. She died from intractable arrhythmias post-operatively when the pathway remained intact. This was a serious setback for the team, though in retrospect, the patient probably had a previously undefined para-septal pathway. Further work by Boineau and Moore served to elucidate the nature of left-sided and multiple anatomic pathways not amenable to correction from the right side using the original epicardial approach. With an increased understanding of the range of atrioventricular connections, Sealy developed external localization and intra-atrial division of left free wall and septal pathways. In 1974, the team reported on the first 20 patients with one death at the American Association for Thoracic Surgery. Left-sided pathways were initially approached through a thoracotomy.

Meanwhile, John Gallagher, who had learned His bundle mapping techniques from Damato at The Staten Island Public Health Hospital, developed greater expertise in catheter electrophysiologic studies. Gallagher was able to identify and localize the accessory pathways preoperatively in the laboratory, which facilitated precise location of the area of excitation during intra-operative mapping. Gallagher added a new dimension to the electrophysiological work at Duke and played a major role in the development of arrhythmia surgery. Catheter studies elucidated other forms of pre-excitation, including Mahaim fibres arising just below the atrioventricular node and connecting directly with ventricular muscle. James' fibres passed directly from the atrium to the His bundle and some pathways were found to conduct only retrogradely. The presence of multiple pathways was recognized and in the first 50 patients operated for tachyarrhythmia, six had more than one Kent bundle.

Early surgical failures occurred in patients with pre-excitation near the crux of the heart and Sealy began to formulate methods to ablate pathways in this difficult area. The use of cardioplegia in 1978 greatly facilitated the more difficult dissections. The WPW operation was standardised, beginning with epicardial mapping then localization of pathways by endocardial studies and intra-atrial transmural dissection. Of the first 20 patients with multiple pathways, 13 underwent complete surgical ablation.

Other teams with the ability to perform detailed electrophysiological studies (including Bentall at Hammersmith Hospital and Wada in Japan) adopted surgery for dysrhythmia. In 1977, the problem of atrioventricular nodal re-entry was addressed by His bundle ablation, using surgical dissection or cryo-ablation. The following year the combination of Ebstein's anomaly an WPW syndrome was corrected by combined valve repair and pathway ablation.

Surgery for ventricular tachycardia

IN THE LATE 1970s, it became apparent that electrophysiological mapping techniques might be applied in the treatment of post-infarction ventricular tachycardia. This problem had previously been addressed by coronary bypass grafting, either alone or in combination with left ventricular aneurysm resection. Undirected attempts were sometimes successful but often disappointing. The potential for guided surgical intervention arose with evidence that re-entry was the mechanism responsible for ventricular tachycardia after myocardial infarction. The re-entry circuits were located in the ischaemic halo between scar and healthy myocardium.

Predicting that the re-entry focus was situated within the visible area of endocardial fibrosis, Gerard Guirudon and colleagues in Paris employed an encircling endocardial ventriculotomy to isolate the fibrosis and dysrhythmia substrate from normal myocardium. The method employed a perpendicular endocardial ventriculotomy incision without intra-operative mapping. Guirudon subsequently modified his technique to perform cryo-ablation rather than sharp dissection. At the University of Pennsylvania, Josephson, Harken and Horowitz used extensive intra-operative mapping and induction of ventricular tachycardia to identify the focus which was then excised. In their first report, 11 of 12 patients survived and ventricular tachycardia could not be induced post-operatively. In 1979, James Cox used the constantly improving mapping techniques at Duke to perform serially the first endocardial encircling ventriculotomy, right ventricular isolation and endocardial resection for ventricular tachycardia at the University Hospital. Cox also worked with Sealy on the WPW programme at Duke from 1980 and in 1981, Sealy and Cox reported on the first 200 consecutive cases of surgery for WPW syndrome at The American Heart Association. Left accessory tracts were most commonly found in the left free wall (45%), with posterior septal pathways being next in frequency. Only 18% of pathways were found in the right free-wall and multiple pathways were noted in 12% of patients overall. Of patients with Ebstein's anomaly, 30% had multiple pathways. Fortunately the first patient, Salter, had a right-sided pathway. If not, the first operation would have failed and the prospect of arrhythmia surgery may have been postponed for several years. Cox subsequently reported 118 consecutive personal cases operated with the endocardial approach and cardioplegic arrest. A more extensive endocardial dissection resulted in a 99% long-term success rate and a reduction in the incidence of complete heart block. By 1987, over 1000 operations for WPW syndrome had been reported worldwide, with important series from Guirudon, Iwa, Harken, Bokeria, Ott, Jatene, Selle and others.

Surgery for atrial tachycardia

COX continued to explore innovative electro-physiological procedures and became Chief of Cardiothoracic Surgery at Washington University. In 1982, he performed the first cryo ablation of the atrioventricular node for re-entrant arrhythmias and following experimental collaboration with Mark Williams, performed the first clinical left atrial isolation procedure. This evolved into the maze operation (Cox procedure) designed to prevent atrial flutter or fibrillation in patients with refractory paroxysmal or chronic atrial fibrillation associated with fatigue, malaise, dyspnoea or recurrent thromboembolism. Patients with paroxysmal atrial flutter or fibrillation manifest similar symptoms to those with other types of supraventricular tachycardia, such as the WPW syndrome and atrioventricular node re-entry.

Progressive improvements in technology have now modified the surgical approach in tachyarrhythmia surgery. The morbidity and mortality of dysrhythmia surgery was principally related to the ancillary techniques of general anaesthesia, cardiopulmonary bypass and myocardial protection. Because of this, Guirudon and colleagues developed methods of ablative dissection of the atrioventricular sulcus without cardiopulmonary bypass or cardiotomy. A dramatic reduction in the need for cardiopulmonary bypass in these operations resulted. Surgery performed on the beating heart also had the benefit of ease of documentation of the electrophysiological changes.

In the late 80s, the emergence of radio frequency catheter ablation (which delivers destructive energy at the site of accessory conduction) virtually eliminated surgery for accessory pathway ablation. For ventricular tachycardia, Guirudon modified his surgical approach by making cryo lesions rather than surgical incisions to isolate arrhythmogenic myocardium. Mesnildrey and his colleagues adopted laser photo coagulation for this purpose. Subendocardial resection at the University of Pennsylvania was associated with an operative mortality of 15% but provided complete ablation of ventricular tachycardia in two-thirds of the patients. Inducible tachycardia, which remained in one-third of patients, was largely abolished when the post-operative patients were restarted on anti-arrhythmic drugs.

To avoid ventriculotomy, Gerald Lawrie and colleagues at Baylor approached the ventricular endocardium via the atrioventricular or aortic valves. Delnar and colleagues attempted intra-ventricular balloon computerized mapping and electric shock ablation of endocardial arrhythmic foci. However, in line with the development of transcatheter ablation of accessory pathways, the widespread early use of thrombolytic agents has dramatically altered the course of acute myocardial infarction and reduced the incidence of ventricular tachycardia.

The implantable defibrillators

THE USE of the implantable defibrillator began in the mid-1980s and has increased steadily, discouraging those somewhat tedious surgical procedures with an uncertain outcome. An estimated 15,000 units were implanted in the United States in 1993; two-thirds in patients with coronary disease. The defibrillators themselves have progressed rapidly, from surgically implanted bulky devices with large epicardial electrodes to pacemaker sized units with endocardial wires. The actuarial incidence of sudden cardiac death after insertion of an implanted cardioverter defibrillator has been reported to be as low as 1% per year. With more than 300,000 episodes of sudden cardiac death considered to be related to ventricular tachycardia or ventricular fibrillation each year, use of the implanted defibrillator will inevitably increase.

Biographies

Claude Schaeffer Beck (1894–1971)

CLAUDE SCHAEFFER BECK was born in Shomokin, Pennsylvania and studied at Franklin and Marshall College (AB, 1916). He went on to study at Johns Hopkins University (MD, 1921), where he was a house officer (1921–22). Beck was Assistant Resident Surgeon at New Haven and Peter Bent Brigham hospitals (1922–23) and Cabot Research Fellow at Harvard (1923–24). He developed closed, punch valvotomy with Elliott Cutler while he was Crile Research Fellow in surgery at Western Reserve University and on the staff of University and Lakeside hospitals, Cleveland (1924–25).

Beck became Professor of Neurosurgery, the second after Cushing, (1940–52) and the first Professor of Cardiovascular Surgery in the United States (1952–65). Beck is known for his clinical studies of the pericardium, the first successful removal of tumours of the heart (1942) and his tireless pioneering of resuscitation of the heart from cardiac arrest. Beck frequently began his lectures by recounting an experience whilst an intern at Johns Hopkins:

> *"The operation was almost complete when the anaesthetist told the surgeon that the patient was pulseless and blue. The surgeon removed his gloves, went to the telephone in the corner of the operating room and called the fire brigade. When the officers arrived some twenty minutes later the pulmotor (resuscitation equipment) was applied but to no avail. The patient was declared dead which left me with the conviction that we were not doing our best for the patient!"*

His first defibrillation of the human heart by opening the chest (1947) solicited the comment from the dean of the medical school of Western Reserve University that Beck "was not a safe man to have on the faculty." He was the first to reverse a fatal heart attack (1955) and was known for his evangelical fervour in "saving hearts that are too good to die, hearts that only need a second chance to beat." Beck, whose writing possesses the clarion quality of the prophet, wrote about improving the circulation of the myocardium:

> *"The contemplation of the period when arterial disease in the heart can be prevented or retarded produces an aura of greatness...Next to food, shelter, and the absence of war there is probably nothing more important."*

Throughout the 30s and 40s Beck occupied himself with experimental efforts to revascularize the ischaemic myocardium. His research was put into clinical practice with the Beck I operation, which sought to stimulate intercoronary collateral circulation by abrasion and talc poudrage on the surface of the heart (Article 5.1, Appendix A). Two observations stimulated Beck to take this course. The first was the demonstration of blood vessels in the fat at the base of the heart; these anastomosed with branches from the aorta. The second was the demonstration of blood vessels in pericardial adhesions. During a previous operation Beck had cut through a band of adhesions extending from the base of the left ventricle to a scar in the pericardium and found that each end of the transected abrasion bled briskly. Beck considered that collateral circulation could be stimulated in experimental animals but it would be necessary to duplicate coronary occlusive disease in order to provide a pressure differential between coronary and extra coronary circulations. This was achieved by placing silver bands around the coronary ostia, flattened, a little at a time, at successive operations, until

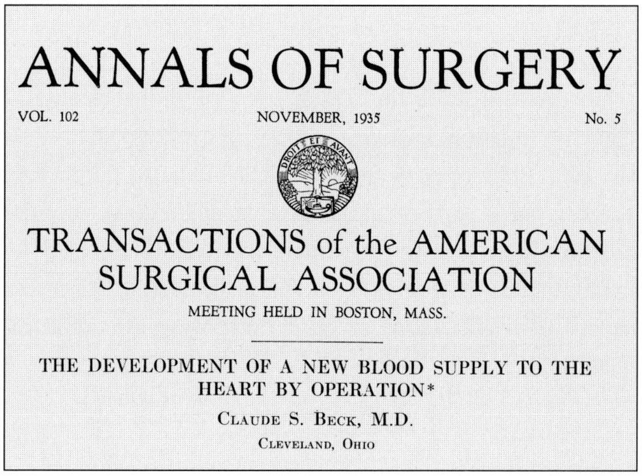

ANNALS OF SURGERY

VOL. 102   NOVEMBER, 1935   No. 5

TRANSACTIONS of the AMERICAN SURGICAL ASSOCIATION

MEETING HELD IN BOSTON, MASS.

THE DEVELOPMENT OF A NEW BLOOD SUPPLY TO THE HEART BY OPERATION*

CLAUDE S. BECK, M.D.
CLEVELAND, OHIO

Figure 5.7. Title page of Beck's 1935 article entitled 'The development of a new blood supply to the heart by operation'. (Reproduced with permission from Annals of Surgery; 102: 801–13.)

complete occlusion of the artery was affected. Using grafts of mediastinal fat, skeletal muscle from the chest wall or omentum brought through the diaphragm, collateral circulation developed sufficiently to protect against coronary occlusion. Ventricular fibrillation sometimes occurred during the tightening of the bands. Beck noticed that this could only be reversed when the bands were removed and the heart reperfused. This experimental work was translated into the Beck I operation but the early mortality was 50%. All patients had advanced coronary sclerosis and accepted the risk because life without improvement was not worthwhile. Beck reduced the operative mortality by selecting patients with less advanced left ventricular damage. Instead of a bilateral approach to the heart with separate parasternal incisions through the costal cartilages, a unilateral pectoral muscle graft was adopted with only one costal cartilage removed. Mechanical scarification of the epicardium by means of a burr caused multiple extrasystoles which could be reduced by applying procaine to the epicardium. Beck subsequently adopted the Beck II operation whereby the coronary sinus was arterialized by a vein graft from the descending aorta. Without circulatory support this was a technically demanding and hazardous operation. However, many of the patients were significantly improved.

Beck followed this lead with further experiments and on 27 January 1948 performed the first Beck II operation on man. He excised a length of brachial artery and used this to join the descending aorta to the coronary sinus; the coronary sinus itself was ligated at its junction with the right atrium. This was a difficult operation and Beck soon changed to a two-stage procedure whereby the graft was inserted first and between 2 and 6 weeks later the coronary sinus was partially ligated. The Beck II operation produced impressive, long-standing intercoronary connections, even though the graft tended to thrombose after a few weeks. However, the operative mortality was 15–20% and this soon brought the procedure into disrepute.

Laurence O'Shaughnessy (1900–1940)

LAURENCE O'SHAUGHNESSY was born in Sunderland, England. He insisted on leaving school at the age of 15 to do war work and studied in coastguards' huts until he was old enough to read medicine at Newcastle Medical School, where he qualified at 21 (FRCS). In 1924, as an inspector in the Sudan Medical Service, he was in charge of a hospital at Omdurman for 7 years. On leaves, he visited Sauerbruch in Berlin where he became interested in thoracic surgery. On his return to England, he received the first Royal College of Surgeons' research fellowship (1931). This allowed him to investigate an artificial blood supply to the heart in cardiac ischaemia and develop a surgical treatment for pulmonary tuberculosis at the newly-opened Buckston Browne Research Farm. As Hunterian Professor, he lectured on surgery of the oesophagus (1933) and lung (1935). He considered his thesis on the mechanism of surgical shock for the Harveian Society Prize a counterbalance to his excessive interest in thoracic surgery.

By 1930, O'Shaughnessy had improved the circulation to the anastomosis after oesophagogastrectomy by using a pedicle wrap of greater omentum. In April 1933, he began to apply omental grafts to the epicardium and found that vascular connections formed quickly with the epicardial blood vessels. When he read that greyhounds were prone to a type of heart failure which might be relieved by this operation, he performed

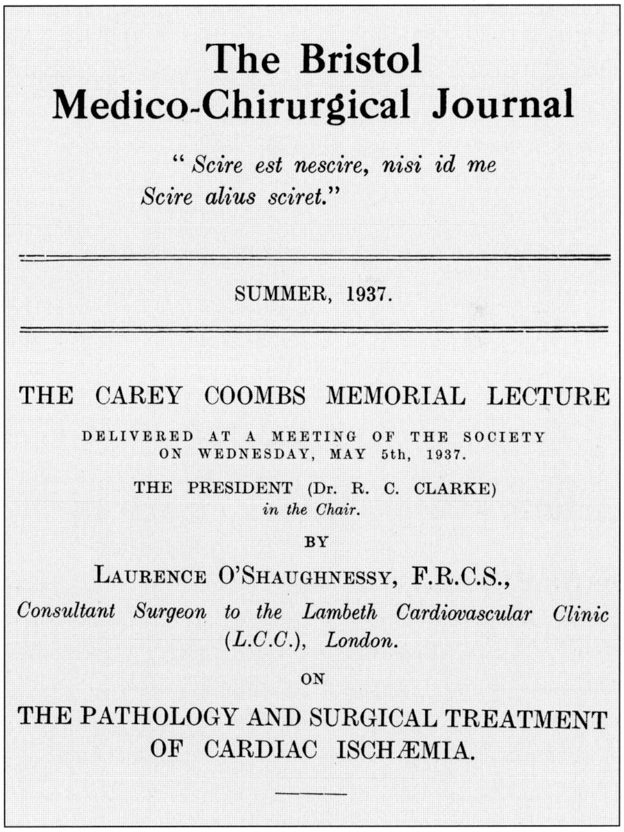

The Bristol Medico-Chirurgical Journal

" Scire est nescire, nisi id me Scire alius sciret."

SUMMER, 1937.

THE CAREY COOMBS MEMORIAL LECTURE

DELIVERED AT A MEETING OF THE SOCIETY ON WEDNESDAY, MAY 5th, 1937.

THE PRESIDENT (Dr. R. C. CLARKE) *in the Chair.*

BY

LAURENCE O'SHAUGHNESSY, F.R.C.S.,

Consultant Surgeon to the Lambeth Cardiovascular Clinic (L.C.C.), London.

ON

THE PATHOLOGY AND SURGICAL TREATMENT OF CARDIAC ISCHÆMIA.

Figure 5.8. Title page of O'Shaughnessy's 1937 article entitled 'The pathology and surgical treatment of cardiac ischaemia. (Reproduced with permission from The Bristol Medico-Chirurgical Journal; *LIV: 109–26.)*

omental grafts to establish a collateral circulation. He then tied off the left coronary artery and showed that the greyhounds could return to the track. This procedure, cardio-omentopexy, (Article 5.2, Appendix A) was improved by applying aleuronat paste between the omental graft and the heart to stimulate formation of adhesions. The first patient to be treated with an omental graft was a 64-year-old man at Lewisham Hospital on 4 January 1936. In 1938, O'Shaugnessy reported improvement in all patients who survived for 6 months or more; those who had been bedridden could walk and those unable to work could do so. O'Shaugnessy's work, for which he was awarded the Hunter Medal by the Royal College of Surgeons in 1937, culminated in the establishment of the cardiovascular clinic at Lambeth Hospital in 1936. Visitors came from all over the world and O'Shaugnessy lectured in France, Germany and the United States.

O'Shaugnessy's published work consists of some 30 papers and book chapters on the oesophagus and diaphragm in Maingot's *Post-Graduate Surgery*. He wrote *Thoracic Surgery* (1937) with Sauerbruch, which popularized this little known field and stressed the necessity of co-operation between physician and surgeon. In collaboration with Walter Pagel and Gregory Kayne, he wrote *Pulmonary Tuberculosis: Pathology, Diagnosis, Management and Prevention*. In a few years, O'Shaugnessy created a new outlook on cardiac surgery and did more to advance this subject than anyone, in England, if not the world. In *Future of Cardiac Surgery*, he pointed out precociously in 1939:

> *"The real key to further advance in the surgical treatment of established cardiac defects will only be provided by some simple and efficient method of maintaining the cerebral circulation while the heart is temporarily out of commission...so long as the surgeon is faced with the certainty of irreparable cerebral damage if he interrupts the circulation for any appreciable period, he has little incentive to devise operative procedures which can never be carried out."*

But for his untimely death, he would have been a leader in the development of cardiac surgery. At the outbreak of World War II, O'Shaugnessy, who believed that chest wounds needed immediate treatment, volunteered to serve at a casualty clearing station with the British Expeditionary Force in Flanders. In a lull, while working on his book on the surgery of the heart, a stray bullet created an open pneumothorax which killed him. "O'Shaugnessy's death," wrote Sir Thomas Holmes-Sellors,

> *"has deprived our profession of a most valuable and rare type: the truly scientific experimental worker. His attitude towards surgery was dominated by a desire to attack problems which had defeated others. If he felt there was a possible solution he would advise and carry out experiment after experiment until his critical mind could find no hindrance to putting his findings into practice in human surgery. In this way, his work on cardiac surgery began. I remember seeing him several years ago at the College of Surgeons Farm at Downe where, surrounded by specimens and data, he defended his thesis triumphantly against friendly but outspoken criticisms from physician, surgeon and pathologist. There he was in his element — forceful, clear-thinking and argumentative, yet with a characteristic generosity that freely admitted the possibility of a weakness in his train of thought."*

Arthur Marie Vineberg (1903–1988)

ARTHUR MARIE VINEBERG was born in Montreal, Quebec and studied biochemistry and medicine at McGill University, (BSc, 1924; MSc 1925; MD, 1928). He trained at the Columbia Division of Bellevue Hospital, New York City (1928–29) and the Royal Victoria Hospital, Montreal (1929–33). After postdoctoral work in the physiology of gastric secretion at McGill University (PhD, 1933), his early publications were devoted to gastric physiology. While teaching anatomy at McGill, Vineberg practised clinical surgery at several hospitals in Montreal. He received The Order of Canada in 1986 at the age of 83.

Vineberg described how he came to develop surgical methods to relieve myocardial ischaemia in 1927:

> *"One of my colleagues, Dr Eric MacNaughton, reminded me of a conversation we had in 1927 in a locker room after a wrestling workout at McGill University. As we dressed, we were talking over a lecture given that afternoon on the pathology of coronary artery disease. The lecturer, Professor Hoerst Ortel, a famous pathologist, had pointed out that coronary artery arteriosclerosis involved mainly the major coronary arteries and surface branches in their epicardial courses, leaving the intramyocardial arterioles comparatively disease-free.*
>
> *Apparently I had said to Eric, if the surface coronary arteries are diseased, why could we not graft another artery into the heart muscle. Eric said that was a good idea, but which artery would you use? Eric reminded me that I had suggested using the left internal mammary artery because of its position close to the*

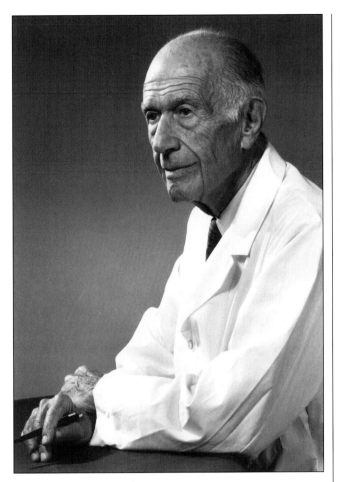

Figure 5.9. Arthur Vineberg.

left ventricle and because its removal from the chest wall would not cause harm to the tissues it supplied. There the idea rested until 1930, when my father, aged 52, suffered an acute myocardial infarction so severe that he required an oxygen tent — a new development at that time. He recovered to become a wheelchair cripple with angina decubitus and night pain. I was living at home at the time and each night when I came home the light was on in his room, where he sat with fear in his eyes. In 1935, he died with a good cardiologist at his bedside. His death renewed my interest in bringing a new artery to the ischaemic left ventricular muscle."

Vineberg continued his research following the death of his father:

"At that time I was instructing in anatomy at McGill University; this gave me the opportunity to examine the left internal mammary artery in many cadavers. I found that in young and old, male and female, tall and short, the left internal mammary artery could be easily dissected free from its

location beneath the costal cartilages and superficial to the sternocostalis muscles, endothoracic fascia, and parietal pleura. It was easy to remove from the chest wall and after the pericardium was opened the freed artery was long enough in most cases to reach not only the anterior left ventricular wall, but to reach the posterior left ventricular wall. Clearly it was possible to bring this artery to the heart in all human bodies dissected; the question remained, how to do it so that it would remain open and supply the ischaemic left ventricular heart muscle with badly needed oxygenated blood."

At the end of World War II Vineberg returned to laboratory research at the Royal Victoria Hospital with the conviction that the internal mammary artery could be grafted successfully into the arteriolar collateral bed of the ischaemic myocardium (Article 5.3, Appendix A).

In 1959, Mason Sones's technique of selective coronary cineangiography gave Vineberg the opportunity to study his patients and prove his theory. Vineberg visited Sones at the Cleveland Clinic but both Sones and his surgical colleague, Donald Effler, expressed doubts about the value of mammary artery implantation. Vineberg nevertheless persuaded Sones to investigate five patients whose angina was relieved by the implant technique. In the first two, the artery was occluded; in the third patient, there was no coronary disease. However, the next two patients both had severe coronary occlusive disease and their internal mammary artery grafts were patent with communications with the coronary circulation. Effler went to

INTERNAL MAMMARY CORONARY ANASTOMOSIS IN THE SURGICAL TREATMENT OF CORONARY ARTERY INSUFFICIENCY*

Arthur Vineberg, M.D. and Gavin Miller, M.D.
Montreal, Que.

THIS paper constitutes a preliminary report of clinical cases which have undergone transplantation of the left internal mammary artery into the left ventricle as a treatment for coronary artery insufficiency. The theoretical and experimental basis on which this procedure is based will be briefly described.

Figure 5.10. Title page of Vineberg's 1951 article entitled 'Internal mammary coronary anastomosis in the surgical treatment of coronary artery insufficiency'. (Reproduced with permission from Canadian Medical Association Journal; 64: 204–10.)

Montreal to study the Vineberg operation and subsequently established a large clinical and arteriographic evaluation of the operation in Cleveland. By 1965, several hundred patients were investigated by coronary angiography, operated on and then restudied.

In 1964, Vineberg had reported 140 operations with 33% mortality, though for the decade 1954–63 the mortality was less than 2%. Of 109 surviving patients, 91 had either no angina or slight pain on effort. The Vineberg procedure was shown to produce worthwhile anastomoses with the native coronary circulation in 70–80% of internal mammary implants.

On the afternoon of 15 October 1965 at the 38th Meeting of the American Heart Association, Effler stated forcefully that Vineberg's concept was valid and confirmed arteriolar connections to patent coronary arteries beyond the site of obstruction. Further proof of the internal mammary artery function was described by other surgeons when Vineberg's patients were subsequently offered direct myocardial revascularization. After the aorta was cross-clamped, persistent coronary flow through the internal mammary artery kept some hearts beating after initial cardioplegic arrest. The heart could only be arrested with the artery occluded. In the audience for Effler's American Heart Association presentation was the surgeon, George E. Green. His paper entitled "*Experimental Microvascular Suture Anastomosis*" demonstrated that vessels 1.0 mm in diameter could be joined successfully under the operating microscope. Green recognized that there was no technical barrier to suturing the internal mammary artery directly to an arteriotomy in the left anterior descending coronary artery. Also, that this procedure should offer substantially more benefit than blind intramyocardial implantation.

Though direct myocardial revascularization techniques had taken centre stage for several years, Vineberg's publications as late as 1975 still offered the mammary implant as the answer to the problems of blocked aortocoronary artery vein grafts. This extraordinary procedure suffered to some extent by having Vineberg as its major protagonist. It became his obsession to prove that the operation was effective and this may have hindered his scientific approach. He added ancillary procedures (the free omental graft, the Ivalon sponge procedure) that had little benefit and weakened his credibility. However, Vineberg remained convinced of his work and just weeks before he died was still vigorously involved in experimental work on omental angiogenic factors that might be used to stimulate cardiac vascularization without the need for more invasive surgical procedures.

William Polk Longmire, Jr. (1913–)

WILLIAM POLK LONGMIRE, Jr. was born in Sapulpa, Oklahoma. He attended the University of Oklahoma (1934) and Johns Hopkins (MD, 1938) where he was Chief Resident to Alfred Blalock (1944–45), to whom he became a close friend. Blalock's superb technician, Vivien Thomas wrote,

> "*Dr Blalock had only done 2 or 3 days of this heavy patient load (for tetralogy of Fallot) when he was scheduled to be out of town for a few days. Dr Longmire took over in the operating room and carried on as if this had been a daily, routine operative procedure for months or years...Dr Longmire was one of the very best to go through the surgical residency programme at Johns Hopkins during the Blalock era. He had superb natural technical skill, his hands moving deftly, smoothly and swiftly and he usually completed the procedure in less time than was required by the Professor.*"

After a brief period in charge of plastic surgery at Johns Hopkins, Longmire was appointed Professor and Chairman of the Department of Surgery at UCLA (1948–76), where he established an outstanding department, housed initially in World War II barracks and described in his book, *Starting from Scratch*. As President of the American College of Surgeons (1964) and the American Surgical Association (1968), he has been a major force in the national affairs of surgery. He was Professor of Surgery at UCLA (1976–84) and is now Emeritus Professor there.

Apart from early coronary endarterectomy and experimental and clinical work in transplantation, Longmire's contributions have been largely in gastrointestinal surgery. His technical skills were advantageously employed in this field: his contributions included the hepatojejunostomy operation for the destroyed common duct; his evaluation of the role of total gastrectomy for gastric cancer; and operative approaches to chronic pancreatitis and hepatic resection.

He wrote to Westaby about the development of coronary endarterectomy (Article 5.4, Appendix A):

> "*In our relatively new Department of Surgery at UCLA, there were two pioneers in the field of vascular surgery: Drs Wiley Barker and Jack Cannon. We also had an active investigative programme in cardiac surgery which had been started by Dr Harry Muller (who later became Chairman of the Department of Surgery, University of Virginia, Charlottesville). These two*

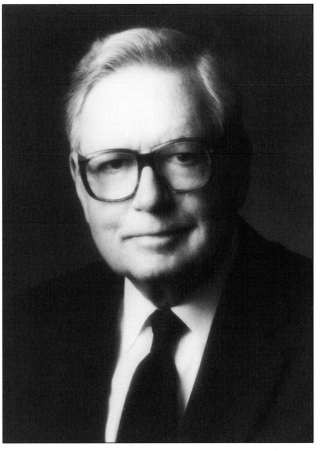

Figure 5.11. William Longmire, Jr.

interests were brought together on the problem of coronary occlusion, with Jack Cannon utilizing his knowledge of endarterectomy and my previous experience in cardiac surgery. We relied entirely on the clinical skill and acumen of Dr Albert Kattus for the selection of patients, and for the medical management and evaluation of patients before, during and after operation. In the early cases, the location of the lesion or lesions in the coronary system was not determined until the beating heart was exposed, as coronary angiography, as developed by Sones, was not available and pump oxygenators were still being improved. Our test to determine if we should continue after the heart was exposed was to see if a vessel that was abnormal to palpation would tolerate temporary complete occlusion. A brief motion picture was made during our fourth case of the removal of a 4 cm core. Interest was immediate and enthusiastic (prematurely so as later experience demonstrated) when the movie was presented at the 1958 meeting of the American Surgical Association during the discussion of Szilagyi's paper on coronary angioplastic procedures."

This must remain one of the most extraordinary operations in surgical history. After studying pathological specimens and with experience gained from endarterectomy of peripheral arteries, these workers performed direct and extensive coronary endarterectomy on the beating heart without cardiopulmonary bypass. The procedure, guided not by coronary angiography

The New England
Journal of Medicine

Copyright, 1958, by the Massachusetts Medical Society

| Volume 259 | NOVEMBER 20, 1958 | Number 21 |

DIRECT-VISION CORONARY ENDARTERECTOMY FOR ANGINA PECTORIS*

WILLIAM P. LONGMIRE, JR., M.D.,† JACK A. CANNON, M.D.,‡ AND ALBERT A. KATTUS, M.D.§

LOS ANGELES, CALIFORNIA

Figure 5.12. Title page of Longmire's 1958 article entitled 'Direct-vision coronary endarterectomy for angina pectoris'. (Reproduced with permission from The New England Journal of Medicine; 259: 993–99.)

(which did not exist) but by direct palpation of the coronary vessels, is also one of the first occasions where a treadmill exercise test was used to assess the response of coronary blood flow to a therapeutic procedure. Even with cardiopulmonary bypass and a heart arrested by cardioplegia, coronary endarterectomy presents difficulties. Years later, coronary endarterectomy remains an important therapeutic option during coronary artery bypass grafting.

Frank Mason Sones, Jr. (1918–1985)

FRANK MASON SONES, Jr. was born in Noxapater, Mississippi. He graduated from the University of Maryland School of Medicine (MD, 1943) and trained in internal medicine, paediatric cardiology and cardiac catheterization at The Henry Ford Hospital. In 1950, he became Director of Paediatric Cardiology and the Cardiac Laboratory at The Cleveland Clinic. Sones seldom missed a chance to insult those who opposed his views of medicine. His distaste for conventional cardiology was acute. He became convinced at the University of Maryland that cardiologists "didn't know what the hell they were doing....I knew back then that all the stuff they were teaching us about managing heart disease was a lot of crap. I decided to dedicate my life to proving that those old guys were full of it." His early work in congenital heart disease produced techniques for right and left ventricular catheterization, subsequently used in adults with valvular heart disease. He was the first to combine cardiac catheterization and selective angiography with high speed x-ray motion photography as a single procedure.

Without a relatively safe diagnostic tool to provide a clear view of the inside of the heart, it was virtually impossible to choose good candidates for cardiac surgery. Selective coronary angiography came about by a nearly catastrophic accident. Sones' former fellow, Royston Lewis, recalled how on 30 October 1958, Sones was doing a left ventriculogram and had pulled the catheter back into the aorta. As was customary, he and Lewis paused for a cigarette while the injector was being reloaded with 40 ml of contrast agent. He intended to photograph the aortogram but the catheter slipped into the right coronary artery before he turned on the camera. Consequently, 40 ml of contrast medium was injected directly into a large dominant right coronary artery, which was visualized superbly with its branches. The patient experienced asystole for 7 seconds. As Sones recounted,

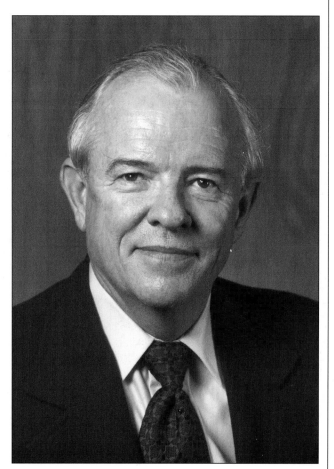

Figure 5.13. Frank Mason Sones.

"I was sure he was going to die, but when I looked over at the oscilloscope the EKG was flat. The guy's heart just wasn't beating at all. Well, I knew there was plenty of blood in the aorta. So I yelled "Cough!!" figuring that would push in the blood and force out the dye. The guy coughed three or four times and his heart resumed beating. There were no defibrillators then. Direct current countershock, developed at about the same time, ensured the safety of this technique."

Sones designed a special tapered coronary catheter for dependable manipulation. This initial experience was repeated on 1020 patients and published nearly 4 years later by Sones,

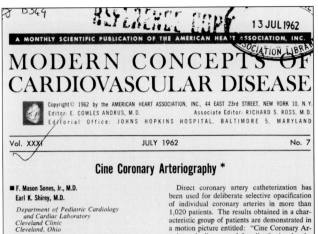

coronary angiography could not have been better timed. His work defined the pathology of coronary artery disease, contributed to an understanding of the natural history of atherosclerosis, and, by providing an accurate diagnosis and pictures that a surgeon could understand, proved to be the stimulus for development of meaningful coronary artery surgery. To quote Floyd Loop, "Collectively all of the cardiological advances in this century pale in comparison with his priceless achievement." Sones went on to make many technical advances by streamlining film processing and projection. He designed the C arm device used in virtually all angiography and devised the catheterization laboratory carousel which permits a large number of patients to be studied expeditiously and safely.

Sones spent his days in a dark room lit by the glow of the projector, clad in a T-shirt and old trousers and puffing on a cigarette. He dictated his findings there, often interrupted by residents and visitors enthralled by his discussions of coronary cineangiographic techniques. At night, he often slept on the catheterization table. René Favaloro recalls taking Sones on a holiday from Marseilles to Verona,

"I think Mason was in direct communication with nature for the first time. It was the end of summer. He was amazed by the wheat prairies, the corn fields, the green valleys, the vineyards and the fruit trees....This giant of modern cardiology was bathed by the sun in the middle of nowhere instead of by the lamps of the cardiac laboratory where he spent all his life."

Before his death from bronchogenic carcinoma at the age of 66, he received many honours, among them the American Medical Association Scientific Achievement Award (1978), the Radiological Society of North America Gold Medal (1979), the Albert Lasker Clinical Medical Research Award (1983) and the Galen Award presented by the Worshipful Society of Apothecaries of London (1985), whereby he became a Freeman of the City of London.

Figure 5.14. Title page of Sones and Earl Shirey's 1962 article entitled 'Cine coronary arteriography'. *(Reproduced with permission from* Modern Concepts of Cardiovascular Disease; *31: 735–38.)*

who, flagrant in verbal abuse, was fastidious about the quality of his published work (Figure 5.14).

Sones' discovery and development of a method for selective

René Geronimo Favaloro (1923–)

RENÉ GERONIMO FAVALORO was born La Plata, Buenos Aires, Argentina, where he accompanied his uncle, a general practitioner, on daily rounds. He graduated from the Medical Science Faculty of La Plata University (MD, 1949) and began postgraduate studies in pulmonary and oesophageal surgery in the Rawson Hospital under Mainetti and the Finochietto

brothers. His studies were interrupted when he joined his brother's small village practice as a general surgeon; this lasted for a decade. Medical journals kept him in touch with advances, particularly with the invention of the Gibbon heart–lung machine. Mainetti advised him to go to the Cleveland Clinic, where George Crile, Donald Effler, Willem Kolff and Mason Sones had established a reputation for cardiac surgery and cardiology.

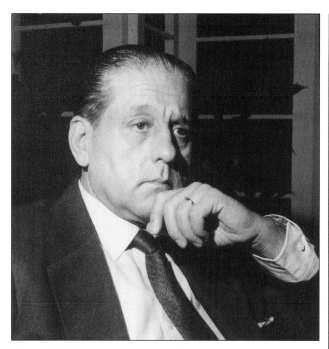

Figure 5.15. René Geronimo Favaloro.

At the Cleveland Clinic, Favaloro developed a unique relationship with Mason Sones which led to the development of coronary bypass surgery. Current adult cardiac surgery has its roots in this development but regardless of his prestigious standing in the United States and the enormous financial rewards, Favaloro returned to his homeland. He returned to visit the Clinic frequently, perhaps the most important occasion being in 1985 when Mason Sones was dying from bronchiogenic carcinoma.

Of his departure from the United States Dwight Harken commented "Rene, whose love and patriotism to his fatherland made the United States lose one of the world's finest surgeons." Favaloro took with him to Argentina not only his fame, prestige and knowledge but also the dream of developing a centre of excellence similar to the Cleveland Clinic. He had learned that such a centre could not exist in the absence of research or an efficient educational system. He quickly established Argentina's most important centre for cardiovascular surgery and developed an intense teaching schedule for cardiac surgeons from all over Latin America.

Andreas Grüntzig (1939–1985)

ANDREAS GRÜNTZIG was born in Dresden, Germany and studied at Heidelberg University (MD, 1964), as well as in England, Switzerland and Germany. His pioneering work was done at the Poliklinik, Zurich University where, in 1979, he became Chief of the Department of Cardiology at the University Hospital. In 1980, he was appointed to the Chair of Medicine and Radiology at Emory University School of Medicine in Atlanta, Georgia. Grüntzig, who died in the same year as Dotter and Sones, was killed with his wife, Margaret, when he was piloting his own plane in bad weather and flew into a mountain near Atlanta, Georgia.

In his work on arterial occlusions in the Department of Angiology at the Poliklinik at Zurich University in 1969, Grüntzig came upon the work of Charles Dotter and Melvin Judkins, radiologists at the University of Oregon Medical School. In 1964, they dilated stenosed leg and pelvic arteries by compressing the blockages with a high pressure balloon. Their first patient was an 83-year-old woman with gangrene in her foot, who refused amputation saying she would "rather die with both feet on." Dotter dilated the narrowed area in 20 minutes. Three irreversibly gangrenous toes sloughed spontaneously but she began to walk for the first time in 6 months and she remained ambulatory until death by heart failure 3 years later. Grüntzig, at the University of Zurich,

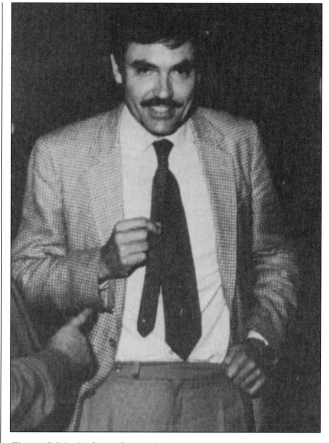

Figure 5.16. Andreas Grüntzig.

devised an inflatable balloon catheter to be pushed in to a blockage and inflated to widen the narrowed part of the artery. This was subsequently used within the much smaller coronary arteries. He first successfully relieved a severe coronary stenosis in a 38-year-old patient with 85% stenosis in the left anterior descending artery, who required only a few days' stay in hospital. Grüntzig recalled his own reaction after he performed the first successful percutaneous transluminal coronary angioplasty: "I was surprised and the patient was surprised over how easy it was." This simple procedure, taking only 30 minutes, re-established circulation and eased the strain on the heart. Grüntzig described its use in a series of 50 patients between 1977 and 1979 (Article 5.6, Appendix A). After its success in Europe, Grüntzig popularised percutaneous transluminal coronary angioplasty in the United States where it had been initially ignored. In 1980, he was appointed to the Chair of Medicine and Radiology at Emory University School of Medicine in Atlanta, Georgia and by 1982, was treating up to five patients a day using this technique.

This alternative to surgery for coronary artery disease rendered a large amount of medical and surgical work obsolete and met with disbelief, resentment and an initial reluctance to hail the brilliance of Grüntzig's breakthrough. Percutaneous transluminal coronary angioplasty and angioplasty of peripheral vessels has had enormous impact on the treatment of vascular disease in general. Angioplasty is preferable to open operation in the treatment of single- and double-vessel coronary disease with discrete stenoses. Variations in the transluminal approach now include coronary atheromectomy, laser techniques, and intravascular stents which might conceivably supersede coronary bypass surgery.

Percutaneous catheter techniques were subsequently adopted for congenital problems, such as coarctation or pulmonary stenosis, and acquired valve problems, such as aortic or mitral stenosis. Percutaneous methods have also been devised to close arteriovenous connections such as patent ductus, aortopulmonary collaterals, cerebral aneurysms and even atrial septal defects.

In 1984, Grüntzig reported the use of an argon laser to recanalize and dilate a superficial femoral artery occlusion. During the ensuing years, several hundred patients have undergone this procedure successfully.

The New England
Journal of Medicine

Volume 301   JULY 12, 1979   Number 2

NONOPERATIVE DILATATION OF CORONARY-ARTERY STENOSIS

Percutaneous Transluminal Coronary Angioplasty

Andreas R. Grüntzig, M.D., Åke Senning, M.D., and Walter E. Siegenthaler, M.D.

Abstract In percutaneous transluminal coronary angioplasty, a catheter system is introduced through a systemic artery under local anesthesia to dilate a stenotic artery by controlled inflation of a distensible balloon.

Over the past 18 months, we have used this technic in 50 patients. The technic was successful in 32 patients, reducing the stenosis from a mean of 84 to 34 per cent (P<0.001) and the coronary-pressure gradient from a mean of 58 to 19 mm Hg (P<0.001). Twenty-nine patients showed improvement in cardiac function during follow-up examination. Because of acute deterioration in clinical status, emergency bypass was later necessary in five patients; three showed electrocardiograpic evidence of infarcts.

Patients with single-vessel disease appear to be most suitable for the procedure, and a short history of pain indicates the presence of a soft (distensible) atheroma likely to respond to dilatation. We estimate that only about 10 to 15 per cent of candidates for bypass surgery have lesions suitable for this procedure. A prospective randomized trial will be necessary to evaluate its usefulness in comparison with surgical and medical management. (N Engl J Med 301:61-68, 1979)

Figure 5.17. Title page of Grüntzig's 1979 article entitled 'Nonoperative dilatation of coronary-artery stenosis'. (Reproduced with permission from The New England Journal of Medicine; 301: 61–68.)

Edvardas Varnauskas (1923–)

EDVARDAS VARNAUSKAS was born in Zaideliai, Lithuania. His medical training at Kaunas, Lithuania was interrupted in 1941 by World War II. However, he continued his studies as a refugee in Sweden at the Karolinska Institute (MD, 1951) and completed residency in internal medicine and cardiology at St Erik's Hospital. As a member of a research team there, he explored total pulmonary and renal haemodynamics in patients with valvular disease and arterial hypertension at rest and during various conditions of stress. Using balloon occlusion of the relevant branch of the pulmonary artery, they were able to show that the pulmonary wedge pressure quite accurately reflected the left atrial pressure. This work culminated in a doctoral thesis on haemodynamics in hypertension (PhD, 1955). Varnauskas gave the Nylin Lecture of the Swedish Medical Society and received the Regnell Prize in 1954. He has received The Sandoz Prize of the Swedish Society of Cardiology and an honorary degree from Vilnius University. He is consultant to the World Health Organization on cardiac rehabilitation, exercise testing, coronary care and the long-term effects of coronary bypass surgery. Varnauskas also advises the Lithuanian Ministry of Health on restructuring the medical care system.

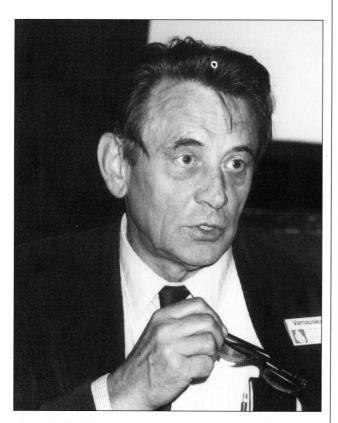

Figure 5.18. Edvardas Varnauskas. (© Patalong Film GmbH, Munich, Germany.)

Upon his return to Sweden from a research fellowship at Johns Hopkins (1955–57), Varnauskas was appointed Head of Cardiology at Sahlgrenska Hospital, Gothenburg (1957–89)

LONG-TERM RESULTS OF PROSPECTIVE RANDOMISED STUDY OF CORONARY ARTERY BYPASS SURGERY IN STABLE ANGINA PECTORIS

European Coronary Surgery Study Group*

Summary   This report presents the final results (follow-up 5–8 years) of a prospective study in 768 men aged under 65 with mild to moderate angina, 50% or greater stenosis in at least two major coronary arteries, and good left ventricular function. 395 were randomised to coronary artery bypass surgery, 373 to no treatment; 1 patient in the surgery group was lost to follow-up. These original groups were compared, whatever subsequently happened to the patients. Survival was improved significantly by surgery in the total population, in patients with three-vessel disease, and in patients with stenosis in the proximal third of the left anterior descending artery constituting a component of either two or three vessel disease, and non-significantly in patients with left main coronary disease. An abnormal electrocardiogram at rest, ST-segment depression $\geqslant 1\cdot5$ mm during exercise, peripheral arterial disease, and increasing age independently point to a better chance of survival with surgery. In the absence of these prognostic variables in patients with either two or three vessel disease the outlook is so good that early surgery is unlikely to increase the prospect of survival. In terms of anginal attacks, use of beta-adrenergic blockers and nitrates, and exercise performance the surgical group did significantly better than the medical group throughout the 5 years of follow-up, but the difference between the two treatments tended to decrease.

*Past and present participants:
   Coordinating centre, Göteborg.*—E. VARNAUSKAS (director of study), S. B. OLSSON, the late E. CARLSTRÖM, THOMAS KARLSSON.
   Participating centres.—Edinburgh: D. G. JULIAN, H. C. MILLER, M. F. OLIVER. Glasgow: A. R. LORIMER, I. HUTTON, R. G. MURRAY, A. TWEDDEL, T. LAWRIE, W. BAIN, the late P. CAVES, D. WHEATLEY. Helsinki: M. H. FRICK, P. T. HARJOLA, M. VALLE. Leiden: B. BUIS, J. DRAULANS, A. G. BROM, H. A. HUYSMANS. London: C. M. OAKLEY, J. F. GOODWIN, W. MCKENNA, H. H. BENTALL, W. P. CLELAND, K. S. C. WONG (Hammersmith Hospital); R. BALCON, M. HONEY, J. E. C. WRIGHT (London Chest Hospital); E. SOWTON, P. ROY, A. C. EDWARDS, J. CRICK, A. YATES (Guy's Hospital). Harefield Hospital, Harefield, Middlesex: M. TOWERS, R. THOMSON, S. A. QURESHI, R. PRIDIE, M. YACOUB. Oslo: S. SIMONSEN, O. STORSTEIN, L. EFSKIND, T. FRÖJSAKER (Rikshospitalet); E. SIVERTSEN, L. MELDAHL, G. SEMB (Ulleval Hospital). Prague: J. FABIAN, the late L. HEJHAL, F. FIRT. Zürich: M. ROTHLINE, A. SENNING, W. MEIER.

Figure 5.19. Title page of the European Coronary Surgery Study Group's 1982 paper entitled 'Long-term results of prospective randomised study of coronary artery bypass surgery in stable angina pectoris'. (Reproduced with permission from Lancet; *November 27; 1173–80.)*

and Associate Professor at Gothenburg University (1957–89), where he established a cardiological division and conducted research on various aspects of cardiovascular pathophysiology. Regulatory mechanisms of pulmonary blood and water volume, as well as gas exchange were investigated in cardiac patients. Beneficial effects of physical training for patients with coronary heart disease were shown to be related to the haemodynamic and metabolic adaptation of peripheral circulation. The use of beta-blocker therapy was shown to improve the clinical condition and working capacity in patients with congestive cardiomyopathy. Electrophysiological studies using recording of monophasic action potential in man opened new avenues for investigation and treatment of arrhythmias.

Between 1970 and 1972 Varnauskas' tenure at Gothenburg was interrupted by a visiting professorship of cardiology at the University of Leiden in the Netherlands, where he designed and started this European study, completed thanks to the research team of cardiologists, surgeons and other personnel of 12 participating centres in six European countries (Article 5.7, Appendix A). In 1993, he felt that surgical revascularization for coronary heart disease was expensive and resources limited in all European and Scandinavian countries; he concurred with opinion of Arnold Relman, who stated that, "We can afford all the care that is medically appropriate according to the best professional standards. We cannot afford all the care a market-driven system is capable of giving."

Charles Richard Conti (1934–)

CHARLES RICHARD CONTI was born Bethlehem, Pennsylvania and studied at Johns Hopkins (MD, 1960), where he fulfilled internship and residency on the Osler Medical

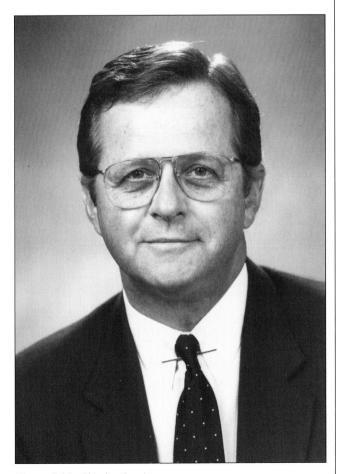

Figure 5.20. Charles Conti.

Service (1960–62). In the cardiology faculty, he was Associate Professor of Medicine and directed the Cardiovascular Diagnostic Laboratory (1968–74). Conti became Professor of Medicine and Chief of the Division of Cardiology at the University of Florida College of Medicine and Gainesville Veterans Administration Hospital (1974), where he now holds an endowed chair. He is also Chairman of the Shands Cardiovascular Center at the University of Florida and Medical Director of the Cardiovascular Clinic.

Conti's clinical, investigative and teaching interests focused on ischaemic heart disease; including unstable angina and myocardial infarction, coronary artery spasm and silent myocardial ischaemia. He is currently Chairman of the Self Study Educational Programs Committee responsible for the development of the American College of Cardiology self assessment programme. Conti was President of the American College of Cardiology (1989–90) and serves on the editorial board of many national and international journals. He is Editor-in-Chief of the American College of Cardiology Learning Center Highlights and Clinical Cardiology.

Conti wrote to us:

"I was privileged to serve as the Chairman of the National Heart, Lung and Blood Institutes sponsored unstable angina trial. The success of this study is directly related to the efforts of the principal investigators in nine myocardial infarction research units. Dr Russell of the University of Alabama unit contributed the largest number of patients to the trial.

The beauty of our study was that it addressed a simple question. What is the best way to treat unstable angina patients in the early phase of their illness? The question arose because at the time it was conventional wisdom to perform catheterization and cardiac surgery on an emergency basis. It became obvious to those of us who were caring for these patients that the operative mortality was not as low as it was in patients with stable angina.

I believe the study answered that question. It showed that it was not necessary to perform emergency coronary artery bypass surgery provided patients were aggressively managed with nitrates, beta blockers and, in many instances, heparin. Aspirin was not routinely used at that time and calcium antagonists were not available in the United States. Despite this limitation, it was shown that emergency surgery did not decrease early

mortality. In fact, the myocardial infarction rate was higher in those who underwent surgery than in those who were treated aggressively with medical management.

The study was not designed to test whether long-term outcome was better with one therapy or the other. However, it became clear that many of these patients had persistent stable symptoms later in their course and eventually many of them went on to bypass surgery electively. We did not address the question of whether or not angioplasty could be used in these patients, since it was not available at the time of study's completion."

John Gordon Coles (1952–)

JOHN GORDON COLES was born in London, Ontario and studied at the University of Western Ontario (MD, 1976). He trained at the University of British Columbia, the Vancouver General Hospital (1976–77) and the University of Western Ontario (1977–80), followed by postgraduate studies at the University of Toronto (1980–81) and the University of

Alabama (1984). In 1982, he qualified as Fellow of the Royal College of Physicians and Surgeons (Canada) and became Chief Resident at Toronto General Hospital (1982) and The Hospital for Sick Children (1983), where he is currently Consulting Staff Surgeon of the Division of Cardiovascular Surgery (1984), Surgical Consultant, Cardiovascular Research Focus (1984), Senior Scientist at the Research Institute (1990) and the Director of the Xenotransplantation Research Program (1992). Coles is also Associate Professor in the Division of Cardiovascular Surgery at The Hospital for Sick Children (1992) and Assistant Professor of Surgery at the University of Toronto (1987). His clinical activities are directed toward the surgical management of complex congenital heart disease.

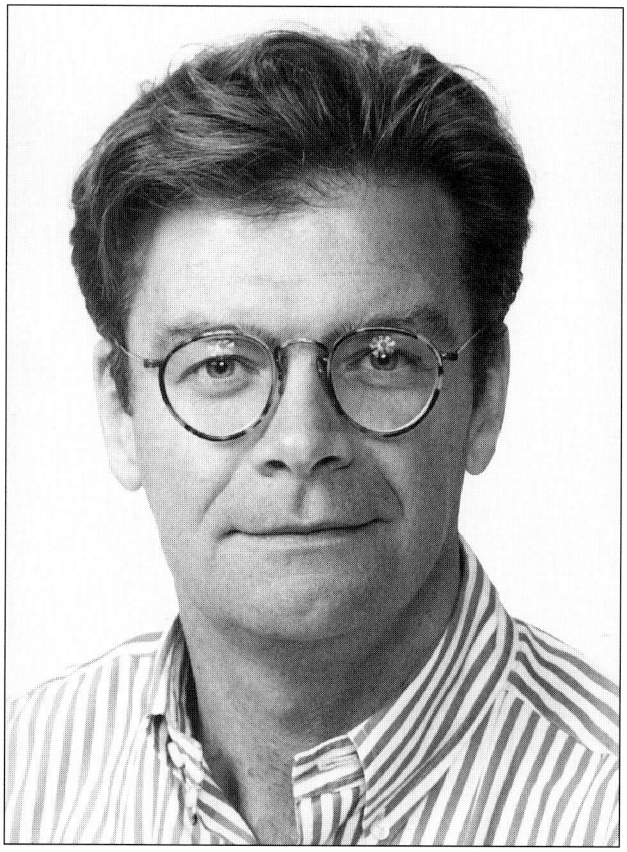

He wrote to us:

"The concept that myocardial ischaemia represents an indication for myocardial revascularization in patients with advanced left ventricular dysfunction, as suggested in our original paper (Figure 5.22), remains valid in contemporary practice. The advent of Thallium and PET scanning techniques currently allows the detection of reversible ischaemia with greater sensitivity and precision than that based solely on the presence or absence of angina and thus helps to refine the indication for revascularization procedures.

These non-invasive diagnostic methods are also being exploited to evaluate the capacity of new pharmacological reagents to favourably modulate the myocardial oxygen supply-demand relationship and thus preserve jeopardized myocardium. Pharmacological approaches appear to be beneficial as an adjunct to surgical revascularization, but are unlikely to be effective as the sole therapy for patients with severe left ventricular dysfunction on an ischaemic basis. More data are needed regarding the effect of therapy, both medical and surgical, on subsequent myocardial function in this subset of patients. Initial clinical experience with innovative techniques

Figure 5.21. John Gordon Coles.

J Thorac Cardiovasc Surg 81:846-850, 1981

Improved long-term survival following myocardial revascularization in patients with severe left ventricular dysfunction

The natural history of patients with coronary artery disease associated with poor left ventricular (LV) function is dismal. This report analyzes the efficacy of myocardial revascularization in this subset of patients with coronary artery disease manifesting severe LV dysfunction on the basis of LV angiography, LV ejection fraction (LVEF), and left ventricular end-diastolic pressure (LVEDP). For the 2½ year period ending November, 1977, 59 consecutive patients with coronary artery disease complicated by severe LV dysfunction underwent aorta-coronary bypass at the University of Western Ontario. All patients had angina refractory to medical therapy. Objective criteria for compromised LV function included the presence of three or more dysfunctional (hypokinetic of akinetic) segments on biplane LV angiography. Eighty-three percent (49/59) of patients had triple-vessel coronary artery disease. The mean LVEF for the series was 0.28 and the mean LVEDP was 18 mm Hg. The duration of follow-up was 24 to 60 months (mean 37 months), with follow-up survival data available on 100% of patients. The hospital mortality was 1.7% (1/59), and there were nine late deaths. The 5 year actuarial survival rate (±SEM) was 80% ± 6%. Of the 44 long-term survivors available for direct assessment, 98% (43/44) report improvement with respect to angina and 66% (29/44) are totally asymptomatic. Eighty percent (28/35) of the long-term survivors under the age of 65 years are currently employed. These results indicate that myocardial revascularization can be performed in patients with severe ischemic LV dysfunction at very low risk and, further, that operation results in a dramatic improvement in survival expectations compared with optimal medical therapy.

J. G. Coles, M.D.,* C. Del Campo, M.D., F.R.C.S. (C),* S. N. Ahmed, M.D.,*
R. Corpus, M.D., F.R.C.S. (C),* A. C. MacDonald, M.D., F.R.C.P. (C),**
M. M. Goldbach, M.D., F.R.C.S. (C),*** and J. C. Coles, M.D., F.R.C.S. (C),****
London, Ontario, Canada

Figure 5.22. Title page of Coles et al. 1981 article entitled 'Improved long-term survival following myocardial revascularization in patients with severe left ventricular dysfunction'. *(Reproduced with permission from* Journal of Thoracic and Cardiovascular Surgery; *81: 846–50.*

such as transmyocardial laser revascularization for patients with diffuse distal coronary artery disease has been promising. However, direct surgical revascularization is technically feasible and effective in the vast majority of patients and can be accomplished with very low risk. Increasing recognition that conventional studies underestimate the typically diffuse and extensive nature of coronary atherosclerosis, as revealed in recent pathological studies, emphasizes the theoretical superiority of prevention compared to medical or surgical treatment of advanced disease."

Chapter 6: Surgery of the thoracic aorta

THE EVOLUTION of cardiac surgery lies in the development of vascular surgical technique. In the history of military surgery, haemorrhage from major blood vessels was always the greatest surgical challenge. The first written account of blood vessel ligation is attributed to the great Indian surgeon Sushruta, between 800 and 600 BC. His textbook, *Sushruta Samhita*, translated from Sanskrit, provides descriptions of the use of hemp fibres to tie blood vessels, application of boiling oil or cautery to stem haemorrhage and guidelines for the performance of amputations. There are also accounts of the use of catgut ligatures by Hindu surgeons of the time. The ancient Greeks were unfamiliar with ligation, but were known to apply various mixtures of verdigris, antimony and lead sulphate directly to bleeding wounds. Amputations were performed in the 4th century BC and Hippocrates advised section through the gangrenous part to avoid bleeding. If haemorrhage was encountered, he advised application of cold compresses to the adjoining limb.

In the 1st century AD, Rufus of Effesus controlled haemorrhage by digital compression, arterial torsion, application of styptics and arterial ligature. He also emphasized the importance of palpation of the pulse for diagnostic purposes. Celsus recognized the importance of cold, suggesting linen pledgets soaked in cold water and packed into the wound to stem bleeding. If this failed, the more damaging and painful vinegar or cautery were used.

The first record of the cause and treatment of aneurysm was by Antyllus in the 2nd century AD. He recognized the difference between traumatic false aneurysms and the cylindrical forms from degenerative or syphilitic disease. The great Oxford physician, Osler, described Antyllus as one of the most daring and accomplished surgeons in history, due to his early operations for proximal and distal ligation of aneurysms with evacuation of the sac. The enormity of his contribution is evident when one considers that the next description of aneurysm surgery came from Rudolph Matas, seventeen centuries later.

Claudius Galen spent three years as a surgeon to the gladiators in ancient Rome. He gained enormous experience in the treatment of haemorrhage and understood the difference between arteries and veins. He used styptics for venous bleeding and ligature for arteries. Both a wide knowledge of anatomy and great technical skill contributed to his success in several different areas of surgery. After his initial appointment in 158 AD, he was reappointed on four further occasions, a record attributed to the fact that he was said to have salvaged all his gladiator patients. Aetius of Amida, on the Tigris river, was one of the great Byzantine medical authors and in one of his sixteen books, he described the treatment of brachial artery aneurysms by proximal ligation. Aetius was probably also the first physician to ligate varicose veins. After this, further accounts of vascular surgical intervention are sparse until the 11th century, when Roger of Palermo utilized the so-called mediate ligature, on a threaded needle, in his efforts to occlude bleeding arteries.

Ambroise Paré

SOME 500 YEARS LATER (1510), Ambroise Paré was born in Mayenne, France. Destined to become the greatest surgeon of the Renaissance period, his training began in a barber's shop and was followed by a residency at the Hotel Dieu between 1536 and 1545. Although the vascular ligature had been described more than 2000 years previously, Paré's greatest influence was in reintroducing this method as the treatment of choice for injured blood vessels. Paré joined the French Infantry at the age of 26 (about the same time that Michaelangelo painted the Sistine Chapel). His first campaign was the invasion of Northern Italy against Charles V in 1536. Apparently, Paré disliked the application of hot iron and boiling oil to wounds, and during the Battle of Chateau de Villaen so many injuries were sustained that the supply of oil was exhausted. Paré then resorted to ligature of bleeding arteries and the use of wound dressings and bandages. He wrote:

"Finally my oil was exhausted and I was forced to apply instead a digestive made of egg yolk, rose oil and turpentine. That night I could not sleep easily thinking that by failure of cauterizing I would find the wounded in whom I had failed to put the oil dead of poisoning. This made me get up early in the morning to visit them. There, beyond my hope, I found those on whom I had used the digestive medication feeling little pain in their wounds, without inflammation and swelling, having rested well throughout the night. The others, on whom I had used the oil, I found feverish, with great pain, swelling and inflammation around their wound. Then I resolved never again to so cruelly burn the poor wounded by gunshot."

Paré subsequently used the ligature in preference to hot iron during amputations:

"Having used this method of closing the veins and arteries in recent wounds several times in case of haemorrhage, I thought that it could be done also in removal of a limb."

Paré's skill and reputation increased progressively during his 30 years as a military surgeon. His presence on the battlefield greatly reassured the soldiers. In the event of wounding, they realized him to be their greatest chance of survival. Paré introduced the first artery forcep, originally used to extract bullets, and then modified it to present an injured artery into the wound for ligation. (Paré's method for vascular ligature remained the treatment of choice for vascular injuries on the battlefield until 1952.) In 1718, the French military surgeon, Petit, developed a screwed tourniquet to facilitate ligation of vessels during amputations on the battlefield.

The earliest attempts at vascular repair with preservation of bloodflow did not occur until the 18th century. In Newcastle-upon-Tyne, Richard Lambert became perturbed by the incidence of secondary haemorrhage after arterial ligation when the ligature eroded through the vessel wall. Civilian arterial injuries became a frequent occurrence when phlebotomy was applied for a wide variety of illnesses. The bloodletter's needle frequently caused arterial laceration, false aneurysm formation or arteriovenous fistula. Direct ligation of the artery proximal to the injury often resulted in gangrene or severe functional impairment. Lambert encouraged his surgical colleague, Hallowell, to attempt arterial repair without compromising the lumen. They used a ½ inch steel pin to lift a lacerated brachial artery into the wound and tied a figure-of-eight stitch around the edges to close the vessel wall. Despite post-operative wound infection, the procedure was clearly preferable to tying off the brachial artery. Some time later, the pin and suture were extruded from the wound and the patient survived with a palpable pulse at the wrist. Lambert related the details of the procedure to William Hunter, who in turn encouraged Lambert to publish the technique.

"It would make the operation for the aneurysm still more successful in the arm, when the main trunk is wounded; and by this method, perhaps, we might be able to cure the wounds of some arteries that would otherwise require amputation or be altogether incurable."

Had it not been for Hunter's enthusiasm, Lambert and Hallowell's operation would have remained in obscurity.

In 1773, Assmann of Kroningen attempted to repair experimental canine femoral arterial lacerations, but the lumen was invariably obliterated, resulting in thrombosis. Assmann's negative report, based on only four unsuccessful attempts, was widely accepted, and further attempts at arterial repair were delayed for another century. In 1774 in Paris, a medical student, LeConte, produced a thesis recording his attempt to preserve the lumen of damaged arteries by wrapping them in a section of a goose quill encircled with a ligature, and sealed with a varnish of turpentine and balm of araeus. The quill was removed after 3 or 4 days, but the artery invariably thrombosed.

William and John Hunter

WILLIAM HUNTER was born in Scotland in 1718 and

from 1736 to 1746 studied anatomy and surgery in Glasgow, Edinburgh and London. During his studies at St George's Hospital, London he became discontent with the quality of anatomical teaching and opened his own school of anatomy in Covent Garden. This was succeeded in 1768 by the Great Windmill Street School of Anatomy. His younger brother, John (born in 1728), studied from 1748 to 1751 at his brother's Covent Garden anatomy school and then served as 'apprentice' to Percival Pott at St Bartholomew's Hospital. In 1753, John Hunter was elected Master of Anatomy at Surgeons' Hall and developed an interest in comparative anatomy. Together, William and John collected different animal species and carefully preserved their dissected specimens. From 1754 to 1756, John Hunter was House Surgeon at St George's Hospital, where he produced comprehensive descriptions of the lymphatic system and placental circulation.

The contribution to vascular surgery for which William Hunter is best known is his description of arteriovenous fistula. Venesection was still common practice and many of Hunter's patients had this same aetiology. A Middlesex Hospital laboratory assistant first presented to Hunter with an 'aneurysmal varix'. Hunter characterized the lesion as containing dilated or varicose veins with a pulsating, 'jarring' motion caused by arterial flow. On auscultation, he described a hissing noise which corresponded to the patient's pulse. In 1757, he produced a manuscript entitled *The History of an Aneurysm of the Aorta with some Remarks on Aneurysm in General*. He became Professor of Anatomy at the Royal Academy of Arts in 1768 and was eventually elected its president.

In 1760, John Hunter joined the British Army under King Frederick and embarked on the Seven Years' War. Experience in Portugal produced the basis for his description of the treatment of gunshot wounds (1794), *A Treatise on Blood, Inflammation and Gunshot Wounds*. He was elected a Fellow of the Royal Society and a Member of the Corporation of Surgeons in 1767. By this time he was already a celebrated teacher. His pupils included William Blissard, John Abernethie, Edward Jenner and Astley Cooper. John Hunter is probably best known for his treatment of popliteal aneurysms. The post-mortem specimen from his first case can still be seen in the Hunterian museum of the Royal College of Surgeons in Lincoln's Inn Fields.

Although ligation of brachial and popliteal aneurysms had been performed before, many patients suffered gangrene or exsanguinating haemorrhage from erosion of the artery. In 1779, Percival Pott condemned ligation for these reasons, but Hunter argued that ligation at a distance from the aneurysm would reduce the chances of secondary haemorrhage, interrupt fewer collateral vessels, and thereby increase the chance of limb preservation. Hunter's most celebrated operation was ligation of the popliteal artery on a 45-year-old London coachman (1785). The events were recorded by Hunter's brother-in-law and archivist, Everard Home, and the paper appeared in the *London Medical Journal* one year later.

"Having disengaged the artery from its lateral connections by the knife, and from the parts behind it by means of the endave thin spatula, a double ligature was passed behind it by means of an ide probe, and the artery tied by both portions of the ligature, but so slightly as only to compress its sides together; a similar application of ligature was made a little lower; and the reasons for passing four ligatures was to compress such a length of artery as might make up for the want of tightness, as he chose to avoid great pressure at the vessel at any one part."

Hunter had clearly learned from experience that over tightening of a vascular ligature would result in erosion of the vessel and secondary haemorrhage. His patient remained in St George's Hospital for a month, but made a straightforward recovery and returned to his job as a coachman. Hunter taught that ligation could be used for aneurysms of the subclavian, carotid and femoral arteries, as well as the popliteal. He recognized that salvage of the distal limb depended upon adequate collateral flow and limitation of damage to surrounding structures. One of Hunter's patients with a popliteal aneurysm survived for 50 years after ligation, and at autopsy the superficial femoral and popliteal arteries were completely fibrosed, with involution of the aneurysm to a small fibrous nodule. Hunter's interest spread widely beyond the realms of vascular surgery. He made contributions to the field of trauma, dentistry, gastric physiology, embryology and venereology, which may well have been his downfall. Speculating on the nature of venereal disease (1767), he inoculated his own penis with a specimen containing *Treponema pallidum* taken from a patient with urethritis.

He consequently developed syphilis, with an ascending aortic aneurysm and central nervous system complications. Towards the end of his life, Hunter suffered debilitating angina, probably from coronary ostial stenoses. He commented that his life was "in the hands of any rascal who chooses to annoy and tease me". Hunter died during a fit of anger and angina during a board meeting at St George's Hospital, when told of the appointment of his successor. Much of his anatomical collection remains in good condition in the Hunterian Museum.

The word aneurysm is derived from the Greek verb meaning to dilate or enlarge. Corvisart described the symptoms and signs which may be encountered in aortic aneurysms in 1806. In an ascending aortic aneurysm, he described the thrill and retromanubrial dullness to percussion, with a whistling sound as the sac compressed the trachea. He pointed out that the diagnosis was difficult to make unless the aneurysm was visible externally. Olive, in 1878, described the sign of tracheal tug with aneurysms of the aortic arch.

Sir Astley Cooper

IT WAS ONE OF HUNTER'S PUPILS, Astley Cooper (Figure 6.1), who became the father of aortic surgery. At the turn of the 19th century, Astley succeeded his uncle, William Cooper, as Senior Surgeon to Guy's Hospital. As a medical student, Cooper had studied the effects of brachial, femoral and carotid arterial ligation in dogs, and in 1805, he performed one of the earliest carotid arterial ligations in humans. The patient, a 44-year-old woman, presented with an enormous aneurysm of the right common carotid artery, which occupied two-thirds of her neck. On 1 November, Cooper ligated the common carotid artery, but the patient died 16 days later from a combination of infection and compression of the larynx and trachea. Cooper attributed the death to expansion of the aneurysmal sac and when the next opportunity arose (in 1808), he doubly ligated and divided the common carotid of his patient, Humphrey Humphries, a 51-year-old porter. Humphries survived until 1821. Cooper obtained the body and reported death due to left-sided cerebral haemorrhage.

The day after Humphries' operation, Cooper ligated the external iliac artery of a 39-year-old man with a large

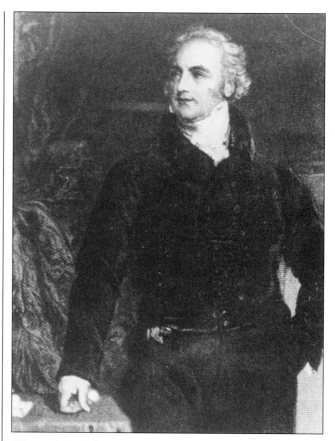

Figure 6.1. Astley Cooper.

femoral aneurysm. Ligations of carotid and external iliac arteries were heroic procedures in Cooper's time, but in 1817, he performed his most notable procedure — that of aortic ligation. The patient, Charles Hutson, a 38-year-old porter, was admitted to Guy's Hospital with a left external iliac aneurysm, which eroded the overlying skin and ruptured with external bleeding. Only 2 days before, Cooper had attempted retroperitoneal exposure of the aorta in a cadaver to explore the surgical possibilities. In Hutson's case of sudden rupture, Cooper exposed the aorta (with the patient still in bed) through a transperitoneal incision and placed a strong silk ligature just above the aortic bifurcation (Figure 6.2). Although Hutson survived for only 48 hours, Cooper's biography by Lord Brock likens the operation to the "Everest ascent of arterial surgery of his day".

Cooper's fame and influence spread rapidly and in 1820, he was summoned to treat King George IV, who was suffering from an infected sebaceous cyst on the head. Cooper commented on this experience, "I feared syphilis as a complication in the post-operative course of my exalted patient, but all went well and I was created a

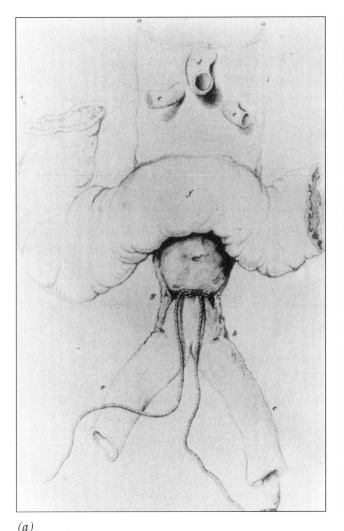 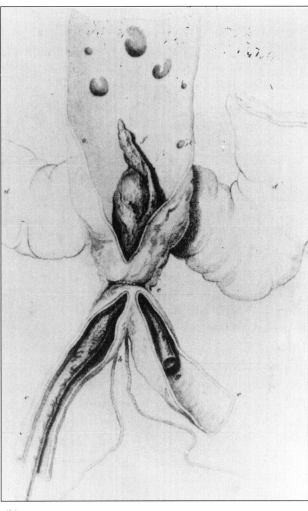

(a)   (b)

Figure 6.2. Astley Cooper's post mortem specimen from Charles Hutson.(a) Anterior view; (b) posterior view.

baronet by His Majesty in 1821". He developed an enormous surgical practice and displayed an unerring scientific approach to clinical problems. He went to great lengths to obtain autopsies on all his surgical patients and once remarked, "There is no man, however great or distinguished, who is likely to avoid my clutches for autopsy, as there is always means of obtaining a body you want". Cooper's other great contributions were in the treatment of hernia, avoidance of amputation in compound fractures, and in the description of non-malignant diseases of the breast. When appointed Examiner to the Royal College of Surgeons of England he commented that his fellow examiners were "a doddering collection of ill-read individuals with lifetime appointments and with little interest in the welfare of the hapless candidates". Cooper became President of the College of Surgeons soon afterwards. In 1840, he deteriorated progressively from congestive cardiac failure and died on 12 February 1841. He is buried in a crypt beneath the chapel of Guy's Hospital.

Valentine Mott

IN THE EARLY 19TH CENTURY, when Cooper was the most renowned surgeon and teacher in Europe, he even attracted Americans as pupils at Guy's Hospital. Valentine Mott travelled there in 1807 to become Cooper's wound dresser. He was present at the ligation for carotid aneurysm and subsequently studied with other great English surgeons, including Henry Klein, William Blissard, Everard Home and John Abernethie.

Mott returned to New York in 1809 and in 1811 became Professor of Surgery at Columbia College. Some 4 years later, he was shown a patient with a subclavian artery aneurysm and proceeded to ligate the innominate artery. The patient exsanguinated following necrosis of the aneurysm, but Mott and his colleagues felt justified in making further attempts. In 1821, he treated a patient with osteosarcoma of the mandible by ligating the carotid artery, followed by mandibulectomy. This was an outstanding feat, performed without access to anaesthesia, antiseptics or blood replacement. Three years later, he performed the first successful hip disarticulation in the United States on a 10-year-old boy who had suffered non-union of a femoral fracture. He went on to perform ligation of the common iliac artery for an external iliac aneurysm, and ligation of the subclavian artery and jugular vein in conjunction with clavicular excision for osteosarcoma. During the American Civil War, he was active in treatment of the wounded and in 1862, reported studies on the treatment of haemorrhage and the use of anaesthetics. In the early 1860s, he suffered increasingly from angina and eventually died in 1865 of a gangrenous leg. His surgical achievements included an innominate artery ligation, eight subclavian arterial ligations, two common carotids, 51 external carotids, one common iliac, six external iliacs, two internal iliacs, 57 femoral and 10 popliteal artery ligations. He is also said to have performed over 900 amputations, many during the Civil War. Mott is accredited with bringing the teaching and principles of John Hunter to the United States and with elevating surgery to the realms of science.

Vascular surgery developed progressively during the mid-19th century. In 1829, James ligated the aortic bifurcation for external iliac aneurysm in a 44-year-old man, though the patient died 4 hours after surgery. Before the end of the 19th century, 10 further cases of aortic ligation were recorded, mostly for syphilitic aneurysms of the iliac arteries in young men. The aortic bifurcation was ligated in eight cases. More proximal occlusions, for instance, at the level of the diaphragm, were performed, but the patients died soon afterwards from haemorrhage or shock. In 1899, Keen performed aortic ligation at the level of the diaphragm for a ruptured abdominal aneurysm. Remarkably, the patient survived for 48 days until the ligature eroded into the lumen.

Rudolph Matas

IN MARCH 1888, a 26-year-old plantation worker was admitted to the Charity Hospital, New Orleans with a brachial artery aneurysm following a gunshot wound to the left upper arm (sustained 2 weeks previously during a hunting accident). Rudolph Matas, an instructor in surgery and anatomy at the hospital at that time, felt that to amputate the limb or perform proximal and distal brachial ligation would render the man an invalid. He therefore attempted to thrombose the aneurysm by tourniquet and mechanical compression. When this failed, Matas performed proximal ligation, but the pulsation within the aneurysm returned 10 days later. He then reoperated and attempted distal ligation, unsuccessfully. Matas proceeded to open the aneurysmal sac and perform endo-aneurysmorrhaphy, which obliterated the mouth of the aneurysm (by direct suture) but preserved onward bloodflow. The patient recovered, with a functional arm, and remained gainfully employed.

Matas described three forms of aneurysmorrhaphy: obliterative, restorative and reconstructive. In the obliterative form, sutures were placed from within the aneurysm sac so as to occlude the proximal and distal artery, together with collateral vessels. Restorative and reconstructive procedures were modifications of the obliterative type, but preserved arterial patency. This was often achieved by placing a catheter in the main arteries and obliterating the aneurysm sac around the catheter with sutures. At this time, the aseptic principles of Joseph Lister were well established and Jassinowsky had introduced small curved needles with fine silk sutures for arterial repair. Gluck then introduced a fine ivory clamp to assist repair of arterial wounds, and Jassinowsky, Burci and Dorfler all demonstrated that arterial wounds could be repaired with preservation of the lumen.

The first attempts to anastomose the transected ends of arteries came at the end of the 19th century. Jaboulay experimentally divided and rejoined the ends of carotid arteries in dogs and monkeys in 1896. He emphasized the importance of approximating intima to intima with interrupted everting U-shaped sutures. Queirolo and Massini produced a rigid glass tube prosthesis through which the divided end of a vessel could be passed, cuffed back and invaginated into the open end of the recipient vessel. This was then secured by a circumferential ligature. In 1897, Nitze introduced the use of small ivory cylinders over which the ends of a transected vessel could be passed to approximate intima to intima. Variations on the non-suture anastomosis became popular, particularly that of Payr, who used small tubes of magnesium over which the divided vessel ends could be passed. It was anticipated that the magnesium ring would be absorbed eventually, leaving a smooth patent lumen. In 1901, Payr removed a segment of femoral artery involved in a tumour and re-established continuity with a graft of saphenous vein secured with his magnesium tube technique. Unfortunately, the patient died from pneumonia on the third post-operative day, but the saphenous vein graft remained patient. Later it was found that the magnesium tubes produced an irritant corrosive substance that led to fibrosis and distortion of the vessel. The use of rubber tubing or paraffin-lined glass tubes was then explored. The young Alexis Carrell, working in Jaboulay's laboratory in Lyons, used rods of caramel as a dissolvable stent over which to suture arteries.

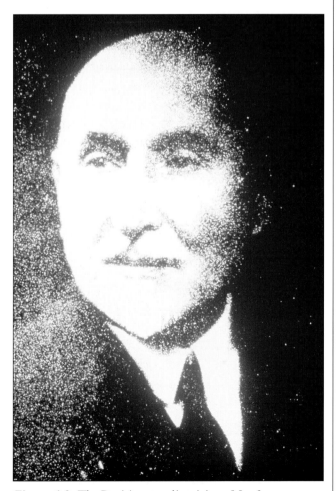

Figure 6.3. The Parisian paediatrician, Marfan.

In 1900, Matas attempted to obliterate an abdominal aortic aneurysm by introducing wire, then an electric current through it. His career was threatened in 1908, when he developed a gonococcal infection of the right eye following surgery on a patient with gonorrhoeal pelvic infection. This led to enucleation of the eye, but he continued to pioneer vascular surgical techniques. In 1923, he ligated the infra-renal aorta proximal to a large abdominal aortic aneurysm, with survival of the patient. In 1940, he reported personal experience of 620 aneurysms to the American Surgical Association; remarkably, the overall mortality was less than 5%. Matas also pioneered the use of intravenous saline to treat hypovolaemia and the use of nasogastric and endotracheal tubes.

In 1896, Marfan (Figure 6.3) reported a skeletal anomaly, characterized by unusually long, slender extremities in a 5-year old girl. Six years later, Archard called this deformity arachnodactyly. In 1929, Erdheim published his description of cystic medial degeneration, characterized by vacuolization of the media and fragmentation of the elastic laminae with aneurysm formation. Baer and associates first reported the association of aortic aneurysms with arachnodactyly in 1943. The lesions present in the aorta in Marfan's syndrome were found to be indistinguishable from Erdheim's cystic medial necrosis. In 1971, Halpern and colleagues noted that dissecting aneurysm was the most serious complication in Marfan's syndrome, accounting for more than half of the deaths.

Alexis Carrell

ALEXIS CARRELL (Figure 6.4) was born in Lyons, France, in 1873 and graduated in medicine from the University of Lyons. His first vascular experiments were performed in the laboratory of Mariel Soulier, Professor of Therapeutics. He created arteriovenous fistulae between the carotid artery and external jugular vein, to induce heart failure in dogs. For this, he developed fine needles and sutures and is said to have taken embroidery lessons to improve his suture technique. Nevertheless, he was unable to pass the exacting clinical examinations to gain a position in the surgical faculty in Lyons, and instead left France in 1904 for Montreal. In Canada, his work on vascular anastomosis was well received, but he and Guthrie used vascular anastomotic techniques to re-implant limbs and transplant kidneys, ovaries, thyroid glands and hearts. Organ preservation became part of their interest and in less than 2 years, Carrell and Guthrie produced 28 scientific papers together. Their collaboration ended in 1906 when Guthrie accepted the position of Professor of Physiology and Pharmacology at Washington University, St Louis. Carrell then joined the Experimental Surgery Department at the Rockefeller Institute in New York, where he made many enormous contributions in the fields of transplantation and vascular surgery.

Carrell considered that the cellular elements of a blood vessel cooled by ice before transplantation had the potential to survive after reperfusion. In contrast, Guthrie, based on histological studies of aortic grafts, concluded that tissue viability was not maintained, but that transplanted blood vessels continued to function as conduits. Carrell used grafts of vena cava to replace segments of the thoracic aorta. Recognizing the dangers of spinal cord ischaemia, he employed paraffin tubes as shunts for distal bloodflow. In 1910, he presented a paper to the American Surgical Association which described mitral valvotomy, ventricular aneurysmectomy and coronary artery bypass. The success of his experimental work was largely attributed to meticulous application of aseptic technique, together with impressive manual dexterity. In 1912 (aged 36), he became the first scientist in America (albeit that he was French!) to be awarded the Nobel Prize for physiology and medicine. In 1913, Carrell was made Knight of the Legion of Honour by the French Government, but whilst in France, World War I broke out and he was

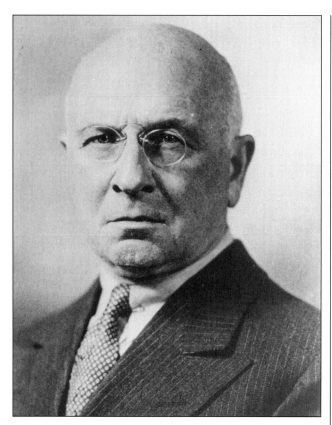

Figure 6.4. Alexis Carrell.

was persuaded by the surgeon, Carl Beck, to accept a position in the Chicago University Department of Physiology. Here he was assigned to work with a recently graduated physiologist, Charles Guthrie. Their experimental work consisted of refining vascular anastomotic technique with the use of vein grafts in the arterial system. The triangulation method of suture anastomosis developed by Carrell in 1902 is still a standard method in modern times (Figure 6.5). Carrell

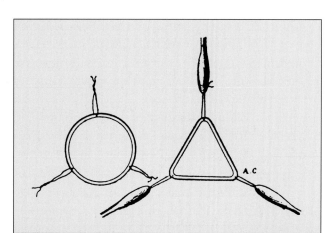

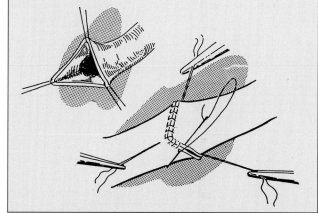

Figure 6.5. Carrell's triangulation method for suture anastomosis.

immediately recruited into the French Army. As a result, he gained considerable experience in the treatment of wounds and prevention of infection. With the help of the chemist, Henry Dakin, of the Rockefeller Institute, hundreds of antiseptic solutions were tested and a means of wound irrigation devised. In 1917, Carrell opened the first mobile army hospital, a forerunner of the American MASH units used in Korea and Vietnam. Carrell was awarded many distinguished honours for his contribution to the war effort.

Between the World Wars

AFTER THE WAR, Carrell returned to New York and resumed his interests in organ preservation. It was in this context that Carrell met and worked with the aviator, Charles Lindberg. Lindberg's sister-in-law had rheumatic heart disease and was progressively deteriorating, causing Lindberg to question why surgery had nothing to offer. When given the answer that the heart could not be stopped for long enough, Lindberg suggested the use of a mechanical pump which might sustain the circulation until the arrested heart could be repaired. He resolved to design such a machine, and after discussing this with a physician friend, was introduced to Carrell at Rockefeller University. Lindberg's ideas immediately caught Carrell's imagination, though he realized the difficulties of oxygenating the blood. The perfusion apparatus which followed was more of a tool to fulfil Carrell's experiments with tissue perfusion than Lindberg's original suggestion for a heart-lung machine. The machine could nevertheless produce pulsatile flow at variable rates and perfusion pressures. Lindberg included floating glass valves which separated individual chambers of the device through which perfusion fluid flowed. It was successfully used in the preservation of hearts, spleens, kidneys and pancreases and probably laid the groundwork for the eventual development of a pump oxygenator and mechanical heart device.

Further developments in arterial repair

PROBABLY the first successful clinical vascular interposition graft was reported by Goyanes in 1906. He implanted a patient's popliteal vein to bridge the defect created by excision of a popliteal artery aneurysm. In 1907, Lexer utilized a long saphenous vein to bridge the defect in a patient's axillary artery. However, ligation remained the mainstay of vascular treatment, particularly for the aorta.

Tuffier first attempted ligation of the thoracic aorta for aneurysm in 1902. The patient had a saccular aneurysm of the ascending aorta and in a particularly daring procedure, Tuffier doubly ligated the neck of the aneurysm with a catgut suture and then attempted to excise it. The operation was eventually abandoned and the patient died on the 30th post-operative day of secondary haemorrhage from necrosis of the aneurysmal sac. Three further attempts at thoracic aortic ligation by Tuffier proved unsuccessful. In 1914, Kummel attempted to salvage a ruptured thoracic aneurysm by oversewing the defect. This attempt also failed.

World War I provided every opportunity to advance the status of vascular surgery, but in general, the results were dismal. The British Army adopted Tuffier's paraffin-lined silver tube method to preserve arterial continuity, whereas the Germans relied on primary arterial suture. With considerable ingenuity, Jaeger and Von Haberer harvested fresh venous and arterial homografts from the fatally wounded and used them for vascular reconstructions. Unfortunately, the repairs invariably thrombosed. Bernheim, who was the first American surgeon to utilize autogenous saphenous vein grafts to bridge an arterial defect, travelled to France with the specific aim of treating arterial injuries by primary repair. He soon became disillusioned and withdrew. Consequently, ligation and amputation remained the approved method of treating arterial injuries. In 1918, McLean, working in Howell's Laboratory, isolated heparin. It was not until 15 years later, however, that a pure form became available and then in amounts so limited as to be unavailable for clinical surgery.

Cystic medial necrosis was first described by Gsell in 1928 before Erdheim who considered this to be the most important cause of ascending aortic aneurysms. There was little progress in aortic surgery between Mattice's successful complete ligation of the aorta in April 1923 and the mid-1940s. Perhaps the highlight of this period was the career of René Leriche, who popularized sympathectomy for ischaemic limbs, attempted autogenous saphenous vein bypasses of occluded iliac arteries and described the syndrome of complete obliteration of the terminal abdominal aorta (1923). Leriche anticipated present day treatment of his syndrome when he wrote, "The ideal treatment of arterial thrombosis is the replacement of the obliterated segment with a vascular graft".

Direct attacks on aneurysms were rare and up until 1940, surgeons such as Blakemore, King, Pearce and Harrison were filling aneurysms with wire. As early as 1939, Page noted the fibrosis-generating effect of cellophane. This property was put into clinical practice by Harrison and Chandy (1942), who introduced cellophane wrapping around aneurysms. This procedure was limited both in scope and success. A somewhat remarkable operation by Alexander and Byron provided a renewed stimulus for further developments. Their patient was a 19-year-old college student with an 8 cm thoracic aneurysm associated with coarctation of the aorta. The aneurysm was ligated proximally and distally and then resected. Remarkably, the patient recovered, with adequate distal perfusion through extensive collateral circulation. The procedure was all the more remarkable because of severe hypertension at the time of surgery.

Congenital heart disease as a catalyst

COARCTATION of the aorta and the palliation of congenital heart disease played a considerable part in the development of vascular surgery in the 1940s. In 1944, Blalock and Park suggested that the left subclavian artery could be used to bypass coarctation and Crafoord first performed resection of coarctation with end-to-end anastomosis. On 19 and 31 October 1944, he resected coarctations in a 12-year-old schoolboy and a 27-year-old farmer, respectively, re-anastomosing the aorta using the triangulation technique described by Carrell. Both patients recovered and in June 1945, Gross repeated the procedure in the US. Realizing the eventuality of not being able to perform end-to-end aortic anastomosis in extended aortic resection, he developed an aortic homograft bank for clinical use. Gross harvested aorta from healthy human subjects dying from trauma and preserved them in a balanced salt solution with 10%

human serum stored at between 1 and 4°C. Fibroblast culture studies showed the homograft arterial wall to remain viable for as long as 37 days after harvest. This proved irrelevant since, as Guthrie pointed out some 30 years previously, tissue viability was not essential for successful implantation. The grafts served only as a bridge for ingrowth of host cells. Indeed, it became apparent that non-viable homografts were preferable because of their lesser tendency to generate an immunological response within the host.

In 1948, Gross reported the use of preserved arterial grafts in humans with both coarctation of the aorta and cyanotic congenital heart disease. The same year, Swann used an arterial homograft to reconstitute the aorta after resection of a thoracic aneurysm in a 16-year-old boy. The previous year, Schumacker had performed aneurysm resection in an 8-year-old boy with coarctation, and achieved end-to-end anastomosis. Nevertheless, it soon became clear that use of a vascular graft was more simple. As the demand for grafts increased, many different hospitals developed their own techniques for sterilizing, preserving and storing homografts. The grafts were immersed in formalin, alcohol glycerine, ethylene oxide or beta propriolactone. They were subject to freeze-drying in liquid nitrogen or irradiated and stored in plastic packets with dry ice.

Aneurysm surgery

IN 1944, Alton Ochsner operated on a 45-year-old man with a suspected mediastinal tumour on chest X-ray, but found a saccular aneurysm of the descending thoracic aorta. He clamped the base of the aneurysmal sac, sutured below this and excised the aneurysm successfully. Given the feasibility of arterial resection and repair, other clinical applications followed rapidly. Dubost, Allary and Oeconomos performed the first successful replacement of an abdominal aortic aneurysm using homograft interposition in 1952. The French surgeon, Jacques Oudot, replaced a thrombosed aortic bifurcation with an arterial homograft in 1952. His patient recovered and Oudot performed four more aortic bifurcation resections with homograft replacement in the next two years. In 1951, Charles Dubost resected an abdominal aortic aneurysm in a 50-year-old man and restored continuity with a thoracic aortic homograft harvested from a young woman three weeks before. Unfortunately, the disadvantages of homografts soon became apparent. Early degeneration could cause suture line dehiscence, possibly through low-grade infection. Eventually, the wall of the homograft became rigid and calcified, though this did not greatly influence its function as a conduit. The need for better arterial substitutes was soon apparent.

DeBakey meets Cooley

MEANWHILE, World War II generated a considerable amount of pathology. But despite the availability of blood transfusion, antibiotics and more efficient methods for evacuating the wounded to surgical treatment stations, the results were only slightly more impressive than during World War I. In a monumental work on vascular trauma, DeBakey and Simeone reviewed 2471 patients with arterial wounds and found only 81 attempts at suture repair, with a 1:3 amputation rate. After arterial ligation, 50% of limbs were lost, and the authors concluded that only a few well localized arterial wounds were amenable to repair:

"From the preceding discussion, it is clear that no procedure other than ligation is applicable to the majority of vascular injuries which come under the military surgeons' observations. It is not a procedure of choice, it is a procedure of stern necessity for the basic purpose of controlling haemorrhage."

DeBakey entered the Army as Chief of the General Surgery Branch of the Surgeon General's office and subsequently became Director of the Surgical Consultants' Division. After the war and a further two years at Tulane University, he was appointed Chairman of the Department of Surgery at Baylor Medical College. As an astute and active politician, he soon became the primary link between the medical profession and Federal Government. Foreseeing the rising interest in cardiovascular surgery, DeBakey invited the brilliant young surgeon Denton Cooley to join the Baylor staff when he returned from Lord Brock's team at the Brompton Hospital. Although they had met briefly during World War II, their first real encounter (11 June 1951) was over a patient with a syphilitic, saccular, aortic arch aneurysm. At the time, the cellophane wrap method to prevent rupture was clearly unsatisfactory and the 48-year-old patient, Joe Mitchell, had a poor prognosis. As DeBakey examined Mitchell during his staff round at the Old Jefferson Davis City County Hospital, he paused to ask Cooley how he would approach this problem. Cooley's reply that he would excise the aneurysm produced a stunned silence, until DeBakey asked Cooley to elaborate. Cooley explained that he would put a clamp across the neck of the aneurysm, remove and oversew it, and that this was the patient's only chance for survival. DeBakey asked if he had done this before, and to everyone's amusement, Cooley responded that he had done it twice.

Cooley's first aneurysms

IN 1945, Cooley was an intern at Johns Hopkins Hospital and, as a particular favourite of Blalock, had the responsibility of administering fluids during the first Blalock-Taussig shunt procedure. One weekend over the Christmas period, Cooley was asked to see a patient who had undergone excision of the sternum for a malignant tumour by Grant Ward, a senior surgeon at Johns Hopkins. The sternum had been replaced with a stellite vitallium plate 10 days before and Cooley found the man in shock. Ward and Cooley returned the patient to the operating room, but removal of the implant caused profuse haemorrhage. It was soon apparent that the metal prosthesis had eroded the aorta, causing a false aneurysm. Ward stemmed the bleeding with a finger in the hole but was himself incapacitated by previous surgery for a spinal-cord tumour. Cooley was obliged to take over. He excised a piece of muscle from the patient's chest wall and sutured it to cover the bleeding point. However, it was clear that the muscle patch would soon give way and alternatives such as cellophane wrapping were inappropriate. When Ward asked Cooley what could be done next, Cooley replied, "I believe I would put a clamp on the side of the aorta and then oversew it." This proved successful, the patient survived and Cooley won great acclaim.

Cooley's second aneurysm operation took place at Johns Hopkins after his return from World War II. In the spring of 1949, Blalock was abroad and Cooley took over the cardiac service. One of Blalock's patients who had undergone resection of coarctation was readmitted to Johns Hopkins with severe chest pains. Chest X-ray showed a massive false aneurysm at the root of the right subclavian artery which Cooley decided to explore. The aneurysm wall was paper thin and clearly about to burst. Cooley had performed coarctation resection before and decided to excise the aneurysm. Again, the operation proved successful. On his return to Baltimore, Blalock remarked that, "If you are confronted with a serious surgical problem that has no proven solution, take a trip to Hawaii and your Resident will handle it." However, whilst Blalock was generous and supportive, the climate in Houston was fiercely competitive.

Two days after Cooley related his experience to DeBakey on the staff round, he operated on Mitchell and removed the aneurysm from the aortic arch (Figure 6.6). This was the first operation of its kind in Houston and probably a world's first. At the Southern Surgical Society the same year, DeBakey presented the case, with Cooley, a non member, sitting in the audience. At that time, the chairman of a surgical department had the option of stamping his name on whatever work emanated from the department. DeBakey was immediately established as the aneurysm surgeon and aneurysm patients were referred from the whole of the US. Baylor soon became the leading centre for vascular surgery and research.

DeBakey, with Cooley, performed the first successful resection and graft replacement of a fusiform aneurysm

of the thoracic aorta on 5 January 1953 using an interposition graft. DeBakey described this case to Viking Björk:

"We were working on aneurysms of the abdominal aorta with homografts and there were several people, other surgeons, who had tried to resect an aneurysm of the descending thoracic aorta and all had failed. The only successful case was the one Dr Ochsner did, almost as an accident, in which he had a sacciform aneurysm of the descending, a small sacciform aneurysm, which he thought was a tumor, and he went in as a tumor and when he got there he found it was a little sacciform aneurysm so he pinched it off at the neck, side-clamped and removed it. So when I had this patient in 1953, I told him that nobody had done this successfully, but I thought the principles were the same as they were in the abdominal aorta. We didn't know at that time, that you ran the risk of spinal cord ischemia, you see. We found that out later. Fortunately he didn't have it. He didn't get it, but he had very, very severe pain. This was eroding the spinal cord, vertebral bodies. He was from Arkansas, a very unusual character, an old Sheriff. He died 15 years later of carcinoma of the lung. He was a pioneer, he became a very successful case."

In August 1962 the patient returned to the hospital with carcinoma of the left lung and on 11 September 1962, DeBakey performed left pneumonectomy. An aortogram made on his admission to hospital showed the aortic homograft functioning well. By July 1955, Cooley and DeBakey had performed 245 aneurysm repairs, far surpassing any other series in volume and success. That August, they toured Europe, lecturing and demonstrating their operations, thus popularizing aneurysm surgery as Blalock, 10 years earlier, had popularized the Blalock-Taussig operation.

Blalock and Cooley published a well-illustrated case report of 1954 introducing the concept of spinal cord protection by hypothermia. An aortic homograft was used to reconstruct the aorta and the safety of cross-clamping of the aortic arch established. By this time the Baylor group had considerable experience of aortic surgery and were pushing back the frontiers almost on a weekly basis. With Cooley, DeBakey published the first Houston experiences with resection of aneurysm in 1954 in the *Journal of the American Medical Association*. The

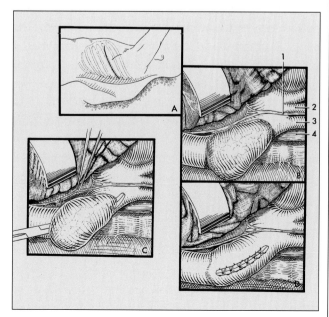

Figure 6.6. Drawings of the first resection of an aneurysm of the distal aortic arch carried out by Cooley in 1953.

Houston reports covered progressively larger series of more complex aneurysms, involving more ingenious reconstructions.

The major challenge of the time was to devise an artificial vascular graft. Whilst homograft replacements of the aorta were initially satisfactory, the incidence of degeneration, thrombosis, aneurysm formation and other problems was too high to be acceptable for peripheral vessels. Previous attempts with Tuffier's paraffin-lined silver tubes, Murray's glass, Blakemore's vitallium and Moore's polyethylene tubes all suffered the same fate of early thrombosis.

The development of vascular grafts

IN 1952, Voorhees, Jaretski and Blakemore made a giant step which opened the door to widespread arterial grafting. Voorhees had graduated from Columbia University in 1946, and following his internship, took a research fellowship with Blakemore. One of his projects in the Spring of 1947 was to work on a potential mitral valve prosthesis constructed from canine inferior vena cava. The valves were stapled into the mitral annulus and silk sutures were used as cordae tendonae. The procedure was performed on a beating dog heart through a left atrial pursestring. Voorhees described his finding as follows:

"During one of the early in vivo trials, I made an error in placing the ventricular suture, with the result that the stitch traversed the central part of the ventricular cavity. It would have been too difficult to correct, but I did make a note of my error, so that several months later at autopsy I took pains to find the misplaced suture. To my surprise, it was coated with what grossly appeared to be endocardium. It resembled a normal corda except for the black core of the stitch. It was a fragile structure which did not withstand microscopic sectioning, but its appearance was sufficiently startling to make me wonder if a piece of cloth might react in a similar way. From there I speculated that a cloth tube, acting as a latticework of threads, might indeed serve as an arterial prosthesis.'

Blakemore was enthusiastic at the prospect and Voorhees

dedicated his time to producing an artificial vascular substitute. To test the hypothesis, a silk handkerchief was first fashioned into a tube and placed into the abdominal aorta of a dog. This functioned for 1 hour, until the animal died from bleeding through the prosthesis.

In 1948, Voorhees was assigned to the Brooke Army Medical Centre in San Antonio, Texas and, whilst working on the development of plasma expanders, continued his work on arterial substitutes. The Union Carbide Company donated a bolt of Vinyon-N cloth, the material from which parachutes were made. Voorhees used this material to construct grafts on a sewing machine and experimentally implanted six more prostheses. One dog survived for 4 weeks and at autopsy the graft was patent. He returned to Blakemore's unit in 1950 to resume his surgical residency and further refined the construction and implantation of Vinyon-N grafts. Histological work, performed in the Department of Pathology at Columbia Presbyterian Medical Center, New York, soon showed that pore size was critical to the ingrowth of fibroblasts and without the latter the formation of a neo-endothelium could not be achieved. In addition, haematoma accumulation around the graft prevented healing.

Jarretski joined the Blakemore team in 1951 and their first report on 15 animal experiments with aortic prostheses appeared in the *Annals of Surgery* in March 1952. Their first human patient was operated on later that year, when an elderly man was admitted to the emergency room at Columbia Presbyterian Medical Center with a ruptured abdominal aortic aneurysm. The homograft bank at New York Hospital was unable to supply a graft and Voorhees used an autoclaved Vinyon-N tube from his lab. The aneurysm was resected and replaced satisfactorily, though the patient succumbed to bleeding and eventual myocardial infarction. The group nevertheless persisted with their human operations. The results were summarized by Voorhees at the American Surgical Society (Cleveland, 1953), and the following year they reported the outcome of Vinyon-N cloth tubes to replace 16 abdominal aortic aneurysms and one popliteal aneurysm. Union Carbide then ceased production of Vinyon-N and laboratories were set up throughout the country to explore the use of different textiles.

Edwards and Tapp introduced graded nylon tubes, some of which were fashioned into bifurcations. Early handsewn synthetic grafts had cuffed edges to avoid fraying. Tapp serendipitously discovered the crimping principle when a braided nylon tube was being soaked in formic acid to weld its fibres together and prevent fraying. In attempting to remove the straight graft from its glass mandril, an accordion pleat was produced which allowed bending without kinking. Sterling Edwards implanted the first human crimped nylon graft to replace a 5 cm segment of femoral artery for arteriovenous fistula (1954). Crimping was employed to prevent kinking of the graft at points of angulation. Cautery was used to seal the ends of the nylon to prevent fraying. Although well tolerated by the tissues, nylon proved to have disappointing durability and degenerated in the face of body fluids. Many grafts fragmented or virtually disappeared after implantation. Other plastic fibres such as Orlon and Teflon were tried, until the discovery of Dacron by DeBakey in a department store in Houston. DeBakey's mother was a seamstress and taught him to sew cloth. As a result, DeBakey was able to construct his own vascular graft including bifurcated prostheses for the distal aorta. After a discussion about knitting vascular grafts with a patient, DeBakey was invited to visit a sock factory in Reading, Pennsylvania in which the patient had half ownership. As the factory had no suitable machine for knitting grafts, DeBakey went to the Philadelphia Textile Institute where Thomas Edman designed and built a knitting machine specifically for DeBakey at a cost of $25,000 paid for by the generous patient. This machine was the forerunner of modern commercial machines used to fabricate Dacron arterial substitutes still used today (Figure 6.7). DeBakey did not patent the knitting machine nor did the commercial producer who, funded by the same patient, subsequently worked full-time for DeBakey and the Baylor Vascular Service.

Oscar Creech, a Baylor patent engineer and necktie factory owner pointed out that crimped Dacron was easily tailored, needed no preparation and formed a perfect lattice for arterial regeneration. He suggested soaking the semiporous Dacron in the patient's own blood in order to fertilize the surface for tissue ingrowth. Several different forms of Dacron were available and the Dacron polyester fibre used by Szilagyi, Julian and Wesoloski proved to be the best. The textile engineers introduced knitting in place of the older methods of braiding, and factors to promote tissue ingrowth and endothelialization of the graft were studied.

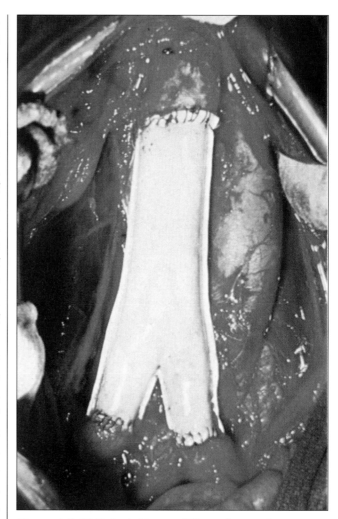

Figure 6.7. DeBakey's Dacron bifurcation graft.

In 1955, Dterling and Rhonslay presented an evaluation of synthetic fabrics for use in vascular reconstruction, and in 1956, a Committee of the Society for Vascular Surgery, which included Creech, Dterling, Edwards, Julian and Schumacker, summarized the status of synthetic prostheses at the time. Whilst recognizing the value of Dacron grafts for aortic replacement, they concluded that no currently available materials appeared adequate for peripheral vascular replacement. In 1956, Norman Rosenberg reported chemical modification of bovine arterial grafts, in an attempt to modify the immunological response to heterograft tissues. Heterograft implantation dated back to Carrell, but in general, had proved disappointing. The autogenous vein graft proposed several decades before was revived by Kunlin's femoro-popliteal bypass operations (1948) and later popularized by Robert Linton in the US. Although the use of saphenous vein as an arterial substitute gained popularity during the Korean War, there was considerable bias against vein graft insertion in the 1950s. Many surgeons were suspicious that insertion of a vein in the arterial system would lead to aneurysm formation. Although this concept was erroneous, it was many years before clinical experience refuted the suggestion.

One of the principal problems, particularly for intrathoracic vascular repair, was control of bleeding. After the introduction of velour knitted grafts by Sauvage, DeBakey and Cooley, attempts were made to standardize the degree of porosity in order to reduce bleeding through the fabric itself. In fully heparinized patients undergoing cardiopulmonary bypass, it was necessary to use tightly woven, low porosity grafts, but these had less desirable handling and suture characteristics than the knitted velour grafts used peripherally. The knitted grafts were pre-clotted to deposit fibrin and occlude the interstices of the fabric. Cooley introduced the method of autoclaving a porous graft soaked with autologous plasma, which rendered it completely impervious to blood. Subsequently, better methods of sealing the grafts became available, including impregnation with bovine collagen or albumen. The handling and suturing characteristics of these grafts used in thoracic aortic replacement are inherently superior.

Dos Santos and thrombo-endarterectomy

IN 1947, Joao Cid Dos Santos evolved the technique of thrombo-endarterectomy. His father, Renaldo Dos Santos, had used the operation of endo-aneurysmorrhaphy for peripheral aneurysms in the early 1940s, and subsequently developed arteriography to study the aorta and its branches. After the introduction of heparin, Joao persuaded his father to use heparin for aneurysm operations in order to extend the safe period of vascular crossclamping. During a femoral artery exploration for embolus, he removed the atheromatous occlusion as well as the thrombus and described the technique as arterial endarterectomy. Joao sent the manuscript to his former teacher, Leriche, who presented it in Dos Santos' name to the French Academy of Surgery (but added a somewhat critical editorial of his own). Dos Santos went on to use separate arterial

incisions and a curette to remove the clot and sequestrum from the intervening artery. He eventually extended the procedure by opening the vessel throughout the entire length of its obstruction. The first operations were performed on iliac vessels, then the axillary subclavian system and the femoral vessels. Freeman and Leeds adopted endarterectomy in the treatment of aortic occlusive disease and aortic aneurysm. They followed Blakemore's lead by using vein grafts within the denuded aortic wall to provide new endothelium. Wylie adopted a different approach by reinforcing the often fragile endarterectomied vessel with a wraparound of fascia lata.

Increasing the scope of vascular surgery

VASCULAR surgery expanded rapidly with the innovations of the 1950s. Technical advances were synchronous with developments in angiography, anaesthesia and critical care medicine. The concept of extra-anatomic revascularization was introduced with the femoro-femoral crossover graft (Freeman, 1952) and axillofemoral bypass (Blaisedell, 1962). Extra-anatomic bypass was performed as an alternative to direct intrathoracic or mediastinal operations for occlusive disease of the aortic arch or its branches. Subclavian carotid bypass was described by Lyons and Galbraith (1956) using a nylon prosthesis.

During the early 1960s, Thomas Fogarty, of the University of Cincinnati, developed the embolectomy catheter and brought about an immediate revolution in the management of arterial embolism. The concept of percutaneous intraluminal dilatation of critical arterial stenosis was conceived in 1963 by Dotter during a post-mortem study of the feasibility of coronary angiography. He discovered that forceful hydraulic balloon inflation injections in a stenotic area led to increased flow. The first transluminal angiography of a femoral artery was performed on 16 January 1964, and later that year, Dotter reported results with the first 15 procedures. He predicted the possibility for angioplasty of the renal, carotid, vertebral and coronary arteries.

In 1974, Grüntzig described his modified flexible balloon catheter (Figure 6.8) and, by 1977, was able to report excellent 3-year patency rates following iliac artery

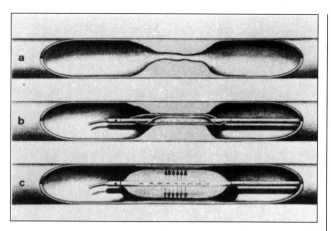

Figure 6.8. Grüntzig's modified flexible balloon cathether.

dilatation. The first four cases of percutaneous transluminal coronary angioplasty were presented at the 1977 Meeting of the American Heart Association. This was a tremendous conceptual advance in the treatment of coronary artery disease and 20 years later, transluminal coronary angioplasty is the first-line treatment for single and two vessel coronary disease. Sadly, Grüntzig and his family died tragically when the plane which he was piloting crashed in bad weather.

Further development of thoracic aneurysm surgery

KAMPMEIER studied the natural history of saccular aneurysms and showed that practically all patients died from rupture within 6–9 months of the onset of symptoms. After the first successful resection of an intrarenal abdominal aortic aneurysm by Dubost in 1951, techniques for resection of both the thoracic and abdominal aorta developed rapidly. In 1954, Ellis first reimplanted a renal artery during aortic aneurysm resection. Later that year, Etherede resected an atherosclerotic thoraco-abdominal aortic aneurysm at the Veterans' Administration Hospital, Oakland, California. He restored aortic continuity with a preserved aortic homograft and directly sutured the superior mesenteric artery and coeliac axis into the graft. The procedure was performed using a 5 mm homemade polyethylene shunt for temporary aortic bypass, and the patient was alive and well 18 years later. Robb (1955) and then DeBakey, Creech and Morris (1956) described resections of thoraco-abdominal aneurysms with

reimplantation of the coeliac, superior mesenteric and renal arteries into the graft. DeBakey provided the first detailed description of four-vessel reimplantation and had undertaken 20 such resections by 1958. Fifteen of his patients had syphilitic aneurysms.

In 1965, Crawford described his method for thoraco-abdominal aneurysm repair by proximal and distal clamping, then suture of the graft from within the aneurysm. He performed side-to-side anastomoses of the origin of each visceral branch, either individually, or in groups if the branches were close enough together on the aortic wall. The aortic wall itself was not excised, but wrapped around the graft to minimize bleeding. In 1964, Joyce and colleagues reported on 107 cases of untreated thoracic aortic aneurysms, noting a 5-year survival of less than 30% in patients with symptoms at the time of diagnosis.

In 1953, Bahnson reported the first successful excision of a saccular aneurysm of the ascending aorta. Cooley and DeBakey (1956) and Bahnson and Spencer (1960) then reported separate series of patients with excision of the entire ascending aorta. In 1960, Muller and associates described the treatment of Marfan's syndrome by excision of the ascending aortic aneurysm and exclusion by direct suture of the non-coronary valve leaflet to restore competence of the aortic valve. Starr (1963) described excision of the incompetent aortic valve in aortic root aneurysm, with replacement by the Starr-Edwards valve and graft replacement of the aneurysmal aorta. The coronary arteries were left *in situ* at this stage.

In 1964, Wheat reported the first successful replacement of the entire ascending aorta (from aortic annulus to the innominate artery) with reimplantation of the coronary ostia and separate replacement of the aortic valve. This was performed by leaving a flap of aortic tissue around the coronary ostia (Figure 6.9). Bentall and DeBono (Figures 6.10 and 6.11) (1968) then reported their technique for complete replacement of the ascending aorta, using a composite valved conduit and reimplantation of the coronary ostia (Article 6.6, Appendix A). This was not a planned procedure but an operation derived in response to pathological findings. Bentall's original intention was to replace the aortic valve and then insert a tube graft in the supracoronary position to replace the aortic aneurysm. When this was not possible, the enduring operation of aortic root replacement was devised and became known as the

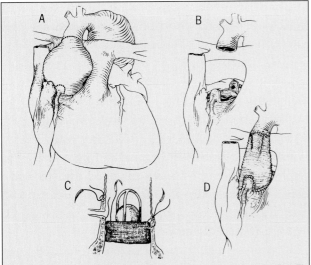

Fig. 4. An illustration of the operative findings and procedure in Case 5 (Table III). *A*, The aortic root aneurysm due to localized dissection; dotted lines indicate lines of excision. The distal dissection is also shown. *B*, Appearance after excision of the aneurysm with the tongues of aortic wall containing the two coronary artery ostia left attached to the aortic annulus. *C*, Close-up drawing of method of suture shows Starr-Edwards valve in subcoronary position; the suture encompasses the aortic annulus, Teflon skirt of the valve prosthesis, and the woven Teflon aortic prosthesis, tying all three together as a unit at the aortic root. *D*, Completed procedure shows tubular aortic prosthesis in place with the tongue of aortic wall containing the right coronary artery ostium sutured into the side of the graft.

Figure 6.9. Wheat's operation for ascending aortic aneurysm.

Bentall procedure. For many years the native coronary ostia were circumferentially anastomosed to holes in the aortic graft but in continuity with the pathological aortic wall. Because the early grafts were porous to some degree, the native aortic wall was then wrapped around the ascending aortic graft to reduce bleeding. This sometimes led to accumulation of blood under tension between the graft and native aorta, and false aneurysm formation if the coronary suture line became partially detached. Cabrol modified the technique by creating a fistula between the wrap around and the right atrial appendage. He also elected to use a Dacron coronary conduit between the ascending aortic graft and the native coronary ostia to prevent tension on these suture lines. With modern impervious grafts, wrap around is now superfluous. It is safer and easier to mobilize the coronary ostia out of the pathological aorta and implant them directly into the graft, a technique popularized by Kouchoukos, Westaby and others. This method has eliminated coronary false aneurysm formation.

Aortic dissection

DISSECTING aneurysms were described by Morgagni

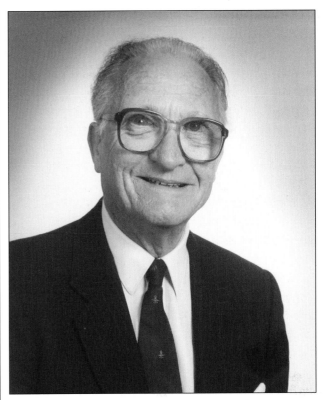

Figure 6.10. Hugh Bentall, Professor of Cardiac Surgery at the Hammersmith Hospital.

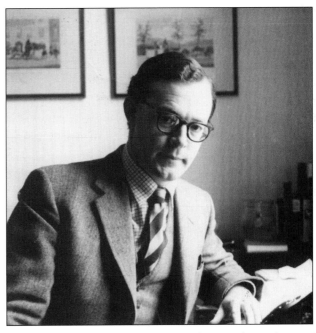

Figure 6.11. Anthony De Bono, subsequently Professor of Cardiac Surgery in Malta.

in 1761. He described the demise of a number of patients who died when blood "forced its way through the aortic wall coming out under the internal coat of the artery". King George II is said to have died from aortic dissection at the age of 76, when his valet discerned a noise "louder than the Royal wind". Laennec (1819) introduced the term aortic dissection (l'aneurysme dissequant). This followed the description by Otto (1824) of the case of a young woman with coarctation of the aorta, bicuspid aortic avlve and acute type A dissection with rupture into the pericardium. Elliotson noted that the most frequent site of origin of aortic dissection was in the ascending aorta. Within a few years, Peacock documented re-entry tears in 19 cases of dissection and regarded these as "an imperfect natural cure of the disease". He also recognized that dissections of the ascending aorta were lethal through the propensity to rupture into the pericardial sac. The first diagnosis of dissection in a live patient was by Latham (1855). The 51-year-old man presented with severe chest pain followed by loss of power in the legs and unconciousness. Leg pulses were absent and at autopsy, aortic dissection was confirmed. In 1920, Krukenberg suggested rupture of the vasa vasorum in the aortic wall as the mechanism predisposing to aortic dissection. Shennan recognized medial degeneration as the defect underlying the dissection process. The first operation for aortic dissection was by Gurin and colleagues (1935), when they attempted localized re-entry in the right external iliac artery for an ischaemic leg. Shaw coined the term 'fenestration', performed by excision of a window from the internal wall of the dissection to allow reperfusion of occluded visceral arteries. In 1955, DeBakey, Cooley and Creech first attempted fenestration in the thoracic aorta. Muller (1960) first introduced resection of the ascending aorta for chronic dissecting aneurysms combined with bicuspidization of the aortic valve to correct aortic regurgitation. Hufnagel and Conrad (1961) introduced the method of Teflon felt buttress to reinforce the friable aortic tissues. Morris and colleagues at Baylor (1963) were the first to repair an acute ascending aortic dissection. This patient was followed with moderate aortic regurgitation until 1977, when elective aortic valve replacement was performed. Remarkably, the false lumen remained patent without aneurysm formation and the patient was well when seen in 1990. In 1965, Wheat emphasized the role of blood pressure control in the medical management of acute aortic dissection. Blood pressure control is the mainstay of treatment prior to surgery for Type A dissection, and

usually the definitive approach for Type B dissection in the absence of complications. By 1965, DeBakey, Cooley and others reported 179 operations for aortic dissection with an overall survival of 79%. The authors classified dissecting aneurysms according to the site of origin of the intimal tear and extent of the dissecting process. In DeBakey Type I dissection, the tear originated in the ascending aorta and extended into the aortic arch or beyond. Type II dissection began and was localized to the ascending aorta, without extension into the arch. Type III originated beyond the left subclavian artery and extended distally for a varying extent, but may also retrogradely involve the arch.

Sorrenson and Olsen (1964) reported the epidemiology of aortic dissection, noting that this was the most common acute catastrophe to involve the aorta, with a frequency of about five episodes per million population per year. They noted a familial predisposition in patients under 40 with Marfan's syndrome, pregnancy or congenital problems, including bicuspid aortic valve and coarctation of the aorta. For patients presenting between the fifth and seventh decades, 90% had a history of hypertension, with an increased incidence in black people. The Stanford classification of acute aortic dissection into Type A and Type B was presented by Daley, Shumway and colleagues in 1970. In this simplified presentation, Type A dissections are those involving the ascending aorta (which may include DeBakey Type I, II or III patients). Type B are dissections which do not involve the ascending aorta (DeBakey Type III without retrograde dissection). This is currently the preferred classification.

In 1971 Halpern and colleagues noted that dissecting aneurysm was the most serious complication in Marfan's syndrome accounting for more than half of the deaths.

In the same year, Wheat and Palmer proposed a mechanism for aortic dissection which includes cystic medial degeneration, hypertension and flexion stresses with repeated motion of the aorta. Sites of maximal stress are on the anterior wall of the ascending aorta and the posterior wall of the descending aorta, just beyond the left subclavian artery. For DeBakey Type III or Stanford Type B patients, Crawford (1973) described direct aortic crossclamping, transection and rapid end-to-end anastomosis. In 1978, Dureau and Ablaza separately reported the use of a ringed intraluminal prosthesis to simplify management of Type B dissection. The rings were placed in the aorta proximally and distally to the point of dissection and secured with tapes about the circumference of the aorta. This method was somewhat unreliable. In the 1970s, mortality for aortic dissection repair was substantial. A landmark paper from Craig Miller and associates at Stanford (19790 showed a hospital mortality of 38% after surgery, though for a selected group managed medically, mortality exceeded 80%.

Aortic arch aneurysms

ANEURYSMS of the aortic arch were recognized in the early 1800s, predominantly due to syphilis. The first attempt to remove a saccular aneurysm of the aortic arch was by Tuffier in 1902. He ligated the base of the aneurysm, but 2 weeks later, ischaemic necrosis resulted in exsanguination. Fifty years later (1952), Schafter and Hardin used a temporary polythene shunt to preserve distal aortic bloodflow whilst resecting a fusiform arch aneurysm; the aorta was replaced by an aortic homograft. This ambitious procedure was complicated by refractory cardiac arrhythmias, which resulted in the patient's death. In 1955, Stranahan reported aortic arch resection with xenograft aortic replacement using a temporary shunt. Again, the patient died from complications, this time from concomitant left pneumonectomy. The first successful operation on an aortic arch aneurysm was by Bahnson in 1955. The saccular aneurysm was clamped and the neck oversewn. Remarkably, the same year, Cooley and DeBakey reported actual aortic arch resection with homograft replacement, employing shunt bypass. The patient survived for 6 days, but did not recover from intraoperative cerebral ischaemia. The following year, Cooley and DeBakey successfully resected a fusiform aneurysm of the proximal aortic arch using cardiopulmonary bypass. A homograft was used to replace the excised segment.

By 1962, DeBakey, Cooley, Crawford and others reported 138 patients operated on for aortic arch aneurysms using temporary Dacron bypass, atriofemoral shunts or total cardiopulmonary bypass with carotid perfusion. Remarkably, their overall mortality was only 22%. They identified increasing age and associated cardiac problems as important risk factors. Cardiac events accounted for 55% of deaths and cerebral ischaemia for 23%. Vincent Gott (1967) designed a vascular shunt to moderate the haemodynamic effects of unprotected aortic crossclamping and to supply the abdominal viscera with bloodflow during descending thoracic aortic operations.

The routine use of cardiopulmonary bypass greatly simplified surgery of the ascending aorta and arch, by offloading the left ventricle and providing direct perfusion of the head vessels. The use of profound hypothermic circulatory arrest for aortic arch surgery was first reported in 1970 by Dumanian, who plicated a traumatic aneurysm of the transverse arch. Five years later, Randall Griepp described complete resection of the aortic arch with graft replacement, using profound hypothermia and total circulatory arrest. He had three survivors from the first four patients. Total circulatory arrest at between 15°C and 18°C provided a bloodless operative field, whilst reducing cerebral metabolic demand to levels where 50 to 60 minutes of ischaemia were tolerable. The Mount Sinai Medical Centre team of Griepp, Ergin and Lansman continued to pursue the scientific evaluation of total circulatory arrest and methods for cerebral protection.

The combination of hypothermic cardiopulmonary bypass and total circulatory arrest provided the basis for a rapid increase in the scope of thoracic aortic surgery. Cooley advocated the open-ended technique for repair of acute type A dissection, which allowed excision or repair of tears in the aortic arch. This, together with the introduction of biological glues by Bachet and others, led to an important reduction in operative mortality. Kouchoukos pioneered the use of circulatory arrest for repair of descending thoracic and thoracoabdominal aneurysms. For full cardiopulmonary bypass through a left thoracotomy, Kouchoukos advocated cannulation of the femoral and pulmonary arteries. As an alternative, Westaby used transjugular cannulation of the right atrium with arterial return to the ascending aorta so as not to interrupt flow to the brain and coronary arteries. For aneurysms that involved the aortic arch and descending thoracic aorta, Borst (Figure 6.12) described the elephant trunk technique to simplify the second stage by leaving a vascular graft within the descending thoracic aneurysm.

The last ten years have witnessed many significant advances in thoracic aortic surgery with improvement or consolidation of operative techniques. In an outstanding series of patients with Marfan's syndrome, Gott demonstrated that elective aortic root replacement, irrespective of symptomatic status, transformed their outlook in contrast to those operated for acute dissection. David and Yacoub independently questioned the need for valve replacement in annulo-aortic ectasia and described aortic root repair and valve conservation in preference to the classic Bentall operation. After extensive anatomical studies, David described the criteria and techniques for root repair which are now widely adopted (Figure 6.13). Both David and Yacoub suggest that the aortic valve may be safely conserved in Marfan's patients. Only time will tell.

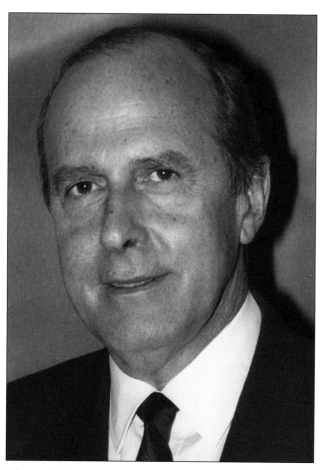

Figure 6.12. Hans Borst.

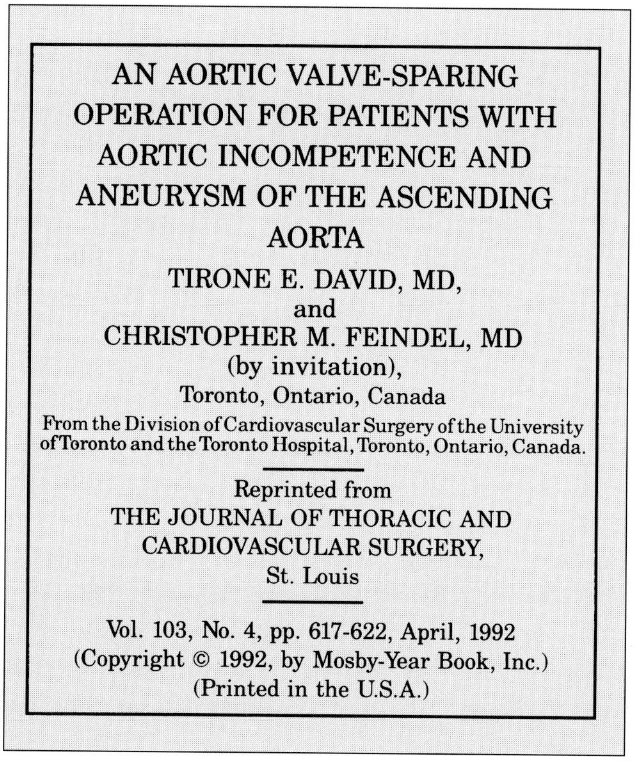

AN AORTIC VALVE-SPARING OPERATION FOR PATIENTS WITH AORTIC INCOMPETENCE AND ANEURYSM OF THE ASCENDING AORTA

TIRONE E. DAVID, MD,
and
CHRISTOPHER M. FEINDEL, MD
(by invitation),
Toronto, Ontario, Canada

From the Division of Cardiovascular Surgery of the University of Toronto and the Toronto Hospital, Toronto, Ontario, Canada.

Reprinted from
THE JOURNAL OF THORACIC AND CARDIOVASCULAR SURGERY,
St. Louis

Vol. 103, No. 4, pp. 617-622, April, 1992
(Copyright © 1992, by Mosby-Year Book, Inc.)
(Printed in the U.S.A.)

Figure 6.13. An aortic valve-sparing operation for patients with aortic incompetence and aneurysm of the ascending aorta. *A 1992 article by Tirone David and Christopher Feindel. (Reproduced with permission from* Journal of Thoracic and Cardiovascular Surgery.)

Biographies

Michael Ellis DeBakey (1908–)

MICHAEL ELLIS DEBAKEY was born in Lake Charles, Louisiana of Lebanese parents. He studied at Tulane University (BS, 1930; MD, 1932), when Rudolph Matas was still operating and Alton Ochsner had just taken over the Department of Surgery. He interned at Charity Hospital, New Orleans (MS, 1934), and went to Strasbourg University to study under René Leriche. Leriche had predicted that the ideal treatment for occlusive disease of the abdominal aorta (since termed 'Leriche's syndrome') would be excision of the diseased segment and its replacement with an aortic graft. It was 30 years later thanks to DeBakey, that this prediction became a reality. Others of DeBakey's generation, including Gene Kuebler who did the first femoral popliteal bypass in 1948, Cid dos Santos and Jean Kunlin, also trained under Leriche.

DeBakey went on to study at the University of Heidelberg under Martin Kirschner (1935–36). He taught at Tulane University and worked at the Ochsner Clinic (1937–48) under Alton Ochsner, with whom he published 71 papers on a wide-range of surgical subjects. In 1934, DeBakey developed a blood transfusion pump, eventually used in Gibbon's heart-lung machine. He was one of the first to recognize the importance of blood banks and the relationship of cigarette smoking to lung cancer.

During World War II, DeBakey was named Director of the Surgical Consultants' Division in the Surgeon General's Office (1942–46) where, with Simeone, he published *Battle Casualties*, an analysis of 2471 battle and other injuries. At DeBakey's suggestion, centres for systematic follow-up of these cases after the war (the Veterans' Administration Medical Center System) were established. DeBakey's capacity to bring his professional knowledge to bear on public policy led to many political posts, such as the three terms he served on the National Heart, Lung and Blood Advisory Council of the National Institutes of Health and as the adviser to almost every president of the United States in the past half-century. Discharged from the army as a colonel in 1946, DeBakey returned to the Oschner Clinic and Tulane University until 1948, when he became Professor and the first Chairman of the Department of Surgery at Baylor University College of Medicine. In 1969, he initiated the medical school's separation

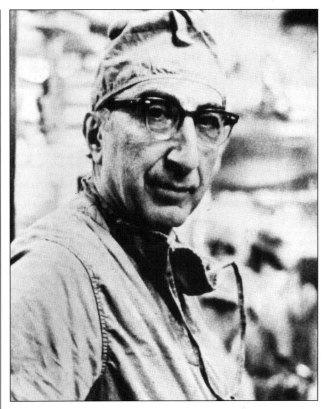

Figure 6.14. Michael Ellis DeBakey.

from Baylor University and became President of the newly-formed Baylor College of Medicine. He has been Chancellor since 1979.

DeBakey presented a paper at the American Surgical Association meeting in 1956 describing the excision and replacement of an aortic aneurysm with a homograft on 19 October 1955 (Article 6.1, Appendix A). DeBakey and his colleagues used a vascular shunt to conduct blood around the cross-clamped segment and thereby minimize the period of distal ischaemia. The method proved satisfactory, though the first patient died from renal failure following more than 100 minutes of aortic cross-clamp time. Excision of the thoraco-abdominal aorta with reimplantation of the visceral vessels was an important surgical landmark and recognized as such by those in the audience. John Gibbon described the operation as one of the most brilliant technical achievements to be

Aneurysm of Thoracoabdominal Aorta Involving the
Celiac, Superior Mesenteric, and Renal Arteries.
Report of Four Cases Treated by Resection
and Homograft Replacement *

MICHAEL E. DEBAKEY, M.D., OSCAR CREECH, JR., M.D., GEORGE C. MORRIS, JR., M.D.**

Houston, Texas

Figure 6.15. Title page of DeBakey's 1956 article entitled
'Aneurysm of thoracoabdominal aorta involving the celiac,
superior mesenteric, and renal arteries.' *(Reproduced with
permission from* Annals of Surgery; *144: 549–72.)*

accomplished in the field of vascular surgery. Forty years later
and despite considerable advances in vascular graft technology,
resection of thoraco-abdominal aneurysms with visceral
reimplantation still generates substantial morbidity and
mortality even in the most experienced hands.

DeBakey went on to improve on this procedure:

*"The highly gratifying immediate and long-term results in this
patient provided us with the conviction that this was the
preferable method of surgical treatment for this type of
aneurysm. Subsequent experience led to a modification of the
procedure that proved to be of great advantage. This
modification consisted of combining the bypass principle with a
permanent replacement. Thus, by attaching a Dacron graft to
the descending thoracic aorta just above the aneurysm and to
the abdominal aorta below the aneurysm, we could maintain
the circulation in each major visceral branch, while sequentially
attaching Dacron grafts from the major bypass graft to one
renal artery and then the other. Attachment of similar grafts to
the superior mesenteric and coeliac axis followed, and then
resection of the aneurysm and suturing of the ends of the aorta.
The period of ischemic arrest in each of these arteries can thus be
minimized to about 10 or 12 minutes, a period which is well
tolerated."*

This operation was simplified by Crawford and co-workers,
who included the graft within the aneurysm and reduced the
hospital mortality to 8 percent.

Aortic homografts were limited in availability and known to
degenerate through calcification. Between 1950 and 1953,
DeBakey developed the Dacron and Dacron-velour artificial
grafts for replacement of diseased arteries (Article 6.2,
Appendix A). DeBakey has described his discovery of Dacron:

*"On my first trip to obtain some of these fabrics from a
department store here (Houston), I found that they only had*

CLINICAL APPLICATION OF A NEW FLEXIBLE KNITTED DACRON
ARTERIAL SUBSTITUTE*

MICHAEL E. DE BAKEY, M.D., DENTON A. COOLEY, M.D., E. STANLEY
CRAWFORD, M.D., AND GEORGE C. MORRIS, JR., M.D.†

Houston, Texas

The direct surgical treatment of various forms of aortic and arterial disease often requires a vascular replacement. Homografts were first employed successfully for this purpose and both technically and functionally have provided highly gratifying results. Their major disadvantage, however, lies in the inconvenience associated with their procurement and preparation and the fact that they are not available in sufficient quantities to meet the increasing demands for their use. For these reasons attention has been directed toward development of a satisfactory arterial substitute for homografts which would be free of these disadvantages. Various materials such as Ivalon, nylon, Orlon, Dacron, and Teflon have been used for this purpose and fashioned into tubes by different methods including heat-sealing, sewing, braiding, knitting, and weaving. In a previous publication we reviewed our experience with these various types of synthetic arterial substitutes based upon observations derived from an analysis of 317 cases in which they were employed.[1] The functional results in this series of cases were generally satisfactory and provided additional evidence that tubular fabrics of these synthetic materials could be used as substitutes for homografts. There were, however, certain disadvantages associated with most of them, particularly in their technical application. For these reasons and with the hope of overcoming some of these objections, efforts were continued toward the development of a more satisfactory arterial substitute.

As a result of these efforts and in cooperation with Professor Thomas Edman of the Philadelphia Textile Institute, a new knitting machine was designed with particular specifications to produce seamless knitted Dacron tubes in different sizes and in the form of bifurcations as well as multi-branch tubes.[2] Various types of synthetic filament yarns were tested from nylon to Teflon, but the most suitable was found to be Dacron texturized on the Flufon process. To achieve greater flexibility a process of cross-crimping the tubular knitted fabric by heat-setting was used. Various means of coating and chemically treating the fabric were tried but were discarded after

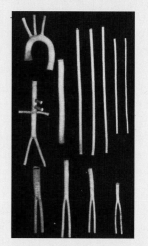

* Supported in part by the United States Public Health Service under Grant H-3137, the American Heart Association, the Houston Heart Association, and Mr. Arthur Hanisch.
† From the Cora and Webb Mading Department of Surgery, Baylor University College of Medicine, Houston, Texas.

FIG. 1. Photograph showing various types and sizes of Dacron grafts for replacement of different anatomic segments of the aorta and peripheral arteries.

862

Figure 6.16. Title page of the 1958 article entitled 'Clinical
applications of a new flexible knitted Dacron arterial
substitute' *written by DeBakey, Cooley, Crawford and Morris.
(Reproduced with permission from* The American Surgeon; *24:
861–69.)*

*some sheets of Dacron. I purchased several yards and cut them
in different sizes to make tubes by sewing on my wife's sewing
machine. I had been taught by my mother as a boy to sew and I
became an expert not only in the use of a sewing machine but
also in the other aspects of sewing. These tubes proved highly
successful in animals, and although we later obtained sheets of
Orlon, Teflon, nylon, and Ivalon, none of these were as good as
the original Dacron fabric. It is rather interesting and an
example of serendipity that the first material we obtained
(Dacron), the only one available in the store at that time,
proved later to be the best material. One of these Dacron grafts
that I had fabricated as a bifurcation graft was used to replace
an aneurysm of the abdominal aorta in September, 1954."*

By 1956, DeBakey had developed flexible arterial substitutes
now used for most vascular replacement or bypass operations.
The DeBakey vascular grafts available in different sizes for

carotid, renal and iliac replacement stimulated the widespread growth of vascular surgery. The pervious nature of the synthetic Dacron material was overcome by the process of pre-clotting until the development of Dacron grafts impregnated with bovine collagen, gelatin or albumen in the late 1980s.

DeBakey performed the first successful carotid endarterectomy on 7 August 1953, and carotid reconstruction by patch-graft angioplasty in 1958. In 1963, he won the Lasker Award for his classification of the segmental nature of occlusive vascular disease. This allowed effective treatment strategies even when the aetiology of vascular disease remained obscure. In 1964, DeBakey and Edward Garrett performed the first successful aortocoronary artery bypass using saphenous vein from the leg. This was not reported until 1972, when the graft was restudied and found patent several years after Favaloro described successful bypass surgery at the Cleveland Clinic (1968). DeBakey's pioneering techniques in vascular surgery are extensively illustrated in his 1979 review article published in *The American Journal of Surgery*.

In the early 1960s, the DeBakey team began testing mechanical heart models in calves. In 1963, he used the first left ventricular assistive device and in 1966, diastolic counterpulsation (a left ventricular bypass pump) successfully. He lined the bypass pump and its connections with Dacron-velour, a concept applied earlier in Dacron arterial grafts. DeBakey's early research into artificial hearts and his testimony before Congress led to federal support of the artificial heart programme. Since its inception, DeBakey has chaired the US–USSR artificial heart programme of the National Heart, Lung and Blood Institute. In February 1994 (at the age of 86), he showed President Clinton a new axial flow impeller pump, developed in collaboration with the National Aeronautics and Space Administration (NASA/DeBakey Heart) using the space agency's expertise in miniaturization pump technology.

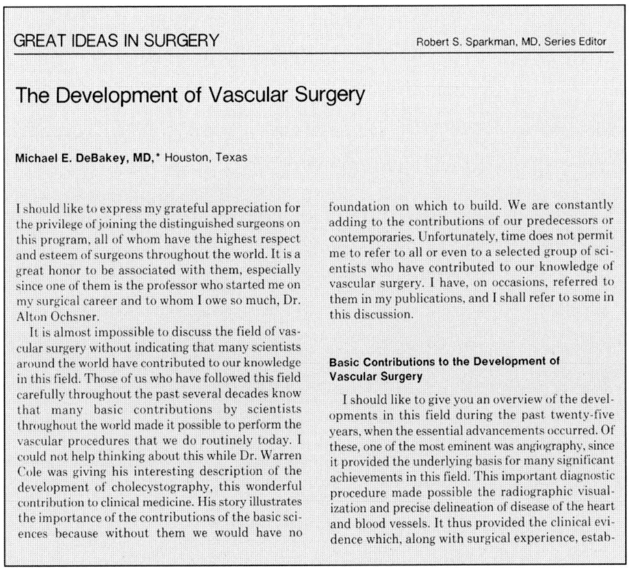

Over an 18-month period beginning in 1968, the DeBakey team performed 12 cardiac transplantations, of which two recipients, Bill Carroll in Phoenix and Duson Vlaco in Belgrade, were still alive in 1971. In an historic multiple-transplantation procedure in 1968, the team transplanted the heart, kidneys and one lung of a donor into four recipients. Because of organ rejection, the transplantation programme was discontinued in 1970 but resumed in 1984 when cyclosporine and other advances made the outcome more predictable.

DeBakey has produced more than 70 surgical instruments or machines used in cardiovascular surgery. He has pioneered many technologies in cardiovascular surgery and trained more than 500 surgeons, who have established the Michael E. DeBakey Cardiovascular Surgical Society, a world-wide organization. In 1980, the Michael E. DeBakey Center for Biomedical Education and Research was established as the headquarters of Baylor's research programmes, encompassing some 300 medical projects of major importance. DeBakey's lifelong scholarship is reflected by more than 1200 articles and books he has written or edited. These include *The Blood Bank and the Technique and Therapeutics of Transfusions, Vascular Surgery in World War II, Christopher's Minor Surgery, Cold Injury, Buerger's Disease, Advances in Cardiac Valves and Factors Influencing the Course of Myocardial Ischemia*. DeBakey has received 32 honorary degrees and 27 awards, including the Prix International Dag Hammarsjold, the Medal of Freedom with distinction from President Lyndon Johnson and the National Medal of Science from President Reagan.

In his late 80's, DeBakey continues to expand the frontiers of cardiovascular research. In 1983, he and Joseph Melnick reported evidence of cytomegalovirus involvement in the arterial walls of some patients with atherosclerosis. As replicating virus was not detected, the study suggested that the occurrence of cytomegalovirus early in life may initiate the lesions that later cause atherosclerosis. Extending this line of investigation, in 1987, DeBakey and colleagues reported that patients with heart disease have higher-than-normal levels of antibodies to cytomegalovirus. DeBakey continues to operate at the age of 87, longer than Rudolph Matas, who stopped at 78. Throughout his long and dignified career DeBakey enjoyed the patronage of Presidents and overseas Royalty. The Duke of Windsor encouraged by his American wife, Wallace Simpson, consulted DeBakey about a suspected aortic aneurysm. Though only 4.5 cm in diameter DeBakey resected the

GREAT IDEAS IN SURGERY   Robert S. Sparkman, MD, Series Editor

The Development of Vascular Surgery

Michael E. DeBakey, MD,* Houston, Texas

I should like to express my grateful appreciation for the privilege of joining the distinguished surgeons on this program, all of whom have the highest respect and esteem of surgeons throughout the world. It is a great honor to be associated with them, especially since one of them is the professor who started me on my surgical career and to whom I owe so much, Dr. Alton Ochsner.

It is almost impossible to discuss the field of vascular surgery without indicating that many scientists around the world have contributed to our knowledge in this field. Those of us who have followed this field carefully throughout the past several decades know that many basic contributions by scientists throughout the world made it possible to perform the vascular procedures that we do routinely today. I could not help thinking about this while Dr. Warren Cole was giving his interesting description of the development of cholecystography, this wonderful contribution to clinical medicine. His story illustrates the importance of the contributions of the basic sciences because without them we would have no

foundation on which to build. We are constantly adding to the contributions of our predecessors or contemporaries. Unfortunately, time does not permit me to refer to all or even to a selected group of scientists who have contributed to our knowledge of vascular surgery. I have, on occasions, referred to them in my publications, and I shall refer to some in this discussion.

Basic Contributions to the Development of Vascular Surgery

I should like to give you an overview of the developments in this field during the past twenty-five years, when the essential advancements occurred. Of these, one of the most eminent was angiography, since it provided the underlying basis for many significant achievements in this field. This important diagnostic procedure made possible the radiographic visualization and precise delineation of disease of the heart and blood vessels. It thus provided the clinical evidence which, along with surgical experience, estab-

Figure 6.17. Title page of DeBakey's 1979 article 'The development of vascular surgery'. (Reproduced with permission from The American Journal of Surgery; 137: 697–738.)

aneurysm and established a friendship with the Royals. His rivals jokingly suggested a new "Duke's" classification of aneurysms. When arch rival Cooley was asked by students "when to resect an aneurysm" his reply became "Now before someone else does!" DeBakey and Cooley have not spoken or corresponded directly since the artificial heart issue in 1969.

DeBakey stepped down as Chairman at Baylor in 1993. He was succeeded in the position by John Baldwin of Stanford and Yale, who is coincidently an authority on the Duke of Windsor.

Denton Arthur Cooley (1920–)

DENTON ARTHUR COOLEY was born in Houston, Texas. He studied at the University of Texas (BA, 1941) and Johns Hopkins (MD, 1944) where he fulfilled internship (1944–45), residency (1945–50) and chief residency with Handelsman (1949–50) under Alfred Blalock. He was senior surgical registrar to Lord Brock at Brompton Hospital (1950–51). In 1951, Cooley was invited by DeBakey to organize a comprehensive heart programme at Baylor Medical College and pursue the development of the heart-lung machine. Cooley became Associate Professor (1954–62) and Professor of Surgery (1962–69) at Baylor. In 1960, he moved his practice from Methodist Hospital across the street to St Luke's Episcopal Hospital and in 1969, he resigned from Baylor Medical College and established The Texas Heart Institute of which he is Surgeon-in-Chief. Cooley has been Clinical Professor of Surgery at the University of Texas Medical School since 1975. He was awarded the René Leriche Prize of the International Surgical Society (1965–67); Billings Gold Medal from the American Surgical Society (1967); Vishnevsky Medal, USSR (1971); and Gifted Teacher Award of the American College of Cardiology (1987).

During Cooley's brief appointment at the Brompton Hospital he demonstrated a formidable administrative capacity. Two months after his arrival, Oswald Tubbs, about to undergo lobectomy for tuberculosis, asked Cooley to ensure that Brock crushed his phrenic nerve (a technique Brock seldom employed) in exchange for which, Tubbs would let Cooley run his department until he recovered. Accordingly, at operation, Cooley reached over Brock's shoulder and crushed the nerve himself. With progress which has since become legendary, Cooley reorganized Tubbs's practice, doubled the operating schedule, pressed the cardiologists for more rapid diagnoses, mobilized post-operative patients sooner and persuaded the operating room personnel to work overtime. When Tubbs returned, the "Cooley method" had won the approval of everyone at Brompton Hospital. Whilst displaying great technical skill in operative surgery, Cooley was less adept with the rigid bronchoscope. One day whilst in difficulties an experienced and humerous operating theatre technician made the legendary suggestion "Mr Cooley, you hold the bronchoscope still and I will thread the patient over it !"

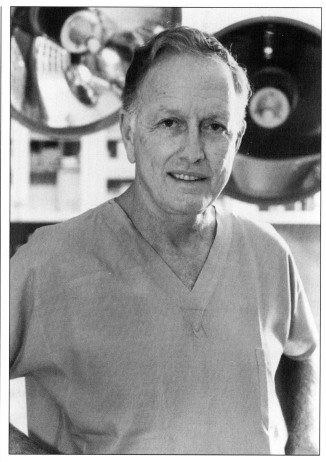

Figure 6.18. Denton Arthur Cooley.

Together with DeBakey, Cooley pioneered the removal of aortic aneurysms by resection with graft replacement. Of his early experience in this field, Cooley wrote:

"While a senior resident at Johns Hopkins, I was confronted with a patient who had previously undergone coarctation repair by Dr Alfred Blalock. The patient was known to have an aneurysm of the aortic arch, involving predominantly the right subclavian artery. The lesion was expanding and had become painful. Dr Blalock was in Hawaii as a visiting professor. I decided to do something which was considered desperate in those days, namely to excise the aneurysm and sacrifice the subclavian artery. The operation was performed successfully in 1950. When Dr Blalock returned from Hawaii, he stated that he was

astonished to see the patient presented at Friday rounds. He simply said that if one has a problem which he does not enjoy facing, he should just leave town and hope the residents could take care of it. Of course, this built my morale to the stars.... Shortly after coming to Houston, the first operation which I performed in July 1951, was removal of a large aneurysm off of the aortic arch involving the root of the innominate artery. Excision of this lesion was successful and without complications. Subsequent to that, I removed about six aneurysms off of the aortic arch by tangential excision. My cases were reported at the Southern Surgical meeting in December, 1951. I recall writing to Dr Blalock after that first operation and told him that I was convinced that excisional therapy of aneurysms of the aortic arch was the treatment of choice. He wrote back and said that the project seemed too strenuous for him but that he would mention it to Hank Bahnson...The surgical treatment of aneurysms became the interest of my chief (DeBakey) and his reputation grew rapidly as an expert in this field and deservedly so...”

In the course of evolving a method for circulatory support, Cooley used hypothermia to repair about 12 atrial septal defects with one death from coronary air embolism in 1951. In 1955, after observing Lillehei's cross-circulation with a human donor, Kirklin's Mayo-Gibbon apparatus, Cooley used an oxygenator powered by a Sigmamotor pump to operate on a patient on 5 April 1956 who died 6 weeks later. In those 6 weeks, five other patients with congenital septal defects survived total correction with this support system and 95 patients by the end of 1956. Later that year, Cooley described the first replacement of the ascending aorta using the pump oxygenator in the *Journal of American Medical Association* (Article 6.3, Appendix A). By this time, Cooley understood that an aggressive approach to aortic aneurysms was justified and necessary. Methods to promote thrombosis by

introduction of foreign material, or extirpation of the lesion without restoration of blood flow were not applicable to ascending aortic aneurysms. The limitation on excisional therapy for aneurysms at the time was a need to maintain cardiac function and continuous blood flow through the ascending aorta and transverse arch. Use of cardiopulmonary bypass with hypothermia transformed quite difficult operations into relatively simple plumbing.

Cooley progressed from using Lillehei's Sigmamotor pump to a roller pump, from the DeWall oxygenator to Vincent Gott's simple collapsible oxygenator with two sheets of plastic, and from low flow rates of 3 to 4 litres to high-volume perfusion advocated by Kirklin. In 1957, Cooley produced a reusable stainless steel bubble oxygenator and by 1961, had incorporated a bloodless prime with 5% dextrose and water for the extracorporeal system, allowing the operation of 542 Jehovah's Witness patients. The cumbersome, reusable extracorporeal circuit, primed with blood for patients with congenital heart defects, was left behind for plastic disposable oxygenators and non-blood prime (except in patients weighing less than 20 pounds). From 1963 to 1969, Cooley devised repair of post-infarction ventricular septal defect, excision of left ventricular aneurysms, embolectomy for massive pulmonary embolism, and a shunt between the ascending aorta and right pulmonary artery for cyanotic congenital heart disease. He transplanted 22 hearts between May 1968 and April 1969 but with consistently poor results, implanted two artificial hearts in 1969 and 1981 and helped design several artificial heart valves. Myocardial revascularization for coronary heart disease dominated the third period (1970–79). From 1980 on, Cooley and Kirklin were the dominant characters in cardiovascular surgery, both performing the complete range of adult and paediatric operations, a repertoire inaccessible for most surgeons. Cooley's rapid accurate operations and laconic wit gave him universal popularity and international acclaim. By 1994, Cooley, had performed 60,000 open-heart operations,

---

J.A.M.A., November 17, 1956

RESECTION OF ENTIRE ASCENDING AORTA IN FUSIFORM ANEURYSM USING CARDIAC BYPASS

Denton A. Cooley, M.D.
and
Michael E. De Bakey, M.D., Houston, Texas

Figure 6.19. Title page of Cooley's 1956 article entitled 'Resection of entire ascending aorta in fusiform aneurysm using cardiac bypass.' *(Reproduced with permission from* The Journal of the American Medical Association; *162: 1158–59.)*

certainly more than any other surgeon. He continues operating and research at the Texas Heart Institute where he is now president.

With Frazier, Reule, Ott and others the department is continuously innovative and at the forefront of cardiac surgery.

Transmyocardial laser revascularisation and mechanical circulatory support have their roots in this department. Cooley remains youthful, innovative, technically brilliant and generous in his patronage.

E. Stanley Crawford (1922–1992)

E. STANLEY CRAWFORD was born near Evergreen, Alabama. He studied at Harvard Medical School (MD, 1946) and served at the Massachusetts General Hospital as surgical intern, resident and Chief Resident (1953–54). His mentors were Edward Churchill, Richard Sweet and Arthur Allen, the last of whom encouraged Crawford to become a vascular surgeon. He joined DeBakey at Baylor College of Medicine in 1954 and practised there for 38 years. Crawford added immeasurably to the understanding of complex diseases of the aorta. Surgeons throughout the United States and abroad visited Houston to see Crawford in action. His highly refined surgical techniques and skilled manual dexterity contributed to his worldwide reputation as a master surgeon. His prodigious scholarly productivity has been documented by more than 300 publications and book chapters. The textbook, *Diseases of the Aorta*, which he co-authored with his surgeon son, John Lloyd Crawford II, has become a standard reference text on aortic surgery. In the Homans Lecture (1991) given to the Society of Vascular Surgery, he sums up the contributions of his chief, DeBakey, to vascular surgery:

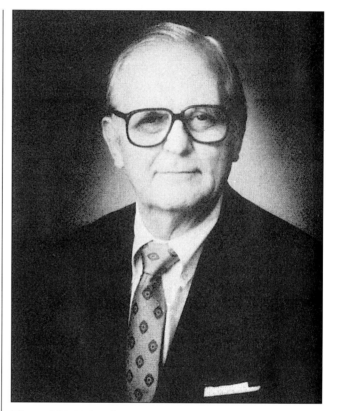

Figure 6.20. E. Stanley Crawford.

"*He was the first to replace an abdominal aortic aneurysm in this country. He and his team performed the first carotid endarterectomy in 1953, the first resection of a descending thoracic aortic aneurysm that same year, and the first graft replacement of the aortic arch with yours truly in 1957. He pioneered the understanding, classification and treatment of dissecting aortic aneurysms and, along with Dr Ed Garrett, performed the first saphenous vein coronary artery bypass procedure in 1967. His development of the roller pump for the bubble oxygenator was a major advance in extracorporeal circulatory technology. Under his leadership, The Baylor College of Medicine and The Texas Medical Center blossomed and gained international prominence in the fields of cardiovascular medicine and surgery...these were indeed exciting times in Houston and in my life.*"

This operation of 21 March 1957 (Article 6.4, Appendix A) took place one year after Cooley's ascending aortic replacement using cardiopulmonary bypass. It was performed at normothermia using cerebral perfusion and cross-clamping of the aorta distal to the left subclavian artery. After excision of the aneurysm, the aorta and roots of the innominate and carotid arteries were reconstituted with an ascending aortic and arch homograft which had the donor innominate and left carotid arteries left *in situ*. The perfusion time was short and the patient woke immediately after the procedure. The surgical team, consisted of DeBakey, Crawford, Cooley and Morris. In practical terms, the aortic homograft was the ideal substitute for this patient, being completely impervious and easy to sew. At the time, other vascular grafts had not been developed. All four surgeons went on to make enormous contributions to the development of vascular surgery in the chest and to pioneer the development of clinically-successful vascular grafts. Crawford was a heavy smoker and died from lung cancer in 1992. He was succeeded in Baylor by his pupil Joseph Coselli who has continued the extraordinarily prolific Baylor aortic practice.

George Cooper Morris, Jr. (1924–)

GEORGE COOPER MORRIS, Jr. was born at Evanston, Illinois. He attended Washington and Lee University (1942–43), Duke University (Navy V-12) (1943–44) and the University of Pennsylvania (MD, 1948). He interned and served residencies in surgical pathology at the University of Pennsylvania Hospital (1948–49) and in general (1950–55) and thoracic surgery (1955–56) at Baylor College of Medicine and Jefferson Davis Hospital. He has been Professor of Surgery at Baylor since 1968. Morris' publications include 300 articles primarily on cardiovascular surgery. He won The Golden Eagle Award (1963) and The Prize Certificate of the American College of Chest Physicians (1964) for the film of the following operation. George Morris wrote:

> "*The patient is now 63 years old, 31 years after the original operation and continues to practice as a surgeon. At the time of my operation, our group had abandoned the Creech re-entry procedure and were not treating this condition surgically. However, I had planned a direct repair for several years if an appropriate patient and opportunity came my way.*
>
> *Interestingly, the patient was a senior fellow with Dr John Kirklin [at the Mayo Clinic] at the time of the catastrophic illness but was on vacation in Louisiana when it occurred [August 1962]. Of further interest, Dr Kirklin, whom I consider the greatest gentleman in American Surgery, was the speaker at the Houston Surgical Society several days after the operation and made rounds with me to visit his assistant.*"

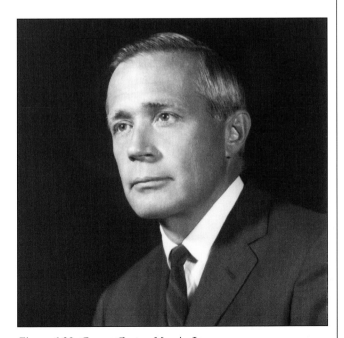

Figure 6.21. George Cooper Morris, Jr.

This case report describes the first successful repair of acute Type A dissection (Article 6.5, Appendix A). The patient was unusually young but did not have Marfan's Syndrome. He presented in August 1962 with severe aortic regurgitation and Morris replaced his aortic valve. In May 1991, the patient was referred back with an abdominal aortic aneurysm and follow-up studies of the thoracic aorta showed a very large ascending aortic aneurysm, with a persistent double lumen in the descending aorta and a saccular dilation at the origin of the hepatic artery. On 3 June 1991, the aortic root (including the previous prosthesis) together with the ascending aorta and proximal aortic arch were resected and replaced with a composite valved conduit by Gerald Lawrie at Baylor. Nine days later Morris resected the hepatic artery aneurysm replacing it with a graft. These events shed considerable light on the natural history of the distal aorta and aortic sinuses after 'successful' surgery for aortic dissection in the acute phase. Persistence of the aortic false lumen with aneurysm formation or free rupture is a common occurrence in the early and late follow-up period.

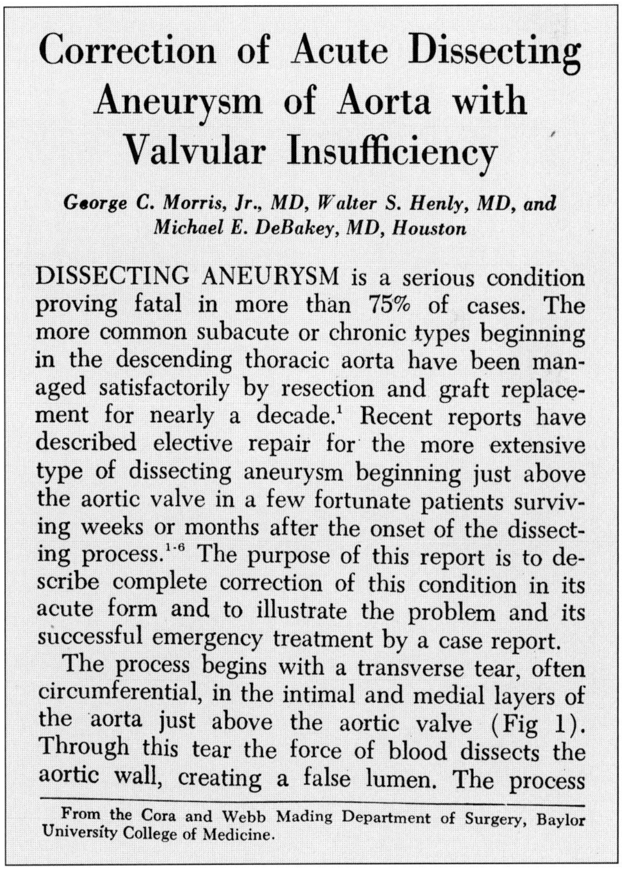

Correction of Acute Dissecting Aneurysm of Aorta with Valvular Insufficiency

George C. Morris, Jr., MD, Walter S. Henly, MD, and Michael E. DeBakey, MD, Houston

DISSECTING ANEURYSM is a serious condition proving fatal in more than 75% of cases. The more common subacute or chronic types beginning in the descending thoracic aorta have been managed satisfactorily by resection and graft replacement for nearly a decade.[1] Recent reports have described elective repair for the more extensive type of dissecting aneurysm beginning just above the aortic valve in a few fortunate patients surviving weeks or months after the onset of the dissecting process.[1-6] The purpose of this report is to describe complete correction of this condition in its acute form and to illustrate the problem and its successful emergency treatment by a case report.

The process begins with a transverse tear, often circumferential, in the intimal and medial layers of the aorta just above the aortic valve (Fig 1). Through this tear the force of blood dissects the aortic wall, creating a false lumen. The process

From the Cora and Webb Mading Department of Surgery, Baylor University College of Medicine.

Figure 6.22. Title page of Morris, Henly and DeBakey's 1963 article 'Correction of acute dissecting aneurysm of aorta with valvular insufficiency.' (Reproduced with permission from Journal of the American Medical Association; *184: 63–64.)*

Myron W. Wheat, Jr. (1924–)

MYRON W. WHEAT, Jr. was born in Sapulpa, Oklahoma. He served as a fighter pilot in the US Air Force (1943–46), earning the distinguished flying cross and the rank of First Lieutenant. He graduated with honours from Washington University Medical School (MD, 1951) and completed his thoracic and cardiovascular surgical internship and residency at Barnes Hospital in St Louis, Missouri in 1958. Wheat became Professor and Chief of Thoracic and Cardiovascular Surgery at the University of Florida College of Medicine (1958–72) and the University of Louisville School of Medicine (1972–75). He was a member of the American Board of Thoracic Surgery (1969–75), Secretary of the American Association for Thoracic Surgeons (1972–78) and Governor of the American College of Surgeons and the American College of Cardiology. His publications include over 100 articles dealing primarily with thoracic and cardiovascular surgery. Since 1975, he has been engaged in the private practice of thoracic and cardiovascular surgery in Clearwater, Florida. Wheat's important contribution on the treatment of dissecting aneurysms (Figure 6.24) was the result of a careful experimental study of the clinical problem and a cumulative effort between physicians and

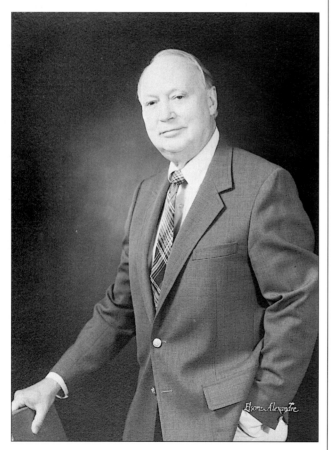

Figure 6.23. Myron W. Wheat, Jr.

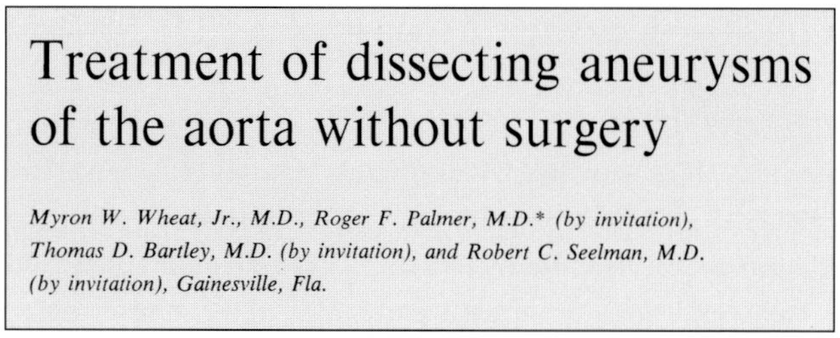

Treatment of dissecting aneurysms of the aorta without surgery

Myron W. Wheat, Jr., M.D., Roger F. Palmer, M.D.* (by invitation), Thomas D. Bartley, M.D. (by invitation), and Robert C. Seelman, M.D. (by invitation), Gainesville, Fla.

Figure 6.24. Title page of Wheat et al. 'Treatment of dissecting aneurysms of the aorta without surgery.' Reproduced with permission from Journal of Thoracic and Cardiovascular Surgery; 50: 364–73.)

pharmacologists. It followed an early bad surgical experience with acute Type A dissection. In Wheat's own words:

"The beginning of intensive drug therapy for acute dissecting aneurysms at the University of Florida in January 1964, was the result of the dismal operative experience with six consecutive patients, all of whom died. Roger Palmer was Assistant Professor of Medicine and Pharmacology. He and I were good friends. One day, I remember walking down the hospital corridor together, shortly after the death of our most recent patient with a dissecting aneurysm. He and I began discussing the problems involved, and as a result of that discussion walking down the hall, the other events followed.

Simpson was in the Veterinary Science Department. We knew of his work in turkeys. This was one of the leading stimuli for us to proceed along the avenues which we did. Certain flocks of turkeys are plagued with naturally occurring dissecting aneurysms. The incidence can be increased by 60% to 75% by adding beta-amino-proprionitrile to the turkey's diet, but this high frequency can be reduced dramatically by the addition of reserpine (0.1 part per million) to the turkey's feed.

Also we were impressed with the natural history of acute dissections. Only 3% of patients died immediately; untreated, the mortality rate rose rapidly to 21% in 24 hours; 60% in 2 weeks. The cause of death was not the intimal tear but the extension of the dissecting haematoma.

The next step was a clinical trial. The next six consecutive patients with acute dissections were treated with an intensive drug regimen. All six survived and were initially reported 1½ years later at the 45th Annual Meeting of the American Association for Thoracic Surgery (1965)."

In a *JAMA* article in 1964, Wheat describes his operation for replacement of the aortic valve and entire ascending aorta including the aortic sinuses — the first aortic replacement before that of Bentall. Only the coronary buttons were left in continuity with the aortic annulus. A Starr–Edwards valve was inserted into the subcoronary position and then a Teflon aortic prosthesis sewn into place over the coronary buttons but around the Teflon skirt of the valve prosthesis. This was the forerunner of aortic root replacement and was also described by Cooley, Bloodwell, Beall, Hallman and DeBakey in 1966.

William C. Roberts (1932–)

WILLIAM C. ROBERTS was born in Atlanta, Georgia, the son of Stewart R. Roberts, Clinical Professor of Medicine at Emory University School of Medicine. He studied at Southern Methodist University in Dallas, Texas (AB, 1954) and Emory University School of Medicine, Atlanta, Georgia (MD, 1958). He interned at Boston City Hospital (1958–59) and served residency in anatomical pathology at the National Cancer Institute in Bethesda, Maryland (1959–62). Roberts pursued further training in internal medicine as assistant resident on the Osler Medical Service at Johns Hopkins Hospital (1962–63). He gained additional experience in surgery (6 months) and cardiology (6 months) at the National Heart Institute (1963–64). He then began his productive career as the cardiovascular pathologist at the National Heart, Lung and Blood Institute, a position which offered him a chance to work closely with the Institute's excellent cardiologists and in return, support the Institute as an excellent spokesman. Roberts holds clinical faculty posts at Georgetown, George Washington, Howard and Hahnemann Universities, as well as other medical institutions in the Washington area. He is currently Chief, Pathology Branch, National Heart, Lung and Blood Institute.

Between October 1960 and June 1991 Roberts gave 1942 lectures in 1180 cities in the United States and abroad; in one 25-year period (July 1966–June 1991), he gave an average of 1½ major lectures a week. He edited *Congenital Heart Disease in Adults* in 1979 and since 1982, has served as Editor-in-Chief of *The American Journal of Cardiology*, where he has written 100 *From the Editor* columns, demonstrating a remarkable ability to push forward any idea he believed in.

Among other awards, Roberts has received The Gifted Teachers Award from The American College of Cardiology (1978) and the Richard and Hinda Rosenthal Foundation Award from The American Heart Association in 1984. He also received The Eugene H. Drake Memorial Award, Maine affiliate, for significant contributions in cardiovascular disease research and treatment. His article published in the *Journal of Thoracic and Cardiovascular Surgery* (1965) is an important and scholarly contribution to the literature on aortic dissection (Figure 6.26). Roberts' skill in correlating pathological and clinical data has created a bridge between pathology and medicine. He has made pathology live for the cardiologist and internist. Relatively few individuals have had Roberts' impact in

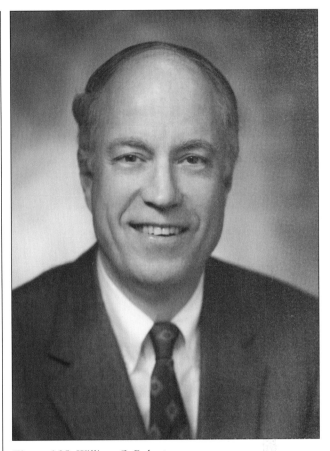

Figure 6.25. William C. Roberts.

CURRICULUM IN CARDIOLOGY

Aortic dissection: Anatomy, consequences, and causes

William C. Roberts, M.D. *Bethesda, Md.*

Despite its recognition at necropsy over 200 years ago and its recognition clinically about 50 years ago, aortic dissection remains a poorly understood condition. Because its anatomic features have received relatively little attention in recent years, this report will focus on them and on the major consequences and causes of aortic dissection.

a single tear serves as both the entrance to and the exit from the false channel. In this circumstance, flow within the false channel may be both retrograde and anterograde.

Once blood under pressure enters the media via the intimal and medial tear, the time required thereafter to dissect the media of the entire length of the aorta appears to be only one or a few seconds.

Figure 6.26. Title page of Robert's 1981 article 'Aortic dissection: anatomy, consequences, and causes.' *(Reproduced with permission from* American Heart Journal; *101: 195–214.)*

this important endeavour. He has studied many aspects of congenital, hypertensive and coronary heart disease, cardiomyopathy and valvular heart disease. He has correlated electrocardiographic and haemodynamic abnormalities with pathologic findings. Roberts gives strong support to modifying risk factors to prevent atherosclerotic coronary disease and advocates the individual's awareness of his weight, blood pressure and blood lipids. Roberts believed that aortic dissection was a "catastrophic cardiovascular event which in the vast majority of patients is entirely preventable by proper treatment of systemic hypertension."

Chapter 7: The beginnings of cardiac transplantation

"Thus sayeth the Lord God, 'A new heart also will I give you, and a new spirit will I put within you; and I will take away the stony heart out of your flesh, and I will give you a heart of flesh'"
(Ezekiel, chapter 36, verse 26)

UNDOUBTEDLY, Ezekiel was speaking metaphorically, but perhaps he had insight into the stony nature of coronary and valve calcification, which produces some of the conditions for which transplantation is the only treatment.

Legend has it that in the 3rd century BC, Pien Ch'iao, a Chinese doctor, slipped a hypnotic potion into the drinks of two soldiers. Whilst they slept, he removed and swapped a number of internal organs, including their hearts. The soldiers awoke 3 days later, none the worse for their experience. Further legendary transplants were carried out by the twin brothers Cosmos and Damian, who after their martyrdom in the 3rd century AD, became the patron saints of surgery (Figure 7.1). The brothers were said to have removed the cancerous leg of a white man and replaced it with the leg of a recently deceased Moor, found in the local cemetery. The following morning, the patient had trouble convincing his colleagues, despite the different colour of his leg. Returning to the Moor grave, they discovered the cancerous leg buried there.

Aristotle considered the heart to be the seat of the soul, emotions and intellect, despite the contrary belief of the Greeks and Romans that this status belonged to the liver. Aristotle's views prevailed into the 20th century, and made it difficult to debate clinical cardiac transplantation dispassionately. Since Barnard's first operation in December 1967, ethical problems, including definition of brain death, age limits and transracial transplantation, have continued to hold the interest of the press.

Carrell and Guthrie

IN 1912, Charles Guthrie, Professor of Physiology and Pharmacology at the University of Pittsburg, opened the chapter on transplantation in his textbook, *Blood Vessel Surgery and its Applications* with the words,

"Transplantation of protoplasm is the widest occurrence in nature. The very existence of the higher plants and animals is proof of this, for it is through transplantation of protoplasm (fertilization, as it is called) that such organisms originate."

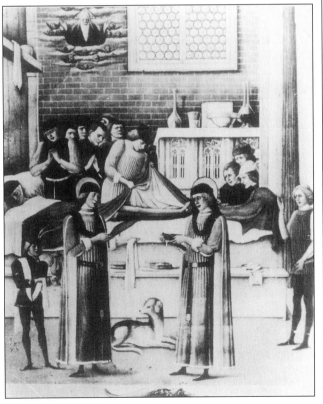

Figure 7.1. Cosmos and Damien: patron saints of surgery.

During the previous 7 years, working with the surgeon Alexis Carrell at the University of Chicago, he had experimentally transplanted a vast array of tissues and organs. They realized that the key to successful transplantation was reliable vascular suture, in order to provide the organ with an adequate blood supply. In 1902, only 21 successful arterial anastomoses had been reported in humans. Suture techniques were largely gut-orientated, using absorbable catgut. When blood vessels required suture repair, small intestinal needles and thin gut were used and the vessels stitched as though they were intestines. The few apparent successes provided little information, as thrombosis of an artery did not always result in death of the tissues, particularly if collateral circulation existed.

In 1905, Guthrie and Carrell perfected vascular suture using small tapered needles of polished steel, together with fine silk thread or human hair. They recognized the need to pass sutures through all coats of the vessel wall and were meticulous in their anastomotic technique. Between them, they transplanted kidneys, adrenals, thyroids, parathyroids, ovaries, legs, arms, loops of intestine, the lower half of a body, the head and neck and the heart. Their aim was to study physiological aspects of transplanted organs in the recipient animal. Fowl and guineapigs gave birth after receiving new ovaries, and cats and dogs lived for several weeks after intra-abdominal transplantation of both kidneys. A successful ovary transplant was also reported by Robert Morris (1906), after the birth of a child to a woman whose ovaries had been removed and replaced with those of a donor 4 years previously.

Experimental cardiac transplantation

GUTHRIE AND CARRELL also performed heart transplants into the necks of recipient animals (1905). These were complicated by the fact that the heart required a blood supply via the coronary arteries, as well as functional flow through the cardiac chambers. They initially joined the aortic stump of the donor heart to the central end of the recipient's transected, common carotid artery, and anastomosed the stump of the donor's superior vena cava to the central end of the recipient's external jugular vein. This provided a coronary blood supply and drained blood entering the right atrium from the coronary sinus. In subsequent experiments, the donor pulmonary veins were joined to the peripheral end of the transected, common carotid artery, and the aorta was joined to the central end of the carotid artery. The vena cava was then anastomosed to the peripheral end of the recipient's cut jugular vein and the pulmonary artery to the peripheral end of the carotid or the jugular vein on the other side of the neck. This arrangement allowed each side of the donor heart to receive an appropriate arterial or venous blood supply, and to work against normal pressures. Circulation was re-established through the donor heart about 75 minutes after removal, and 20 minutes later, the coronary circulation resumed. An hour after the operation, the donor ventricles were contracting at 80 beats per minute, compared with the recipient's rate of 130 per minute. The experiment ended 2 hours later, when blood began to clot in the donor heart chambers.

Their final experiment was to transplant the lungs and heart of a one-week-old kitten into the neck of an adult cat. Carrell wrote of this venture,

"The aorta was anastomosed to the peripheral end of the carotid, and the vena cava to the peripheral end of the jugular vein. The coronary circulation was immediately re-established and the auricles began to beat. The lungs became red and the ventricles began to contract strongly; oedema of the lungs soon appeared and the right heart became distended. Owing to infection, the examination was discontinued 2 days later."

Carrell and Guthrie realized from their success with autotransplants that the rapid destruction of the grafted tissues (despite an intact blood supply) was due not to severance of the nerve supply but to some toxic effect of the host's blood on the graft tissues. They considered rejection of the transplanted organs to be due to 'biotoxins', and believed that a preliminary process of immunization of the donor or recipient, or both, might overcome this problem. The importance of blood groups for blood transfusion had been established by Landsteiner many years before. Nevertheless, it was not until 1944 that Peter Medawar demonstrated that the rejection of skin grafts was due to an immunological reaction. By the end of the 1950s, the same mechanism was shown to be a cause of rejection of the transplanted organs.

Cornea and bone were transplanted without vascular

anastomosis in the early part of the century, but there were only a few abortive attempts to transplant animal kidneys into human patients before the discovery of immunosuppressant drugs in the 1960s. The stimulus for renal transplantation began with the remarkable achievements of Wilhelm Kolff, who developed renal dialysis during the Nazi occupation of Holland in 1944. Kolff constructed an artificial kidney using a dialysing membrane of sausage skins. Once the technical imperfections of the machine were overcome, haemodialysis was used to improve the general condition of endstage renal failure patients prior to transplantation, a use later applied to the artificial heart. It also provided a safety net, should the kidney fail or be rejected.

Mann's incidental discoveries

IN 1933, Frank Mann of Rochester, Minnesota, stimulated further interest in cardiac transplantation whilst researching a denervated heart model with Makovitz from Georgetown University. Their aim was to eliminate the role of the central nervous system during research on the chronotropic action of drugs such as thyroxine. They transplanted canine hearts into the carotid-jugular circulation, using methods similar to those of Carrell and Guthrie. Mann emphasized the importance of restoring the coronary circulation as quickly as possible. If reperfusion was delayed, the heart muscle lost its tone and the valves failed to function. He managed to achieve an ischaemic time of less than 5 minutes between disconnection of the coronary circulation in the donor's body and re-implantation in the recipient. He found that if the donor aorta was joined to the peripheral end of the recipient's carotid artery (rather than the central end, as Carrell had done), the donor heart performed better, without incompetence of the aortic valve. Only the right side of the heart was made functional by anastomosing the donor pulmonary artery to the recipient's jugular vein. The blood ejected by the right ventricle then came from coronary sinus return.

In successful experiments, cardiac action started at once with a constant rate of between 100 and 130 beats per minute. This was seen to increase by 15 beats per minute on exercise. Mann's longest surviving transplant recipient lasted for 8 days; the average survival was 4 days. Though transplantation was incidental to his experimental aims, Mann's findings were a landmark in transplantation research.

Failures early after transplantation were usually due to distension of the heart before a regular rhythm could be established. The mode of failure after 4 days was characteristic. The rhythm became irregular, followed by fibrillation and cardiac arrest. Histological examination of the excised hearts showed mottling and ecchymoses, infiltration with lymphocytes, large mononuclear cells and polymorphonuclear leucocytes. Oedema fluid collected around the transplanted heart, and (if transplanted with the pericardium intact) required drainage. Mann postulated that a 'biological factor' was the cause of death and correctly described the cytological basis of acute organ rejection.

Interest in cardiac transplantation, as distinct from the denervated heart as a model, resumed in 1951, when Marcus, Wong and Luisada, working at the Chicago Medical School, reported their experience with a modified Mann preparation:

> *"The problem which we are attempting to explore can be stated as follows: Can a combination of highly specialized tissues, the heart, be grafted in a mammalian animal? Can such a graft live in an homologous environment? Can such a graft actually function by receiving and delivering blood? Whether it might so function as to replace its counterpart in the host is a matter of fantastic speculation for the future."*

Marcus focused on the problem of donor organ preservation. He performed bilateral cervical vagotomy and cocaine injection into the pericardium prior to harvesting the heart, in an attempt to reduce dysrhythmias and ventricular distension. Realizing that an ischaemic period was harmful, he elaborated a system of 'interim parabiotic perfusion'. The results were disappointing, with only 10 survivors from 22 technically successful transplants, and a maximum survival time of 48 hours. In 1953, the same workers modified the Mann preparation again, so that the donor left ventricle would act as a pump. In this preparation, the proximal end of the divided recipient common carotid artery was anastomosed to the donor's left atrium, and the recipient's distal common carotid to the donor's innominate artery. In this way, the donor's left ventricle supplied blood to its own coronary arteries and to the recipient's cerebral circulation. Although maximum survival with this technique was still only 48 hours, this experimental preparation remained a valuable tool for evaluating the transplanted heart.

The intrepid Demikhov

MEANWHILE, unbeknown to the West, Vladimir Demikhov performed many remarkable transplant experiments at the Moscow State University. In the 1940s, he began transplanting hearts into the inguinal region using Carrell's technique of blood-vessel suture. His efforts were halted by World War II, but he resumed in 1946, and decided to transplant the heart into the thorax as an auxiliary pump. Between February 1946 and July 1958, Demikhov carried out 250 experiments in 24 different ways. His aim was to determine the best vascular connections to achieve filling of both sides of the transplanted heart. To accommodate the new heart in the chest he removed different parts of the recipient dog's lungs. A lobe of the donor lung was sometimes included to reduce the number of anastomoses. The longest survivor was a dog named Borzoi, who received a second heart on 4 October 1956. Although myocardial infarction occurred in the transplant several days after surgery, Borzoi survived to resume an active life and ECGs taken at the expected time of rejection showed no alteration. The dog was eventually put down at 32 days when the transplanted heart started to fibrillate.

Demikhov persisted in the face of substantial early operative mortality. He had no heart–lung machine or other support techniques and attributed his success to effective anaesthesia, controlled respiration and the maintenance of systemic blood pressure. For the latter he used temporary compression of the aorta and intra-arterial transfusion. He was perturbed by the length of time needed for multiple anastomoses as this led to cerebral hypoxia. He therefore embarked on a second series of experiments in which the heart and lungs were transplanted as a unit. With two animals lying side-by-side, he used rubber tubes and temporary anastomoses in such a way that the operation could be carried out without interrupting the circulation to either the recipient animal or the donor organs. Fifteen attempts were needed before Demikhov could sustain an animal throughout the whole procedure. His first success was in

October 1946, when the recipient lived for 2 hours supported by its new heart and lungs. In 1951, after 67 operations, he achieved a post-operative survival of 6 days in a bitch called Damka. The most common causes of death were thrombosis and embolism from the heart or infection in the transplanted lungs. The high incidence of pulmonary infection eventually caused Demikhov to restrict transplantation to the heart. Dogs have more pulmonary veins than humans, and to overcome the problem of individual venous anastomosis, he separated the left atrium from the right and left the whole of the recipient's left atrium in its body.

As well as cardiac transplantation, Demikhov performed a series of notorious operations by transplanting puppies' heads and necks onto the necks of adult dogs. The transplanted heads apparently reacted normally to their surroundings and would lap up water when thirsty. When the donor preparation included the four legs, these sometimes gave running movements. The longest survival in this bizarre undertaking was 29 days. Demikhov also transplanted the kidneys, adrenals, the whole of the gastrointestinal tract, the pancreas and the liver. He transplanted the lower half of the body, which he believed offered the opportunity to transplant all the organs in one operation. Because of language and other barriers, Demikhov's work was unknown in the West until 1962, when his book (first published in Russian in 1960) was translated into English. By this time, Western scientists had overtaken many of his principles of transplantation. David Wheatley, Professor of Cardiac Surgery in Glasgow (but a student in Cape Town at the time [1962]) recalls sitting in the surgeon's changing room when a report of Demikhov's head transplant appeared in the Cape Argos newspaper. The news was conveyed to Christiaan Barnard who was clearly put out. He stormed out with the retort that anything those Russians can do we can do too. The same afternoon Barnard transplanted the head of a dog onto a recipient dog, which survived for several days. Animal rights protestors were incensed and the medical students built a papier mâché two-headed dog for their rag parade. Barnard had already walked the tight rope between genius and vulgarity.

The Marcus operations

MARCUS, meanwhile, continued to refine his transplants

by crossmatching the blood of donor and recipient animals to reduce the risk of rejection. In the Marcus II operation, the anastomoses were arranged to provide bloodflow through both sides of the heart. The left ventricle could then sustain a blood pressure sufficient to perfuse its own coronary arteries. His first 22 experiments with this technique were all successful, though none of the donor hearts continued to beat for more than 48 hours (due to acute rejection). With increasing experience and improved technique they eventually managed to prolong graft survival for up to 6 days.

The Marcus III procedure was more ambitious still, as it involved transplantation of the donor heart and lungs into the lower abdomen. The donor trachea was led to the surface through a hole in the recipient's abdominal wall, and this allowed artificial respiration to be carried out. This remarkable arrangement was able to sustain life in the recipient animal, even when its own heart and lungs were excluded from circulation. The maximum survival time (in eight experiments) was 9 hours. Marcus had avoided ischaemia in the transplanted organs by parabiotic perfusion. This employed a third animal to supply a temporary blood supply to the graft. Contact between the donor heart and the tissues of the recipient was prevented by wrapping the heart in non-irritant cellophane. This made no difference to the outcome.

The 1950s brought great interest in hypothermia as a therapeutic technique, largely due to the pioneering efforts of Bigelow. Before this, experimental cardiac transplantation had been predominantly heterotopic. Orthotopic transplantation awaited a solution to the problem of ischaemic necrosis during the critical transfer period (between donor heart excision and implantation). Before cardiopulmonary bypass, the potential orthotopic recipient could not be maintained for the duration of surgery.

Simplified surgical methods

FOR ORTHOTOPIC CARDIAC TRANSPLANTA-TION, a simplified surgical method was required to avoid the multiple anastomoses of pulmonary veins and venae cavae. By 1952, Brian Cookson, Wilford Neptune and Charles Bailey were able to use systemic hypothermia to stop an animal's circulation completely for 30 minutes without harm. If the animal's organs were

mobilized before the circulatory arrest, it was possible to perform exchange of organs in less than 15 minutes. This group performed three animal experiments in which dogs were cooled to temperatures between 21 and 25°C in a beverage cooler. The entire heart–lung block was then transplanted to avoid multiple pulmonary venous anastomoses. The aortas were anastomosed first and then the superior venae cavae. These were temporarily joined by sliding them over a polyethylene tube, thereby restoring partial circulation. An endotracheal tube was inserted for artificial respiration, and the inferior venae cavae were temporarily connected in the same way as the superior venae cavae. This restored the complete circulation and, with the new heart beating satisfactorily, tracheal and vena caval anastomoses were performed by direct suture. The first two animals died shortly after the operation, but the third dog lived for 6 hours with its new heart maintaining the circulation. Spontaneous respiration was resumed, the ECG was normal (at 24°C) and the reflexes returned. The cause of death was never established.

Bailey's claim that this was the first time a transplanted heart had fully supported the recipient's circulation irritated Demikhov, who failed to understand why knowledge of his work had not reached the West. By 1955, Demikhov had performed 67 orthotopic transplants of the heart–lung block without cardiopulmonary bypass or hypothermia. He also anastomosed the donor aorta first, followed by the superior and inferior venae cavae. The pulmonary artery was anastomosed end-to-side to the recipient and the inferior pulmonary veins of the donor were joined together and anastomosed to the recipient's left atrial appendage. When all anastomoses were complete, the proximal aorta and pulmonary artery of the recipient were ligated, and the recipient's left atrium closed by a pursestring suture at the atrioventricular groove. Once the recipient's heart had been excluded, it was excised. Demikhov had only two survivors (up to 15 hours) with a circulation supported entirely by the transplanted heart.

In 1957, Webb and Howard reported on *Restoration of function of the refrigerated heart*. They demonstrated that canine hearts, heparinized and flushed with potassium citrate, could survive for prolonged periods at low temperatures (4°C), and subsequently regain function when transplanted heterotopically (Marcus II technique). Anticipating long-distance heart procurement, Webb and Howard commented that when the problems of immunology were solved and transplantation became a clinical possibility, it would presumably take several hours to obtain the heart, prepare the recipient and perform re-implantation. Consequently, their methods for myocardial protection seemed to render clinical cardiac transplantation feasible, as far as the time element was concerned.

Introduction of cardiopulmonary bypass by Gibbon then greatly increased the feasibility of cardiac transplantation. In Puerto Rico, a group led by the head of Bailey's research laboratory, Gumersindo Blanco, employed a pump oxygenator to sustain the transplant recipient and elective potassium citrate arrest of the donor heart during the ischaemic period. Their anastomotic technique was similar to that of Cookson's, and soon after restoring coronary bloodflow, the transplanted heart began to beat vigorously. Six of eight operations were completed and in these cases, the new heart worked effectively for a few hours. Again, the cause of failure was not understood. Nevertheless, activity in the field intensified, resulting in an ever increasing number of papers on every aspect of cardiac transplantation.

In 1958, Goldberg, Burman and Akman, at the University of Maryland, reported on three experimental orthotopic cardiac transplants. Their major contribution was to transect the left atrium and circumvent the need to individually anastomose each of the pulmonary veins. The recipient heart was excised, leaving a posterior cuff of left atrium which contained the openings of all four pulmonary veins. Consequently, only one relatively simple left atrial anastomosis was required. The venae cavae were reconnected with synthetic tubes and the aorta and pulmonary arteries re-anastomosed by direct suture. The recipient animal's circulation was maintained with cardiopulmonary bypass during the transfer of the donor heart, which was arrested with potassium citrate prior to excision. The ischaemic times ranged from 25 to 35 minutes and hypothermia was not employed. The maximum duration of circulatory support by the transplanted heart was 20 minutes.

In 1959, Webb, Howard and Nielly accomplished 12 successful orthotopic transplants, using hypothermia to preserve the donor heart and the pump oxygenator to maintain the recipient. They first sutured the aortic and pulmonary anastomoses. The individual pulmonary veins were then joined using vascular couplers, but they also suggested that the pulmonary venous anastomoses could be facilitated by leaving an atrial cuff around all four veins.

Also in 1959, Ross and Brock, of Guy's Hospital in London, described six different methods of cardiac excision and replacement. This work was significant as it included the method by which the native heart was separated from both the venae cavae and pulmonary veins by sectioning the walls of the atria. This formed both right and left atrial cuffs, and was the first method to reduce the multiple pulmonary venous and venae caval anastomoses to two atrial anastomoses.

Lower and Shumway

THE FOLLOWING YEAR, Lower and Shumway published the cardinal paper on orthotopic cardiac transplantation, in which advances in surgical technique, recipient support and donor organ preservation were integrated into a single approach. The recipient animal underwent cardiopulmonary bypass with moderate hypothermia (30°C), induced by surface cooling. Hypothermia was also employed for donor heart preservation by rapidly immersing the excised heart in iced saline (4°C) for 5 minutes. The heart was implanted using direct suture anastomoses for every aspect, with ischaemic times averaging 1 hour. Ischaemia was minimized by combining the pulmonary venous and venae caval suture lines into two atrial cuff anastomoses. Of eight consecutive dog transplants, five recipients survived between 6 and 21 days. All were functionally restored to eat and exercise normally. This was the first description of a simple and reproducibly successful technique for mammalian orthotopic cardiac transplantation that enabled the recipient animals to return to normal activity. No immunosuppressive agents were given, so that death occurred from rejection and rapid myocardial failure. Histology showed massive infiltration by lymphocytes and interstitial haemorrhage. Lower and Shumway proposed that if the immunological system of the host could be prevented from destroying the heart, in all likelihood it would continue to function adequately for the normal lifespan of the animal. The Stanford surgeons paid no attention to breed when selecting their dogs, and made no attempt to alter their immunological status. At first their animals lived for only a few hours, but this soon became days and in 1961, a dog lived for 21 days.

In tandem with the research on homograft hearts, a great deal of work was performed on autotransplanted hearts, which were excised and then replaced in the same animal. With autotransplantation, the effects of the transplant (e.g. denervation) could be studied without the intrusion of rejection. Nevertheless, autotransplant survivors still suffered complications, supposedly due to interruption of the nerve supply and lymphatic connections. Eventually, autotransplant animals survived for 1, 2 and then 5 years, with normal cardiac function and even evidence of autonomic re-innervation.

The advent of immunosuppression

WITH THE ADVENT of immunosuppressive therapy for renal transplantation, attempts were soon underway to prolong the survival of transplanted hearts. Keith Reemtsma, of Tulane University School of Medicine, increased the survival time for recipients of cardiac grafts in the neck from 10 days in untreated (control) animals to 27 days in those treated with methotrexate at the first sign of rejection. Two years later in 1964, he performed heterotopic transplants, inserting the donor heart (in parallel) into the recipient animal's chest. With elective azathioprine immunosuppression, the treated animals lived for up to 32 days, whilst those without treatment lived for less than 10 days. David Blumenstock, of Cooperstown, New York, obtained a 42-day survivor with methotrexate therapy after an orthotopic transplant, though his report in 1963 made no mention of control animals, or the fact that 42 of the 50 dogs died within 24 hours.

Adrian Kantrovitz and co-workers in Maimonides Hospital, Brooklyn, performed orthotopic transplants in 3-month-old puppies and achieved remarkable survival times of 213 days without immunosuppression. This somewhat unexpected and conflicting result was attributed to the relative immunological incompetence of very young animals. When the pump oxygenator was used there were no long-term survivors. In contrast, deep hypothermia without bypass proved to be remarkably successful. The difference was probably due to the adverse effects of cardiopulmonary bypass on the immature animal. Kantrovitz noted that the hearts of long-term survivors showed no histological evidence of rejection, and they steadily grew in size with time, keeping pace with the growth of normal puppies. This was encouraging data for the eventual application of heart transplants in infants. Although others adopted Kantrovitz's methods, none achieved comparable results and attention was focused on immunosuppressive therapy.

In the early 1960s, the range of drugs was limited and the experimental results discouraging. Among the best were those of Richard Lower, who had moved from Stanford to the University of Virginia. In 1967, he described long-term survival of orthotopic transplanted hearts in dogs using methotrexate (up to 15 months). A transplanted bitch even gave birth to a litter of healthy puppies, the father of which also had a heart transplant. Lower and Shumway used the prolonged survival of human renal transplant recipients to justify their cardiac homografts. Shumway commented, "Enough has been achieved in fact to provoke expression of the concept that only the immunological barrier lies between this day and a radical new era in the treatment of cardiac diseases."

By the mid-1960s, cardiopulmonary bypass techniques, myocardial protection and post-operative care had improved considerably. Methods for diagnosing and treating rejection were increasingly available. The basis for clinical cardiac transplantation was therefore established, though the legal and logistic issues were unexplored. That which Brock had considered a 'fantastic dream' in the late 1950s was about to become reality.

Clinical cardiac transplantation

THE FIRST HUMAN CARDIAC TRANSPLANT took place in 1964 at the University of Mississippi Medical Centre, Jackson. James Hardy and his team felt that progress in transplantation research overall justified a planned approach towards cardiac transplantation in humans. However, the first human recipient did not receive a human heart. Hardy was expecting the donor heart to be obtained from a relatively young patient dying of brain damage; the recipient was a patient with terminal myocardial failure. The key issue was how soon after cardiac standstill could the donor's heart be removed? If this was not done promptly, irreversible ischaemic damage might occur.

In an attempt to avert irreversible ischaemic damage, Hardy planned to insert catheters into the donor's femoral vessels and begin total body perfusion as soon as death was pronounced. He presumed that if the relatives were willing to donate the heart for transplantation, they would not object to heparinization and insertion of perfusion catheters under local anaesthetic just prior to death. The logistics of the time clearly did not include the concept of brain death: only cardiorespiratory arrest constituted legal demise. Consequently, unless the donor's clinicians were willing to suspend mechanical support, it was exceedingly unlikely that a potential donor would die within the limits during which a patient could be kept alive on a pump oxygenator. Since Hardy and his colleagues were unwilling to turn off the donor's ventilator, they formulated a contingency plan to use the heart of a lower primate.

Hardy had spent many years in basic animal research and had performed mock operations on human cadavers so that his team was prepared. He had performed the first human lung transplant (on 11 June 1963) and had also gained experience with immunosuppression using both drugs and cobalt radiotherapy. The transplanted lung worked well, but the patient died 18 days later from pre-existing renal failure. Post-mortem showed no evidence of pulmonary rejection and this relative success, together with knowledge of Reamer's use of primate kidneys for renal heterotransplants, gave Hardy confidence that a chimpanzee heart would provide suitable backup should homotransplantation fail.

Their first potential transplant recipient (January 1964) was a 36-year-old man whom we would now consider completely unsuitable. He presented one year after surgical closure of a left ventricular knife wound, having suffered recurrent cerebral emboli, permanent right hemiplegia, severe mental impairment and urinary and faecal incontinence. Amputation of the left leg for gangrene was followed several months later by amputation of the right leg. He had also suffered a recent intra-abdominal catastrophe. Hardy had already purchased two large chimpanzees for possible use as kidney donors when no human kidney was available. The cardiac output of the largest chimpanzee was 4.25 litres/min. The legless patient weighed 33.1 kg and the chimpanzee weighed 43.5 kg. Eventually, this patient did not undergo transplantation, but soon afterwards a second potential candidate was referred.

This was a 68-year-old man with hypertension and lower leg gangrene. He had been admitted, pulseless and comatose, but was resuscitated. Further management included tracheostomy, mechanical ventilation, femoral embolectomy and below-knee amputation. Elsewhere in the hospital, a young patient was dying of irreversible brain damage, but not quickly enough for this transplant. The team were therefore faced with the same legal and logistic problems as before. The chances that both prospective donor and recipient would enter terminal decline simultaneously were very slim. Eventually, the prospective recipient went into shock and it was obvious that if a heart transplant was to be performed, it should be done at once. The condition of the prospective donor had not yet deteriorated to the state where death was imminent. Consequently, the recipient was placed on cardiopulmonary bypass and the larger chimpanzee was anaesthetized in an adjacent operating room. Shumway's transplant guidelines were used, apart from the fact that donor graft preservation was obtained by retrograde coronary sinus perfusion with chilled oxygenated blood. The transplant itself was technically satisfactory, but the monkey's heart was unable to maintain the circulatory load. The patient died approximately one hour after discontinuing cardiopulmonary bypass, despite vigorous attempts at circulatory support. The outcome of this operation was never widely discussed.

In 1966, Lower performed mirror-image experiments of Hardy's transplant, whereby human cadaver hearts were resuscitated after kidney harvesting and implanted in baboons. In one such experiment, the resuscitated heart provided satisfactory circulatory support in the monkey for several hours. This was never reported in the medical literature, but Shumway and others were aware of Lower's experiments, which confirmed that the heart could be stopped, removed, resuscitated and successfully transplanted.

By the summer of 1967, Shumway considered that the three most crucial problems associated with cardiac transplantation had been addressed and solved. These were the development of a workable surgical procedure, cardiopulmonary bypass to maintain the recipient's circulation and a therapeutic regime to moderate the body's immunological response. In an interview for the *Journal of the American Medical Association*, Shumway stated that the time was right for human heart transplantation, if a potential recipient and compatible donor could be found simultaneously. Indeed, Shumway had a 35-year-old man with endstage cardiac disease in hospital and awaiting transplantation at the time. This patient had undergone extensive radiotherapy for Hodgkin's disease and already had a depressed immunological system. Shumway was eagerly awaiting a donor. The interview was published in November and shortly afterwards Adrian Kantrovitz in New York sent out 500 telegrams in search of a donor. Nevertheless, it was Christiaan Barnard who was first past the post with his transplant on 9 December 1967.

Barnard and the operation in Cape Town

PRIOR TO the first successful transplant, Chris Barnard and his brother Marius had studied the Shumway method of preserving as much of the atria and interatrial septum as possible in the recipient animal. Chris had also spent some time with Lower before his first human transplant and had already performed a kidney transplant.

In 1967, South African law allowed organ removal if the donor was declared dead by two doctors, one of whom should have been qualified for more than 5 years. Neither of the doctors could be in the transplant team. Death itself was not defined and it was possible to use the concept of irreversible brain damage. Permission was obtained from either the relatives or the coroner. Barnard was well prepared for the operation and chose a potential recipient, Louis Waskansky, with endstage cardiac failure not amenable to conventional treatment. In fact, Waskansky's angiograms had been sent to the Cleveland Clinic for an opinion on the feasibility of coronary grafting and he had been deemed inoperable. This philosophy was slightly different from that in the US, where surgeons anticipated cardiac transplantation for an on-table surgical failure. Barnard elected not to use either a black donor or recipient because of potential criticism.

The donor for the first transplant was a 25-year-old ledger machinist, Denise Anne Darvall. She was shopping in Cape Town with her mother, when a car left the road and hit both women. Mrs Darvall was killed immediately. Denise sustained serious head injuries and was admitted to a local hospital, resuscitated and transferred to the neurosurgeons at Groote Schuur Hospital.

The recipient, Louis Waskansky, was a 54-year-old diabetic who had sustained three previous myocardial infarctions in 1959, 1960 and 1965, which had irreparably damaged the left ventricle (Figure 7.2). He was now in intractable heart failure and readily agreed to transplantation. In many respects, he was a poor candidate, because of diabetes, gross ascites and *Pseudomonas* cellulitis, where metal Southay's cannulae had been inserted into the groin to drain oedema. However, donor and recipient blood groups were compatible and Denise Darvall had a similar leucocyte antigen pattern to Waskansky's.

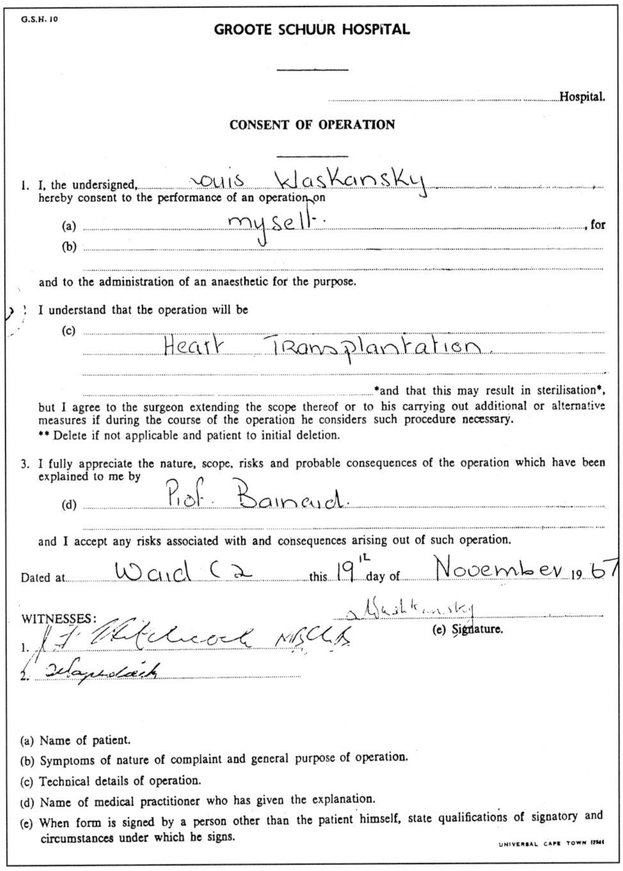
G.S.H. 10

GROOTE SCHUUR HOSPITAL

............Hospital.

CONSENT OF OPERATION

1. I, the undersigned, Louis Waskansky hereby consent to the performance of an operation on
(a) myself, for
(b)
and to the administration of an anaesthetic for the purpose.

2. I understand that the operation will be
(c) Heart Transplantation.
and that this may result in sterilisation, but I agree to the surgeon extending the scope thereof or to his carrying out additional or alternative measures if during the course of the operation he considers such procedure necessary.
** Delete if not applicable and patient to initial deletion.

3. I fully appreciate the nature, scope, risks and probable consequences of the operation which have been explained to me by
(d) Prof. Barnard.
and I accept any risks associated with and consequences arising out of such operation.

Dated at Ward C2 this 19th day of November 1967

WITNESSES:
1.
2.

(e) Signature.

(a) Name of patient.
(b) Symptoms of nature of complaint and general purpose of operation.
(c) Technical details of operation.
(d) Name of medical practitioner who has given the explanation.
(e) When form is signed by a person other than the patient himself, state qualifications of signatory and circumstances under which he signs.

UNIVERSAL CAPE TOWN

Figure 7.2. Louis Waskansky's consent form for the first human heart transplantation operation.

In the early hours of the morning (3 December 1967), Waskansky was taken to the operating room, anaesthetized and his chest opened. Direct examination of the heart confirmed that nothing other than transplantation could help him. Meanwhile, Denise Darvall was taken to the adjoining operating room, after a neurosurgeon had stated that her brain injuries were irreversible and fatal. At an appropriate time, her ventilator was disconnected and as soon as the heart fibrillated, supportive cardiopulmonary bypass and cooling were established by femoral cannulation. Body temperature was lowered to 26°C. With the chest open, the aorta was clamped, the heart cooled to 16°C and then excised and placed in a bowl of physiological saline at 10°C. The donor organ was transferred to the adjacent operating room and reperfused with blood, after an ischaemic time of only 4 minutes. Meanwhile, Waskansky was placed on cardiopulmonary bypass, but the line pressure in the femoral arterial cannula was very high. Barnard (assisted by Terry O'Donovan and Roger Hewitson) decided to transfer the cannula to the ascending aorta, but in the excitement of the moment, the arterial line was clamped without stopping the bypass machine. When disconnected, the arterial line sprayed blood throughout the whole room. Some air was pumped when the system was reconnected, and worse still, the sino-atrial node of the donor heart was damaged by ligation of the superior vena cava-right atrial junction. The donor heart required pacing and it took three attempts to wean it from cardiopulmonary bypass. Nevertheless, the operation was completed successfully (Figure 7.3).

The donor heart had arrived in the operating room at 3.01 a.m. and at 6.13 a.m. the procedure was concluded with a satisfactory cardiac output. The medical superintendent of the hospital was informed of the event some time later, with the short sentence, "Sir, we have just transplanted a heart and the patient is well."

Waskansky's post-operative care was meticulous. Immunosuppression was started on the day of surgery with corticosteroids and azathioprine. Cobalt irradiation was applied to the heart on the fifth, seventh and ninth

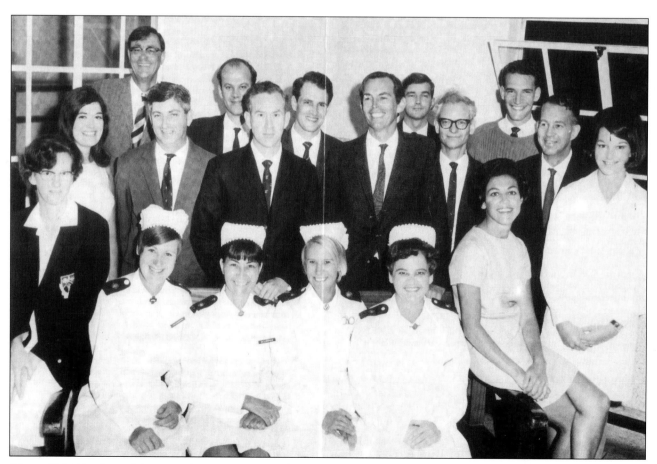

Figure 7.3. Members of the transplant team for Waskansky's operation.

post-operative days. He was kept in isolation within the same operating room in order to minimize the infection risk. In practice, it was difficult just to keep the reporters out.

Waskansky's response to the transplant was remarkable, in that the signs of heart failure disappeared rapidly after a substantial diuresis (Figure 7.4). The grossly oedematous legs returned to their normal shape by the third post-operative day and the liver involuted to normal size. The diabetes was easier to control. Inevitably, the media response was enormous and not always complimentary (Figure 7.5). In a BBC broadcast, the interviewer asked Barnard whether he had performed the first transplant in Cape Town to improve the bad image of South Africa. Others suggested that Barnard had stolen both the idea and surgical methods from Shumway. This was unfair, since all of the principles of cardiac transplantation had been published previously in medical journals and Barnard had performed numerous experiments in preparation for the technical aspects of the transplant. Three days after the Waskansky operation, Kantrovitz found an encephalic infant donor and transplanted its heart into a 2-day-old baby. This was a 9-hour operation and the tiny recipient died on the operating table.

Waskansky started to show signs of pneumonia 13 days after the operation. This worsened and caused his death on 21 December. The transplanted heart maintained a good cardiac output until the last moment. The post-mortem findings were reported in the *British Medical Journal* by James Thompson, Professor of Pathology at Groote Schuur Hospital.

> "*Necropsy on the first heart transplantation in man confirmed that death was due to extensive bilateral pneumonia and not to rejection of the heart. Signs of rejection, however, were demonstrated histologically, but were of a low order compared to those seen in the transplanted dog heart. How far the mildness of the rejection signs is to be ascribed to species' differences, immunosuppressive drugs and procedures, post-operative rest and nursing and medical care, or to the good matching leucocyte antigens, cannot at the moment be assessed.*"

Even before Waskansky's death, an international panel of prominent cardiac surgeons was convened in The

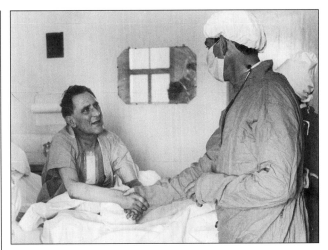

Figure 7.4. Barnard talking to Waskansky after the operation.

Plaza Hotel, New York, to discuss the ethical implications. Bailey, who in the early 1950s had caused controversy by his hospital-to-hospital rush to perform a successful mitral valvotomy, declared the South African transplant to be 10 years premature. Jacob Zimmerman, a colleague of Bailey's at New York's St Barnabas Hospital, agreed adding, "It is medically and morally wrong for doctors to stand by a dying patient's bedside, hoping he will get it over with quickly so we can grab his heart." In contrast, Donald Ross, a fellow South African and former classmate of Barnard's, and the Swiss surgeon Åke Senning, both said that they would perform transplants, and they were optimistic that heart banks would be established where organs could be stored. In Houston, DeBakey established his own committee to deliberate the question and concluded that heart transplants were as yet untenable. On learning of this decision, Cooley doubled his own efforts to find a donor.

Barnard was encouraged by the first transplant and not perturbed by the fatal outcome. On 2 January 1968, he transplanted a heart into a 58-year-old Cape Town dentist, Philip Blaiberg. On this occasion, the donor was a 24-year-old factory worker (Clive Haupt) who had suffered a massive subarachnoid haemorrhage whilst sunbathing on a Cape Town beach. When his condition was declared hopeless, he was transferred from Victoria Hospital to Groote Schuur Hospital, pending the transplant. The operation transformed Blaiberg from a breathless 'cardiac cripple' to an independent man, able to drive a car and swim in the sea. He spent 73 days in hospital, but then lived for 18 months before dying of chronic rejection.

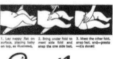

Figure 7.5. The Cape Argus newspaper after the first human heart transplant.

Shumway and the first transplant at Stanford

ON 6 JANUARY 1968 (4 days after the Blaiberg transplant), Shumway put into effect his many years of experimental preparation when he transplanted the heart of 43-year-old Virginia May White into a 54-year-old steelworker, Mike Casparak. Mrs White had collapsed with a cerebral haemorrhage whilst celebrating her 22nd wedding anniversary and Kasperak was dying from chronic viral myocarditis. Misfortune dogged the operation from the start. The diseased heart was so large that after excision the pericardial cavity was almost three times the size of the donor heart. This resulted in technical problems, and 5 hours after the operation, Kasperak was taken back to the operating room with bleeding and tamponade. Two days later, the liver and kidneys failed and Casparak suffered diffuse gastrointestinal haemorrhage. He required a vast volume of transfused blood (288 pints at a total cost of $7200) and then peritoneal dialysis. On the 8th post-operative day he underwent cholecystectomy under local anaesthesia, but lapsed into hepatic coma and died on 21 January. The hospital bill for this operation was $28,845, almost $2000 per day for the 15 post-operative days. This expenditure brought a barrage of criticism from many who felt that the money could have been better spent.

Kantrovitz attempted a further transplant 3 days after the Kasperak operation. This operation lasted for 9 hours, the patient survived for 6 hours only and Kantrovitz withdrew from the transplant scene. Shortly afterwards, Sen in Bombay lost a transplant patient on the operating table, and Cabrol, at the Hôpital de la Pitié in Paris, transplanted a truck driver who died without regaining consciousness.

Ross, at the National Heart Hospital, London, and Cooley, at St Luke's in Houston, performed their first transplant on the same day (3 May 1968). Ross' operation was undertaken on 45-year-old Frederick West, a patient with chronic, severe, congestive heart failure. The previous day, a 26-year-old building worker had sustained serious head injuries during a fall and, despite craniotomy at King's College Hospital, could not be salvaged. In the afternoon of the 3rd, when Ross discovered the donor, the body was rushed across London in an ambulance, with the circulation maintained by external cardiac massage. The recipient survived for 45 days.

Cooley and cardiac transplantation

AFTER THE INITIAL INTENSITY of the media coverage, the press interest was directed towards clinical justification of this expensive high-risk procedure, and whether all the surgeons and hospitals who were attempting heart transplants were equipped to do so. Another revelation to the public was that surgeons were actively working in competition with each other, partly on behalf of their patients, but certainly for the gratification of their own egos. In his forthright and honest manner, Cooley summarized his feelings on the matter:

> *"My first concern was saving the lives of sick people, but it would be untrue to say that I was not eager to take part in this, the most exciting development in cardiac surgery. The delay of my entry into heart transplantation is easily explained. We couldn't find any donors, and we suspected that they were being purposely denied us."*

Transplantation began in Houston in May 1968, and would soon overtake the combined experience of all other centres. Cooley's first patient was 47-year-old Everett Thomas, who had been bedridden for 5 months with rheumatic disease and needed triple valve replacement. He also had paralysis and blindness following cerebral emboli. Triple valve replacement was scheduled for 3 May, but on 1 May a 15-year-old female donor, with a gunshot wound of the brain, was referred as a transplant donor. Coincidentally, Cooley had operated on the girl for coarctation of the aorta at the age of 9 and she had a hypotrophied left ventricle. Cooley explained to Thomas and his family that the chances of surviving triple valve replacement were small and that a potential heart donor was available. He suggested valve replacement followed by transplantation if Thomas could not be weaned from cardiopulmonary bypass. The donor and potential recipient were moved to adjacent operating rooms and when it was established that Thomas' heart was irreparable, Cooley's colleague Grady Hallman harvested the donor heart. No cooling or myocardial protection were used. The detached heart continued to beat and was implanted directly. The actual transplant procedure took 35 minutes, a fraction of the time of previous operations, and the heart functioned well.

Within 72 hours Cooley had performed two further transplants. The next donor was the 15-year-old son of a personal friend of Cooley and the recipient a hospital administrator whose cardiac problem had been deemed inoperable a few months earlier. The third donor was a homicide victim and the County Medical Examiner refused permission because of the potential difference between assault and murder charges. Cooley argued that the victim met the legal criteria for brain death and proceeded. The second patient died from sepsis on day 3, and the third from hepeto-renal failure on day 7, but Thomas survived and became the first 'successful' transplant in the United States.

By the middle of August 1968, Cooley had performed nine transplants, but despite large numbers of accidents and homicides in Houston, donors were scarce. St Luke's Hospital and surrounding motels soon filled with patients awaiting transplants and on one occasion Cooley, in desperation, transplanted a sheep's heart in a 48-year-old man. This rejected acutely on the operating table without giving time for replacement with a backup pig's heart. On 17 August, Cooley transplanted the heart of an 8-year-old boy with severe head injuries into a 5-year-old girl with congenital heart disease. This was the first paediatric transplant, though the patient survived for less than a week.

DeBakey enters the arena

AT METHODIST HOSPITAL, DeBakey's colleague Ted Diethrich orchestrated a multiple transplant from a single teenage suicide victim. On 31 August, the donor heart, a single lung and both kidneys were harvested and transplanted into four separate recipients. The newspaper headlines read, "DeBakey team of 60 performs multiple transplant". The DeBakey team followed with a second cardiac transplant on 5 September, though the patient died a week later. On 14 September, Cooley took the heart and lungs from a 1-day-old anencephalic baby and transplanted them en bloc into a 2-month-old infant with complex congenital anomalies. This child died 14 hours post-operatively. In less than a month, Cooley's team had performed 10 transplants and the DeBakey team five. Cooley's longest survivor, Everett Thomas, returned to St Luke's in November with severe rejection and was retransplanted only to survive for 3 days.

During the 12 months after Barnard's first operation, over 100 transplants were performed in almost 50 centres. The results were discouraging: almost 60 patients dead by the 8th post-operative day and a mean survival of less than 30 days. Cooley presented his experience at the Society of Thoracic Surgeons' (USA) meeting in January 1969, and in discussion, John Callahan pointed out that 71 of the first 100 recipients were already dead. Enthusiasm amongst the medical profession waned rapidly and the number of operations decreased. Most physicians considered that the procedure should be limited to centres with a record of transplant research and established renal transplantation. Such departments could provide tissue typing and immunosuppressive therapy, together with facilities for prevention of infection and rejection. These criteria favoured Shumway's unit at Stanford, Lower's unit in Richmond, Virginia, and both the Texas Heart Institute and Baylor.

Heterotopic transplantation

BARNARD persisted in Cape Town and explored the use of heterotopic transplantation, considering two hearts to be better than one. Experimental work by Reemtsma and Johansson (of the Karolinska Institute) showed that an auxiliary heart implanted in the thorax could support the circulation whilst the native heart was made to fibrillate. Barnard first used heterotopic transplantation clinically in 1974 and by 1981, reported 30 transplants without an operative death. One-year survival rate was 60% and a small number of patients survived for 5 years. This operation allowed an element of recovery in the diseased heart and, paradoxically, allowed hearts which were less than ideal for orthotropic transplantation to be used. The function of donor hearts with prolonged ischaemic times gradually improved in the heterotopic position. Rejection of the heterotopic graft did not result in death of the patient, though severely diseased native hearts or rejected heterotopic transplants were a source for cerebral embolism. Cooley's group considered heterotopic transplantation to be a suitable option for a select group of high-risk patients with pulmonary hypertension, where there was substantial weight mismatch between recipient and donor, or when the viability of a donor heart was in doubt.

The technical details of both orthotopic and heterotopic cardiac transplants were not difficult to master, but several logistic problems prevented progress. Fundamental to the transplant process was the concept and definition of brain death. Failure to resolve this issue led to difficulties. Shumway commented,

"It should be underlined that no one can transplant a dead heart. The hearts which have been transplanted by surgeons all over the world could have been resuscitated in the donors and the chests could have been closed leaving these hopelessly brain injured persons to the fate of infection or peripheral vascular collapse. Death of the donor is a diagnosis which must be made by the neurological and neurosurgical team."

The treatment of rejection

THE SECOND PROBLEM was the diagnosis and treatment of rejection. Early immunosuppressive regimes were based on hydrocortisone, prednisone, azathioprine and cobalt irradiation. The protocol used at Stanford consisted of azathioprine (2 mg/kg iv) administered immediately prior to surgery, followed by oral treatment starting on the first post-operative day and maintained at a level of between 1 and 2 mg/kg (dependent on avoiding leucopenia or thrombocytopenia). Immediately following surgery, 500 mg methylprednisolone was administered intravenously, followed by 125 mg/day until oral intake could be resumed. Prednisone was then started at a dose of 1.5 mg/kg/day, reducing to a maintenance level of 1 mg/kg at about 2 months post-operatively. Further gradual reduction of the daily dose was continued until a level of approximately 0.25 mg/kg/day was achieved, usually at about 1 year post-transplant.

The immunosuppressive potential of heterologous antibodies against lymphocytes was first demonstrated by Woodruff and Anderson in 1963. The use of anti-lymphocytic serum was soon superseded by the use of a globulin fraction containing the active antibodies (anti-lymphocytic globulin). Such preparations were used clinically by Starzl in renal and liver transplants. The success of the Stanford cardiac transplant programme has been partially ascribed to the use of home produced, rabbit anti-human thymocyte globulin, which was injected intramuscularly at a dose of 2.5 mg/kg. Anti-thymocyte globulin was given daily for the first 3 days, and then every other day in order to reduce the T cell number in peripheral blood samples to less than 5% of the circulating lymphocytes (normally over 60%), and to maintain this low level for at least the first 3 weeks post-transplant. With these regimes, the patient was susceptible to infection and elaborate precautions were used to minimize the risk. In the pre-operative period, the patient was washed daily with hexachlorophene soap. Swabs were taken from the skin, nose, throat, mouth and rectum and potential pathogens treated with appropriate antibiotics. Nurses and medical staff in contact with the patient had swabs taken from the nose, throat, mouth and rectum. Apparatus to be used in proximity to the patient, were carefully cleaned and disinfected. In the post-operative period, the patient was kept in an isolation room with an air lock at the entrance. All attending staff wore caps, masks, overshoes and sterile gowns. Ventilators and other equipment were carefully cleaned and disinfected. Every second day swabs were taken from the patient for bacteriological examination and daily blood cultures were obtained. Any positive cultures were treated aggressively with an appropriate antibiotic.

Initially, there were only clinical markers for rejection, including leucocyte response, deterioration in cardiac output, elevation of serum enzyme levels, (indicating myocardial damage) and changes in the R wave voltage of the electrocardiogram. The greatest early advance in the diagnosis of rejection was the introduction of transvenous endomyocardial biopsy in 1972. Philip Caves from Glasgow worked as a research fellow at Stanford and was instrumental in devising the biotome (though Konno had previously produced such a device in Japan). This was introduced through an internal jugular vein and into the right ventricle of the transplanted heart to obtain a biopsy, approximately 1.5 mm in diameter. Routine biopsies, together with histological confirmation of rejection during a clinical episode, have remained the standard means with which to monitor immunosuppressive therapy. Caves returned to Glasgow as Professor of Cardiac Surgery but had a strong family history of hypercholesterolaemia and coronary disease. In his mid-30s, he suffered a fatal acute myocardial infarction whilst playing squash. Another advance from Stanford, which followed the introduction of anti-thymocyte globulin, was T cell monitoring. This test provided a functional method to assess the dose of an immunosuppressive agent before it had produced toxic effect.

The introduction of cyclosporine

THE INTRODUCTION of cyclosporin A had a major impact on the survival rate after all types of transplantation. The substance was first isolated from two fungal strains (*Cylindrocarpon lucidium* and *Trichoderma polysporum*) in soil samples in Switzerland by the Microbiology Department of Sandoz Laboratories. Crude metabolic mixtures were prepared from the fungal hyphae and were found to possess a number of anti-fungal properties. In 1973, Borel identified the immunosuppressive potential of these fungi and the structure of cyclosporin A was elucidated by x-ray crystallography. Green and Alison at the Medical Research Council Clinical Research Centre in England showed that cyclosporin A possessed a potent anti-lymphocyte activity, thereby inhibiting humoral immunity. It was toxic for human lymphoblasts of both T and B cell origin but not for resting lymphoblasts, resting lymphocytes or bone marrow cells. This finding suggested that cyclosporin A might be able to eliminate clones of lymphocytes responding to a specific antigenic challenge, whilst leaving intact clones of lymphocytes able to respond to other challenges such as viral infections. Roy Calne and colleagues in Cambridge demonstrated the ability of cyclosporin A to prevent rejection of transplanted hearts in pigs and found it sufficiently non-toxic to suggest clinical investigation in patients. The drug was first used in human renal transplantation in 1978, improving graft survival by 10–20%. Through its specific inhibition of interleukin-2, whilst sparing much of the remainder of the body's immune system, cyclosporin A was a distinct improvement over other agents. This, together with improvements in preservation of the donor organ, the feasibility of distant organ procurement and improvements in pre- and post-operative care emanating from Stanford and other major centres, acted as a stimulus for widespread adoption of cardiac transplantation. The Registry of the International Society for Heart Transplantation shows that in 1988,

2450 known heart transplant operations were performed in 118 centres in the US, 61 in Europe and 23 in other parts of the world. Hospital mortality dropped below 10% and 5-year actuarial survival increased to almost 75%. Centres carrying out more than 50 transplants per year showed lower mortality figures, and patients treated with cyclosporin A, azathioprine and steroids had a 5-year survival of 80%.

Heart and lung transplantation

EXPERIMENTAL preparations of heterotopic heart and lung transplants were described by the pioneers Carrell, Demikhov and Marcus before the advent of cardiopulmonary bypass. Marcus described a particularly ingenious experiment where the heart and lung preparation was anastomosed to the distal aorta and inferior vena cava in the abdomen, with ventilation of the trachea through a fistula to the skin (Marcus III procedure). With the donor heart and lung block working satisfactorily, Marcus entered the chest of the host animal, occluded the main pulmonary artery and allowed the left side of the heart to empty. The host heart could then be opened with an incision in the left atrial appendage, which allowed inspection and manipulation of the mitral valve. After 7 minutes, the atrium was closed and the heart allowed to fill and eject. Marcus had devised a somewhat complicated method for open intracardiac surgery using a donor heart and lungs as pump oxygenator and concluded that a transplanted heart or heart/lung preparation might be used for replacement of the diseased organ.

In 1957, Webb and Howard used the pump oxygenator to perform heart–lung transplantation in dogs with survival of up to 22 hours. They also performed auto transplantation of the heart and lungs, discovering that the heart functioned well but the animals were unable to breath. They concluded that cardiopulmonary denervation was not well tolerated and that the operation was unlikely to succeed due to respiratory paralysis. Blanco and colleagues in 1958 reported eight attempts at orthotopic heart–lung transplantation and whilst spontaneous respiration was restored in two animals, none survived for more than 5 hours. In 1961, Lower and Shumway attained spontaneous respiration in six animals and demonstrated the need to preserve the recipient's phrenic and vagus nerves. In those dogs that resumed spontaneous respiration, the pattern was altered with increased tidal volume and slow respiratory rate, and two animals survived up to 4 days post-operatively. In an extensive study of heart–lung transplantation in dogs, Longmire introduced the concept of a single inflow anastomosis of the right atrium instead of two vena-caval anastomoses.

The importance of species selection in experimental animals was highlighted by exhaustive experiments from Nake and colleagues. They found that whilst dogs and cats subject to cardiopulmonary orthotopic transplantation and mediastinal denervation died from respiratory failure, primates could resume adequate spontaneous respiration. Castanada (1972) confirmed this finding by performing cardiopulmonary orthotopic transplants on baboons. Attaining six long-term

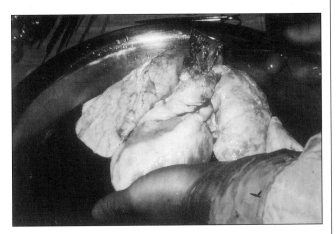

Figure 7.6. Heart and lung graft from the donor.

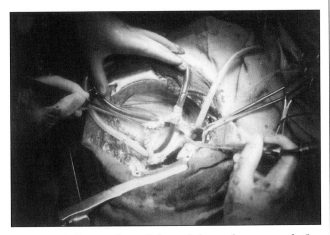

Figure 7.7. Empty chest of the recipient after removal of the heart and lungs.

survivors (some for several years), they found pulmonary ventilation, perfusion and circulatory haemodynamics to be essentially normal. Castenada then predicted that heart–lung transplantation could be successful in patients. At Stanford, Bruce Reitz achieved long-term survival with orthotopic transplants in monkeys and then obtained cyclosporin A for allograft experiments. In a landmark paper in the *Journal of Thoracic and Cardiovascular Surgery* (1980), Reitz described prolonged survival (exceeding 140 days) of allograft heart–lung transplants in primates. Cyclosporin proved effective in preventing rejection and the overall experience suggested the feasibility of heart–lung transplants in humans. Several of Reitz' monkeys went on to live for more than 5 years. It was initially thought that rejection episodes affected both heart and lungs similarly so that endomyocardial biopsy might be sufficient to monitor progress of the heart–lung bloc. Clinical experience would subsequently prove that pulmonary rejection could occur in the absence of cardiac rejection.

Up until this time there had been three unsuccessful clinical attempts. Cooley had transplanted a 2½-month-old child with an atrioventricular canal defect and pulmonary hypertension in 1968; the infant died within 24 hours. The following year, Lillehei transplanted the heart and lungs of a 50-year-old woman into a 43-year-old man with end-stage respiratory problems. This patient was extubated on the first post-operative day and was able to walk around the hospital before dying at 8 days from bronchial pneumonia. Barnard performed the third operation in 1981, with survival for 23 days before dehiscence of the tracheal anastomosis and intractable bronchial pneumonia. This initial experience confirmed that heart–lung denervation did not preclude patient survival, as was suggested by canine experiments.

Heart–lung transplants began at Stanford in March 1981 when the Food and Drugs Administration approved the use of cyclosporin A as an investigational drug. The first patient was a 45-year-old female with end-stage pulmonary hypertension. For this first procedure, the donor was brought to the transplant theatre so that the organs could be harvested and implanted with minimal ischaemic time (Figures 7.6 and 7.7). The first operation was a technical success and the patient was extubated in less than 48 hours. An acute rejection episode occurred at 10 days and required reventilation. After this, recovery was straightforward and the patient was well 5 years later. The second patient with Eisenmenger's syndrome and a large premembranous ventricular septal defect was transplanted several months later with long-term success. Four out of the first five Stanford heart–lung transplants were long-term survivors and results continue to improve with increasing experience of pre- and post-operative care, immunosuppressive therapy and the preservation of donor organs. Data from the International Society for Heart Transplantation showed that more than 200 patients receiving a heart–lung transplant in 1988 had a less than 20% 30-day mortality. Calculated one-year actuarial survival was 55% between 1981 and 1986, rising to more than 60% in 1988. The serious problem of obliterative bronchiolitis then led to a somewhat pessimistic long-term outlook, in the same way that accelerated coronary atherogenesis has blighted cardiac transplantation. Both of these problems are likely to be immune-related and have been managed by re-transplantation.

The widespread adoption of cardiac transplantation

Progressive improvements in immunosuppressive techniques and diagnosis of rejection at Stanford caused renewed interest internationally. Surgeons were forced to realise that cardiac transplantation was not just a relatively simple but glamorous operation; it was rather a complex immunological challenge best managed by experts in the field. In England, Terrence English (at Papworth) and Magdi Yacoub (at Harefield) developed highly successful and productive transplant programmes. Sir Terrence went on to be President of the Royal College of Surgeons of England, then President of the British Medical Association and Master of St Catherine's College Cambridge (Figure 7.8). Yacoub accrued the greatest number and variety of transplants in the world and also received a knighthood. In Europe, Cabrol (Paris), Hetzer (Berlin) and Korfer (Bad Oyenhausen) were prolific though the availability of donor organs restricted transplant numbers. Paediatric cardiac transplantation was developed by Leonard Bailey and his colleagues at Loma Linda. This group achieved success even in the neonatal period for infants with hypoplastic left heart—mechanical bridge to transplantation became an important precursor of the transplant operation in affluent units who could afford the devices. Frazier (Texas Heart Institute), Griffiths (University of Pittsburgh), McCarthy (Cleveland Clinic) and Rose (Columbia Presbyterian Medical Centre) were prolific in this respect and showed that patients who were rehabilitated by a Left Ventricular Assist Device had improved outcome.

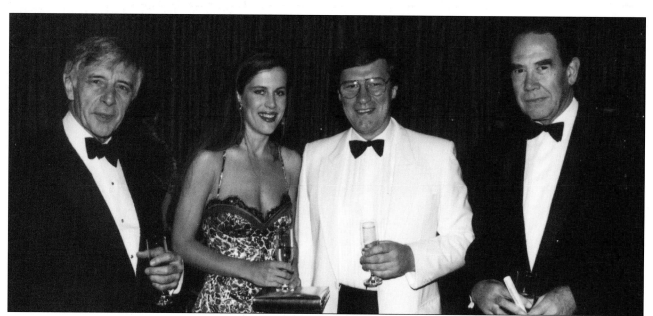

Figure 7.8. Robert Frater, Mrs Christiaan Barnard, Stephen Westaby and Sir Terrence English at the Ball in Cape Town to celebrate the 25th anniversary of the first heart transplant.

Biographies

Christiaan Neethling Barnard (1922–)

CHRISTIAAN NEETHLING BARNARD, the son of a Dutch Reform minister, was born in Beaufort West, Cape Province, South Africa. He studied at the University of Cape Town (MB; ChB, 1946, MMed (Medicine); MD, 1953) and the University of Minnesota under Lillehei and Varco (MS; PhD, 1958). He returned to South Africa in 1958 and joined Groote Schuur Hospital as Cardiothoracic Surgeon and the University of Cape Town as lecturer and Director of Surgical Research under Professor Louw. He became Head of Cardiothoracic Surgery of the Cape Town University teaching hospitals (1961), Associate Professor (1962) and Professor of Surgical Science, (1968–83). He has received more than 75 international awards for his work on heart transplantation and is the author of 14 books in the medical field including *Surgery of Common Congenital Cardiac Malformations* with Schrire (1968) and an autobiography, *One Life* (1969). He has been Emeritus Professor at The University of Capetown since 1983.

Since only extracorporeal support allowed survival of a transplanted heart for longer than a few hours, Barnard named Wangensteen the 'fairy godmother' of the first human heart transplant. Just before Barnard left the University of Minnesota, Wangensteen, in a 2-minute telephone conversation, asked the US government for $2000 for a bypass machine for Barnard to take back to South Africa, and $2000 a year financial support for 3 years. With his pump, Barnard progressed steadily toward transplantation from the time he returned to South Africa. He transplanted a second head onto a dog (1960) and visited the Soviet Union to discuss other transplants. In 1965, he started an experimental renal and heart transplant programme, employing the Cass and Brock (1959)/Lower and Shumway (1960) technique to preserve as much as possible of the atrial and interatrial septum in the recipient. In early 1967, Barnard visited David Hume, who was working on kidney transplantation, and Richard Lower, who was practising transplantion of animal hearts, at the Medical College of Virginia. He also saw Thomas Starzl in Denver, involved in the use of the immunosuppressant, antilymphocyte serum. He returned to Capetown in September 1967 to

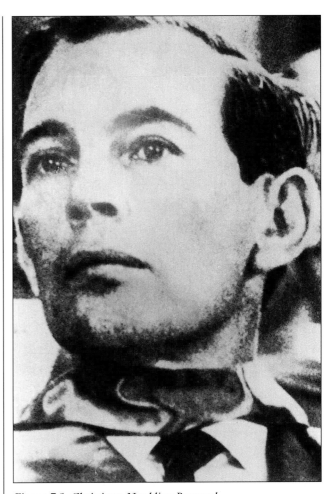

Figure 7.9. Christiaan Neethling Barnard.

transplant a kidney in a patient who subsequently lived for more than 20 years.

Barnard's 48 animal heart transplants, added to Shumway and Lower's 90% success rate in more than 300 transplants in dogs, convinced him that a human heart could be transplanted with minimal risk. On 3 December 1967, he put the heart of Denise Darvall, a 25-year-old ledger machinist, killed in a car accident, into Louis Waskansky, a 54-year-old grocer, whose extensive coronary artery disease and three myocardial infarctions had left him with intractable heart failure (Article 7.1, Appendix A). Thirteen days after transplantation, Waskansky showed signs of pulmonary infection which caused

THE OPERATION

A HUMAN CARDIAC TRANSPLANT: AN INTERIM REPORT OF A SUCCESSFUL OPERATION PERFORMED AT GROOTE SCHUUR HOSPITAL, CAPE TOWN

C. N. BARNARD, M.D., M.MED., M.S., PH.D., D.SC. (HON. CAUSA), F.A.C.S., F.A.C.C., *Department of Surgery, University of Cape Town and Groote Schuur Hospital, Cape Town*

On 3 December 1967, a heart from a cadaver was successfully transplanted into a 54-year-old man to replace a heart irreparably damaged by repeated myocardial infarction.

This achievement did not come as a surprise to the medical world. Steady progress towards this goal has been made by immunologists, biochemists, surgeons and specialists in other branches of medical science all over the world during the past decades to ensure that this, the ultimate in cardiac surgery, would be a success.

THE OPERATION

As soon as it had become obvious that, despite therapy, death was imminent in the donor, the recipient was anaesthetized and the saphenous vein and common femoral artery were exposed through a right groin incision. The saphenous vein was cannulated and this cannula was used for intravenous fluid administration and venous monitoring. The heart of the recipient was exposed through a median sternotomy incision. The pericardium was opened and the superior and inferior venae cavae and ascending

Figure 7.10. Title page of Barnard's 1967 describing the first human cardiac transplantation at Groote Schuur Hospital. (Reproduced with permission from The South African Medical Journal; *41: 1271–74.)*

his death on 21 December. The transplanted heart maintained good circulation without rejection.

Barnard's operation aroused hostility in the United States because it appeared to preempt Shumway's careful and systematic work published since 1959. The profession complained that the immunological difficulties had not been resolved, that Barnard's first human heart transplant was premature, flamboyant and irresponsible. James Hardy, who transplanted a chimpanzee's heart to man (1964), reflected the chagrin of many Americans:

"I confess my disappointment was enormous, though not so much for myself personally, for I knew that Shumway's group at Stanford had done the most extensive and best work in the field. We had long been waiting for them to transplant a heart in man, following which we planned to transplant another. Hanlon's group in St Louis had also been in the field, as had Blumenstock at Cooperstown, New York, and other groups. Then why had none of us performed another heart transplant following our first, 3 years earlier? The reason was public and professional opinion in the United States, along with the national governmental committees within committees, protecting the public from "experimentation." These had become so burdensome and severe that we simply could not risk another transplant: should the patient fail to live at least a few weeks, as well he might under the American strictures of not being able to remove a still-beating heart and requiring a terminally-ill recipient, the results could prove disastrous, both professionally and with regard to grant support from Washington, upon which all of us were heavily dependent."

However, Cooley, DeBakey, Kantrowitz and even Shumway, welcomed his achievement and quickly followed suit. DeBakey said:

"Barnard has broken the ice. It is a real breakthrough in the whole field of heart replacement. It is a great achievement. There were at least 20 medical centers in the world where there was skill and knowledge enough to perform transplants. What we've all been waiting for is the right circumstances — the right donor and the right recipient. Dr Barnard had the right circumstances and he did it. They took the first step. We will do it too."

Christiaan Barnard was responsible for the first heterotopic transplant in man with long-term survival. The implantations of heterotopic hearts on 25 November and 31 December 1974 provided the first long-term survivors (Figure 7.11). He wrote:

"When we discussed the possibility of a heterotropic transplant with the cardiologists they pointed out that in many patients, the right heart failure is secondary to the left heart failure and not due to intrinsic disease of the right heart. It was therefore only necessary to support the left heart in these cases.

The result was that in the first two heterotropic transplants, we did not join the donor's pulmonary artery to that of the recipient, but connected it to the recipient's right atrium just to take care of the coronary sinus venous return.

Our first patient lived for only 70 days but the second patient was a long-term survivor and allowed us to observe the danger of this approach. He developed attacks of ventricular fibrillation of his own diseased heart. During these periods he was in real trouble, as the pulmonary circulation then depended solely on the increase in venous pressure. For this reason we abandoned this procedure and from then on bypassed both right and left ventricles."

Left Ventricular Bypass

C. N. BARNARD,   J. G. LOSMAN

SUMMARY

The removal of the patient's own diseased heart in order to perform a total cardiac transplantation has several disadvantages. A new technique for bypassing the patient's diseased left ventricle by using a cardiac allograft has been developed in our laboratory and applied clinically in 2 patients. This technique carried no direct surgical mortality, and no complications resulting from the patient's own heart being left *in situ* have been observed thus far. The presence of a second heart lying partly in the anterior mediastinum and partly in the right pleural space appeared to have no deleterious effects. Several advantages over the conventional transplant have been noted and are discussed.

transplant, the most important being that the transplanted normal right ventricle will not be burdened by increased pulmonary vascular resistance. With this goal in mind, we developed a surgical technique in baboons in our experimental laboratory, which has now been applied clinically in 2 patients. This article reports our early clinical experiences.

SURGICAL TECHNIQUE

Donor

The surgical technique for the removal of the donor heart is only slightly different from that originally reported

Figure 7.11. Title page of Barnard's 1975 article entitled 'Left ventricular bypass'. (Reproduced with permission from The South African Medical Journal; *49: 303–12.)*

Adrian Kantrowitz (1918–)

ADRIAN KANTROWITZ was born in New York City. His early interest in science was encouraged by his father, a general practitioner in the Bronx, his mother, who told him he was going to be a doctor when he was three and his brother, a physicist who was interested in electronics. The young brothers designed and built an electrocardiograph from old radio parts. Kantrowitz studied mathematics at New York University (BA, 1940) and medicine at what is now the State University of New York Downstate Medical Center (MD, 1943). After the war, he was resident in surgery at Mount Sinai Hospital in New York City (1946), assistant resident in surgery (1948) and pathology (1949) at Montefiore Hospital in the Bronx. In 1964, Kantrowitz achieved the longest experimental transplant survivors without immunosuppressive drugs. His use of 3-month-old puppies with weaker immune response and deep hypothermia without a pump-oxygenator, allowed survival of 24 of 40 puppies for more than a day. One died after 57 days and one was still living 112 days after operation, showing no evidence of rejection, and growing steadily with signs of gradual reinnervation. Kantrowitz's transplant of a heart to an infant on 6 December 1967 was the first attempt in the United States and the second in the world (just 3 days after Barnard's).

Kantrowitz conceived intra-aortic balloon counter-pulsation (IABP) while teaching cardiovascular physiology at Western Reserve University School of Medicine (1951–52) under Carl Wiggers. Kantrowitz and his brother, Arthur, then in the Cornell Physics Department and at AVCO Corporation, performed experiments to demonstrate the principles of diastolic augmentation. Kantrowitz's research group at Maimonides Hospital in Brooklyn, together with AVCO-Everett Research Laboratory in Massachussetts, then developed a permanent mechanical assist device to provide diastolic augmentation for the relief of chronic left ventricular failure. In 1966, after several

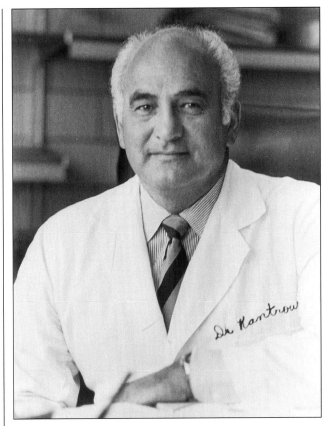

Figure 7.12. Adrian Kantrowitz.

years of animal studies, they implanted the pump into the aorta of two patients with chronic, terminal, left ventricular failure. One patient survived 24 hours, the second, 11 days, when she died of a cerebral embolus. The haemodynamic support of this device was impressive and pointed to further problems that had to be overcome before a permanent left ventricular assist device could become a reality. They decided that it would be easy to produce a temporary assist device based on the principles of diastolic counterpulsation.

Moulopolous, Topaz and Kolff had reported their early experiments with an intra-aortic balloon pump in 1962, as did Clauss and his colleagues, using a latex balloon (condom) on a small plastic catheter driven by carbon dioxide. However, latex was too distensible and could damage the aorta whilst carbon dioxide as the shuttle gas probably moved too slowly through the narrow catheter. After the initial papers, there were no further studies.

By 1967, Kantrowitz had enough experimental experience to show clearly the advantages of a non-distensible polyurethane balloon. The use of helium as the shuttle gas gave sufficient transit speed to assure appropriate timing. Kantrowitz believed that there was sufficient evidence to warrant a clinical trial in a small number of patients in cardiogenic shock which, at that time, was inevitably fatal (Figure 7.13). In 1969, Kantrowitz received inquiries from colleagues eager to try the IABP. To get a clear-cut answer about its clinical usefulness, he wanted to organize a co-operative trial in which a considerable number of patients could be treated under a common protocol. Cardiologists and surgeons from nine hospitals and university medical centres in the eastern United States prepared a clinical trial and obtained approval from their respective institutional research committees. The Maimonides Committee, however, doubted that the balloon pump really worked and vetoed the protocol. Maimonides Hospital, as Kantrowitz pointed out, was already stressed by being the site of the first heart transplantation in the United States (Kantrowitz's) and of the first implantation of a permanent left ventricular assist device (Kantrowitz's) and the risk of IABP was too much. In 1970, Kantrowitz took his research group and some of the surgical residency staff (25 in all), to the Sinai Hospital, Detroit to begin a co-operative study of IABP, supported by the John A. Hartford Foundation. Two and a half years after the publication of this article, several groups reported poor results

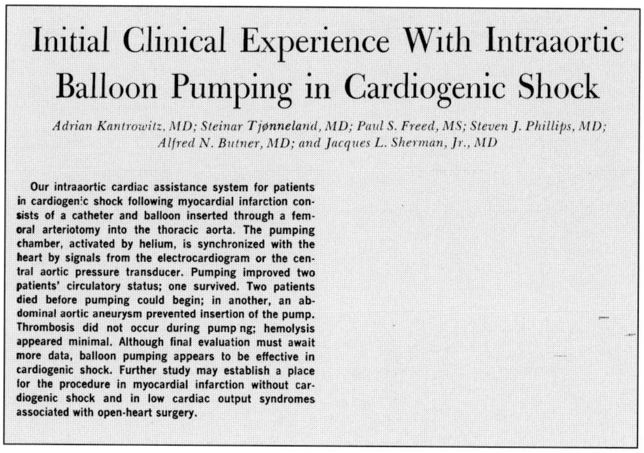

Initial Clinical Experience With Intraaortic Balloon Pumping in Cardiogenic Shock

Adrian Kantrowitz, MD; Steinar Tjønneland, MD; Paul S. Freed, MS; Steven J. Phillips, MD; Alfred N. Butner, MD; and Jacques L. Sherman, Jr., MD

Our intraaortic cardiac assistance system for patients in cardiogenic shock following myocardial infarction consists of a catheter and balloon inserted through a femoral arteriotomy into the thoracic aorta. The pumping chamber, activated by helium, is synchronized with the heart by signals from the electrocardiogram or the central aortic pressure transducer. Pumping improved two patients' circulatory status; one survived. Two patients died before pumping could begin; in another, an abdominal aortic aneurysm prevented insertion of the pump. Thrombosis did not occur during pump ng; hemolysis appeared minimal. Although final evaluation must await more data, balloon pumping appears to be effective in cardiogenic shock. Further study may establish a place for the procedure in myocardial infarction without cardiogenic shock and in low cardiac output syndromes associated with open-heart surgery.

Figure 7.13. Title page of the 1968 article by Kantrowitz et al. entitled 'Initial clinical experience with intraortic balloon pumping in cardiogenic shock'. *(Reproduced with permission from* Journal of the American Medical Association; *203: 135–40.)*

in early clinical experience. It was not clear why the balloon pump effort did not disappear except that the beneficial haemodynamic effects of IABP promised to be useful in other acute low-output circulatory problems.

That the IABP was not aborted in its infancy is a tribute to the remarkable support from the National Institutes of Health, the Hartford Foundation, from many research staff and from independent-minded colleagues and investigators. Some 23 years later, approximately 70,000 IABP implants are performed annually. More formidable than technical difficulties were the institutional political agendas and their obstructive policies. In 1990, Kantrowitz acknowledged his gratitude to the *Journal of the American Medical Association* for publishing this paper despite the meagre clinical experience of only three patients.

Norman Edward Shumway (1923–)

NORMAN EDWARD SHUMWAY was born in Kalamazoo, Michigan and studied at Baylor and Vanderbilt Universities (MD, 1949). A 5-year surgical training programme at the University of Minnesota, interrupted by the Korean War (1951–53), resulted in a thesis, *Experimental surgery of the heart and great vessels under hypothermia* (PhD, 1956). Shumway declined chief residency in Wangensteen's service to take up private practice in California (1957). After a year, he sought academic posts in San Francisco at the University of California. The head of surgery, Leon Goldman, fell asleep

during Shumway's interview but he was hired to run the kidney dialysis machine at Stanford-Lane Hospital. Ann Purdy, the wife of Emil Holman asked Shumway to operate the heart–lung machine with Roy Cohn at Children's Hospital. At Stanford-Lane, Shumway, with Raymond Stofer, worked out an extraordinarily unadorned and simple perfusion system with a minimum of gauges and monitors to watch, clean or repair. The simplicity of this system became the hallmark of Shumway's surgical advances. In Cohn's absence, the heart–lung machine was transported to Children's Hospital for paediatric operations. Stanford-Lane then moved to Palo Alto and became the Stanford University Medical School where

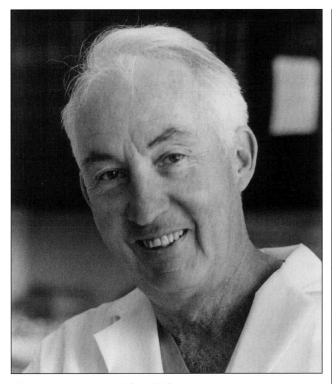

Figure 7.14. Norman Edward Shumway.

Shumway became Professor and Chairman of the Department of Cardiovascular Surgery in 1974.

In 1958, while studying topical hypothermia as a means of protecting the heart during surgery, Shumway and Lower spent some time performing cardiac allografts. Shumway wrote:

> *"When I started work at Stanford, the idea (cardiac transplantation) grew out of our local cooling experiments since we had 1 hour of aortic cross-clamping during cardiopulmonary bypass. Accordingly, we decided to remove the heart at the atrial level and then to suture it back into position. After several of these experiments, we found it would be easier to remove the heart of another dog and do the actual allotransplant. Something like 20 to 30 experiments were performed before we had a survivor. All of this was done before chemical immune suppression was available."*

Shumway's first clinical transplantation of a heart on 6 January 1968 at Stanford Medical Center was the fourth in the world. The patient, Mike Kasperak, a 54-year-old steel worker, was near death from cardiomyopathy. Kasperak lived for 15 days with, as Shumway said, "a fantastic galaxy of complications": kidney failure, liver failure and three major operations, a situation which offered "some hope" for the future of heart transplantation. Nevertheless, this initiated the Stanford clinical programme, the culmination of a decade of experimental laboratory work. Over the next 15 years, the Stanford team was the most active of all transplant groups and responsible for many developments in transplant patient care.

On 3 December 1970, the third anniversary of clinical heart transplantion, the only place in America where enthusiasm remained for the procedure was Stanford University. Nine transplant patients were still alive out of the first 26 Shumway had performed.

The problem of rejection was addressed by serial cardiac biopsy described below (Article 7.2, Appendix A) and then cyclosporine therapy. Philip Caves and Margaret Billingham's percutaneous transvenous endomyocardial biopsy technique for monitoring heart allograft rejection (1972) was the most significant clinical advance of this decade. This technique offered many advantages including minimal discomfort to the patient (with the use of only small amounts of local anaesthetic), direct passage of the bioptome into the apex of the right ventricle, repeated entry into the vein through the sheath, absence of bleeding and preservation of a patent vein for subsequent biopsy. By 1993, the Caves–Schultz bioptome was the one most frequently used. Cardiac biopsy had progressed from a crude operative intervention (exposing the patient to considerable risk), to a safe and reliable percutaneous technique, performed as an outpatient procedure.

Shumway's systematic, carefully followed cardiac transplantations continued and outdistanced all other series in number, quality of results and yield of scientific information. Without Shumway's persistence and scientific efforts, which inspired others such as English and Yacoub, cardiac transplantation would have been abandoned for many years. Shumway is responsible for modern cardiac transplantation and its steadily improving results and made many other major contributions in the surgery of valvular and congenital heart disease. The old Stanford team of Shumway, Ed Stinson, Bruce Reitz, Craig Miller, Bill Baumgartner and Phil Oyer developed one of the most formidable cardiac units in the United States. The transplant surgeons, Bruce Reitz and Bill Baumgartner left Stanford for Johns Hopkins in Baltimore. Reitz subsequently returned to Stanford as Chief of Cardiac Surgery when Shumway retired. Baumgartner remained at Hopkins as Chief.

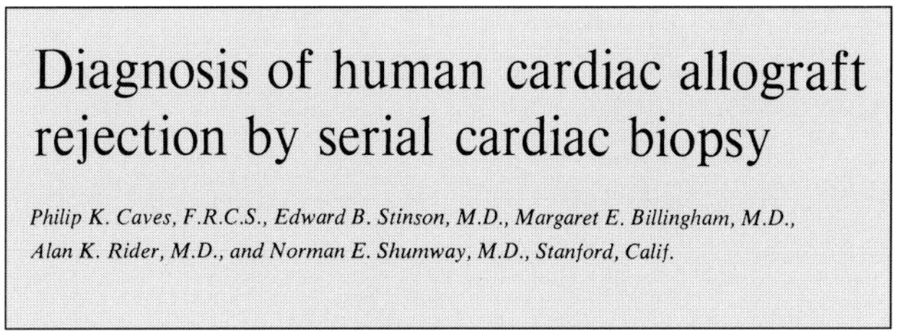

Diagnosis of human cardiac allograft rejection by serial cardiac biopsy

Philip K. Caves, F.R.C.S., Edward B. Stinson, M.D., Margaret E. Billingham, M.D., Alan K. Rider, M.D., and Norman E. Shumway, M.D., Stanford, Calif.

Figure 7.15. Title page of the 1973 report describing the use of serial cardiac biopsy to monitor allograft rejection. (Reproduced with permission from Journal of Thoracic and Cardiovascular Surgery; 66: 461–66.)

Donald C. Watson (1945–)

DONALD C. WATSON was born in Fairfield, Ohio and received his early education in the northeastern United States. He graduated from Lehigh University after majoring in mechanical engineering and applied science (BSc, 1969). After receiving a masters degree in mechanical engineering from Stanford University, he completed his medical training at Duke University in 1972. Because of a keen interest in cardiac transplantation, Watson continued his training at Stanford University (1972–80) under the direction of Norman Shumway, punctuated by laboratory experience at the National Heart and Lung Institute (1974–76). After completion of training at Stanford, he joined the faculty at George Washington University and worked principally at Children's Hospital National Medical Center in Washington, D.C. In 1984, Watson joined the faculty at the University of Tennessee in Memphis where he is now Chairman of Cardiothoracic Surgery, Residency Training Program Director, and Director of Thoracic Organ Transplants in the Memphis Affiliated Transplant Hospitals Program. He is also Professor of Surgery and Pediatrics and works principally at LeBonheur Children's Medical Center.

Donald Watson wrote to us:

"This landmark work was produced in an environment which facilitated the expression of new ideas at the margin of our understanding in the treatment of a specific medical problem. It was brought about by a unique coalition of energetic and creative people under the direction of a world eminent surgeon, Norman Shumway. The techniques had been well described and this paper (Article 7.6, Appendix A) was merely an extension to allow an improved donor pool. Many experimental efforts had shown that the myocardium could be safely preserved for hours and even preserved for up to 72 hours while maintaining life-sustaining function in animals during the early post-operative phase. Refinement in the techniques described have allowed improved results over the past one and a half decades. Efforts persist at increasing the donor pool. Xenografts, presumed consent and non-heart beating cadaveric donors currently represent exciting and diverse alternatives. Many new landmarks in cardiac surgery will come from these efforts."

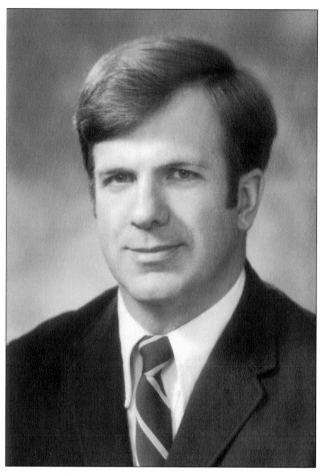

Figure 7.16. Donald C. Watson.

Distant heart procurement for transplantation

Donald C. Watson, M.D., Bruce A. Reitz, M.D., William A. Baumgartner, M.D., Aidan A. Raney, M.D., Philip E. Oyer, M.D., Edward B. Stinson, M.D., and Norman E. Shumway, M.D., *Stanford, Calif.*

Between January 1, 1977, and September 15, 1978, 39 cardiac transplants were performed on 38 patients. Twenty donor hearts were removed at Stanford University Hospital, and 19 donor hearts were removed at distant hospitals. The characteristics of recipients and donors in both groups were similar. The only significant difference between donor hearts was the mean ischemia time (154 ± 30 minutes in distant hearts and 52 ± 12 minutes in local hearts, P < 0.001). As of February 1, 1979, the total mortality rate was 32% for the distant heart donors and 40% for the local heart donors. No difference between the two groups was present in immediate myocardial function, the need for postoperative inotropic support, the mortality rate within the first 90 days after operation, the mean maximum serum enzyme levels, the occurrence of rejection or infection, and the histological appearance of the hearts, both early and late. The results of cardiac transplantation when hearts are removed at distant hospitals are entirely comparable to the results with hearts removed on site with a minimum ischemic time. Distant heart procurement provides an expanded donor pool for potential cardiac recipients.

From the Department of Cardiovascular Surgery, Stanford University Medical Center, Stanford, Calif.

Figure 7.17. 'Distant heart procurement for transplantation'. *A paper by Watson et al. published in 1979. (Reproduced with permission from* Surgery; 86: 56–59.)

Bruce A. Reitz (1944–)

BRUCE A. REITZ was born in Seattle, Washington. He studied at Stanford (BSc, 1966) and Yale Universities (MD, 1970) and completed internship at Johns Hopkins University Medical School (1970–71) and residency in cardiovascular, vascular, thoracic, general and cardiac transplantation surgery at Stanford University Medical Center (1971–78). He held an appointment as clinical associate at the National Heart and Lung Institute, Bethesda, Maryland (1972–74). He was Chief Resident and Instructor in Surgery (1977–78) and Assistant and Associate Professor of Cardiovascular Surgery (1978–82) at Stanford before he became Professor and Director, Division of Cardiac Surgery at Johns Hopkins University School of Medicine, Cardiac Surgeon-in-Charge at Johns Hopkins Hospital (1982–92) and attending cardiac surgeon, Sinai Hospital, Baltimore. In succession to Shumway, he is now Professor and Chairman of Cardiothoracic Surgery at Stanford University School of Medicine.

The first successful heart–lung transplantation was performed after nearly 4 years testing in primates. Encouraged by the animal work, Reitz and his team looked for potential recipients. Mary Gohlke, his first patient, contacted Reitz after reading a newspaper account of his work. According to Reitz, she served as an inspiration for many subsequent patients facing the ordeal of heart–lung or lung transplantation. She described the course of events in her autobiography, *I'll Take Tomorrow*, beginning with her first question to Reitz about how many heart–lung transplants he intended to do that year. "10", he said. "Fine," she replied "I'd like to be number 10 anyhow, after you've got your act together and everything straightened out." Gohlke was in fact the first in the series of heart–lung transplants (Article 7.4, Appendix A). This operation was performed only hours after the Food and Drug Administration was persuaded to legalize the use of cyclosporin A (a known carcinogen) by the efforts of Gohlke herself, Max Jennings (editor of the *Mesa Tribune*) and DeConcini, then senator of Arizona. Gohlke died an accidental death due to trauma a little over 5 years after the successful procedure.

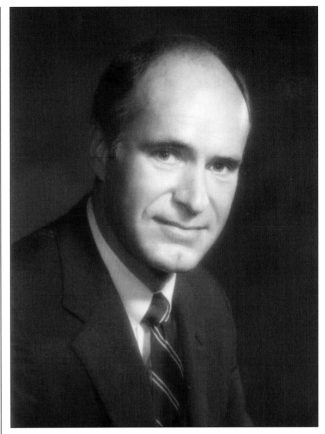

Figure 7.18. Bruce Reitz.

The New England
Journal of Medicine

©Copyright, 1982, by the Massachusetts Medical Society

Volume 306   MARCH 11, 1982   Number 11

HEART-LUNG TRANSPLANTATION

Successful Therapy for Patients with Pulmonary Vascular Disease

BRUCE A. REITZ, M.D., JOHN L. WALLWORK, M.B., CH.B., SHARON A. HUNT, M.D., JOHN L. PENNOCK, M.D., MARGARET E. BILLINGHAM, M.B., PHILIP E. OYER, M.D., PH.D., EDWARD B. STINSON, M.D., AND NORMAN E. SHUMWAY, M.D., PH.D.

Abstract We report our initial experience with three patients who received heart-lung transplants. The primary immunosuppressive agent used was cyclosporin A, although conventional drugs were also administered.

In the first patient, a 45-year-old woman with primary pulmonary hypertension, acute rejection of the transplant was diagnosed 10 and 25 days after surgery but was treated successfully; this patient still had normal exercise tolerance 10 months later. The second patient, a 30-year-old man, underwent transplantation for Eisenmenger's syndrome due to atrial and ventricular septal defects. His graft was not rejected, and his condition was markedly improved eight months after surgery. The third patient, a 29-year-old woman with transposition of the great vessels and associated defects, died four days postoperatively of renal, hepatic, and pulmonary complications.

We attribute our success to experience with heart-lung transplantation in primates, to the use of cyclosporin A, and to the anatomic and physiologic advantages of combined heart-lung replacement. We hope that such transplants may ultimately provide an improved outlook for selected terminally ill patients with pulmonary vascular disease and certain other intractable cardiopulmonary disorders. (N Eng J Med. 1982; 306:557-64.)

Figure 7.19. Title page of the 1982 article by Reitz et al. entitled 'Heart–Lung Transplantation'. (Reproduced with permission from The New England Journal of Medicine; 306: 559–64.)

Chapter 8: Mechanical circulatory support

CONVENTIONAL cardiac transplantation has always been limited by donor availability, the need for continuous immunosuppression and the dangers of infection or malignant disease. Less than one-third of potential recipients ever receive a transplant, a worsening situation as motor vehicle safety measures improve. Although the problem of donor availability has been addressed by research into xenotransplantation, this remains an unattractive proposition through enhanced immunological problems and the risk of virus transmission. The goal for artificial heart protagonists is an effective mechanical cardiac substitute, which can be taken from the shelf during normal working hours and implanted with the need for little more than anticoagulation. The artificial heart has always captured the imagination of cardiac surgeons, the media and the patient with heart disease. The prospects for long-term mechanical cardiac support are now improving rapidly, with the probability of increasing the availability of treatment for patients with end stage heart disease of all age groups. The relatively recent history of mechanical hearts is fascinating and has generated controversy exceeding that of cardiac transplantation in the late 1960s.

Early blood pumps

WITH THE DEVELOPMENT of the pump oxygenator came the possibility of using this device as a treatment in its own right. Clarence Dennis of New York was the first surgeon to employ the apparatus solely to support the failing heart. On 1 November 1954, he was asked to see a 54-year-old woman in cardiogenic shock due to end stage rheumatic valve disease. He took her to the operating room and established mechanical circulatory support. Venous drainage was obtained via the left femoral vein (with a cannula introduced through the saphenous vein) and the blood was returned to the left brachial artery. During the next 4 hours of left heart bypass, her pulmonary oedema and pleural effusions resolved, and orthopnoea disappeared. This improvement lasted for 10 days, after which her condition steadily deteriorated again.

Dennis suggested that by treating patients with severe mitral stenosis in this way, it might be possible to improve their symptoms and reduce operative mortality. At the time, mortality was 40% for mitral valvotomy in NYHA class IV patients, and between 5 and 10% for NYHA class III patients. Dennis then considered the possibility for cardiac support in selected patients with acute myocardial infarction. He chose patients in cardiogenic shock with a blood pressure of less than 80 mmHg and signs of progressive deterioration. The plan was to support the circulation and rest the heart until surviving muscle was able to sustain cardiac output unaided. With local anaesthetic, a catheter was inserted through the saphenous vein into the common iliac vein. The blood drained was then pumped through a disc oxygenator with a bubble trap and returned to the brachial artery. A heat exchange coil in a waterbath was incorporated into the circuit to maintain body temperature. The first clinical attempt (27 February 1957) was on a 52-year-old man, in cardiogenic shock following myocardial infarction 12 hours before. Extracorporeal support was used for 3 hours, but discontinued when haemoglobin appeared in the urine, indicating excessive haemolysis. Although this patient slowly recovered (because, or in spite of treatment), the next two patients died. It soon became apparent that the pump oxygenator was unsuitable for prolonged circulatory support.

Dennis and Senning then concentrated their efforts on left heart bypass (1962). Using a dog model, they passed a catheter through the internal jugular vein, into the right atrium, and then through the interatrial septum to the left atrium. Blood was withdrawn through this catheter, and pumped back into the body through a femoral artery. The method seemed to work, and the hole between the atria usually healed within 3 months. The procedure was attempted in one patient with post-infarction rupture of the interventricular septum. Signs of cardiogenic shock disappeared after about 3 hours on the machine and he was taken to the operating room for surgical repair. He subsequently died from left ventricular failure.

The early artificial hearts

AT THE TIME, few surgeons had considered physical replacement of the heart with a mechanical pump. Perhaps the first was the intrepid Vladimir Demikhov, who designed an artificial heart in Moscow (1937). His device, about the same size as a normal heart, consisted of two membrane pumps side-by-side, primed with physiological saline solution. Demikhov inserted the two inflow cannulae of the apparatus through the atrial appendages of a dog and tied them in place with ligatures. The outflow cannulae were then introduced into the aorta and pulmonary artery with clamps. Ligatures were tied tightly around the base of each ventricle and the ventricles excised as the pump was switched on. The machine was driven by an electric motor outside the body, with the drive shaft of the pump passing through the chest wall. Demikhov carried out three experimental implantations of this device in dogs during 1937 and five more in 1938. The longest survival was 5½ hours, during which time the dog's cerebral perfusion and respiration were maintained. Demikhov considered this a unique method for maintaining the organs of a dead donor pending preparation of a transplant recipient.

In 1958, Yukihiko Atsumi and colleagues, of Tokyo University School of Medicine, developed a hydraulically driven plastic heart, which could maintain a dog's circulation for up to 6 hours. Two years later, they successfully provided biventricular support for 13 hours, with a completely different roller pump driven by a miniature motor. The main problem with these early machines was thrombosis. The Japanese team attempted to avoid this by building a bellows type of pump lined with silicone rubber. With this, they succeeded in

keeping one dog alive for 27 hours, though the majority of animals died from pulmonary oedema or cerebral embolism.

Atsumi soon identified the complex problems of achieving a physiological circulation with a mechanical pump. In particular, the human heart itself does not influence venous return or systemic arterial pressure, but accommodates changes in both. He identified the need for a sophisticated control system in an artificial device, so that appropriate mechanical responses could accommodate hormonal, biochemical and pressure changes.

In the US, Willem Kolff, the pioneer of renal dialysis, also worked on an artificial heart. In 1959, his team, including the Japanese engineers Tetsuzo Akutsu and Yukihiko Nose (Figure 8.1, page 299), implanted a pendulum type of artificial heart into a dog. The ventricles of this pump emptied alternately. The animal breathed spontaneously for 2 hours after chest closure and retained both corneal and tendon reflexes. The device maintained a blood pressure greater than 80 mmHg for 5 hours, after which the experiment was concluded. There was no pulmonary oedema at post-mortem.

Three days later, the Kolff team implanted a different type of biventricular roller pump device, which had a valve on each side corresponding to the aortic and pulmonary valves. Again, the ventricles emptied alternately. The team persisted with their work and by 1965 had developed a one piece, four chamber heart. This was implanted orthotopically into the pericardial sac of a calf, which lived for 31 hours. After the development of clinical cardiac transplantation, Kolff's aim was to provide short-term support for patients waiting for donor hearts. (Figures 8.2 to 8.4, page 299)

Liotta and the Baylor programme

IN 1958, Domingo Liotta, from Argentina, developed an interest in the artificial heart during postgraduate surgical training in Lyons, France. He returned to Argentina as Assistant Professor of Surgery at the University of Cordoba (1960) and established his own artificial heart research programme. With plastics obtained from the Fabrica Militar de Iviones (an aeroplane factory run by a group of immigrant German generals), Liotta and his brother Salvador constructed one of the world's first implantable heart pumps. They obtained financial backing from the Cordoba Public Health Ministry, and with Thomas Taliani, an Italian engineer who had retired from the directorship of the Archimedes Institute in Rome, Liotta undertook hundreds of experiments on dogs and calves.

Their third prototype mechanical heart was so successful that the Dean of the University, Juan Martin Alendez, persuaded Liotta to present the work to the American Society for Artificial Organs. When Liotta presented his paper on mechanical cardiac replacement in Atlantic City, Kolff was so impressed that he invited him to continue the work at the Cleveland Clinic. However, Kolff had difficulty in attracting research funds and when DeBakey learned of Liotta's device, he offered him financial backing and extensive laboratory facilities. Liotta then transferred his plastic hearts to Houston and organized the first artificial heart programme at Baylor.

DeBakey considered complete cardiac replacement to be too problematic and wished to concentrate on left ventricular support with an implantable device. Liotta reluctantly set aside the total artificial heart (TAH), but obtained a substantial grant from the American Heart Association to work with Cooley and Beall on left ventricular bypass. Their first prototype took blood from the left atrium to the ascending aorta. The second model took blood from the left atrium to the descending aorta using a tube-type pump, and was both safer and easier to insert. The device consisted of a silastic tube, reinforced with Dacron, with ball-type valves at each end to direct flow. Surrounding this tube was a second one, connected to an external source of compressed air. The volume of air pumped into the outside tube could be adjusted (from 0 to 60 ml per stroke), and the pump console was driven electronically in synchrony with the R wave of the electrocardiogram. Compressed air in the outside tube squeezed the blood onwards in synchrony with the cardiac cycle. The apparatus was used to support the left ventricle of experimental animals for weeks or months, without significant blood damage. In 1963, DeBakey reported the use of the left ventricular assist device (LVAD) in a 42-year-old man with severe calcific aortic stenosis and left ventricular failure, who had undergone aortic valve replacement with a Starr–Edwards valve. The morning after valve replacement, he suffered a cardiac arrest and needed internal cardiac massage. Although he had clearly sustained hypoxic cerebral damage and was in pulmonary oedema, the DeBakey team decided to use the LVAD. The device was inserted by Stanley Crawford and performed continuously over the next 4 days, until the patient was declared brain dead.

Harken and diastolic counterpulsation

WHILST the DeBakey team worked on left ventricular assistance, Harken in Boston explored the concept of diastolic counterpulsation. A pump was designed to aspirate blood from the aorta during systole and pump it back into the circulation during diastole. The physiological aim of this novel process was to reduce the cardiac afterload (resistance against which the heart must pump), then augment blood flow during diastole, which improved coronary and myocardial perfusion.

Harken's pump was a large extracorporeal device. The exchange of blood occurred through a cannula inserted into the aorta, via the femoral, iliac or left subclavian artery. It was this type of device that the DeBakey team next employed in 1966. The patient was a 65-year-old coalminer with rheumatic mitral stenosis, who underwent mitral valve replacement with a Starr–Edwards ball valve. Pre-operatively, he had severe pulmonary hypertension and DeBakey decided to use the counterpulsation device during weaning from cardiopulmonary bypass. The relatively small pump was situated by the bedside and connected by tubes passed through the chest wall into the aorta. Augmented circulation was sustained for several days, but was insufficient to prevent death.

'The first success'

LATER THAT YEAR, DeBakey returned to his original pulsatile LVAD, which was modified (lining it with velour cloth) to prevent clotting. On 8 August 1966, the pulsatile tube device was used in a 37-year-old female who was critically ill with rheumatic aortic and mitral valve disease and left ventricular failure. She underwent double valve replacement, but her heart could not be weaned from cardiopulmonary bypass. On this occasion, the LVAD was inserted with great success. The pump maintained a physiological bloodflow, and on several occasions when the heart failed again, pump flow was increased with impressive results. After 10 days of support, the patient's own heart could sustain a satisfactory cardiac output without the LVAD. It was removed, and 18 days later she was discharged from hospital to resume a normal life.

Encouraged by this result, the team next supported a 16-year-old female for 4 days after mitral valve replacement (October 1967). Venous drainage was taken from the left atrium and returned via the right axillary artery. Again, the outcome was successful. Beall presented the three patients at a symposium in New York (1967) and emphasized that this type of support should be used only when the cardiac muscle was potentially recoverable.

Sticky politics and media attention

THE FIRST clinical cardiac transplant in Cape Town that same year provided an additional stimulus for expansion of the artificial heart programme. Whilst refining the LVAD in DeBakey's unit, Liotta persisted with his ambition to design an implantable TAH. The research funds at Baylor were wholly inadequate and Liotta's co-worker, William Hall, resigned from the programme following an argument with DeBakey about selling experimental animals to raise money. From then on, Liotta had no collaborator in the laboratory and the research ground to a halt.

Until the cardiac transplants, the Cooley–DeBakey rivalry was amicable to a degree, and mutually productive. Cooley had effectively separated from DeBakey with the development of the Texas Heart Institute (1963), shortly before Crawford implanted Liotta's LVAD in a patient. Further developments in Houston took place against a background of intense competition between the two teams, fuelled by media attention. At the Pan–Pacific Surgical Congress of 1963, Cooley had predicted the advent of heart transplantation and implantable artificial hearts. With Cooley's dramatic entry into the transplant race in 1968, the publicity focus, which had previously centred on the Baylor artificial heart programme, shifted to Cooley and the Texas Heart Institute. The gulf between the two

surgeons widened, until their only communication consisted of press releases.

DeBakey commended Barnard's first transplant as "a real breakthrough in the whole field of heart replacement". He established a heart transplant committee at Baylor, which did not include Cooley. After Cooley's first three transplants in May 1968, DeBakey, through *Medical World News*, declared that "the artificial heart would prove the answer to cardiac replacement". Cooley's reply, through *Universal Press*, was that "the permanent artificial heart was closer to science fiction than reality".

By August 1968, the Cooley team had overtaken all other units, including Cape Town, with nine transplants. The DeBakey team then performed their first. In September 1968, when heart donors were scarce, Cooley announced his intention to build a TAH, different to that of DeBakey. His aim was to produce the total replacement device with Liotta. However, Liotta was still funded from the National Heart Institute with Federal grants secured by DeBakey. Consequently, before human trials could be undertaken with devices from Liotta's research, DeBakey's permission was necessary. Cooley was still a full professor at Baylor at that time, and had access to the research laboratories, provided that he personally funded any experiments which were not part of a formal College programme. Liotta decided not to resign from the Federally funded programme, but to work with Cooley on the TAH in his spare time. Liotta had not seen or heard from DeBakey in 3 months, and the Baylor–Rice LVAD programme was at a low ebb. Because of the rivalry between Cooley and DeBakey, Liotta realized that DeBakey would disapprove of their collaboration and decided not to inform him.

The Liotta total artificial heart

LIOTTA had a design for an implantable TAH driven by carbon dioxide gas, pulsed through tubes from a control console. A local company, Texas Medical Instruments, already manufactured a suitable power console, but the company's specialist in this field, William O'Bannon, was a participant in the Baylor–Rice artificial heart programme through his position as Professor of Engineering at Rice University. However, O'Bannon was also a large stockholder in Texas Medical Instruments, and Cooley, who believed in the activating force of profit, persuaded Liotta that some sort of arrangement could be made. Cooley met with O'Bannon at Rice University and explained the design for an implantable device that could pump 6 litres of blood per minute, and thereby keep a patient alive pending access to a human heart donor. O'Bannon expressed concern about conflict with the Baylor–Rice programme, but Texas Medical Instruments was in financial difficulty and the prospect of an implantable TAH was commercially compelling. After consultation with David Hellums, Chairman of the Department of Engineering at Rice, it was agreed that O'Bannon should work on the power console in his own time. The project was undertaken in his garage at home and the seeds were sewn for the greatest interpersonal dispute in the history of surgery. On 30 January 1969, Liotta began a series of TAH implants in calves. Initially, there were problems with the bulk of the device and inability to provide blood and airtight seals between human tissue and plastic. Also, there was no satisfactory valve system until Cooley obtained a consignment of Wada–Cutter valves. Several problems were identified and eliminated during the first four calf implants. The fifth modification of the device, together with the new valve system, resulted in a 40% increase in efficiency. The next calf implant proved successful, until one of the rubber diaphragms ruptured, causing acute failure and further redesign. Clotting on the fabric of the heart presented problems and 60 different fabrics were tested before a synthetic material with relatively low thrombogenicity was found. It then seemed that the last major problem had been overcome.

The Liotta TAH consisted of two air-driven, diaphragm-type, reciprocating pumps constructed from dacron impregnated silastic with a reticular dacron fabric lining. The pumps were activated by two external power units with a pulse timer to determine ventricular rate. Uni-directional flow was regulated by Wada–Cutter hingeless valves.

The first total artificial heart operation

ON 5 MARCH 1969, a prospective patient, Haskell Karp, was admitted to St Luke's Hospital with severe coronary disease and a large left ventricular aneurysm. He required a transvenous pacing wire for heart block. The initial plan was to resect the left ventricular aneurysm, but Cooley regarded this as a high-risk operation and considered using the Liotta TAH as a bridge to transplantation. (Karp was not prepared to undergo transplantation as a primary procedure). Accordingly, O'Bannon delivered the filing cabinet sized control console and attached two cylinders of carbon dioxide. The white silastic heart was immersed in water in a stainless steel sink to test the system. The console and heart functioned well for 3 days (Figure 8.5, page 299).

On Wednesday, 2 April, Cooley asked Henry Reinhard, the Administrator of the Texas Heart Institute and Cooley's transplant programme, to produce a special consent form for Karp's aneurysmectomy followed by mechanical TAH implantation and transplantation should the need arise. On the afternoon of the 3 April, Cooley explained the plan to Mr and Mrs Karp and obtained consent. Realizing the extent of media interest, Liotta, Cooley and Reinhard prepared the following answers to predictable questions:

Q1: Which individuals are to be credited with the design and development of the device?
Answer: The intrathoracic pump was developed by Dr Liotta and Dr Cooley at Baylor. The control system was developed by off-duty engineers, Hardy Bourland and Bill O'Bannon at Rice University in conjunction with Texas Medical Instruments and Mr John Maness. (The emphasis on off-duty was important because of the pending NIH grant application from Dr DeBakey involving Rice University).

Q2: How long did it take to develop this particular model of the heart device?
Answer: The device was the product of years of research by investigators throughout the world; the result of accumulated knowledge as it was shared among the membership of such organizations as the American Society for Artificial Internal Organs. The particular model was constructed and tested over a 4-month period by Dr Cooley and Dr Liotta.

Q3: When did research on this particular device begin?
Answer: The device is a refinement of a prototype first

reported by Dr Liotta from his research in Argentina in 1959.

Q4: What institutional company is credited with the development or construction of the equipment?

Answer: The intrathoracic device was constructed at Baylor University College of Medicine. The control console was developed by Texas Medical Instruments.

Q5: Where was the intrathoracic device built?

Answer: At Baylor and the control console at Texas Medical Instruments.

Q6: To what extent has this device been tested in animals?

Answer: The present device was the result of years of testing many different designs and models.

Q7: How long did it sustain life in an animal?

Answer: The post-operative problems of maintaining an animal after implantation of the device are considerably more complex than in a human being. For this reason one should be cautious about assigning too great a value to the length of animal survival. This particular device had sustained a calf for 47 hours at the end of which time the device was functioning adequately when the animal was sacrificed.

Q8: Where were the animal experiments carried out?

Answer: Baylor University College of Medicine.

Q9: Is the artificial heart in any way similar to the left ventricular bypass pump used previously by the DeBakey team?

Answer: The device was built on an entirely different concept.

Q10: How is the artificial heart attached to the patient?

Answer: The intrathoracic device is attached in the same manner as a transplanted human donor heart. The device is connected externally to the control console by two polyethylene tubes through which carbon dioxide is pulsed to supply the pumping action.

On the evening of 3 April, Cooley met with Liotta and O'Bannon to make final checks on the equipment and with the operating room nurses, Barbara Lichty and Gwynn Baumgartner, to explain the sequence of events. Karp's operation was scheduled for around midday Good Friday, 4 April, after six other patients.

The following day the surgical team comprised the anaesthetist, Arthur Keats, with the perfusionist, Euford Martin, and surgical assistants, Robert Bloodwell and Bruno Messmer; Liotta was the third assistant. Karp's own heart was extensively scarred and could not be separated from bypass. Accordingly, the native heart was excised and replaced with the mechanical TAH. There were technical difficulties with the suture line between the friable atrial tissues and the dacron sewing cuff of the mechanical device but these were eventually overcome. With the artificial heart pumping at 6 litres/min, Karp was successfully weaned from cardiopulmonary bypass. Soon afterwards the team began the search for a transplant donor.

Problems

IRONICALLY, DeBakey had left his office at 4.30 p.m. the same day to attend an artificial heart meeting at the National Institutes of Health, Washington. He was informed of the event by Ted Diethrich, then a staff surgeon at the Methodist Hospital. Meanwhile, Karp was kept within the operating room, but regained consciousness and was extubated in the early evening. There were immediate, though bizarre, offers of transplant donors that same night in response to media coverage. One was a 31-year-old housewife who suffered amniotic fluid embolism during childbirth but had been dead for at least 30 minutes when the body arrived by ambulance at the emergency room of St Luke's Hospital.

In the meantime, Karp developed acute renal failure following prolonged cardiopulmonary bypass and the haemocrit fell progressively due to haemolysis. By Easter Sunday, (6 April) Karp's condition had deteriorated with pulmonary infiltrates requiring reventilation. There was a further offer of a donor, but a conscious young Jehovah's Witness dying from uterine bleeding was considered too controversial to accept. The same day, DeBakey's team, in his absence, performed a lung transplant at the Methodist Hospital but Cooley was denied access to the donor's heart. At 3.00 p.m. the same afternoon, a female patient in Massachusetts was declared brain dead after an accident during electroconvulsive therapy for depression. The patient's relatives asked that she should be kept on a ventilator and considered as a donor for Karp. A Lear jet was despatched from Houston to collect the ventilated donor, together with her eldest daughter and the referring physician. They set off to return to Houston at 12.25 a.m. but 90 minutes into the flight with the donor's condition deteriorating progressively, the aircraft's hydraulic system failed and the plane lost altitude. The pilot made an emergency landing at a closed Air Force base near Shreveport, Louisiana, without breaks or flaps. Almost simultaneously the ventilator ran out of oxygen. An oxygen cylinder was provided by the infirmary and 15 minutes later a second Lear jet arrived from Houston to continue the journey.

During transfer between Houston's airport and St Luke's Hospital the donor suffered a cardiac arrest but was resuscitated. The transplant began at 7.00 a.m. with cardiopulmonary bypass established from the femoral artery and venae cavae. The artificial heart was easily removed and, since Cooley had already performed 19 cardiac transplants, the procedure went smoothly. Nevertheless, 32 hours later (Tuesday, 8 April) the transplanted heart failed and Karp died.

This was the beginning of the most extensive series of investigations and litigations the medical profession had ever known. Cooley and Liotta's stance was that they had independently built and tested a new artificial heart using private funds with the help of engineers from Texas Medical Instruments. DeBakey's argument was that Cooley had intentionally made secret arrangements to obtain a substantial duplicate of the artificial heart which was being developed under the NIH grant in DeBakey's laboratory at Baylor. DeBakey, backed by the Central Judiciary Committee of the American College of Surgeons, claimed that Cooley had deliberately planned to use the artificial heart prior to the operation on Karp and that Cooley actively participated in immediate and extensive publicity afterwards. Cooley insisted that the artificial heart developed by himself and Liotta was used in an emergency for bridge to transplantation in a patient who would otherwise have died on the operating table.

The aftermath

The dispute was greatly inflated by incessant media coverage, resulting in Cooley's resignation from Baylor. During the same week, the American College of Surgeons voted to censure Cooley over the event but invited him to present the Karp case at a meeting (attended by Barnard and Shumway) to publicise their annual congress. In August 1969, Cooley was invited to a private audience with Pope Paul, whilst operating in Rome. The Pope is said to have favoured the artificial heart in contrast to human heart transplants because of the difficulty in definition of brain death.

This and other controversies are addressed in Cooley's biography by Harry Minetree, an ex-patient with a thoracic aneurysm. In the *Hospital Tribune* 14 July 1969, Kolff, inventor of the artificial kidney, wrote

> *"The implantation of an artificial heart in Houston, Texas, on April 4th, was a step forward in medical history. Dr Denton Cooley, Dr Domingo Liotta and others kept a patient alive for 64 hours with a mechanical heart before he received a natural heart transplant. While the patient eventually died of complications from having the second operation, the important fact is that the Houston doctors proved that an artificial heart can indeed replace a natural one in man".*

The intra-aortic balloon pump

MEANWHILE, away from the public eye, other programmes worked towards the goal of mechanical cardiac support from a different standpoint. In the early 50s, the brothers, Adrian and Arthur Kantrovitz studied diastolic augmentation of coronary blood flow at Western Reserve University. They calculated that if peak arterial pressure could be achieved during diastole, the coronary blood flow could be augmented by 20–40%. Harken recognized the importance of diastolic augmentation whilst working with the heart-lung machine as a support device in closed chest situations. At a meeting on extracorporeal circulation in September 1957, Harken clearly predicted the benefit that might result from diastolic counterpulsation.

> *"In short, it seems likely that the returned arterialized blood should be returned during diastole when the aortic valve is closed. This would probably offer less resistance to the ailing heart's systolic effort and therefore, presumably, less cause for myocardial work which is of course our objective".*

Harken went on to predict that synchronized oscillation of blood flow could be obtained through synchrony with the QRS complex of the electrocardiogram. Adrian Kantrovitz moved to New York University in Brooklyn and continued experimenting with methods to augment diastolic perfusion. In one of his experiments, a piece of diaphragm with an intact phrenic nerve and blood supply was wrapped around the distal thoracic aorta of dogs in such a way that the contained aortic segment could be constricted by phrenic nerve stimulation. Measuring carotid artery pressure and flow during diastolic stimulation, this auxiliary heart was seen to reduce left ventricular stroke work and add energy to the forward propulsion of blood in the descending aorta. Soon afterwards, Harken and co-workers described their ingenious electronically controlled arterial counter-pulsator which enabled blood to be withdrawn from the abdominal aorta during systole and returned in diastole. This mechanism increased diastolic pressure and off-loaded the left ventricle in systole with potential benefits for the treatment of heart failure.

Harken and the Kantrovitz brothers had different aims: the first to diminish left ventricular workload and the second to augment coronary blood flow. In tandem, their work demonstrated that both objectives could be achieved by diastolic augmentation, the concept of which formed the basis for intra-aortic balloon counter-pulsation. In 1962, Kolff's group at the Cleveland Clinic and Roy Klaus, working with Harken, both devised a balloon catheter which could be introduced into the aorta and inflated during diastole to produce counter-pulsation. Adrian Kantrovitz and colleagues in Brooklyn adopted this device, though it was 5 years before clinical use was reported. Kantrovitz, working with Yukihiko Nose (Figure 8.6), tested different types of balloon pump. The first was a silastic bulb within a lucite casing, which was compressed by air in ventricular diastole via an R wave electrocardiographic control mechanism. The bulb was tested experimentally by anastomosis end-to-end with the abdominal and thoracic aorta and proved most effective in close proximity to the heart. The second model, a valveless tube within a lucite casing was inflated by the same mechanism, and afforded the best cardiac support in the animal model. It was first applied to a patient with severe heart failure in 1966. The auxiliary ventricle was implanted by division and suture closure of the aorta and provided a stroke volume of about 40 ml at a rate of 80 inflations/min before the patient died.

In 1968, Adrian Kantrovitz and colleagues described their clinical experience with balloon pumping in five

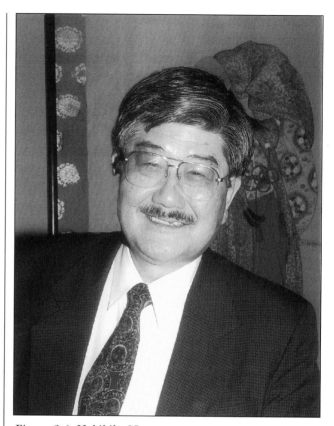

Figure 8.6. Yukihiko Nose.

patients with cardiogenic shock treated during June and July 1967. All patients were improved and one was discharged from the hospital. Nevertheless, acceptance of the method was slow and the balloon mechanism was modified on several occasions to employ single- or double-chambered balloons. A multi-centre trial of the pump in cardiogenic shock (1969) recruited only 87 patients from 10 institutions when reported in 1973. However, the results were encouraging and intra-aortic balloon pumping was widely adopted thereafter. The variable results were soon found to depend on the indication for use and the timing of intervention. In 1972, Mortimer Buckley and associates, at Massachusetts General Hospital, described the use of balloon counterpulsation to wean patients from cardiopulmonary bypass. Eighteen of 27 patients left the operating room and 13 were long-term survivors. Kantrovitz's use of the balloon in patients with unstable angina resulted in 90% survival, but only 12% survived its use in cardiogenic shock after myocardial infarction. It was 1979 before David Bregman described a single-chambered balloon that could be inserted percutaneously through the femoral artery by the Seldinger technique. By this time, many studies had shown intra-aortic balloon pumping to decrease left ventricular workload, myocardial time tension index, end diastolic pressure and mean pulmonary wedge pressure. Both cardiac output and coronary diastolic flow were increased.

Second generation blood pumps

IN 1967, William Pierce and Glen Morrow designed an LVAD in the form of an implantable roller pump. The device, powered by a DC motor, consisted of two rollers encased in an anodized aluminium and polycarbonate housing, designed to bridge between the left atrium and descending aorta. The motor was driven by an external power source, with only an electric wire and pressure catheter traversing the chest wall. The output of the pump was regulated through an electronic servo system based on left atrial pressure. The pump was implanted in calves and functioned for several days before failure of the electric motor. Pierce then left the National Heart Institute to join John Waldhausen's group at Pennsylvannia State University in Hershey. Here they developed an external air driven roller pump device used with a closed chest technique via catheters between the left atrium and carotid artery. Their experiments were similar to those of Clarence Dennis and Åke Senning in the early 1960s. Pierce progressed to design implantable, flexible blood pumps driven by an external electronic R wave synchronization unit, together with the pneumatic Baylor–Rice power unit. The most successful artificial ventricle comprised a thin walled blood sac of segmented polyurethane in a polysulphate housing. A membrane bisected the mid-part of the spheroidal shaped casing, and was inflated and deflated by a pneumatic drive and control unit synchronized with the electrocardiogram. The Pennsylvania State device was used clinically by withdrawing blood either from the apex of the left ventricle or from the left atrium, with return to the aorta. For right ventricular assistance, the inflow cannula was placed in the right atrium and the outflow graft anastomosed with the pulmonary artery. Between 1976 and 1982, Pierce's group employed left ventricular assistance in 22 patients, right ventricular assistance in two, and bi-ventricular support in six. Fourteen patients were successfully separated from the pump, with nine

survivors. With improvements in design and technique, 10 of the last 16 patients were successfully weaned, with seven survivors. Bleeding around anastomic sites was a common problem in the early experience and contributed to mortality.

The total artificial heart revisited

SEVERAL other North American groups worked towards the goal of an implantable TAH in the early 60s. Gerald Rainer and associates, at St Joseph's Hospital in Denver, produced a bi-ventricular model with simultaneously contracting ventricles and inflow and outflow valves mounted in a lucite chamber. These were opened and closed by synchronized compressed air corresponding with the systolic and diastolic phases of ventricular contraction. At the University of Indiana, Burns, Shumacker and colleagues began an intensive programme to develop a totally implantable electrically powered TAH based on a closed loop hydraulic system, with alternate compression of separate right and left flexible silastic ventricles within a semi-rigid casing. Several different systems of motor, pump and valves were tested. The power source was external with a transcutaneous wire to rechargeable external batteries, though the aim of this team was to create transthoracic energy transfer. The device was tested in calves and large dogs, with orthotopic replacement of the excised heart with the bi-ventricular unit. This was connected by short, large bore, plastic tubes to the electrohydraulic unit situated in the upper abdomen. The device functioned adequately for up to 18 hours without the development of pulmonary oedema or thrombo-embolism. Free haemoglobin levels were low and there was no excessive heat production from the device. The early models were too large for clinical intrathoracic placement. Later models were suitable for extraperitoneal abdominal implantation, with inflow and outflow grafts passing through the diaphragm to the great vessels.

In Europe, Felix Ungar of Innsbruck developed an air driven double ventricular replacement unit in the 1970s. At the Cleveland Clinic, Kolff's group, which included Akutsu (Figure 8.7), designed an electromagnetically driven heart with two encased sac-type polyurethane ventricles with leaflet valves. Kolff also developed a

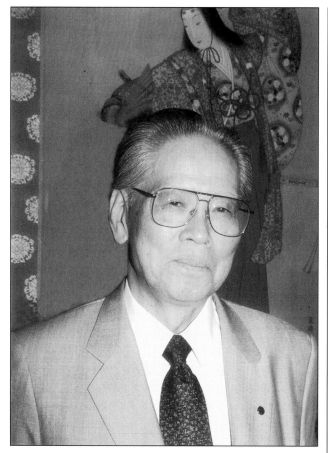

Figure 8.7. Tetsuzo Akutsu.

rotating roller that compressed two collapsible ventricles and ejected blood into the systemic and pulmonary circulations. After their initial experience with intrathoracic motors, which generated heat but limited power, Kolff's team redirected their efforts towards air-driven hearts with trans-thoracic airlines connected to an external power and control system. Silastic was used for the ventricular sacs instead of polyurethane. In one design, a diaphragm was pushed during systole by an air-driven piston and returned to the diastolic position by a spring within each ventricle. Electronic timers were used to determine pulse rate. With increasing experience, the pump design, control and power systems improved but survival times in recipient animals were limited.

At Tokyo University, Atsumi and associates constructed plastic bag ventricles surrounded by water within a casing. Two alternating bellows, operated by a cam controlled lever, compressed the ventricles and ejected blood during systole. There were many problems, including leakage of air into the ventricular

bags. Atsumi went on to develop a bi-ventricular sac-type heart with two air-driven bellows with inlet and outlet valves. The control system employed a phototransistor and light source for a pulse generator, which rotated a pulse motor forward and backward to move the piston and lever control bellows. By 1981, the Tokyo team obtained survival in experimental animals of up to 9 months.

The second total artificial heart operation

AKUTSU then joined Cooley in Houston and developed a bi-ventricular, polyurethane, hemispherical, diaphragm blood pump with Björk–Shiley valves. This heart was air driven by an external electrical power supply and a drive console with a sophisticated monitoring system. Measured inflation pressure then vacuum were supplied separately to each ventricle, but with a controlled common rate and duration of systole. In addition to the ordinary electrical supply, a battery powered system was available for emergency situations.

Cooley implanted this artificial heart into a patient on 23 July 1981 (Figure 8.8, page 300). On this occasion, the patient had undergone coronary artery bypass but required intra-aortic balloon pumping to wean from cardiopulmonary bypass. Despite increasing inotropic support, the patient deteriorated inexorably with eventual cardiac arrest requiring re-entry and internal cardiac massage. When intractable ventricular fibrillation ensued, he was returned to the operating room and placed again on cardiopulmonary bypass. The fibrillating heart was excised and replaced with the artificial heart. The heart maintained a cardiac output of between 3.5 and 4 litres/min and urine flow remained satisfactory. An initial diffuse coagulopathy was eventually brought under control. Next, the device compressed the left-sided pulmonary veins, causing pulmonary oedema and hypoxia. This responded to veno-venous bypass and membrane oxygenation pending acquisition of a donor heart. The transplant was performed during the early hours of 25 July, after about 6 hours of mechanical support. Seven days later the patient developed multiple organ failure with Gram-negative infection and died (2 August). By this time, artificial heart programmes had developed in a dozen laboratories in Argentina, Austria,

China, Czechoslovakia, France, Germany, Italy, Japan, the US and Russia.

Functional criteria for a total artificial heart

THE TAH had to be small enough to fit within the mediastinum, yet of sufficient size to support the whole body. There should also be the facility to vary the rate of pump flow according to metabolic requirements. It should be durable and readily sterilized. Last, and of greatest importance, the device must not cause red cell destruction and haemolysis or be prone to thrombotic complications. Clearly, this was a tall order. For a dual chamber device the output of the right ventricle must equal that of the left and for moderate exercise the resting cardiac output (5–6 litres/min) must double. The TAH should be responsive to the increased volume and pressure of blood returning to the heart with exercise and increase its output correspondingly. Because of the complexity of the physiological responses to activity, the National Aeronautic and Space Administration (USA) participated in the development of a computer-based control system that regulated the output of the artificial heart according to various physiological conditions, including atrial pressure (1963). Congress allocated money for an artificial heart programme under the guidance of the National Heart, Lung and Blood Institute. Other organizations joined in the assessment of artificial heart technology, the problems associated with its development and the clinical need for such a programme.

Because of early difficulties with dual chamber hearts of the sac-type, Pierce tried to work with only a left ventricle. The right ventricle was bypassed with a shunt from the vena cava to the pulmonary artery, similar to the Fontan circulation for uni-ventricular hearts. This proved unsuccessful. Attempts were made to develop nuclear powered hearts with programmes jointly funded by the National Heart, Lung and Blood Institute with the Atomic Energy Commission. The plan was to develop a fully implantable artificial heart that would operate for 10 years without external support. The various prototype systems utilized heat from the radioactive isotope plutonium 238 to run an engine of the Sterling Cycle, Rankine or Thermocompressor type.

The engine, in turn, drove a blood pump pneumatically, hydraulically or mechanically. The nuclear powered artificial hearts had only limited success (Figure 8.9, page 300).

Kolff and the Utah programme

IN THE EARLY 70s, the feasibility of a TAH remained in doubt. Kolff left the Cleveland Clinic in 1967 for the University of Utah. Here, together with Clifford Kwan-Gett, he worked on a new design with a diaphragm pumping element. The Kwan–Gett heart was mechanically durable and free from haemolysis, and supported animals for 2 weeks. Unfortunately, the smooth silicone rubber surfaces caused excessive clotting, platelet consumption and uncontrolled bleeding. To overcome this problem, dacron fibre was glued to the silicone rubber surface in an attempt to stimulate a fibrin coating. The aim of this counter intuitive approach to thrombosis was to encourage seeding by endothelial cells in order to achieve a biocompatible surface. In practice, the dacron fibres produced a build up of fibrin at the blood interface and this became so thick that it impaired filling and blocked the motion of the diaphragm. Nevertheless, the textured surface approach would eventually prove successful in the Thermo Cardio Systems Incorporated (TCI) LVAD (Figure 8.10). Nose attempted to address the biocompatibility issue with his so-called biolized heart, where the blood–foreign surface interface was lined by biological surfaces, such as pericardium. These were gluteraldehyde fixed in the same way as a biological valve. In 1973, a heart of this kind functioned in a calf for 17 days.

The Jarvik heart

IN 1970, Robert Jarvik joined the artificial heart programme at Utah. Jarvik's interest in medical engineering stretched back to his high school years, where he worked on automatic surgical staplers. Having first enroled at the Syracuse University School of Architecture, Jarvik switched to premedical studies after his father was operated on for an aortic aneurysm. He

(a)

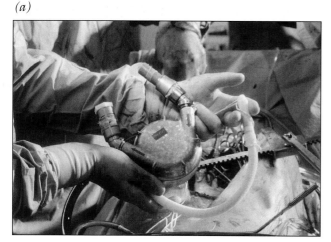

(b)

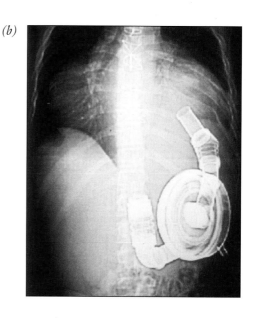

Figure 8.10. (a) Thermo Cardio Systems Inc (TCI) left ventricular assist device. (b) Chest X-ray of the device in situ.

went to medical school at the University of Bologna (Italy) before completing a Master's Degree in biomechanics at New York University. The Utah team switched their emphasis from electrically driven hearts to pneumatically powered devices, with an intensive programme to refine design, biocompatibility and durability. Selection of the experimental animal and details of operative technique became increasingly important when potentially satisfactory devices failed through poor fit to the natural anatomy (Figure 8.11, page 300). The result was kinking and obstruction of the native circulation, with early failure through thrombosis or haemolysis. The Jarvik 3 heart was designed to overcome some of these problems and raised the maximum time of survival in the animal model. By 1977, the longest survival time of calves with pneumatic powered sac-type hearts was 60 days. The main technical problem encountered was linear tearing of the blood sacs. The Jarvik 3 heart was fitted with a highly flexible three layered diaphragm made of smooth polyurethane (earlier hearts had a single layer diaphragm of polyurethane which ruptured too easily). This modified diaphragm soon increased survival time. Meanwhile, with different devices the Cleveland Clinic increased animal survival to 5 months and the Berlin group to 6½ months. With further refinement the Jarvik 7 heart was fabricated to conform to human anatomy but was implanted experimentally in the calf, which has substantial anatomical differences. Despite this, survival of 221 days was achieved and the calves grew to a size far beyond the capacity for which the device was designed (Figure 8.12, page 300).

The Jarvik 7 TAH consisted of two ventricles made of polyurethane supported on an aluminium base. Rings of polycarbonate supported Björk–Shiley disc valves (Figures 8.13 and 8.14). For the animal implants, the natural ventricles were excised and polyurethane cuffs sutured to the atrial remnants, the transected aorta and the main pulmonary artery. The procedure essentially mimicked cardiac transplantation with a mechanical device. The separate right and left ventricles of the device were then snapped onto the polyurethane cuffs and connected to an external driving system by means of two tubes traversing the thoracic wall. In the longest surviving calf, the heart sustained growth from a weight of 200 lbs at implantation to more than 350 lbs several months later. The calf was able to walk on a treadmill for an hour even after it had grown to twice the size of an intended recipient human. Biochemical parameters remained normal for most of the calf's existence. One potential problem was the autopsy finding of panus ingrowth at the suture lines. Tissue spread across the inflow opening at atrial level, reducing its size and eventually limiting cardiac output. This finding was rarely seen in patients given prosthetic valves and was attributed to the fact that the calf was growing rapidly. The University of Tokyo used fully grown goats as experimental animals for TAH implants and no panus formation was found in animals who survived up to 8 months.

In January 1981, Jarvik described the progress in development of the TAH in *Scientific American*. Towards the end of the article he wrote:

"How long will it be before total artificial hearts are routinely implanted in human beings? Probably at least a decade, although clinical trials on a small scale may begin sooner. The experience of six laboratories that have maintained animals on an artificial heart for 5 months or more is encouraging. The devices themselves, the surgical techniques and the post-operative care have all been highly developed. Certainly the feasibility of an artificial heart has been demonstrated. When such hearts were first implanted in animals more than 20 years ago, it was hypothesised that the heart functions solely as a mechanical pump and that an appropriate artificial device could sustain that function for long periods of time, maintaining the recipient in good condition. Today these concepts can be considered facts rather than hypotheses. Why then will it be so long before artificial hearts are routinely implanted? The answer is to be found mainly in ethical considerations and in the allocation of the limited money available for research on the artificial heart. The pneumatically powered artificial hearts that have proved successful in animals are not portable. The animal is confined to a cage, tethered to a large drive system and exercised only on a treadmill. Such conditions would be unacceptable for human beings. Even if compressed air drives were made portable, the large pneumatic tubes that enter the chest would be uncomfortable and would carry a high risk of infection at the points of entry. Perhaps many people would accept such limitations if the alternative was death. It should be evident from this account that substantial technical problems remain to be solved before a total artificial heart can be routinely utilized in human patients. Ethical, social and economic considerations must also be dealt with. When the artificial heart has been perfected, it must be made available in sufficient quantity to serve a large number of people. The criteria for selecting recipients must be defined clearly and objectively to ensure a short period of hospitalization and a rapid recovery for a high percentage of the recipients. Patients will need sociological and psychological counselling to help them adapt to a situation new in human experience. Nowhere else will the dependence of life on technology and machines be more apparent. If the artificial heart is ever to achieve its objective, it must be more than a pump. It must be more than functional, reliable and dependable. It must be forgettable."

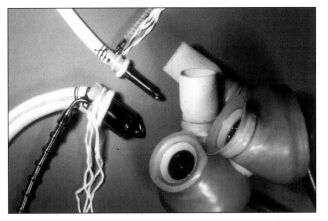

Figure 8.13. The Jarvik 7 heart, compared with adult and paediatric Jarvik 2000 impeller pumps.

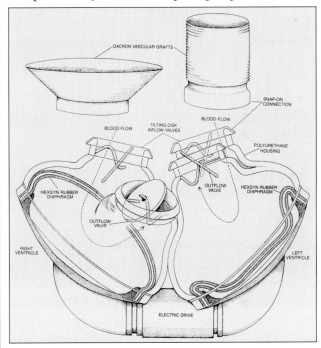

Figure 8.14. Diagram of the Jarvik 7 heart. (Reproduced with permission from Jarvik R. E. The total artificial heart. Scientific American 1981; 244: 74–80.)

The human Jarvik 7 implants

IN DECEMBER the following year (1982), after more than $160,000,000 in Federal funds had been invested in the development of an artificial heart, the University of Utah team performed the first operation to deliberately replace a human heart with a permanent mechanical device. The patient, 61-year-old Dr Barney

Clarke, was a lifelong smoker with chronic obstructive airways disease and severe congestive heart failure. Atrial fibrillation with a rapid ventricular response was poorly controlled by medical therapy. The echocardiographic left ventricular end diastolic diameter was 7.0 cm and ejection fraction less than 15%. Multiple hospital admissions were required for medical management. Six weeks before the operation, Clarke was admitted to hospital with low output failure requiring intravenous dobutamine and intensive diuretic therapy. He was severely debilitated with fatigue, dyspnoea, nausea, ascites and weight gain of 10 kg and on maximal medical therapy (digoxin 0.375 mg daily, frusemide 80 mg twice daily, captopril 50 mg or 100 mg on alternate days, prednisone 20 mg daily and oral azathioprine 50 mg twice daily). He was anticoagulated with warfarin. When increasing doses of dobutamine caused ventricular tachycardia, use of the artificial heart was considered. Clarke was not a candidate for conventional cardiac transplantation and both he and his family were keen for the implant to proceed.

The operation was carried out by William Devries and his team at the University of Utah (Figure 8.15, page 300). A report of the event was published in the *New England Journal of Medicine*. Cardiopulmonary bypass was initiated and the ventricles excised, leaving the atria intact. The pre-clotted pulmonary arterial and aortic grafts were anastomosed to these vessels, then the prosthetic atrial cuffs trimmed to an appropriate size and anastomosed to the atria. Great care was used to achieve haemostasis. The left-sided pneumatic drive line was then tunnelled through the thoracic cavity, the abdominal musculature and the skin just left of the umbilicus. This air line was attached to the left heart drive console and the prosthetic ventricle snapped into position. The atrial cuffs were approximated and air removed from the ventricles. Left ventricular pumping was initiated first, and then the same steps undertaken for the right ventricle. With both sides of the heart appropriately situated and functioning, cardiopulmonary bypass was progressively discontinued and the drive pressures from the self-contained portable Utah drive system adjusted for optimum pumping action. The system delivered regular bursts of compressed air through the drive lines to inflate the polyurethane diaphragm of each ventricle. Inflation ejected blood through the aortic and pulmonary valves, whilst passive filling occurred through the mitral and triscuspid valves causing collapse of the diaphragm and forcing air back through the controller unit for measurement and computer analysis. The diastolic period was then followed by a further systole. With the drive lines secured by skin bonds, haemostasis was checked and an attempt made to close the sternum, leaving pressure lines in both atria and the pulmonary artery. Sternal closure was complicated by the friability of Clarke's atrial tissues and bleeding problems, so the chest was left open (Figure 8.16, page 301). When the pump was started, there was dysfunction of the prosthetic mitral valve which required replacement of the mechanical left heart. Despite these problems, cardiopulmonary bypass was eventually discontinued with the artificial heart producing satisfactory cardiac output. Total cardiopulmonary bypass time was 4 hours and 9 minutes, and the overall duration of the operation was over 7 hours. At the end of the operation the chest could still not be closed over the device. Despite this, Clarke regained consciousness in 3 hours, moved all extremities on command and opened his eyes. He remained sufficiently conscious to communicate with his family and after eventual chest closure, was extubated on the second post-operative day (Figure 8.17, page 301). A brisk diuresis occurred in response to the improved cardiac output.

The following day, progressive subcutaneous emphysema was noted which required surgical exploration. Two ruptured bullae were identified and ligated on the right lung. On the 4th and 5th days, haemoglobinuria and progressive renal failure were apparent. This failed to respond to volume loading and diuretics, and was addressed by increasing the cardiac output of the TAH to 12 litres/min. Epileptic convulsions occurred shortly afterwards and were treated with phenytoin. The postictal coma abated gradually over the next 2 weeks. On day 13, the rapid onset of pulmonary oedema heralded acute mechanical left heart failure, following strut fracture of the Björk–Shiley mitral valve. Clarke was returned to the operating room and the valve replaced. On day 24, a sudden increase in pulmonary artery pressure was noted in association with a fall in left heart filling pressures. Mechanical ventilation was resumed and this unexplained phenomenon gradually resolved over the next 48 hours. The acute tubular necrosis resolved and by the 32nd day a continuing diuresis resulted in an overall improvement.

The mechanical heart continued to function satisfactorily and Clarke's cerebral status lightened with less confusion and increasing periods of lucid thought.

Attempts to provide 3000 calories per day in order to compensate for his cachectic pre-operative state then resulted in fluid overload and pulmonary oedema. Renal function deteriorated again following aggressive medical management of pneumonia and amphotericin therapy for fungal superinfection. More antibiotics for a urinary tract infection and epididymitis contributed to the development of pseudomembranous colitis and on the 92nd post-operative day, diarrhoea and projectile vomiting caused aspiration pneumonia. Mechanical ventilation was resumed with gradual improvement until the 109th day, when rapidly progressive renal failure led to anuria. Haemodynamic instability and circulatory shock (due to the colitis) exacerbated the situation and Clarke died with low cardiac output on the 112th post-operative day. Autopsy showed healing around the suture lines of the artificial heart, and no significant thrombus or infection (Figure 8.18, page 301). The outcome suggested that Jarvik's caution, less than 2 years previously, was appropriate. The case caused considerable controversy, both in the medical profession and the media. Although for a limited period Clarke was conscious and retained his sense of humour, his quality of life was poor, and the venture massively expensive.

In the midst of controversy, Devries realized that further implants at the University of Utah were unlikely and moved to the private Humana Hospital in Louisville, Kentucky. Whereas Federal grants were available for animal research, funding was not forthcoming for human operations at the University. In contrast, the Humana organization offered to fund the first 100 implants at their hospital in Kentucky. In fact, only three further implants were undertaken, the first on 25 November 1984. William Schroeder was a diabetic already cachectic through end stage coronary disease. On this occasion, the procedure was well rehearsed and proceeded far more smoothly than Clarke's operation. Though the initial progress of the three patients was satisfactory, their activities were restricted through tethering to a large console via the transthoracic tubes, and they were beset by complications. Schroeder lived for more than 2 years, but the overall experience was considered unacceptable and no further permanent implants of a TAH were undertaken in the US. More than 160 Jarvik 7 hearts have been implanted clinically, mostly for bridge to transplantation. The largest series of Jarvik 7 implants was by Christian Cabrol in Paris, and of 40 consecutive patients, more than half were successfully transplanted. One female patient was sustained for 620 days with a TAH. However, on 8 January 1990, the Food and Drug Administration (FDA) prevented further implantation of the Symbion heart, apparently because of inadequate record keeping by the company.

Many of the advances in heart and heart-lung transplantation and the development of mechanical cardiac support systems have been criticised by both the medical profession and the lay public. Many regard the patients subject to these great advances as unfortunate guinea pigs. Some of these criticisms can be put in perspective by the comments of Barney Clarke before implantation of his artificial heart. Clarke told his attendants that he had given up fishing several years before because "I cannot stand seeing the fish gasping for breath on the dock, like I do". When shown the calves with artificial hearts in situ in the laboratory, he said "These calves cannot speak, but I believe they feel a lot better than I do." We should remember that without the consent of many courageous patients, the great advances described in this text could not occur.

Mechanical bridge to transplantation

ATTENTION focused on ventricular assist devices as a bridge to cardiac transplantation. Shortly after the Cullen Cardiovascular Laboratories were established at the Texas Heart Institute in 1969, Cooley and colleagues devised a pneumatically activated polyurethane bladder within a titanium housing as a LVAD. This was provided with silicone rubber disc valves to ensure unidirectional flow between the apex of the left ventricle and the infrarenal abdominal aorta. The pump was designed to be implanted in the abdomen to avoid pulmonary compression and to enable removal of the system without thoracotomy. Only the inflow tube traversed the diaphragm for connection to the left ventricular apex. This type of device was first implanted in a patient on 9 February 1978 by Cooley and Norman. The patient could not be weaned from cardiopulmonary bypass after aortic and mitral valve replacement and repair of a ruptured sinus of Valsalva aneurysm following bacterial endocarditis. Despite the assist device, marked dilatation of the right ventricle prevented sternal closure. When the patient was returned to the operating room 2 days later for sternal closure, both ventricles were seen to be dilated and non-functional. Renal failure progressed to complete anuria and after combined cardiac and renal transplantation on 14 February 1978, the transplanted kidney failed and the patient died. Nevertheless, the LVAD provided adequate circulatory support for 5 days and showed that the circulation could be maintained without right ventricular support during bridge to transplantation. The Cooley team persisted with this device, which was eventually used in 22 patients at the Texas Heart Institute, and 17 children at Children's Hospital Medical Centre in Boston. Although survival was uncommon, the device itself functioned well without mechanical difficulties for between 3 and 7 days. Three of the Texas Heart patients recovered sufficient left ventricular function to be weaned from the device. These were the first examples of mechanical bridge to myocardial recovery.

Norman Shumway's group at Stanford University worked on transcutaneous transfer of energy. In 1973, they described a fully implantable pump placed in the left chest of experimental animals with the solenoid in the left extraperitoneal space; the transcutaneous electric power source was external. This device worked well for up to 43 days. In 1978, the same group described a microprocessor controlled energy converter with a dual pusher plate, sac-type artificial heart — a predecessor of the Novacor system. The pump was driven by a magnetically latched spring couple pulsed solenoid energy converter, with two symmetric pivoting armatures. An attached electronic control system provided electrocardiographically triggered counter-pulsation or fixed rate pumping. The device could be used for single or biventricular assistance but was not translated into clinical practice.

By 1980, cardiac transplantation had reached a watershed. After notable advances in immuno-suppression and the impressive results of Bailey, Gundry and colleagues (Loma Linda, CA) in the paediatric age group, progress decelerated through lack of availability of donor organs. In the US, data from the United Network for Organ Shairing (1993) showed that a male with type O blood group, weighing more than 200 lb would wait a mean of 595 days for a donor heart. At least one-third of the highly selected patients under 60 years of age died on the waiting list. Whilst transplantation markedly improved quality of life for the select group of recipients, outcome remained limited by the side-effects of chronic immunosuppression, opportunistic infection and the development of allograft coronary artery disease, which required retransplantation in 40% of patients by 6 years. Many countries could not develop transplantation for reasons of religion or lack of a definition for brain death. In Japan, Wada performed a single transplant, but was accused of murdering the donor and forced to move to another hospital. So far no one in Japan has taken the same risk again.

Prior to the advent of cyclosporine, all bridge to transplant attempts met with infection and multiple organ failure. Less invasive methods were explored and the first successful outcome came with the use of the intra-aortic balloon pump by Reemtsma in 1978. The balloon pump soon became the most commonly used method for dealing with the potential transplant recipient who develops cardiogenic shock. Hardesty, Griffith and colleagues at the University of Pittsburg showed that patients requiring balloon pump support for cardiogenic shock had similar outcomes to those transplanted electively (1986). Pennington at St Louis University then introduced veno/arterial extracorporeal membrane oxygenation to support moribund potential transplant recipients.

Devices for long-term implantation

IN 1980, the National Heart, Lung and Blood Institute, invited submissions towards the development of an implantable electrically powered left heart assist system that would enable unrestricted mobility for the patient. The major goals in the development of this LVAD were mechanical durability and reliability (exceeding 2 years) with a tether-free system. Contracts were awarded to several institutions, including Thermo Electron, Aero Jet together with the Cleveland Clinic, Andros (currently Novacor), Avco Everett (currently Abiomed) and the Texas Heart Institute with Gould Incorporated. Subsequently, further contracts were awarded to four groups in 1984. These included Victor Poirier of

ThermoCardio Systems and Peer Portner of Novacor (Figure 8.19, page 301), both of whose LVADs are now used for prolonged bridge to transplantation.

One of the major problems in designing an implantable electrically powered moving diaphragm type pump for long-term use was the means to compensate for changes in air volume within the motor housing. Unless the system could be satisfactorily vented, a negative pressure could form behind the pumping diaphragm and prevent its movement. Venting can be achieved by a trancutaneous vent tube open to the atmosphere, or an implantable compliance chamber where air is displaced into a bag within the thoracic cavity. Implanted compliance chambers were tested in animals during the 1970s, but failed when fibrous tissue encapsulated the exterior of the chamber and decreased its flexibility. Gas within the chamber gradually escaped, resulting in failure of the system within 200 days.

O. H. Frazier (Figure 8.20) and colleagues at the Texas Heart Institute achieved consistent survival in calves to beyond 200 days with an improved compliance chamber, but the system was too problematic for clinical studies. The reliability of the pumping device was far superior to that of the compliance chamber. Frazier then collaborated with Poirier at TCI to develop an externally vented pusher plate LVAD with a portable power source. The first device was air driven (pneumatic model) through a line attached to a 73 lb console which the patient could push on a cart. Engineers at TCI then developed an electrically powered version that could be used with a battery pack small enough to be worn by the patient. The current electrically powered version (Figure 8.10), under development since 1973, has a pumping chamber identical to that in the pneumatic device. The electric motor drives the pusher plate through a pair of nestled helicle cams and the low speed torque motor sits in a chamber below the flexible diaphragm and makes one revolution for each heart beat. The device has a percutaneous line for the electrical control system and vent. It weighs 900 g and measures 11.2 cm in diameter and 4 cm in thickness. The pneumatic model of the same dimensions is lighter (600 g) but the external console is cumbersome and restricts the patient to hospital.

The first successful bridge with an implantable LVAD

ON 5 SEPTEMBER 1984, Oyer and colleagues at Stanford University implanted Portner's 'Novacor' electric left ventricular assist system into a 51-year-old man with ischaemic cardiomyopathy. The patient was transplanted 9 days later and survived a stormy post-operative course to become the first successful bridge to transplant with an implantable LVAD. On 6 September,

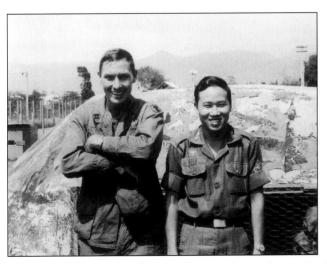
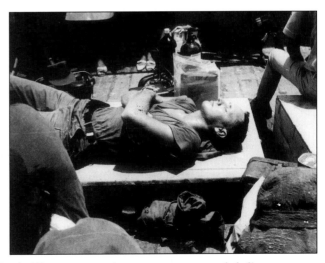

Figure 8.20. O.H. Frazier photographed during his service in the Vietnam war. As a surgeon on assault helicopters, Frazier was concerned about the high mortality rate of his medical colleagues. When told that flight surgeons were good for the men's morale, Frazier suggested that Marilyn Monroe would be better still!

Hill, at Pacific Medical Centre, San Francisco, used the external pneumatic Pierce/Donachy LVAD from Thoratec Laboratories to support a 47-year-old patient with post-infarction cardiogenic shock. The man was transplanted and again, after a protracted and complicated course, survived as the first success with an external LVAD. On 6 March 1985, Vaughan and Copeland excised a failed orthotopic transplant from a 33-year-old man and used the Jarvik 7 TAH for 36 hours prior to a second transplant. The patient, who was dying from heart failure, succumbed to bleeding and pulmonary oedema. However, on 29 August the same team used the Jarvik 7 TAH as bridge to transplant for a 25-year-old man with cardiomyopathy and cardiogenic shock. The Jarvik 7 TAH was used for 9 days, the transplant was successful and the patient became the first to leave hospital after implantation of an orthotopic TAH.

In 1986, the FDA gave permission for the pneumatic TCI LVAD to be used in patients. By 1992, 164 patients in the United States had been treated with the pneumatic TCI LVAD for bridge to transplant; 106 of these received a donor heart. On 9 May 1991, the electric TCI LVAD was first implanted by Frazier at the Texas Heart Institute.

On 3 September 1991, the electric TCI device was implanted into a young cardiomyopathy patient who was supported successfully for 505 days. Chronic heart failure resolved completely by the 3rd post-operative week and the patient was able to resume near normal activity within the hospital environment. Under the terms of the investigational agreement, the patient was restricted to the hospital grounds, but was employed in computer work within the hospital. Because of a previous pulmonary embolism and large heart size, he was anticoagulated with warfarin. Depressed by his restricted activities, warfarin was discontinued abruptly by the patient on 11 January 1992 and he died of a massive stroke 7 days later. When the device was switched off, the patient's own heart continued to support circulation, showing a remarkable degree of recovery. When the LVAD was removed it was free from thrombus or pannus formation and there was a thin pseudo-endothelial layer over the blood containing surfaces.

In 1992 and 1993, the United Network for Organ Sharing (USA) gave the mean waiting times for donor hearts (of all blood types) as 208 and 245 days, respectively. Long waiting times were often fatal, particularly for large patients with blood type O. Patients who waited many months for transplant in an intensive care unit proved extremely expensive. Whilst the costs of an LVAD and maintenance were considerable, this proved less than a median wait time of 75 days in intensive care. In the US, Frazier (Texas Heart), Rose (Columbia Presbyterian Medical Center), McCarthy (Cleveland Clinic) and Griffiths (University of Pittsburg) soon showed dramatic physiological rehabilitation and reduction in mortality for patients awaiting transplantation with an LVAD. Resolution of renal and hepatic failure increased the patient's physical capacity and quality of life. As experience with bridges to transplant grew, it became more obvious that post-transplant survival of patients treated with an LVAD was better than survival of those who waited without a device. As LVAD patients improved progressively to Class I status, they were transferred out of the intensive care unit to a regular floor and eventually discharged from the hospital to wait at home for their transplant (Figure 8.21, page 302). This experience was paralleled by that of Hetzer (Berlin), Korfer (Bad Oyenhausen) and Loisance (Paris). Survival to 505 days with the TCI 'Heartmate' and beyond 2 years with the Novacor confirmed the ability of these devices to support the circulation artificially for extended periods.

This major advance had important implications for thousand of end-stage heart failure patients who failed to qualify for transplantation or for whom a donor heart was not available. Current estimates in the United States suggest that between 35,000 and 60,000 patients could benefit from temporary or permanent circulatory support each year. With only 2000 donor hearts available, transplantation fulfils only about 3% to 6% of this need. A reliable LVAD may therefore provide an acceptable alternative for deteriorating heart failure patients with no other options. Increasingly optimistic reports of out-patient LVAD use in the United States led to intentionally permanent LVAD implants by Wallwork (Novacor) and Westaby (TCI) in the UK (Figure 8.22, page 302). Medical ethics determined the selection of very sick patients who were deemed unfit for cardiac transplantation. Whilst this limited the success of this approach, the implants nevertheless stimulated renewed interest in permanent artificial hearts and were soon followed by FDA approved trials of LVAD versus medical

Skeletal muscle cardiomyoplasty

SKELETAL MUSCLE was first introduced into cardiac surgery when DeJesus used the pectoralis major muscle to repair a penetrating cardiac injury in 1931. Two years later, Leriche and Fontan applied well vascularized pectoralis major muscle grafts to the surface of infarcted canine myocardium in order to reinforce the myocardial scar. The muscle flaps remained viable and became incorporated into the surrounding tissues. In 1959, the versatile Russian pioneer, Petrovsky, used diaphragmatic pedicle grafts to replace myocardial scar in patients with left ventricular aneurysms. The diaphragmatic muscle was sutured directly to the epicardial surface of the left ventricle in such a way as to flatten out and obliterate the aneurysm. The two muscles became firmly adherent and may have improved the myocardial blood supply through collateral circulation. Whilst the operative mortality approached 20%, one-third of patients were relieved of dyspnoea and chest pain.

The concept of skeletal muscle electrical stimulation began in 1959, when Kantrowitz and McKinnon wrapped pedicle grafts of canine left hemidiaphragm around the heart and stimulated the phrenic nerve in synchrony with cardiac systole. Contraction of the diaphragmatic muscle increased left ventricular pressure, though the effect was transitory (15 min) through muscle fatigue. Nakamura and Glenn pursued similar principles in 1964 when they incorporated pedicled grafts of diaphragm in the right atrial wall and stimulated the graft via the phrenic nerve. Schepherd (1969), using diaphragmatic grafts to the canine right ventricle, showed that long-term stimulation of the nerve supply could prevent denervation atrophy.

Experiments with the latissimus dorsi began in 1966, when Termet wrapped the muscle around the heart and after an 8 months' delay, stimulated the thoraco-dorsal nerve and fibrillated the dog's heart. Contraction of the latissimus dorsi provided aortic ejection with systolic pressures up to 80 mmHg, but the effect lasted only 10–15 minutes due to muscle fatigue.

An implantable synchronous pacemaker was first used by Macoviak in 1980 to stimulate skeletal muscle grafts. Innervated and vascularized pedicle grafts of canine diaphragm were used to replace portions of the right ventricular free wall and were stimulated through the intact phrenic nerve. Synchronous graft and cardiac contraction were obtained with supra maximal voltage stimulation. After similar experiments using latissimus dorsi pedicled grafts to replace full thickness portions of the right and left ventricle in goats, Carpentier and Chachques described the first successful use of synchronously stimulated skeletal muscle for ventricular assist in man. A Medtronic DDD-type cardiac pacemaker was used to sense the heart and then stimulate the skeletal muscle. Medtronic then developed a cardiomyostimulator that sensed the cardiac R-wave and delivered a burst of stimuli to the muscle graft in order to increase the force of the latissimus dorsi contraction. In 1986, Magovern and associates performed the first dynamic cardiomyoplasty in the United States.

The basis for the clinical application of this technique was the ability to electrically condition skeletal muscle as replacement for myocardium. Salmons (1969) showed that the stimulation pattern of a nerve determines the muscle fibre type. A fast twitch muscle could be transformed into a slow twitch muscle by delivering the frequency pattern normally received by slow twitch myocytes to the fast twitch nerve. Several weeks of electrical stimulation were required to make this transformation and resistance to fatigue developed through biochemical and morphological changes in the recipient myocyte. Stephenson, working with Edmunds in Philadelphia, became the driving force behind the use of fatigue-resistant muscle for cardiac replacement or assist in the US (Figure 8.23, page 302.).

Clinical trials of synchronously paced latissimus dorsi wrapped around the left ventricle after preconditioning have shown subjective symptomatic improvement in many patients, yet little evidence of improved systolic function. The 1-year survival rate of 70% was no better than that of medically treated New York Heart Association Class III heart failure patients (the target population for this procedure in light of the unacceptably high peri-operative mortality rate in Class IV patients). Whilst reports from Carpentier and others showed an average increase of 1.5 in the New York Heart Association Classification for heart failure, the mechanism is not augmentation of systolic function.

Sophisticated experimental analysis of the contribution of the latissimus dorsi to left ventricular performance using magnetic resonance imaging (MRI), showed a very limited contribution by the skeletal muscle wrap. There is also evidence of increasing stiffness of the latissimus dorsi over time, which suggests that the primary benefit may be to limit progressive ventricular dilation by a girdling effect. If this hypothesis is correct, similar benefit could be achieved with passive prosthetic material.

Mechanical bridge to myocardial recovery

PARADOXICALLY, the critical shortage of donor hearts, resulted in prolonged ventricular offloading and the crucial finding that in some patients the myocardium showed the propensity to recover. In 1968, Burch had shown that with maximal reduction in the workload of the dilated heart by prolonged bedrest, a degree of left ventricular recovery could be acheived in patients with congestive heart failure. Subsequently, medical treatment with angiotensin converting enzyme (ACE) inhibitors and nitroglycerine were also shown to attenuate left ventricular enlargement after myocardial infarction, suggesting that reduction in wall stress may promote ventricular remodelling. In contrast to modest pharmacological reductions in left ventricular filling pressure, mechanical blood pumps provide complete offloading and the capacity to rest the left ventricle whilst the patient remains active. The improved haemo-dynamics with LVAD support reverse multisystem organ failure, so that patients can resume physical activity and adopt an exercise programme.

In the US, committal to LVAD bridge to transplant carried the legal necessity for transplantation. At the time of cardiac transplantation, it was apparent to Frazier, McCarthy and others that the hearts of some patients, particularly with idiopathic cardiomyopathy, had reverted towards normal size and weight. In some patients, the indices of left ventricular function approached normal by the time a donor organ became available. Detailed studies of ventricular recovery suggested that chronic offloading of the left ventricle could lead to regression of myocyte hypertrophy, normalization of fibre orientation and resolution of the

metabolic changes of heart failure. Bridge to myocardial recovery was pursued by Hetzer, resulting in four adults with dilated cardiomyopathy and two children with viral myocarditis undergoing elective explant of an LVAD with prolonged survival (1995–7). Clearly the scope for mechanical bridge to myocardial recovery is substantial. When the pacemaker was designed to treat problems of heart rhythm during cardiac surgery in the 1950s, the widespread application of the technology was unforseen. It is only a matter of time before a blood pump emerges as a substitute for the left ventricle and becomes the mechanical equivalent of the pacemaker for heart failure.

Efforts are now directed towards the design of improved LVADs for widespread use in the various settings of acute and chronic heart failure. Currently, the most promising of these is the Jarvik 2000 axial flow impeller pump (Figure 8.24), which is inserted into the apex of the failing left ventricle (Figure 8.25, page 302). An impervious dacron graft conveys blood from the ventricle to the descending thoracic aorta. The

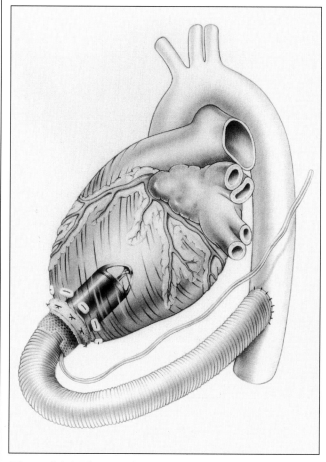

Figure 8.24. The Jarvik 2000 impeller pump inserted into the apex of the left ventricle.

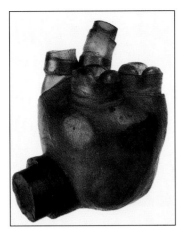

Figure 8.1. Polyvinyl chloride heart designed by Willem Kolff and Tetsuzo Akutsu in 1957. This heart kept a dog alive for 90 minutes.

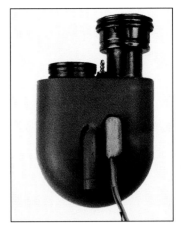

Figure 8.2. Yukihiko Noses's 1965 steel heart covered with Teflon. The device contained two silicone rubber sacs which damaged red blood cells but kept a sheep alive for a record 50 hours in 1969.

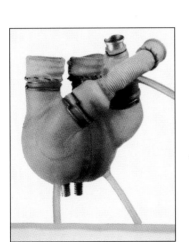

Figure 8.3. Clifford Kwan-Getts flexible heart was the first to be pumped by a diaphragm without causing haemolysis. It sustained a calf for 2 weeks.

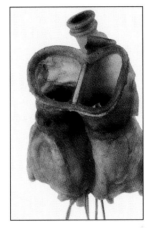

Figure 8.4. Early four chambered heart from Kolff and the Utah team.

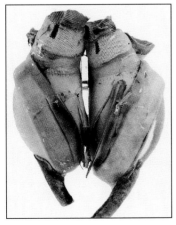

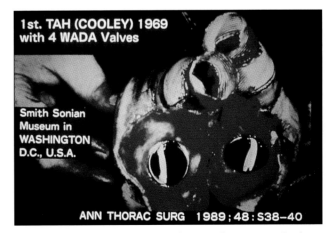

Figure 8.5. This 1969 heart designed by Domingo Liotta was the first to be implanted into a human by Denton Cooley. The patient was sustained by the device for 3 days but lived for only 36 hours after transplantation. The patients widow accused Cooley of making her husband the "unfortunate victim of human experimentation".

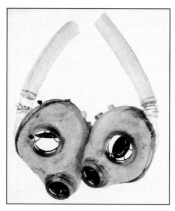
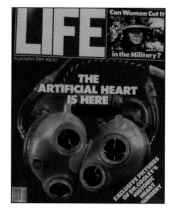

Figure 8.8. *This is the heart implanted into Willebrordus Meuffels in July 1981. The engineer Tetsuzo Akutsu had placed prototypes in more than 100 calves and 20 human cadavers. The event was widely covered in the media though LIFE's caption may have been more appropriate as 'Here is an artificial heart'. Akutsu's heart was not used again.*

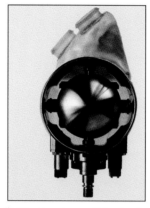
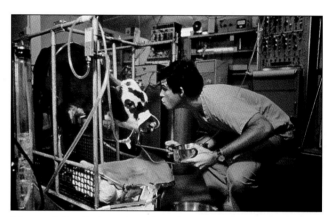

Figure 8.9. *In 1965 scientists at Wastinghouse and the University of Utah completed a prototype for a nuclear powered heart. Designed to free the recipient from external machines it was never implanted because of controversy over its radioactive power source plutonium 238.*

Figure 8.11. *Robert Jarvik and a calf with an early implant of the Jarvik 2 model in Salt Lake City (1972).*

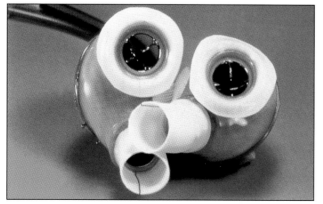
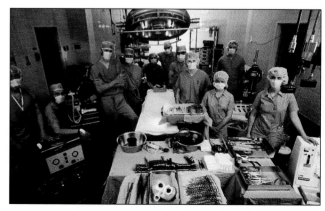

Figure 8.12. *The Jarvik 7 heart designed by Robert Jarvik and the Kolff team at the University of Utah. This device was first used clinically as a permanent artificial heart in 1982 then for bridge for cardiac transplantation.*

Figure 8.15. *William Devries and the artificial heart team after the Barney Clarke operation (1982).*

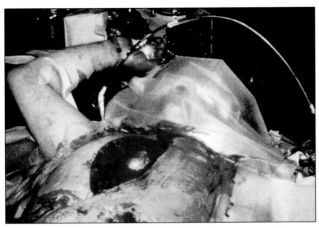

Figure 8.16. Barney Clarke with his chest splintered to accommodate the total artificial heart.

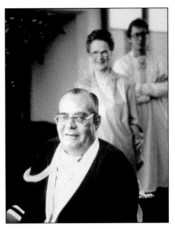

Figure 8.17. Clarke with Mrs Clarke after his initial recovery.

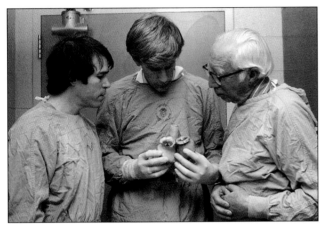

Figure 8.18. Jarvik, DeVries and Kolff examine Clarke's mechanical heart at autopsy (1983).

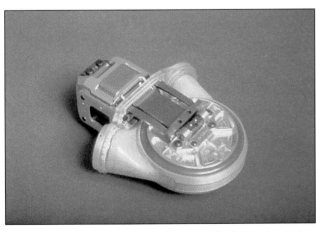

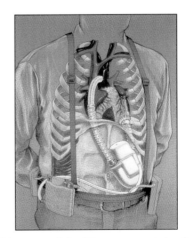

Figure 8.19. (a)The Novacor left ventricular assist device (LVAD). (b) Diagram of the Novacor pump in situ.

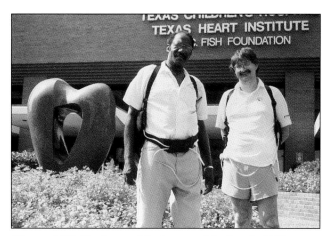

Figure 8.21. Patients with the portable electric TCI LVAD at the Texas Heart Institute.

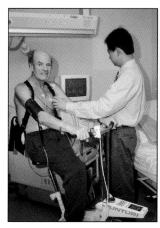

Figure 8.22. The TCI as a permanent artificial heart in Oxford. Detailed echocardiographic follow-up of the native heart with dilated cardiomyopathy showed recovery of left ventricular function as early as six weeks postoperatively.

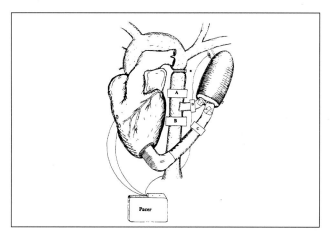

Figure 8.23. Stephenson's drawing of a skeletal muscle ventricle.

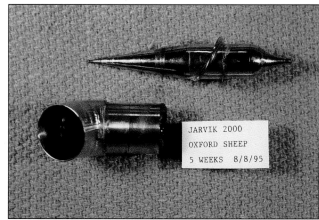

Figure 8.25. The impeller of the Jarvik 2000, which rotates at speeds up to 18,000 r.p.m. without causing haemolysis.

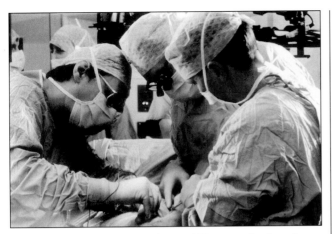

Figure 8.26. Westaby, Frazier and Taggart during the first permanent TCI LVAD implant in Oxford.

electromagnetic pump consists of a rotor with impeller blades encased in a titanium shell and supported at each end by tiny blood-immersed ceramic bearings less than 1 mm in diameter. The adult model measures only 2.5 cm in diameter by 5.5 cm in length, with a weight of 85 g and a displacement volume of 25 ml. Jarvik worked with Westaby in Oxford to produce a system with power delivered through a fine, percutaneous wire conveyed through a pyrolite carbon button secured to the skull. The combination of immobility and highly vascular scalp skin was known to resist infection in a percutaneous system for artificial hearing. Meanwhile, Frazier, funded by the National Institute of Health, pursued a fully implantable electric system based on transcutaneous power through induction coils. The potential for a compact, user-friendly, axial flow impeller pump is recognized by other groups, as reflected by the NASA/DeBakey and NIMBUS/Pittsburg programmes. It is only a matter of time before this type of technology provides a long-term substitute for the left ventricle. Mechanical blood pumps can then be used electively (much earlier then transplantation) to provide an exciting new treatment for advanced heart failure.

Biographies

Domingo Liotta (1924–)

DOMINGO LIOTTA was born in Diamante, Entre Rios, Argentina. He studied at the National College of Uruguay (BSc, 1942) and interned (1949–52) at the National University of Cordoba (MD, 1949; DMS, 1952). He fulfilled residency in surgery (1952–55) and thoracic and cardiovascular surgery (1956; 1958–59) at the University of Lyon, France, where he became interested in developing an artificial heart. In Argentina, Liotta and his brother constructed the first implantable heart pumps from plastic in an airplane factory (1960). His third plastic heart, presented to the American Society for Artificial Organs, so impressed Willem Kolff that he invited Liotta to continue research at the Cleveland Clinic. Together they made "the earliest successful laboratory attempts at replacing the heart with an artificial intrathoracic pump."

DeBakey's interest in a mechanical substitute for the heart began in the late 1950s. Early attempts to devise an artificial heart proved discouraging and in the opinion of Theodore Cooper, Head of the National Heart and Lung Institute, premature. Aiming to create a ventricular bypass assist device DeBakey offered Liotta, shortly after his arrival in Cleveland, more financial support and better facilities at Baylor College of Medicine. In July 1961, Liotta became assistant to William Hall, Director of the first cardiac device programme focused, not on total replacement with an artificial heart, but on a ventricular bypass pump. In 1963, the Baylor–Rice Artificial Heart Program acquired an National Heart Institute (NHI) grant of $4.5 million dollars.

Whilst refining the left ventricular assist device between 1961 and 1968, Liotta's ambition to design an implantable artificial heart persisted despite DeBakey's and the NHI's reluctance. By August 1968, however, the Baylor–Rice Artificial Heart Program had ground to a halt: research funds had become wholly inadequate and Hall, following arguments with DeBakey about selling

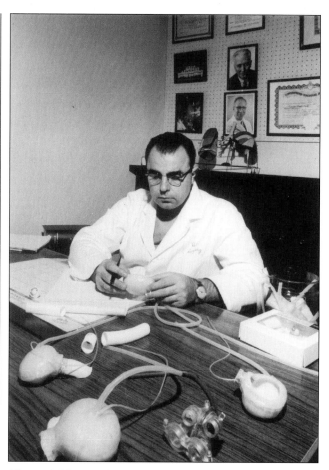

Figure 8.28. Domingo Liotta.

experimental animals to raise funds, resigned, effective 1 January 1968, and ceased his involvement in the laboratory programme in August 1968. The Saturday before Christmas, 1968, Cooley and Liotta met to discuss the possibility of Liotta's joining Cooley's clinical staff for a few months to allow Liotta to work half-time in the lab and begin operating again. Cooley who, in Barnard's wake, had transplanted nine hearts by 31 August 1968, announced that because donors were so scarce, he was going to build an artificial heart. He joined with Liotta to complete this project at his own expense. Liotta did not resign from the NHI programme or DeBakey's administration, but, unknown to both, spent spare time, building and testing the artificial heart. The console pump for Cooley's artificial heart, a duplicate of the one used in the Baylor–Rice Program, was built by a member of the Baylor–Rice Program, William O'Bannon. He was a Texas Medical Instruments specialist in power consoles and Professor of Engineering at Rice University. It was built in his garage to avoid conflicting with the federal grant for the Baylor–Rice Program at a cost of $20,000 to Cooley. The artificial heart, now in the Smithsonian Museum, was eventually implanted on Good Friday, 4 April 1969; it maintained the life of Cooley's patient, Haskell Karp for 64 hours. At the same time DeBakey was publishing a report describing the design of the artificial heart built in the Baylor Laboratories and the testing of 10 cows by The Baylor–Rice Artificial Heart Program, beginning on 31 January 1969 (Liotta's technical assistance is acknowledged at the end of the article). It proved that the plastic heart was not sufficiently successful in cows for it to be risked in a human.

Cooley's implantation of a heart, necessarily similar to DeBakey's, received prolonged attention from the media and the medical profession. Baylor College of Medicine set up formal investigations, partly in response to inquiries from the National Heart Institute, who had funded the ventricular bypass pump and had a vested interest in its tangential developments. Baylor University insisted that henceforth all faculty members must sign a letter adhering to the decision of a peer review board before clinical trials. Cooley refused to sign and resigned from Baylor Medical College (1969). On 14 October 1969, The American College of Surgeons, with C. Rollins Hanlon as President and William Longmire as Chairman of the Board of Regents, voted to censure Cooley for one year. Mrs Karp, whose husband died following implantation of the transplanted heart, brought a $4,500,000 malpractice suit against Cooley for experimenting on her husband. The charges were dismissed by a federal court in July 1972 and the decision was upheld by the United States Supreme Court. Liotta left Houston for Spain, where he developed a laboratory for artificial heart research and co-ordinated an exchange programme between the Texas Heart Institute and the University of Madrid Hospital. He later returned to his native Argentina to set up a heart institute.

Postscript

"What is the future? We need a steady supply of new ideas, the courage to apply them and tenacity of purpose in our difficulties. Difficulties are in plenty all along the way; all of us know the heartache and despair that can beset us and the black moments that come from a series of failures. In these black moments it is essential for the surgeon to hold to his plans and policies and program, provided he has confidence that he is in the right. I remember at an early stage of our development of the surgery of mitral stenosis we had had four successive deaths in our women's ward. Despair stalked before us and everyone's morale was low. I remember saying to my team that we could do only one of two things; give up or go on; it was impossible to give up as we were certainly in the right; the only thing, therefore, that we could do was to go on. We did continue and had 30 consecutive successful cases.

In this need for tenacity of purpose I am reminded of Drake's prayer. Although Francis Drake was English, and in fact very specially English, he has some connection with America. You may remember that on his famous voyage around the world he sailed up the west coast of America, what is today California. As is often the case it was foggy and so he sailed past the Golden Gate. Perhaps if it had not been foggy and he had sailed through the Golden Gate into San Francisco Bay, who knows that he might not have changed the history of the world!

His so-called prayer was not spoken as such by him but was composed from a sentence in a letter he wrote when he lay outside Cadiz harbor before going in to set fire to and destroy the Spanish ships.

"O Lord God, when thou givest to thy servants to endeavour any great matter, grant us also to know that it is not the beginning, but the continuing of the same unto the end, until it be thoroughly finished, which yieldeth the true glory."

That should be our guiding thought and it has certainly been exemplified in what we have heard in this symposium."

Lord Russell Claude Brock
Henry Ford Hospital
International Symposium on Cardiovascular Surgery
Detroit, Michigan, US
March 1955

Appendix A: Original articles

Chapter 1

1.1.   R. Matas. Traumatic aneurism of the left brachial artery. *Medical News* 1888; 53: 462–6. [See pp. 311–15]

1.2.   L. L. Hill. A report of a case of successful suturing of the heart, and table of thirty-seven other cases of suturing by different operators with various terminations and the conclusions drawn. *Medical Record* 1902; 62: 846–8. [See pp. 316–18]

1.3.   D. E. Harken. Foreign bodies in, and in relation to, thoracic blood vessels and heart. I. Techniques for approaching and removing foreign bodies from chambers of heart. *Surgery, Gynecology and Obstetrics* 1946; 83: 117–25. [See pp. 319–23]

1.4.   C. Walton Lillehei, V. L. Gott, P. C. Hodges, D. M. Long, E. E. Bakken. Transistor pacemaker for treatment of complete atrioventricular dissociation. *JAMA* 1960; 172: 76–80. [See pp. 324–8]

Chapter 2

2.1.   F. J. Lewis, M. Taufic. Closure of atrial septal defects with the aid of hypothermia: experimental accomplishments and the report of one successful case. *Surgery* 1953; 33: 52–9. [See pp. 329–36]

2.2.   J. H. Gibbon. Application of mechanical heart and lung apparatus to cardiac surgery. *Minn Med* 1954; March: 171–85. [See pp. 337–47]

2.3.   D. G. Melrose, B. Dreyer, H. H. Bentall, J. B. E. Baker. Elective cardiac arrest. *Lancet* 1955; July 2: 21–2. [See pp. 348–9]

2.4.   C. E. Drew, I. M. Andeson. Profound hypothermia in cardiac surgery. *Lancet* 1959; April 11: 748–50. [See pp. 350–2]

2.5.   B. G. Barratt-Boyes, M. Simpson, J. M. Neutze. Intracardiac surgery in neonates and infants using deep hypothermia with surface cooling and limited cardiopulmonary bypass. *Circulation* (Suppl.1) 1971; May: 26–30. [See pp. 353–7]

2.6.   J. K. Kirklin, S. Westaby, E. H. Blackstone, J. W. Kirklin, D. E. Chenoweth, A. D. Pacifico. Complement and the damaging effects of cardiopulmonary bypass. *J Thoracic Cardiovasc Surg* 1983; 86: 845–57. [See pp. 358–70]

2.7.   W. Van Oeveren, N. J. G. Jansen, B. P. Bidstrup, D. Royston, S. Westaby, H. Neuhof, C. R. H. Wildevuur. Effects of aprotinin on hemostatic mechanisms during cardiopulmonary bypass. *Ann Thorac Surg* 1987; 44: 640–5. [See pp. 371–6]

Chapter 3

Chapter 4

Chapter 5

5.1.   C. S. Beck. The development of a new blood supply to the heart by operation. *Ann Surg* 1935; 102: 801–13. [See pp. 525–37]

5.2.   L. O'Shaugnessy. The Carey Coombs Memorial Lecture. The pathology and surgical treatment of cardiac ischaemia. *Br Med Chir J* 1937; 545: 109–26. [See pp. 538–42]

5.3.   A. Vineberg, G. Miller. Internal mammary coronary anastomosis in the surgical treatment of coronary artery insufficiency. *Can Med Assoc J* 1951; 64: 204–10. [See pp. 543–9]

5.4.   W. P. Longmire Jr, J. A. Cannon, A. A. Kattus. Direct-vision coronary endarterectomy for angina pectoris. *New Engl J Med* 1958; 259: 993-9. [See pp. 550–6]

5.5.   R. G. Favaloro. Saphenous vein autograft replacement of severe segmental coronary artery occlusion. *Ann Thoracic Surg* 1968; 5: 334–9. [See pp. 557–62]

5.6.   A. R. Güntzig, Å Senning, W. E. Siegenthaler. Nonoperative dilatation of coronary-artery stenosis. Percutaneous transluminal coronary angioplasty. *New Engl J Med* 1979; 301: 61–8. [See pp. 563–9]

5.7.   European Coronary Surgery Study Group. Long-term results of prospective randomised study of coronary artery bypass surgery in stable angina pectoris. *Lancet* 1983; November 27: 1173–80. [See pp. 570–7]

Chapter 6

6.1.   M. E. DeBakey, O. Creech, G. C. Morris. Aneurysm of thoracoabdominal aorta involving the celiac, superior mesenteric and renal arteries. Report of four cases treated by resection and homograft replacement. *Ann Surg* 1956; 144: 549–72. [See pp. 578–99]

6.2.   M. E. DeBakey, D. A. Cooley, E. S. Crawford, G. C. Morris. Clinical application of a new flexible knitted dacron arterial substitute. *Am Surg* 1958; 24: 862–9. [See pp. 600–7]

6.3   D. A. Cooley, M. E. DeBakey. Resection of entire ascending aorta in fusiform aneurysm using cardiac bypass. *JAMA* 1956; 162: 1158–9. [See pp. 608–9]

6.4.   M. E. DeBakey, E. S. Crawford, D.A. Cooley, G. C. Morris. Successful resection of fusiform aneurysm of aortic arch with replacement by homograft. *Surgery, Gynecology and Obstetrics* 1957; 105: 657–64. [See pp. 610–18]

6.5.   G. C. Morris, W. S. Henly, M. E. DeBakey. Correction of acute dissecting aneurysm of aorta with valvular insufficiency. *JAMA* 1963; 184: 185–6. [See pp. 619–20]

6.6.   H. H. Bentall, A. De Bono. A technique for complete replacement of the ascending aorta. *Thorax* 1968; 23: 338–9. [See pp. 621–2]

Chapter 7

7.1.   C. N. Barnard. The operation. A human cardiac transplant: an interim report of a successful operation performed at Groote Schurr Hospital, Cape Town. *S Afr Med J* 1967; 30th December: 1271–4. [See pp. 623–6]

7.2.   P. K. Caves, E. B. Stinson, M. E. Billingham, A. K. Rider, N. E. Shumway. Diagnosis of human cardiac allograft rejection by serial cardiac biopsy. *J Thoracic Cardiovasc Surg* 1973; 66: 461–6. [See pp. 627–32]

7.3.   E. B. Stinson, P. K. Caves, R. B. Griepp, P. E. Oyer, A. K. Rider, N.E. Shumway. Hemodynamic observations in the early period after human heart transplantion. *J Thoracic Cardiovasc Surg* 1975; 68: 264–70. [See pp. 633–9]

7.4.   B. A. Reitz, J. L. Wallwork, S. A. Hunt, J. L. Pennock, M. E. Billingham, P. E. Oyer, E. B. Stinson, N. E. Shumway. Heart–Lung transplantation: successful therapy for patients with pulmonary vascular disease. *New Engl J Med* 1982; 306: 557–64. [See pp. 640–6]

ORIGINAL ARTICLES.

TRAUMATIC ANEURISM OF THE LEFT BRACHIAL ARTERY.

Failure of direct and indirect pressure ; ligation of the artery immediately above tumor ; return of pulsation on the tenth day ; ligation immediately below tumor ; failure to arrest pulsation : incision and partial excision of sac ; recovery.

BY RUDOLPH MATAS, M.D.,
VISITING SURGEON CHARITY HOSPITAL, ETC., NEW ORLEANS, LA.

NOTWITHSTANDING the fact that in these latter days the integrity of the brachial artery has ceased to be endangered by the practice of venesection, still, traumatic aneurisms of this vessel are sufficiently common and amenable to ordinary treatment to merit for the records of such cases no other than a commonplace interest. The exceptional features presented by this case, as indicated by the heading, are sufficiently instructive and interesting, it is hoped, to commend this report to the attention of the reader.

The patient, Manuel H., colored, laborer, native of Louisiana, æt. twenty-six, was admitted into Ward 2, Charity Hospital, April 30, 1888. The history given by patient was, to the effect, that two months before admission he was accidentally shot with a rifle, the whole load, consisting of fine bird shot, being distributed in the scapular, posterior acromial, and humeral regions of the left side, the gun having been fired at a distance of about fifteen feet from the patient. Two weeks after the shooting and when he believed himself completely recovered from the effects of the injury, he noticed a swelling on the inner and posterior aspect of the arm, nearly midway between the bend of the elbow and the lower border of the armpit. This swelling "throbbed" and rapidly increased till it attained its present dimensions.

Condition on admission.—Patient is a robust, tall, and very muscular negro, to all appearance perfectly healthy, outside of the local trouble for which he seeks relief, and without any history of hereditary or acquired taint. On stripping the patient, the left arm presents a marked contrast to the opposite member; it is decidedly larger as shown by the most superficial inspection, presenting an elongated, fusiform swelling which pulsates. On closer inspection it is also noticed that the skin over the scapular, acromial, and posterior humeral regions is closely sprinkled with small dark cicatricial dots which indicate the points of entrance of the small shot; an opinion which is confirmed by the ready detection, by palpation, of the shot as they lie, for the most part, encysted, subcutaneously, at the very point of entrance. It is found that the prominence of the tumor begins, above, about three inches from the lower border of the pectoralis major and terminates below at a point one and one-half inches from the bend of the elbow. The circumference of the affected arm at the most prominent part of the tumor is fourteen and five-eighths inches that of the healthy arm at the same point being twelve inches.

Inspection reveals pulsation which is confirmed by palpation. A marked thrill is also detected in the most prominent and apparently thinnest part of tumor; a decided purring murmur is heard on auscultation, and it is noticed that the pulsation is diffused, characteristically expansive, and synchronous with the radial beat. Pulsation, thrill, and all the active phenomena manifested by the tumor are immediately arrested by pressure over the axillary lower third, or subclavian, above clavicle. Pressure on axillary, sufficient to arrest radial pulsation, causes marked diminution in size of tumor, but this reduction is best marked after application of the Esmarch bandage, under which the circumference of the arm is quickly reduced to twelve and six-eighths inches.

Diagnosis is, plainly, traumatic aneurism of the brachial artery.

Treatment.—In view of the readiness with which the circulation in the tumor was controlled by pressure, the Esmarch was applied; but this had to be removed ten minutes after application owing to the intolerable pain and almost agony that it produced. The patient protested so emphatically against this method of treatment (Reid's method) that it was not repeated.

The next day, April 1, the patient was put to bed,

the diet was reduced, veratrum viride, potass. iod., and ergot were administered, and the Massachusetts General Hospital compressor was carefully adjusted to the brachial, just above the aneurism. At the same time, the forearm was tightly flexed on the arm. The patient bore the compressor, screwed sufficiently tight to arrest the radial pulsation, for forty minutes, when the pain became intolerable and the pressure had to be diminished. The compressor was subsequently applied, only lightly enough, however, to slacken the circulation in the tumor and weaken the radial pulsation.

April 22. The compressor has been alternately compressed and relaxed but kept on the artery all day and all night under the supervision of Mr. Sherck, the *interne* of the service. The patient gives evidence of having passed a wretched and sleepless night owing to pain from the compression. On removing the compressor, the tumor pulsates most vigorously and the arm measures now fifteen inches in circumference, showing an increase of three-eighths inch since the beginning of treatment.

23d. The compressor has been kept moderately adjusted, the forearm flexed on the arm and the arm on shoulder; the arm being kept in this position of forced flexion by a well-adjusted bandage which fixes it to head. The patient, who is anxious to get well and is willing to do all in his power to facilitate a cure, has stood with fortitude the ordeal imposed upon him, though an occasional hypodermatic injection of morphia has been required to help him, especially at night-time. The tumor, in the meantime, has not been in the least affected by the therapeutic measures thus far instituted. It pulsates more vigorously than ever, the arm has gained one-eighth inch more in circumference, and the sac is apparently becoming much thinner on the inner aspect of the arm where it threatens to rupture. In view of the unfavorable outlook, it was decided to ligate the brachial in its upper third, just below the superior profunda and immediately *above* tumor. This was done under careful antiseptic precautions, and without difficulty; the artery being ligated with a Kocher's catgut No. 9 (juniper oil), the ligatures cut short, and the incision closed without drains.

Immediately after ligation the pulsation and all the active phenomena in the aneurism were arrested. The tumor became hard, the radial pulse imperceptible. The arm shrank one and one-half inches at maximum circumference of tumor.

30th. Dressing removed, union by first intention throughout wound. Tumor does not pulsate, but has shrunk very little since day of operation.

May 2. In examining the case, my attention was directed to a slight localized pulsation in the tumor, by one of the students in attendance. This pulsation became more marked the next day and progressively continued until it was almost as pronounced, and the tumor as painful, as when patient was first seen.

6th. I decided to ligate the distal end of artery *immediately below tumor* at bend of elbow, and in case of failure to control the pulsation thereby, to apply the Esmarch and lay open the sac and seek for the intermediary nutrient branches.

Operation.—A catgut ligature (Kocher's, 9) was applied to the brachial at the bend of the elbow without the slightest perceptible effect on the pulsation or size of the aneurism. The Esmarch was then applied and an incision was made along the whole length of the tumor extending from the primitive incision for the ligation of the brachial, close to the lower border of the axilla, to the bend of the elbow, about six and one-half inches. The sac was at once exposed, and, with the hope of extirpating it, a close though rapid dissection was begun which succeeded in isolating both ends of the sac and the major portion of its anterior and internal aspect; it was found impossible, owing to intimate connection of the sac with the important and deeper structures of the arm, especially with the biceps and brachialis anticus, to continue the dissection toward the humerus.

The dissection and isolation of the sac were therefore stopped and a large incision made throughout its whole length; at the same time an elliptical piece of sac, representing its exposed portion, was excised, and the clot which was partially laminated, but mostly passive, in its central parts, was turned out in larger quantities, the whole cavity being constantly and thoroughly irrigated with a 1 : 2000 acid sublimate solution (Laplace's). By this means three orifices were readily detected at the bottom of the sac, two of these being large enough to admit readily a No. 8 gum catheter; the middle orifice only offering some resistance to the catheterization.

The gum catheter was first passed into the orifice nearest the axilla and it readily passed upward inside of the artery until it stopped at the point where the first ligature had been applied sixteen days previously, proving clearly that that was the proximal axillary end of the aneurism. A catgut ligature was once more applied while the catheter was *in situ*, the catheter, which served as a perfect guide, being withdrawn as the ligature was tightened. The introduction of the catheter into the lower orifice led at once to the bend of the elbow, where it was arrested at the point where the ligature had just been applied. It remained now to close the third or middle orifice, which was smaller and apparently had no connection with the two preceding; this orifice I presumed to be the orifice of a much dilated inferior profunda. This orifice was completely sealed by passing four fine interrupted silk sutures (for want of fine catgut) through its lips. The Esmarch constrictor was then relaxed and I was considerably surprised to notice a decided flow of blood from the other two orifices notwithstanding the fact that the vessels with which they communicated had been apparently controlled by previous ligature at the proximal and distal extremities of the sac; this showed plainly that there must be some important collaterals which communicated with the vessels between the points of ligature and the internal or aneurismal orifices. In view of this I immediately stitched the lips of the orifices with *fine* sublimated silk, by which means the openings were sealed completely and not a drop of blood entered the sac henceforth. A strip of acid sublimated gauze (Laplace's) was then left in the sac instead of a drain and deep interrupted sublimated silk and catgut sutures applied.

In addition to the usual antiseptic dressing the whole arm was wrapped up in cotton wadding and hot bottles were kept to the forearm and hand.

7th. Patient has passed a restless night and suffered great pain at site of wound. Temperature 102° F.

In view of this, dressings were removed under antiseptic precautions, and the cause of the trouble discovered to be an intense erythema and *complete* vesication of the edges of the wound, owing to the overzealous application of the too strong and caustic 1 : 500 acid sublimate gauze. The trouble could have been obviated by using a weaker gauze, or previously protecting the skin with a layer of Lister's protective or iodoform gauze.[1] A milder gauze (1 : 1000) was substituted and the wound dressed otherwise as usual. From that date onward the wound gave no further trouble; it granulated without further suppuration and the patient was discharged completely cured and with only a linear cicatrix to indicate the site of the aneurism, May 21, 1888.

Remarks.—An eminent authority[2] has written: "Deligation of the brachial, or of the lower part of the axillary artery for aneurism is so very generally successful and is so slight an operation that but a small number of cases are published." It is to the fact that the case under consideration proved so marked an exception to the general rule thus stated that it owes its main interest. It will be noticed that (1) after the failure of the various measures that had been instituted to diminish the circulation in the sac, (2) the brachial was ligated at what might be called the point of election in the upper third of the arm, just below the origin of the superior profunda and immediately above the sac; that (3) apparent cure followed the deligation of the artery at this point, (Anel's operation); that (4) pulsation returned on the tenth day, and with it all the other aneurismal symptoms; (5) that four days after the return of the aneurismal symptoms a ligature was applied to the brachial at the distal end of the sac; (6) that notwithstanding this ligature the tumor still pulsated and its size remained totally unaffected; (7) that after incising at the same sitting and clearing the sac (old operation) the orifices of three arteries of supply were readily discovered and the inefficiency of the ligatures easily explained, as will be readily understood by referring to the accompanying diagram; (8) the ease and the thoroughness with which the bleeding orifices of the nutrient vessels were sealed by the method employed, viz., *suture;* (9) lastly, the rapid recovery of the patient and the equally prompt healing of the wound in spite of the extensive traumatism inflicted.

Tripier, an excellent authority, states in a valua-

---

[1] Vide article on "Corrosive Sublimate" by Dr. F. W. Parham, New Orleans Medical and Surgical Journal, June, 1888.

[2] Barwell, Ashhurst's Encyclopædia of Surgery, 1883.

ble contribution on the pathology of the brachial artery[1] that "in all cases of circumscribed traumatic

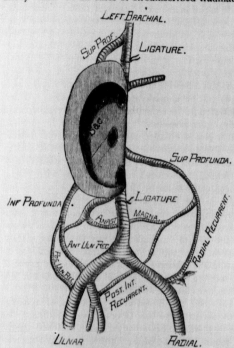

LEFT BRACHIAL.

SUP PROF

LIGATURE.

SUP PROFUNDA.

INF PROFUNDA.

LIGATURE

ANAST MAGNA

RADIAL RECURRENT.

ANT ULN REC

POST. INT. RECURRENT.

ULNAR   RADIAL.

Schematic representation of the collateral circulation in the case of M. H.

aneurism we should always try indirect digital compression if it is possible to apply it. If it does not succeed, then we must chose between the ancient method and that of Anel. The ancient method is of more *difficult execution*, but it is incomparably more certain in its results, as it more positively guards against relapses and hemorrhages. It is certain, however, that by Anel's method some very good results have been obtained; but in a certain number of cases it has failed and the surgeon has had to appeal to the ancient method. Several instances of this sort have been recorded. The most complete and instructive [thus far, 1869] having been that of Brodie, who in 1820, in a case of brachial aneurism resulting from an unfortunate venesection, applied a ligature to the brachial about seven centimetres above the tumor. The aneurism returned about five months after; a second ligature about three centimetres above the aneurism was now applied [and the sac opened.—R. M.]; the tourniquet was removed and hemorrhage followed from the sac. A fresh ligature was now placed immediately below the sac; the tourniquet was again removed, and another gush of blood followed from

the sac; then a fourth ligature was placed *immediately* above the tumor and this did finally control the hemorrhage."

This was certainly an obstinate case; but energetic as were the procedures adopted by Brodie they would have failed with the aneurism now reported, as, in this instance, the ligature immediately *above* and *below* the sac completely failed to check the circulation in the tumor. It is plain that no other method would have succeeded but that which was adopted, *i. e.*, the free opening of the sac and *the closure of the orifices of supply in the sac itself*. It is in accomplishing this last result that we have an opportunity of observing the advantages gained by the improved technique of the present day.

It is doubtless greatly due to the difficulties formerly experienced in attempting to secure the nutrient orifices in the sac that Tripier and the majority of contemporary writers who appreciate the thoroughness and great merits of the Antyllian operation for aneurisms of the extremities, still regard it as of "more difficult execution." In the light of my recent experience, I feel convinced, however, that this is one of the difficulties of the operation which is most easily surmounted. It will be remembered that Boyer, Günther, and other older surgeons already recommended the introduction of bougies or catheters into the aneurismal openings in order more readily to isolate and secure the proximal and distal ends of the artery. By this means they succeeded readily enough in securing the distal and proximal end of the tumor, but only beyond the limits of the sac, so that the intermediary branches, which, as in the case here recorded, are sometimes so troublesome, were not intercepted by the ligature and continued to bleed in spite of it. In order to secure these collaterals, which communicate with the main vessel between its immediate extra-aneurismal portion and its proper opening, or mouth, in the sac, the method recently suggested and practised by Annandale offers great and positive technical advantage.[1] This method consists "in introducing a bougie of suitable size into the openings from the side of the sac, in making a small incision through the wall of the sac on each side of the bougie, and in passing an aneurism needle through these round the vessel, the ligature being tightened as the bougie is carefully withdrawn."

In the present instance the bougies were only used to apply ligatures outside of the sac; the bleeding orifices within the sac having been thoroughly sealed by a few fine sutures. This procedure served me so satisfactorily, that I cannot but heartily recommend it to those who may be placed in similar circumstances.

[1] Article "Brachiale," Dechambre's Dictionnaire Encyclopedique des Sciences Médicales.

[1] Vide Edinburgh Medical Journal, February, 1886; also, Editorial, in THE MEDICAL NEWS, May 29, 1886.

In addition to this important detail, we might add that the complete ischæmia of the limb which is solely obtainable by the Esmarch bandage, which so readily adapts the parts to the difficult and delicate dissections sometimes required in the practice of this operation; also the introduction of the animal ligature, which has so thoroughly revolutionized the practice or, at least, the principles of arterial deligation to such a degree indeed that, in future, the so-called spontaneous or idiopathic aneurisms will, in many cases, be treated with the ligature in as close a proximity as the purely traumatic. Again, the superiority of the antiseptic practice which totally suppresses or greatly minimizes the risks of suppuration, risks that were so unavoidable and disastrous in the older days; and, finally, that greatest and grandest of the advantages of the modern surgeon —anæsthesia—which allows the operator to cut with a calm and deliberation that were denied his ancestors, are all circumstances which are conspiring to return to the "old" operation the prestige which has been necessarily denied it for so many years.

A REPORT OF A CASE OF SUCCESSFUL SUTURING OF THE HEART, AND TABLE OF THIRTY-SEVEN OTHER CASES OF SUTURING BY DIFFERENT OPERATORS WITH VARIOUS TERMINATIONS, AND THE CONCLUSIONS DRAWN.

By L. L. HILL, M.D.,
MONTGOMERY, ALA.,
SURGEON TO THE HILL INFIRMARY.

HENRY MYRICK, negro, thirteen years of age, of rather delicate appearance, was stabbed at five o'clock Sunday afternoon, September 14, 1902. About six hours after the injury Drs. Parker and Wilkerson were called, and, perceiving the nature of the case, advised that I should be sent for, and upon my arrival I urged an immediate operation. To this the parents readily consented, and I was assisted in the operation by Drs. Wilkerson, Parker, Michel, R. S. Hill, Robinson, and Washington. The knife blade entered the fifth intercostal space about a quarter of an inch to the right of the left nipple, and penetrating the apex of the heart passed into the left ventricle. The wound was about three-eighths of an inch in length, and from it came a stream of blood at every systole. There was no external bleeding, but his general condition was very unfavorable. The radial pulse was almost imperceptible, and the heart sounds were heard with difficulty. There was a triangular-shaped area of dulness. He had dyspnœa, and was very restless. His extremities were cold, as were his lips and nose. When aroused, he answered questions intelligently, though his countenance showed great distress. Securing two lamps, I removed the boy from his bed to a table, at one o'clock at night, eight hours after the stabbing, and proceeded to cleanse the field of the operation, and place the patient in as favorable a condition as my surroundings in the negro cabin would allow. Commencing an incision about five-eighths of an inch from the left border of the sternum, I carried it along the third rib for four inches. A second incision was started at the same distance from the sternum and carried along the sixth rib for four inches. A vertical incision along the anterior axillary line was made, connecting them. The third, fourth, and fifth ribs were cut through with the pleura. The musculo-osseous flap was raised, with the cartilages of the ribs acting as the hinges. There was no blood in the pleural cavity, but the pericardium was enormously distended. I enlarged the opening in the pericardium to a distance of two and one-half inches, and evacuated about ten ounces of blood. The pulse immediately improved, and was commented upon by Dr. L. D. Robinson, who so successfully and skillfully administered the chloroform. I had my brother, Dr. R. S. Hill, to pass his hand into the pericardial sac and bring the heart upward, and, at the same time, steady it sufficiently for me to pass a catgut suture through the center of the wound in the heart and control the hemorrhage. I cleansed the pericardial sac with a saline solution, and closed the opening in it with seven interrupted catgut sutures. The pleural cavity was also cleansed with a saline solution, and drained with iodoform gauze. The musculo-osseous flap was brought down and stitched in position. The operation lasted forty-five minutes. The patient's pulse on reaching his bed was 145° and respiration 56. I injected strychnine hypodermically, and employed hypodermoclysis and autotransfusion. The following morning, September 15, the boy's pulse was 130° and temperature 102°, and he was slightly delirious. On September 16 there was but slight

Nov. 29, 1902] MEDICAL RECORD. 847

change in the temperature and pulse, though the delirium was much worse. On September 17 he commenced to improve, and his recovery has been uninterrupted. I allowed him to sit up on the fifteenth day. Dr. E. C. Parker, who assisted me in the subsequent management of the case, examined the urine frequently, but was only able to find once a trace of albumin.

Wounds of the heart may be either non-penetrating or penetrating, injuring the cardiac wall or opening a cavity. The chief dangers from the former are shock and injury to a coronary artery. Ninety per cent. are penetrating, and of these only 19 per cent. are immediately fatal. The right ventricle is most frequently injured, and the left auricle is least so. Auricular wounds are more fatal than ventricular ones, and injuries to the apex are less dangerous than either. A needle puncture will rarely cause hemorrhage from a ventricle, but excessive bleeding, which is mostly systolic, is liable to follow a like injury to an auricle. A wound inflicted during diastole is less dangerous than a similar injury during systole, perpendicular wounds are more fatal than diagonal, and those of the right heart bleed more profusely than those of the left. The presence of the foreign body in the heart, the size of the wound, the location of the wound, the number of wounds, the connecting cavities, the attending syncope, and the involvement of Kronecker's coordination center are important factors in determining the outcome. Pericarditis, myocarditis, endocarditis, cerebral embolism, and empyema are frequent secondary complications. When the wound heals there is a possibility of cicatricial stretching, and

	OPERATOR AND YEAR.	LOCATION OF EXTERNAL WOUND.	CHAMBER WOUNDED AND SIZE OF WOUND.	TIME OF OPERATION AFTER INJURY.	ANÆSTHETIC.	RESULTS AND REMARKS.
1	Farina 1896	Just above the margin of the left sixth rib, near the sternum.	R. V.; ½-inch; 3 stitches	....	....	Death on sixth day, from broncho-pneumonia.
2	Cappelen 1896	Fourth left intercostal space in mid-axillary line.	L. V.; ⅜-inch.	1 hour.	....	Death after several days; from pericarditis: branch coronary artery cut.
3	Rehn. 1896	Fourth left intercostal space near sternum.	R. V.; 3 stitches.	Following evening.	....	Recovery; empyema.
4	Parozzani ... 1897	Seventh left intercostal space in mid-axillary line.	L. V.; ¾-inch: 4 stitches.	5 hours.	None.	Recovery
5	Parozzani	Third left intercostal space.	L. V.; ⅜-inch; 2 stitches.	½ hour.	None.	Death on second day from anæmia(?) Interventricular septum had been cut.
6	Fummi 1898	Under left nipple.	Apex; cavity not opened; 1 stitch.	Several hours	....	Recovery; empyema.
7	Ninni........ 1898	Fifth left intercostal space.	L. V.; 3 stitches.	Quickly.	None.	Death on table.
8	Parlavecchio 1898	Fifth left intercostal space.	L. V.; 1½-inch; apex: 4 stits.	8 hours.	Chloroform	Recovery.
9	Giordano 1898	Second left intercostal space	L. V.; ½-inch; 4 stitches.	½ hour.	None.	Death on nineteenth day from empyema; abscesses of right lung.
10	Nicolai 1899	Fourth left intercostal space, middle way between margin of sternum and nipple	R. V.	1½ hour.	Y .	Death after twelve hours.
11	Tuzzi.	Fourth left intercostal space.	Two wounds; one non-penetrating.	....	None.	Death on twenty-second day from empyema; pericarditis.
12	Longo.	Fifth left intercostal space; ⅜-inch internal to nipple.	L. V.; 3 stitches.	At once.	None.	Death in fifteen minutes.
13	Ramoni..........	At third left cartilage; ⅜-inch from sternum.	R. V.; two wounds; one non-penetrating; 4 stitches.	....	None.	Recovery.
14	Marion 1899	Shot through breast.	R. V.; catgut sutures.	....	....	Death.
15	Rosa 1899	Fifth intercostal space.	L. V.; ⅜-inch; not certain it penetrated ventricle.	....	None.	Recovery.
16	Horodynski . 1899	....	R. V.; 1½ cm. long.	....	....	Death.
17	Maliszewski 1899	....	....	....	....	Death.
18	Maliszewski . 1899	....	....	....	....	Death.
19	Bufnoir. 1899	Sixth left intercostal space.	R. V.; gunshot, 22 caliber.	....	....	Death; necropsy showed perforation of ventricle and the anterior opening only had been sutured.
20	Pagenstecher. 1899	Fourth left intercostal space beneath the nipple.	L. V.; 1⅜ inch; near apex; 3 celluloid stitches.	16 hours.	None.	Recovery.
21	Nanu. 1900	Third intercostal space, 4 cm from edge of sternum.	R. V.; 2 cm. long; 2 interrupted sutures.	....	....	Death on fifth day from infection of pericardium and pleura.
22	aselli 1900	Below and internal to left nipple, cutting sixth rib.	L. V.; near apex; 2 stitches.	1½ hours.	None.	Death in twelve hours.
23	Fontan...... 1900	Six wounds with scissors between third and seventh ribs in cardiac regioa	L. V.; 12 mm. long; continuous catgut sutures; 3 stitches.	6 hours.	Chloroform.	Recovery.
24	Nietert 1901	....	R. V.; penetrated; 3 silk sutures.	....	....	Death after thirty-six hours.
25	Vaughan 1901	Fifth left costal cartilage divided.	L. V.; 2½ cm. long; continuous silk sutures; 7 stitches	¾ hour.	Ether.	Death on table from hemorrhage about completion of operation.
26	Nietert 1901	Left of sternum.	L. V.; not sure cavity was penetrated; 2 stitches.	....	....	Recovery.
27	Nini. 1901	Left of sternum.	R. A.	....	....	Death in four days; sepsis.
28	Mignon et Sieur 1901	....	R. V.	....	....	Death.
29	Fontan 1901	....	L. V.; catgut sutures.	....	....	Recovered; had empyema.
30	Brenner 1901	Left of sternum, near sixth cartilage.	R. V.; 7 cm.	Following day.	Yes.	Death on table; degenerate heart muscle.
31	Watten 1901	Fourth right intercostal space.	R. V.; 3.5 to 4 cm.	....	....	Recovery; right pleura wounded; pneumothorax.
32	Lastaria 1901	....	L. V.	....	....	Died soon.
33	Zulehner. ... 1901	....	L. V.; ½ cm. long.	....	....	Suture tore out at once, and patient bled to death on table; heart showed fatty degeneration.
34	Zulehner. ... 1901	....	R. V.; 1 cm. long; sutured with catgut.	....	....	Recovery.
35	Stern. 1901	....	L. V.; pistol shot; unable to suture on account of location of wound on posterior surface; closed the opening with gauze.	....	....	Death in thirty minutes.
36	Launay.* 1902	....	L. V.; anterior and posterior walls; pistol shot; catgut sutures in each.	....	....	Recovery; no complications.
37	J. H. Gibbon. 1902	....	R. V.; one suture.	....	....	Died on table.
38	L. L. Hill 1902	Fifth intercostal space, a little to the right of left nipple.	L. V.; ⅜-inch; one catgut suture.	8 hours.	Chl'form.	Recovery.
39	Stewart. 1902	Fourth intercostal space, half-inch to left of sternum.	L. V.; ⅜ of an inch; six catgut sutures.	At once.	Ether.	Death on third day.

848   MEDICAL RECORD.   [Nov. 29, 1902

subsequent rupture, as in a case reported by Izzo, of a man stabbed in the left ventricle, who was conveyed to the hospital, from which he was discharged cured on the twenty-eighth day; a few hours afterward, while lifting a heavy body, he fell and quickly died. At the autopsy the cicatrix of the left ventricle was found ruptured. In addition to injuries of the heart caused by bullets, daggers, knives, needles, and various implements of war, it may be wounded by a fractured rib, by a foreign body that has perforated the œsophagus, or by blows upon the chest. Traumatic ruptures are more frequent after a full meal, as the distended stomach pushes the heart upward and forward, and causes a large area of the organ to be in contact with the thoracic wall and receive the impact.

Newton and Gamgee have collected forty-five cases in which traumatisms caused rupture of the heart without opening the pericardium. All were fatal. Only one of Gamgee's cases survived the injury fourteen hours. The fatality is easily understood, for, there being no exit, as soon as the accumulation of blood exceeds the limit of pericardial distensibility, the cardiac movements are mechanically stopped. The surgeon not only would be justified, but it is his bounden duty to operate upon every one of these cases, for it is more important, if possible, to rescue a drowning heart than to relieve a strangulated hernia. It is possible for a foreign body, as a gun missile, to remain quiescent for years in the myocardium, as in the case of a British officer, reported by Stevenson, who carried a bullet encapsuled for eleven years, or the still more remarkable case of Beers (*Cincinnati Lancet-Clinic*, 1898), of an American soldier who survived the lodgment of a bullet in the wall of the left ventricle for thirty-seven years.

Symptoms.—There is no certain cardinal sign by which an injury of the heart can be denoted, but when we consider the location of the external wound, and the usually profuse hemorrhage from it, if it is large, in connection with other signs and symptoms, it can generally be recognized. The pulse is weak, irregular, and intermittent, and often imperceptible in the extremities. There are pain, pallor, restlessness, and general dyspnœa. Frequent attacks of syncope are common. The mind is clear, but the countenance depicts an anxiety and distress that seemingly would welcome death, with the wintry sterility of the grave, as a sympathizing friend. If there is much blood in the pericardium the heart sounds are indistinct, and percussion elicits increased dulness. With the pulsation of the heart a foreign body, as a needle, may be seen to move under the skin.

I have adopted the convenient tabular form of Prof. Vaughan in presenting the following thirty-nine cases, one of which was not sutured, but Professor Stern attempted to close the opening with gauze. Nine were collected by Professor Vaughan, seven by Professor Sherman, and the remainder by myself, chiefly from Italian literature.

From my own experience, and a careful review of the cases reported above, I have drawn these conclusions:

First.—That any operation which reduces the mortality of a given injury from 90 to about 63 per cent. is entitled to a permanent place in surgery, and that every wound of the heart should be operated upon immediately.

Second.—Whenever the location of the external wound and the attending symptoms cause suspicion of a wound of the heart, it is the duty of the surgeon to determine the nature of the injury by an exploratory operation, as is recommended by Professor Vaughan.

Third.—Unless the patient is unconscious, and corneal reflex abolished, as in Pagenstecher's case, an anæsthetic should be given, and preferably chloroform. Struggling is liable to produce a detachment of a clot, and renew the hemorrhage, as occurred in Parlavecchio's patient.

Fourth.—Never probe the wound, as serious injury may be inflicted upon the myocardium.

Fifth.—Rotter's operation renders access to the heart extremely easy, and should be generally adopted.

Sixth.—Steady the heart before attempting to suture it, either by carrying the hand under the organ and lifting it up, or, if the hole is large enough, introduce the little finger, as Parrozzani did, which will serve the double purpose of stopping the bleeding and facilitating the passage of the stitches.

Seventh.—Catgut sutures should be used, as wounds of the heart heal in a remarkably short time. The sutures should be interrupted, introduced, and tied during diastole, not involve the endocardium, and as few as possible should be passed, commensurate with safety against leakage, as they cause a degeneration of the muscular fiber with its tendency to dilatation and rupture.

Eighth.—In cleansing the pericardium it should be sponged out, and no fluid poured into the sac.

Ninth.—It hardly seems necessary to accentuate the fact of the necessity of perfect cleanliness in these operations whenever the urgency of the case does not require instant intervention, as in the patients of Longo and Ninni.

Tenth.—The wound in the pericardium should be closed, and should symptoms of compression arise, reopen the wound and drain as Rehn did.

FOREIGN BODIES IN, AND IN RELATION TO, THE THORACIC BLOOD VESSELS AND HEART

I. Techniques for Approaching and Removing Foreign Bodies from the Chambers of the Heart

DWIGHT E. HARKEN, M.D., Lieutenant Colonel, M.C., A.U.S., Brookline, Massachusetts

THE purpose of this short discussion is to outline briefly a few aspects of the problem of foreign bodies in relation to the thoracic blood vessels and heart. Principal attention will be given: first, to the location of the missiles, second, to some reasons for the surgical removal of such bodies, and third, to the technique of approaching and removing fragments from the chambers of the heart. The necessity for brevity will dictate certain dogmatism and even the use of unsupported statements. Further clarification and support are to be presented (1, 2).

During the past 10 months with the thoracic unit of the 160th General Hospital 78 missiles were removed from within or in relation to the great vessels, at least 3 of which were embolic. During the same period 56 foreign bodies in, or in relation to, the heart have been removed, 13 of which were in the chambers of the heart. The great vessel series of 78 cases and the cardiac group of 56 cases, represent a total of 134 patients and 139 operations. There have been no deaths. A more precise breakdown in the distribution of these missiles is as follows: pericardial, 26; involving pericardium but principally pulmonary, 17; intracardiac, 13; on great vessels (and in walls), 35; intravascular (3 embolic), 7; on great vessels but principally pulmonary, 17; mediastinal but not directly on great vessels, 19, a total of 134, with no deaths.

The first diagram (Fig. 1) is a scale drawing of the heart and great vessels presenting the approximate size and location of a few of the foreign bodies first removed in the Unit. The gray shading represents a position impinging on the indicated structure, cross-hatching signifies an embolus and black indicates removal of foreign body from within the structure designated.

A current diagram (Fig. 2) has been prepared but in representing 129 missiles it has been neces-

sary to use point localization only. The same key to location is used in the margin, gray for foreign bodies impinging on the structure, cross-hatching for the embolic missiles and solid black for those lying within the structure outlined.

About all that such a gross method of localization conveys, is that the foreign bodies occupied a variety of positions, diffusely distributed about the mediastinum but that only one was found to lie in the left ventricle and none within the lumen of the thoracic aorta. It is, therefore, assumed that the direct entrance of foreign bodies of surgical size into either of these structures is rarely sur-

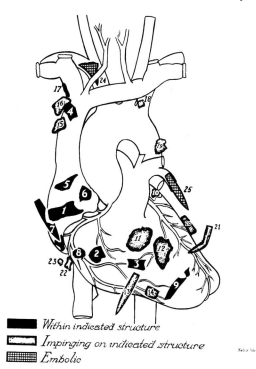

Within indicated structure

Impinging on indicated structure

Embolic

Fig. 1. A scale drawing of some of the first missiles removed in this clinic. Gray shading, impinging position; cross hatching, an embolus; black, within structure designated.

From the 160th General Hospital.
Presented at meeting of the Association of Surgeons of Great Britain and Ireland, May 2, 1945.

I

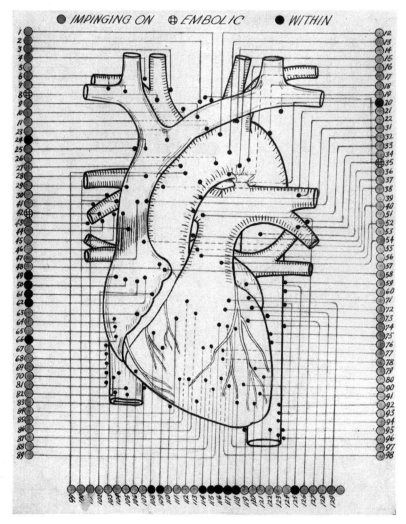

Fig. 2. Gross localization of foreign bodies presented in this discussion. Gray, impinging; cross hatching, embolic missiles; black within structure.

vived. It is further suggested that fragments small enough to enter the left ventricle as migrating missiles are swept along by the high systemic pressure in contrast to those arriving at the right ventricle.

FOREIGN BODIES IN OR ON GREAT VESSELS

The danger of erosion and suppuration attending large retained missiles in relation to thoracic blood vessels is real. Three deaths from massive hemorrhage due to erosion have come to our attention. Furthermore, approximately 15 per cent of the thoracic vessel foreign bodies in our series have been associated with abscess formation, just over 30 per cent were associated with other foreign material such as cloth or bone and 67 per cent showed pathogenic bacteria on culture. It is therefore, our policy to remove all foreign bodies measuring one or more centimeters in two dimensions, at times smaller missiles are taken out. The technical aspects of finding such fragments at operation are insignificant. We have failed in only one instance and that, the third case in this clinic. The fact that there have been no deaths supports our contention that removal is safer than retention.

In passing, attention is called to the three foreign bodies that have been established as embolic;

one was from the liver to the left pulmonary artery, another traveled from the heart to lodge in the innominate artery, and the third shifted from the left to the right pulmonary artery. All of these were removed without incident and with restoration of vascular continuity. These will be reported in detail separately (1).

FOREIGN BODIES IN OR ON THE HEART

Of the 56 foreign bodies in, or in relation to, the heart 13 have been removed from the chambers of the heart. The locations of the missiles in the chambers of the heart are indicated in the photograph (Fig. 3). Four were in the right auricle, 7 were in the right ventricle, 1 was in the left auricle and 1 was in a small cystic myocardial hernia of the left ventricle.

One fragment listed as within the right auricle lay in the interauricular septum and was associated with systemic embolus producing hemiplegia. Another fragment, described as in the right ventricle, was more evasive than the others (LeR.R. in Fig. 3). At the first operation with the patient in the dorsal decubitus position, the fragment wriggled from the grasping forceps and migrated to the right auricle just over the opening of the inferior vena cava. Three months later at the second cardiotomy the missile, though surgically exposed and visualized fell from the auricle into the right ventricle—the direction of fall being influenced by the patient's left lateral decubitus position. Finally at the patient's request a third cardiotomy was performed and the fragment was trapped in the apex of the right ventricle and successfully removed. The patient is now apparently in robust health. The last operation was recorded in colored moving pictures which demonstrate the firmly healed cardiotomy of the

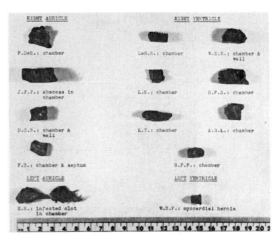

Fig. 3. Photograph of intracardiac missiles that have been removed.

first operation and an area of damaged wall over the last intracardiac resting place of the migrating missile. This case demonstrates that even migrating foreign bodies can damage the overlying heart wall.

In spite of isolated reports of asymptomatic foreign bodies lodged in the heart, there is also evidence in the medical literature that some do cause death. These reports together with experimental evidence were the early basis for a policy of surgical intervention. It was found that foreign bodies placed inside the hearts of animals were associated with subsequent bacterial endocarditis. With such a background it was elected to remove 13 of 28 intracardiac foreign bodies. *It was felt that certain foreign bodies should be removed:* (1) to prevent embolus of the foreign body or the associated thrombus; (2) to reduce the incidence of

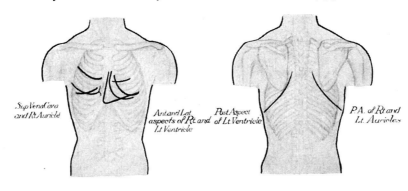

anterior view   posterior view

Fig. 4. Some of the incisions, indicating the variety of approaches used to obtain adequate direct exposure.

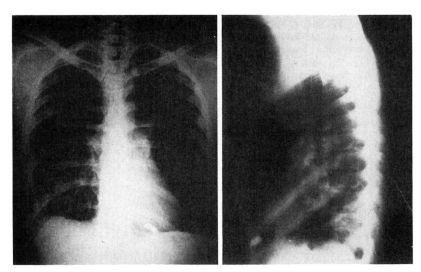

Fig. 5. Anteroposterior and lateral views of a foreign body in the chamber of the right ventricle. The right hemithorax was cleared of an infected hemothorax by decortication before these pictures were taken.

bacterial endocarditis; (3) to avoid recurrent pericardial effusions; and (4) to diminish the danger of myocardial damage with subsequent rupture or myocardial aneurysm.

It is now fair to say that this rationale originally borrowed from the medical literature and partially confirmed by personal animal experimentation, has been clinically established. The evidence cannot be reviewed here, but will be further elaborated in a later publication (2).

Inevitably size and location are factors influencing surgical intervention. Small foreign bodies are probably less hazardous as they may be associated with less myocardial damage, they are

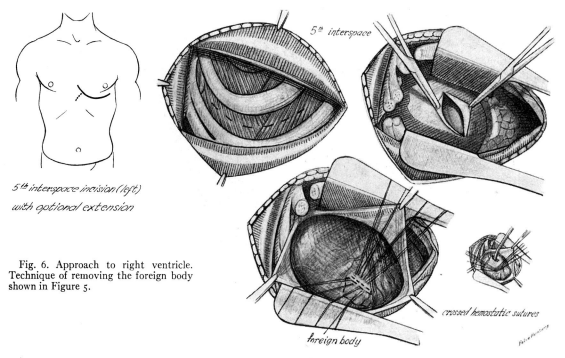

5th interspace incision (left)
with optional extension

Fig. 6. Approach to right ventricle. Technique of removing the foreign body shown in Figure 5.

5th interspace

foreign body

crossed hemostatic sutures

HARKEN: FOREIGN BODIES IN RELATION TO THORACIC BLOOD VESSELS 5

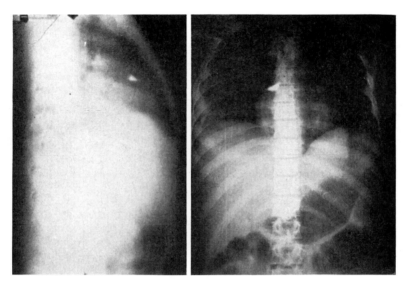

Fig. 7. A missile is shown to lie in the right auricle.

more readily and more firmly encapsulated and, finally, small foreign bodies are technically more difficult to remove. Accordingly in this clinic, the retention of 15 foreign bodies apparently in the heart has been regarded as less hazardous than their surgical removal. In short, Figure 3 illustrates the foreign bodies that we have elected to remove. Size alone dictated removal of some of these, whereas, attending clinical manifestations influenced the decision to intervene in others.

Once the decision to remove a missile from the heart is made, the technical considerations are contingent upon surgical exposure and safe removal at cardiotomy.

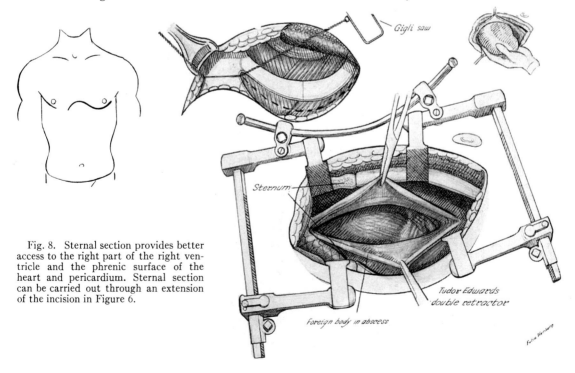

Fig. 8. Sternal section provides better access to the right part of the right ventricle and the phrenic surface of the heart and pericardium. Sternal section can be carried out through an extension of the incision in Figure 6.

J.A.M.A., April 30, 1960

TRANSISTOR PACEMAKER FOR TREATMENT OF COMPLETE ATRIOVENTRICULAR DISSOCIATION

C. Walton Lillehei, M.D., Ph.D., Vincent L. Gott, M.D., Paul C. Hodges Jr., M.D., David M. Long, M.D.
and
Earl E. Bakken, B.E.E., Minneapolis

A transistor pacemaker (fig. 1) and bipolar electrode has been developed for use in patients with complete atrioventricular dissociation and an inadequate cardiac output. This pacemaker is designed for either short-term or long-term ventricular stimulation by means of an internally implanted myocardial electrode.[1]

Complete atrioventricular dissociation is likely to occur in about 10% of patients who have undergone surgical repair of septal defects located in the vicinity of the atrioventricular node and the common bundle of His, and this method of internal stimulation was developed originally to meet this need.

Temporary or permanent complete heart block is not, however, a rare complication of many diverse types of myocardiopathy, sometimes idiopathic or induced by arteriosclerosis, infection, or drug administration; therefore this method of internal stimulation has found a place also in the treatment of selected patients with complete block from these causes.

At first the significance of surgically induced complete heart block rested in its high mortality. Of the first seven patients with septal defects in whom this complication of open-heart surgery developed in 1954-55, all died in the immediate postoperative interval despite the use of epinephrine, ephedrine, atropine, sodium lactate, and the external electric pacemaker; death was clearly a result of an insufficient cardiac output owing to the acutely slowed ventricular rate. The condition was further aggravated by the increased metabolic needs in the immediate postoperative interval, so that cardiac rates below 70 per minute were usually incompatible with life. Moreover, as we have previously pointed out [1a] the widespread adoption by many surgeons of the practice of arresting the heart with potassium citrate and prolonged anoxia during surgical repair of septal defects significantly increases the incidence of complete heart block.

Attention then turned to the use of isoproterenol hydrochloride,[2] and this drug was effective in reducing the mortality to about 40% by increasing cardiac rhythmicity and rate.[3]

Treatment was not satisfactory, however, until the combined use of an electric pacemaker and a fine electrode implanted into the heart muscle was developed.[4] The ventricles in block are very respon-

From the Department of Surgery and the Variety Club Heart Hospital, University of Minnesota Medical School.

The pacemaker here described has been used in 66 patients to correct complete heart block. In most cases the block followed surgical procedures, but it also occurred in some nonsurgical patients. The pacemaker consists of three parts: a 9.4-volt mercury cell battery as the source of power; a transistorized oscillator transformer to generate the pulses needed to stimulate the heart; and a unipolar or bipolar electrode in the form of a wire anchored by stitches to the myocardium. The myocardium of the right ventricle has usually been chosen as the most convenient site. Nonsurgical patients incapacitated by complete heart block with low cardiac output have had their conditions maintained on continuous stimulation for up to 15 months by means of this equipment.

sive to repetitive electric stimuli, and only low currents, which are imperceptible to the patients, are needed. With this treatment the mortality of heart block occurring as a complication of cardiac surgery has fallen greatly, and this, together with other developments, has been one of the important factors reducing the over-all risk of operation for septal defect to low levels.[5]

In addition, a simple technique has recently been developed for percutaneous insertion of a myocardial electrode [1a] which should prove equally lifesaving for certain nonsurgical patients with this problem and in whom emergency treatment may be required.

Advantages of Internally Implanted Transistor Pacemaker

The pacemaker is compact, being only slightly larger than a package of cigarettes. Its small size, light weight, and self-contained power source allow for complete patient mobility. A light, washable shoulder "holster-type" sling, made of cotton with snap fasteners, has been developed to allow ambulant patients who require continuous stimulation to wear their pacemaker conveniently while leading an active life. Because it is battery-operated, patient safety and efficiency of patient care are greatly improved. The patient is not in danger of electrocution should a short circuit develop, as he is with equipment operated by alternating current, nor is he at the mercy of a power line failure or an accidentally pulled power cord.

Several recent developments in electronics make this practical and reliable pacemaker possible; namely, the transistor, improved mercury cell batteries, and miniature components, together with advances in plastics and insulating materials. The transistor offers several advantages over the vacuum tube in pacemaker application. These advantages have resulted in high reliability and long life expectancy, greater battery efficiency, elimination of need for warm-up time, and much smaller size. Also, the transistor adapts well to the low-voltage, low-resistance, high-current circuits necessary for artificial cardiac stimulation.

Method of Operation.—The battery used in this pacemaker is a 9.4-volt mercury battery. This battery has a high capacity-to-size ratio and flat voltage-discharge curve, so that for a given setting of the pacemaker stimulation is relatively constant throughout the useful life of the battery. The pacemaker output chosen was a 2-msec. square wave-current pulse, variable in amplitude from 1 to 20 ma. into a 1,000-ohm load. A 2-msec. pulse length was used, since this is far enough out on the strength-versus-duration stimulation curve to evoke a systole with a reasonably small current and yet far short of that capable of triggering ventricular fibrillation. A special blocking oscillator transformer was developed to secure the proper pulse width at the voltage used and yet have a low core loss. Because experience has shown that heart circuit resistances seldom run below 350 ohms, the pacemaker is calibrated in milliamperes for this load

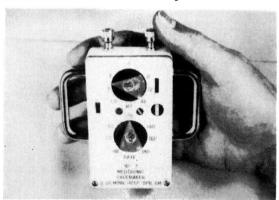

Fig. 1.—**Transistor pacemaker with self-contained battery for use in treatment of complete atrioventricular dissociation.**

plus a liberal margin, since it is current density at the cathodal lead that initiates a self-propagating excitation wave in the myocardium. The blocking oscillator repetition rate is variable from 60 to 180 pulses per minute. A neon flasher is incorporated on the face of the pacemaker to indicate the stimulating pulse frequency.

Location of Electrodes.—The pacemaker stimulus is delivered directly to the heart by means of an electrode implanted in the ventricular myocardium. This myocardial electrode is a braided tantalum (or stainless steel) wire (copper wires being less satisfactory because of fatigability and increased reaction about the electrode) insulated with poly-

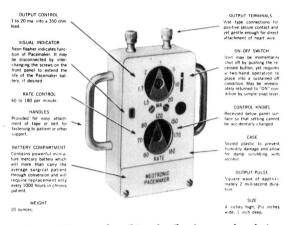

Fig. 2.—**Diagram describing details of pacemaker design, construction, and operation.**

tetrafluoroethylene (Teflon). A semicircular needle, swedged onto the end of the wire, facilitates rapid and easy insertion. The electrode is anchored in the myocardium with several silk sutures; the wire is brought out through a tiny stab incision in the chest wall and connected to the negative pole of the pacemaker. A flat metallic electrode is inserted into the subcutaneous tissue of the chest wall and connected to the indifferent pole of the pacemaker (fig. 3, *top*). An alternative method, frequently used, has been bipolar stimulation by means of two myocardial electrodes, in which case the indifferent electrode is unnecessary (fig. 3, *center*). More recently a bipolar electrode, as a single unit, with the two terminals 5 mm. apart, has been developed (fig. 3, *bottom*). This is advantageous when long-term stimulation is contemplated, since only a single small wire needs to emerge through the chest wall. We also use this single bipolar electrode routinely now in our surgical patients.

In our experimental work there have been no appreciable differences in demand for current or cardiac function with regard to whether unipolar or bipolar ventricular stimulation has been used. It appears that in patients the ventricles are slightly more responsive to bipolar as compared to unipolar stimulation and slightly more responsive to endocardial as contrasted with myocardial stimulation. While it should be obvious that in the presence of complete heart block the electrode must be placed within the ventricular myocardium, it makes no difference [6] where in the ventricles the electrode(s) is implanted. Thus, the right ventricle is usually chosen as the most convenient site, and in surgical patients the diaphragmatic surface of the right ventricle away from the cardiotomy incision is recommended.

In medical patients or in other emergency situations, pacemaker stimulation can be instituted by

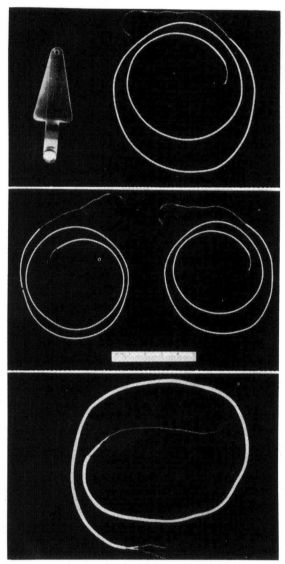

Fig. 3.—Myocardial electrodes used with pacemaker for direct cardiac stimulation. *Top*, braided tantalum electrode with Teflon insulation. Swedged-on needle facilitates implantation into myocardium, after which needle is cut off and electrode wire secured in place with several silk stitches. Triangular indifferent electrode is placed subcutaneously in thorax over left apex beat as indifferent electrode. *Center*, alternative method of bipolar stimulation, with use of two electrodes implanted directly into myocardium. *Bottom*, recently developed bipolar electrode combined into single unit. End implanted into myocardium has two terminals, 5 mm. apart. Swedged-on needle facilitates implantation, after which excess distal wire is cut off flush with myocardial surface. This electrode consists of two fine braided stainless steel wires coated individually with polytetrafluoroethylene insulation and then combined into single sheath of a nonreactive silicon plastic (Silastic).

percutaneous insertion [14] of a wire in the myocardium. Insulation of the electrode is not necessary. However, where long-term stimulation is contemplated, we believe it is preferable to expose a small area of the right ventricle myocardium and insert an insulated bipolar electrode directly. This may be done by means of a small incision in the fourth interspace just to the left of the sternum, with the patient under local anesthesia, without entering the pleura.

Timing and Degree of Stimulation.—In cardiac surgical patients, the electrode is inserted without delay at the time of thoracotomy if complete atrioventricular dissociation is noted or even suspected. If complete block is obvious, it has proved advantageous to institute stimulation before taking the patient off the heart-lung machine. The pacemaker stimulus is used as long as the patient remains in complete heart block. The rate of stimulation is usually 100 to 120 per minute, or roughly equivalent to what the patient would be expected to have under similar conditions were complete heart block not present.

About two-thirds to three-fourths of the surgical patients regain sinus rhythm within the first two to three weeks of continuous electrical stimulation. When the patient reverts to sinus rhythm, the pacemaker is turned off and careful monitoring of the pulse rate is instituted. (A companion transistorized monitor, with alarm, has been developed. This monitor uses the myocardial electrode to augment sensitivity and reliability. The monitor is inserted into the same circuit with the pacemaker to activate the pacemaker automatically should the patient's rate suddenly fall below a predetermined level.) After several days, if sinus rhythm has been maintained, the myocardial electrode is removed by gentle traction.

Those surgical patients who remain in complete block after this time may usually be weaned from the pacemaker gradually by progressive lowering of the rate of stimulation, supplemented by use of rectally or orally given isoproterenol hydrochloride as previously described.[7] If other factors indicate a need, there is no contraindication to the use of digitalis in patients on pacemaker stimulation.

The transistor pacemaker in combination with the myocardial electrode has been used in 66 patients at the University of Minnesota Hospitals to date. Most of the patients have had complete heart block secondary to surgical procedures, but an increasing number of nonsurgical patients with Stokes-Adams syndrome have been restored to useful activity.

The longest interval of continuous stimulation of a patient's heart by means of a bipolar electrode and the equipment herein described has been 15 months. This patient is still under stimulation, and the resistance through the electrode gradually rose to about 500 ohms in the first six weeks and has not changed appreciably since.

In another patient, a 38-year-old engineer who was unable to work since 1957 because of idiopathic heart block and is now able to return to work, the resistance measured through his bipolar electrode six days after insertion was 230 ohms and the heart was driven by less than 2.5 ma. One month later, these measurements were 366 ohms and less than 3 ma. respectively.

Comment

Since the initial description of a patient with complete heart block after closure of a ventricular septal defect who, in 1957, was successfully treated by use of a myocardial electrode and an artificial pacemaker,[8] this method has been universally adopted by cardiac surgeons faced with this complication.

The miniaturized equipment here described, as well as the bipolar electrode, has been thoroughly tested and found to facilitate the use of this method by increasing safety and reliability and by providing the possibility of ambulatory treatment. The latter advantage has been particularly useful in extending the benefits of this form of treatment to those nonsurgical patients who sustain complete heart block secondary to coronary arteriosclerosis, drug therapy, or one of the other diverse causes of Stokes-Adams syndrome. In these persons the indication for use of electrical stimulation has been limited to those who are incapacitated despite the conventional forms of medical treatment by either intermittent attacks of syncope or a cardiac output which remains consistently so low that useful work and physical activity have become impossible. Not only has the threat of sudden death in these patients been removed, but their physical and emotional rehabilitation has been dramatic. Further miniaturization of equipment for such patients is entirely feasible. Moreover, experimental work in dogs has indicated the feasibility of implantation of a tiny coil within the myocardium and the use of electromagnetic waves through the intact chest wall from a transmitter on the skin surface. This latter method of stimulation by electromagnetic induction has not yet reached the state of practicality necessary for clinical use.

With regard to the clinical use of direct myocardial stimulation, two facts are worthy of mention. First, the ventricles with a reduced cardiac output due to a slow rate secondary to complete atrioventricular dissociation respond extremely well to repetitive electric stimuli of small magnitude delivered directly to the myocardium. On the other hand, an inadequate cardiac output due to a failing myocardium, e. g., from anoxia or any of innumerable causes, will not respond to electrical stimuli.

Even though complete heart block may be present in such patients, it is clearly secondary to the cause of the myocardiopathy and not the primary problem.

Secondly, in patients in whom complete block is the primary problem, even though the heart rate and cardiac output are readily restored to adequate levels by internal stimulation, the fact that the induced ventricular and the natural atrial contractions are asynchronous means that the heart is less efficient than it would be under comparable conditions with normal sinus rhythm. This reduction in efficiency is not great but it is similar to that which occurs with atrial fibrillation and has been estimated to be about 15%. In the usual patient this reduction is not significant because of the large reserve that exists. In a few surgical patients with complete heart block, however, such as those with a ventricular septal defect and severe pulmonary hypertension due to extensive arteriolar vascular narrowing or in patients with tetralogies with a very hypoplastic pulmonary artery, this reduction in cardiac efficiency might be a decisive factor in the immediate postoperative interval before readjustments have had time to occur. Thus, we have considered the possibility of using the patient's own P wave to trigger the ventricular stimulus, according to a system which has been described.[9] The practical difficulties, aside from the additional complexity of the equipment needed, have been due to the fact that, in the immediate postoperative interval when such a method has its greatest value, the P-wave rate is often unreliable, showing extremes in both directions. For the more usual patient, therefore, use of a P-wave pick-up and amplification to synchronize atrial and ventricular contractions does not seem necessary.

The question of how long stimulation can be maintained appears to be related to electrode materials, design, and technique of implantation. Suffice it to say that, with the present electrodes, continuous stimulation for periods well over one year has been achieved, without appreciable increase in the impedance after the first six weeks. Since these patients are still under stimulation, it is not possible to provide, at this time, an estimate of the average functional interval to be expected with a single electrode. If an electrode does fail, another may be implanted. We recently have implanted two of the single bipolar electrodes in nonsurgical patients in whom long-term stimulation is anticipated. One is brought out through the skin immediately to be used for stimulation, and the other is left buried in the subcutaneous tissue where it can be easily located should the first fail.

The possibility of infection along the wire exists, but we believe that this danger can be minimized by tunneling the wire for some distance before bringing it out through the skin.

Summary

In complete heart block the ventricles are extremely responsive to repetitive electrical stimuli of small magnitude delivered by an electrode implanted in the ventricular myocardium. This method has proved to be the most effective method of managing this complication of open-heart surgery and has been universally adopted by cardiac surgeons.

A light-weight transistorized pacemaker, with a self-contained battery of long life, has been developed to facilitate continuous electrical stimulation of the heart. This pacemaker may be worn by the patient, making ambulatory treatment practical. Safety to the patient has been increased by this unit, since sources of difficulty due to power failure or electrocution due to short circuits are obviated by the use of a battery power source.

A single bipolar braided stainless steel electrode, with good duration of function characteristics, has also been described.

Nonsurgical patients incapacitated by complete heart block with low cardiac output have been maintained on continuous stimulation for up to 15 months by means of this equipment. It would appear that a small portable pacemaker such as the one herein described may improve the prognosis of many patients afflicted with incapacitating complete atrioventricular dissociation associated with an otherwise adequate myocardium. Various refinements and improvements of this equipment are possible, feasible, and under study.

This study was supported by research grants from the graduate school of the University of Minnesota; the Minnesota Heart Association; the Life Insurance Medical Research Fund; the National Heart Institute; donors to Minnesota Surgical Research Fund and the Anthony R. Barnett Memorial Fund.

Mr. C. W. Norman supplied the braided tantalum and stainless steel electrodes with swedged-on needles. The polytetrafluoroethylene insulation was supplied as Teflon by Medtronic Laboratories, Inc., Minneapolis 818, who manufactured the pacemaker, cardiac alarm, and electrodes used in this study.

References

1. (*a*) Allen, P., and Lillehei, C. W.: Use of Induced Cardiac Arrest in Open Heart Surgery: Results in 70 Patients, Minnesota Med. **40:**672-676 (Oct.) 1957. (*b*) Weirich, W. L.; Gott, V. L.; and Lillehei, C. W.: Treatment of Complete Heart Block by Combined Use of Myocardial Electrode and Artificial Pacemaker, S. Forum **8:**360-363, 1958. (*c*) Weirich, W. L.; Gott, V. L.; Paneth, M.; and Lillehei, C. W.: Control of Complete Heart Block by Use of Artificial Pacemaker and Myocardial Electrode, Circulation Res. **6:**410-415 (July) 1958. (*d*) Thevenet, A.; Hodges, P. C.; and Lillehei, C. W.: Use of Myocardial Electrode Inserted Percutaneously for Control of Complete Atrioventricular Block by Artificial Pacemaker, Dis. Chest **34:**621-631 (Dec.) 1958.

2. Nathanson, M. H., and Miller, H.: Effect of 1-(3, 4, Dihydroxyphenyl)-2 Isopropylaminoethanol (Isopropylepinephrine) on Rhythmic Property of Human Heart, Proc. Soc. Exper. Biol. & Med. **70:**633-636, 1949.

3. Lillehei, C. W.: Discussion, Surgery for Ventrical Septal Defect, J. Thoracic Surg. **33:**57-59 (Jan.) 1957.

4. Reference 1*a*, *b*, and *c*.

5. DeWall, R. A.; Warden, H. E.; and Lillehei, C. W.: Helix Reservoir Bubble Oxygenator and Its Clinical Application, in Garott, A. J.: Extracorporeal Circulation, Springfield, Ill., Charles C Thomas, Publisher, 1958, pp. 41-46.

6. Reference 1*b* and *c*.

7. Barnard, C. N.; DeWall, R. A.; Varco, R. L.; and Lillehei, C. W.: Pre- and Post-Operative Care of Patients Undergoing Open Cardiac Surgery, Dis. Chest **35:**194-211 (Feb.) 1959.

8. Reference 1*a* and *b*.

9. Folkman, M. J., and Watkins, E.: Artificial Conduction System for Management of Experimental Complete Heart Block, S. Forum **8:**331-334, 1957.

CLOSURE OF ATRIAL SEPTAL DEFECTS WITH THE AID OF HYPOTHERMIA; EXPERIMENTAL ACCOMPLISHMENTS AND THE REPORT OF ONE SUCCESSFUL CASE

F. JOHN LEWIS, M.D., AND MANSUR TAUFIC, M.D., MINNEAPOLIS, MINN.

(From the Department of Surgery, University of Minnesota Medical School)

IN THE past the use of general or regional refrigeration in clinical medicine has been disappointing. Despite the fact that Fay,[13] a number of years ago, stimulated interest in the therapeutic potentialities of hypothermia when he reported on its use as a palliative method for treating patients with advanced cancer, little evidence developed to show that his method was better than the more simple treatments for incurable cancer, and it was never widely used. A little later, regional refrigeration, used as a preservative and anesthetic agent in treating gangrenous or severely wounded extremities, received consideration[9, 10] and many articles were published concerning the technique, but this method seems no longer to be of interest. Other anesthetic agents are better.

Despite these failures, it might still be expected that the production of greatly lowered body temperature would find use in medicine. The strikingly reduced metabolic rates associated with states of hibernation or artificially induced hypothermia[1, 3, 4] offer intriguing possibilities for the performance of operations requiring relatively prolonged vascular occlusion. A rewarding exploration of some of these possibilities has been undertaken by Bigelow,[2, 4] who has experimentally demonstrated the potentialities of hypothermia as an aid in cardiac surgery. He showed that during profound hypothermia in the dog, a longer cardiac inflow occlusion was possible than was tolerated without danger at normal body temperature. This maneuver made possible a cardiotomy in a dry field allowing examination of the interior of the heart for a number of minutes without the aid of complicated pumps or shunting procedures. With the body temperature reduced to 20° C., 51 per cent of his dogs, including 11 which had a cardiotomy during the operation, survived a fifteen-minute period of total cardiac inflow occlusion.

Boerema[6] also has used body cooling in dogs for the performance of intracardiac operations. In a number of animals the circulation was interrupted for ten to twenty minutes and in four dogs portions of the atrial septum were removed.

It has been our purpose to continue in this direction, using hypothermia experimentally as an aid for the production and correction of intracardiac defects under direct vision. We have tried to make the technique simple and safe enough so that its use for the closure of similar defects in human beings

This work was supported, in part, by a grant-in-aid from the Graduate School of the University of Minnesota and by a grant from the Minnesota Heart Association.

Received for publication, Sept. 15, 1952.

52

would be possible. Our experimental efforts to date have been concerned with the production and closure of atrial septal defects. It is sensible to work with this lesion first, for of the various intracardiac lesions which demand some kind of plastic repair for their correction it is probably the simplest to deal with. Experience gained in treating this lesion might later be directed toward the more difficult ventricular septal and aortic valve defects. Furthermore, ability to correct atrial septal defects in human beings would have great practical value, for this is a frequent and disabling congenital cardiac defect.[12, 18]

Atrial septal defects have been closed experimentally by a number of blind techniques[8, 14, 16-18, 20] and some of these methods have been used in clinical cases. Closure of the defect under direct vision, a more deliberate approach, has been attempted clinically at this hospital with a heart lung apparatus, but the patient did not survive.[11]

EXPERIMENTAL METHODS

It was planned to submit each of the adult mongrel dogs used in these experiments to two operations. At the first operation a large atrial septal defect was made under direct vision, then after a recovery period of a week or longer, the heart was re-entered and the defect was closed.

Production of Defects.—For each operation, either to make or to close the defects, the same cooling technique was used. The dog was first anesthetized with Pentothal Sodium and then cooled by wrapping the entire animal in rubberized blankets through which flowed a cold alcohol solution.* The trachea was intubated and, when respiration became shallow, artificial respiration was started, utilizing an automatic respirator. The rectal temperature and the pulse rate fell gradually over a period of one to two hours from a normal temperature of 38° C. and a pulse rate of 160 to 180 down to a temperature of 26 to 28° C. and a pulse rate of 50 to 70.

At that point the blankets were partially removed and the chest was entered through the right fourth interspace. The azygos vein was ligated and the inferior and superior venae cavae were isolated and each was encircled with a double loop of heavy silk. Though Procaine or no local anesthetic had been used earlier, later in the series, 3 to 4 c.c. of 1 per cent butacaine sulfate (Butyn Sulfate) was injected into the pericardial sac and allowed to remain there for five minutes before direct manipulation of the heart was begun, as has been recommended by Bill and Wagner.[5] After this the pericardium was opened. When we were ready to open the right atrium, the loops of silk were tightened occluding both cavae and, during more recent operations, a Satinsky vena cava clamp was applied to the base of the heart occluding the pulmonary artery, the aorta, and the origins of both coronary arteries. This was accomplished by inserting one blade of the clamp through the transverse sinus of the heart.

The right atrium was opened through a longitudinal incision, any remaining blood was evacuated, and the interior was explored. Then the greater part of the membranous septum was removed, creating a large defect through which

---

*The cooling apparatus, similar to the one used by Bigelow,[2] was made by the Therm-O-Rite Products Corporation, Buffalo, N. Y.

the index finger could be introduced with ease. Following this, the heart was closed with a running stitch of 000 silk and as this stitch was being placed, at least in all but the earlier operations, the heart was filled rapidly with saline through a polythene catheter which was left in the atrium as the stitches were drawn up. Filling of the heart in this manner allowed evacuation of all the air remaining within the chambers. Essential to this method of removing the air during closure was the occlusion of all cardiac outflow with the Satinsky clamp. Without occlusion of the outflow channels, a foam of air and liquid would be ejected into the great vessels during closure of the atrium even though a rapid filling of the heart with blood or saline was attempted just before the atrial wall was approximated.

Closure of Septal Defects.—Actually these precautions against air embolism seemed to be more essential during closure of atrial septal defects than they were during production of the defects. When the defects were closed, the right atrium was opened through the same wound which had been used previously and then the defect was identified and closed with a running stitch of 000 silk. During this closure, the polythene catheter was introduced through the defect into the left atrium for the purpose of injecting saline rapidly into this chamber to wash out any residual air. This was an important step, for even a very small amount of air remaining within the left atrium after its closure seemed to find its way into the coronary arteries when circulation was restarted. The result of that accident was usually fatal.

After completion of the operation either for production or closure of a septal defect, the animal was rewarmed with the same apparatus which had been used to cool him. For rewarming, the alcohol solution was heated before it was pumped through the rubberized blankets. Lately, in other cooling experiments not reported here, we have rewarmed the dogs by immersing them in hot water.

At varying periods following the second operation the animals were sacrificed so that observations on the healing of the septal wounds could be made.

RESULTS

Production of Septal Defects.—Production of atrial septal defects was attempted in thirty-nine animals and of these twenty-seven survived the procedure, an immediate mortality rate of 31 per cent. Of these twenty-seven survivors, one died two days postoperatively with a hemiplegia but the remaining twenty-six lived and were subjected to a second operation for closure of their septal defects. The results are summarized in Table I.

TABLE I. PRODUCTION AND CLOSURE OF ATRIAL SEPTAL DEFECTS

| | | | | CAUSE OF DEATH | | |
	NUMBER OF DOGS	SURVIVORS	DEATHS	VENTRICULAR FIBRILLATION	TECHNICAL ERROR	INDEFINITE
Production	39	27	12	8*	2	2
Closure	26	18†	8	4‡	3	1

*Coronary air embolism occurred in five of these dogs.
†In one of these the defect had closed spontaneously; seven recovered from ventricular fibrillation.
‡Coronary air embolism occurred in two of these dogs.

Ventricular fibrillation occurring during surgery was a prominent cause of death among the twelve animals which failed to survive the operations for the production of atrial septal defects, for eight of the twelve died of this complication. In five animals the ventricular fibrillation was associated with coronary air embolism while in the other three no air was noticed in the coronary arteries. Two animals died because of technical errors and the remaining two deaths occurred during and shortly after surgery, apparently due to cardiac standstill. Among the eight animals which suffered ventricular fibrillation, cardiac massage was effective in restoring a regular beat temporarily in six, but none of them recovered. Electrical defibrillation was not used on these animals.

Closure of Septal Defects.—Twenty-six dogs with atrial septal defects then became candidates for the more difficult operation of closing the defect. Of these, one which had had its septal defect made two and one-half months earlier was found to have a healed defect at the second operation, hence the heart was closed without attempting further surgery. Spontaneous closure of the defect was not noted in the remaining animals, probably because the interval between operations was purposefully kept short. Four dogs died during anesthesia or cooling before the heart was opened, thus leaving twenty-one animals which actually had their septal defects closed. Seventeen of these survived the surgery. Among the eight operative deaths, technical errors were responsible for three, one dog died of indefinite causation, and four died of ventricular fibrillation. In two of the four which succumbed to ventricular fibrillation there was coronary air embolism.

Regarding the problem of ventricular fibrillation, it is of further interest that seven other animals which developed ventricular fibrillation during surgery survived. In two of these the fibrillation was brought on by coronary air embolism while in five no air was present in the coronary arteries. Electrical defibrillation was important in the recovery of two of the dogs, while the other five recovered after periods of massage lasting from five to thirty-five minutes.

Most of the deaths in the series occurred early before the technique now used was evolved. Lately the operations have been quite safe; among the last ten attempts at the production of a septal defect there was only one death and similarly only one death among the last ten operations for closure of the defects.

When the animals were finally sacrificed, the septal defect was found to be soundly healed in every case. In the early postoperative period a small firm thrombus would be found over the wound but later there would be only a smooth endothelial-covered scar. A healed atrial wound is shown in Figs. 1 and 2.

DISCUSSION

The low mortality rate for the operations performed recently is attributable largely to the gradual development of a better technique. The success of the present technique appears to be based primarily on its ability to prevent the accident of coronary air embolism, a frequent cause of ventricular fibrillation early in the series. In developing the operative procedure, we have also been concerned with the occurrence of ventricular fibrillation not related to air

Fig. 1.

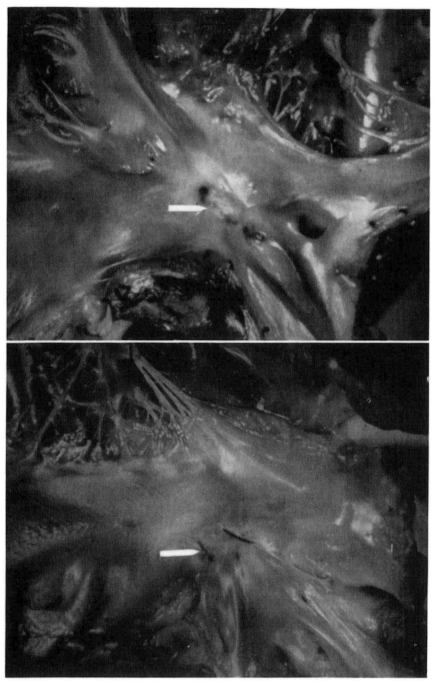

Fig. 2.

Fig. 1.—The atrial wall, viewed from the right atrium, two and one-half months after the defect was closed with a continuous silk stitch. The scar is seen just to the left of the coronary sinus.

Fig. 2.—The same heart shown in Fig. 1 viewed from the left atrium. From this side the endothelial-covered stitches are visible.

embolism. In preventing this type of fibrillation we have not, as yet, been completely successful, but its treatment with electrical defibrillating shocks has often been lifesaving.

Air Embolism.—Air embolism is very likely to occur during or immediately after any operation in which the heart is opened. Though small amounts of air are tolerated by the pulmonary circulation without difficulty, even a minute amount remaining within the left heart may find its way into the coronary arteries with fatal results. The difficulty and importance of avoiding this complication during open intracardiac surgery has been emphasized by other investigators.[7, 17, 19] If success is to be achieved, methods must be developed to avoid coronary air embolism during open intracardiac surgery whether it is performed with refrigeration or by any other technique.

The use of a Satinsky clamp to occlude the outflow of the heart while it is open, as previously described, has been successful in almost completely eliminating air embolism when operating upon the atrial septum. Though it occurred seven times in the first twenty-nine operations, during which the heart was opened either to make or close defects, coronary air embolism happened only twice in the last thirty operations performed with use of the Satinsky clamp. These two failures occurred when the outflow clamping method was first used; later, with better application of the clamps, there has been less danger. In fact, there has been no coronary air embolism during the last twenty-one operations. Proper application of the occluding clamp seems to be important; it should be applied low enough to occlude the coronary arteries if possible. Occlusion of the aorta alone beyond the origin of the coronary arteries was not always adequate to prevent coronary air embolism even though the heart was well filled at the time of closure. In this case air probably escaped beyond the aortic valve while the heart was still open.

Ventricular Fibrillation Not Associated With Air Embolism.—Even when air embolism is eliminated, ventricular fibrillation may still occur. Once started this type is more easily interrupted than that associated with air embolism, but prevention has been difficult. We have tried to reduce its incidence by avoiding the profound reduction in body temperature used by Bigelow[2, 4] and by the use of local anesthetics within the pericardium.

The temporary anoxia which occurs during inflow occlusion supplemented by the cardiac trauma which occurs during manipulation may be sufficient to cause fibrillation in these cases, but there is, in addition, the possibility that cold itself is a further predisposing cause. Bigelow's work suggests that this may be true at least for body temperatures of 20° C. or lower,[2, 4] and another investigator has concluded that cold increases the sensitivity of the ventricles to fibrillation.[15] A study of the effects of various degrees of hypothermia on ventricular irritability has not been done, but, nevertheless, we felt that it would be safer to use somewhat higher body temperatures than Bigelow did. Even at the temperatures we used, a cardiac inflow occlusion is tolerated for a sufficient length of time to allow the performance of intracardiac procedures under direct vision.

Butacaine sulfate applied topically has been advocated as a more effective agent than procaine for reducing the irritability of the heart muscle.[5] Though we have no controlled data concerning butacaine's effectiveness, in our experience fibrillation has occurred only following its use, when topical application has been difficult due to the rent in the pericardium made at previous surgery.

CLOSURE OF AN ATRIAL SEPTAL DEFECT IN A CLINICAL PATIENT

This is a preliminary report on the successful closure of an atrial septal defect in a 5-year-old child using the same technique we have employed in dogs. When we felt that the method had reached the stage where clinical trial was justified, Dr. R. L. Varco kindly sought and found a suitable candidate for the operation.*

The patient (University Hospital No. 843410) was an underdeveloped, sickly, 29½ pound, 5-year-old girl in whom the diagnosis of an atrial septal defect had been established by cardiac catheterization. On Sept. 2, 1952, she was anesthetized with Pentothal Sodium and curare and the trachea was intubated. She was then wrapped in the refrigerated blankets until, after a period of two hours and ten minutes, her rectal temperature had fallen to 28° C. (82° F.). At this point the blankets were removed and the chest was entered through the bed of the right fifth rib. The cardiac inflow was occluded for a total of five and one-half minutes and during this time a septal defect measuring approximate'y 2 cm. in diameter was closed under direct vision, in the manner described in the section on experimental method. In one respect the procedure was easier than it had been in dogs, for the right atrium was more dilated and hence roomier to work in. When the Satinsky clamp and ligatures had been removed, the pulse promptly regained its strength.

At the conclusion of the operation, which lasted fifty-eight minutes, the patient's rectal temperature was 26° C. (79° F.). To rewarm her she was placed in hot water kept at 45° C. (113° F.), and after thirty-five minutes her rectal temperature had risen to 36° C. (96.8° F.) at which time she was removed from the bath. Recovery from the anesthesia was prompt and her subsequent postoperative convalescence has been uneventful. She left the hospital on the e'eventh postoperative day. Her cardiac murmur is gone.

SUMMARY

1. In dogs, atrial septal defects were made and subsequently closed under direct vision with the aid of hypothermia. Body temperature of the animals was reduced to 26 to 28° C. rectally. With the right atrium open, a dry field was obtained by temporarily occluding the superior and inferior venae cavae for periods of time up to eight minutes.

2. Production of atrial septal defects was attempted in thirty-nine animals and there were twenty-seven survivors. Among the last ten attempts there were nine survivors. Twenty-six of the survivors had operations for closure of the defects, and in seventeen the defects were successfully closed and the animals survived. In nine of the last ten attempts at closure the animals lived.

3. The occurrence of ventricular fibrillation was the most harassing complication encountered. Its incidence has been reduced by the adoption of measures designed to prevent the development of coronary air embolism during the surgery.

*The authors wish to acknowledge their appreciation of Dr. R. L. Varco's sympathetic and helpful interest in the project.

4. The successful closure under direct vision of an atrial septal defect in one clinical case is reported. For this case the same technique as that used in the dogs was employed.

APPLICATION OF A MECHANICAL HEART AND LUNG APPARATUS TO CARDIAC SURGERY

JOHN H. GIBBON, Jr., M.D.

Philadelphia, Pennsylvania

IT IS A PLEASURE to be here and to talk about a subject in which I have been interested for many years. The ultimate objective of my work in this field has been to be able to operate inside the heart under direct vision. From the beginning, I have not only been interested in the substitution of a mechanical device for the heart, but also for the lung. We have always considered congenital abnormalities of the heart the most suitable lesions for operative repair. Many of these abnormalities are septal defects. In the presence of a septal defect, shunting the flow of blood around one side of the heart with a pump, will not provide a bloodless field for operative closure of the defect. An apparatus which embodies a mechanical lung, as well as pumps, enables you to shunt blood around both the heart and lungs, thus allowing operations to be performed under direct vision in a bloodless field within the opened heart. Furthermore, an apparatus which embodies a mechanical lung enables you to provide partial support to either a failing heart or failing lung where a major operative procedure is not contemplated. Such an apparatus can also be used as an adjunct during the course of a major operative procedure. This partial support of the cardiorespiratory functions consists in removing venous blood from some peripheral vein continuously, oxygenating the blood and getting rid of the carbon dioxide in it and then injecting the blood continuously in a central direction in a peripheral artery. Of course, such partial circulation, or cardiorespiratory support, requires the use of a mechanical lung in the circuit.

I shall not describe in detail the entire apparatus. I shall merely discuss six aspects of the problem which I consider of fundamental importance. Four of these concern the apparatus itself, and two concern problems which arise on opening the heart and operating within it under direct vision.

The first feature of a mechanical heart-lung

apparatus is a suitable pumping mechanism to move the venous blood from the subject, through the apparatus, and back into an artery of the subject. There is no real problem about a pumping apparatus. There are many ways of moving blood through tubing without producing significant amounts of hemolysis. We have used for many years a roller type of pump which does not contain any internal valves. Such pumps are extremely simple. Because of the absence of valves, the blood circuit is easy to clean and there are no stagnate regions where fibrin might be apt to form. There are many other advantages in this type of pump such as the simple and rapid control of the rate of blood flow. The pumps cause no significant hemolysis. In human patients in which we have used the apparatus, hemolysis has always been well below 100 mg. of free hemoglobin per 100 ml. of plasma. In animal experiments, hemolysis is similarly minimal.

The second main feature of a mechanical heart-lung apparatus is the mechanical lung itself. This presents far more difficulties than pumping blood. I am sure that the most efficient apparatus for performing the functions of the lung has not yet been devised. Our present mechanical lung, however, provides a reasonably satisfactory working solution to this problem. The mechanical lung performs the gas exchange required for respiratory function by filming blood on both sides of screens which have a somewhat larger mesh than ordinary fly screens. These screens are made of stainless steel wire and are suspended vertically and parallel in a plastic chamber. As the blood flows over these screens, it takes up oxygen and gives off carbon dioxide. It should be remembered that it is equally important to remove carbon dioxide from the blood as it is to add oxygen. It is easy to observe that sufficient oxygen is being picked up in the apparatus, as the blue blood entering the oxygenator becomes red as it leaves. This can be determined more accurately, of course, by intermittent sampling or by continuous reading with a Wood cuvette and oximeter. On the other hand, there is no way of estimating the carbon dioxide tension by observing the color of

Presented in the Symposium on Recent Advances in Cardiovascular Physiology and Surgery, University of Minnesota, Minneapolis, September 16, 1953.

Dr. Gibbon is Professor of Surgery and Director of Surgical Research, The Jefferson Medical College, Philadelphia, Pennsylvania.

the blood. We have solved this problem by reading continuously the pH of the blood as it leaves the oxygenator. As there is no significant increase in fixed acids in the blood in the course of these experiments, the pH changes are due practically entirely to changes in carbon dioxide tension. We have an automatic control which keeps the carbon dioxide tension at the desired normal level and which is operated by any change in the continuously recorded pH level of the blood.

A third important feature of any apparatus which temporarily performs the function of the heart and lungs is constancy of fluid volume. The apparatus should at all times hold a constant volume of blood at any rate of blood flow. If the apparatus is not designed so as to hold a rigid volume of blood at all rates of blood flow, blood might accumulate in the apparatus with consequent depletion of the subject's vascular system and a dangerous drop in the subject's blood pressure. Similarly, if the apparatus should hold less blood at any time, there would be an excessive amount of blood in the subject's vascular system. Obviously the tubing in the blood circuit will always hold a constant amount of blood. There are two places in the circuit, however, where the blood volume might vary. One is in the blood reservoirs at the bottom of the plastic chambers which draw venous blood from the subject, and the other is in the thickness of the film of blood on the screens in the oxygenator. Rigid control of the volume of blood at the bottom of these plastic chambers has been obtained by an electronic device invented by Dr. B. J. Miller in our laboratory. This electronic device senses the level of the blood in these chambers and automatically operates the pumps which draw blood from the chambers. Thus when the level of blood tends to rise, the pump automatically operates at a faster rate. When the level falls the pump automatically is slowed. This electronic circuit has proven eminently satisfactory and maintains a rigid volume of blood in these chambers.

In the second place where blood might accumulate, on the screens of the oxygenator, a very simple way to avoid such an increase is by inserting an additional pump in the circuit which draws not only from the bottom of the mechanical lung but also from the tubing carrying venous blood from the subject. This additional pump operates at a rate which is always greater than the rate of blood flow from the venae cavae of the subject. As this pump operates at a fixed rate, the thickness of the blood on the screens in the oxygenator does not vary.

The fourth important requirement of any mechanical heart and lung apparatus is that the apparatus should remove all of the blood returning to the heart through the venae cavae and yet should not apply too great a negative pressure to the orifices of the cannulae because the venae cavae would then be collapsed around the orifice of these cannulae. We have found that the simplest way of obtaining such a smooth blood flow from the cavae is to interpose a suction chamber between the pump and the cannulae in the venae cavae. The degree of negative pressure can be easily regulated in this chamber and a smooth uniform flow of blood is easily obtained.

In summary, then, every mechanical heart-lung apparatus devised to take over temporarily the entire functions of the heart and lungs must comprise four essential features. First, there must be a good method of pumping blood through the circuit which does not cause hemolysis, which can be quickly and easily adjusted to varying flow rates and finally which enables the blood circuit to be easily and thoroughly mechanically cleaned. Second, the mechanical lung must not only fully saturate the blood with oxygen but must maintain the carbon dioxide tension of the blood at a normal level. The latter requirement may be taken care of by an automatic apparatus which continuously reads the pH of the blood leaving the mechanical lung and adjusts the carbon dioxide tension accordingly. Third, the apparatus must hold a constant amount of blood at all rates of blood flow. This can be accomplished by electronic control of the pumps removing blood from plastic chambers so that the pumps operate always to maintain a constant level of blood in the reservoirs at the bottom of the chambers. The thickness of the blood film on the screens in the oxygenator is kept constant by an extra pump which always circulates a constant flow of blood over the screens. Fourth such an apparatus must be able to remove smoothly all the venous blood returning to the heart through the venae cavae without collapsing these veins. We have found the simplest way of accomplishing this is to interpose a negative pressure chamber between the pump and the cannulae in the venae cavae.

There are two problems concerning operations upon the open heart which merit discussion. The first consists in the disposal of the blood returning to the chambers of the heart even though all the

Air embolism must be avoided when the heart is opened. If there is no septal defect, operations upon the right side of the heart can be performed without any great danger from air embolism. It

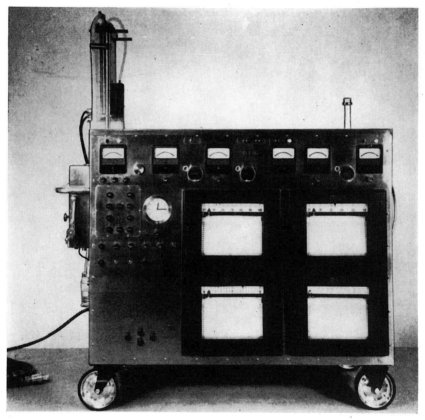

Fig. 1. Front view of apparatus showing the recording and control instruments and the lung suspended above the cabinet on the left.

blood flow from the venae cavae is diverted to the apparatus. The second problem is the avoidance of air embolism when the heart is opened.

The first problem is not difficult to solve. When the entire functions of the heart and lungs are taken over temporarily by the mechanical heart-lung apparatus, the myocardium continues to receive its normal flow of oxygenated blood by way of the coronary arteries. This blood is returned to the interior of the heart by way of the coronary sinus and the Thebesian veins. This blood must be disposed of so that the operative held can be clearly visualized when the heart is opened. We have accomplished this by aspirating this blood into a special plastic chamber in which any air aspirated is dissipated. The blood collects at the bottom of this chamber and is pumped back into the main extracorporeal circuit free of air.

is easy to flood the chamber of the heart with blood or salt solution after the operation is completed so as to avoid air embolism. Small amounts of air in the pulmonary arteries are probably not significant. On the other hand, operations on the left side of the heart, or on the right side of the heart in the presence of a septal defect, present a real problem in the prevention of air embolism into the ascending aorta. The immediate result of such air embolism is usually blockage of the coronary arteries with ventricular fibrillation and death. Our solution of this problem is to insert a small plastic catheter through a stab wound in the apex of the left ventricle. Suction is applied to this plastic catheter during the course of the open cardiotomy so that any air or blood entering the left ventricle takes the path of least resistance out through this plastic catheter instead of being

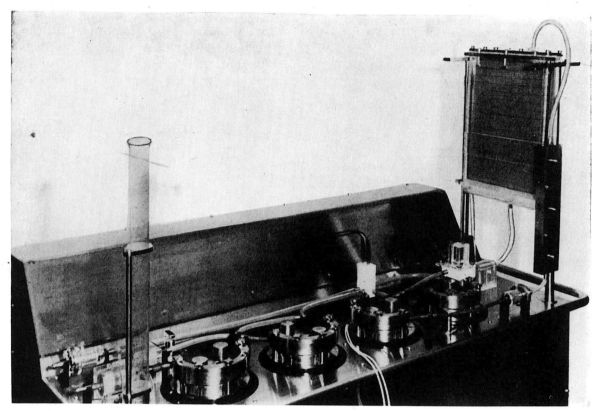

Fig. 2. Oblique rear view of apparatus showing the rotary blood pumps and the battery-type screen lung suspended above the cabinet on the right side.

ejected into the aorta. This plastic catheter is also connected to the debubbling chamber which receives the cardiac venous blood aspirated from inside the heart. Thus this blood is also returned to the circuit, and so to the subject, after the air bubbles are removed. After the wound in the heart is closed, and no further bubbles of air appear in the tubing connected to this catheter, it is removed and the small stab wound in the left ventricle closed by suture. Since employing this method in both animals and patients, we have had no instances of air embolism.

Figure 1 shows the front view of the apparatus which I have described, with the recording and control devices on the front panel. Figure 2 shows the rear view with the roller type pumps on top of the cabinet. Two rollers on a revolving arm pass over the rubber tubing which is clamped in a semicircular position. The rollers move the blood through the tubing and the blood cannot flow back because there is always a roller compressing the tube. To the right of Figure 2 is the mechanical lung which consists of vertical screens suspended in parallel in the plastic case.

Blood passes onto the screens through slits at the top of the lung. The blood collects in the bottom of the plastic case as it leaves the screens. The pump returning the oxygenated blood to the subject is automatically controlled by the electronic device which senses the level of the blood at the bottom of the plastic case, through which the blood passes. The lucite block near the oxygenator contains glass and calomel electrodes which continuously measure the pH of the blood. The filter consists of a screen with wires 150 microns in diameter and a 300-micron mesh. We do not know whether such a filter is necessary before returning the blood to the subject. However, we regard it as a good safety precaution in human patients. The tube at the end of the apparatus returns the blood to the patient through a cannulae directed in a central direction in an artery. In human patients we employ the central end of the divided left subclavian artery. The other two tubes are connected with cannula which are inserted into the superior and inferior venae cavae.

Oxygen is blown over the screens suspended

in the plastic case. Thus the blood film on the screens is exposed to an atmosphere of pure oxygen. The lung shown in Figures 1 and 2 has six screens. We have a larger mechanical lung with eight screens which are of longer length and which we have used on adult patients. An additional pump draws blood both from the bottom of the oxygenator and from the tubing containing the venous blood coming from the patient. The pump maintains a constant rate of flow through the oxygenator so that there is no variation in the thickness of the films on the screens. The electronic control circuit maintains the blood level in the bottom of the plastic case constant at all rates of flow. The pump removing the blood from this chamber is controlled by this electronic device.

There are two plastic negative pressure chambers. One of them collects the blood from the venae cavae and the other (Fig. 3) is the debubbling chamber in which the blood from the cardiac veins and from the left ventricle is collected. As the blood passes down the sides of this plastic chamber any bubbles of air are dissipated. Last spring we reported the successful repair of interatrial septal defects in animals using a flap of pericardium. We have been prepared to use such a flap of pericardium in human patients. We found, however, as Swan has, that it is quite easy to close such defects with a continuous suture in the open heart under direct vision and that consequently a pericardial graft is not needed.

The inferior vena cava is cannulated by a "tygon" tube passed into the inferior vena cava by way of the right atrial appendage. The superior vena cava is cannulated by a "tygon" tube passed through a stab wound in the right atrial wall. Oxygenated blood from the apparatus is pumped into the aorta through the divided central end of the left subclavian artery. Ligatures passed around the superior and inferior venae cava are tied over the enclosed cannulae. This diverts all the venous blood to the extracorporeal blood circuit. In addition to closing atrial septal defects in dogs with the pericardial graft, we have successfully closed interventricular defects in dogs by direct suture. The defect is exposed by an incision in the anterior wall of the right ventricle parallel to the left anterior descending coronary artery.

There has been a progressive decline in operative mortality in successive series of animals operated upon in our laboratory. Three years ago we had an 80 per cent mortality. In the most recent series this mortality has declined to 12 per

CARDIAC VENOUS BLOOD COLLECTING APPARATUS

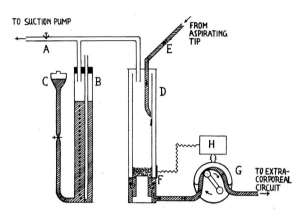

Fig. 3. Diagram of the cardiac venous blood collecting apparatus. The diagram is self-explanatory. The rotary pump G returns the blood to the main extracorporeal circuit after it has dissipated its bubbles in the inner chamber of cylinder D.

Reprinted from The Medical Clinics of North America (Volume 37, page 1615) with permission of the publishers.

cent. By operative mortality we mean any death which could be attributed to the operation and any death occurring the first month after operation. We have successfully temporarily taken over the entire blood flow through the heart and lungs of a dog for as long as one hour and forty minutes with prolonged survival in a healthy condition.

The average saturation of the venous blood entering the apparatus is 63 per cent. We regard a normal saturation of venous blood with oxygen as the best indication of an adequate blood flow to the tissues. If the saturation of venous blood with oxygen falls to low levels it is obvious that there is an inadequate blood flow to the tissues. We have been successful in maintaining the pH in a normal range. The hemolysis in this group of experiments averaged 35 mg. of free hemoglobin per hundred ml. of plasma. You are all aware that this is an insignificant amount of hemolysis and that a similar degree of hemolysis can occur if blood is forced rapidly through a fine needle. There is only slight increase in the fixed acids, generally in the neighborhood of three millimoles per liter which is within the normal diurnal variation.

Now I suppose what you are all interested in is not how many animals we have successfully operated upon but how many humans we have operated upon. The details of our animal experiments have appeared in two articles recently published. The human patients we have operated upon, using the apparatus, have not yet been reported.

We have used the apparatus to carry temporarily the entire cardiorespiratory functions of four human patients. The first was operated upon a year and one-half ago, and the last in July, 1953, of this year. We have one surviving patient who is quite well in every way with complete closure of an atrial septal defect. The three deaths have all been due to human error and not to failure of the apparatus.

The first patient, who was operated upon a year and one-half ago, was a fifteen-month-old baby that weighed eleven pounds and was in severe congestive cardiac failure. Attempts at cardiac catheterization in this baby were unsuccessful. It was the opinion of everyone who saw this baby that the cardiac abnormality was an interatrial septal defect. We explored the right side of the heart using the apparatus and discovered that no atrial septal defect existed. The child died after operation and at postmortem was shown to have a huge patent ductus arteriosus which had not been recognized at the time of operation. This, of course, illustrates the importance of complete exploration of every heart which is operated upon. We might have saved this child's life if we had closed the ductus.

The second patient was operated upon May 6, 1953. She was an eighteen-year-old girl who had a large interatrial septal defect proved by cardiac catheterization. The patient had been symptom free until about six months before operation, when she began to show symptoms of right- sided heart failure. She was hospitalized three times in these six months. Every time she returned to ordinary activity, she had symptoms of heart failure. Cardiac catheterization revealed an atrial septal defect with a left to right shunt through the defect amounting to nine liters per minute. The patient was connected with the apparatus for forty-five minutes and for twenty-six minutes all cardiorespiratory functions were maintained by the apparatus. She had a large interatrial septal defect which was quite easily closed with a continuous silk suture. The patient's postoperative convalescence was uneventful. She was readmitted to the hospital in July, 1953. At this time, cardiac catheterization showed that the septal defect was completely closed and that there was no evidence of any shunt. The cardiac murmur had completely disappeared and she was in good health. We believe that a transverse incision extending from one axilla to the other opening both pleural cavities through the fourth interspace, and dividing the sternum, gives the best exposure for this type of cardiac operation. The chest wound heals quite solidly and results in an inconspicuous scar beneath the breasts.

The last two patients were operated upon in July, 1953. They were both underdeveloped girls aged five and one-half years. Each of them weighed only about thirty pounds. The first child had a large interatrial septal defect proved by cardiac catheterization. Cardiac arrest occurred after we had opened the chest but before we had cannulated any vessels. The heart became blue and dilated as the chest was being explored. We tried for one hour to establish normal cardiac contractions but were unable to do so. We then rather reluctantly cannulated the superior and inferior venae cavae and the left subclavian artery while an assistant massaged the heart. As soon as the patient was connected with the apparatus the heart action became strong and the color of the heart pink. We then opened the right atrium and repaired five separate defects in the interatrial septum. After the defects were closed and the heart wound sutured, the ligatures around the venae cavae were cut allowing the heart to take over part of the circulation. Whenever we stopped the artificial support by the machine, the heart dilated and began to fail. Partial support by the extracorporeal blood circuit was maintained for three or four hours at the end of which time the cannulas were withdrawn and the chest was closed. The patient's heart, however, dilated and cardiac arrest occurred. Death, of course, in the patient cannot be attributed in any way to the use of the heart-lung apparatus as cardiac failure occurred prior to the use of the apparatus. Perhaps the dilatation of the heart and cardiac arrest was the result of a reversal of the shunt through the interatrial defect due to blood transfusion which was given during the early part of the operation.

The second five and one-half-year-old child had a proven interatrial septal defect by cardiac catheterization. It proved impossible, however, to pass the catheter into the right ventricle. On clinical grounds an interventricular septal defect was thought to exist in addition to the interatrial defect. It was known that the patient had a left superior vena cava which was somewhat larger than the right superior vena cava. The child turned out to have not only a huge interatrial septal defect but also a large interventricular septal defect and a small patent ductus arteriosus. Cannulation proceeded normally in this child and when we opened the right atrium we found it to be flooded with bright red blood returning to the atrium through the tricuspid valve. Ae we could not get a clear field to work and the flow of bright red blood was so excessive, we closed the atrium and removed cannulae. The child died after the operation. which was to be expected due to our failure to correct any of the cardiac defects.

(Motion picture shown)

This motion picture was taken during the course of the operation in which the five separate interatrial defects were sutured. It illustrates the value of being able to visualize the interatrial septum. It seems to me that the four smaller defects might have been missed by the employment of indirect blind methods. The film clearly shows how simple it is to keep the operative field clear of blood and that the heart appears of normal color and is beating well because the myocardium is receiving oxygenated blood from the apparatus through its coronary vessels.

In conclusion, I would like to say that I think the work I have reported is some of the early work in this field and that there is considerably more work to be done. It seems to me that there will always be a place for an extracorporeal blood circuit because it permits a longer safe interval for opening the heart than can ever be obtained by any of the hypothermia methods.

Discussion

DR. F. D. DODRILL, Detroit, Michigan—You have just heard an excellent review of the mechanical heart work by the leading pioneer in this country. Dr. Gibbon has had vastly more experience than the rest of us in this field, and I am envious of his vast accomplishments in this work.

When I first began this work several years ago, it was not definitely known, nor is it now definitely known, just how this can best be done. It was originally thought by those working in the field one could not bypass either side of the heart without completely bypassing the entire heart and lungs at the same time. As time has gone on and various workers have made definite contributions along this line, it is now apparent that either the right side or the left side of the heart may be bypassed while the opposite side of the heart and lungs continue to perform their functions.

We began a few years ago, therefore, to explore the possibilities of the following types of procedures: (1) bypass of the right heart, (2) bypass of the left heart, (3) bypass of both sides of the heart using the lungs for oxygenation, and (4) bypass of the heart and lungs using the mechanical oxygenator. We have performed more than 100 operations on the experimental animal doing one of these various procedures.

Our apparatus is so constructed that it can perform any or all of these functions. Insofar as the mechanical heart itself is concerned, I feel there are three factors which are important. These are: (1) it should be strong, sturdy and not subject to breakdown, (2) it should be so constructed that all parts coming in contact with the blood can be sterilized by ordinary autoclaving, and (3) it should produce and maintain a pulsatile flow in the vascular system.

Bypass of the Right Heart.—Our experimental work in bypass of the right heart has been highly successful in the experimental animal. This consists in taking the blood from the superior and inferior vena cava, passing it through the right side of our mechanical heart and back into the pulmonary circuit through the artery to the right lower lobe of the lung. By this method, the right side of the heart can be bypassed while the opposite side and the lungs continue to perform their functions. Also, if one wishes, the blood may be taken from the right atrial appendage. By this method not only the superior and inferior vena cava flow, but the coronary sinus flow,

as well, can be completely diverted from the right side of the heart. These connections depend upon the type of procedure and the exposure which one is attempting.

In our experimental work on the right-sided bypass, we encounter severe hypotensive reflexes. These hypotensive reflexes are greatly increased by even the slightest degrees of anoxia. This reflex has been referred to as the Bainbridge reflex but it may be possible that additional reflexes may be present. It is my impression that a great deal of physiological investigation is needed along this line. On the left side, however, these hypotensive reflexes are much less acute and oftentimes in the experimental animal we see no evidence at all of a decrease in the blood pressure during a left-sided bypass. Using such a procedure, any purely right-sided heart disease may be exposed and corrected under direct vision. The examples of such conditions are pure pulmonary stenosis with an intact cardiac septa and diseases of the tricuspid valve also with an intact septa. Figure 1 illustrates the pulmonary valve in a patient with pure pulmonary stenosis during a right-sided bypass. This valve was exposed for a period of twenty-five minutes while the mechanical heart pumped approximately 4½ liters of blood per minute. The left side of the heart continued to perform its function as did the lungs. While the right-sided bypass of the heart seems to be a rather practical procedure, it should be pointed out that there are not many pathological conditions of the right side of the heart alone in which such a procedure can be used. The great majority of patients with pulmonary stenosis have a defect in either the intratrial or interventricular septum and in such a patient a unilateral bypass is, of course, out of the question. There are rare instances of large emboli lodging in the right side of the heart which give some warning before death and it is possible that such large emboli could be removed during a right-sided bypass.

A right-sided bypass is a practical procedure for patients with pure right-sided disease. There is no need at all for bypassing the lungs as well for exposure of a purely right-sided defect. The main advantage of using the mechanical lung along with the mechanical heart is that the connections of the apparatus to the anatomical structures are much easier. However, with a right-sided bypass, the connections are likewise easy and should present no obstacle at all to the operating surgeon. Of all these various procedures which can be done in the way of

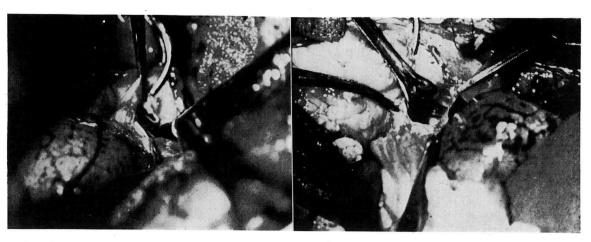

Fig. 1. Stenotic pulmonary valve in a seventeen-year-old boy.

Fig. 2. Open left strium exposing the mitral valve in a fifty-year-old woman.

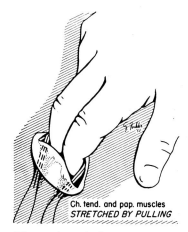

Ch. tend. and pop. muscles
STRETCHED BY PULLING

Fig. 3. A method of elongating the chordae tendineae in a patient with mitral regurgitation.

bypassing the entire heart or a portion thereof, I strongly feel that a right-sided bypass alone is a practical procedure which will be useful in years to come. The pathological conditions, however, are rather limited for this type of a procedure.

Bypass of the Left Heart.—A great deal of animal experiments have been done on the left-sided bypass. This consists in taking the blood from the pulmonary veins, passing it through the left side of the mechanical heart and back into the aorta which is its ultimate destination. The experimental work on dogs is extremely gratifying. We have been able to expose the mitral valve in dogs for fifteen consecutive times without a fatality. During the left-sided bypass, the right side of the heart and the lungs continue to perform their functions. During such a procedure, it is necessary to maintain a sufficient systemic blood pressure and preferably to maintain it by a pulsatile flow. The hypotensive reflex which is rather acute on the right side, especially if there exists any degree of anoxia, is not so acute on the left side. In

numerous animal experiments, we have not encountered such a reflex at all. We have applied this procedure to a few patients. Figure 2 illustrates the open left atrium with the mitral valve in the depths of the cavity. This patient made an uneventful recovery and is much improved from the surgical procedure. It seems logical to assume that if the mitral valve can be exposed, there is more apt to be an opportunity to improve valve function especially in mitral regurgitation. Figure 3 illustrates the elongation of the chordae tendineae in a patient with mitral regurgtation during a left-sided bypass. Although, the valve and the chordae were not visualized, the arterial pressure pattern shows conclusively that the mechanical heart was completely maintaining the systemic circulation. It has now been over one year since this patient was operated and he is vastly improved, even to the point of almost a complete disappearance of his loud murmur. One additional patient has also been treated in a similar manner with encouraging results. There are several factors in the production of mitral insufficiency; however, the most important one seems to be the shortening of the chordae tendineae and sometimes the papillary muscles as well. The valve leaflet itself may be nearly normal, and if the chordae can be lengthened to the point where it permits valve closure, the regurgitation is markedly diminished or corrected. Oher types of procedures have been done during a left-sided bypass. The aortic valve may be manipulated by inserting a finger into the left atrial appendage down through the mitral valve and upwards through the aortic valve. A patient with aortic stenosis has been so treated and the valve was easily fractured with the finger. Whether or not this procedure will be better than the method of going directly through the left ventricle remains to be seen.

Bypass of Both Sides of the Heart.—A bypass of both sides of the heart using the lungs for their natural functions is a more difficult procedure from the technical standpoint. We have been able to do this, however, quite satisfactorily in experimental animals and have applied it to one patient. Both sides of the heart were completely taken over by the mechanical device. A stenotic pulmonary valve was corrected and the interventricular septum was exposed. Unfortunately, this patient had, in addition to the pulmonary stenosis, marked infundibular stenosis and could not be sufficiently corrected. During the course of the procedure, the systemic blood pressure as well as respiratory function were quite satisfactory. Unfortunately, the patient succumbed on the fourth postoperative day from atelectasis and pneumonitis.

A Combination of Hypothermia and the Mechanical Heart.—These various procedures which I have shown you have been done solely with the mechanical heart. We are now working along the lines of the combination of hypothermia and the mechanical heart. Whether or not various types of intracardiac surgery will be done under hypothermia alone, using the mechanical heart alone or a combination of these two methods remains to be seen. The advantage of combining hypothermia with the mechanical heart is that during hypothermia, the circulating blood volume is markedly reduced and the work of the mechanical heart is vastly decreased. Moreover, with the circulation of such a small volume of blood, only one lobe of the lung needs to be used for respiration. Such a small quantity of blood can be easily circulated through one lobe of the lung while the rest of the lungs are at rest. This vastly minimized the technical difficulties with the use of the mechanical heart alone. It is easy to cannulate one of the upper pulmonary veins, to pass the blood through the left side of the mechanical heart and back into the aorta. The right-sided connections for such a procedure are similar to a complete bypass of the heart and lungs and consists simple of cannulating the superior and inferior vena cava and passing the blood back into the pulmonary circuit. The lung is a very intricate organ. It is not known but that it may perform other functions aside from the uptake of oxygen and the release of carbon dioxide. It seems as though a good hard attempt should be made at using the lung for its natural function before we completely discard it.

———

DR. CLARENCE DENNIS, Brooklyn, New York.—After Dr. Maurice D. Visscher and Dr. Owen H. Wangensteen jointly suggested to me, late in 1945, the undertaking of a project to develop an artificial heart-lung apparatus, I very quickly became aware of the activities of Dr. John H. Gibbon, Jr., and his group in Philadelphia. I consulted him at that time, and was very cordially received, shown protocols, shown the apparatus as it had developed up to that time, and welcomed into the group of those working on this project. Between that time and this, there have been associated in the research project with Dr. Karl E. Karlson and me approximately eighteen physicians. Work has been carried out first at the University of Minnesota and more recently at the State University of New York, and has been supported by the United States Public Health Service, the Graduate School of the University of Minnesota, the State University of New York, the Life Insurance Medical Research Fund, and private sources. In our search for an answer to this problem, my associates and I have come to have the very highest regard for the ingenuity, integrity, and cordiality of Dr. Gibbon and his associates. Success could not have come to finer people.

Dr. Gibbon has very carefully listed the qualifications of a satisfactory artificial heart-lung apparatus. We have

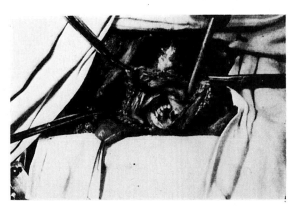

Fig. 1. Closure of inter-atrial septal defect, May, 1951. Closure was easily performed with interrupted silk sutures under direct vision. The patient suffered air embolism before opening the atrium, a consequence of human error in failure to switch on an automatic control mechanism. She died of complication of air embolism after several hours of partial support by the machine.

been concerned with an additional qualification, namely, the ability to render the whole apparatus absolutely free of bacterial contamination. The reason for our preoccupation with this qualification arises from the work of Dr. Russell M. Nelson, who was a member of our research group three years ago. Dr. Nelson showed that our apparatus at that time was contaminated with the paracolon bacillus, and that injection intravenously into normal dogs of a re-suspended fourteen-hour culture of this organism resulted in a symptom complex which had been responsible for most of the deaths prior to that time. This symptom complex developed rapidly and killed some dogs in less than three hours. The affected dogs showed a rapidly progressive metabolic acidosis, an incoagulable state of the blood, development of effusions into the serous cavities, massive gastrointestinal hemorrhage, and death in shock.[3] Satisfactory sterilization of the apparatus removed this symptom complex from our list of problems. The machine which we formerly used could not tolerate autoclaving, and sterilization by formaldehyde proved fairly regularly to be incomplete. Nevertheless, it was possible for us to do a long series of animal perfusions with this old apparatus, with no more than a 10 per cent mortality attributable to the perfusion *per se*.[1]

We gained so much confidence with this apparatus that, in conjunction with Dr. Richard Varco, we perfused two patients in efforts to achieve satisfactory closure of inter-atrial defects.[2] We were unsuccessful in salvaging either of these patients, but it was the consensus that the failure was not due to any intrinsic defect in the apparatus, but rather to human errors. The repair which was accomplished in the second patient is shown in Figure 1. This patient was lost as a consequence of human error, namely, failure to turn on the automatic control apparatus, which had been designed and proven adequate to maintain the desired blood level in the reservoir of the oxygenator. Air embolism oc-

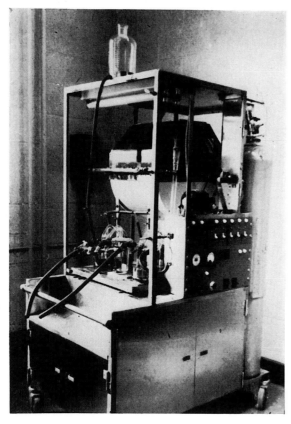

Fig. 2. The present pump-oxygenator apparatus. The entire blood-bearing unit can be autoclaved after assembly. Oxygenation is accomplished by filming on steel mesh discs which are mounted on a rotating horizontal shaft. The pumps are a modification of the Dale-Shuster pattern. Risk of human error has been reduced by use of largely automatic controls.

curred because of this oversight. The patient survived approximately eight hours after the procedure, but only by virtue of partial support by the pump-oxygenator, and the closure at the time of autopsy was perfectly adequate. Dr. Gibbon's observation is in agreement with ours, namely that the margins of most inter-atrial septal defects in clinical patients are thick, and firm, and silk closure, therefore, is not usually difficult of accomplishment. Closure in this instance, in the summer of 1951, was very easily accomplished.

Because of our concern over the occurrence of human errors and because of our concern with regard to absolute sterility, we have spent the past year and a half in the construction of a new apparatus, the blood-bearing portion of which can be assembled and autoclaved as a unit. This apparatus is not yet complete, but has reached a stage of construction which has permitted us to employ it for approximately two dozen trial perfusions.

The apparatus in question is indicated in Figure 2. In this apparatus, oxygenation is accomplished by the filming of blood near the center of a 50 cm. disc of stainless steel mesh which is mounted on a slowly rotating horizontal shaft. It will oxygenate 500 to 600 cc. of blood per minute from half saturation to full saturation and has a volume content of approximately 65 cc. of blood at any given moment. The pumps are a modification of the Dale-Shuster pattern. They are activated by hydraulic pressure, which is produced by a mechanical cam and bellows arrangement below the surface of the table. The apparatus as a whole will handle about 5 liters of blood per minute. It has been calculated that it should be capable of adding in excess of 350 cc. of oxygen per minute and in perfusions in large dogs has been measured to add 210 cc. per minute. We now regularly observe sterile blood cultures at the end of perfusion, and hemolysis produces approximately 1 mg. per cent of plasma hemoglobin per minute of perfusion.

There are many problems which remain and which are the source of considerable concern at the present time. It has been found that our greatest problem is that of postoperative hemorrhage. A technique of protamine titration, which has been employed over a period of several years in our laboratory, indicates that the addition of protamine to the animal is effective for only an hour or two and that additional protamine thereafter must be added until approximately six hours have passed. The platelet count is not appreciably lowered, and this, therefore, is not the reason for our hemorrhagic difficulties. It is suspected that there is excessive trauma to the blood which may be responsible for the degree of hemorrhage which we have experienced, but the low plasma hemoglobin concentrations cast a doubt even on this suggestion. Preliminary studies suggest fibrinolysin as the offender.

Perhaps our major remaining problems with the new machine rotate around the completion of satisfactory automatic controls. We have, at times, utilized the suggestion of Professor Dogliotti of Turin, Italy, that the pumping of blood from the machine to the arterial system of the subject be governed entirely by the arterial blood pressure of the subject. At other times, we have maintained a constant volume in the extra-corporeal circuit. The latter appears to be the preferable arrangement. As far as controls are concerned, the removal of blood from the venae cavae has been simplified by setting the apparatus up in such fashion that the pumps fill by gravity from the vena cava.

There remain several metabolic problems that have to be studied. An occasional perfusion is characterized by a profound loss of circulating plasma sodium. An occasional perfusion is also complicated by development of marked metabolic acidosis, even when there is a negative blood culture. Finally, there is occasionally a profound disappearance of circulating protein, which, as yet, we have not been able satisfactorily to explain.

It is likely that Gibbon has better solutions to many of these problems than we, but all of them must be painstakingly resolved before utilization of pump-oxygenators in clinical surgery can become general.

References

1. Development of a pump-oxygenator to replace the heart and lungs; an apparatus applicable to human patients, and application to one case. Dennis, Clarence; Spreng, Dwight S., Jr.; Nelson, George E.; Karlson, Karl E.; Nelson, Russell M.; Thomas, John V.; Eder, Walter P., and Varco, Richard L. Ann Surgery, 134:709 (Oct.) 1951.

2. Acute metabolic changes associated with employment of a pump-oxygenator to supplant the heart and lungs. Dennis, Clarence; Spreng, Dwight S. Jr.; Young, LaVonne; Nelson, George E.; Karlson, Karl E., and Pereyma, Constantine. Pages 165-171 in Surgical Forum: Clinical Congress of American College of Surgeons. Philadelphia: W. B. Saunders Company, 1952.

3. Nelson, Russell M.: Metabolic effects of paracolon bacteriemia. Ann. Surgery, 134:885 (Nov.) 1951.

Preliminary Communication

ELECTIVE CARDIAC ARREST

THE goal of cardiac surgeons must be the unhurried correction of cardiac abnormalities under direct vision. Toward this end are being developed many techniques for working within the bloodless heart and for excluding the possibility of air embolism after such interventions. Among these measures against air embolism is the induction of ventricular fibrillation in order to prevent the ejection by the heart of any air that may be within its cavities [1] and the alternative of closing the cardiac wound under saline.[2] A most valuable contribution to this problem and indeed to the whole problem of intra-cardiac surgery would be made if the heart could be arrested and re-started at will, suffering no damage during periods of arrest and cessation of coronary blood-flow.

Ringer [3] drew attention in 1883 to the effect of the different cations on the heart-beat, and Hooker [4] in 1929 suggested that potassium inhibition induced by an excess of potassium chloride could be used to stop the heart when its beat was disorganised by ventricular fibrillation. He recommended a solution of calcium chloride as an antidote to potassium when re-starting the heart. This work has been revived by Montgomery et al.[5] in order to reverse ventricular fibrillation in hypothermic patients. We have not been able fully to substantiate these findings but have, by modifying this basic technique, succeeded in evolving a reliable method of stopping and re-starting the heart at both normal and reduced body-temperatures.

METHODS AND RESULTS

Initial Experiments

Thirty-three adult dogs, anæsthetised with thiopentone and ether, were used to determine whether the induction of cardiac arrest by chemical means was a practical measure. While the vital centres were protected by perfusion with a heart-lung machine [6] or by reduction of the general body-temperature, cardiac arrest was induced by an injection of potassium citrate into the coronary circulation. Blood was excluded from the heart by ligating the venous inflow tracts and also the pulmonary artery and aorta. The injection of potassium citrate in concentrations varying from 25 to 100 mg.

1. Senning, A. *Acta chir. scand.* 1952, suppl. 171.
2. Swan, H., Zeavin, I., Holmes, J. H., Montgomery, A. V. *Ann. Surg.* 1953, **138**, 360.
3. Ringer, S. *J. Physiol.* 1883, **4**, 29.
4. Hooker, D. R. *Amer. J. Physiol.* 1929, **91**, 305.
5. Montgomery, A. V., Prevedel, A. E., Swan, H. *Circulation,* 1954, **10**, 721.
6. Melrose, D. G. *J. Physiol.* 1955, **127**, 51P.

per ml., was made into the root of the aorta. Arrest in diastole followed within five seconds. When this was accomplished a token operation was performed within the left atrium or ventricle. The heart was quite flaccid and could be freely handled, making the elimination of air an easy task when resuturing the cardiac wound. In no instance did air embolism occur. While the heart was stopped without coronary blood-flow for at least fifteen minutes, the heart remained pink and serial oxygen determinations on blood obtained from the coronary sinus showed that a negligible amount of oxygen was being utilised. When the period of arrest had exceeded fifteen minutes blood was allowed to re-enter the heart, and efforts were made to restore a normal beat. Cardiac massage, combined with the injection of calcium chloride, and in some cases of adrenaline and neostigmine, always restored muscle tone, and this was followed in almost every case by ventricular fibrillation: Electrical defibrillation was successful in only 70% of experiments and the restoration of normal activity was not reliable. These results were unsatisfactory and it was felt that the questions of duration and reversability of action of potassium citrate, and the need for stimulants, might profitably be studied further on isolated-heart preparations.

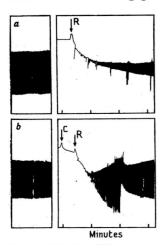

Perfused rabbit heart, 37°C : ventricular recording (systole downwards).

(a) Left, normal beat. Right, resumption of beat by re-starting perfusion ; cardiac arrest 6 min. previously by stopping perfusion.

(b) Left, normal beat. Right, resumption of beat by re-starting perfusion ; cardiac arrest previously by potassium citrate ; perfusion stopped for 15 min.

R = restoration of perfusion with Locke's solution. C–R = change-over from citrated to normal solution.

Isolated Perfused Hearts

Coronary perfusions of hearts from five rabbits, a guineapig, a kitten, and a puppy were made with oxygenated Locke's solution by the Martin-Langendorff method of aortic cannulation. The apparatus maintained the chosen cardiac temperature, usually 37°C, even in the absence of any coronary flow.[7] A few experiments were made between 23° and 37°C. Heart-beats were recorded by a spring-loaded lever attached by thread to the ventricles.

The injection of 10–40 mg. of potassium citrate in 0·2–0·4 ml. close to hearts with coronary flows of 10–20 ml. per minute stopped the beat. By perfusion with Locke's solution with previously added potassium citrate, 1 mg. per ml. was found to be the least which could stop the heart ; but in some a just-discernible auricular movement persisted. However, 5 mg. per ml. always caused complete arrest, and concentrations of up to 20 mg. per ml. were used to determine the dosage safety-margin. Diastolic cardiac arrest always occurred within ten to twenty seconds of injection of the solutions, and could be maintained as long as the heart contained them. During this period coronary flow was stopped for fifteen minutes without cardiac damage appearing subsequently. Spontaneous beating started again usually within ninety seconds of perfusion with pure Locke's solution, but with the highest concentrations of potassium citrate this interval doubled. The heart-rate was normal in under a

7. Baker, J. B. E. *Ibid*, 1951, **115**, 30P.

minute, and force was almost fully recovered in a further two to three minutes. This series of events was perfectly repeatable, and the time of arrest could be prolonged ; one fair recovery followed even fifty-five minutes of induced arrest without perfusion. By contrast, hearts in which the beat was stopped by asphyxia, induced by stopping the coronary flow without the addition of potassium citrate, recovered very slowly and then only partially after only five minutes of arrest (see figure). No hearts fibrillated as a result of the potassium citrate combined with coronary arrest—not even the puppy heart which had originally to be defibrillated as soon as it was set up—and on no occasion did a heart so treated fail to resume normal beating after perfusion with pure Locke's solution.

Final Experiments

Encouraged by the results of isolated heart perfusions we modified the initial experiments in the intact animal and established the following technique.

In dogs weighing about 30 lb., 2 ml. of a 25% solution of potassium citrate, diluted to 20 ml. by aspiration of blood into the syringe, was injected through a catheter into the ascending aorta, which was occluded distal to the tip of the catheter. After cardiac arrest for fifteen minutes oxygenated blood was driven through the coronary arteries from the heart-lung machine by release of the aortic clamp. This effectively restored a normal environment to the heart, which responded by a resumption of strong and regular contractions. In an animal protected by a reduction of the body-temperature to 25°C, coronary perfusion was achieved by connecting the catheter in the aorta to a bottle containing fresh oxygenated blood under pressure, without release of the aortic clamp. In this instance a single electric shock was required to restore normal rhythm.

CONCLUSIONS

Cardiac arrest in diastole inevitably results from an injection of potassium citrate into the root of the aorta so that the bulk of it enters the coronary arteries.

The dose of potassium citrate is critical in that a minimum coronary blood-level of 1 mg. per ml. is required to stop the heart, but as yet no upper limit for safety has been determined.

Arrest is maintained as long as an adequate level of potassium citrate remains in the coronary arteries.

Normal beat is restored when simple perfusion of the coronary circulation reduces the level of potassium citrate.

The method is effective both at normal body-temperature and at temperatures down to 26°C, while the perfused isolated heart is responsive at temperatures down to at least 23°C.

The addition of stimulants, such as calcium chloride or adrenaline, is unnecessary and may be dangerous.

The oxygen consumption of the quiescent heart is very low, and at normal body-temperature cessation of the coronary circulation for over fifteen minutes does not endanger such a heart.

Although a great deal of further work remains to be done, this method may offer an opportunity for useful surgery on the motionless heart, without the danger of air embolism.

D. G. MELROSE
M.A., B.M. Oxfd

B. DREYER
M.D. Cape Town, F.R.C.S.

Department of Surgery,
Postgraduate Medical School
of London

H. H. BENTALL
M.B. Lond., F.R.C.S.

Department of Physiology,
Charing Cross Hospital Medical
School, London

J. B. E. BAKER
M.A., B.Sc., B.M. Oxfd

PROFOUND HYPOTHERMIA

C. E. DREW
M.V.O., F.R.C.S.

ASSISTANT SURGEON, WESTMINSTER HOSPITAL, LONDON, S.W.1;
THORACIC SURGEON, ST. GEORGE'S HOSPITAL, S.W.1

G. KEEN
M.B. Lond., F.R.C.S.

SURGICAL RESEARCH ASSISTANT, WESTMINSTER HOSPITAL

D. B. BENAZON
M.R.C.P., F.F.A. R.C.S.

RESEARCH ASSISTANT, DEPARTMENT OF ANÆSTHETICS,
WESTMINSTER HOSPITAL

AT the present time visual intracardiac surgery may be achieved by the use of either a pump-oxygenator or hypothermia. A combination of the two methods, with cooling to 30°C, has been tried experimentally by several investigators, and clinically by Sealy et al. (1958). Hypothermia lessens the demand on the pump-oxygenator during cardiopulmonary bypass, because the body's oxygen requirements are smaller and can be met by a lower blood-flow.

When hypothermia is used by itself the customary limit of cooling is 28–30°C. At this level of temperature circulatory arrest and open heart surgery is possible for eight to ten minutes only: after this time there is considerable risk of permanent cerebral damage. Cooling to lower temperatures has been regarded as unwise because it often causes irreversible ventricular fibrillation. The use of antifibrillation drugs has not yet improved the position. There is much experimental evidence, however, to show that mammals (non-hibernating as well as hibernating) can survive profound hypothermia.

Anjus and Smith (1955) cooled rats to 1°C and rewarmed them to recovery. Smith et al. (1954) showed that golden hamsters can survive supercooling to −5·5°C, despite partial crystallisation of body fluids, and complete arrest of recordable body function for some hours. Gollan et al. (1955) combined the use of a pump-oxygenator and a heat-exchanger to cool dogs to 0°C with survival.

In dogs subjected to surface cooling, Bigelow et al. (1950) showed that, down to the point of cardiac arrest, which was usually between 18° and 22°C, the relation between oxygen consumption and temperature was almost linear. At 20°C oxygen consumption was 15% of normal. By extrapolation of the curve they deduced that somewhere between 10° and 12°C oxygen consumption would be minimal. At these low temperatures circulatory arrest might be tolerated for a long time, provided both the body temperature and circulation could be restored.

Niazi and Lewis (1958) have recently reported the case of a woman with widespread malignant disease whose temperature was reduced to 9°C by surface cooling, with cardiac arrest for forty-five minutes, and who recovered her normal body temperature without harm.

Investigation

This paper describes some of our work on profound hypothermia in dogs. It arose out of some experiments—at first unconnected with hypothermia—in which we studied the feasibility of bypassing the left ventricle during operations on this chamber.

To achieve this, a cannula was inserted in the left atrium, and blood was collected by siphon drainage into a reservoir, from which it was pumped into the femoral artery. Cooley and DeBakey (1957) have used a similar method to bypass aortic aneurysms during resection and graft replacement.

We considered the effect of producing cardiac arrest under these conditions. Would blood, returning to the right atrium, flow through a non-functioning right ventricle, through the low-pressure pulmonary vasculature, and, aided by the pumping effect of artificial respiration, find its way into the left atrium? We tested this by cooling the blood in its extracorporeal course, because we knew that hypothermia eventually stops ventricular function because of fibrillation or asystole. In a small series of experiments, fibrillation occurred at about 22°C as recorded in the pharynx; left atrial return was variable, sometimes ceasing very quickly, sometimes continuing for several minutes before gradually decreasing in amount. We also hoped that, if the load on the left ventricle was diminished, by its partial bypass, the heart might continue to beat regularly at lower temperatures. This was not so.

It appeared that, to achieve profound hypothermia by blood-stream cooling, it would be necessary to take over the function of both ventricles by mechanical means, particularly when fibrillation or asystole had occurred. In this way we might be able to (1) establish a satisfactory pulmonary and systemic circulation; (2) continue the cooling process in the presence of a non-functioning heart; (3) rewarm when desired; and (4) restore normal heart action.

Experimental Method

The extracorporeal circuit (fig. 1) contained two reservoirs—one to collect pulmonary venous blood from the left atrium,

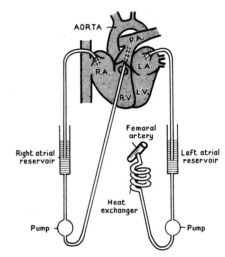

Fig. 1—Diagram of experimental circuit.

and the other to collect systemic venous blood from the right atrium.

Blood from the pulmonary venous or left-atrial reservoir passed through a cooling coil, and then returned to a femoral artery through one head of a 'Sigmamotor' pump unit. Blood from the sytemic venous or right-atrial reservoir was pumped through the other head into the pulmonary artery, via a cannula inserted through a stab incision in the infundibulum of the right ventricle. Systemic venous blood was not cooled. The heat-exchanger consisted of 100 ft. of polyvinyl ethylene chloride tubing (¼ in. internal diameter)—poor material for heat exchange, because of its low conductivity, but easy to obtain and convenient to use. This was immersed in a refrigerant mixture of methyl alcohol and carbon-dioxide snow maintained at 2–4°C. The apparatus was primed with 2–3 pints of fresh heparinised blood.

In half the experiments in which this circuit was used, a stainless-steel filter and a bubble trap were placed proximal to the femoral cannula.

Surgical Technique

Mongrel dogs of 8–15 kg. were used. Each was anæsthetised with thiopentone and succinylcholine, and maintained on nitrous oxide and oxygen from an automatic respirator. In later experiments a mixture of 95% oxygen and 5% carbon-dioxide was used. The femoral artery was first mobilised but not cannulated. The chest was opened by bilateral trans-sternal thoracotomy or median sternotomy. Heparin, 1·5 mg. per kg., was given, and the femoral artery cannulated.

A catheter as large as possible was inserted into the left atrium and connected by the pulmonary venous line to the left-atrial reservoir. The appropriate pump was then started, with partial left-ventricular bypass and cooling. Cooling was so rapid that the right atrium required immediate cannulation, and connection to the systemic venous line and right-atrial reservoir. The pulmonary-artery cannula was inserted as soon as left-atrial drainage began to diminish at the onset of heart-failure, and the pulmonary circulation was begun. Systemic flow could be varied by means of the pump transmitting blood into the femoral artery. This pump was calibrated before each experiment. The arterial flow determined the amount of systemic venous return, and the pulmonary flow could be adjusted to keep the reservoir levels constant. Little adjustment was needed once the levels were stabilised, and this was quickly achieved. Regurgitation through the pulmonary valve with the cannula in situ did not occur.

Twelve experiments were carried out, with flow-rates varying from 50 to 70 ml. per kg. per minute. In ten experiments rewarming was started as soon as a pharyngeal temperature of about 10°C was reached: in two others a period of circulatory arrest of thirty minutes was allowed. For rewarming, water at 40–44°C was substituted for the refrigerant solution. When the pharyngeal temperature had risen to about 30°C a single electric shock was sufficient to restore regular rhythm in the fibrillating heart, and at this stage right-ventricular bypass was discontinued. Shortly afterwards left-ventricular bypass was stopped, and the cannulæ were withdrawn. Protamine sulphate was then given, 3 mg. per kg., to neutralise the effect of heparin. Surface cooling and warming was not used, and no attempt was made to control room temperature.

The following data were obtained:

1. Central aortic pressures were recorded via a catheter introduced into the femoral artery. Continuous tracings with an electro-encephalograph (E.E.G.) and electrocardiograph (E.C.G.) were made.

2. Pharyngeal, rectal, mediastinal, and intraperitoneal temperatures were recorded with thermistors and a multichannel recorder.

3. Blood analyses included arterial and venous oxygen saturation, and estimation of plasma hæmoglobin and electrolyte concentrations.

Results

The significance of some observations is speculative, but some are worthy of note.

It was always possible to cool from 37° to 8°C (pharyngeal temperature) in about twenty-five to thirty minutes. Rewarming was a little slower (fig. 2). In a separate experiment to investigate the relationship between pharyngeal and cerebral temperature, an animal was cooled to a pharyngeal temperature of 8°C, with thermistors placed as before, but with an additional needle electrode in the brain. In this experiment the temperature fell more slowly than usual (fig. 3). The brain temperature lagged 4°C behind the pharyngeal temperature above 21°C, but at lower temperatures this difference fell to between 2° and 2·5°C. This showed that the brain was not excluded from the cooling process. The difference in brain and pharyngeal temperature may be attributable to hæmatoma formation around the needle thermistor in a heparinised animal. In another experiment, where the brain needle was placed in the subdural space between the cerebral hemispheres, the gradient was about 1°C.

Plasma-electrolyte changes were not significant. Arterial oxygen saturation was always in the region of 98%, and venous

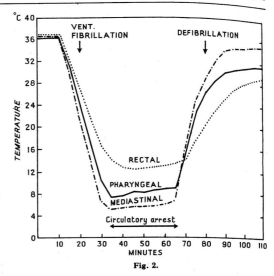

Fig. 2.

oxygen saturation increased with cooling to as much as 85% at 8°C.

The mean blood-pressure was usually between 80 and 130 mm. Hg with flows of 50 to 70 ml. per kg. per minute. The E.E.G. became isoelectric at about 20°C, and the E.C.G. underwent changes characteristic of cooling, bradycardia being followed by varying degrees of heart-block culminating in ventricular fibrillation. Atrial fibrillation was not observed; occasionally the atria continued to beat at a slow rate in the presence of ventricular fibrillation.

Two animals died because of our inexperience with the method. Of the others all recovered to the point of normal respiration and reflexes, and some to consciousness. All but two, however, died up to twenty-four hours later. The two survivors had a total period of ventricular fibrillation lasting about one hour, during which time the pumps maintained a circulation. They made complete recoveries without evidence of neurological damage. In the others no cause of death was apparent at postmortem examination, but, whereas the survivors had plasma-hæmoglobin values of 40 and 45 mg. per 100 ml., the non-survivors had levels above 100 mg.

Comment

The high mortality in this series was disappointing, but the survivors were proof that, using the method

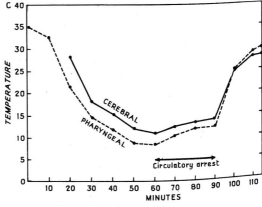

Fig. 3.

described, it is possible to cool a dog to 8°C, and rewarm it, without harm.

The deaths were similar to some we had seen following cardiopulmonary bypass using the pump-oxygenator of Lillehei and de Wall, and were probably associated with cerebral damage which might have been produced in several different ways. It may have resulted from defects in the extracorporeal circuit causing gaseous or particulate emboli—although at necropsy the cerebral vessels appeared to be normal, and contained no obvious gas bubbles. A hundred feet of plastic tubing in the heat-exchanger was a considerable resistance to blood-flow: on one occasion this exceeded 750 mm. Hg, and was clearly undesirable.

In some experiments a fall in blood-pressure had been observed when partial left-ventricular bypass and cooling were started. Although this was eventually corrected, such a period of hypotension in the early stages of the experiment, when the body temperature was normal, would affect the final results. As the flow-rates used would have been adequate at normal body temperature during cardiopulmonary bypass using a heart-lung machine, the deaths are unlikely to have been due

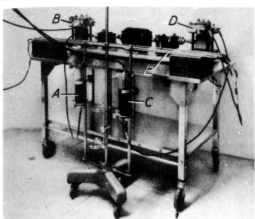

Fig. 4—The apparatus.

(A) Right atrial reservoir. (Systemic venous blood enters at top.) (B) Roller pump transmitting blood from this reservoir to pulmonary artery. (C) Left atrial reservoir. (Pulmonary venous blood enters at top.) (D) Roller pump transmitting blood from this reservoir to aorta via (E) stainless steel tubes arranged in parallel. (These are normally suspended in a trough through which hot or cold liquids are passed to effect heat exchange.)

to an inadequate circulation. The high systemic venous oxygen saturations at low temperature seem to show that flow was adequate; on the other hand there could be some interference with oxygen utilisation apart from the effect of cold. The ideal flow-rate was difficult to assess. It seemed logical to suppose that it could be decreased as the temperature fell, in step with the fall in tissue demand for oxygen. Under the conditions of these experiments, however, the circulating blood was discharging an additional function—that of a secondary refrigerant. A flow-rate exceeding the body's requirements may have been used in some phases of the experiment, because of the necessity for rapid cooling and rewarming.

Some features of the work encouraged us; although difficult at first in small hearts, the cannulations became easy with experience: cannulation of the left atrium is the most difficult, while that of the pulmonary artery is the easiest. There was no difficulty in getting venous return to the reservoirs, or in effecting a balance between the levels.

There were no postoperative lung complications, even minor ones; this is in contrast to our experience with cardiopulmonary bypass, when we frequently observed bloodstained

bronchial secretion (Drew et al. 1957). There was never any difficulty in restoring the heart to normal rhythm. There was no plasma-electrolyte disturbance.

Further Experiments

In the next series of experiments the apparatus was modified as follows (fig. 4):

The heat-exchanger consisted of four stainless-steel tubes ($^1/_4$ in. internal diameter), each of which was five feet in length and highly polished on the inside. They were arranged in parallel, and connected together with Y-shaped stainless-steel connectors and short lengths of polyvinyl ethylene chloride tubing. This arrangement was preferred to a coil because it offered less resistance and the straight tubes were easy to clean. The tubes were suspended in a trough through which cooling or warming liquids were passed from two reservoirs. The temperatures of these were kept at 2° and 45°C.

The sigmamotor pump-heads were discarded in favour of others of DeBakey type, which were designed and constructed in our laboratory. In-vitro experiments (to be published) showed that these gave consistently low hæmolysis-rates. It was decided to discard the filter.

To prevent sudden hypotension at the onset of partial left-ventricular bypass, an adjustable clip was placed on the pulmonary venous line, so that drainage from the atrium could be controlled by the surgeon. The flow of chilled blood into the aorta was started slowly, and increased to its maximum of 50–70 ml. per kg. per minute at the onset of right-ventricular bypass. The rate of increase in flow through the extracorporeal circuit was governed by the blood-pressure which was kept at an arbitrary mean of 80 to 100 mm. Hg.

Results

In four experiments cooling was carried out to 15°C, followed by a period of complete circulatory arrest lasting twenty to forty-five minutes before rewarming. Two animals survived without evidence of neurological damage.

One died after six hours from hæmorrhage, but, after operation had stood upright, and appeared to be normal neurologically. The fourth animal was hypertensive before operation, failed to recover consciousness, and at necropsy was found to have enlarged and grossly diseased kidneys.

In three of the four experiments, plasma-hæmoglobin was so little in amount that there was no difference in colour between samples taken before and after the experiment. This showed that the extracorporeal circuit was improved, and resolved previous fears that the fragility of red blood-cells might increase unduly if they were exposed to trauma at temperatures as low as 2°C, and as high as 45°C.

Summary and Conclusions

A small number of experiments was sufficient to show that, using simple apparatus, it is possible to induce profound hypothermia in a dog, followed by complete circulatory arrest for thirty minutes, and then to rewarm it with recovery.

Many colleagues helped in this investigation. Our thanks are due to Dr. Percy Cliffe, Mr. D. M. Forrest, and Mr. John Gooden for the design and construction of the pumps used in the latter part of this work; to Mr. R. E. Trotman who devised the temperature recording apparatus; and to Mr. W. S. James, our laboratory technician. Miss Joan Smith provided unstinted secretarial help. Dr. Peter Hansell of the photographic department was responsible for the illustrations.

REFERENCES

Anjus, R. K., Smith, A. U. (1955) *J. Physiol.* **128**, 446.
Bigelow, W. G., Lindsay, W. K., Harrison, R. C., Gordon, R. A., Greenwood, W. F. (1950) *Amer. J. Physiol.* **160**, 125.
Cooley, D. A., DeBakey, M. E. (1957) *Ann. Surg.* **146**, 473.
Drew, C. E., Cliffe, P., Scurr, C. F., Forrest, D. M., Pearce, D. J., King, P. A., Coles, H. M. T., Leveaux, V. M., Zilva, J. F. (1957) *Brit. med. J.* ii, 1323.
Gollan, F., Phillips, R., Grace, J. T., Jones, R. M. (1955) *J. thorac. Surg.* **30**, 626.
Niazi, S. A., Lewis, F. J. (1958) *Ann. Surg.* **147**, 264.
Sealy, W. C., Brown, I. W., Young, W. G. (1958) *ibid.* p. 603.
Smith, A. U., Lovelock, J. E., Parkes, A. S. (1954) *Nature, Lond.* **173**, 1136.

P2

Intracardiac Surgery in Neonates and Infants Using Deep Hypothermia with Surface Cooling and Limited Cardiopulmonary Bypass

By Brian G. Barratt-Boyes, M.B., Ch.M., M. Simpson, M.B., Ch.B., and John M. Neutze, M.D.

SUMMARY

In an attempt to achieve safe intracardiac surgery in severely ill babies with congenital heart defects, a technique of deep hypothermia with surface cooling and limited bypass has been used. Under halothane anesthesia, these infants were cooled to a nasopharyngeal temperature of 26 C on a circulating water blanket and the temperature was lowered further to 22 C by a short period of total body perfusion. After a period of circulatory arrest which averaged 48 minutes at 22 C, during which the intracardiac repair was carried out, rewarming to 32 C was achieved by 20 minutes of total body perfusion and final rewarming to 36 C by surface means.

Thirty-three of 37 infants under 10 kg in weight, with correctable lesions, survived this procedure, including 25 aged 8 days to 12 months. Conditions corrected were transposition (13), tetralogy of Fallot (9), total anomalous pulmonary venous connection (6), ventricular septal defect (6), and atrioventricular canal (3). The technique gave ideal operating conditions and is believed to have wide application in the neonatal and infant group.

Additional Indexing Words:

Circulatory arrest	Bypass rewarming	Ventricular septal defect
Cyanotic heart disease	Transposition of great vessels	Tetralogy of Fallot
Pulmonary circulation	Total anomalous pulmonary venous connection	

INTRACARDIAC surgery for congenital heart disease in neonates and infants by conventional cardiopulmonary bypass techniques has carried a high mortality and morbidity, particularly for complex prolonged procedures. This has been due in part to metabolic disturbances and pulmonary complications which are difficult to manage in this age group. In addition, with total body perfusion caval cannulation, which can be technically difficult, is usually required. Moreover, this technique tends to be associated with the presence of some intracardiac blood and with incomplete myocardial relaxation,

both of which hinder rapid accurate repair of complex defects within these tiny hearts.

These disadvantages can be avoided by a technique of deep hypothermia and circulatory arrest, which is designed to limit the duration of total body perfusion to an absolute minimum, does not require caval cannulation, and provides a completely bloodless, relaxed heart.

Technique

The infant is placed supine on a cooling blanket and is anesthetized with equal parts of nitrous oxide and oxygen, halothane (0.5% to 1%), and intravenous d-tubocurarine (1 mg/kg). Plastic bags of crushed ice are positioned to cover the trunk, the upper parts of the limbs, and the crown of the head, avoiding contact with peripheral parts. At 26 C nasopharyngeal, the ice

From the Cardio-thoracic Surgical Unit, Green Lane Hospital, Auckland, New Zealand.

Supplement I to Circulation, Vols. XLIII and XLIV, May 1971

bags are removed and the chest opened through a sternal splitting incision. No important cardiac arrhythmia has occurred during the cooling phase. After systemic heparinization the cavae are taped and a single venous cannula is inserted into the right atrial appendage, followed by an arterial cannula into the ascending aorta. These are connected to an infant bypass circuit incorporating a disc oxygenator and an efficient heat exchanger. The machine is primed with 2 units of fresh, heparinized whole blood containing an additional 2 mEq of potassium chloride and 5 mEq of sodium bicarbonate.

A short period of cardiopulmonary bypass is now usually, but not always, required to carry the temperature down to 22 C, a temperature which appears to allow a safe period of circulatory arrest in these infants, lasting from 60 to 70 minutes. The arterial line is then clamped and the venous blood allowed to drain freely into the machine. The aorta is cross-clamped and the caval tapes tightened. The intracardiac repair is carried out in a totally bloodless, completely relaxed heart.

When the repair has been completed and air has been evacuated from the heart, cardiopulmonary bypass is restarted to rewarm the infant rapidly to 32 C. The heart has usually begun beating spontaneously within moments of the start of perfusion, but if ventricular fibrillation has occurred it has easily been reverted electrically. At 32 C to 34 C, bypass is stopped and the chest closed. Final rewarming to 36 C is completed by surface means.

These events are depicted in graphic form in figure 1. Their duration was as follows: surface cooling 153 minutes (98 to 217 minutes); bypass cooling 9 minutes (2 to 18 minutes); circulatory arrest 48 minutes (30 to 69 minutes); bypass rewarming 21 minutes (11 to 34 minutes); and total operating time 5⅓ hours (4 to 7 hours).

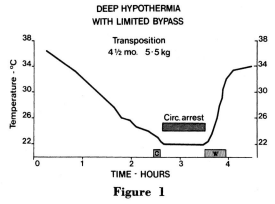

**DEEP HYPOTHERMIA
WITH LIMITED BYPASS**

Figure 1

Temperature graph during operation in an infant with transposition. C = cooling bypass; W = warming bypass.

Carbon dioxide (2½%) has been added to the respiratory gases (including the extracorporeal circuit) at temperatures below 30 C, and 10 mEq of sodium bicarbonate and 2 mEq of potassium chloride to the machine blood at the commencement of rewarming bypass. The procedure has been associated with a metabolic acidosis only slightly greater than that seen in adults using heart/lung bypass.[1, 2]

Results

Forty-one infants with congenital heart disease under two years of age and under 10 kg in weight have been operated upon by this technique during the first year of our experience, which commenced in July 1969. In four instances the defects encountered were uncorrectable (two with aortic stenosis and endocardial fibroelastosis and two with hypoplastic right-heart syndrome). These infants died within 24 hours of operation and are not considered further. The remaining 37 infants with correctable lesions are best considered in two categories.

**(a) Left-to-Right Shunt
and High Pulmonary
Blood Flow**

There were six infants with a large ventricular septal defect, three with partial atrioventricular canal (table 1), and six with total anomalous pulmonary venous connection (table 2). The associated defects listed in the tables were corrected along with the main lesion, including all the complex anomalies present in case 11 (table 2).

Fourteen of the 15 infants in this category were under one year of age, and in all but cases 10, 11, and 14 the weights were under the third percentile for their age. All had been in congestive heart failure and case 4 (table 1) required assisted ventilation for 24 hours preoperatively to control pulmonary edema.

Complete correction was successful in all but one infant (case 12) who, after a smooth initial course, died 36 hours postoperatively from a pneumothorax produced as the chest tube was removed. All others survived operation and have shown dramatic disappearance of heart failure and improvement in weight.

Assisted ventilation was necessary postoperatively in six infants (tables 1 and 2), and in

Table 1

Ventricular Septal Defect and Atrioventricular Canal

Case no.	Age (months)	Weight (kg)	Other defects	Outcome	IPPB
			Large ventricular septal defect		
1	2½	2.9	ASD, PDA	Alive	No
2	3	3.4	(Coarctation)*	Alive	No
3	3	3.5	ASD, dextrocardia	Alive	Yes (3 days)
4	4	3.9	Nil	Alive	Yes (18 hours)
5	4	3.7	PDA	Alive	No
6	7	5.8	PDA	Alive	No
			Partial atrioventricular canal		
7	6	4.7	Nil	Alive	No
8	9	4.4	Nil	Alive	No
9	20	7.2	Common atrium	Alive	No

*Repaired at one month of age.

IPPB = intermittent positive-pressure breathing postoperatively; ASD = atrial septal defect; PDA = patent ductus arteriosus.

Table 2

Total Anomalous Pulmonary Venous Connection

Case no.	Age	Weight (kg)	Type	Outcome	IPPB
10	8 days	3.3	Infradiaphragmatic + PDA	Tracheal stenosis; late death	Yes† (4 days)
11	9 days	3.2	Coronary sinus*	Alive	Yes (2 days)
12	3 months	2.5	RSVC	Hospital death	Yes (12 hrs)
13	3¾ months	4.8	Coronary sinus	Alive	No
14	4½ months	5.7	LSVC	Alive	Yes† (15 days)
15	10 months	6.8	Coronary sinus	Alive	No

*Additional defects present (interrupted aortic arch, large patent ductus arteriosus, and large ventricular septal defect).

†Tracheostomy required.

RSVC, LSVC = right and left superior venae cavae; PDA = patent ductus arteriosus; IPPB = intermittent positive-pressure breathing postoperatively.

cases 10 and 14 tracheostomy was required. Case 10, eight days old at operation, developed a subglottic stenosis and died at four months of age from this complication, despite a perfect repair (confirmed by autopsy). This baby's chest radiographs are shown in figure 2 and are representative of the dramatic improvement which has followed operation in this group. Case 14 developed pulmonary edema postoperatively which gradually resolved completely, although assisted ventilation was necessary for 19 days. These two

infants are the only patients with important morbidity in the entire series.

(b) Cyanotic Heart Disease

There were 22 infants in this category (table 3). The nine with tetralogy of Fallot required surgery because of cyanotic spells, and complete correction under deep hypothermia was chosen in preference to a palliative shunt. The youngest was aged 2 months and the oldest 18 months. Four had important hypoplasia of the pulmonary ring and main pulmonary artery and required an

Supplement 1 to Circulation, Vols. XLIII and XLIV, May 1971

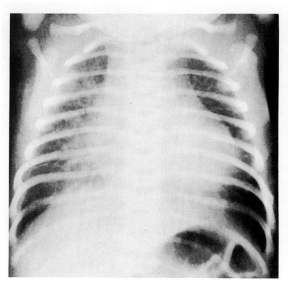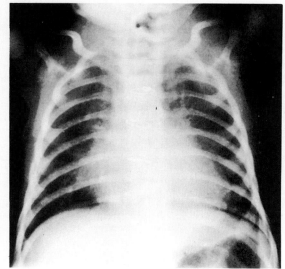

Figure 2

Chest radiographs of an infant with infradiaphragmatic total anomalous pulmonary venous connection (case 10, table 2). (Left) Preoperative; (right) three weeks postoperative.

outflow pericardial patch; one, aged four months, had a complete pulmonary atresia associated with a patent ductus arteriosus and large ventricular septal defect, and here the pulmonary trunk was completely reconstructed with pericardium. There was no morbidity or hospital mortality in these patients. Only one required assisted ventilation for 24 hours. One of these infants has recently died five months postoperatively of epidemic diarrhea, and autopsy showed an excellent repair.

The remaining 13 infants with complete transposition of the great vessels had a Mustard atrial baffle repair[3] following initial palliation by balloon septostomy. In three, aged 2, 4, and 14 weeks, the transposition was complex, as all had a large ventricular septal defect, two had a patent ductus arteriosus, and in one there was a hypoplastic distal aortic arch which had been partially corrected at a preliminary operation when the baby was one week old. All three were in severe congestive heart failure with marked cardiomegaly and corrective surgery, which included ventricular septal defect and duct closure, was urgently required. Two of the three died, one from technical error during operation and one from left-lung collapse which developed

during operation and was initially unrecognized. The remaining infant has progressed well.

In ten infants the transposition was not complicated by other cardiac defects, apart from a large patent ductus in one. All were cyanosed and came forward to operation, usually electively, at varying intervals following balloon septostomy. The youngest was 11 days old and the oldest 20 months. One, aged 6 months, died 24 hours after operation, probably of anoxia with a low cardiac output, while the other nine made a complete and uncomplicated recovery. None in this group received assisted ventilation postoperatively.

In summary, there have been 37 infants with correctable lesions operated upon with this technique, with 4 hospital deaths, all of which have occurred among the 29 infants

Table 3

Cyanotic Heart Disease

	0–12 months	13–20 months	Hospital deaths
Tetralogy of Fallot	7	2	0
Complex transposition	3	0	2
Transposition	5	5	1

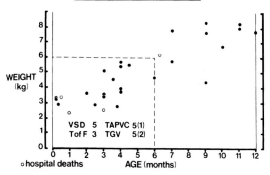

DEEP HYPOTHERMIA IN INFANCY

Figure 3

Age and weight of infants operated upon under one year of age. T of F = tetralogy of Fallot; TGV = transposition of the great vessels; TAPVC = total anomalous pulmonary venous connection; VSD = ventricular septal defect.

References

1. HARRIS EA, SEELYE ER, BARRATT-BOYES BG: Respiratory and metabolic acid base changes during cardiopulmonary bypass in man. Brit J Anaesth **42**: 912, 1970

2. SEELYE ER, HARRIS EA, SQUIRE AW, BARRATT-BOYES BG: Metabolic effects of deep hypothermia and circulatory arrest in infants during cardiac surgery. To be published in Brit J Anaesth

3. MUSTARD WT, KEITH JD, TRUSLER GA, FOWLER R, KIDD L: Surgical management of transposition of the great vessels. J Thorac Cardiovasc Surg **48**: 953, 1964

4. HIKASA Y, SHIROTANI H, SATOMURA K, ET AL: Open heart surgery in infants with an aid of hypothermic anesthesia. Arch Jap Chir **36**: 495, 1967

5. MOHRI H, DILLARD DH, CRAWFORD EW, MARTIN WE, MERENDINO KA: Method of surface-induced deep hypothermia for open-heart surgery in infants. J Thorac Cardiovasc Surg **58**: 262, 1969

6. BELSEY RHR, DOWLATSHAHI K, KEEN G, SKINNER DB: Profound hypothermia in cardiac surgery. J Thorac Cardiovasc Surg **56**: 497, 1968

7. BAUM D, DILLARD DH, MOHRI H, CRAWFORD EW: Metabolic aspects of deep surgical hypothermia in infancy. Pediatrics **42**: 93, 1968

8. DAICOFF GR, MILLER RH: Congestive heart failure in infancy treated by early repair of ventricular septal defect. *In* Cardiovascular Surgery 1969, edited by EB Mahoney. American Heart Association Monograph 30. Supplements to Circulation **41** and **42** (suppl II): II-110, 1970

Complement and the damaging effects of cardiopulmonary bypass

Postoperative cardiac, pulmonary, renal and coagulation dysfunction, along with C3a levels, were studied prospectively in 116 consecutive patients undergoing open cardiac operations and 12 patients undergoing closed operations in the same time period. The level of C3a 3 hours after open operation was high (median value 882 ng · ml⁻¹ plasma) and was related to the C3a level before cardiopulmonary bypass (CPB) (p = 0.03), the level at the end of CPB (p < 0.0001), elapsed time of CPB (p = 0.07), and older age at operation (p < 0.0001). It was inversely related to the cardiac output as reflected by the strength of the pedal pulses (p = 0.006). In contrast, C3a levels did not rise in patients undergoing closed operations. The probability of postoperative cardiac dysfunction after open operations (present in 27 of 116 patients) was predicted by C3a levels 3 hours after operation (p = 0.02), the CPB time (p = 0.02), and younger age (p < 0.0001). The same risk factors pertained for postoperative pulmonary dysfunction (present in 41 of the 116 patients); renal dysfunction (present in 24 of the 116 patients) except that CPB time was not a risk factor here; abnormal bleeding (present in 2L of the 116 patients); and important overall morbidity (present in 26 of 116 patients). As regards important overall morbidity, the C3a level effect became evident at about 1,900 ng · ml⁻¹ (a level reached by 9% of patients); the effect of increasing time of CPB became evident at about 90 minutes of CPB time; and the effect of young age became evident as age decreased from 10 to 4 years. This study demonstrates the damaging effects of CPB, relates them in part to complement activation by the foreign surfaces encountered by the blood, and supports the hypothesis that the mechanisms of the damaging effects include a whole-body inflammatory reaction.

James K. Kirklin, M.D. (by invitation), Stephen Westaby, F.R.C.S.* (by invitation),
Eugene H. Blackstone, M.D. (by invitation), John W. Kirklin, M.D.,
Dennis E. Chenoweth, M.D. (by invitation), and Albert D. Pacifico, M.D.,
Birmingham, Ala., and San Diego, Calif.

Cardiopulmonary bypass (CPB) with maintenance of the circulation by a pump oxygenator has become an established modality for support of the patient during cardiac operations. However, whether or not damage to the patient results from its use and, if so, the mecha-

nisms underlying the damage, remain contentious.

Changes in plasma proteins, including those of the coagulation system, have been shown to result from the contact of blood with foreign surfaces, including blood-gas interfaces, during CPB.[1-4] Complement levels fall,[5] and the complement degradation products C3a and C5a are elaborated during CPB.[6] C3a and C5a have physiological effects similar to those observed in many patients after CPB, including vasoconstriction and increased capillary permeability.[7,8] Previous work from this institution has evolved the hypothesis that a whole-body inflammatory reaction of variable magnitude develops as a result of CPB and that a transient damaging effect results.[9]

This clinical study was undertaken to investigate further the possibility that CPB has a damaging effect and that certain phenomena, including complement activation on the foreign surfaces of the pump oxygenator, may be related to its magnitude.

From the Department of Surgery, School of Medicine and Medical Center, University of Alabama in Birmingham; the Alabama Congenital Heart Disease Diagnosis and Treatment Center; and the Department of Pathology, University of California School of Medicine, San Diego, Calif.

Supported in part by Research Grant No. HL27440, National Heart, Lung and Blood Institute, U.S. Public Health Service.

Read at the Sixty-third Annual Meeting of The American Association for Thoracic Surgery, Atlanta, Ga., April 25-27, 1983.

Address for reprints: James K. Kirklin, M.D., Department of Surgery, University of Alabama School of Medicine and Medical Center, Birmingham, Ala. 35294.

*Current address: Royal Postgraduate Medical School, Hammersmith Hospital, London, England.

Material and methods

Patients. A prospective study was made of all patients undergoing closed or open cardiac operations on two cardiac surgical services at the University of Alabama Hospital in Birmingham between Feb. 24, 1981, and April 10, 1981. A total of 118 patients were operated upon with the use of CPB and 28 patients by closed methods. Twenty-seven of the closed operations were for congenital heart disease, as were 40 of the open operations. All patients were studied except 18 with congenital heart disease, two treated by the open technique and 16 by the closed technique. The 16 patients in the closed series who were excluded did not have an indwelling arterial or venous catheter large enough for sampling. Thus the study group consisted of 116 patients having open (11 deaths) and 12 having closed (no deaths) operations. This experience may not be a representative one, since in the calendar year 1981, among 892 patients undergoing open operation on these services, 59 died (6.6%, CL* 5.8% to 7.6%) and among 148 patients undergoing closed operations of all types, including thoracic aneurysm procedures, 11 died (7%, CL 5% to 10%).

Protocols and methods. The study protocol included collection of blood for measurement of plasma C3a levels, tabulation of intraoperative data about the details of CPB, recording of routine postoperative laboratory and clinical measurements relating to the performance of each subsystem of the patients, and observation and categorization of a number of clinical events indicating abnormal convalescence.

Blood samples for C3a determination, anticoagulated with ethylenediaminetetracetic acid, were obtained from large-bore indwelling venous catheters as near to the cutaneous puncture site as possible to avoid artifactual activation of complement by plastic tubing. In five closed operations, only an arterial line was available for sampling. R. B. Stewart, S. Westaby, and J. K. Kirklin (unpublished data) have shown that no differences exist between arterial and venous C3a levels before, during, or after CPB. Samples were obtained before CPB (before the skin incision, in closed operations), just prior to the termination of CPB from the venous port of the oxygenator (in closed operations, just after closure of the chest), 3 hours after termination of bypass (in closed operations, 3 hours after arrival in the intensive care unit), and at 5 A.M. on the first postoperative morning. All samples were promptly centrifuged and the supernatant plasma stored at $-80°$ C until analyzed.

Levels of human C3a antigen were quantitatively

*Throughout the text, CL refers to 70% confidence limits.

determined by radioimmunoassay.[10] The mean quantity of plasma C3a (ng $\cdot$ ml^{-1}) was defined from duplicate measurements by means of linear standard curves (Bo/B versus concentration C3a standard) whose correlation coefficients were >0.98. These values for plasma levels of C3a were used directly in the analysis, not corrected for hemodilution.

Abnormal convalescence among patients undergoing open operations was assessed by identification of cardiac, pulmonary, and renal dysfunction and abnormal postoperative bleeding. Death was deliberately avoided as an end-point of the study because of lack of specificity of the event. To assess cardiac performance, routine indices of cardiac function were observed and recorded in each patient for the first 48 hours after operation, including cardiac index measured by indicator-dilution methods, atrial pressures, strength of pedal pulses, pedal skin temperature, and presence or absence of inotropic support. Cardiac performance was considered normal when pedal pulses were Grade 3 or 4 (4 being normal), pedal skin temperature was tepid or warm, cardiac index was 2 L $\cdot$ min^{-1} $\cdot$ m^{-2} of body surface area (BSA) or greater, and no inotropic support more than dopamine 2.5 mg $\cdot$ min^{-1} $\cdot$ kg^{-1} was employed. Cardiac performance which was considered normal or mildly depressed on the basis of all available information was graded 0, moderately depressed cardiac performance graded 1, and severely depressed cardiac performance graded 2.

Pulmonary performance was considered normal (and graded 0) when tracheobronchial secretions were absent or minimal, gas exchange was good, and extubation was accomplished within 24 hours of operation. Postoperative pulmonary dysfunction during the first 48 postoperative hours was graded 1 when secretions were moderate or large in amount, but prolonged (>24 hours) intubation was not required. The dysfunction was graded 2 if prolonged (>24 hours) intubation was required because of pulmonary dysfunction. However, four patients with prolonged intubation were considered to have pulmonary dysfunction Grade 1, because in two of them the intubation was prolonged only because of low cardiac output and in two intubation was required preoperatively because of severe hypoxia, shock, and acidosis; in these latter two, pulmonary dysfunction postoperatively seemed no greater than that preoperatively.

Renal performance was considered normal (and graded 0) when the urine was free of gross evidence of blood or hemoglobin, urine flow was equal to or greater than 15 ml $\cdot$ hr^{-1} $\cdot$ m^{-2} BSA, and serum creatinine was less than 2 mg $\cdot$ dl^{-1}. Renal dysfunction during the first 48 hours was judged to be Grade 1 if the urine was red, Grade 2 if oliguria (<15 ml $\cdot$ hr^{-1} $\cdot$ m^{-2} BSA) was

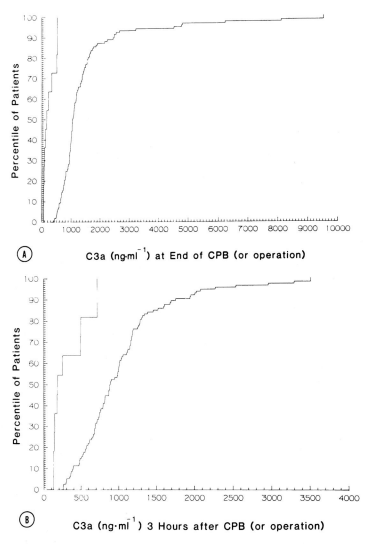

Fig. 1. Percentile distribution of patients according to C3a levels. The steep *vertical line* on the *left* represents closed cases and that on the *right*, cases in which cardiopulmonary bypass *(CPB)* was used. *A*, End of CPB (or end of operation in closed cases). *B*, Three hours after CPB (or end of operation in closed cases).

present in 2 consecutive hours, Grade 3 when serum creatinine was greater than 2 mg · dl⁻¹, and Grade 4 when peritoneal dialysis was used.

Abnormal bleeding, or bleeding more than is usually seen after CPB, was considered to be present if a greater than usual bleeding diathesis in the operating room was described by the surgeon (11 patients); if the patient was reentered for bleeding within the first 24 postoperative hours and the bleeding was found to be diffuse (four patients); or if the patient was not reentered but excessive bleeding postoperatively was nonetheless considered to be present by the observing nurse clinician and confirmed by review of his/her notes and of the amount of chest drainage (eight patients). Two patients

had abnormal bleeding both intraoperatively and postoperatively, but without reentry. Four patients had extreme diffuse bleeding in the operating room, one patient required two reentries (5 and 8 hours after operation), and one patient continued to bleed excessively from all incisions after reentry 25 hours postoperatively. These six were judged to have abnormal bleeding Grade 2. All others (15 patients) were considered to have abnormal bleeding Grade 1.

All clinical observations were recorded by one group of nurse clinicians, trained specifically for this task.

An overall appraisal of important postoperative morbidity in individual patients was made. Important morbidity was considered to be present if cardiac dysfunc-

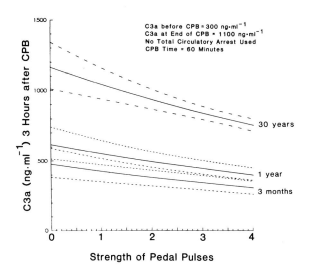

C3a before CPB = 300 ng·ml⁻¹
C3a at End of CPB = 1100 ng·ml⁻¹
No Total Circulatory Arrest Used
CPB Time = 60 Minutes

Fig. 2. Nomogram from the multivariate analysis of variables associated with the C3a levels 3 hours after CPB (Table I). It shows the shape of the relation between the pedal pulses at that time and the C3a level, for ages 3 months, 1 year, and 30 years.

Table I. *Variables associated with higher C3a levels 3 hours after CPB*

Variable	Coefficient ± SD	p Value
C3a level before bypass (ln)	0.12 ± 0.051	0.03
C3a level at the end of bypass (ln)	0.32 ± 0.079	<0.0001
Total elapsed time of bypass (min)	0.0019 ± 0.00103	0.07
Strength of pedal pulses (0-4) 3 hr after CPB	−0.11 ± 0.039	0.006
Age at operation (ln yr)	0.19 ± 0.034	<0.0001

Intercept: 3.4 ± 0.57.
Legend: CPB, Cardiopulmonary bypass. SD, Standard deviation. ln, Logarithm.
Note: If total circulatory arrest was used, add 0.63 ± 0.171 (p = 0.0004) to intercept and remove variable "age at operation."

tion was Grade 2 and/or pulmonary dysfunction Grade 2 and/or renal dysfunction Grade 3 or greater and/or abnormal bleeding Grade 2 were present.

Data analysis. Inspection of the sorted data, simple contingency tables, and comparisons of means were used for initial analysis of the data. Multivariate linear regression[11] and logistic regression[12] analyses were then added.

For the multivariate linear regression analysis of C3a levels, the following variables were entered: age, weight, BSA of the patient with and without logarithmic transformation and the squaring of these variables to test for quadratic effects, and preoperative serum creatinine levels. Dichotomous variables entered were history of an allergy, congenital heart disease, primary operation, preoperative renal dysfunction by history, and preoperative pulmonary dysfunction by history. The additional factors considered in the analysis of C3a levels at the end of CPB included: surgical service A versus B; pre-CPB methylprednisolone (30 mg · kg⁻¹); Bentley versus Shiley oxygenator; elapsed time of CPB (elapsed time between start of CPB and end of CPB, including low flow and circulatory arrest time); use of total circulatory arrest; surface cooling; total circulatory arrest time; perfusion time (elapsed time of CPB minus total circulatory arrest time); use of low flow (≤0.5 L · min⁻¹ · m⁻² BSA); and prebypass C3a concentration. C3a level at the end of bypass and the strength of pedal pulses 3 hours after CPB were also considered for analysis of C3a level 3 hours after bypass. In the analysis of C3a level on postoperative day 1, the following factors

also were considered: the C3a level 3 hours after bypass; strength of pedal pulses 3 and 5 hours after CPB and at 5 A.M. on postoperative day 1; cardiac index approximately 5 hours after CPB and on the first postoperative morning; and the presence of abnormal postoperative bleeding. In all instances the logarithmic transformation of the various C3a levels was employed in these analyses due to their more normal distribution.

All these variables were also used in the multivariate logistic regression analysis of postoperative subsystem dysfunction. Since subsystem dysfunction was graded (polychotomous) rather than considered merely present or absent (dichotomous), the particular generalization of logistic regression for polychotomous data suggested by Walker and Duncan[12] was employed. The assumption of their method is that the same risk factors and logistic regression coefficients apply to all patients, and only the intercept is altered for the various severities; this assumption is considered valid since the same risk factors and not demonstrably different coefficients were estimated for each severity level by analyzing the data according to the more general polychotomous model suggested by Hosmer and co-workers.[13]

In analysis of nomograms of the multivariate logistic analysis, the effect of an incremental risk factor (variable) was considered evident (p value about 0.1) when the upper 70% CL of the lowest probability of event was no longer overlapped by the lower 70% CL of the probability as the strength of the risk factor increased. For these analyses we utilized a C3a level of 250 ng · ml⁻¹, 30 minutes of CPB, and age 70 or 10 years as the reference points for determining evident differences.

Results

C3a levels. Among the 116 patients undergoing open operation, the median value (and the fifteenth and

Table II. *C3a levels (ng · ml⁻¹) in operations for congenital heart disease*

Time	Closed operations (n = 11)			Open operations (n = 38)			p Value
	n	Mean*	CL	n	Mean*	CL	
End of CPB	10	160	70-370	38	1140	620-2,110	<0.0001
3 hrs after CPB	9	200	90-490	36	710	350-1,440	<0.0001
5 A.M. on postop. day 1	9	220	130-370	36	270	140-510	0.4

Legend: CPB, Cardiopulmonary bypass (operation, in closed cases). CL, Confidence limits (equivalent to ± one standard deviation of the observations).

*Geometric mean.

Table III. *Cardiac dysfunction after open operations (n = 116; 27 patients had events)*

Variable (incremental risk factor)	Logistic coefficient ± SD	p Value
[Higher] C3a levels (ng · ml⁻¹) 3 hr after CPB	0.0010 ± 0.00042	0.02
[Longer] Elapsed time of CPB (min)	0.014 ± 0.0058	0.02
[Younger] Age at operation (ln yr)	−0.60 ± 0.138	<0.0001

Intercepts: Grade ≥1 = −2.3 ± 0.71; Grade 2 = −4.1 ± 0.82.

Legend: Standard deviation. CPB, Cardiopulmonary bypass. ln, Logarithm.

Table IV. *Pulmonary dysfunction after open operations (n = 116; 41 patients had events)*

Variable (incremental risk factor)	Logistic coefficient ± SD	p Value
[Higher] C3a levels (ng · ml⁻¹) 3 hr after CPB	0.0025 ± 0.00094	0.008
[Longer] Elapsed time of CPB (min)	0.025 ± 0.0111	0.02
[Younger] Age at operation (ln yr)	−1.17 ± 0.183	<0.0001
C3a levels × CPB time	$-0.015 \cdot 10^{-3} \pm 0.0086 \cdot 10^{-3}$	0.08

Intercepts: Grade ≥1 = −0.5 ± 1.01; Grade 2 = −3.7 ± 1.12.

Legend: SD, Standard deviation. CPB, Cardiopulmonary bypass. ln, Logarithm.

eighty-fifth percentile values) for C3a preoperatively, at the end of CPB (Fig. 1, *A*); 3 hours later (Fig. 1, *B*), and at 5 A.M. on postoperative day 1 was, respectively, 304 (150 to 691), 1,052 (684 to 1,726), 882 (486 to 1,390), and 288 (167 to 450) ng · ml⁻¹ (p < 0.0001).

By multivariate analysis, the C3a level at the end of CPB was correlated only with that before CPB (p = 0.005). The C3a level 3 hours after CPB was correlated not only with the previous C3a levels, but also with the elapsed time of CPB, the strength of pedal pulses (Fig. 2), and the age at operation (Table I). Total circulatory arrest was associated with increased C3a levels 3 hours after CPB and absence of an age effect. By the multivariate analysis, the C3a levels on postoperative day 1 were correlated only with those 3 hours after CPB (p < 0.0001) and with the presence of abnormal postoperative bleeding (p = 0.001).

Among patients having closed operations, C3a levels before operation, at the end of operation, 3 hours postoperatively, and on postoperative day 1 were not dissimilar (p for difference = 0.5) (Fig. 1, *A* and *B*). Thus, among patients with congenital heart disease, C3a levels were higher in those having open operations than in those having closed ones at the end of CPB (or operation) and 3 hours later, but not the next morning (Table II).

Postoperative cardiac performance in patients having open operations. Cardiac dysfunction was present during the first 48 postoperative hours in 27 (23%, CL 19% to 28%) of the 116 patients. Of these, 17 (15%) had moderate (Grade 1) cardiac dysfunction and 10 (9%) had severe (Grade 2) dysfunction. Higher C3a levels 3 hours after CPB, longer elapsed time of CPB, and younger age at operation were incremental risk factors for postoperative cardiac dysfunction, according to the multivariate logistic analysis (Table III).

Postoperative pulmonary performance in patients having open operations. Pulmonary dysfunction was present in the first 48 postoperative hours in 41 (35%, CL 30% to 40%) of the 116 patients. Pulmonary dysfunction was Grade 1 in 30 (26%) of the patients and Grade 2 in 11 (9%). The incremental risk factors for postoperative pulmonary dysfunction were the same as those for cardiac dysfunction (Table IV). In patients 1 year of age, undergoing 60 minutes of CPB, the effect of higher levels of C3a on the probability of important

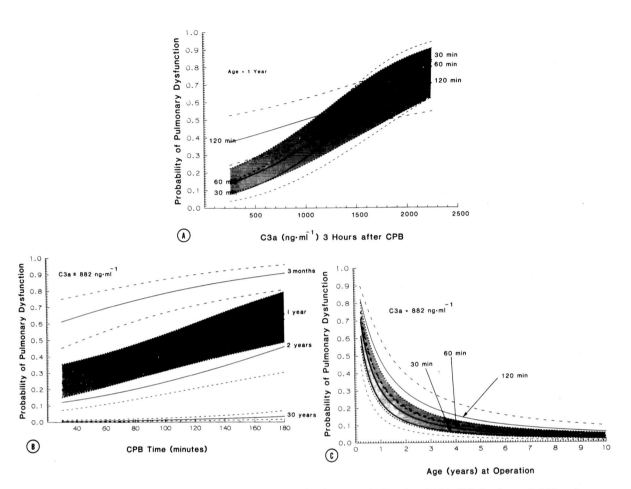

Fig. 3. Nomogram from the multivariate analysis of pulmonary dysfunction (Table IV) for the probability of important (Grade 2) postoperative pulmonary dysfunction, represented by the solid line. The *dashed lines* enclose the 70% confidence limits. *A,* The relation of C3a levels 3 hours after CPB and CPB time to the probability, when age is 1 year. The *shaded area* indicates the 70% confidence limits for 60 minutes of CPB. *B,* The relation of CPB time and age to the probability, when the C3a level is 882 ng · ml⁻¹. The *shaded area* indicates the 70% confidence limits for age 1 year. *C,* The relation of age and CPB time to the probability, when the C3a level is 882 ng · ml⁻¹. The *shaded area* indicates the 70% confidence limits for 60 minutes of CPB. In *C,* the age at which an evident difference in pulmonary dysfunction occurs, compared to the age at the far *right* of the scale, is indicated for each CPB time by the point of the *arrows.*

(Grade 2) postoperative pulmonary dysfunction was evident (see Material and methods) at a level of 916 ng · ml⁻¹ (Fig. 3, *A*). Forty-seven percent of patients had this or a higher level (Fig. 1, *B*). The effect of longer time of CPB on the probability of pulmonary dysfunction in patients with C3a levels of 882 ng · ml⁻¹ (the median value for the 116 patients) was evident at 118 minutes in patients aged 1 year (Fig. 3, *B*). The effect of young age was evident when age was reduced from 10 years to 4 years when CPB time was 60 minutes and C3a level was 882 ng · ml⁻¹ (Fig. 3, *C*).

The interrelated effects of the three variables (C3a levels, CPB time, and age) on the probability of pulmonary dysfunction are shown in Table V; either

high C3a levels or long CPB times increased the probability of pulmonary dysfunction, but the effect of both was greatly reduced in adult patients.

Postoperative renal performance in patients having open operations. Renal dysfunction was present early postoperatively in 24 (21%, CL 17% to 25%) of the 116 patients undergoing open operations. Grade 1 dysfunction was present in five (4%) of the patients, Grade 2 in eight (7%), Grade 3 in six (5%), and Grade 4 dysfunction in five (4%). The incremental risk factors for postoperative pulmonary dysfunction, determined by multivariate logistic regression analysis, were higher levels of C3a 3 hours after CPB and younger age at operation (Table VI).

Table V. *Pulmonary dysfunction Grade 2 after open operations*

Elapsed time of bypass (min)	C3a levels (ng · ml⁻¹)	Estimated probability of pulmonary dysfunction							
		3 mo*		12 mo*		5 yr*		30 yr*	
		P	CL	P	CL	P	CL	P	CL
30	400	37%	23%-54%	10%	6%-19%	1.8%	0.8%-3.7%	0.2%	0.08%-0.6%
	800	57%	41%-72%	21%	13%-32%	4%	2%-7%	0.5%	0.2%-1.1%
	1,600	87%	74%-94%	58%	39%-74%	17%	9%-30%	2.5%	1.2%-5.3%
60	400	51%	37%-66%	17%	11%-26%	3.1%	1.7%-5.6%	0.4%	0.2%-0.9%
	800	67%	54%-78%	28%	20%-39%	6%	3%-9%	0.7%	0.4%-1.5%
	1,600	88%	77%-94%	59%	43%-73%	18%	11%-28%	2.6%	1.4%-4.9%
120	400	77%	63%-87%	40%	27%-54%	9%	5%-15%	1.2%	0.6%-2.6%
	800	82%	70%-89%	47%	35%-59%	12%	8%-18%	1.6%	0.9%-3.1%
	1,600	89%	79%-94%	60%	47%-72%	19%	13%-27%	2.8%	1.6%-5.0%

Legend: P, Probability expressed as percent. CL, 70% confidence limits.
*Age at operation.

Table VI. *Renal dysfunction after open operations (n = 116; 24 patients had events)*

Variable (incremental risk factor)	Logistic coefficient ± SD	p Value
[Higher] C3a levels (ng · ml⁻¹) 3 hr after CPB	0.0009 ± 0.00036	0.02
[Younger] Age at operation (ln yr)	−0.70 ± 0.142	<0.0001

Intercepts: Grade ≥1 = −0.5 ± 0.47; Grade ≥2 = −0.9 ± 0.47; Grade ≥3 = −1.6 ± 0.50; Grade 4 = −2.6 ± 0.60.
Legend: SD, Standard deviation. CPB, Cardiopulmonary bypass. ln, Logarithm.

Table VII. *Abnormal bleeding after open operations (n = 116; 21 patients had events)*

Variable (Incremental risk factor)	Logistic coefficient ± SD	p Value
[Higher] C3a levels (ng · ml⁻¹) 3 hr after CPB	0.0006 ± 0.00037	0.10
[Longer] Elapsed time of CPB (min)	0.017 ± 0.0059	0.005
[Younger] Age at operation (ln yr)	−0.24 ± 0.133	0.07

Intercepts: Grade ≥1 = −3.2 ± 0.78; Grade 2 = −4.7 ± 0.89.
Legend: SD, Standard deviation. CPB, Cardiopulmonary bypass. ln, Logarithm.

Abnormal bleeding in patients having open operations. Fifteen (13%, CL 10% to 17%) of the 116 patients had abnormal bleeding Grade 1, whereas bleeding was Grade 2 in another six (5%, CL 3% to 8%). The risk factors for abnormal bleeding were higher levels of C3a 3 hours after CPB, longer elapsed time of CPB, and younger age at operation (Table VII). The effect of higher C3a levels in patients 1 year of age undergoing 60 minutes of CPB was evident at 2,300 ng · ml⁻¹ (Fig. 4, A), a level reached by 4% of patients. The effect of longer bypass times in patients 1 year of age with C3a concentration of 882 ng · ml⁻¹ was evident at 92 minutes (Fig. 4, B). The effect of younger age was evident when age was reduced from 70 years to 1½ years, with C3a concentration of 882 ng · ml⁻¹ and with CPB time of 60 minutes (Fig. 4, C).

Important postoperative morbidity in patients having open operations. Among the 116 patients, 26 (22%, CL 18% to 27%) had important postoperative morbidity (see Material and methods for definition) within the first 48 hours postoperatively. The incremental risk factors assocated with this were higher levels of C3a 3 hours after CPB, longer elapsed time of CPB, and younger age at operation (Table VIII). In patients 1 year of age undergoing 60 minutes of CPB, the effect of C3a was evident at a level of 1,900 ng · ml⁻¹, a level reached by 9% of patients (Fig. 5, A). Even when complement levels were very high, the length of CPB remained associated with morbidity, as did young age (Table IX). The effect of CPB time in patients aged 1 year with a C3a level of 882 ng · ml⁻¹ became evident when it exceeded 82 minutes (Fig. 5, B). When age at operation decreased from 10 years, the effect of young age became evident at age 4 years (Fig. 5, C) when the C3a concentration was 882 ng · ml⁻¹ and the CPB time was 60 minutes. The interrelated effects of the three

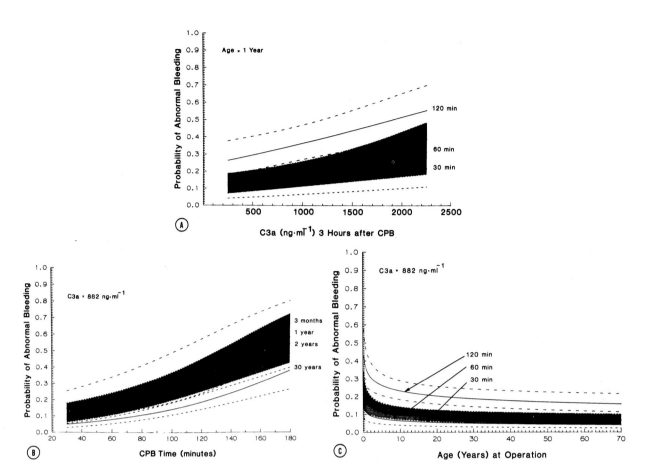

Fig. 4. Nomogram from the multivariate analysis (Table VII) of abnormal bleeding (Grades 1 or 2). The presentation, including *A, B,* and *C,* is as in Fig. 2. The *shaded areas* indicate the 70% confidence limits for 60 minutes of CPB *(A),* age 1 year *(B),* and 60 minutes of CPB *(C).*

Table VIII. *Important morbidity after open operations (n = 116; 26 patients had events)*

Variable (incremental risk factor)	Logistic coefficient ± SD	p Value
[Higher] C3a levels (ng · ml−1) 3 hr after CPB	0.0006 ± 0.00033	0.07
[Longer] Elapsed time of CPB (min)	0.017 ± 0.0048	0.0004
[Younger] Age at operation (ln yr)	−0.71 ± 0.131	<0.0001

Intercept: −2.0 ± 0.60.
Legend: SD, Standard deviation. CPB, Cardiopulmonary bypass. ln, Logarithm.

variables (Table IX) are such that when CPB time is increased from 60 to 120 minutes, there is an evident difference in the probability of morbidity at all ages and all C3a levels.

Discussion

Study methods. A study of postoperative morbidity is open to the criticism that many of the observations of subsystem dysfunction are subjective and affected by observer bias. In an attempt to meet this criticism, the observations were made by one group of nurse clinicians rather than by the physicians responsible for the patients, and objective data were recorded for each patient during the real time of his convalescence.

The methodology for measurement of C3a levels appears to be reliable and accurate. Plasma levels were used as measured, and ignoring the hemodilution that occurred at the onset of bypass and to some extent during it may result in as yet unknown errors of interpretation.

In an effort to avoid discarding possibly useful information, we retained variables in the multivariate

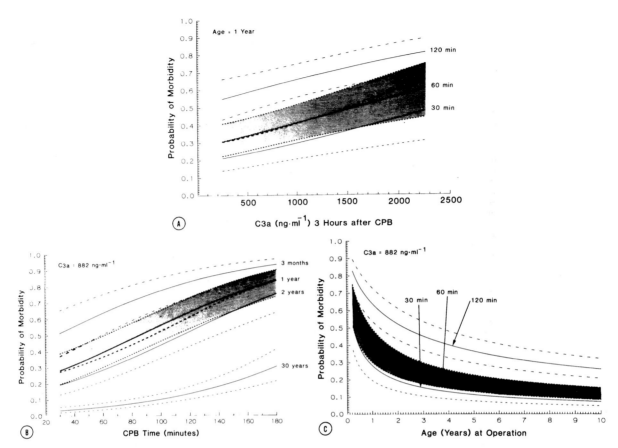

Fig. 5. Nomogram from the multivariate analysis (Table VIII) of important postoperative morbidity. The presentation, including *A, B,* and *C,* is as in Fig. 2. The *shaded areas* indicate the 70% confidence limits for 60 minutes of CPB *(A),* age 1 year *(B),* and 60 minutes of CPB *(C).* In *C,* the age at which an evident difference in morbidity occurs, compared to the age at the far *right* of the scale, is indicated for each CPB time by the point of the *arrows.*

analysis if the p value was less than 0.2, as is the usual practice in this and other institutions.[14] It could be argued that elimination of variables with a p value less than 0.05 would be more appropriate, but this would increase the likelihood of type II errors. In any event, the data presented must be interpreted in light of the p values.

C3a levels. Complement activation has been shown to occur during hemodialysis for renal failure, and this is believed to be due to contact of blood with the foreign surfaces of the dialysis unit.[15] This activation is postulated to contribute to the pulmonary dysfunction that sometimes occurs after this type of treatment. A previous study from this institution demonstrated activation of complement during CPB in man with the production of its degradation products C3a and C5a.[6] In the current study, C3a did not increase in patients undergoing closed operations without CPB. It did increase in patients undergoing open operations with CPB, and it was still considerably elevated above normal 3 hours

after CPB. This supports further the idea that complement activation is occurring as a result of contact of blood with the foreign surfaces of the pump-oxygenator system. However, in as yet an unknown and unquantified manner, certain pharmacologic interventions such as administration of heparin and/or protamine may play a role,[16-18] as may other immunologic and inflammatory processes within the patient.

The previous study[6] and this one suggest a continuing complement activation during CPB, with the levels of C3a 3 hours after CPB being associated, among other things, with the duration of CPB. An alternative hypothesis is that mechanisms for inactivating or metabolizing C3a are impaired by CPB.

The demonstrated association between higher C3a levels and the use of total circulatory arrest is not easily interpreted. It may result from the prolonged exposure of blood only to the pump oxygenator during the circulatory arrest (most of the blood is drained out of the patient into the machine as the circulatory arrest is

Table IX. *Important morbidity after open operations*

Elapsed time of bypass (min)	C3a levels $(ng \cdot ml^{-1})$	Estimated probability of important morbidity											
		3 mo*		6 mo*		12 mo*		24 mo*		5 yr*		30 yr*	
		P	CL	P	CL	P	CL	P	CL	P	CL	P	CL
30	400	44%	31%-58%	33%	22%-45%	23%	15%-32%	15%	10%-22%	9%	6%-13%	2.6%	1.5%-4.3%
	800	50%	36%-64%	38%	27%-51%	27%	19%-38%	19%	13%-26%	11%	7%-16%	3%	2%-5%
	1,600	62%	46%-76%	50%	35%-65%	38%	26%-52%	27%	18%-39%	16%	11%-24%	5%	3%-8%
60	400	57%	43%-69%	44%	33%-56%	33%	24%-43%	23%	17%-31%	13%	10%-19%	4%	3%-6%
	800	63%	49%-74%	51%	39%-62%	38%	29%-49%	28%	21%-36%	17%	12%-22%	5%	4%-8%
	1,600	73%	59%-84%	62%	49%-74%	50%	38%-63%	38%	28%-49%	24%	18%-33%	8%	6%-12%
120	400	78%	67%-86%	69%	57%-78%	57%	46%-68%	45%	35%-55%	30%	23%-38%	11%	7%-15%
	800	82%	72%-89%	74%	63%-82%	63%	53%-72%	51%	42%-60%	35%	28%-43%	13%	10%-18%
	1,600	88%	80%-93%	82%	72%-89%	74%	63%-82%	63%	53%-72%	47%	38%-56%	20%	15%-26%

Legend: P, Probability expressed as percent. CL, 70% confidence limits.
*Age at operation.

induced), or from an increased inflammatory reaction from tissue hypoxia during the arrest period, or from a deleterious effect of the circulatory arrest on the mechanisms for inactivating or metabolizing C3a.

The inverse relationship between strength of pedal pulses and C3a levels 3 hours after bypass suggests that C3a may be more rapidly "cleared" in the presence of good circulatory performance. However, it may merely reflect poorer cardiac performance associated with higher levels of C3a.

The explanation for the association between older age and higher levels of C3a is not evident.

Subsystem dysfunction in patients undergoing open operations. Cardiac,[19-22] pulmonary,[23-27] renal,[28, 29] and coagulation[2-4, 30-32] dysfunction after CPB have been described in many studies. Subsystem dysfunction was also noted in the present study and, when analyzed separately or together as morbidity, was probably accentuated by higher C3a levels after CPB, younger age, and longer CPB times. Since the mortality experienced during the study period was higher than that for all other patients during the calendar year for the two services (see Patients), and thus possibly not representative of results in a larger sample, a more realistic estimate of the probability of subsystem dysfunction in a larger sample of similar patients in similar circumstances might be achieved by using the lower 70% CL.

The probable association found in this study between the level of C3a 3 hours after CPB and subsystem dysfunction suggests that complement activation and generation of the anaphylatoxins C3a and C5a, along with other phenomena, may play a role in producing a whole-body inflammatory response. Furthermore, the subsystem dysfunction may be the result of the inflammatory reaction, with vasoconstriction, increased capillary permeability, and other phenomena involving formed and unformed blood elements.[8, 9]

In the lungs, for example, increased interstitial water is a nearly uniform accompaniment of CPB.[23] Activation of the alternative pathway of complement produces C5a as well as C3a.[8] Polymorphonuclear leukocytes have specific binding sites for C5a,[33] and transpulmonary sequestration of these leukocytes has been demonstrated during partial bypass.[6] In sheep, white blood cells play an important role in the development of interstitial pulmonary edema following microembolization.[34] Such a mechanism may play a role in the pulmonary dysfunction following CPB.

The incremental risk of young age for dysfunction was noted in all four subsystems studied. Turley, Mavroudis, and Ebert[35] reported no such effect in neonates operated upon in their first week of life as long as the elapsed time of CPB was short, but they observed a high mortality when it was 130 minutes. These observations are not inconsistent with the findings of the current study, nor are the excellent results in young infants reported by Castaneda and colleagues.[36] Good results have been achieved with many types of open operations in infants, particularly in recent years,[36-41] but special efforts and expertise are required, and this present study suggests that this is because of an apparent increased sensitivity of the young to the damaging effects of CPB.

In this study, longer CPB time was an additional risk factor for the presumed damaging effects of CPB. This has been the intuitive opinion of many surgical groups and emphasizes the importance of performing open heart operations in as time-efficient a manner as possible consistent with an accurate and complete repair.

A combination of relatively short CPB times, skillful operations, a patient not already affected by advanced or long-standing heart failure, and attention to the details of intraoperative and postoperative care can largely neutralize the presumed damaging effects of CPB, as many excellent experiences have shown. Even under these circumstances, however, an otherwise unexplainable subsystem dysfunction occasionally occurs. Further investigation is required for elucidation of the underlying mechanisms and development of methods for complete neutralization of these damaging effects.

The Nurse Clinicians, Ms. Marjorie Land, Ms. Deborah O'Connell, Mr. Joseph Knight, Ms. Zenaida Bavez, and Mr. Charles McCook, of the Cardiovascular Surgery Intensive Care Unit participated in an invaluable way in making and recording the clinical observations utilized in this study. Ms. Kathy Peterson, Mr. Jack Acton, Mr. William Tracy, and Ms. Nona Andrews organized the logistics of the study, compiled the data, and handled the blood samples. Ms. Carol Soderberg assisted in performing the C3a radioimmunoassays. Mr. Robert Brown and Dr. David Naftel, Department of Biostatistics and Biomathematics, assisted in data preparation and analysis. Dr. Edwin Bradley, Department of Biostatistics and Biomathematics, assisted us in developing the concepts of "evident differences." Ms. Sandy O'Brien assisted with the artwork, and Ms. Nancy Ferguson typed the manuscript.

REFERENCES

1 Lee WH Jr, Krumbhaar D, Fonkalsrud EW, Schjeide OA, Maloney JV Jr: Denaturation of plasma proteins as a cause of mobidity and death after intracardiac operations. Surgery 50:29-39, 1961

2 Kalter RD, Saul CM, Wetstein L, Soriano C, Reiss RF: Cardiopulmonary bypass. Associated hemostatic abnormalities. J Thorac Cardiovasc Surg 77:427-435, 1979

3 McKenna R, Bachmann F, Whittaker B, Gilson JR, Weinberg M Jr: The hemostatic mechanism after open-heart surgery. II. Frequency of abnormal platelet functions during and after extracorporeal circulation. J Thorac Cardiovasc Surg 70:298-308, 1975

4 Woods JE, Kirklin JW, Owen CA Jr, Thompson JH Jr, Taswell HF: Effect of bypass surgery on coagulation sensitive clotting factors. Mayo Clin Proc 42:724-735, 1967

5 Parker DJ, Cantrell SW, Karp RB, Stroud RM, Digerness SB: Changes in serum complement and immunoglobulins following cardiopulmonary bypass. Surgery 71:824-827, 1972

6 Chenoweth DE, Cooper SW, Hugli TE, Stewart RW, Blackstone EH, Kirklin JW: Complement activation during cardiopulmonary bypass. Evidence for generation of C3a and C5a anaphylatoxins. N Engl J Med 304:497-503, 1981

7 Dias da Silva V, Eisele JW, Lepow IH: Complement as a mediator of inflammation. III. Purification of the activity with anaphylatoxin properties generated by interaction of the first four components of complement and its identification as a cleavage product of C3. J Exp Med 126:1027-1048, 1967

8 Muller-Eberhard HJ: Complement. Ann Rev Biochem 44:697-724, 1975

9 Blackstone EH, Kirklin JW, Stewart RW, Chenoweth DE: The damaging effects of cardiopulmonary bypass, Prostaglandins in Clinical Medicine: Cardiovascular and Thrombotic Disorders, KK Wu, EC Rossi, eds., Chicago, 1982, Year Book Medical Publishers, Inc., pp 355-369

10 Hugli TE, Chenoweth DE: Biologically active peptides of complement techniques and significance of C3a and C5a measurements, Future Perspectives in Clinical Laboratory Immunoassays: Clinical Laboratory Techniques for the 1980's, RM Nakamura, WR Dito, ES Tucker III, eds., New York, 1980, Alan R. Liss, pp 443-460

11 Draper NR, Smith H: Applied Regression Analysis, ed 2, New York, 1981, John Wiley & Sons, Inc.

12 Walker SH, Duncan DB: Estimation of the probability of an event as a function of several independent variables. Biometrika 54:167-79, 1967

13 Hosmer DW Jr, Wang CY, Lin IC, Lemeshows S: A computer program for stepwise logistic regression using maximum likelihood estimation. Comput Programs Biomed 8:121-134, 1978

14 Kempthorne O: Of what use are tests of significance and tests of hypothesis. Comm Stat Theor Meth A5:763-777, 1976

15 Craddock PR, Fehr J, Brigham KL, Kronenberg RS, Jacob HS: Complement and leukocyte-mediated pulmonary dysfunction in hemodialysis. N Engl J Med 296:769-774, 1977

16 Lakin JD, Blocker TJ, Strong DM, Yocum MW: Anaphylaxis to protamine sulfate mediated by a complement-dependent IgG antibody. J Allergy Clin Immunol 61:102-107, 1978

17 Rent R, Ertel N, Eisenstein R, Gewurz H: Complement activation by interaction of polyanions and polycations. I. Heparin-protamine induced consumption of complement. J Immunol 114:120-124, 1975

18 Siegel J, Rent R, Gewurz H: Interactions of C-reactive protein with the complement system. I. Protamine-induced consumption of complement in acute phase sera. J Exp Med 140:631-647, 1974

19 Brody WR, Reitz BA, Andrews MJ, Roberts WC, Michaelis LL: Long-term morphologic and hemodynamic evaluation of the left ventricle after cardiopulmonary bypass. J Thorac Cardiovasc Surg 70:1073-1085, 1975

20 Buckberg GD, Olinger GN, Mulder DG, Maloney JV Jr: Depressed postoperative cardiac performance. Prevention by adequate myocardial protection during cardiopulmonary bypass. J Thorac Cardiovasc Surg 70:974-988, 1975

21 Kirklin JW, Theye RA: Cardiac performance after open intracardiac surgery. Circulation 28:1061-1070, 1963

22 Laks H, Standeven J, Blair O, Hahn J, Jellinek M, Willman VL: The effects of cardiopulmonary bypass with crystalloid and colloid hemodilution on myocardial extra-

vascular water. J THORAC CARDIOVASC SURG **73**:129-138, 1977

23 Cooper JD, Maeda MD, Lowenstein E: Lung water accumulation with acute hemodilution in dogs. J THORAC CARDIOVASC SURG **69**:957-965, 1975

24 Geha AS, Sessler AD, Kirklin JW: Alveolar-arterial oxygen gradients after open intracardiac surgery. J THORAC CARDIOVASC SURG **51**:609-615, 1966

25 Ratliff NB, Young WG Jr, Hackel DB, Mikat E, Wilson JW: Pulmonary injury secondary to extracorporeal circulation. J THORAC CARDIOVASC SURG **65**:425-432, 1973

26 Rea HH, Harris EA, Seelye ER, Whitlock RML, Withy SJ: The effects of cardiopulmonary bypass upon pulmonary gas exchange. J THORAC CARDIOVASC SURG **75**:104-120, 1978

27 Olinger GN, Becker RM, Bonchek LI: Noncardiogenic pulmonary edema and peripheral vascular collapse following cardiopulmonary bypass. Rare protamine reaction? Ann Thorac Surg **29**:20-25, 1980

28 Abel RM, Buckley MJ, Austen WG, Barnett GO, Beck CH Jr, Fischer JE: Etiology, incidence, and prognosis of renal failure following cardiac operations. Results of a prospective analysis of 500 consecutive patients. J THORAC CARDIOVASC SURG **71**:323-333, 1976

29 Gailiunas P Jr, Chawla R, Lazarus JM, Cohn L, Sanders J, Merrill JP: Acute renal failure following cardiac operations. J THORAC CARDIOVASC SURG **79**:241-243, 1980

30 Hope AF, Heyns A duP, Lötter MG, van Reenen OR, de Kock F, Badenhorst PN, Pieters H, Kotze H, Meyer JM, Minnaar PC: Kinetics and sites of sequestration of indium 111–labeled human platelets during cardiopulmonary bypass. J THORAC CARDIOVASC SURG **81**:880-886, 1981

31 Tamari Y, Aledort L, Puszkin E, Degnan TJ, Wagner N, Kaplitt MJ, Peirce EC II: Functional changes in platelets during extracorporeal circulation. Ann Thorac Surg **19**:639-647, 1975

32 Lambert CJ, Marengo-Rowe AJ, Levenson JE, Green RH, Thiele JP, Geisler GF, Adam M, Mitchel BF: The treatment of postperfusion bleeding using ε-aminocaproic acid, cryoprecipitate, fresh-frozen plasma, and protamine sulfate. Ann Thorac Surg **28**:440-444, 1979

33 Chenoweth DE, Hugli TE: Demonstration of specific C5a receptor on intact human polymorphonuclear leukocytes. Proc Natl Acad Sci USA **75**:3943-3947, 1978

34 Flick MR, Perel A, Staub NC: Leukocytes are required for increased lung microvascular permeability after microembolization in sheep. Circ Res **48**:344-351, 1981

35 Turley K, Mavroudis C, Ebert P: Repair of congenital cardiac lesions during the first week of life. Circulation **66**:Suppl I:214-219, 1982

36 Castaneda AR, Lamberti J, Sade RM, Williams RG, Nadas AS: Open-heart surgery during the first three months of life. J THORAC CARDIOVASC SURG **68**:719-731, 1974

37 Kirklin JK, Blackstone EH, Kirklin JW, McKay R, Pacifico AD, Bargeron LM Jr: Intracardiac surgery in infants under age 3 months. Incremental risk factors for hospital mortality. Am J Cardiol **48**:500-506, 1981

38 Barratt-Boyes BG, Neutze JM, Clarkson PM, Shardey GC, Brandt PWT: Repair of ventricular septal defect in the first two years of life using profound hypothermia–circulatory arrest techniques. Ann Surg **184**:376-390, 1976

39 Rizzoli G, Blackstone EH, Kirklin JW, Pacifico AD, Bargeron LM Jr: Incremental risk factors in hospital mortality rate after repair of ventricular septal defect. J THORAC CARDIOVASC SURG **80**:494-505, 1980

40 Studer M, Blackstone EH, Kirklin JW, Pacifico AD, Soto B, Chung GKT, Kirklin JK, Bargeron LM Jr: Determinants of early and late results of repair of atrioventricular septal (canal) defects. J THORAC CARDIOVASC SURG **84**:523-542, 1982

41 Piccoli G, Pacifico AD, Kirklin JW, Blackstone EH, Kirklin JK, Bargeron LM Jr: Changing results and concepts in the surgical treatment of double outlet right ventricle. Am J Cardiol (in press)

Discussion

DR. RICHARD M. ENGELMAN
Springfield, Mass.

I rise to support the results presented by Dr. Kirklin and associates and to further define this phenomenon of complement activation by data of our own. In a sequential group of 11 patients undergoing routine coronary revascularization, C5a and C3a inhibitors, enzymes which inactivate chemotactic factor and anaphylatoxin, were assayed quantitatively before, during, and after bypass. The C3a inhibitor falls precipitously within 5 minutes of the institution of CPB and does not reach control levels until after 6 hours. Sometime between 6 and 24 hours, this value appears to return to normal. The inhibitor for the C5a appears to stay within control limits throughout the duration of bypass.

These data serve to define as least one mechanism whereby C3a activity, the inverse of the inhibitor activity just described, measureably increases during routine CPB, whereas C5a and C5a inhibitor remain unchanged. From previous studies one is aware of that.

Dr. Kirklin, do you believe it will be possible to conduct CPB without complement activation and, if so, what techniques might be employed?

DR. RAY CHU-JENG CHIU
Montreal, Quebec, Canada

In our own study, which will appear in *The Annals of Thoracic Surgery*, we also found rapid consumption of both C3 and C4 right after the start of CPB. This phenomenon could not be accounted for by hemodilution alone and thus indicates acute complement activation. However, we did not detect further consumption in serial sampling of C3 and C4 after protamine administration, even though protamine, and especially protamine-heparin complex, are known to be strong activators of complements in vitro, and had been thought to play a role in protamine hypotension encountered not infrequently in cardiac operations.

Dr. Kirklin, did you see futher complement activation after protamine injection in your series, and, if you did, could you correlate it both in timing and in magnitude with the hemodynamic changes associated with protamine administration? I recall you made some comments on this subject at the previous meeting of the Association.

MR. JOHN R. KEATES
London, England

We also see the postperfusion syndrome, which includes hemorrhagic diathesis, systemic inflammatory reaction, and diffuse organ dysfunction. A retrospective analysis of the last 1,500 bypasses at King's College Hospital revealed 10 florid examples of this syndrome which could not be explained by low cardiac output or infection. Five of the 10 patients subsequently died. We also feel that complement activation could be implicated in this syndrome.

Our efforts at studying complement have included analysis of C3d, release of which is accepted by immunologists as being unequivocal evidence of complement activation. We studied 10 patients undergoing routine coronary artery bypass. We noted that there was a progressive rise in C3d throughout the perfusion, that there was no extra rise after the administration of protamine, and that the levels fell rapidly to near normal but remained slightly elevated up to the fifth day.

Although these patients made an uneventful recovery, we would suggest that the degree of complement activation found, which is in excess of that found in severe disseminated lupus, is disturbing, particularly in view of the correlation found by Dr. Kirklin between C3a release and organ dysfunction. Moreover, we suggest that these types of investigations represent a potentially highly sensitive yardstick for the evaluation of all components of the extracorporeal circuit in respect to their potential production of diffuse organ damage.

Finally, has Dr. Kirklin any data incriminating particular parts of the bypass circuit in complement activation?

DR. J. K. KIRKLIN *(Closing)*

I would like to thank the discussers for providing very important and interesting additional information to this material.

Dr. Engelman's data are extremely interesting. In response to his specific question regarding whether CPB can be conducted without complement activation, there are some preliminary studies which suggest that it may be possible. However, although certain components of the oxygenator system, for example, the nylon components, are known to be powerful activators of complement, the mere presence of complement activation is perhaps not the most important thing. We view this as a mere window through which we can get some glimpse into a very much more complicated process of an overall inflammatory effect of CPB. The other components of what is called the humeral amplification system, which includes the coagulation system, fibrinolytic system, kallikrein system, and the complement system, are probably all very important and closely interrelated. I think the problem is much more complicated than whether or not we can prevent complement activation.

Regarding protamine, in this particular study we did not serially follow measurements of plasma C3a levels after the administration of protamine. We do have other unpublished data, however, which suggest very strongly that protamine or the protamine-heparin complex is a powerful activator of complement, not via the alternative pathway, as is true with CPB, but via the classical pathway involving C4a. We do have some studies regarding patients receiving protamine in a prospective manner. However, as you know, protamine reactions are extremely rare. These studies were carried out in patients having routine coronary artery bypass grafting, and no patients manifested an adverse reaction to protamine. In the preliminary data, we have seen marked changes in hemodynamics or pulmonary or systemic vascular resistance with protamine. Of course, that says nothing about the situations in which there is a profound protamine reaction.

Regarding the components of the bypass circuits, we know that multiple components of the bypass circuit activate complement in vitro. Nylon has been shown in a previous study to markedly activate complement; but, again I think the solution is much more complicated than merely removing nylon from the circuit. Thus many aspects of the CPB circuit need to be thoroughly investigated both in vitro and in vivo.

In answer to Dr. Spencer's question about any other operations studied: These are the first data that we have accumulated regarding closed operations. We have not yet studied noncardiac procedures, but certainly other situations, such as trauma, in which multiple blood products are given, merit investigation.

Regarding the possible role of cardiotomy suction on complement activation, we currently have no data to answer this question.

Regarding the membrane oxygenator, I believe there is no secure evidence at present relating to complement activation in the membrane versus the bubble oxygenator system, but certainly this is an area which needs to be actively investigated.

Effects of Aprotinin on Hemostatic Mechanisms during Cardiopulmonary Bypass

Willem van Oeveren, M.Sc., Nicolaas J. G. Jansen, M.D., Ben P. Bidstrup, M.D., Dave Royston, M.D., Steven Westaby, M.D., Heinz Neuhof, M.D., Ph.D., and Charles R. H. Wildevuur, M.D., Ph.D.

ABSTRACT Cardiopulmonary bypass (CPB) is associated with activation of humoral systems, which results in the release of proteases. These proteases may affect platelets and stimulate granulocytes. In the present study, the protease inhibitor aprotinin was given in high doses to 11 patients to achieve plasma concentrations of more than 150 kallikrein inactivator units per milliliter during CPB. At such concentrations, kallikrein and plasmin are effectively inhibited. This treatment resulted in platelet preservation during CPB. Platelet numbers were virtually unaffected, and thromboxane release was prevented in the aprotinin-treated group in contrast to the control group. Postoperatively, hemostasis was significantly better preserved after aprotinin treatment (blood loss of 357 ml in the treated group versus 674 ml in the untreated group; $p < 0.01$). Since tissue-plasminogen activator activity was similar in both groups, the improved hemostasis most likely should be attributed to platelet preservation. Furthermore, aprotinin lessened neutrophilic elastase release, which might contribute to decreased pulmonary dysfunction in patients at risk.

The damaging effects of cardiopulmonary bypass (CPB) continue to contribute to the morbidity and mortality of cardiac procedures, particularly in patients at risk. The so-called postperfusion syndrome, comprising fever of noninfective origin, pulmonary and renal dysfunction, leukocytosis, and abnormal bleeding, has recently been interpreted as a "whole-body inflammatory response" possibly initiated by contact of blood with the nonbiological materials of the extracorporeal circuit [1]. The stimulus for this sequence of events is thought to be activation through the Hageman factor (Factor XII) of the closely interrelated humoral systems: complement, coagulation, fibrinolytic, and kallikrein/kinin. In addition, the alternative pathway of complement can be activated by C3b binding on the surface of the allegedly biocompatible polymers of the extracorporeal circuit [2]. Particularly through the activation of the fibrinolytic and complement systems, the generalized inflammatory reaction may also affect platelets and leukocytes, and this result might contribute in a major way to postbypass complications such as impaired hemostasis and pulmonary dysfunction. To identify the importance of the fibrinolytic and complement systems in this regard, patients undergoing CPB were treated with aprotinin, which in high doses inhibits plasmin. The effect of aprotinin was determined by differences in platelet and leukocyte numbers and their release products in treated and nontreated patients. The clinical relevance of platelet preservation was indicated by the hemostatic capacity, expessed as postbypass blood loss and blood requirements.

Material and Methods

Informed consent was obtained from 22 otherwise healthy patients undergoing elective coronary artery bypass grafting. Eleven patients were randomly assigned to aprotinin treatment during CPB; the other 11 served as controls. Aprotinin (Trasylol) was supplied by Bayer AG (West Germany) in bottles containing 50 ml of saline solution without any additives or preservatives, each milliliter containing 10,000 kallikrein inactivator units (KIU).

The study protocol was approved by the ethical committee. The following dosage regimen was used in the treatment group. At the start of anesthesia, an infusion of $2 \cdot 10^6$ KIU (200 ml) was given over a 20- to 30-minute period. Thereafter a continuous infusion of $0.5 \cdot 10^6$ KIU (50 ml) per hour was administered until the end of the operation after the last blood sample had been collected. To each liter of transfused whole blood given during the operation, an additional $0.5 \cdot 10^6$ KIU (50 ml) of Trasylol was administered by a separate bolus infusion. Patients with a history of allergy, acute pancreatitis, hemorrhage due to fibrinolysis, or a possibility of previous exposure to aprotinin were not admitted to the study.

The anesthesia management, operative procedure, and conduct of bypass were standardized. All operations were done with the same surgeon (B. P. B.), anesthesiologist (D. R.), and perfusionist. The extracorporeal circuit consisted of a bubble oxygenator either Dideco Hiflex D700 (Dideco S.P.A., Mirandola, Italy) or Optiflo II Model 42-221 (Cobe Laboratories, Inc., Lakewood, CO). A Dideco cardiotomy reservoir was used, and the circuit had polyvinyl chloride tubing except for the roller pump tubing, which was silicone rubber. The extracor-

From the Department of Cardiopulmonary Surgery, University Hospital, Groningen, The Netherlands, The Department of Cardiopulmonary Surgery and Anaesthetics, Hammersmith Hospital, London, England, and the Department of Internal Medicine, University Hospital, Giessen, West Germany.

Accepted for publication July 24, 1987.

Address reprint requests to Dr. Wildevuur, Department of Cardiopulmonary Surgery, Research Division, University Hospital, Oostersingel 59, 9713 EZ Groningen, The Netherlands.

poreal circuit was primed with 2,000 ml of Hartmann's solution and 25 mmol of $NaHCO_3$, and also contained $1 \cdot 10^6$ KIU (100 ml) of Trasylol in the treated group.

Bovine lung heparin (300 IU per kilogram of body weight) was given intravenously before cannulation of the aorta and right atrium. When the activated clotting time was shorter than 400 seconds, additional heparin (100 IU/kg) was given. Protamine sulfate (1 mg/100 IU of heparin) was administered within 5 minutes after the end of perfusion. The perfusion flow rate was 2.4 L/min/ m^2, and the patient's nasopharyngeal temperature was reduced to 27°C during bypass.

Cardioplegia was achieved after aortic cross-clamping with an ice-cold isotonic solution containing 3.253 gm of $MgCl_2$, 1.193 gm of KCl, and 272.8 mg of procaine hydrochloride per liter. One liter of cardioplegic fluid was used in each patient, and the solution was returned to the circulation.

Blood Samples

Blood samples (25 ml) were taken from the radial artery after induction of anesthesia, 5 minutes before CPB, and 30 minutes after protamine administration. Samples were taken from the venous inlet of the oxygenator 5 and 30 minutes after the start of CPB and at the end of CPB. In addition, blood was collected 5 minutes before and 5 minutes after release of the aortic cross-clamp.

Biochemical Analysis

HEMATOLOGICAL STUDIES. Two milliliters of blood was used for hematocrit and blood cell counts were done using a Coulter counter (model s 4+; Coulter Electronics, UK). Platelet and leukocyte numbers were corrected for hemodilution with reference to the pertinent hematocrit values during CPB. Total leukocyte number and polymorphonuclear cells (PMN) were counted manually.

APROTININ CONCENTRATIONS. Citrated blood (5 ml containing 0.3% sodium citrate) was taken for determination of the aprotinin levels in the treated group. This blood was centrifuged within two hours (15 minutes, 4°C, 1,500 g). The aprotinin concentration was determined according to the technique of Mueller-Esterl and co-workers [6].

FIBRIN(OGEN) DEGRADATION PRODUCTS. Citrated blood (2.5 ml) was sampled for determination of plasma levels of fibrin(ogen) degradation products with an enzyme immunoassay using monoclonal antibodies [7].

THROMBOXANE B_2. Indomethacin-EDTA blood (5 ml) was used for measuring the generation of thromboxane B_2 as a metabolite of thromboxane A_2 released by the activated platelets. Thromboxane B_2 was determined by a specific radioimmunoassay (Amersham, UK)

TISSUE-PLASMINOGEN ACTIVATOR ACTIVITY. Citrated blood (2.5 ml) was collected to determine plasminogen activator activity of euglobulins [8].

COMPLEMENT ACTIVATION. Three milliliters of blood was anticoagulated with EDTA and centrifuged, and the plasma was stored at −70°C until C3a and C4a assays were performed. Plasma levels of C3a antigen and C4a antigen were determined by radioimmunoassay (The Upjohn Company, Kalamazoo, MI) according to the manufacturer's instructions.

ELASTASE. Citrated (0.1 mol/L) blood (3 ml) was taken for elastase assay to monitor the release of proteases by activated granulocytes [9].

Statistical Analysis

Statistical analysis was performed with the Wilcoxon two-sample or the Wilcoxon signed rank test. Results are expressed as the mean ± the standard error of the mean. A p value of less than 0.05 was considered significant.

Results

The mean age of the patients in the control group and the aprotinin-treated group was 57.5 ± 5.1 years and 56.2 ± 3.9 years, respectively. The CPB procedure lasted for 66.4 ± 3.5 minutes in the controls and 65.0 ± 3.0 minutes in the aprotinin-treated group, and the duration of aortic cross-clamping was 42.6 ± 3.0 and 39.4 ± 1.3 minutes, respectively. Differences were not statistically significant.

Aprotinin Concentrations

Before the onset of CPB, aprotinin levels in plasma were 185 ± 19 KIU/ml. At the onset of CPB, hemodilution by the circuit-priming solutions reduced the levels to 150 ± 20 KIU/ml. During complete bypass with the heart and lungs out of circulation, the levels remained around 150 KIU/ml. With the release of the aortic cross-clamp and the return of cardiac ejection, the heart and lungs were reperfused and the aprotinin level fell to 80 KIU/ml.

Fibrin(ogen) Degradation Products

A small but significant ($p < 0.05$) rise in fibrin(ogen) degradation products was observed in the control group 30 minutes after the onset of perfusion. Another rise followed immediately after the beginning of the rewarming phase, a time at which the kinetics of biochemical reactions increases after hypothermic perfusion. No increase in fibrin(ogen) degradation products was detected in plasma from aprotinin-treated patients throughout CPB (Fig 1). After the discontinuation of CPB, fibrin(ogen) degradation products were detected in 5 of the treated patients. These 5 patients also received 1 unit of donor blood after bypass.

Platelets

In the untreated patients, platelet numbers decreased significantly ($p < 0.05$) in the rewarming phase (Fig 2). In contrast, the aprotinin-treated patients maintained platelet numbers at a remarkably constant level throughout CPB. After the termination of CPB, a dramatic fall in platelet numbers occurred in both groups of patients (p

642 The Annals of Thoracic Surgery Vol 44 No 6 December 1987

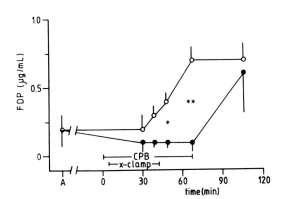

Fig 1. Fibrin(ogen) degradation products (FDP) were not generated in the aprotinin-treated patients (●) during cardiopulmonary bypass (CPB). In the rewarming period, these products increased significantly in untreated patients (○). Thereafter significant differences between both groups were observed. (* = p < 0.05, ** = p < 0.01.)

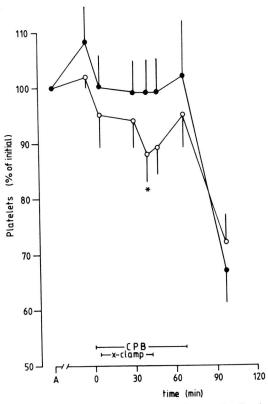

Fig 2. Platelet numbers fell in both groups at the onset of cardiopulmonary bypass (CPB). Thereafter, the numbers remained stable in aprotinin-treated patients (●) until the administration of protamine sulfate. During rewarming, platelet numbers decreased significantly in the untreated patients (○). (* = p < 0.05.)

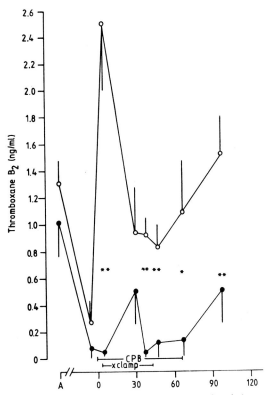

Fig 3. Thromboxane B_2 concentration increased significantly (p < 0.01) in the control group (○) after 5 minutes of cardiopulmonary bypass (CPB) and remained elevated as compared with prebypass values. In the aprotinin-treated group (●), thromboxane B_2 release was virtually inhibited. (** = p < 0.01; * = p < 0.05.)

< 0.01). This corresponded to the administration of protamine.

Thromboxane B_2

Five minutes after the onset of bypass, a tenfold increase in thromboxane B_2 levels was found in the untreated patients (Fig 3). Thromboxane concentrations remained high during CPB and increased again after protamine administration. In aprotinin-treated patients, thromboxane generation during bypass was significantly lower than that in untreated patients. The thromboxane B_2 concentrations in samples from both groups obtained just after the induction of anesthesia were high. These samples were taken before heparinization. After heparinization but prior to CPB, thromboxane levels were found to be in the normal range.

Postoperative Bleeding

The measured blood loss and the transfusion requirement were significantly lower in the aprotinin-treated patients compared with the untreated patients (p < 0.01 and p < 0.05, respectively) (Fig 4). In addition, a difference in hemostasis was noted by the surgeon during

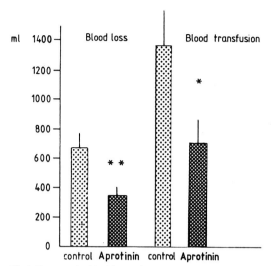

Fig 4. *Postoperative blood loss and requirement for blood transfusion were significantly decreased in the aprotinin-treated patients, compared with the controls. (** = p < 0.01; * = p < 0.02.)*

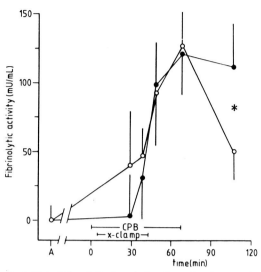

Fig 5. *Fibrinolytic activity dependent on tissue-plasminogen activator (t-PA) activity of euglobulins in untreated (○) and aprotinin-treated patients (●). In the treated group, t-PA activity increased later during cardiopulmonary bypass (CPB) but developed similar values compared with the untreated group. After bypass, highest t-PA activity was measured in the plasma of aprotinin-treated patients. (* = p < 0.05.)*

operation. In particular, the sternum side was unusually "bone-dry" in the aprotinin-treated patients.

Tissue-Plasminogen Activator Activity

Tissue-plasminogen activator (t-PA) activity increased during the rewarming phase of CPB in both groups and developed peak values after 60 minutes of CPB (Fig 5). Following protamine administration, t-PA activity decreased significantly in the control group, but remained high in the aprotinin-treated patients.

Complement Activation

In both groups, plasma C4a anaphylatoxin levels (classic pathway activation) were raised to 500 ng/ml following induction of anesthesia. They fell before the onset of perfusion and remained low throughout CPB (mean, 200 ng/ml). Neutralization of heparin by protamine caused further generation of C4a to levels of approximately 600 ng/ml in all patients. Levels of C4a were higher in aprotinin-treated patients, though not significantly so.

Plasma C3a levels (mainly alternative pathway activation) were similar in both groups. During the first 30 minutes of bypass, C3a levels remained moderate (mean, 400 ng/ml), but thereafter increased to 1,000 ng/ml before and after release of the cross-clamp. At the end of bypass, C3a levels remained elevated following protamine infusion.

Polymorphonuclear Leukocytes

Initial PMN numbers did not differ significantly between the two groups (mean, 5.4 and range, 4.1 to 9.1 · 10⁹/L in the controls; mean, 5.7 and range 4.0 to 8.4 · 10⁹/L in the aprotinin-treated group). In both groups, the numbers of PMNs decreased equally at the onset of CPB (mean, 5.1 and range, 3.4 to 8.0 · 10⁹/L and mean, 5.6 and range,

3.7 to 8.3 · 10⁹/L in the controls and aprotinin-treated group, respectively) and remained low with release of the aortic cross-clamp and rewarming from hypothermia. Then an identical and progressive rise in PMNs in central venous blood of both groups occurred (mean, 10.0 and range, 4.5 to 16.9 · 10⁹/L and mean, 10.3 and range, 5.3 to 13.5 · 10⁹/L in the controls and aprotinin-treated group, respectively, at the end of bypass).

Plasma Elastase

Elastase-α₁–proteinase inhibitor complexes were significantly raised in the plasma of both groups after 30 minutes of bypass. A further significant increase in elastase levels occurred after release of the aortic cross-clamp and during rewarming in the control group (p < 0.01) but not in the aprotinin-treated group (Fig 6). Thereafter, elastase levels remained lower in the treated group.

Comment

The potential therapeutic benefits of protease inhibitors during CPB relate to their interaction with the proteolytic enzymes that are released during bypass. Aprotinin is a known inhibitor of plasmin and kallikrein, both of which are likely generated by CPB as part of the whole-body inflammatory reaction. The most potent activator of plasminogen, t-PA, is released during CPB procedures [10], as was documented in both groups of patients in our study. In addition, activated Factor B (Bb) of the complement system [11] and activated Hageman factor (Factor XIIa) [12] can cleave plasminogen. Both these plasminogen activators are generated in the fluid phase,

644   The Annals of Thoracic Surgery   Vol 44   No 6   December 1987

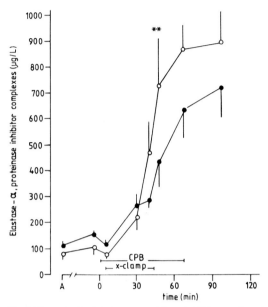

Fig 6. Plasma levels of elastase-α_1-proteinase inhibitor complexes increased similarly in both groups until 30 minutes of cardiopulmonary bypass (CPB). After release of the aortic cross-clamp and during rewarming, elastase levels increased significantly in the untreated patients (○). In the aprotinin-treated patients (●), no significant increase was observed at that time (p = 0.1). (** = p < 0.01.)

Bb by activation of the complement system and Factor XIIa through a positive feedback mechanism of the contact system with kallikrein.

The increase in fibrin(ogen) degradation products during CPB in the untreated patients proves that plasmin was generated. In the aprotinin-treated group, fibrin(ogen) degradation products were not generated, a finding that implies successful inhibition of plasmin throughout the procedure by the concentration of about 150 KIU/ml of plasma. The beneficial effect of aprotinin on platelets suggests that plasmin does play an important role in the impairment of platelets during CPB. This is indicated by the observation that, in the treated patients, platelet numbers remained constant during CPB and thromboxane B_2, mainly released by platelets [13], was inhibited. Furthermore, the hemostatic mechanism in these patients in terms of postbypass blood loss and blood requirements improved significantly compared with the controls.

We observed that oozing of blood from the sternum during operation was almost absent in the aprotinin-treated patients. This indicates that platelets were protected by aprotinin during bypass against pathological stimuli, but functioned normally on a physiological basis. A similar observation was made in vitro with the protease inhibitor leupeptin, which could prevent platelet aggregation elicited with thrombin and trypsin, but not with collagen [14].

Based on our findings, we postulate that the deleterious effects of proteases on platelets, as exerted by plasmin, might be explained by their action on platelet receptors. Two main platelet receptors are to be considered: the von Willebrand receptor for adhesion and the fibrinogen receptor for aggregation. The von Willebrand receptor (GPIb) can be removed by plasmin [15]. The importance of von Willebrand factor–platelet interaction during CPB was provided by Salzman and associates [16], who showed improved hemostasis after CPB by increasing the amount of endothelial von Willebrand factor, which probably compensates for the decreased number of platelet receptors [17].

The fibrinogen receptor (GPIIbIIIa) is exposed by a variety of platelet agonists such as adenosine diphosphate, thromboxane A_2, and proteolytic enzymes, all of which can be released during CPB [18]. Exposure of platelet receptors is accompanied by release of thromboxane A_2 [19]. After receptor exposure, fibrinogen molecules connect platelets by interacting with the receptor through the D-domains of each end of the fibrinogen molecule; this causes platelet aggregation. Plasmin may remove the bound fibrinogen from platelets, thus preventing aggregation [20] and resulting in ineffective postoperative platelet function. Evidence for loss of GPIb and GPIIbIIIa during CPB is given by George and colleagues [21].

Since aprotinin inhibited the release of thromboxane A_2, most likely the exposure of platelet receptors was effectively prevented in the treated patients. This suggests that the impaired postoperative hemostasis in the untreated patients has to be attributed to impaired platelet adhesion and platelet aggregation, whereas aprotinin appeared to have a protective effect on these specific platelet receptors. Though aprotinin inhibited fibrin(ogen)olysis during CPB, it is not likely that it did so postoperatively [22]. In the aprotinin group, t-PA levels were significantly higher than levels in the nontreated group, thereby indicating potentially even higher fibrinolytic activity, while aprotinin levels were lower than effective plasmin inhibitory concentrations at that time. Therefore, it is not likely that the improved postoperative hemostasis was due to decreased fibrinolytic activity.

Aprotinin seems not to have an important effect on complement activation during CPB, since C3a and C4a levels were similar in the treated and untreated group. Consequently, leukopenia caused by complement-dependent PMN aggregation and adhesion [23] was similar in both groups. Nevertheless, PMN elastase release was higher in the untreated group. This might be explained by the higher thromboxane generation in this group, since arachidonic acid metabolites can stimulate elastase release [24]. This inhibition of elastase release by aprotinin may be important to reduce pulmonary dysfunction after CPB, since elastase might affect the endothelial cells of the alveolar capillaries [25].

We conclude that aprotinin infusion has important

platelet-preserving effects during CPB, thus leading to a better hemostatic mechanism and consequently reducing postoperative blood loss and blood requirement. This finding implies that the inflammatory reaction during CPB has an important impact on the hemostatic mechanism. The postulated hypothesis is consistent with the findings in this study, but should be verified in a prospective study including determinations of the platelet receptors. Since the inflammatory reaction during CPB seems to have multiple effects, studies should be designed to identify its role in various clinical symptoms, such as pulmonary dysfunction, which is known to contribute to morbidity after CPB. In this study, all patients were otherwise fit adults with ischemic heart disease, and no pulmonary dysfunction was experienced. However, in a population of patients including those having reoperation, the very young, the elderly, and the very sick, or in case of a long perfusion time, aprotinin infusion might markedly reduce morbidity.

This study was supported by Grant 84040 from the Dutch Heart Foundation and by Bayer AG, Wuppertal, West Germany.

Thanks are due to Dr. E. J. P. Brommer, Mrs. M. M. Barrett-Bergshoeff, and Mrs. E. Hoegee-de Nobel of the Gaubius Institute TNO, Leiden, for assay of fibrinolytic activity and fibrinogen degradation products.

We are indebted to Dr. W. Mueller-Esterl for determination of the aprotinin plasma levels. Prof. H. Fritz and Dr. F. Schumann made an important contribution in reviewing and correcting the manuscript. Charles G. B. Wildevuur, Jr, is gratefully acknowledged for collecting and processing blood samples and data.

References

1. Kirklin JK, Westaby S, Blackstone EH, et al: Complement and the damaging effects of cardiopulmonary bypass. J Thorac Cardiovasc Surg 86:845, 1983
2. Fishelson Z, Pangburn MK, Muller-Eberhard HJ: Characterization of the initial C3 convertase of the alternative pathway of human complement. J Immunol 132:1430, 1984
3. Boonstra PW, Vermeulen FEE, Leusink JA, et al: Hematological advantage of a membrane oxygenator over a bubble oxygenator in long perfusions. Ann Thorac Surg 41:297, 1986
4. Boonstra PW, van Imhoff GW, Eysman L, et al: Reduced platelet activation and improved hemostasis after controlled cardiotomy suction during clinical membrane oxygenator perfusions. J Thorac Cardiovasc Surg 89:900, 1985
5. Fritz H, Wunderer G: Biochemistry and applications of aprotonin, the kallikrein inhibitor from bovine organs. Arzneimittelforsch 33:479, 1983
6. Mueller-Esterl W, Oettl A, Truceit E, Fritz H: Monitoring of aprotinin plasma levels by an enzyme-linked immunosorbent assay (ELISA). Fresenius Z Anal Chem 317:718, 1984
7. Koppert PW, Huysmans CMG, Nieuwenhuizen W: A monoclonal antibody, specific for human fibrinogen, fibrinopeptide-A containing fragments and not reacting with free fibrinopeptide A. Blood 66:503, 1985
8. Verheyen JH, Mullaart E, Chang GTG, et al: A simple, sensitive spectrophotometric assay for intrinsic (tissue-type) plasminogen activator applicable to measurements in plasma. Thromb Haemost 48:266, 1982
9. Neumann S, Jochum M: Elastase-α1-proteinase inhibitor complex. In Bergmeyer HU et al (eds): Methods of Enzymatic Analysis, ed 2. Weinheim, Verlag Chemie, 1984, vol 5, pp 184–195
10. Stibbe J, Kluft C, Brommer EJP, et al: Enhanced fibrinolytic activity during cardiopulmonary bypass in open-heart surgery in man is caused by extrinsic (tissue-type) plasminogen activator. Eur J Clin Invest 14:375, 1984
11. Sundsmo JS, Wood LM: Activated factor B (Bb) of the alternative pathway of complement activation cleaves and activates plasminogen. J Immunol 127:877, 1981
12. Goldsmith GH, Saito H, Ratnoff OD: The activation of plasminogen by Hageman factor (Factor XII) and Hageman factor fragments. J Clin Invest 62:54, 1978
13. Faymonville ME, Deby-Dupont G, Larbuisson R, et al: Prostaglandin E$_2$, prostacyclin and thromboxane changes during nonpulsatile cardiopulmonary bypass in humans. J Thorac Cardiovasc Surg 91:858, 1986
14. Ruggiero M, Lapetina EG: Protease and cyclooxygenase inhibitors synergistically prevent activation of human platelets. Proc Natl Acad Sci USA 83:3456, 1986
15. Adelman B, Michelson AD, Loscalzo J, et al: Plasmin effect on platelet glycoprotein Ib–von Willebrand's factor interaction. Blood 65:32, 1985
16. Salzman EW, Weinstein MJ, Weintraub RM, et al: Treatment with desmopressin acetate to reduce blood loss after cardiac surgery. N Engl J Med 314:1402, 1986
17. LaDuca FM, Bettigole RE, Bell WR, Robson EB: Platelet-collagen interaction: inhibition by ristocetin and enhancement by von Willebrand factor-platelet binding. Blood 68:927, 1986
18. Peerschke EIB: The platelet fibrinogen receptor. Semin Hematol 22:241, 1985
19. Bennett JS, Vilaire G, Burch JW: A role for prostaglandins and thromboxanes in the exposure of platelet fibrinogen receptors. J Clin Invest 68:981, 1981
20. Peerschke EIB, Wainer JA: Examination of irreversible platelet-fibrinogen interactions. Cell Physiol 17:C466, 1985
21. George JN, Pickett EB, Saucerman S, et al: Platelet surface glycoproteins: studies on resting and activated platelets and platelet membrane microparticles in normal subjects, and observations in patients with adult respiratory distress syndrome and cardiac surgery. J Clin Invest 78:340, 1986
22. Popov-Cenic S, Urban AE, Noë G: Studies on the cause of bleeding during and after surgery with a heart-lung machine in children with cyanotic and acyanotic congenital cardiac defects and their prophylactic treatment. In McCorn R (ed): Role of Chemical Mediators in the Pathophysiology of Acute Illness and Injury. New York, Raven, 1982, pp 229–242
23. Gerard C, Chenoweth DE, Hugli TE: Response of neutrophils to C5a: a role for the oligosaccharide moiety of human C5a desarg-74 but not of C5a in biologic activity. J Immunol 127:1978, 1982
24. Naccache PH, Showell HJ, Becker EL, Sha'afi RI: Arachidonic acid–induced degranulation of rabbit peritoneal neutrophils. Biochem Biophys Res Commun 87:292, 1979
25. Smedly LA, Tonnesen MG, Sandhaus RA, et al: Neutrophil-mediated injury to endothelial cells. J Clin Invest 77:1233, 1986

SURGICAL LIGATION OF A PATENT DUCTUS ARTERIOSUS

REPORT OF FIRST SUCCESSFUL CASE

ROBERT E. GROSS, M.D.

AND

JOHN P. HUBBARD, M.D.

BOSTON

The continued patency of a ductus arteriosus for more than the first few years of life has long been known to be a potential source of danger to a patient for two reasons: First, the additional work of the left ventricle in maintaining the peripheral blood pressure in the presence of a large arteriovenous communication may lead eventually to cardiac decompensation of severe degree. Second, the presence of a patent ductus arteriosus makes the possessor peculiarly subject to fatal bacterial endarteritis. While it is true that some persons have been known to live to old age with a patent ductus of Botalli, statistics have shown that the majority die relatively young because of complications arising from this congenital abnormality. Dr. Maude Abbott [1] presented a series of ninety-two cases which came to autopsy in which it was shown that the patient had had a patent ductus arteriosus without any other cardiovascular abnormality. Of these patients, approximately one fourth died of bacterial endarteritis of the pulmonary artery and an additional one half died of slow or rapid cardiac decompensation. The average age of death of patients in this series was 24 years.

The complications arising from the persistence of a patent ductus arteriosus would seem to make surgical ligation of this anomalous vessel a rational procedure, if such a procedure could be completed with promise of a low operative mortality. Dramatic results have previously been obtained in persons with cardiac enlargement and decompensation resulting from a peripheral arteriovenous aneurysm when the short-circuiting vessels have been ligated or excised. [2] On similar theoretical grounds, future cardiac embarrassment should be averted if a shunt between the aorta and the pulmonary artery could be removed. It would also seem plausible to expect that the shutting off of the anomalous stream of blood pouring into the pulmonary artery would lessen the formation of the thickened endothelial plaques within the pulmonary artery, which are so likely to be the seat of later bacterial infection. The surgical approach to the aortic arch and pulmonary conus having been studied previously in animal experimentation, [3] it seemed within reason that a patent ductus could be adequately exposed in man and possibly ligated without undue danger. It was therefore decided to undertake the operation in a child who presented the classic signs of a patent ductus arteriosus. At the age of 7 years she already had cardiac hypertrophy, which developed presumably from the embarrassment resulting from the anomalous communication. It was to be expected, therefore, that she would have increasingly severe disability in the future, aside from the danger of having bacterial endarteritis develop.

From the Surgical and Medical Services of the Children's Hospital and the Departments of Surgery and Pediatrics of the Harvard Medical School.

1. Abbott, Maude E.: Atlas of Congenital Heart Disease, New York, American Heart Association, 1936, pp. 60-61.

2. Holman, Emile: Arteriovenous Aneurysm, New York, Macmillan Company, 1937, pp. 169-178.

3. Gross, R. E.: A Surgical Approach for Ligation of a Patent Ductus Arteriosus, New England J. Med., to be published.

REPORT OF CASE

History.—L. S., a girl aged 7½ years, entered the hospital Aug. 17, 1938, for study of her cardiac condition. The family history was irrelevant. She was born normally at full term. No cyanosis was noted at birth or during the postnatal period. The records of the hospital where she was born give no information about an examination of the heart at that time. At the age of 3 years she was seen in the cardiac clinic of another hospital, where it was found that she had physical signs suggesting congenital malformation of the heart. At that time she had a precordial thrill and a loud murmur. The carotid pulsations were abnormally marked, and pistol shot sounds could be heard over the brachial and femoral arteries. The blood pressure was recorded in both arms as 104 mm. of mercury systolic and 0 diastolic. There was definite cardiac enlargement, as shown by teleoroentgenograms. The diagnosis made at that time was "congenital malformation of the heart with a patent ductus arteriosus."

During the next four years she was seen in several different hospitals, where the same diagnosis was made. At no time

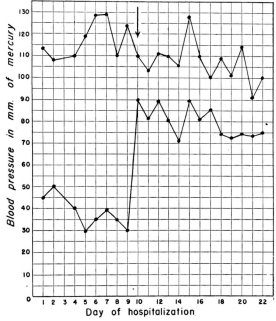

Daily blood pressure readings of the patient with a patent ductus arteriosus before and after operation. Prior to operation the large ductus opening from the aorta produced a low diastolic pressure. Following operative closure of the ductus, the diastolic pressure rose to twice its former level. The average daily diastolic pressure preoperatively was 38 mm. of mercury. The average diastolic pressure postoperatively was 80 mm. of mercury. The arrow points to the time of operation.

had cyanosis been observed. Dyspnea developed after moderate exercise, and her physical activities had been limited accordingly. She had never had peripheral edema or other evidence of cardiac decompensation. Frequently the child had been conscious of "something wrong in the chest" and her mother spontaneously offered the information that she had heard a "buzzing noise" in her daughter's chest when standing nearby.

Physical Examination.—At the time of admission, the patient was slender and undernourished. The pulsations of the carotid arteries were abnormally forceful. The radial pulse was of the Corrigan type, and a capillary pulsation was readily seen. The veins over the chest were somewhat prominent. There was a precordial bulge. The heart was definitely enlarged by percussion, the enlargement being for the most part to the left. Over the entire precordium there was a prominent coarse thrill which was most intense in the third interspace to the left of the sternum. This thrill was continuous but was accentuated during systole. There was a rough "machinery" murmur heard with maximal intensity over the pulmonic area to the left of the sternum in the second and particularly in the

third interspace. It was continuous throughout the cardiac cycle but like the thrill was greatly accentuated during systole. It was transmitted to the left along the third interspace and into the axilla with only slightly diminished intensity. The systolic element was heard faintly over the vessels of the neck and could be heard clearly in the right axilla and over the mid-thoracic region posteriorly. Blood pressure readings were respectively right arm 115/40, left arm 110/50, right leg 150/55, left leg 140/40 mm. of mercury. There was no clubbing of the fingers and no evidence of peripheral edema. The liver edge was palpable at the costal margin. The examination in other respects was negative.

Laboratory Data.—A 7-foot x-ray film of the chest showed the transverse diameter of the heart to be 11.7 cm., compared to an internal diameter of the chest of 20 cm. There appeared to be definite enlargement of the left ventricle. There was questionable prominence of the pulmonary artery. A mottled increased density around the lung hili was interpreted as representing circulatory congestion. Fluoroscopic examination showed a "hilar dance." An electrocardiogram was normal, showing no deviation of the axis. The red blood count was 5,080,000 cells per cubic millimeter and the hemoglobin was 85 per cent (Sahli). Circulation time with dehydrocholic acid was 10 and 8 seconds, respectively, on two tests.

Operation.—August 26, operation was undertaken (by R. E. G.) under cyclopropane anesthesia. The approach to the mediastinum was made through the left pleural cavity anterolaterally. Incision was made through the left third interspace, cutting the third costal cartilage, and the third rib was retracted upward. As the left lung was allowed to collapse inferiorly, an excellent view was gained of the lateral aspect of the mediastinum. The parietal pleura covering the aortic arch and left pulmonic artery was then incised and these structures were directly exposed. A large patent ductus arteriosus was found, which was from 7 to 8 mm. in diameter and from 5 to 6 mm. in length. A palpating finger placed on the heart disclosed a continuous and very vibrant thrill over the entire organ, which was increasingly prominent as the finger reached up over the pulmonic artery. A sterile stethoscope was employed and an extremely loud continuous murmur was heard over the entire heart. When the stethoscope was placed on the pulmonary artery there was an almost deafening, continuous roar, sounding much like a large volume of steam escaping in a closed room.

A number 8 braided silk tie was placed around the ductus with an aneurysm needle, and the vessel was temporarily occluded for a three minute observation period. During this time the blood pressure rose from 110/35 to 125/90. Since there was no embarrassment of the circulation, it was decided to ligate the ductus permanently. The ductus was too short to tie double and divide, so that ligation alone was resorted to. When the thread was drawn up tight the thrill completely disappeared. The chest was closed, the lung being reexpanded with positive pressure anesthesia just prior to placing the last stitch in the intercostal muscles.

Postoperative Course.—The child underwent the operative procedure exceedingly well and showed no signs of shock. Prior to operation blood had been taken from a donor in order to have it ready whenever needed, but the patient's condition was so good that it was not given. There was only mild discomfort on the afternoon of the day of operation, and on the following morning the child was allowed to sit up in a chair. By the third day she was walking about the ward. When the skin sutures were removed on the seventh day the wound was well healed, but because of the interest in the case the child was detained in the hospital until the thirteenth day. After the dressing was removed and the chest could be examined adequately the thrill had completely disappeared, there was a faint systolic murmur in the left third interspace which was not transmitted over the precordium, and no murmur could be heard in the axilla, in the neck or over the back. The daily blood pressures which had been taken prior to operation and subsequent thereto showed a striking change in the diastolic levels, as is shown by the accompanying chart. The average of the daily pressures prior to operation had been 114 systolic and 38 diastolic as contrasted with a postoperative daily average of 108 systolic and 80 diastolic.

VOLUME 112
NUMBER 8

RABIES—HART AND EVANS

SUMMARY

A girl aged 7½ years had a known patency of the ductus arteriosus and beginning cardiac hypertrophy. In the hope of preventing subsequent bacterial endarteritis and with the immediate purpose of reducing the work of the heart caused by the shunt between the aorta and the pulmonary artery, the patent ductus was surgically explored and ligated. The child stood the operative procedure exceedingly well. The most objective finding, which indicated that the serious loss of blood from the aorta into the pulmonic artery had been arrested by operation, was a comparison of the preoperative and postoperative levels of the diastolic blood pressure. Prior to operation the daily blood pressure showed an average diastolic level of 38 mm. of mercury as compared with a postoperative diastolic level of 80 mm. of mercury. This is the first patient in whom a patent ductus arteriosus has been successfully ligated.

THE SURGICAL TREATMENT OF MAL- FORMATIONS OF THE HEART

IN WHICH THERE IS PULMONARY STENOSIS OR PULMONARY ATRESIA

ALFRED BLALOCK, M.D.

AND

HELEN B. TAUSSIG, M.D.

BALTIMORE

Heretofore there has been no satisfactory treatment for pulmonary stenosis and pulmonary atresia. A "blue" baby with a malformed heart was considered beyond the reach of surgical aid. During the past three months we have operated on 3 children with severe degrees of pulmonary stenosis and each of the patients appears to be greatly benefited. In the second and third cases, in which there was deep persistent cyanosis, the cyanosis has greatly diminished or has disappeared and the general condition of the patients is proportionally improved. The results are sufficiently encouraging to warrant an early report.

The operation here reported and the studies leading thereto were undertaken with the conviction that even though the structure of the heart was grossly abnormal, in many instances it might be possible to alter the course of the circulation in such a manner as to lessen the cyanosis and the resultant disability. It is important to emphasize the fact that it is not the cyanosis, per se, which does harm. Nevertheless, since cyanosis is a striking manifestation of the underlying anoxemia and the compensatory polycythemia, a brief discussion of the causes of cyanosis and the factors operative in congenital malformations of the heart is essential in order to understand the principles underlying the present operation.

Cyanosis is due to the presence of reduced hemoglobin in the circulating blood. It is a well established fact that there must be at least 5 Gm. of reduced hemoglobin per hundred cubic centimeters of circulating blood for cyanosis to become apparent. It has long been recognized that one of the principal factors in the production of cyanosis in malformations of the heart is the direct shunting of venous blood into the systemic circulation. Lundsgaard and Van Slyke[1] in their classic studies on the causes of cyanosis showed that there were four important factors in the production of cyanosis: the height of the hemoglobin, the volume of the venous blood shunted into the systemic circulation, the rate of utilization of oxygen by the peripheral tissues and the extent of the aeration of the blood in the lungs. Their studies demonstrated the great importance of pulmonary factors. The extent of the oxygenation of the blood in the lungs clearly depends on the vital capacity of the individual, the rate of the flow of blood through the lungs, the partial pressure of the oxygen in the inspired air and also on specific pulmonary factors, which these authors designated as the a factor. These investigators showed that in most, if not in all, cases in which there was a pronounced polycythemia, secondary changes occurred in the lungs of such a nature that all of the blood that passed through the lungs was no longer in effective contact with the oxygen in the

alveoli. The importance of this factor can be demonstrated by the prolonged inhalation of oxygen. In almost every case in which there is polycythemia, cyanosis can be greatly lessened by the prolonged inhalation of oxygen. The fact that all of the blood which circulated through the lungs is not fully oxygenated made it seem improbable that if more blood circulated through the lungs a larger proportion of the blood would be oxygenated. Thus the demonstration of the a factor completely overshadowed another vitally important factor, namely the volume of blood which reaches the lungs for aeration.[1a]

Expressed in the simplest terms, the circulation of the blood through the lungs after birth is essential for life; any one deprived of such circulation dies. Indeed there is a point at which, even though none of the other pulmonary factors are operative in the production of cyanosis and all of the blood that passes through the lungs is fully oxygenated, the volume of blood that reaches the lungs for aeration and hence the volume of oxygenated blood returned to the systemic circulation is insufficient for the maintenance of life. For example, in all cases of pulmonary atresia in which the circulation to the lungs is by way of the ductus arteriosus the closure of the ductus arteriosus renders the condition incompatible with life.

Undoubtedly the importance of the diminution of flow of blood to the lungs has not been fully appreciated, mainly because studies on the nature of cyanosis have been made on older children and young adults, and it is only when this factor is not of vital importance that the individual has survived to that age. All infants with pulmonary atresia with or without a right ventricle and with or without dextroposition of the aorta, in whom the closure of the ductus arteriosus cuts off the circulation to the lungs, die at an early age. In cases of complete pulmonary atresia death occurs before the complete cessation of circulation of blood through the lungs; hence in such cases there is always slight patency of the ductus arteriosus. In cases of a tetralogy of Fallot with an extreme pulmonary stenosis, the ductus arteriosus may become entirely obliterated before death.

There are two different types of congenital malformations which illustrate the importance of the volume of the pulmonary circulation in the production of cyanosis. The first is that of a single ventricle with a rudimentary outlet chamber in which it is common to find that one great vessel is given off from the common ventricle and one from the rudimentary outlet chamber. Usually the vessel which arises from the common ventricle is of normal size and that from the rudimentary outlet chamber is diminutive in size.[2] If the great vessels occupy their normal positions, the aorta arises from the common ventricle and is of large caliber, whereas the pulmonary artery which arises from the rudimentary outlet chamber is of small caliber. Under such circumstances a large volume of blood goes to the systemic circulation and only a small volume of blood goes to the lungs. Consequently a large volume of unoxygenated blood is mixed with a small volume of oxygenated blood and cyanosis is intense.[3] When, however, the great vessels are transposed and the pulmonary artery is large and the aorta is small, a large volume of blood goes to the lungs for aeration. Under these circumstances a large

Read before the Johns Hopkins Medical Society March 12, 1945.
Aided by a grant from the Robert Garrett Memorial Fund for the Surgical Treatment of Children.
From the Departments of Surgery and Pediatrics of the Johns Hopkins University and the Johns Hopkins Hospital and the Cardiac Clinic of the Harriet Lane Home.

1. Lundsgaard, C., and Van Slyke, D. D.: Cyanosis, Medical Monographs, vol. 2, Baltimore, Williams and Wilkins Company, 1923.

1a. The relative importance of this factor and of the a factor will be discussed in a forthcoming paper by Taussig and Blalock.
2. Taussig, H. B.: Clinical Analysis of Congenital Malformations of the Heart, to be published by the Commonwealth Fund, New York.
3. Taussig, H. B.: A Single Ventricle with a Diminutive Outlet Chamber, J. Tech. Meth. & Bull. I. A. M. M. **19**: 120-127, 1939.

volume of oxygenated blood is mixed with a relatively small volume of venous blood and cyanosis is minimal or absent, as in the case reported by Glendy and White.[4]

The same phenomenon is also seen in cases of truncus arteriosus. When the pulmonary arteries are given off directly from the aorta there is adequate circulation to the lungs, and cyanosis is minimal or absent. In contrast to this, if the pulmonary artery fails to arise from the heart or connect with the aorta and the circulation to the lungs is by way of the bronchial arteries only a small volume of blood reaches the lungs for aeration, and cyanosis is intense.[5]

The importance of adequate circulation to the lungs is further illustrated in the anomalies of the venous return in which all of the pulmonary veins drain into the right auricle; consequently within this chamber there is complete admixture of venous and arterial blood. In such cases a large volume of blood goes to the lungs for aeration and a large volume of oxygenated blood is

Sup Vena Cava
Phrenic Nerve
Azygus V.
Bulldog clamp on Innominate A.
R Common Carotid A.
R Subclavian A.
AORTA
Posterior sutures in anastomosis
Bulldog clamps on R. Pulmonary. A.
INCISION in third intercostal space

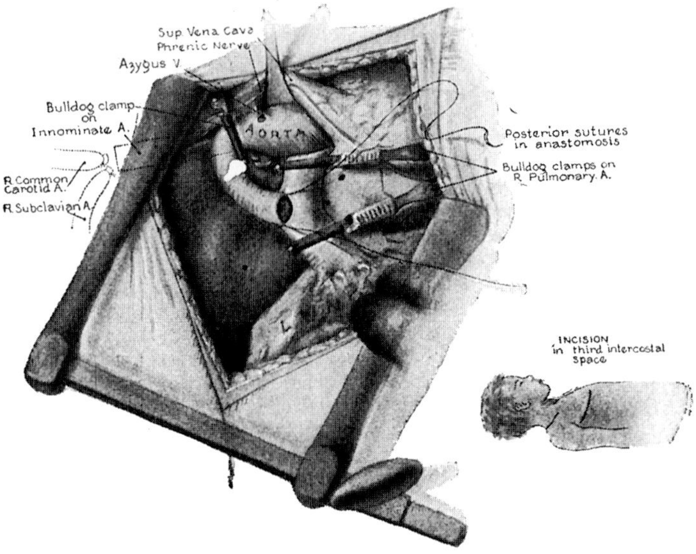

Fig. 1.—General exposure of the operative field on the right side. The end of the innominate artery is being anastomosed to the side of the right pulmonary artery. The posterior row of sutures is complete. The anterior row has not been inserted.

returned to the right auricle. There is great right-sided cardiac enlargement but no cyanosis until the terminal collapse of the circulation.[6]

These observations clearly indicate that many gross malformations of the heart are compatible with life provided there is adequate circulation to the lungs, and furthermore that lack of circulation to the lungs is the primary cause of death in many infants with congenital malformations of the heart. Furthermore, one of us (H. B. T.) has seen several infants with pulmonary stenosis in whom cyanosis was not apparent until the ductus arteriosus closed. In other words, there was no "visible" cyanosis while the circulation to the lungs was adequate. It was an appreciation of these facts (H. B. T.), together with an extensive previous experience with the experimental use of large arteries for the purpose of conducting blood to sites not usually

supplied by such vessels, that led to the development of the clinical work recorded in this paper.

The feasibility of anastomosing a systemic artery to one of the pulmonary arteries in experimental animals has been demonstrated by Levy and Blalock.[7] As far as we are aware, this was the first time that both the course and the function of a large artery were altered. Similar experimental alterations were produced subsequently by Eppinger, Burwell and Gross[8] and by Leeds.[9] Blalock and Park[10] have reported the suturing of the severed proximal end of the subclavian artery to the aorta as a means for conducting blood beyond the point of an experimental coarctation of the aorta. In unreported observations by Kieffer and Blalock the divided proximal end of the splenic artery has been connected to the distal end of the divided left renal artery and there has been no evidence of renal failure even though the right kidney was removed. In other words, arterial anastomoses have been performed in animals for the purpose of conducting blood to sites other than those ordinarily supplied by these vessels.

Before undertaking the operations on patients, many experiments were performed in an effort to produce pulmonic stenosis in dogs. This work met with little success. Finally, in an effort to cause a significant decrease in the oxygen saturation of arterial blood, one or more lobes of the lungs were removed from each side of the chest, and the main arteries and veins of these lobes were connected end to end by suture. In other words, bilateral pulmonary arteriovenous fistulas were produced. These procedures resulted in some instances in a pronounced reduction in the oxygen saturation of the arterial blood. As the result of an artificial patent ductus arteriosus made in two such experiments, there was a significant increase in the arterial oxygen saturation. Although this experimentally produced condition is quite different from that seen in patients, it is of interest that the making of an anastomosis between systemic and pulmonary arteries caused an increase in the oxygen saturation of the arterial blood despite the fact that several lobes of the lungs had been removed.

Since the present operation was devised to compensate for an inadequate flow of blood to the lungs, it seemed desirable that the anastomosis be made in such a manner that the blood from the systemic artery would be able to reach both lungs. It is obvious that the suture anastomosis could not be made to the main pulmonary artery since occlusion of this vessel for more than a few minutes causes death. It appeared, therefore, that the anastomosis should be made just distal to the division of the main pulmonary artery and, furthermore, that the side of the chosen vessel should be used in order that the blood might flow to both lungs.

It was our original idea that the subclavian artery would be the ideal systemic vessel and that after division

4. Glendy, Margaret M.; Glendy, R. E., and White, P. D.: Cor Biatriatum Triloculare, Am. Heart J. **28**: 395-401, 1944.
5. Taussig, H. B.: Clinical Findings in Cases of Truncus Arteriosus, to be published.
6. Taussig, H. B.: Clinical and Pathological Findings in the Anomaly of Venous Return in Which All of the Pulmonary Veins Drain into the Right Auricle, to be published.

7. Levy, S. E., and Blalock, A.: Experimental Observations on the Effects of Connecting by Suture the Left Main Pulmonary Artery to the Systemic Circulation, J. Thoracic Surg. **8**: 525-530, 1939.
8. Eppinger, Eugene C.; Burwell, C. Sidney, and Gross, Robert E.: The Effects of the Patent Ductus Arteriosus on the Circulation, J. Clin. Investigation **20**: 127-143 (March) 1941.
9. Leeds, S. E.: The Effects of Occlusion of Experimental Chronic Patent Ductus Arteriosus on the Cardiac Output, Pulse and Blood Pressure of Dogs, Am. J. Physiol. **139**: 451-459 (July) 1943.
10. Blalock, A., and Park, E. A.: The Surgical Treatment of Experimental Coarctation (Atresia) of the Aorta, Ann. Surg. **119**: 445-456 (March) 1944.

of this artery its proximal end should be anastomosed to the side of the left pulmonary artery. The fortunate experience to be reported in regard to the second patient has led us to prefer the use of the innominate artery in patients with a severe degree of anoxemia. This patient had a right aortic arch, and the innominate artery was directed to the left side of the chest and neck.

Although there were slight variations in each of the operations, the major features were as follows: Light general anesthesia was produced by the inhalation of ether or cyclopropane. The patient was placed on the table on his back with a slight elevation of that side of the chest which was to be exposed. The patient's arms were strapped in place along his sides. The operation was performed on the right or left side depending on the position of the great vessels and the artery to be used in the anastomosis. The incision was made in the third interspace and extended from the lateral border of the sternum to the axillary line. The pleural cavity was entered and the third and fourth costal cartilages were divided. A rib spreader was introduced and a good exposure of the upper half of the pleural cavity was obtained. This area is shown in figure 1. The right or left pulmonary artery was then exposed and the vessel was dissected from the adjacent tissues for as great a distance as possible. This was more difficult on the right side than on the left and it was necessary to ligate and divide the azygos vein and to retract the superior vena cava medially. Nothing further was done to the pulmonary artery at this time. Attention was then focused on the systemic artery which was to be anastomosed to one of the pulmonary arteries. The subclavian or innominate artery was dissected free of the adjacent tissues and the vessel chosen was occluded temporarily at the point where it arose from the aorta by the use of a bulldog arterial clamp. In cases in which the innominate artery was chosen, its branches (subclavian and common carotid) were ligated at their origins and the innominate artery was cut across just proximal to the ligatures. In the 1 case in which the left subclavian artery was used for the anastomosis to the pulmonary circulation it was necessary to divide the thyrocervical trunk, the vertebral artery and the internal mammary artery in order to gain access to a sufficient length of the vessel. After the removal of some of the adventitia from the systemic vessel the pulmonary artery was further prepared for the anastomosis. A bulldog arterial clamp was placed on the left or right pulmonary artery just distal to the point of division of the main pulmonary artery. A second bulldog arterial clamp was placed on the left or right pulmonary artery just proximal to the point where the vessel gave off a branch to the upper lobe of the lung. A transverse opening was made into the side of the pulmonary artery approximately midway between these two arterial clamps. This opening was of about the same diameter as that of the end of the systemic vessel which was to be anastomosed to it. It must be emphasized that the pulmonary artery was

not occluded until all preparations for the anastomotic procedure had been made.

The anastomosis between the end of the systemic artery and the side of the pulmonary artery was carried out in the following manner: Fine silk on a curved needle was used as suture material. Before placing the posterior row of sutures, a stay suture was placed at one end. This was followed by the insertion of a running suture, which was not drawn taut until the greater part of the posterior row had been placed. The stay suture was then tied and the running suture was in turn tied to the stay suture. The posterior row was completed and was tied to another stay suture. The anterior row consisted of a simple through and through

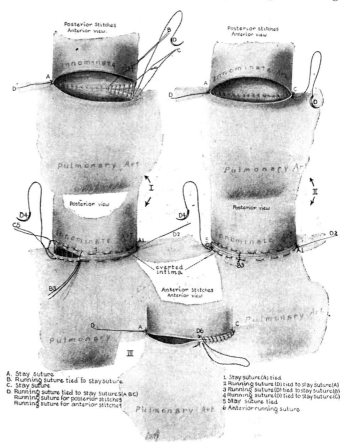

A. Stay suture.
B. Running suture tied to stay suture.
C. Stay suture.
D. Running suture tied to stay sutures (A B C)
   Running suture for posterior stitches
   Running suture for anterior stitches

1. Stay suture (A) tied
2. Running suture (D) tied to stay suture (A)
3. Running suture (D) tied to stay suture (B)
4. Running suture (D) tied to stay suture (C)
5. Stay suture tied
6. Anterior running suture

Fig. 2.—Details of the method by which the end of a systemic artery is anastomosed to the side of one of the pulmonary arteries.

continuous suture which approximated intima to intima. The anastomosis is shown diagrammatically in figure 2. The bulldog clamps were then removed from the pulmonary artery, and this was followed by removal of the clamp from the systemic vessel. If bleeding from the suture line did not cease spontaneously, it was stopped by the use of additional sutures. The lung was reexpanded and the incision in the chest wall was closed. Two encircling sutures of braided silk were used for approximating the third and fourth ribs. The soft tissues of the chest wall were closed in multiple layers with interrupted silk sutures.

There follows a detailed report of the 3 cases in which such an operation has been performed.

REPORT OF CASES

CASE 1.[11]—*History.*—E. M. S., a girl, was born prematurely in the obstetric service of the Johns Hopkins Hospital on Aug. 3, 1943. Her birth weight was 1,105 Gm. A systolic murmur was noted shortly after birth. Slight cyanosis was noted on the fourth and fifth days of life; this subsequently disappeared. The baby gained weight slowly and was finally discharged at 4 months of age weighing 2,900 Gm. After discharge the baby was followed in the dispensary. She was at first thought to have a simple interventricular septal defect, because the heart was normal in size and there was no cyanosis.

At 8 months of age the baby had her first attack of cyanosis, which occurred after eating. It was then for the first time that we thought she had a tetralogy of Fallot and not a simple interventricular septal defect. It soon became evident that cyanosis was increasing. It seemed probable that this increase in cyanosis was due to the fact that the ductus arteriosus was undergoing obliteration and thereby lessening the circulation to the lungs. By March 1944 it was obvious that the baby had a serious congenital malformation of the heart. After eating she would become deeply cyanotic, roll up her eyes, lose consciousness and appear extremely ill. Fluoroscopy showed that the heart was slightly enlarged; there was no fulness

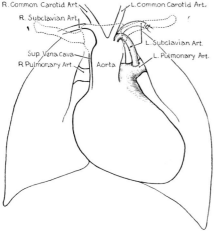

Fig. 3 (case 1).—Procedure used. The end of the left subclavian artery was anastomosed to the side of the left pulmonary artery.

in the region of the pulmonary conus. In the left anterior oblique position the right ventricle appeared slightly enlarged and the pulmonary window was abnormally clear. The clinical diagnosis was tetralogy of Fallot with a severe degree of pulmonary stenosis.

On June 25, 1944 she was first admitted to the Harriet Lane Home. Physical examination showed that she was poorly nourished and poorly developed. She had a glassy stare. Her lips were cyanotic. The heart was slightly enlarged and there was a harsh systolic murmur best heard along the left sternal border. The liver was at the costal margin. The baby was given oxygen and phenobarbital but remained very irritable and would become intensely cyanotic when taken out of the oxygen tent. During her three weeks' stay in the hospital she gained 200 Gm. and weighed 4.66 Kg. on discharge. She was sent home because it was felt that her condition was hopeless.

She was followed in the cardiac clinic for three months, during which time she showed increasing cyanosis and failed to gain weight. She was readmitted on October 17 because of increasing spells of cyanosis, coma and great venous distention of the head and body.

The weight on admission was 4.6 Kg. The venous distention was so great that the possibility of a subdural hydroma or hematoma was considered. Subdural tap was performed, with

11. This case was discussed briefly at the meeting of the Southern Surgical Association, Dec. 5, 1944, in a paper by Dr. Arthur Blakemore.

the removal of 8 cc. of clear fluid from the right side and a small amount of bloody fluid from the left.

The size of the heart as seen in the anteroposterior view was essentially the same as noted previously. There was still a harsh systolic murmur. In the left anterior oblique position the contour of the heart appeared as a little round ball with a narrow aorta and a clear pulmonary window (fig. 4); this, we believe, is characteristic of a very severe tetralogy of Fallot with a functional pulmonary atresia, that is, a pulmonary stenosis which is so extreme that the condition is not long compatible with life.[2] It was questioned at that time whether in addition to the malformation of the heart she suffered from mental retardation.

During the next six weeks she refused most of her feedings; she lost weight and just before operation weighed only 4 Kg. The red blood cell count, which had been 7,000,000 on admission, had fallen to 5,000,000. Cyanosis was proportionally less conspicuous; indeed, at times while lying quietly, cyanosis was not visible. The clinical diagnosis was again tetralogy of Fallot which was so severe that the baby's condition was becoming critical.

Operation.—This was performed on November 29. The procedure consisted in the anastomosis of the divided proximal end of the left subclavian artery to the side of the left pulmonary artery, as shown diagrammatically in figure 3. The anesthetic agent was administered by Dr. Merel Harmel.

Under ether and oxygen anesthesia, administered by the open method, an incision was made on the left side of the chest extending from the edge of the sternum to the axillary line. The pleural cavity was entered through the third interspace. The left lung appeared normal. No thrill was felt on palpating the heart and pulmonary artery. The left pulmonary artery was identified and was dissected free of the neighboring tissues. It appeared to be of normal size. The superior pulmonary vein, on the other hand, seemed considerably smaller than normal. The left subclavian artery was identified and was dissected free of the neighboring tissues. In order to secure access to a sufficient length of this vessel it was necessary to ligate and divide the vertebral artery, the internal mammary artery and the thyrocervical axis. A bulldog arterial clamp was placed on the subclavian artery at a point just distal to its origin from the aorta. The subclavian artery was ligated distal to the point at which the thyrocervical trunk had been ligated and divided, and the vessel was cut across just proximal to this ligature. Two bulldog clamps were placed on the left pulmonary artery, the first clamp being placed at the origin of the left pulmonary artery and the second clamp being placed just proximal to the point where the pulmonary artery entered the lung. There was ample space between these two clamps for our purpose. A small transverse incision was made in the wall of the pulmonary artery at a point approximately equidistant between the two clamps. By the use of china beaded silk on fine needles an anastomosis was performed between the end of the left subclavian artery and the side of the left pulmonary artery. There was practically no bleeding following the removal of the clamps.

From a technical point of view the anastomosis seemed to be satisfactory. The main cause for concern was the small size of the left subclavian artery. It was somewhat disturbing that one could not feel a thrill in the pulmonary artery. We were confident, however, that the anastomosis was patent. A small quantity of sulfanilamide was placed in the left pleural cavity and the incision in the chest wall was closed. The patient was given 200 cc. of isotonic solution of sodium chloride and 50 cc. of blood during the operative procedure. The operation required slightly less than an hour and a half and the left pulmonary artery was occluded for approximately thirty minutes. The patient's condition at the end of the operation seemed moderately good.

Postoperative Course.—This was stormy. The patient's left arm and hand were observed frequently. The radial pulse was not palpable and this extremity was cooler than the opposite one, but it was apparent that the circulation was adequate to maintain life of the part. The child suffered from repeated bilateral pneumothoraces, and frequent aspirations were required.

Probably the pneumothorax on the right was due to the use of too great pressure in the reexpansion of the left lung at the completion of the operative procedure. As it was found to be a positive pressure pneumothorax, constant suction was exerted through a needle inserted into the right pleural cavity. Had it not been for the excellent care given by the pediatric house staff, particularly Dr. Kaye, Dr. Whitemore, Dr. Steinheimer, Dr. Hammond, Dr. Gilger and Dr. Helfrick, in all probability the child's life would not have been saved.

The child's condition began to improve two weeks after operation. Thereafter further aspirations of the pleural cavity were not required. The occasions on which the patient would become cyanotic became less frequent. Otitis media developed and responded to treatment. The systolic murmur became somewhat louder, but a continuous murmur could not be heard in the pulmonary area.

The patient was discharged from the hospital on Jan. 25, 1945, almost two months after the day of operation. Her condition was considerably better than it had been before operation. More recent follow-up studies have shown that she is gaining weight and that she is only occasionally cyanotic. If the cyanosis increases, it may be necessary to perform a similar operation on the opposite side. Roentgenograms of the patient's heart both before and after operation are shown in figure 4.

It is unfortunate that we do not have a quantitative degree of improvement such as might have been afforded by determinations of the oxygen saturation of the arterial blood. In view of the small size of the child we did not feel warranted in doing arterial punctures. The clinical improvement, however, has been striking. The baby takes her feedings well, is alert and active and has gained a kilogram in weight (that is, 25 per cent of her former body weight).

CASE 2.—*History.*—B. R., a white girl born July 9, 1933, was first seen at the Harriet Lane Home at 9 years of age, referred by Dr. Dexter Levy of Buffalo. The patient was cyanotic at birth. The birth weight was 6½ pounds (2,955 Gm.). She was breast fed for six months. In infancy she gained extremely slowly. She had erysipelas at 1½ years of age, a septic sore throat at 4½ years of age, chickenpox at 7 years, measles at 8 years and mumps at 9 years.

The patient was first seen in the Harriet Lane Home on Feb. 13, 1943. She was intensely cyanotic, became dyspneic on slight exertion and would constantly squat to get her breath. There was intense cyanosis and clubbing of the fingers and the toes. The buccal mucous membranes were of a deep mulberry color. There was suffusion of the conjunctiva. The chest was barrel shaped. Her heart was within normal limits in size. There was no thrill over the precordium. On auscultation there was a harsh systolic murmur which was maximal low down in the third and fourth interspaces. The murmur was much louder in the recumbent position than in the erect position, and louder when she bent forward than when she tried to sit erect. The murmur was not widely transmitted and was not audible in the back. The second sound at the base was pure. The lungs were clear. The liver was at the costal margin and the spleen was not palpable. The femoral arteries were readily palpable. The extremities, as previously mentioned, showed intense cyanosis and pronounced clubbing. At this time she climbed half a flight of stairs and walked, almost ran, leaning forward, 60 feet to her room, and then fell forward on the bed and lay in a knee-chest position, panting heavily and without speaking for half an hour.

The red blood cell count was 8,700,000; the hemoglobin was 25 Gm.; the hematocrit reading was 78.

The electrocardiogram showed a normal sinus mechanism, PR interval of 0.16 second, normal upright T waves in all four leads, and considerable right axis deviation.

X-ray examination and fluoroscopy showed the heart to be of normal size with a concave curve at the base to the left

of the sternum (fig. 6). To the right of the sternum the superior vena cava cast a wide ribbon-like shadow. After the administration of barium, the aorta was seen to indent the esophagus to the left on its right margin. Examination in the left anterior oblique position showed that the right ventricle was not greatly enlarged; indeed, the left ventricle appeared larger than the right ventricle. The esophagus was seen to be indented by the aorta in the left anterior oblique position; in the right anterior oblique position its descent was independent of the aorta. There was no enlargement of the left auricle.

The clinical diagnosis was an extreme tetralogy of Fallot with a right aortic arch.

On Jan. 6, 1945 the patient returned for a check-up and because her parents wished to discuss the possibility of operation. The physical findings were essentially the same as previously noted but she was even more severely incapacitated. She could not walk 30 feet without exhaustion, and she panted when she moved from a wheel chair to the examining table. The fluoroscopic findings were essentially the same as noted previously except that the shadows at the hili of the lungs were more conspicuous. There were, however, no pulsations visible in this region.

The patient returned on January 29. Studies on the arterial blood are recorded in table 1.

A sample of venous blood showed that the red blood cell count was 7,500,000, the hemoglobin was 24 Gm., the hematocrit

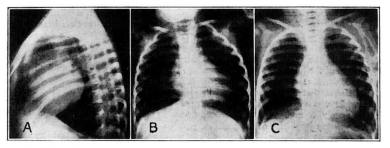

Fig. 4 (case 1).—Appearance before and after operation: *A,* left anterior oblique view before operation; *B,* anteroposterior view before operation; *C,* anteroposterior view after operation.

reading was 71 (Wintrobe) and the white blood cell count was 5,200. The electrocardiogram was essentially the same as that taken in 1943. A roentgenogram of the heart showed a small heart with a right aortic arch. The maximal right diameter was 4 cm. and the maximal left was 7 cm. The total transverse diameter was 26 cm. The cardiothoracic ratio was 42.4.

Operation.—This was performed on February 3. The procedure consisted in anastomosing the divided proximal end of

TABLE 1.—*Studies on Arterial Blood (Case 2)*

Dates	Arterial Oxygen Content, Volumes per Cent	Arterial Oxygen Capacity, Volumes per Cent	Arterial Oxygen Saturation, per Cent	Arterial Carbon Dioxide Content, Volumes per Cent
2/ 1/45	11.7	32.3	36.3	34.9
2/ 3/45	Innominate artery anastomosed to left pulmonary artery			
2/12/45	20.3	27.5	73.8	37.8
3/ 1/45	19.8	23.9	82.8	37.2

the innominate artery to the side of the left pulmonary artery. This is shown diagrammatically in figure 5. The anesthetic agent was administered by Dr. Austin Lamont.

Cyclopropane with a high percentage of oxygen was administered through an endotracheal tube. The incision extended from the left costal margin to the anterior axillary line. The pleural cavity was entered through the third interspace. There were no adhesions between the lung and the chest wall, and the lung looked normal. Although the surgeon had been informed by his pediatric colleague that this patient almost certainly had a right aortic arch, no special thought was given to the fact, and it caused some surprise when it was noted that the aorta was not on the left side. It was fortunate, however, that the incision had been made on the left because this allowed the use of the innominate artery rather than the subclavian artery. There was a very tortuous artery, which

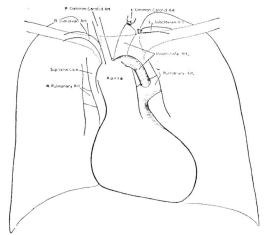

Fig. 5 (case 2).—Procedure used. The patient had a right aortic arch, and the innominate artery was directed to the left. The end of the innominate artery was anastomosed to the side of the left pulmonary artery.

was lying anterior to the vertebral column and which appeared to run from the region of the hilus of the lung toward the upper part of the left pleural cavity. Compression of this vessel indicated that the blood was flowing from above downward. It is believed that this vessel was a large accessory bronchial artery. It was estimated that the lumen of this artery was approximately 3 mm. in diameter. Still another abnormal finding was the large size of the posterior portions of the intercostal arteries. It seems likely that these vessels were also supplying blood to the hilus of the lung. The evidence of extensive collateral circulation led us to believe that we were probably dealing with a case of complete pulmonary atresia.

The innominate artery was located and dissected free of the surrounding tissues. The encouragement of the first assistant, Dr. William Longmire, played no small part in the continued effort to find a large systemic artery. A bulldog arterial clamp was placed on the innominate just distal to its origin from the aorta. The subclavian and common carotid arteries were ligated near their points of origin from the innominate. The innominate artery was divided just proximal to these ligatures. It was estimated that the diameter of the lumen of the innominate artery was approximately 1.3 cm. The left main pulmonary artery was then prepared for the anastomosis. A bulldog clamp was placed just distal to the origin of this vessel from the main pulmonary artery, and a second clamp was placed proximal to its entrance into the lung. A transverse opening was made into the lumen of the vessel midway between the two clamps. A suture anastomosis was performed between the end of the innominate artery and the side of the left pulmonary artery. The length of time that the left pulmonary artery was occluded was fifty to sixty minutes. The bulldog clamps were removed. There was bleeding from one point, which was controlled by an additional suture. An easily palpable thrill was felt in the pulmonary artery both proximal and distal to the anastomosis. The pulmonary artery seemed to be considerably larger than before this new current of systemic blood was admitted to it. The systemic arterial pressure was 110 systolic and 70 diastolic at the time that the arterial clamps were removed. Immediately following the removal of the clamps the systemic pressure declined 30 mm. of mercury. There followed a rise in systolic pressure of 20 mm. of mercury, but the pressure then declined gradually during the next thirty minutes until it reached 60 systolic and 30 diastolic. The pulse rate during this time rose from 72 to 120 per minute.

After the completion of the anastomosis and the removal of the clamps, several grams of sulfanilamide were placed in the pleural cavity. The left lung was partially inflated by the use of positive pressure, and the incision in the chest wall was closed. The patient was given a slow continuous intravenous drip of isotonic solution of sodium chloride during the operation and her condition at the end of the operation appeared to be satisfactory.

The operation required two hours and forty minutes. A considerable part of this time was consumed in studying the tortuous vessel which was seen above the hilus of the lung and also in trying to locate the innominate artery.

The patient awakened from the anesthesia a short time after the closure of the incision. She could move the left arm without difficulty. The left arm and hand were slightly cooler than the right, but it was evident that the circulation was adequate to maintain life. There was no evidence of a cerebral disturbance as the result of the ligation of the common carotid. No pulse could be felt in the left arm or the left side of the neck and face.

Postoperative Course.—This was smooth. There was no vomiting following operation, and fluids were taken by mouth. She was placed in an oxygen tent. The administration of penicillin was started immediately after operation and was continued for nine days. The left pleural cavity was aspirated twenty-four hours after operation; 250 cc. of air and 70 cc. of blood were removed. There were no other thoracenteses. Although a thrill was palpable at the site of the anastomosis immediately on release of the bulldog clamps, no murmur was audible immediately after the chest was closed. By the second evening a faint diastolic murmur was audible over the base and at the apex. By the third postoperative day an extraordinarily loud continuous murmur was audible throughout the chest on both the right and the left side. The oral administration of dicumarol was begun on the fourth postoperative day; 50 to 200 mg. was given daily for several weeks. Prothrombin determinations were performed daily. The dose of dicumarol was such as to keep the clotting time of the patient's blood approximately twice that of the normal control.

Femoral arterial punctures were performed on the ninth and twenty-sixth postoperative days. The results of the analyses are given in table 1. Before operation the red blood cell count was 7,500,000, the hemoglobin 24 Gm. and the hematocrit reading 71. Three days after operation the red blood cell count had decreased to 6,000,000, the hemoglobin to 19 Gm. and the hematocrit reading to 61. By the twenty-first day the red blood cell count was 6,000,000, the hemoglobin was 17.5 Gm. and the hematocrit reading was 55.

A roentgenogram of the heart taken ten days after operation showed that the heart had increased in size; that taken twenty-one days after operation revealed no further increase in size.

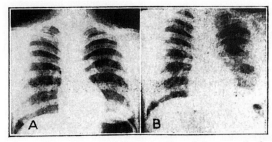

Fig. 6 (case 2).—Heart *A*, before operation and *B*, one month after operation.

Indeed, the heart was a trifle smaller than on the previous date. Roentgenograms of the heart before and after operation are shown in figure 6. Before operation the cardiothoracic ratio was 42.4 and three weeks after operation it was 44.7. The electrocardiogram showed no change (fig. 7). The stethocardiogram showed a continuous murmur (fig. 8). There was a significant increase in the pulse pressure. The preoperative arterial pressure had been 110 systolic and 90 diastolic. On the thirty-seventh postoperative day the arterial pressure was 98 systolic and 66 diastolic.

An appreciable diminution in the cyanosis of the lips and fingernails was apparent several days after operation. The patient was allowed to walk, beginning two and a half weeks after operation. This exercise resulted in a slight increase in the cyanosis, but it was evident that cyanosis was much less than it had been preoperatively. By the end of the third week she could walk 60 feet in an erect posture without panting, whereas before operation, stooping and leaning forward, she could walk only 30 feet and would then stop and pant. There has been a slow but steady recession of the clubbing of the fingers and toes. The patient was discharged from the hospital on the thirty-eighth postoperative day.

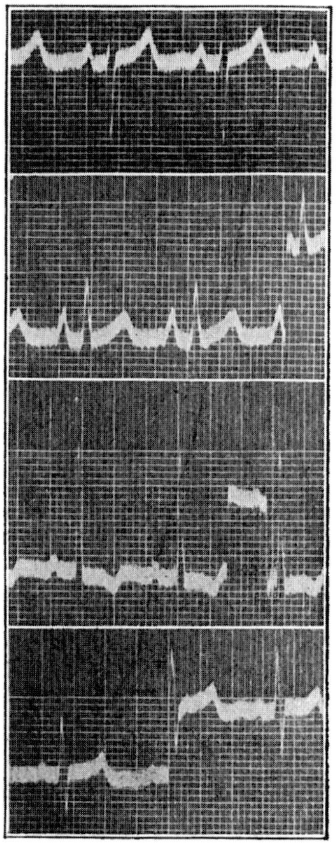

CASE 3.—*History.*— M. M., a boy born July 15, 1938, was first seen at the Harriet Lane Home at 8 months of age with the complaint of heart trouble.

The family history is of importance in that the maternal grandfather was known to have heart trouble and had had a heart murmur throughout his life. The mother's brother and sister are both reported to have dextrocardia; both have refused examination.

The past history stated that the patient was a full term baby. The birth weight was 6½ pounds (2,955 Gm.). Development was slow; he held his head up at 5 months and sat alone at 6½ months. At 8 months the patient weighed 13½ pounds (6 Kg.). When lying quietly he showed slight persistent cyanosis, which became intense when he cried. On examination of the heart there was no thrill but a very definite systolic murmur, which was audible all over the precordium and well heard in the back. Fluoroscopy showed that the heart was within normal limits in size. There was a wide shadow above the heart which was interpreted as a large thymus. There was no fulness of the pulmonary conus, and the shadow at the base of the heart was concave. The clinical diagnosis was tetralogy of Fallot.

The patient was followed in the cardiac clinic until January 1940, when the family moved to California. They returned to Baltimore in the fall of 1944 and the patient was again brought to the clinic on September 29. At that time the boy, 6 years of age, was thin and undernourished, intensely cyanotic and dyspneic on slight exertion. The temperature was 99.2 F., weight 34½ pounds (15.6 Kg.), height 42 inches (107 cm.), pulse 140, respirations 20 and blood pressure 90 systolic and 60 diastolic.

There was manifest suffusion of the conjunctiva. The lips were purple and the buccal mucous membranes were a deep mulberry color. The teeth were in bad condition; the tonsils

Fig. 7 (case 2).—Electrocardiogram.

were not unduly enlarged. The chest was barrel shaped. The increase in the size of the heart was in proportion to the growth of the child. There was a systolic thrill at the apex and a harsh systolic murmur, which was maximal along the left sternal border in the third interspace. The second sound at the base of the heart was clear but not accentuated. The lungs were clear. The liver was at the costal margin; the spleen was not palpable. The femoral arterial pulsations were easily felt. The extremities showed deep cyanosis and pronounced clubbing. Although the patient had learned to walk by November 1944, he was so incapacitated that he was unable to walk and even refused to try to take a few steps. The diagnosis was tetralogy of Fallot with a severe degree of pulmonary stenosis.

The patient was referred to the dental clinic, where several teeth were extracted. Sulfadiazine was given for two days. One month later the patient returned to the cardiac clinic with a rectal temperature of 100.4 F. and with numerous petechiae on his legs, which the mother said were of two days' duration. A blood culture taken at this time was sterile and no further petechiae appeared.

TABLE 2.—*Studies on Arterial Blood (Case 3)*

Dates	Arterial Oxygen Content, Volumes per Cent	Arterial Oxygen Capacity, Volumes per Cent	Arterial Oxygen Saturation, per Cent	Arterial Carbon Dioxide Content, Volumes per Cent	Comment
2/ 8/45	7.3	31.2	23.4	27.5	Patient struggling
2/ 9/45	10.7	30.2	35.5	29.3	Patient quiet
2/10/45	Innominate artery anastomosed to right pulmonary artery				
2/19/45	17.7	22.2	79.7	37.4	Patient crying
3/ 6/45	17.7	21.1	83.8	35.2	Patient quiet

The family was desirous of prompt operation and the patient was admitted to the hospital on Feb. 7, 1945. The results of analyses of blood obtained by arterial puncture are shown in table 2. With venous blood the red blood cell count was 10,000,000, the hemoglobin 26 Gm. and the hematocrit reading 81. The patient continued to have a daily elevation of temperature.

An electrocardiogram showed a normal sinus mechanism, a normal PR interval of 16, high P waves in L_2, and normal upright T waves in leads 1, 2 and 4, and T_3 inverted and an apparent right axis deviation.

X-ray examination (fig. 10) showed that the maximal right diameter of the heart was 2.1 cm., the maximal left 7 cm. and the total transverse diameter 18.8 cm.; the cardiothoracic ratio was 47.5. There was no fulness of the pulmonary conus. Fluoroscopy showed that the aorta descended on the left, and there were no visible pulsations in the lung fields.

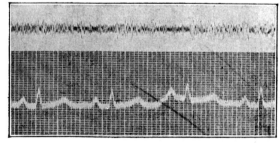

Fig. 8 (case 2).—Stethocardiogram.

Operation.—This was performed on February 10. The procedure consisted in anastomosing the divided proximal end of the innominate artery to the side of the right pulmonary artery. This is shown diagrammatically in figure 9. The anesthetic agent was administered by Dr. Merel Harmel.

Anesthesia was produced by cyclopropane with a high concentration of oxygen. It is of interest that the patient's color was much better under anesthesia than it had been previously.

This patient did not have a right aortic arch. In view of the great improvement in the second case we wished to use the innominate artery, and therefore the incision was made on the right side. There were no adhesions between the lung and the chest wall, and the lung appeared normal. The right upper lobe was retracted downward and the azygos vein was visual-

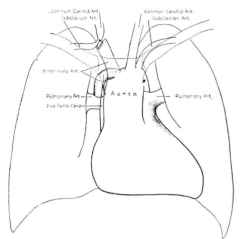

Fig. 9 (case 3).—Procedure used. The end of the innominate artery was anastomosed to the side of the right pulmonary artery.

ized. It was doubly ligated and divided. The superior vena cava and phrenic nerve were retracted medially, and the artery to the right upper lobe of the lung was seen. This was followed medially and the main right pulmonary artery was exposed. This exposure was considerably more difficult than that on the left side. Attention was then turned to the innominate artery. By dissecting under and medial to the superior vena cava the innominate artery was exposed and was dissected free of the surrounding tissues. This vessel was occluded temporarily by the use of a lung tourniquet which was equipped with a catheter overlying a piece of braided silk. The subclavian artery and the common carotid artery were ligated just distal to their origins from the innominate artery. The innominate artery was cut across proximal to these ligatures. Two bulldog clamps were placed on the right main pulmonary artery, and a transverse incision was made into the vessel between these clamps. The proximal bulldog clamp was not of sufficient length to secure entire control of the flow of blood. This resulted in a moderate loss of blood, and another clamp was substituted.

With 5-0 silk on a small curved needle an anastomosis was made between the divided proximal end of the innominate artery and the side of the right main pulmonary artery. This anastomosis was more difficult than that in the previous cases because the exposure was less satisfactory. Following the removal of the bulldog clamps from the pulmonary artery there was a rather copious flow of blood from one point along the anterior row of sutures. The clamps were reapplied, and this opening was closed with a mattress suture. Subsequent removal of the clamps did not result in further bleeding. The patient's condition up to the time of this blood loss had been excellent. Occlusion of the right pulmonary artery had not seemed to increase the cyanosis. There was an increase in the cyanosis and a decline in pressure when this loss of blood occurred. It was estimated that at least 250 cc. of blood was lost.

The anastomosis seemed to be a satisfactory one. An easily palpable thrill could be felt in the pulmonary artery both proximal and distal to the anastomosis. It was estimated that the lumen of the innominate artery was slightly less than 1 centimeter in diameter. The right lung was partially inflated and the incision in the chest wall was closed.

The patient received 500 cc. of a mixture of isotonic solution of sodium chloride and glucose and 200 cc. of plasma during the operative procedure. The operation required a total of three hours, the greater part of this time being consumed in making the anastomosis. It was obvious that a better instrument for occluding the pulmonary artery proximal to the site of the anastomosis is needed. The right pulmonary artery was occluded for approximately ninety minutes.

The patient's condition at the completion of the operation was very good. He was conscious a few minutes after the incision had been closed, was asking for water and was moving his right arm. This arm was slightly cooler than the left. Pulsations could not be felt in the right arm or in the right side of the neck and the face. There was, however, no evidence of cerebral damage, and it was obvious that the circulation of the arm was adequate to maintain life.

Postoperative Course.—This was remarkably smooth. The patient was placed in an oxygen tent for several days. The circulation to the right arm remained adequate. Aspiration of the chest was not necessary. Immediately after operation the child's color improved. It was seen on the fourth postoperative day when the administration of oxygen was discontinued that the cyanosis of the lips had disappeared. The cyanosis of the fingertips decreased more slowly. The administration of penicillin was started the day before the operation and was continued for three weeks postoperatively. Dicumarol was given by mouth, beginning on the third postoperative day. The usual daily administration was 25 mg. Prothrombin determinations were performed daily, and the drug was continued for three weeks.

Although a thrill was palpable at the site of the anastomosis after the arterial clamps had been released, no murmur was audible immediately after the chest had been closed. By the first evening a faint murmur was audible, which gradually increased in intensity. By the fourth postoperative day a continuous murmur was audible over the site of the anastomosis and posteriorly throughout both lungs.

The child's compensation has remained excellent. In contrast to a preoperative arterial pressure of 85 systolic and 65 diastolic, the arterial pressure postoperatively was usually 106 systolic and 52 diastolic. The heart increased somewhat in size during the first ten days after operation, but there did not appear to be a further increase in the subsequent two weeks. Roentgenograms of the heart both before and after operation are shown in figure 10.

Arterial punctures were performed on the 9th and 24th postoperative days. The results of the analyses are given in table 2. On comparing the preoperative studies with those performed twenty-four days after operation, samples of venous blood showed that the red blood cell count decreased from 10,000,000 to 6,000,000, the hemoglobin from 26 to 20 Gm. and the hematocrit reading from 81 to 53 (Wintrobe).

The patient had had a preoperative daily elevation of temperature to 100 F., and this continued for three weeks after operation. For this reason he was not allowed out of bed

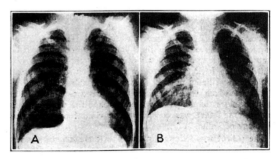

Fig. 10 (case 3).—Heart *A*, before operation and *B*, two weeks after operation.

despite his vigorous protests until three and a half weeks after operation. When permitted to do so, the child walked 40 feet with ease. He was then allowed to be up for several hours each day and has walked and played in his room. He did not develop either cyanosis or dyspnea on this activity. The patient was discharged from the hospital on the thirty-eighth postoperative day.

COMMENT

Each of these 3 patients suffered from such a severe degree of pulmonary stenosis that there was inadequate circulation to the lungs. Although the three operations differed in detail, in each instance the operation greatly increased the volume of blood which reached the lungs.

In the first case the end of the left subclavian artery was anastomosed to the side of the left pulmonary artery. As the baby was small and weak, extensive laboratory studies were not performed. Before operation the baby had been steadily losing ground. She had ceased to be able to sit alone; she had refused her feedings and had lost weight. The red blood cell count had declined from 7,000,000 to 5,000,000; consequently the cyanosis had diminished considerably. After operation her clinical improvement was remarkable. The appetite improved, she gained weight and she is now starting to learn to walk.

The second patient had a right aortic arch; hence it was possible to anastomose the innominate artery to the left pulmonary artery. The patient was deeply cyanotic and severely incapacitated and could not walk 30 feet without panting. Two and a half weeks after operation she walked 60 feet, rested a short time and walked 60 feet back to her room and sat down quietly. The seriousness of her condition and the extent of the improvement are shown by the changes in the oxygen saturation of the arterial blood, which was 36.3 per cent before operation and which rose to 82.8 per cent three weeks subsequently. The red blood cell count dropped from 7,500,000 to 6,000,000, the hemoglobin from 24 Gm. to 17.5 Gm. and the hematocrit reading from 71 to 55.

The success of the second operation led us to perform the same operation in the third case. Since the aorta was in the normal position, in order to use the innominate artery the operation was performed on the right side. The end of the innominate artery was anastomosed to the side of the right pulmonary artery. The patient was younger, and improvement was even more dramatic. Before operation he was intensely cyanotic, the lips were a dark purple, and the child was unable to take even a few steps. The day after operation he lay in an oxygen tent with cherry red lips. When taken out of the tent his color remained good. His disposition has changed from that of a miserable whining child to a happy smiling boy. We were slow to permit him to walk because of a persistent low grade fever, but at the end of the third postoperative week he could walk 40 feet without panting and without becoming cyanotic. The oxygen saturation of the arterial blood rose from 35.5 to 79.7 per cent in nine days, and it reached a saturation of 83.8 per cent twenty-four days after operation. The red blood cell count fell from 10,000,000 to 6,000,000; the hemoglobin decreased from 26 Gm. to 20 Gm. and the hematocrit reading from 81 to 53.

There are a number of features of the operative procedure which merit discussion. We were fearful that an intensely cyanotic child would not tolerate a long operative procedure in which it was necessary to open the pleural cavity and to occlude temporarily one of the pulmonary arteries. For this reason our first clinical attempt to increase the circulation to the lungs was postponed almost a year after it was decided that the procedure was a sound one, with the hope that some method of administering oxygen in addition to inhalation might prove satisfactory. This seemed particularly important since it was obvious that a new and untried procedure should be performed first on patients with a severe degree of anoxemia whose outlook without aid of some sort was hopeless. Although the use of intravenous oxygen has been reported by Ziegler[12] and may prove to be of benefit in this operation, it was impossible during wartime to procure the necessary equipment. Therefore this method could not be studied.

From our limited experience it appears that this type of patient can tolerate the use of inhalation agents for general anesthesia. We have been fortunate in this respect in that the anesthetic agents were chosen and administered expertly by Dr. Austin Lamont and Dr. Merel Harmel.[13] The first of these 3 patients was only 14 months of age and weighed less than 9 pounds. Ether by the open drip method was used during the major part of the procedure for the reason that a sufficiently small closed system was not available. In the anesthetization of the second and third patients, cyclopropane with a high concentration of oxygen was employed. Fortunately the administration of oxygen apparently increased the oxygen content of the arterial blood and cyanosis was definitely lessened. Although in only 1 patient was there any serious hemorrhage, the precaution was taken of having both blood and plasma readily available. Indeed, a slow continuous drip of plasma is advisable so that at a moment's notice if necessary the patient can be given large quantities of plasma. With these precautions no great difficulty was encountered in spite of the fact that two of the three operations required three hours.

The next question which arose was whether a patient who was already suffering from a severe degree of anoxemia would tolerate the occlusion of one of the main pulmonary arteries for the period during which the anastomosis was being performed. These periods of occlusion were approximately thirty, sixty and ninety minutes in the three operations. It is a remarkable fact that the cyanosis did not appear to be greatly increased during the occlusion period. It may be that the decreased flow of blood to the lungs caused by the congenital deformity rendered it possible for the opposite artery and lung to utilize this reduced volume almost as effectively as could the two lungs. Be that as it may, the 3 children tolerated occlusion of the left or the right main pulmonary artery for periods ranging from approximately thirty to ninety minutes.

Another question which arose was whether ligation and division of the left subclavian artery or the innominate artery would result in serious impairment of the circulation to the arm and the brain. In most instances heretofore these vessels have been occluded because of preexisting disease such as aneurysm, and it is possible under such circumstances that there has been a prolonged stimulus for the formation of collateral arterial pathways. It was gratifying, therefore, to note in our patients that there was little evidence of impairment of circulation to the parts deprived of their major arterial pathway. It is true that the pulse was absent for some time postoperatively and the part was slightly cooler than that of the opposite part of the body, but immediately after operation it was evident that the circulation was adequate to maintain life of the part. It may prove desirable to perform an upper dorsal sympathectomy at the time of operation. This would not add to the gravity of the operative procedure, since one has an excellent exposure of this region in perform-

12. Ziegler, E. E.: Intravenous Administration of Oxygen, J. Lab. & Clin. Med. **27**: 223-232 (Nov.) 1941.
13. Drs. Lamont and Harmel will deal with this subject in a subsequent communication.

ing the arterial anastomosis. In future cases the circulation of the arm will be studied more carefully.

The operation has not been attempted before on patients and there are many operative as well as clinical features which are still under investigation. The first of these is concerned with the type of anastomosis which is to be performed. This will undoubtedly depend on many factors, especially the age of the patient and the degree of anoxemia. As stated previously, in our patients the anastomosis was performed between the end of the subclavian artery or innominate artery and the side of the left or right pulmonary artery. This type of anastomosis appears to be sound in that it allows the blood to flow from the systemic circulation to both lungs. The fact that the continuous murmur which results from the operation is readily audible on both sides of the chest indicates that the anastomosis does direct blood to both lungs. It was this type of anastomosis which was used by Eppinger, Burwell and Gross [8] in their studies on the cardiac output of dogs with an artificial ductus arteriosus.

The easiest of the end to side arterial anastomoses in this region is that between the end of the left subclavian artery and the side of the left pulmonary artery. On the other hand, the subclavian artery is so small in an infant that the chances of the occurrence of thrombosis at the anastomotic site are great. This is particularly true if the patient has extreme polycythemia. Even though the anastomosis remains patent, the size of the vessel is a limiting factor in the flow of blood to the lungs which may not be sufficient to overcome the high degree of anoxemia from which some of these patients suffer. In an older patient with only a moderate degree of cyanosis the subclavian artery would appear to be the ideal vessel. The left common carotid is somewhat larger than the left subclavian artery, and its employment under some circumstances seems to be warranted. When dealing with the degree of anoxemia which was present in our patients, the innominate artery is much to be preferred to the left subclavian artery or the left common carotid artery. The performance of the anastomosis is not very difficult when the left pulmonary artery can be used. The anastomosis of the innominate artery to the left pulmonary artery is possible only in patients with a right aortic arch and hence an innominate artery on the left. With the innominate artery in its normal position the anastomosis of this vessel to the right pulmonary artery is more difficult because so much of the latter artery lies behind the aorta and the superior vena cava. Improvements in the designs of instruments will facilitate this procedure.

It is important to bear in mind that the degree of impairment in the flow of blood to the lungs varies from patient to patient, and the selection of the vessel to be used depends on the extent of the need of the patient for an increase in the circulation to the lungs. Experimental observations and clinical trial and error will undoubtedly shed additional light on this subject. It is obvious that the vessel chosen and the size of the anastomosis itself should not be larger than is necessary for the relief of anoxemia because of the danger associated with excessive shunting of blood to the lungs.

There are other methods in addition to union of an end of a systemic artery to the side of a pulmonary artery by which an anastomosis between the two circulations may be made. Included among these are (1) anastomosis of the divided proximal end of one of the vessels which arise from the aortic arch (innominate,

left common carotid, left subclavian) to the divided distal end of one of the two pulmonary arteries, (2) anastomosis of the divided proximal end of the subclavian artery or the common carotid artery to the divided proximal end of the pulmonary artery to an upper lobe of one of the lungs, (3) anastomosis of the side of the aorta to the side of the left pulmonary artery and (4) anastomosis of the side of the aorta to the side of the left pulmonary artery. These will be considered in the order in which they are enumerated.

The results of the use of the first method, in which the divided proximal end of the left subclavian artery is anastomosed to the divided distal end of the left main pulmonary artery, were reported in 1939 by Levy and Blalock.[7] It was stated that "dogs which have been observed for several months following this procedure appear entirely normal. The left lung was aerated and the respiratory movements were unaltered. The systemic arterial blood pressure was not affected by this operation. The blood pressure in the pulmonary artery only a short distance beyond the anastomosis was less than half of that in the systemic arteries. This was due to the relatively low peripheral resistance in the pulmonary bed. Since only arterial blood entered the left lung, the quantity of oxygen consumed by this lung was very small. However, when anoxemia was caused, a larger quantity of oxygen was taken up by the incompletely oxygenated arterial blood. The left lung appeared pinker than the right on gross examination during life. Microscopic examination revealed no noteworthy alteration in either the left pulmonary artery or lung." Some of these animals have now been observed over periods ranging up to six years. The only disturbing finding has been that a few of the animals at autopsy have shown a thickening of the left pulmonary artery. It was noted by Dr. Arnold Rich that this was found only in instances in which the anastomotic site was partially occluded as a result of thrombosis. The discrepancy in the size of the left subclavian artery and that of the left pulmonary artery may have accounted in part for this finding. Furthermore, this discrepancy in size may be responsible in part for the sudden diminution in the arterial pressure just beyond the point of anastomosis. At any rate, it is improbable that the anastomosis of the subclavian artery to the end of the left pulmonary artery would be the procedure of choice in the treatment of pulmonic stenosis. If this type of anastomosis should be performed, the innominate artery would be a better choice than the subclavian because it is more nearly the size of the pulmonary artery. It may be found that an end to end anastomosis is more apt to remain patent than an end to side one; certainly it is technically easier to perform. If, in the process of performing an anastomosis between the end of the innominate artery and the side of one of the pulmonary arteries, the latter vessel should be torn beyond repair, it should be borne in mind that an anastomosis may still be performed between the end of the innominate and the distal end of the pulmonary artery. Experimental studies are being carried out on the relative virtues of end to end and end to side anastomoses.

A second alternative method consists in anastomosing the proximal end of the divided subclavian or carotid artery to the proximal end of the divided pulmonary artery to one of the upper lobes. Since it is technically easier to perform an end to end than an end to side anastomosis, one may consider the advisability of using this procedure for a patient with only a slight degree of cyanosis. The proximal end of the pulmonary artery is specified because this would conceivably allow blood to gain access to all the lobes except the one supplied by the artery which was used for the anastomosis. This procedure has been performed in the laboratory and is not difficult.

The third possible operative procedure is concerned with an anastomosis of the side of the aorta to the side of the left pulmonary artery. That such a procedure is possible in dogs has been shown by Leeds [9] in his studies on patent ductus arteriosus. We considered the use of this method in our patients but were discouraged by the experience of Blalock and Park [10] in studies on experimental coarctation of the aorta. In these experiments the aorta was divided just distal to the ligamentum arteriosum, the two ends of the aorta were closed, the left subclavian artery was divided at some distance from the arch of the aorta, and the proximal end of the divided subclavian artery was anastomosed to the side of the distal end of the aorta just below the point at which it had been divided. Thus the subclavian artery was used for the conduction of blood beyond the point of division of the aorta. The discouraging feature of these experiments was that in approximately half of the animals the hind legs were paralyzed at the completion of the operative procedure. In 1 dog in which we occluded the aorta for forty minutes for the purpose of making an anastomosis between the side of the aorta and the side of the left pulmonary artery the hind legs became paralyzed. It is impossible to make an accurate anastomosis between the aorta and the left pulmonary artery without interrupting temporarily the circulation through the two vessels. We were fearful of causing a paralysis of the lower extremities and hence did not use this method with our patients. Another difficulty associated with the use of the aorta is that its walls are thick and rather friable and it is difficult to obtain an accurate approximation of the intimal surfaces.

The fourth method to be considered is that of an anastomosis of the aorta and the main pulmonary artery. It is obvious that occlusion of these vessels for the length of time that is required for an open suture anastomosis would result in death. If such a union was to be secured, it would have to be done by some other method. Fortunately the first portions of the medial walls of the aorta and the pulmonary artery are intimately adherent to each other. The ascending aorta and the main pulmonary artery are contained within the pericardial cavity and are enclosed in a tube of serous pericardium common to the two vessels. We have been able to produce a fistula between the two vessels in dogs by inflicting a stab wound in this region. The knife blade was introduced through the opposite free wall of the pulmonary artery, the walls of the pulmonary artery and aorta which were in intimate contact were pierced, the knife was withdrawn, and the opening in the free side of the pulmonary artery was closed by sutures. The establishment of the fistula required only a few seconds. This method is mentioned because it may be necessary to use the major blood vessels and to employ considerable speed if newborn infants with pulmonary stenosis or atresia are to be saved. It would not be at all surprising if this experimental method should prove to be a useful one in patients.

It remains to be proved whether a communication between the two circulations should be brought about by direct anastomoses between blood vessels such as

we have employed or by the use of tubes such as those devised for other purposes by Blakemore, Lord and Stefko.[14] It is our impression that the suture method is preferable when it can be accomplished without undue tension. This method obviates the necessity for leaving a large foreign body in the tissues; furthermore, there is at least a possibility that the opening will increase in size with the growth of the child. Studies on the latter point are in progress. These comments are in no sense a criticism of the Blakemore method, which is of great value in those instances in which part of a blood vessel has been destroyed and the ends cannot be united by direct suture.

One of the possible complications which causes concern is the danger of thrombosis at the anastomotic site. The improvement of our 3 patients indicates that thrombosis has not occurred. Furthermore, in cases 2 and 3 loud continuous murmurs developed after operation. As mentioned previously, partial occlusion of the anastomotic site has been found in some of the dogs in which such anastomoses were performed. Partial occlusion of the opening and emboli in the lungs were found at autopsy in 1 animal in which the end of the subclavian artery had been anastomosed to the side of the left pulmonary artery. This experiment was complicated by the previous creation of bilateral pulmonary arteriovenous fistulas. The sizes of the vessels used and the size of the communication between the two vessels are, of course, of prime importance in the determination of whether or not the opening will remain patent. This consideration is another point in favor of using a large vessel such as the innominate artery. Because of the difference in pressure on the two sides of the anastomotic site between the systemic and pulmonary circulations, it would be more likely that such an anastomosis would remain open than communications of similar size between two systemic arteries or two systemic veins.

As previously stated, most patients with the type of malformation of the heart under consideration have a decided polycythemia and an increased viscosity of the blood. This condition undoubtedly increases the danger of thrombosis. Indeed, cerebral thromboses are of not infrequent occurrence in these patients. Therefore the question arose as to whether these patients should receive heparin shortly after the termination of the operation. After much deliberation it was decided that the possible dangers were greater than the possible advantages. This opinion, however, is subject to change. By way of compromise, it was decided to give dicumarol during the period of convalescence. Therefore, beginning respectively on the fourth and third postoperative days the second and third patients were given dicumarol in small quantities. Prothrombin determinations were made daily and the dose of dicumarol was regulated so as to keep the clotting time approximately double that of the normal control. This medication was continued for a period of approximately three weeks. It is impossible to state whether this therapy has been of importance in the maintenance of the patency of the fistulas.

In order to understand the changes produced by the operation and its application to other malformations, it is essential to understand the nature of this malformation and the course of the circulation. The four features which constitute the tetralogy of Fallot are pulmonary stenosis, dextroposition of the aorta, an inter-

14. Blakemore, A. H.; Lord, J. W., Jr., and Stefko, P. L.: Restoration of Blood Flow in Damaged Arteries: Further Studies on Nonsuture Method of Blood Vessel Anastomosis, Ann. Surg. 117: 481-497, 1943.

ventricular septal defect and right ventricular hypertrophy. The pulmonary stenosis consists in a narrowing of the pulmonary orifice, and it is usual to find that the constriction also involves the pulmonary conus of the right ventricle. Dextroposition of the aorta means that the aorta rises from the left ventricle and partially overrides the right ventricle. Whenever this occurs, the aortic septum cannot meet the ventricular septum; consequently there is a high ventricular septal defect. Such is the nature of an interventricular septal defect in the tetralogy of Fallot. The malformation renders it difficult for the blood to be expelled from the right ventricle; hence there is hypertrophy of that chamber. The structure of the heart and the course of the circulation are diagrammatically shown in figure 11.

The degree of incapacity in a tetralogy of Fallot depends on the severity of the pulmonary stenosis and the degree of the overriding of the aorta. It is well known in cases in which the pulmonary stenosis is not extreme that the malformation is compatible with relative longevity. However, with extreme degrees of pulmonary stenosis and greatly diminished circulation to the lungs, the condition causes severe incapacity and death occurs at an early age.

The anastomosis of the innominate artery to the pulmonary artery directs a large volume of blood from the systemic circulation into the pulmonary circulation. By this means the volume of blood which reaches the lungs for aeration is increased; it follows that a greater volume of oxygenated blood is returned by the pulmonary veins to the left auricle and the left ventricle; consequently a greater volume of oxygenated blood is pumped out into the systemic circulation. As some blood from the aorta is diverted to the pulmonary circulation, the volume of blood to the systemic circulation is decreased and less blood is returned to the right auricle and the right ventricle. Thus the volume of blood which is returned to the right ventricle is lessened and that which is returned to the left side of the heart is increased. The alteration in the course of the circulation as influenced by the operation is shown in figure 12.

In short, the operation enables some blood to bypass the obstruction to the pulmonary circulation. Hence the operation should be of value in all malformations in which the primary difficulty is due to lack of adequate circulation of the blood to the lungs; that is, in all cases

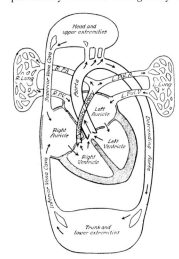

Fig. 11. Diagram of the course of the circulation in the tetralogy of Fallot. In this malformation there is pulmonary stenosis, the aorta is dextroposed and hence receives blood from both ventricles, the ductus arteriosus undergoes normal obliteration and the foramen ovale is closed. The blood from the right auricle flows into the right ventricle; hence part of the blood is pumped through the stenosed pulmonary orifice into the pulmonary artery and part of the blood is pumped directly into the aorta. Only that portion of the blood from the right ventricle which is pumped into the pulmonary artery goes to the lungs for aeration and is returned to the left auricle and the left ventricle. All of the blood from the left ventricle and some of the blood from the right ventricle is pumped out into the aorta to the systemic circulation and is returned by the superior vena cava and the inferior vena cava to the right auricle. There the cycle starts again.

of the tetralogy of Fallot and complete pulmonary atresia, in cases in which the right ventricle is absent or defective in its development, in cases of truncus arteriosus with bronchial arteries, or even a single ventricle with a rudimentary outlet chamber in which the pulmonary artery is diminutive in size.

Complete pulmonary atresia is, of course, compatible with life only as long as the ductus arteriosus remains open unless the bronchial arteries dilate and establish sufficient collateral circulation for the maintenance of life. This, we believe, happened in case 2, as at operation large aberrant vessels were found in the region of the hilus of the left lung. However, in the great majority of cases of pulmonary atresia the closure of the ductus arteriosus is so rapid that adequate collateral circulation does not develop and consequently the condition is fatal in early infancy. In all such cases the operation, if performed early, may be life saving. The same is true in cases of a defective development of the right ventricle in which all of the blood from the right auricle is directed to the left auricle and hence to the left ventricle and out by way of the aorta, and the only circulation to the lungs is by way of the ductus arteriosus.[15] The operation should be equally valuable in cases of truncus arteriosus with bronchial arteries because the bronchial arteries never become sufficiently large to provide adequate circulation to the lungs.

In every instance there is, of course, an admixture of venous and arterial blood. It would be impossible, therefore, to bring the oxygen saturation of the arterial blood to normal; nevertheless, it is conceivably possible to bring the oxygen saturation of the arterial blood sufficiently high so that there would be no "visible" cyanosis. Certainly in the 2 older children there has been an increase in the oxygen content of the arterial blood, a decrease in the oxygen capacity, an increase in the oxygen saturation of the arterial blood, a decrease in the red blood cell count, a diminution in the hemoglobin and the hematocrit reading, a striking decrease in the patients' disability and a great improvement in the patients' ability to exercise.

In cases of the tetralogy of Fallot the heart is either normal in size or relatively small. Following the creation of an artificial ductus, the increased volume of blood which reaches the pulmonary circulation undoubtedly increases the work of the left side of the heart. In our patients the heart has definitely increased in size but compensation thus far has remained excellent. Sir Thomas Lewis[16] has emphasized that in cases of coarctation of the aorta prolonged overwork does not cause cardiac failure. Palmer[17] in his studies on cardiac enlargement showed that, in essential hypertension, cardiac enlargement occurs with the gradual rise in blood pressure and that progressive enlargement does not easily occur after the blood pressure level has become stabilized. Therefore it is our hope and expectation that in this operation, although the heart immediately increases in size in response to the altered blood flow, the condition will not lead to progressive cardiac enlargement. It is encouraging that in both cases 2 and 3, although the heart increased in size in the first ten days, there was no further increase in the second ten days.

15. Taussig, H. B.: The Clinical and Pathological Findings in Congenital Malformations of the Heart Due to Defective Development of the Right Ventricle Associated with Tricuspid Atresia or Hypoplasia, Bull. Johns Hopkins Hosp. **59:** 435-445, 1936.
16. Lewis, T.: Material Relating to Coarctation of the Aorta of the Adult Type, Heart **16:** 205-261, 1933.
17. Palmer, J. H.: The Development of Cardiac Enlargement in Disease of the Heart: A Radiological Study, Medical Research Council Special Report Series, No. 222, 1937.

It is important to emphasize that the operation is not of value to all patients with persistent cyanosis. It is of value only in malformations in which the primary difficulty is lack of circulation to the lungs. The operation would be of no use in cases of complete transposition of the great vessels or in the so-called "tetralogy of Fallot of the Eisenmenger type" and probably not in aortic atresia.

In complete transposition of the great vessels the pulmonary artery arises from the left ventricle and the aorta from the right ventricle. The blood from the left ventricle is pumped out through the pulmonary artery to the lungs and is returned by the pulmonary veins to the left auricle and thence to the left ventricle. The blood from the right side of the heart is pumped out into the aorta to the systemic circulation and is returned by the superior vena cava and the inferior vena cava to the right auricle and the right ventricle. The primary difficulty in this malformation is not in the volume of blood which reaches the lungs but in the mechanism by which the blood which has been oxygenated in the lungs can reach the systemic circulation.

In the Eisenmenger complex cyanosis appears to be due to secondary changes in the alveolar wall or in the pulmonary vascular bed of such a nature as to hinder the aeration of the blood as it passes through the lungs; it is even possible that the high pressure in the lesser circulation may increase the right to left shunt and thereby increase the volume of reduced hemoglobin in the arterial blood. In any event, in this malformation there is no lack of circulation to the lungs and, furthermore, only rarely, if ever, is there deep cyanosis in early childhood.

In aortic atresia[18] not only is there difficulty in pumping blood to the systemic circulation but also the blood which does reach the systemic circulation is pumped through the ductus arteriosus before it has been to the lungs for aeration. Under such circumstances the creation of an additional ductus arteriosus would act to direct a larger volume of blood to the body; but it must be borne in mind that this blood has the same oxygen content as that directed to the lungs.

It is worthy of note in almost all patients with much polycythemia that all of the blood which circulates through the lungs is no longer fully oxygenated. Whether the size of the capillary bed in the lungs varies with the plasma volume and not with the number of red blood cells is not known, but there is clear evidence to show that even in patients in whom the primary difficulty is lack of circulation to the lungs the oxygen saturation of the arterial blood can be appreciably raised by the prolonged inhalation of a high concentration of oxygen. The potency of this factor was demonstrated by the great improvement in the peripheral cyanosis during operation when the patients were receiving oxygen. The importance of the volume of blood which reaches the lungs for aeration is demonstrated in our patients by the extent of the rise in the oxygen saturation of the arterial blood which resulted from the operation; in 1 instance it rose from 36.3 to 82.8 per cent and in the other from 35.5 to 83.8 per cent.

It may be that, with prolonged meager flow of blood to the lungs, secondary changes occur so that the pulmonary capillary bed is no longer capable of complete expansion and restoration to normal. Our 6 year old child showed prompter improvement than did the 12

year old girl. Hence the operation may prove less beneficial to older persons than to young children. For this reason the ideal age for operation appears to be after the systemic pressure has risen sufficiently high to permit the continuous flow of blood from the aorta to the pulmonary artery and before the condition has persisted long enough to cause irreversible changes in the lungs. We believe that the optimal age of patients is probably between 4 and 6 years; however, in all cases in which the closure of the ductus arteriosus renders the malformation incompatible with life the operation must be performed in early infancy.

Since the operation should be of value to all patients in whom the primary difficulty is lack of circulation to the lungs, it behooves the clinician to recognize this condition.[19] The two outstanding features, both of which should be present, are (1) roentgenographic evidence that the pulmonary artery is diminutive in size and (2) clinical and roentgenographic evidence of absence of congestion in the lung fields.

The size of the normal pulmonary artery is not difficult to determine by roentgenography. The striking feature in the roentgenogram is the absence of the fulness of the normal pulmonary conus. The shadow at the base of the heart to the left of the sternum is concave and not convex. A concave shadow in this region in patients with persistent cyanosis always means that the pulmonary artery is misplaced, absent or diminutive in size.[2] When the pulmonary artery is absent or diminutive in size, there is the additional finding in the left anterior oblique position of an abnormally clear pulmonary window.[2]

Absence of clinical and x-ray evidence of congestion in the lungs is highly important in reaching a decision. When circulation to the lungs is inadequate, the diminished blood flow to the lungs lessens the chances of congestion in the lungs and congestion rarely occurs.[2] When congestion does occur, it suggests that the circulation to the lungs is adequate or excessive. The operation should never be attempted when x-ray exam-

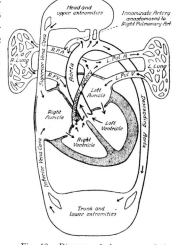

Fig. 12.—Diagram of the course of the circulation in the tetralogy of Fallot after the anastomosis of the innominate artery to the pulmonary artery. Under these circumstances the blood from the right auricle flows into the right ventricle and, as before, part of the blood from the right ventricle is pumped directly into the aorta. Now, in addition to the blood which is pumped through the pulmonary orifice into the pulmonary artery, some of the blood from the aorta is diverted through the anastomosis to the lungs. Thus the volume of blood which reaches the lungs is increased and the volume of oxygenated blood which is returned to the left auricle and the left ventricle is proportionately increased. All of the blood from the left ventricle and also some blood from the right ventricle is pumped into the aorta. Some of the blood from the aorta is directed to the lungs, and the remainder goes to the systemic circulation and is returned by the superior vena cava and the inferior vena cava to the right auricle. Thus the left ventricle receives more blood than before operation and the right side of the heart receives less. The operation has bypassed the obstruction in the circulation of the blood to the lungs.

18. Taussig, H. B.: Clinical and Pathological Findings in Aortic Atresia or Marked Hypoplasia of the Aorta at Its Base, Bull. Johns Hopkins Hospital, to be published.

19. The following discussion is based mainly on original unreported observations which are dealt with in detail in chapters II and III of Taussig's forthcoming book on "The Clinical Analysis of Congenital Malformations of the Heart," to be published by the Commonwealth Fund.

ination shows a prominent pulmonary conus or when there are pulsations at the hili of the lungs. These pulsations should be looked for by careful fluoroscopic examination after one's eyes are fully accommodated.

Virtually the only malformation in which there is absence of the normal shadow cast by the pulmonary artery in the presence of adequate circulation to the lungs is complete transposition of the great vessels. In this condition the pulmonary artery lies behind the aorta; therefore, in the anteroposterior view there is a narrow aortic shadow and a concave curve at the base of the heart to the left of the sternum. In the left anterior oblique position the two vessels lie side by side; hence the shadow cast by the great vessels increases in width [20] and the pulmonary window is not abnormally clear. The condition does not cause pulsation at the hili of the lungs but frequently leads to congestion in the lung fields. These observations, together with evidence of relatively rapid progressive cardiac enlargement,[2] should aid in the establishment of the correct diagnosis.

The operation should be performed on the right or left side, depending on which vessel is to be used and on which side the aorta descends. Furthermore, it is important to bear in mind that the occurrence of a right aortic arch is by no means rare in congenital malformations of the heart which cause persistent cyanosis. Bedford and Parkinson [21] have shown that the determination of the course of the aorta is not difficult, provided fluoroscopy is carefully performed and the esophagus delineated with a barium opaque mixture. Normally the aortic knob is visible on the left, the esophagus lies in the midline and is indented by the aorta on the left margin, and in the right anterior oblique position the esophagus is seen to be slightly displaced backward by the aorta. In cases of a right aortic arch the aortic knob frequently is hidden within the shadow cast by the superior vena cava. In the anteroposterior view the esophagus is indented on the right and is displaced backward in the left anterior oblique position.

It remains to be seen whether these patients will develop heart failure. Even if this occurs, the intervening period appears to be one of great clinical improvement. It may well be that, if more patients with congenital malformations of the heart survive, more will develop subacute bacterial endocarditis. Certain it is that there is nothing in persistent cyanosis which renders an individual immune from subacute bacterial endocarditis. The condition is less frequently encountered in cyanotic persons only because a comparatively small number of patients survive long enough to be liable to contract the disease. The fear of subacute bacterial endocarditis in the future is no justification for allowing a patient to die of anoxemia in the present. Even the possibility of future cardiac failure does not weigh heavily against present extreme incapacity and the danger of early death from anoxemia or cerebral thrombosis.

SUMMARY

An operation for increasing the flow of blood through the lungs and thereby reducing the cyanosis in patients with congenital malformations of the heart consists in making an anastomosis between a branch of the aorta and one of the pulmonary arteries; in other words, the creation of an artificial ductus arteriosus. Thus far the

procedure has been carried out on only 3 children, each of whom had a severe degree of anoxemia. Clinical evidence of improvement has been striking and includes a pronounced decrease in the intensity of the cyanosis, a decrease in dyspnea and an increase in tolerance to exercise. In the 2 cases in which such laboratory studies were performed there has been a decline in the red blood cell count, in the hemoglobin and in the hematocrit reading, an increase in the oxygen content of the arterial blood, a fall in the oxygen capacity, and most significantly a decided rise in the oxygen saturation of the arterial blood.

The types of abnormalities which should be benefited by this operation are the tetralogy of Fallot, pulmonary atresia with or without dextroposition of the aorta and with or without defective development of the right ventricle, a truncus arteriosus with bronchial arteries, and a single ventricle with a rudimentary outlet chamber in which the pulmonary artery is diminutive in size. The operation is indicated only when there is clinical and radiologic evidence of a decrease in the pulmonary blood flow. The operation is not indicated in cases of complete transposition of the great vessels or in the so-called "tetralogy of Fallot of the Eisenmenger type," and probably not in aortic atresia. It must be emphasized that the operation should not be performed when studies reveal a prominent pulmonary conus or pulsations at the hili of the lungs.

———————

20. Taussig, H. B.: Complete Transposition of the Great Vessels, Am. Heart J. **16**: 728-733, 1938.
21. Bedford, D. E., and Parkinson, J.: Right-Sided Aortic Arch, Brit. J. Radiol. **9**: 776-798, 1936.

BRITISH MEDICAL JOURNAL

LONDON SATURDAY JUNE 12 1948

PULMONARY VALVULOTOMY FOR THE RELIEF OF CONGENITAL PULMONARY STENOSIS

REPORT OF THREE CASES

BY

R. C. BROCK, M.S., F.R.C.S.

Surgeon to Guy's Hospital

The surgery of the heart may be said to have begun in 1896 when Rehn (1897) first successfully sutured a wound of the heart. Until a short time before this a semi-mystical, mediaeval attitude prevailed in relation to the heart, which was generally thought to be untouchable surgically. Thus even as late as 1883 Billroth declared that the surgeon who attempted to suture a wound of the heart would lose the respect of his colleagues. Rehn's epoch-making operation demonstrated conclusively that the heart of man was, in some measure at any rate, tolerant of interference. Surgeons were quick to profit by this lesson, so that within ten years Rehn was able to collect reports from the literature of 124 cases of a wound of the heart treated by suture.

The early promise of the development of direct cardiac surgery engendered by Rehn's success was not fulfilled; development there has been, but most of the progress has been by indirect methods. Operations have been conducted upon the surface of the heart and upon the great vessels near the heart, but very few indeed have been done upon the actual substance or internal structure of the heart except for injury or removal of retained foreign bodies.

The successful ligation of the patent ductus arteriosus by Gross and Hubbard (1939) and resection of aortic coarction by Crafoord and Nylin (1945) were followed by the brilliant work of Blalock and Taussig (1945) in the treatment of *morbus caeruleus*. By anastomosing a systemic artery to the pulmonary artery Blalock was able to relieve cyanosis in those cases of " blue babies " in which an inadequate supply of blood was going to the lungs—usually those in which a pulmonary stenosis was present. Even this carefully thought out and brilliantly executed operation, which has brought relief to so many hundreds of sufferers otherwise doomed to disability and death, is an indirect operation and not a direct one upon the substance or structure of the heart itself. It is in the nature of a by-passing operation to avoid the stenotic zone.

Earlier Operations for Valvular Stenosis

In 1913 Doyen tried to divide what was thought to be a stenosed valve in a patient aged 20 suffering from pulmonary stenosis. He did this by introducing a small tenotomy knife into the right ventricle; the patient died several hours later, and necropsy showed that a subvalvular rather than a valvular stenosis existed. About the same time Tuffier (1913) dilated a stenosed aortic valve with his finger by invaginating the wall of the aorta, but he did not open the heart or the aorta; the patient was said to be improved. Souttar (1925) used a method of direct digital dilatation of the mitral valve and his patient survived, although it appears from the case report that no true mitral stenosis was present.

The most sustained effort to solve the problem of relief of valvular stenosis by direct attack on the valves was made by Cutler and his associates (Cutler and Beck, 1929); they used a tenotome in their first three cases and a cardiovalvulotome in four others. Their first patient survived four and a half years and was thought to have been improved; six other patients died soon after operation, as also did single cases reported by Allen and Graham (1922) and Pribram (1926).

These early efforts were succeeded by a long period of inaction, and in the minds of many these operations of a quarter of a century ago seem to have proved that direct surgical attack on the diseased valves of the heart is too dangerous to be practicable.

Now, we must remember that these attempts were indeed made nearly a quarter of a century ago. Since that time there have been great advances in surgery and anaesthesia. Enormous developments have been made in the whole field of intrathoracic surgical technique; great strides have been made in pre-operative and in post-operative care, particularly in regard to blood transfusion and oxygen administration; and, more recently still, chemotherapy has heralded a new era. With our present knowledge and experience of intrathoracic operations we can understand the difficulties in the way of these early pioneers. It is no discredit to them that they did not succeed; they deserve only the greatest credit and recognition for their courageous efforts. At the same time it is important to realize that this accumulated experience and development of the last 25 years has entirely altered the prospects of success, and he would be blind who did not realize that the time has now come to try the matter again. When one examines the heart post mortem in patients dying of valvular disease and contemplates the minute size of the orifice through which the whole life-blood of the body has to be forced it is impossible not to feel that this simple mechanical obstruction must be capable of relief by surgery. The relief of such mechanical derangements is one of the oldest functions of surgery, and surgery is wanting in some part until it has been able to relieve cardiac valvular stenosis. It should require no special imagination to grasp this—even a student in training could postulate it.

Objections continue to be raised that even if the stenosed valve is successfully dealt with the secondary alterations in cardiovascular mechanics may prove disabling or fatal. This is no fundamental objection to the operation; it is merely a potential difficulty that has to be assessed or overcome. By timorous meditation we arouse fear and postpone success. Meditation and planning are essential, but in such circumstances as this, faced with a problem beset with so many and obvious hazards, the first step must be to

4562

assess the essentials. The essential fundamental is the stenosed valve which holds up the passage of blood; the relief of this stenosis must be the ideal to be aimed at. Relief by indirect methods has its place and may prove ultimately to be the wisest and best course to adopt, but until proved otherwise, relief by direct attack must be our goal.

The day must surely come when direct operations upon the substance and structure of the heart will be as firmly established and as successfully conducted as operations upon the lungs, brain, and other major systems and viscera that for so long defeated our efforts. There can be little doubt that there will be fundamental changes in technique, such as possibly those associated with temporary discontinuance of the circulation through the heart while it is being operated upon. In the meantime we must attack the problem and begin the development of a technique for intracardiac operations, for unless begun the task can never proceed.

It is with this justification, therefore, that I record three cases in which a direct operation was performed upon the pulmonary valves in an attempt to relieve a pulmonary stenosis; these three patients are alive and their cardiac condition has been improved. It is not suggested that these three cases provide the solution to the problem, but they would appear to be of sufficient importance to deserve description at this time. So far as I know, apart from the earlier attempts mentioned above, they are the only recorded examples of successful direct operations upon the heart to relieve disease within the heart, apart from the repair of injuries and the removal of foreign bodies.

I am indebted to my cardiological colleague, Dr. Maurice Campbell, for his unstinted enthusiasm, co-operation, and medical and moral support in this most difficult venture; the selection of suitable cases would not have been possible without his knowledge, skill, and partnership.

The Problem of Congenital Pulmonary Stenosis

The postulate of the Blalock–Taussig or "blue-baby" operation is that an inadequate supply of blood is going to the lungs and that by joining a systemic artery to the right or left pulmonary artery an additional amount of blood can be delivered to the lungs for oxygenation. The stenosed area is thus by-passed. The immediate results of this operation can be dramatically successful and can usually be described as excellent. It is so far not possible to assess the late results, since Blalock's first operation was done only as recently as November, 1944. Two possible drawbacks to the procedure immediately suggest themselves. First, that the fistulous communication may not grow *pari passu* with the child and thus will prove ineffective in later years: observations upon growing animals and upon patients dying after several years should provide the answer to this. Secondly, an arteriovenous leak or artificial ductus arteriosus is created—a condition for the relief of which, when it occurs as a congenital maldevelopment, an operation has been considered necessary. To this objection Blalock rightly replies that the fear of complications in the future is no justification for allowing a patient to die of anoxaemia in the present; he also believes that the existence of the patent interventricular septum, which is present in most of these patients as a part of the tetralogy of Fallot, may modify the usual drawbacks that a patent ductus arteriosus entails.

The relief of the obstruction itself by direct operation would certainly answer the second and greatest objection: an increased supply of blood would be provided to the lungs without the disadvantages of an arteriovenous leak and the doubtful ultimate prognosis that this condition carries.

It is usually stated that the stenosis in these cases is almost invariably subvalvular or infundibular and is therefore not amenable to relief. In fact this is not so; a proportion of cases of Fallot's tetralogy have a valvular stenosis either with or without a subvalvular stenosis; in addition a further proportion of cases of *morbus caeruleus* occur in which a pure pulmonary valvular stenosis is present. It is not as yet possible to state with certainty the exact proportion of cases in which a valvular or diaphragmatic type of stenosis exists; there can be no doubt, from my observations so far, that the incidence is far higher than has been supposed. Investigations are proceeding to decide this more exactly.

When a valvular stenosis exists it is of a diaphragmatic nature; the fused valves form, as it were, a septum which in time, as the patient gets older, is forced by the blood stream into a nipple-like projection with a tiny hole in its summit. It projects into the pulmonary artery much as the cervix projects into the vagina. Its formation and structure show at a glance that it is eminently suitable for relief by division; moreover, a much larger hole could be made in a very short time, in exactly the right place, than is possible with the Blalock operation, in which a long and tedious dissection is necessary to secure a systemic artery of adequate size.

Before attempting to relieve a valvular stenosis it is clearly desirable first to diagnose its presence. This diagnosis should consist of a pre-operative assessment by clinical and various accessory methods and an actual final assessment at operation. This is not the place to enlarge upon the problem of pre-operative diagnosis, which will be dealt with in a later communication.

A great deal can be learned at operation, although experience is as yet too limited for dogmatism. Time and further experience can alone provide greater efficiency. At present it must suffice to say that much can be learned from direct cardiac examination.

Direct Cardiac Examination at Operation

One disadvantage of the Blalock operation, especially if it is done from the right-hand side, is that only very limited examination of the heart is made. In most cases all that is done is that the great vessels are exposed, dissected free, and an anastomosis performed. The completeness of the pre-operative diagnosis can only be assumed, unless the patient dies and the heart can be inspected.

Clearly the best way to assess the state of the valves is to inspect them under direct vision. This formed the first problem that was dealt with. A cardioscope to allow inspection of the interior of the heart was designed and described by Allen and Graham (1922); the principle of contact visualization is used in which the blood is displaced and the instrument rests directly upon the structure to be viewed. Using an operating cardioscope constructed for me by Mr. Schrantz, of the Genito-Urinary Manufacturing Company, with his usual superb skill, I have made a number of direct inspections in living patients.

One problem is the route of cardioscopy. Passage of the instrument through the ventricular wall has such apparent disadvantages that an alternative was sought. Study of the anatomy suggested the possibility of using the left pulmonary artery, for this structure normally forms an almost direct line with the main pulmonary trunk and provides a direct route to the valves. Left pneumonectomy provided excellent opportunities to test this, and it was shown to be a practical procedure. The instrument could be passed without difficulty and the valves inspected, although the vision in a normal patient is naturally limited by the constant movement of the cusps.

The first patient with congenital pulmonary stenosis, a young man of 17, was operated upon in May, 1947. The chest was opened through a left postero-lateral incison, as this approach is necessary in order to introduce the straight instrument into the heart. The valves were inspected and were seen to be normal; the stenosis was clearly subvalvular. A Blalock operation was performed by anastomosing the left subclavian artery to the left pulmonary artery, using the hole made for the passage of the cardioscope. The whole procedure meant that the pulmonary artery was occluded for a very much longer time than is usual in the Blalock operation, and this was largely responsible for the patient's death 12 hours later. Necropsy confirmed the presence of a Fallot's tetralogy with a severe infundibular stenosis and normal valves.

The next patient, a girl of 19, sent to me by Dr. East, was diagnosed pre-operatively as having a pure pulmonary valvular stenosis; the heart was very large, chiefly due to hypertrophy of the right ventricle. At operation in November, 1947, the left pulmonary artery was found to be very small and, owing to the great size of the right ventricle, which had caused gross dilatation, it arose from the main trunk at a right-angle so that it was not possible to pass the cardioscope. Neither was it possible to perform a Blalock operation. No ill effect followed the operation. The patient died of heart failure several months later and, most unfortunately, no post-mortem examination could be made.

A third patient, a girl aged 20, had severe pulmonary stenosis, which was diagnosed clinically as being of a pure valvular type. She had had several attacks of heart failure, had gross albuminuria and oedema, and had a very large heart. She was considered unsuitable for operation, but at the express entreaty of herself, her parents, and her doctor it was agreed to make the attempt. A left postero-lateral thoracotomy was done, the pericardium was opened to permit more direct examination of the heart as in the other cases, and a confident diagnosis of valvular stenosis was made. A short pause was made while the operating cardioscope was assembled, and when one turned again to the heart it was found to have stopped. It was eventually started again by massage and injection of adrenaline, but gradually failed again. It was again revived and again began to fail. It was decided to perform cardioscopy: the instrument was passed and the presence of a diaphragmatic valvular obstruction of characteristic nipple-like shape was easily observed. The heart, however, had again stopped and could not be revived. Necropsy confirmed a pure valvular stenosis with an almost pin-hole orifice of such minute size that it was astonishing that she could have supported life for so many years; very gross hepatic cirrhosis was present from back-pressure; the kidneys showed similar gross changes from chronic passive congestion.

From the experience of these cases, and in particular of the last one, it was felt that the approach through the left pulmonary artery was unsatisfactory, or at any rate was sufficiently unsatisfactory to be discarded for the time being in order to assay the ventricular route. It is clear that in certain of these patients with a valvular stenosis occlusion of the left pulmonary artery for even a short time may not be tolerated; in addition it was felt that the conical shape of the valve made rapid and precise division from above uncertain. These experiences with three patients had shown, however, that it was possible to diagnose pulmonary valvular stenosis with some degree of confidence at operation.

In addition to direct inspection of the valves much other valuable and significant information can be obtained by direct critical external examination of the heart. Even before the pericardium is opened a tentative diagnosis can be made. When a valvular stenosis is present the stem of the pulmonary artery immediately distal to the obstruction is often dilated and forms a thin-walled aneurysm-like bulge; this can be seen through the intact pericardium and a thrill of characteristic nature can be readily felt. If the pericardium is opened a much more useful examination can be made. The sac should be incised longitudinally for

some 5-8 cm. just anterior to the phrenic nerve, and by means of an additional transverse incision at each end a flap is turned forwards; by grasping the corners of this flap with haemostats it is also possible to manipulate the heart. Attention should first be directed to the region of the sinuses of Valsalva; if the sinuses are present and fully formed it is almost certain that the valve cusps are normal. Conversely, when a valvular stenosis is present there is either a continuous collar of dilated artery just above the valve-level, or the artery shows a larger, aneurysm-like dilatation resembling the bulb-like swelling of a young onion. The lesser degree of dilatation is usually associated with a smaller pulmonary artery of lower tension, and I suspect that it implies the existence of a subvalvular stenosis as well, although as yet insufficient observations have been made to confirm this. The greater degree of dilatation suggests a more powerful jet of blood coming through the stenosis. Palpation of the first part of the artery is most suggestive of this; the thrill is quite characteristic, and is of a fine high-pitched frequency, very strictly localized at a level just above the origin of the artery, and, most significant of all, can actually be felt to be extremely localized within the central portion of the lumen. Indeed, it feels as if it were caused by a thin but very powerful jet of fluid being forced through a tiny hole; and this is exactly how it is formed. If the thin-walled dilated artery is gently compressed between the fingers the precise, localized nature of the thrill becomes more obvious, and it is even possible to feel the conical valve momentarily between each heartbeat. If the finger is now passed down on to the surface of the right ventricle it will be found that the fine, purring thrill rapidly fades.

When a subvalvular stenosis is present no such characteristic localized thrill is felt in the first part of the pulmonary artery. The thrill is coarser, as if of a lower frequency, and although it can be felt by a finger placed on the artery this is because it is conducted towards it; it is felt more strongly just below the level of the valves, and altogether its localization is less precise; it is felt over a somewhat wider area. The infundibulum may also present as a thin-walled, aneurysm-like dilatation with a coarse thrill palpable at its base and conducted distally along the pulmonary arteries. Further information should be obtainable by means of direct pressure readings at different levels, but so far this has not been done successfully on the unopened heart.

Direct external examination of the heart in this way, coupled with pre-operative assessment, should provide enough information to decide whether a valvular stenosis exists.

The final observation should be direct valvuloscopy through the wall of the ventricle, and it is intended to do this. It had been planned in the three cases next to be described, but at the actual operation it was felt to be wiser to omit it, chiefly on account of the uncertainty of how the heart would tolerate the extra manoeuvre. It is, after all, a serious and anxious step to perform a cardiotomy, and until one is more familiar with what these abnormal hearts will tolerate in the way of manipulation and interference it seems wiser to proceed cautiously step by step. With an operation of this sort one makes certain plans beforehand, but in the tension of the most critical phase of the operation it may be found easier not to attempt too much. It is nevertheless definitely desirable to include direct cardioscopy in the operative assessment.

Although the cardioscope is provided with a cutting knife which can be advanced under direct vision it was decided to use a special valvulotome for division of the stenosed valve in these first cases. This enables the stenosis to be located and divided almost instantaneously, whereas the operating cardioscope might well entail considerable fumbling and uncertainty. The valvulotome used has a gently curved shaft ending in a blade shaped like a spearhead and carrying a short probe-end ; the two edges proximal to the probe-end are cutting ; the shoulders and the retreating edges are blunt. This instrument was also made for me by Mr. Schrantz. A pair of gently curved dilating forceps with fine blades, rather like a curved sinus forceps, are also used after the valvulotome.

Case 1

Miss D. N., aged 18, had been cyanosed from birth. She walked and talked at a normal age, but always had great disability in getting about, and during the winter could not walk at all outside the house ; in the summer, unless it was too hot, she could sometimes walk as much as 200 to 300 yards, although in recent years she could rarely manage more than 50 yards. She squatted as soon as she learnt to walk, and continued the habit when older, although her mother tried to stop it. She found that nothing relieved her discomfort so quickly after walking, and needed to do this in the x-ray room after feeling exhausted when standing up for screening.

Her cyanosis was fairly severe, Grade III, though it did get less with complete rest on a warm day. It would get worse with emotion as well as with exertion, and was changed greatly by a minor effort like undressing. The nails showed Grade III clubbing. She had fairly severe cyanotic attacks as a child after feeding ; and at 15 she spent a period of many months in bed, when her colour was exceptionally bad and her doctor thought she was not likely to survive.

The heart was not enlarged ; there was a rough systolic murmur down the left side, loudest in the pulmonary area, and a faint systolic thrill ; the pulmonary second sound was faint. Screening showed clear lung fields, a left-sided aorta, and no increased pulsation in the lung roots ; the heart was not generally enlarged. Electrocardiograms revealed extreme right ventricular preponderance. Blood pressure was 110/85. A blood count showed : red cells, 7,400,000 ; Hb, 127%. The arterial oxygen saturation at rest (Dr. Zak) was 90.9%.

A diagnosis of Fallot's tetralogy was made.

Operation (Feb. 16, 1948)

Intratracheal cyclopropane was given by Dr. E. H. Rink, and an intravenous infusion of plasma (one bottle) was administered. A left inframammary incision was made and the chest was opened through the second left interspace with division of the second costal cartilage ; many collateral vessels were met with. As soon as the chest was opened the heart's action became very feeble and slow—less than 50 ; the general condition was poor and gave considerable anxiety. The left pulmonary artery was small, thin-walled, and of low tension, and the anaesthetist felt that the patient would not tolerate its occlusion for a Blalock operation.

Palpation of the pulmonary artery area revealed a thrill suggestive of a valvular stenosis. The pericardium was opened and the pulmonary artery was seen to be slightly dilated in its first part and showed no sinuses of Valsalva. The thrill was of a jetlike character and was situated exactly in the position of the pulmonary valves ; moreover, what appeared to be a conical valve could be felt through the vessel wall. No thrill could be felt lower down. It was decided to perform valvulotomy.

Two rows of three interlocking mattress sutures of linen thread were inserted in the wall of the right ventricle, which was then incised between them ; the pressure within the ventricle was 24 cm. of saline. The wall was 1.25 cm. thick. The mattress sutures were crossed and held by an assistant so as to control haemorrhage from the incision. The curved valvulotome was inserted and passed effortlessly into the pulmonary artery ; a dilating forceps was then passed and opened fully. Very little blood was lost. The heart wound was closed by two linen-thread mattress sutures and the pericardium sewn to it ; the heart was frequently moistened with 1% procaine solution throughout the operation.

The thrill persisted, but its character changed from a fine jet-like nature to a coarser one of lower frequency ; the pulse-wave could be clearly seen within the pulmonary artery. The colour was poor at the end of the operation in spite of a good respiratory exchange.

Post-operative Course

The patient's condition was grave after the operation and her colour was bad even with oxygen. She showed little improvement until Feb. 20, when her colour was better and her blood pressure had slowly risen to 120/80. The heart was very large on Feb. 18, suggesting grave dilatation, possibly due to profound alteration in mechanics ; it was much smaller by Feb. 21 and her colour had improved further. A systolic murmur could still be heard.

She made steady improvement as regards her heart, but on the evening of Feb. 24 she complained of sudden severe pain in both legs with loss of movement and sensation. Unfortunately the full significance of this was not appreciated, and I was not informed until more than 24 hours later. By this time the right leg had improved, but the left leg was cold, pulseless, pale, painful, and insensitive. It was clear that an arterial occlusion was present, probably embolic, but it was considered to be too late to justify exploration. Further improvement occurred in the legs, and all peripheral pulses could be felt on the right but not on the left. Two or three superficial ulcers appeared around the left ankle ; these have since healed. The condition of the legs delayed her getting up, but her colour remained good except for occasional mild cyanosis with emotion and when she first began to get out of bed. She was allowed home on March 18, at which time her red cell count was 6,200,000, Hb 119%, and arterial oxygen saturation 79.6%.

She was seen on April 10 and had made good progress. There was no cyanosis, the finger-nails were pink, and she walked about the room without dyspnoea although there was a slight suggestion of cyanosis. She no longer squats. Her relatives are most emphatic that the relief of cyanosis and of dyspnoea is impressive. They emphasize especially the absence of dyspnoea, which had always been a marked feature even at rest.

Comment.—It is as yet too early to assess the results of operation completely in this case. The condition of the left leg has prevented full test of activity. It would appear that a sharp watch must be kept in these cases for symptoms suggesting arterial embolism and prompt action taken. There has been definite improvement in the cardiac condition, although less than hoped for. The prognosis in these older patients is less certain, and from her behaviour under anaesthesia she might not have tolerated a Blalock's operation. She would appear to be an example of Fallot's tetralogy with a valvular stenosis, although probably some degree of subvalvular stenosis exists as well.

Case 2

Gwenda B., aged 11, the youngest of eight children, had been obviously cyanosed at 6 months, though blue lips had been noted before this. She walked at 1 year and squatted as soon as she walked ; she was never able to walk more than 100 yards without distress, although she could sometimes manage as much as half a mile by getting very breathless. Cyanosis was extreme, ranging from Grade III to Grade IV ; the fingers showed Grade III clubbing. She was well developed physically and could walk about the ward without getting breathless.

The heart was sabot-shaped, with the apex raised off the diaphragm. The aorta was right-sided. A faint thrill was felt in the pulmonary area on one occasion ; a loud systolic murmur was maximum in the pulmonary area and widely conducted. The blood pressure was 95/65 ; electrocardiograms showed gross right ventricular preponderance. The lung fields were clear and there was no pulsation. Red cells, 8,700,000 ; Hb, 156% ; haematocrit, 77.5%.

A diagnosis of Fallot's tetralogy was made.

Operation (Feb. 19, 1948)

Intratracheal cyclopropane was given by Dr. Helliwell, and one bottle of plasma was infused intravenously. A left infra-mammary incision was made and the chest was opened through the second left intercostal space with division of the second costal cartilage. There were numerous collateral vessels ; the left pulmonary artery was small. The pericardium was opened and the main pulmonary artery was also found to be small, being about 1.25 cm. in diameter ; it was of low tension and there were no sinuses of Valsalva. A fine faint thrill could be felt in the position of the valves but not in the subvalvular position. After some deliberation it was decided to perform valvulotomy.

The right ventricle was opened and the valvulotome passed ; it met with definite resistance at the valves, and slight pressure carried it into the pulmonary artery ; dilating forceps were passed and opened widely. Free bleeding occurred from the heart, and during manipulations the pulse became poor in quality but soon improved. The cardiotomy incision was closed with four sutures ; the pericardium was sewn down over the suture line. The general condition was fair, although the colour was poor ; it had been poor at the beginning of the operation. The blood pressure was 85/55, as opposed to 90/60 at the beginning.

Post-operative Course

The patient was very blue, even in the oxygen tent, for the first 24 hours ; her colour then began to improve very slowly but steadily, and by Feb. 27 was reasonably good. Her progress was then rapid, and in fact by March 1 she was out of bed and visited the next ward, where she sat at table for a birthday party with other children without any distress. She was very soon able to walk freely about the ward and even come down to the x-ray department, and maintained her good pink colour. This was in marked contrast to her constant cyanosis before operation. The arterial oxygen saturation (March 22) was 81%, but she was crying and distressed during the arterial puncture.

She was discharged home on March 25, the blood count at that time being : red cells, 6 millions ; Hb, 116% ; haematocrit, 56. She had ceased to squat.

She was seen on June 4, when she looked well and was a good colour ; her mother said that her exercise tolerance was greatly improved and she was now able to run, a thing she could never do before the operation. The mother particularly remarked upon the normal colour of the nails, which had always been blue. The child walked normally to the x-ray department for screening, but although she showed no dyspnoea a slight tinge of cyanosis could be seen in the cheeks. This is not uncommon on exercise after a successful Blalock operation.

Comment.—This would appear to be a case of Fallot's tetralogy with a valvular stenosis ; the hypoplasia of the pulmonary artery strongly suggests that a degree of sub-valvular stenosis is present as well. Nevertheless, the result of valvulotomy has been most encouraging. The colour and clinical improvement are as good as after a successful Blalock operation.

Case 3

Miss R. C., aged 23, had been cyanosed since birth and did not walk until 3 years old. She was never allowed to go to school and dyspnoea had always been extreme. As a child she was able to play with other children, but had to rest frequently by squatting. She has always squatted, and even sleeps propped up with her legs curled up. Until the age of 18 she was able to walk perhaps 50 yards without stopping and could go considerably further with frequent rests. About five years ago, however, she became much worse quite suddenly, and found she could do very little without extreme distress. In fact, until October, 1947, she remained almost wholly in bed or on a couch, moving only from bedroom to sitting-room ; any effort, even moving in bed, provoked dyspnoea and pain across the chest. In October, 1947, she spent five weeks in the National Heart Hospital, and with encouragement found she was able to do a little more ; for instance, she could just about walk the length of the ward and could sit up for meals.

She was poorly covered ; finger clubbing was Grade I and cyanosis Grade I (i.e., not cyanosed at rest in bed) ; there was

extreme dyspnoea with rapidly developing cyanosis on walking ; the blood pressure was 115/70. The heart was not enlarged, although the apex was raised a considerable distance from the diaphragm, suggesting right ventricular hypertrophy ; a definite rounded shadow in the region of the " conus " suggested a minor degree of aneurysmal dilatation of the pulmonary artery. Perhaps a slight thrill could be felt in the pulmonary area ; a harsh systolic murmur, loudest in the pulmonary area, was audible all over the praecordium and also at the back of the left chest. On screening, the lung fields were clear and showed no pulsation. Red cells, 6,500,000 ; Hb, 128% ; haematocrit, 56. Circulation time (Dr. Allanby) : arm to tongue, 10.5 seconds ; arm to lung, 8.4 seconds (indicates right to left shunt).

Cardiac catheterization (Drs. Zak and Hollings): pressure in right ventricle, 53 mm. Hg ; pressure in pulmonary artery, 13 mm. Hg. Oxygen saturation in superior vena cava, 56% ; in right pulmonary artery, 67% ; in femoral artery, 77%. This was taken to indicate pulmonary stenosis with a right to left shunt.

A diagnosis of Fallot's tetralogy was made, although the presence of an associated valvular stenosis was considered probable.

Operation (March 23, 1948)

Intratracheal cyclopropane was given by Dr. Helliwell. Two bottles of plasma were infused, followed by one bottle of blood. A left inframammary incision was made and the chest opened through the second interspace, with later division of the second and third costal cartilages ; a considerable number of collateral vessels were encountered.

As soon as the heart was exposed the smooth globular dilatation of the pulmonary artery within the pericardium was seen ; a fine jetlike thrill could also be felt. The pericardium was opened ; the pulmonary artery was now seen to be dilated to a diameter of about 2.5 cm. and was thin-walled, with dark blood easily seen through it. The artery beyond the dilatation was small, lax, showed no visible pulsation, and was rather less than 1.5 cm. in diameter. There were no sinuses of Valsalva. Careful palpation again confirmed the jetlike nature of the thrill, which seemed to arise from the level of the valves ; moreover, at times it seemed as if one could actually see the white cone of the valvular stenosis through the thin wall.

In addition to applying swabs wet with procaine solution to the heart 1 ml. was injected into the wall of the ventricle. A double row of mattress sutures was inserted and a small incision made to allow a curved cannula to be introduced. The pressure in the ventricle was only 5 cm. of saline, and was the same in the pulmonary artery ; it was felt that this low pressure was the result of manipulation of the heart. A probe 3 mm. in diameter was now passed into the ventricle, and was felt to catch on the valves, suggesting a diaphragmatic stenosis. It was decided not to pass a cardioscope in view of the low blood pressure.

The valvulotome was now inserted, and was felt to catch on the valves and then to pass on into the pulmonary artery. After a pause the valves were further dilated with forceps. A pressure reading was again taken ; this showed a mean of 15 cm. of saline in both the ventricle and the pulmonary artery, with obvious fluctuation in systole and diastole. The incision was now closed with three mattress sutures ; the pericardium was not sewn to it.

The general condition at the end of the operation was satisfactory ; the systolic blood pressure was 70 mm. Hg.

Post-operative Course

Although the patient began to come round at the end of the operation she became very drowsy the same evening, and on the next morning was still drowsy and had a complete left-sided hemiplegia. She was slightly blue even in the oxygen tent. Dr. McArdle, who saw her, thought the hemiplegia might be due to an embolism rather than to thrombosis.

Her general condition steadily improved and her colour became and remained a good pink. The paralysis showed no sign of improvement for over three weeks. By April 22 she was able to move the upper arm, elbow, hip, and knee, but hand and foot movements were still absent. At that time she was up most of the day in a chair with no distress. Red cells,

4,600,000 ; Hb, 92% ; haematocrit, 48. On April 27 arterial oxygen saturation was 88.5%.

Comment.—There seems little doubt that there has been considerable improvement in the cardiac condition, and the fall in blood count and haematocrit reading (both of which are now normal) and the rise in the oxygen saturation percentage are most encouraging. Unfortunately the persistence of the hemiplegia makes it impossible to assess the actual functional improvement. It is thought that the paralysis will soon improve enough to allow the patient to move about by herself.

Conclusion

These three cases are by no means precise, but the results are considered to be encouraging enough to be recorded in this preliminary communication. They serve, at any rate, to show that pulmonary valvulotomy is a feasible operation, and all three patients have survived the procedure. The result in the first may be classed as moderately successful so far ; in the second the result is good ; in the third it would appear to be good, but is as yet indeterminate functionally.

Two of the patients were of an age when the prognosis is ordinarily poor and when any operation carries a grave risk ; both were very severely disabled. There can be no doubt that far better results are to be anticipated in younger patients, but it has not yet been possible to extend the operation to the younger age groups, although it is intended to do so.

The vascular complications in the first and third cases are disturbing and disappointing. The first case teaches us that a careful watch must be kept for signs of peripheral arterial embolism after cardiotomy so that immediate embolectomy can be considered. Arterial thrombosis, even to the extent of hemiplegia, occurs with the Blalock operation just as often. Presumably it is most likely to occur when the blood pressure falls to a low figure for some time, especially in the presence of polycythaemia.

Much still remains to be done in the development of this operation in the treatment of " blue children " suffering from pulmonary stenosis, but the results in these three cases are encouraging enough to justify proceeding further with it. It should be made clear that it is not suggested that this operation is meant to supplant the Blalock operation. As it stands at present it is of use in only a small proportion of cases ; until a method can be found to relieve the subvalvular stenosis (if indeed this is possible), the Blalock operation must continue to take precedence. However, unless the Blalock operation is considered to have solved the problem of *morbus caeruleus* completely, it is essential to try to develop new and alternative measures.

I am indebted to Dr. Maurice Campbell, under whose care all these patients were, for most of the case histories, which are made from his own notes.

REFERENCES

Allen, D. S., and Graham, E. A. (1922). *J. Amer. med. Ass.*, **79**, 1028.
Blalock, A., and Taussig, H. B. (1945). Ibid., **128**, 189.
Crafoord, C., and Nylin, G. (1945). *J. thorac. Surg.*, **14**, 347.
Cutler, E. C., and Beck, C. S. (1929). *Arch. Surg.*, **18**, 403.
Doyen, E. (1913). *Pr. méd.*, **21**, 860.
Gross, R. E., and Hubbard, J. P. (1939). *J. Amer. med. Ass.*, **112**, 729.
Pribram, B. O. (1926). *Arch. klin. chir.*, **142**, 458.
Rehn, L. (1897). Ibid., **55**, 315.
Souttar, H. S. (1925). *British Medical Journal*, **2**, 603.
Tuffier, T. (1913). *Trans. Internat. Cong., Med. Sect.*, **7**, Pt. 2, p. 249. London.

The British Red Cross Society has published a neatly illustrated pamphlet (price 1s., by post 1s. 1½d.) by Air Marshal Sir Harold Whittingham, entitled *ABC of First Aid Treatment*. It is suitable as a short manual of reference or for refreshing the first-aider's memory.

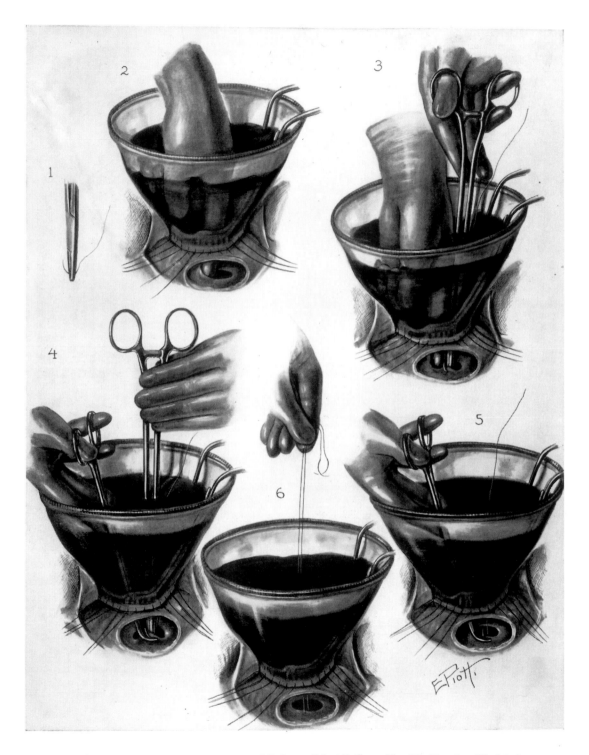

A Method for Surgical Closure of Interauricular Septal Defects.—Robert E. Gross, Elton Watkins, Jr., Alfred A. Pomeranz, and Edward I. Goldsmith.

(Legend on opposite page.)

SURGERY

GYNECOLOGY AND OBSTETRICS

VOLUME 96   JANUARY, 1953   NUMBER 1

A METHOD FOR SURGICAL CLOSURE OF INTERAURICULAR SEPTAL DEFECTS

ROBERT E. GROSS, M.D., F.A.C.S., ELTON WATKINS, JR., M.D.,
ALFRED A. POMERANZ, M.D., and EDWARD I. GOLDSMITH, M.D.,
Boston, Massachusetts

OPENINGS in the interauricular septum allow shunting of blood from the left to the right atrium, thereby increasing the flow through the right side of the heart and through the pulmonary circulation. Although the condition is frequently encountered as the sole cardiac abnormality, its influence on longevity is poorly documented. In the average run of cases, there seems to be little doubt that a septal defect reduces life expectancy. While there is no direct correlation between the size of a septal opening and the duration of life, in general the smaller defects are known to be compatible with a long and active existence, while the larger openings are very apt to bring about right-sided heart failure or fatality in childhood or early adult years. If possible, it is highly desirable to find some surgical means whereby the larger defects can be closed and

From the Surgical Service of The Children's Hospital and the Department of Surgery, Harvard Medical School.

These investigations were aided by grants from the American Heart Association, Inc., the National Heart Institute of the United States Public Health Service, the Oregon Heart Association, and the Dazian Foundation for Medical Research.

cardiac invalidism or fatality thereby be prevented. With careful clinical evaluation and with the use of modern ancillary diagnostic methods, it should be possible to select those humans who have atrial defects of considerable size and who might logically be expected to be in considerable danger from the abnormality. Such patients would constitute a group who should be greatly benefited by an adequate corrective procedure.

Described is a method devised for the closure of interauricular septal defects. Investigations in the Laboratory for Surgical Research have permitted development and perfection of the technique; experiences gained from surgical undertakings in humans indicate that the method is of practical value for treatment of interauricular septal defects in man.

METHODS PREVIOUSLY ADVOCATED FOR CLOSURE OF INTERAURICULAR SEPTAL DEFECTS

To date, various methods have been suggested, or have been attempted, for closure of interauricular septal openings; they fall

Fig. 16. Method of placing sutures in the edge of a septal defect, working through an atrial well. 1, Atraumatic needle carrying No. 000 Deknatel silk. Position of needle in needleholder. 2, Left index finger exploring the septal defect and identifying its margin. 3, With the right hand, a 10 inch long, diamond-jawed needle holder carries the needle into place, grasping 3 or 4 millimeters of the septal edge. 4, The needle holder is given to an assistant who keeps upward traction on it. The presenting point of the needle is palpated with left index finger and grasped with a right angle clamp. 5, Original needle holder removed, right angle clamp still grasping the needle. 6, Needle recovered. When a septal closure is to be made by direct suture, the 30 inch threads should carry an atraumatic needle at either end to facilitate placement of suture through both sides of the septal margins.

1

into four general categories: (1) external trans-fixion of the auricles with mattress sutures placed in the plane of the septum; (2) invagi-nation of atrial appendages, or lateral wall of an auricle, to plug the defect; (3) introduction of plastic material to cover the orifice; (4) closure of the opening under direct vision while the septum is isolated from the circula-tion by a special clamp or while blood is diverted from the opened heart.

1. Murray has passed large mattress sutures of silk through the heart, placing these approx-imately in the plane of the atrial septum. Snugging up of these sutures compresses the heart anteroposteriorly, and in some cases partially diminishes the size of the atrial opening. Certainly, the method gives no promise of closing a septal defect completely. Although clinical improvement has been re-ported in several patients subjected to this procedure, no decisive evidence has been pre-sented yet to show that the shunts have actu-ally been reduced.

2. Various workers have devised methods for invaginating the atrial appendages or the lateral wall of an auricle to occlude a septal opening. Swan and his co-workers have in-verted both the right and left auricular ap-pendages to the septum, occluding the defect by holding the inverted appendages in this position with mattress sutures which pass through both of the appendage tips. The use of this procedure in humans has been aban-doned by Swan, because of the danger of par-tially obstructing orifices of the pulmonary veins. Santy and his associates reported the plugging of a small septal opening by inverting the tip of an auricular appendage through it. Cohn has suggested inversion of the right auricular wall toward the septum, anchoring it in this position by sewing it to the septum with sutures which have been introduced from the exterior of the heart. Bailey has modified this by introducing a finger through the auricular appendage, so that the digit inside of the auricular cavity could guide the place-ment of the sutures around the edges of the septal defect. While these various techniques of inversion of an auricular wall (or append-age) to the septum might be highly satisfac-tory for closure of centrally placed defects, it

is well to remember that many of the septal openings in humans are located very high, very low, or very far forward, so that the in-version of an appendage (or auricular wall) to occlude them would almost certainly give partial obstruction of the superior vena cava, the inferior vena cava, the coronary sinus, the tricuspid valve, or the pulmonary veins.

3. Experimentally produced atrial defects have been closed successfully with appliances made of plastic materials. Hufnagel and Gillespie have accomplished this in animals through an incision in the atrial appendage (controlled by a pursestring suture), intro-ducing a two piece button which is manipu-lated into such a position that it occludes the defect. One disc is placed on the left of the septum and the other on the right side; then the two can be screwed to each other by a simple and ingenious handle, the discs being anchored into place by grasping edges of septum around the periphery of the septal opening. The secure placement of such but-tons requires a rim of septal tissue around a considerable portion of the circumference of the defect—a condition which is all too fre-quently absent in the naturally occurring malformations.

Martin and Essex have described the intro-duction of sheets of plastic material into the heart of dogs through an incision made in the atrial wall. Sutures are attached to this pros-thesis. The plate is secured in place by passing the threads from within the atrium to the external surface of the heart approximately in the plane of the septum. It is obvious that the edge of a defect near the annulus of the tri-cuspid valve could not be firmly closed by this method. No accurate method is suggested for placement of the sutures, or for positioning the prosthesis. We are convinced that it is impossible to accomplish either of these ma-nipulations in a reasonably satisfactory way by palpation through a thickened lateral wall of an auricle.

4. In attempts to close septal defects in dogs under direct vision Swan and his co-workers and Martin and Essex have tem-porarily occluded the caval inflow and have opened the heart for short periods of time while the circulation was thus interrupted.

This drastic maneuver, while tolerated temporarily, cannot be continued for more than a few minutes; it would certainly seem to be impractical for the closure of large defects. Furthermore, it is quite doubtful (in the presence of septal openings) whether it would be possible to prevent embolization of air into the systemic arteries.

A simple method for the repair of septal defects under direct vision has been suggested by Dodrill, who constructed a special ring-shaped clamp for temporary compression of the lateral walls of both atria against the septum. Although it is possible to incise the auricular wall within the ring of this clamp and have a bloodless field, the operative area is small and is entirely limited to the central portion of the septum; the method will probably have little use for closure of septal defects in man. Furthermore, serious arrhythmias and heart failure were observed during the temporary applications of such a clamp.

Considerable information has been accumulated regarding the technical designs and capabilities of various mechanical pump-oxygenators which could divert blood from the heart while the organ is temporarily open. Little information is yet available concerning the use of these appliances during actual intracardiac operations on humans. Dennis and his associates have reported experiences in the use of a mechanical heart-lung machine attached to a human, with an attempt at suture of an atrial defect under direct vision after opening the heart. To date, no successful repair has been reported by this method. While enormous strides have been made in the perfection of machines for temporary diversion of blood from the heart, there is yet much to be learned concerning the various problems dependent upon the use of these during intracardiac operations in humans.

Summary. The various methods listed which have been suggested or have been tried for the obliteration of auricular septal openings in man have focused attention of surgeons on the problems at hand. Obviously, some of the techniques will not be of practical value. Others will be found to be very satisfactory for treatment of certain kinds of openings but ineffective or hazardous for others. It is evi-

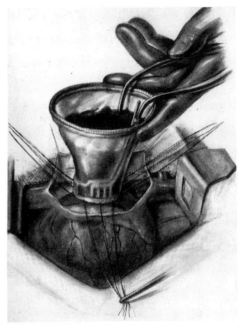

Fig. 1. Type of small, rubber atrial well attached to the right auricle of a dog. From the opened auricle, blood rises up into the rubber well.

dent that a more versatile method must be developed if we are to be able to treat all variations of septal anomalies which are known to occur in humans.

LABORATORY STUDIES IN THE DEVELOPMENT AND PERFECTION OF AN ATRIAL WELL

As a new approach to the problem of surgically closing interauricular septal apertures, it seemed to us that it might be possible to attach temporarily to the heart some sort of a hollow cylinder, into the base of which the auricle could be opened. Blood would rise up into the receptacle for a distance equal to the intra-auricular pressure, which should not be more than a few centimeters. If it were possible to couple such an appliance to the heart, it might then be feasible to work through this pool of blood in a blind manner, but deliberately with the guidance of exploring fingers, so that a septal opening could be approached and could be occluded by some appropriate means. Our initial experiences involved considerable trial and error evaluation of various ways of securing a rubber cylinder or "well" to the side of the auricle, locating a well in the

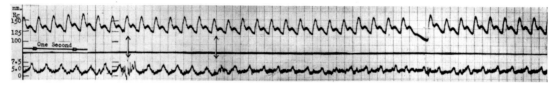

Fig. 2. Continuous pressure recording during the opening of the right atrium of a dog. Top tracing is carotid arterial pressure; lower tracing is effective right atrial pressure. A rubber well has already been sutured to the side of the right atrium. At the first arrow, the atrial clamp was released; by the time of the second arrow, the atrial well was widely open. Note the absence of any important influence on carotid arterial pressure or atrial pressure.

best possible location for giving the optimum access to the atrial septum, and of studying methods for prevention of coagulation of blood in the appliance.

To attach a piece of rubber to the surface of the heart in a leakproof manner, it was hoped that a union could be made with rubber cement or other adhesive material, but all of these were found to be ineffectual. Without enumerating the various methods which we found to be unreliable, it was eventually discovered that it was possible to join a hollow rubber bag to an auricle with a number of interrupted stitches of No. 0000 Deknatel silk, as indicated in Figure 1. The coupling together of the two structures required no more than 10 to 15 minutes; the junction could be made watertight.

Numerous designs for a rubber well were tried before evolving the one which seemed to be most suitable for the purposes we had in mind. For work on dogs, a satisfactory form is shown in Figure 1. It is made of latex rubber, is 0.38 millimeter thick, is 10 centimeters high, has an upper orifice 10 centimeters in diameter, this opening being held expanded by a circular stainless steel spring incorporated into the rubber. The lower orifice is 3 centimeters in diameter and its rim has been reinforced to a thickness of 1 millimeter to withstand the piercing of sutures and the stretching to which it is subjected.

Two special instruments were required. One was a clamp, to pinch off and isolate a small segment of the atrium while the well was being attached. The second was a self-retaining retractor for insertion into the slit in the atrial wall (at the base of the well) so that the auricular opening could be spread to an adequate diameter for allowing fingers to pass into the auricle.

Early in the studies, it became evident that it was easier to approach the septum through the right atrium than through the left one, because a larger surface of atrial wall was available, a better angle of approach was afforded, the septum lay higher in the surgical field, and finally, the venae cavae would be available if at any time it seemed desirable to occlude them temporarily.

Exposure of the heart and attachment of a well. One hundred and fourteen adult mongrel dogs, ranging in weight from 17 to 26 kilograms, were employed to develop a method of attachment of an atrial well and also to become proficient in the performance of the

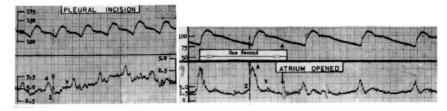

Fig. 3. Observations on circulatory dynamics at opening of pleura and at opening of an atrium. Top tracing is of carotid arterial pressure; lower tracing is effective right atrial pressure. At the time of opening of the right pleura, the interatrial pressure at first rises (as suction effect of negative intrathoracic pressure is lost). The carotid arterial pressure shows a slight rise. At the time of opening the atrium there is a fall in the effective atrial pressure and there is no change in the carotid arterial pressure.

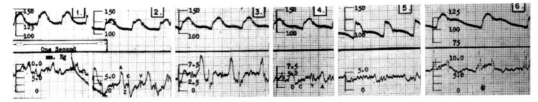

Fig. 4. Carotid arterial pressure (above) and effective right atrial pressure (below) during various phases of an atrial well operation on a dog. 1, Preoperative tracing, following nembutal anesthesia. 2, After incision of chest wall, but before opening of pleura. 3, Thirty minutes after opening of right pleural sac. The atrial pressure has risen. 4, Thirty seconds after opening right atrium into a rubber well. The effective atrial pressure and the carotid arterial pressure have fallen slightly. 5, After creation of an inter-atrial septal defect and then closure of it by the suture onlay of a plastic disc. By now the well had been open 45 minutes. There has been some fall in arterial pressure, but it is still at an adequate level. 6, After completion of operation. The atrial well has been removed, the pericardium closed, the lung expanded, and the chest closed. Following this restoration of subatmospheric intrathoracic pressure, the effective atrial pressure has been raised and the arterial pressure has become stabilized at a higher level.

maneuvers. Anesthesia was induced with intravenous nembutal. Atropine was given to minimize any deleterious reflex reactions. Lung aeration was provided by a mechanical insufflator during the thoracotomy. Oxygen was given after the cardiac manipulations were started. In the latter part of the series, all animals received transfusions of unmatched whole dog blood in amounts which were sufficient to replace that which had been lost from the circulation.

The right pleural space was entered through the fifth or sixth intercostal muscles. Ten cubic centimeters of 2 per cent solution of procaine hydrochloride were injected into the pericardial sac, which was then entered parallel and anterior to the phrenic nerve. The lung was packed away by gauze pads. The posterior flap of opened pericardium was pulled upward with traction sutures, a maneuver which helped to raise the heart in the operative field and make it more accessible.

The best exposure of all parts of the septum was obtained by the placement of a well very low on the right atrial wall. A segment of the auricle was isolated by the application of an atrial clamp. The isolated portion was then incised and the well was secured around its periphery with interrupted stitches. The strands of silk were left long to facilitate traction and manipulation of them during the opening of the well. The inner surface of the well was moistened with heparin solution and the atrial clamp released so that the blood could flow up into it. At this point, traction on the anterior and posterior silk sutures at the base of the well pulled open the auricular orifice and this facilitated insertion of the self-retaining retractor into it. Both the retractor and the rubber well could then be supported by one hand of an assistant.

In the earlier experiments, animals were completely heparinized to prevent clotting of blood in the open well. There was a prohibitive mortality from postoperative hemothorax, despite careful hemostasis and the administra-

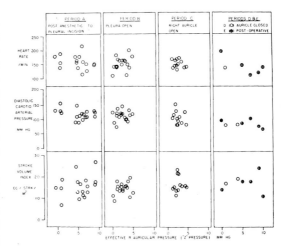

Fig. 5. Observations on heart rate, carotid diastolic arterial pressure, and the stroke volume index during various periods of atrial well operations on dogs. Fifty-five observations from 8 animals have been plotted. Period A, Following induction by nembutal anesthesia. Period B, Following opening of pleural sac to atmospheric pressure. Period C, Following opening of the right auricle into a rubber well. Period D, Following closure of the auricle and, Period E, following closure of the chest. The significant finding is the absence of any important deviation from the general levels of the pulse rate, arterial pressure, and stroke volume during period C when the well is open.

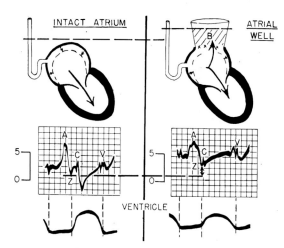

Fig. 6. Influence of an atrial well on the dynamics of ventricular filling. Left, With the intact atrium, the atrial pressure is at a low level but the contraction of atrial systole is effective in propelling blood into the relaxed ventricle. Right, With an atrial well in place, the atrial pulse wave is damped, because masses of blood fluctuate in and out of the well during each atrial contraction. An elevation of end-diastolic atrial pressure (Z) compensates for the loss of effectual atrial contraction. At the bottom, a schematic ventricular pulse is shown for purposes of orientation to the components of the atrial pressure pulse.

tion of adequate amounts of protamine sulfate after operation. It was soon found that blood could be prevented from clotting in a well by merely adding to it every few minutes a few cubic centimeters of 0.01 per cent heparin solution in 0.9 per cent sodium chloride. No animal received more than 20 milligrams of heparin. Following operation, it was not necessary to inactivate any small amount of heparin which had entered the general circulation. Pulmonary embolization was not observed in any instance.

Intracardiac manipulations. With the well open it was possible to introduce exploring fingers into an auricular cavity and to identify easily and accurately the caval orifices, the tricuspid valve, the coronary sinus, and the entire septum including the fossa ovalis and the limbus. The eustachian valve was difficult to identify in those animals where it was thin or rudimentary.

Removal of atrial well; closure of atrium. After intracardiac exploration or manipulations had been carried out, the well could be very simply removed by withdrawing the self-retaining retractor, replacement of a clamp

across the auricle to shut off the base of the well from the general auricular cavity, and then cutting the various silk sutures which had anchored the rubber appliance to the heart. There was no difficulty in repairing the auricle with interrupted figure-of-eight stitches of No. 0000 Deknatel silk. After lavage of any blood from the pericardial sac, the latter could be closed loosely.

PHYSIOLOGIC STUDIES OF CARDIOVASCULAR SYSTEM WHILE AURICLE WAS OPENED INTO AN ATRIAL WELL

Operative manipulations on the wall of an auricle frequently set up extrasystoles. Serious disorders of rhythm were extremely rare after completion of the attachment and during the time when the appliance was being left open. Studies on the cardiovascular dynamics were conducted on a small group of animals. Pressures were measured[1] in the carotid artery, the right atrium, and the right pleural space (Figs. 2, 3, 4, and 5). From these data, various calculations could be made. It was found that: (a) After opening the well, the wave of atrial systole (designated *A* on the tracings) is damped but is not abolished. (b) The other components of the atrial pulse are also damped. (c) There is a rise of mean atrial pressure and end-diastolic pressure after the well has been open for several minutes. The end-diastolic pressure (designated *Z*) is the pressure in the atrium at the end of ventricular diastole and is an important determinant of the volume of ventricular filling. The observed elevation of end-diastolic pressure is thought to be a compensatory mechanism whereby the animal maintains ventricular

[1]The pressure measurements were made with capacitance manometers and a two-channel direct-writing oscillograph. The hydraulic and recording systems demonstrated a satisfactory frequency response during square wave impact experiments. Atrial and pleural pressure pulses were calibrated frequently with a saline manometer graduated directly in equivalent mercury pressures and corrected to a zero point at the uppermost wall of the right atrium as measured at each operation. The value, *effective atrial pressure*, was calculated as the difference between the pressure within the atrium and the pressure outside the atrium in the closed heart, e.g. the pleural pressure, thereby correcting for variations in subatmospheric intrathoracic pressure. The pleural pressure was assumed to equal atmospheric pressure when the chest was open. All atrial pressure observations reported are typical values recorded late in expiration or late between insufflator blasts. Stroke volume indices were calculated by the modified Hamilton-Remington arterial pulse contour method (9) using enlarged camera obscura tracings of the carotid pulse.

filling in the absence of competent atrial pulsation. (d) Following the time that blood had been allowed to escape up into a well, there was a tendency for the peripheral arterial pressure to fall slightly. Undoubtedly, this was due to the loss of blood from the circulation by the segregation of it into the atrial well but in addition there must have been the influence of those factors which prevail during any long and complicated thoracotomy. The peripheral arterial pressure could be kept at a satisfactory level by the intravenous transfusion of blood shortly after a well had been opened.

We could find no precise relationship between preoperative atrial pressure and the height to which blood would rise in the open well at operation. When effective atrial pressure was low after induction of nembutal anesthesia, no fall of pressure occurred when the pleural sac was opened, but when effective atrial pressure was maintained after barbiturate administration, an appreciable drop of atrial pressure occurred as the chest was opened. This phenomenon resulted in wide variations of preoperative effective atrial pressure falling into a narrow low range by the time the well was to be opened. Consequently, fluid levels in the well were never disturbingly high.

There was no evidence of cardiac decompensation in the dogs as a result of well operations. In Figures 4 and 5 it can be seen that during successive periods of the operation, the response of the myocardium does not alter, since arterial pressure and stroke volume values late in the operative procedures are comparable to those during early periods of the operation. This was observed in spite of the fact that the well was kept open for periods up to 1 hour. It is likely that in these animals the wells could have been left open for much longer intervals without deleterious effects.

CREATION OF INTERAURICULAR DEFECTS

By working through atrial wells, interauricular septal openings were created. After a small opening was made in the center of the fossa ovalis by puncture with a hemostat, the edges around this wound could be grasped

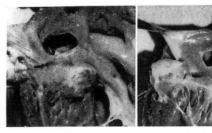

Fig. 7. Interauricular defects made in dogs, working through an atrial well and cutting out portions of the septum. Left, Defect 22 days after operation, the opening measures 2.0 centimeters in maximum dimensions. Right, Auricular septal defect 3 months after its establishment. The opening measures 1.5 centimeters in diameter. Probe lies in the coronary sinus.

with a curved hemostat, elevated, and the defect enlarged by peripheral excision of tissue. The excised substance was always held in the hemostat so that tissue embolization did not occur. Defects could be made, varying in size up to 2.5 centimeters in diameter. Creation of an opening was followed by the appearance of arterialized bright red blood in the well, without an appreciable change in the level of blood within the well.

Recent publications have emphasized the difficulty of making septal orifices in laboratory animals which will remain open permanently. There is rather general agreement that artificially made holes of small size can close spontaneously and rather promptly. However, we believe that this is not entirely true when openings of great size are made. While it is evident that there is some cicatrization in the surrounding septum and a definite diminution in the size of the septal opening large windows will remain for considerable periods of time (Fig. 7).

STUDY OF METHODS FOR CLOSURE OF INTERAURICULAR SEPTAL DEFECTS

By carrying out manipulations through atrial wells, attempts were made to close artificially made atrial defects in 68 dogs. Four general methods for obliteration were studied: (1) by sewing over the defect pieces of animal tissue, such as an excised atrial appendage, a plaque of pericardium, or a segment of vein; (2) by the application of Hufnagel double disc plastic buttons; (3) by the onlay of a sheet of plastic material which

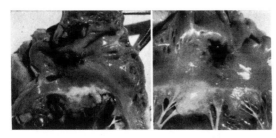

Fig. 8. Experimental closure of artificially made inter-auricular septal defect by sewing a piece of free auricular appendage over the opening. Left, Appearance in right auricle 14 days after operation. There is complete closure of the defect by the graft. Right, View in the left atrium.

was sutured to the surrounding septum; (4) by direct stitching and approximation of the septal edges.

1. *Atrial appendage graft.* A resected portion of atrial appendage presents many desirable characteristics when used as an intra-cardiac graft. It is organic tissue and it is easily available in the operative field. Its bulk makes for ease of handling. In 22 animals auricular appendage grafts were used to close septal defects. Eleven of these were autologous. For the other 11 experiments, atrial appendages were removed from donor dogs under aseptic conditions, sealed in sterile plastic envelopes, and stored in carbon dioxide ice deep-freeze at −76 degrees C. for periods between 3 and 14 weeks. In each experiment a piece of appendage of appropriate size was sutured to the interauricular septum in such a manner as to close over and plug the existing artificially made defect.

Surface thrombus formation on these grafts rarely exceeded a millimeter or two in thickness and was usually most prominent in the

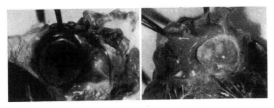

Fig. 9. Experimental closure of artificially made inter-auricular septal defect by application of Hufnagel double disc buttons. Left, Showing button in place, covering the septal opening. Dog sacrificed at end of operation. Right, Heart from an animal sacrificed 12 weeks after insertion of buttons. The button is completely incorporated within the substance of the septum and is entirely covered by endothelium.

declivities between the trabeculae carneae of the graft and at the junctions between graft and septum. In successive weeks, keeping pace with organization of the graft, there was gradual contraction of the graft to approximately one third of its original size. Within a few weeks the graft became covered with a smooth coat of endothelium, presenting an irregular but smooth interior to the auricle (Fig. 8). When examined beyond 3 months, the identity of the graft was completely lost and the region was represented by a small contracted scar, with smooth surfaces.

Histologic examination of such grafts at different times after their placement showed certain changes. In about a week the muscle fibers were becoming pale, homogeneous, and eosinophilic; there was disappearance of the nuclei and loss of muscle striations. These findings persisted and progressed for several weeks until the muscle was replaced by connective tissue. At no time was there any tendency to fragmentation or disintegration of the graft substance. Instead, its unity was maintained, in spite of progressive loss of its histologic elements, and the entire structure gradually became completely replaced with fibrous tissue and formed an integral part of the septum. Endothelization was usually complete in 10 to 14 days. Beyond 3 months there was a decrease in local vascularity, a condensation of the connective tissue, and a greater deposition of collagenous substance. In scattered areas the deposition was extremely dense and consisted of whorls of deeply basophilic material. In some grafts, small deposits of calcium were seen.

There was little difference in the overall results from the autologous and the homologous appendage grafts, excepting that in the latter the process of healing was slower by several weeks; the same end result being eventually achieved.

Vein or pericardial graft. Segments of external jugular vein (turned inside out) or sections of pericardium were utilized as free grafts for closure of septal defects in 4 dogs; they were sewed into place. Thrombus formation was negligible. Most of these tissues underwent progressive histologic regression, were replaced by scar tissue which became a part of the septum, and became smooth covered by endothelium. However, there were important disadvantages in the use of either of these materials. First, veins of sufficient size were not obtainable for closure of very large defects. Second, pericardium was troublesome to work with because it was so thin and limpid that it was difficult to place a number of stitches around its periphery and through the septal wall without producing a hopelessly twisted mass of strings before all of these sutures could be tied when the graft was pushed down into the depths of the auricle.

2. Plastic buttons. Paired plastic buttons, fashioned after those described by Hufnagel and Gillespie were machined from lucite or kel-F and were used for occlusion of septal openings in 6 dogs. The plastic buttons were put into place with the handle devised by Hufnagel. One disc of the button was placed on the left side of the septum and its mate introduced on the right. The buttons were then screwed together, being held firmly apposed to each other by virtue of the central threaded stem and core which they possess (Fig. 9). Within a few minutes such plastic buttons were covered with a layer of fibrin or a sheet of thrombus less than a millimeter in thickness. This overlying fibrinous clot rapidly became organized and then covered by a continuous layer of endothelium within 2 or 3 weeks. The buttons were tolerated extremely well and became incorporated into the septum in an amazing way.

The greatest value of buttons is derived from the speed with which they can be inserted. All of the intracardiac manipulations could be completed within a few minutes. For their use, it was essential to have a complete margin of tissue around the septal opening for the prosthesis to grasp and hold on to.

3. Onlay of plastics, sewed into place. In 30 dogs, septal defects were closed by the onlay of discs or sheets of plastic materials which were sewed to the surrounding septum with silk sutures. Materials studied were nylon (0.13 mm. and 0.81 mm. thick), polyethylene (0.51 mm. and 1.52 mm. thick), and lucite (3.17 mm. thick). The meagerness of tissue reaction to these substances, when pure, has been described (6).

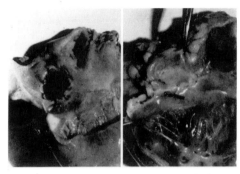

Fig. 10. Experimental closure of interauricular septal defect by the onlay of a sheet of nylon sutured into place with silk sutures around its periphery. Left, Photograph of plastic sheet sewed into place, animal sacrificed at the end of operation. Right, Animal sacrificed 16 weeks after closure of a septal defect by a sheet of nylon, 0.8 millimeter thick. The foreign material is well tolerated by the septum and is completely covered by fibrous tissue and endothelium.

Both nylon and polyethylene film are sufficiently soft and pliable to be cut readily by scissors and shaped to desired size at the operating table, yet stiff enough to be easily manageable. The alignment of numerous sutures around their periphery can be maintained. These materials are easily pierced with needles. Sutures are not cut by the edge of the plastic. Because of their extreme hardness, discs of lucite must be prepared before operation; they have to be machined to appropriate sizes; holes must be drilled around the edges of the plates to receive sutures.

After these various plastics were sewed onto septums, the rapidity with which they were covered was striking. The observed changes were closely similar for each of the substances.

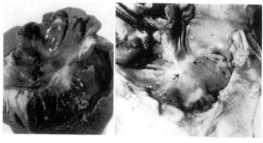

Fig. 11. Experimental closure of interauricular septal defects in dogs by direct suture of a septal opening. Left, Opening closed with interrupted silk stitches, animal sacrificed at end of operation. Right, Specimen from dog sacrificed 5 weeks after closure of interauricular septal defect by direct suture. Between the arrows is an irregular scarred area indicating the operative site. Silk sutures are completely incorporated within the substance of the septum.

Within a few hours after operation there was a fine layer of thrombus, less than a millimeter thick, on both sides of the foreign material. This thrombus was loosely adherent to the plastic but was tightly enmeshed in the sutures and the suture knots. Several dogs sacrificed 1 week after operation showed a slight increase in the thickness of the thrombus, usually not greater than 2 millimeters. By then the clot was generally compact, glistening, and smooth. After 2 weeks there was a rapid conversion of the thin purple-red thrombus to a fibrous covering, this change starting at the periphery and progressing toward the center. Endothelization was always complete in 2 or 3 weeks. Beyond 6 to 12 weeks plastics were encased in a tough, white fibrous membrane, which blended imperceptibly with the adjacent septal tissue. The plastic materials always became sequestrated within the septum; in no instance was there any formation of cyst around them.

The only disturbing reaction to plastics was the tendency for more pronounced thrombus formation on the plates of 0.81 millimeter nylon. These were solitary, sessile, rounded masses of clot as large as a centimeter in diameter. In a few months these became contracted, hard nubbins of scar tissue 2 to 4 millimeters in diameter, well covered by endothelium and firmly adherent to underlying structures. Embolization from these lesions was never demonstrated. Such a reaction might have been due to the presence of foreign substances (plasticizers) in the lot of nylon which was employed.

Our conclusions regarding these plastic materials (sewed into place) were as follows: All of the substances are tolerated very well and become covered over in an amazing way. *Lucite* is not practical because its great hardness requires that it be machined and also drilled beforehand. Furthermore, it is too rigid and will not adapt itself to those septa which do not have a flat contour. *Nylon* sheet is very satisfactory, can be cut with scissors at the operating table, and can be easily pierced with needles. The sheets 0.081 millimeter thick caused some reactions which, while apparently not harmful, might be best to avoid. Thinner sheets did not produce the

reaction and were very satisfactory. *Polyethylene* sheeting was highly satisfactory; the 1.52 millimeter thickness was unnecessarily heavy, while the 0.51 millimeter thickness had all the desirable characteristics. It could be cut easily, could be pierced with needles, had enough substance so that it did not flop or fold over, but yet would bend sufficiently to adapt itself to any irregularity of septal contour to which it was applied. It had sufficient body and stiffness so that it could easily be palpated and guided into place with fingers in the auricle. This material appeared to be overwhelmingly the one of choice for onlay closure of septal defects.

4. *Suture closure.* In 6 dogs, septal defects were closed by direct approximation of the septal borders with interrupted silk sutures. The animals were sacrificed at varying times up to 6 months. For the first few days there was a regional, fine layer of thin thrombus overlying the operative site. This gradually became organized and merged with the substance of the septum. The sutures always became buried in this cicatrix. Within 3 or 4 weeks the region was endothelialized and was represented solely by irregular, contracted scar, which was smoothly covered.

To suture septal defects, working through an atrial well might seem to present formidable problems of technique. We were surprised to find that with a little practice it was possible to carry out the manipulations of placement and tying of stitches in the depths of a pool of blood. It was not necessary to design special instruments for holding needles. A good holder is 10½ inches long and had diamond jaws which prevent a needle from turning. The needle is grasped as shown in Figure 16, 1. With the left index finger the margin of the septal defect can be palpated; with the needle holder in the right hand, the needle can be made to grasp and pierce the septal tissue, 3 or 4 millimeters back from its edge. The needle holder is then transferred to an assistant who carefully maintains the impalement of the needle by upward traction. The point of the needle can then be grasped with a right angle clamp, following which the original needle holder is released and removed. The right angle clamp can then draw the

GROSS ET AL.: CLOSURE OF INTERAURICULAR SEPTAL DEFECTS   11

needle out of the wound. It is highly important to use only atraumatic needles since this insures that (if lost) they can be instantaneously retrieved by pulling up on the silk thread which emerges from the well.

There is no clear-cut separation of defects into those which can or cannot be closed by direct stitching. In general, smaller openings (less than a centimeter in width) which have thick and firm substance in the adjacent septum can be sutured with a reasonable expectancy of obtaining a complete and permanent closure. Conversely, defects which are larger than 1 or 1.5 centimeters in width, which have only thin substance surrounding them, or which have incomplete rims of tissue, should not be sutured because too much tension will be placed on the stitches, some of the threads will tear out, and incomplete closures will result.

Summary. Attempts at obliteration of artificially made septal defects were carried out in 68 dogs, working through right atrial wells. The animals were sacrificed at varying periods of time up to 6 months after operation. Complete closures were observed in 60 animals at autopsy; in 8 dogs there were small residual holes ranging up to 4 millimeters in diameter. These incomplete closures almost certainly resulted from tearing out of stitches or the poor placement of sutures. Without doubt, success in the obliteration of septal defects is closely related to the extent of the operator's experience and his manual dexterity when working with a heart; in the last 30 of our attempts to repair septal apertures, the opening was found to be completely occluded at subsequent autopsy examination.

SURGICAL CLOSURE OF SEPTAL DEFECTS IN HUMANS

After laboratory experimentation with the atrial well approach to the interior of an auricle, it was felt justifiable to attempt closure of interauricular septal openings in humans. To date, 7 subjects have been operated upon. We are greatly indebted to Dr. Alexander S. Nadas and Dr. Walter Goodale for aid in study and care of these patients.

Believing that the atrial pressures to be encountered in man with cardiac anomalies

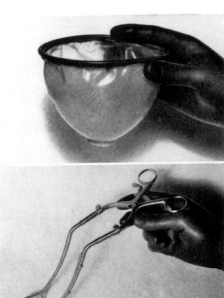

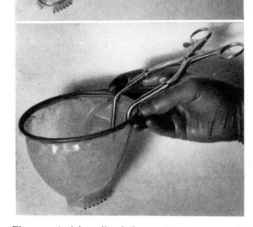

Fig. 12. Atrial well of large size, constructed for application to human hearts. Above, Photograph of the rubber well. Middle, Self-retaining retractor for insertion into the well and spreading of its neck. Below, Showing method of placement of retractor into the well so that its neck can be appropriately spread. An assistant can support both the retractor and the well as shown.

might be higher than those which had been found in normal dogs, a new and larger rubber well was designed to care for this contingency. A well was constructed which had a height of 15 centimeters, an upper orifice 13 centimeters in diameter, a lower orifice 5 centimeters in diameter, and a rather capacious contour which would admit an entire hand (Fig. 12). To accompany this, an atrial clamp was de-

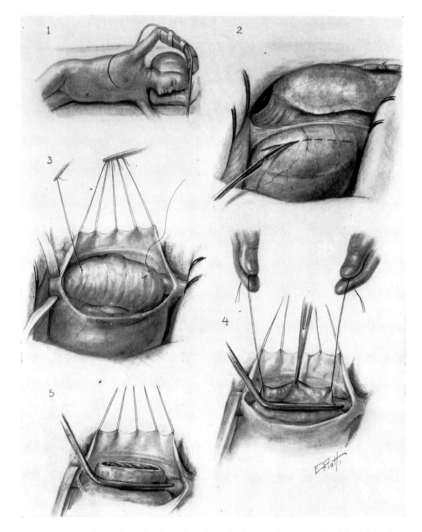

Fig. 13. Method of application of well to the human heart. 1, Position of patient on table. Surgical approach through the fifth interspace. 2, Lung falls toward the patient's back, pericardium being opened along the dotted line. 3, Flap of pericardium held upward and backward. Traction on this helps to raise heart into the operative field. Two traction sutures being applied to the greatly enlarged right atrium. 4, Segment of right atrium being held up while an atrial clamp is put into place to isolate this segment from the auricular cavity. 5, The isolated segment of atrium cut open.

vised, the jaws of which were 6 centimeters in length and which were prominently knurled so that they would not slip. Next, a self-retaining retractor of greater depth and with larger jaws was manufactured. When subsequently used on human patients, these devices were all found to be completely satisfactory.

At first, we were somewhat concerned about the height of columns of blood which would be encountered in human atrial wells, feeling that there might be little correlation with pressures which had been observed at pre-operative catheterization. In the 7 patients, the right atrial pressures before operation were 4, 8, 14, 8, 14, 15, and 7 centimeters of saline respectively. Generally, heights of blood columns in the wells at operation were much lower than these figures.

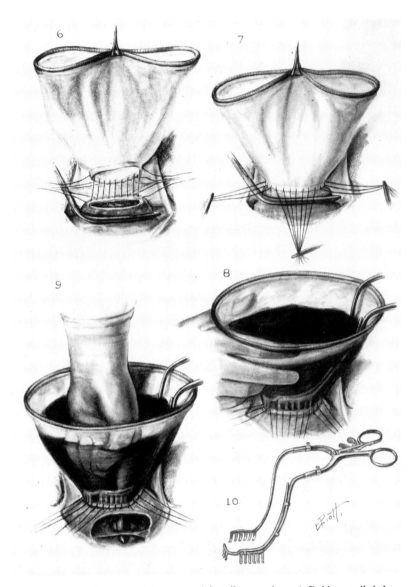

Fig. 14. Continuation of human atrial well operation. 6, Rubber well being brought into place and attached to atrial wall with interrupted silk sutures around the periphery of its lower rim. 7, Attachment of well to atrium completed. 8, Atrial clamp removed, allowing blood to flow up into the well. 9, Exploring hand run down through the pool of blood so that a finger can feel the interauricular septal defect and estimate the size and position of the septal opening as well as the nature of its edges. 10, Type of self-retaining retractor which holds open the atrial wall. An orifice 5 or 6 centimeters in diameter is sufficient to permit unhindered intracardiac manipulations.

Operation in each instance was under general anesthesia with ether by use of a tracheal tube and a closed system. Exposure was made throughout the entire length of the right fifth interspace, the sixth and seventh ribs being divided posteriorly and the fifth, fourth, and third cartilages cut near their sternal junctions. A wide opening of the chest wall was found to be essential. Techniques of applying and using a right atrial well are illustrated in

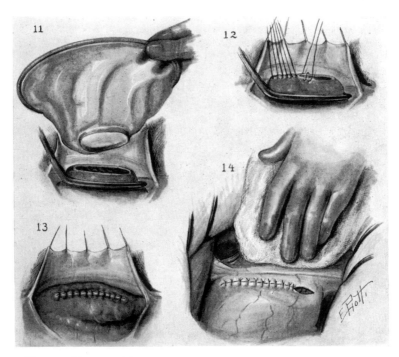

Fig. 15. Human atrial well operation, continued. Method of removal of the well at completion of operation. 11, The atrial clamp reapplied, after which the rubber well is cut away from the heart. 12, Closure of the atrial wall with interrupted figure-of-eight silk sutures. 13, Closure of auricle completed. Atrial clamp removed. 14, Closure of pericardial sac.

Figures 13, 14, and 15. In every case there was a greatly enlarged right auricle (as determined by roentgenographic study before operation and as confirmed at the operating table) so that there was plenty of auricular surface for attachment of the rubber appliance to the heart wall.

Because of the large flow of blood through the pulmonary circuit, the presenting right lung was always found to be heavy with blood, always had a distinct thrill in its central vessels, and had enormously distended and tense pulmonary veins where they could be seen behind the heart.

In 5 of the patients, 8 to 10 cubic centimeters of 2 per cent procaine were injected into the pericardial sac before opening it; in the other 2 this substance was not used. We are inclined to think that such use of procaine is not of real value in reducing the irritability of the heart. In some instances it seemed to depress the cardiac activity and to produce a mild fall in the peripheral arterial pressure.

We now prefer to omit the use of procaine as a routine measure and to bathe it onto the surface of only those hearts which seem to be irritable as an atrial well is being attached to it. In only 1 case was pronestyl employed.

After the pericardium was opened, it was dissected away from the terminal portion of the inferior vena cava, to make certain that this region was freed so that the atrial well could be placed as far inferiorly and posteriorly on the auricular wall as possible, thus to facilitate and give the best possible positioning for the transauricular approach to the septum.

Linen tapes were always passed around the inferior and the superior vena cava so that if a defect should be found very low or very high in the septum and near the orifice of either vena cava, the cava could be pulled forward and the plastic plate which was to be used for occlusion of the septal defect could be run up against and attached to the auricular wall just *medial* to the orifice of the cava. This would make sure that all caval blood would be diverted into the right atrium. The lower cava could be encircled with a tape either inside or outside of the pericardium. For the superior vena cava, it was found that encirclement of the structure within the pericardium gave irritation of the nearby sinoauricular node and produced disturbing extrasystoles. Therefore, it was best to run the tape around the superior vena cava just above the pericardium.

There was no difficulty in any instance attaching a rubber well to the auricular wall. This could be made completely leakproof. It took from 15 to 20 minutes to sew the appliance in place.

Before allowing blood to run up into a well, its interior was flushed with 0.04 per cent heparin in 0.9 per cent sodium chloride. After blood entered the well, a few cubic centimeters of this material were added by an assistant every few minutes. In no instance was there clotting. From time to time the operator's gloves were rinsed with heparin solution.

The wells were all tolerated in an extraordinary manner. In some cases there were a few extrasystoles during attachment of the rubber bag and the handling of the atrial well. These were never troublesome. The wells were left open for times varying from 12 minutes up to 2 hours and 5 minutes! There seemed to be no doubt that cardiovascular adjustments to the appliance could be made without difficulty, even in patients who previously had been in failure, and that there need be no haste during the intracardiac manipulations. It was possible to make deliberate and careful examination of the interior of an auricle and to carry out the various steps for closure of the defects which were found.

Regarding the use of transfusions during operation, three general rules were employed: (1) Immediately after opening the auricle into a rubber well, blood was given intravenously to compensate for that which had been "lost" into the rubber sac. This varied from 1 to about 300 cubic centimeters in amount. (2) From here on throughout that portion of the operation while the well was open, relatively small volumes of blood were infused, using only amounts which would be reasonable for an intrathoracic procedure of the given duration, throughout which very little blood was being lost. (3) After closure of the atrium, the blood which remained in the well (usually several hundred centimeters) was discarded and the patient was *not* transfused with a similar amount. By using these general guides, but altering them somewhat in relation to the patient's pulse rate and peripheral arterial pressure, there was no difficulty in any case in keeping the patient in a very satisfactory state during the operative procedure.

After removal of an atrial well, there was no problem in attaining a tight closure of the lateral wall of the auricle, this being accomplished with interrupted figure-of-eight stitches of silk. The pericardial sac was only loosely closed, so that any excess subsequent collection of fluid could escape into the pleural cavity. It was mandatory to drain the pleural sac for several days after operation so that any accumulation of blood (which might possibly arise from oozing from the chest muscles after the use of heparin) could be quickly evacuated. In all cases, examination of the clotting time showed this to be normal within a few hours after operation.

The appearance in all of the surviving patients of a peculiar postoperative syndrome of transient right-sided heart embarrassment suggests that for some reason there is a period of diminished function of the right ventricle, in spite of the fact that a large burden has been removed from the pulmonary circulation. The mechanism of this phenomenon is obscure and needs further study. It might be related to a hypervolemia, salt retention, or other fluid or electrolyte imbalance of a temporary sort. It tends to correct itself, but doubtless the readjustment could be hastened by appropriate measures if the exact nature of the disturbance were known.

Three general methods for closure of septal defects have been attempted in these patients: (1) by the use of Hufnagel double-disc buttons; (2) by the onlay of plastic sheets to cover septal openings; (3) by direct suture of smaller defects.

1. In 3 patients, with septal openings from 2.5 to 5 centimeters in diameter, lucite or

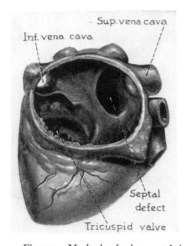 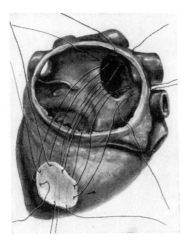 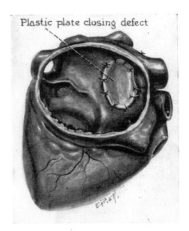

Fig. 17. Method of closure of interauricular septal defect in Case 4, by the application of a nylon sheet. Left, Showing the defect in the superior, posterior portion of the septum, there being an excellent rim of septal tissue inferiorly, but none at the base of the superior vena cava. Middle, All sutures in place. Wherever there is an edge of septal tissue to grasp, sutures are taken through it. Where no such edge exists, sutures are passed out through the atrial wall. Right, Plastic sheet securely anchored into place with silk sutures around its periphery. Where marginal sutures have been placed around the defect, these are tied within the atrium. Where there had been no rim of septal tissue, the sutures which pierce the auricular wall are anchored externally.

kel-F double disc buttons, varying in size from 3 to 4.5 centimeters in diameter, were employed. These choices all proved to be unwise ones. In these first human subjects there was some feeling of haste, and it seemed undesirable to keep the hearts open very long. It was felt that the quick application of a double disc button might put the least strain on the heart, each one of which was known to have had some degree of embarrassment before operation. There was an incomplete rim, or else there was only a very thin substance, around the periphery of the defects; it was impossible to place the buttons in such a way that good tissue could be grasped around their entire circumference. However, it was thought that possibly there was enough available tissue at least to anchor a button in place and provide a baffle which, while not completely occluding the orifice, would greatly cut down the size of the shunt and, therefore, be helpful. As a result of these improper decisions, death occurred in every case. The buttons all worked loose; one fell into the left auricle, another into the right auricle, and one still retained some anchorage at an edge but dropped over into the orifice of the tricuspid valve which it obstructed. In the first 2 cases cited, there was fatality within a few days. In the one

wherein the button had obstructed the tricuspid valve there was a rise of pressure in the right auricle which gave a right-left type of shunt through the persisting auricular defect, producing cyanosis (which had not been present before operation). At a second exploration 3 weeks later, the button was retrieved from the interior of the heart and the septal defect closed by direct suture. While the chest was being repaired the patient died. Such disasters would seem to make it evident that the use of these double disc buttons (which can be used so successfully for the occlusion of septal defects in dogs where there is a good rim around the entire periphery of the opening) will probably have very little usefulness in man where septal defects notoriously have incomplete margins and will, therefore, not hold buttons firmly in place.

2. In 3 subjects a septal defect was covered over with a sheet of nylon or polyethylene, sewed to the surrounding structures with interrupted silk stitches. In one of these, the plastic plate was made too large. It completely covered the septal opening but extended too far down over the annulus of the tricuspid valve. The plate had been well anchored posteriorly, superiorly, and anteriorly, but was not tightly tied down to the septum in the

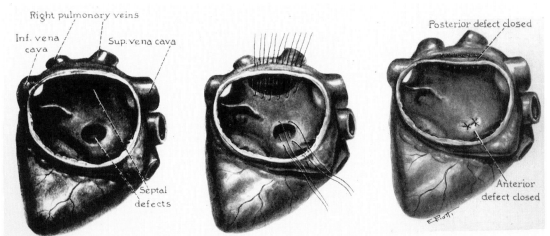

Fig. 18. Closure of interauricular septal defects in patient 5. Two openings were found. Left, There is a long narrow defect toward the posterior portion of the septum, there being no ridge of tissue along the posterior auricular wall. The smaller defect appears in the anterior part of the septum, there being good substance around its entire periphery to allow placement of sutures. Middle, Silk sutures appropriately placed for closure of the two defects. Right, All sutures snugged up and tied, for closure of the two openings.

region just above the annulus. Beneath this raised portion of the plastic plate, there was formation of a blood clot which then propagated downward into the orifice of the tricuspid valve, thereby partially occluding it and leading to death on the third day. In 2 other patients, polyethylene plates of suitable size and shape were fashioned and brought into place to cover the opening completely; they could be accurately held down around their peripheries with interrupted silk stitches (Fig. 17). These 2 children have had extremely satisfactory postoperative courses. Subsequent catheter studies have been performed in 1 of them; it shows the septum to be completely closed.

3. In patient 5, two septal apertures were found (Fig. 18). Because of the relatively small size or narrowness of these, it was decided to attempt primary suture. Various silk stitches were placed as shown in the sketches. Around the smaller anterior opening the tissues were very thin and there was some reason to believe that these might have been torn as the sutures were being tied. With the long, posterior defect there was no rim along the back wall of the atrium. It, therefore, seemed best to grasp the thick margin of septum and to pass the needles out of the back wall of the

auricle in a mattress stitch fashion, bringing these sutures to lie just to the right of the right pulmonary veins. Snugging up of these sutures pulled the septal edge backward and also indented the posterior wall of the auricle in a forward direction; the combination apparently completely closed off the area (when examined with an exploring finger). This child has had an amazing recovery. Whereas before she had been in chronic, right-sided heart failure, had marked limitation of activity, an enlarged liver, required digitalization, low salt diet, and other supportive measures, she now appears to be transformed into a different individual. The liver has receded almost to the costal margin. The child greatly enjoys playing tennis, which is an entirely new experience for her.

CASE REPORTS

CASE 1. D.K., an 8 year old girl, was admitted for treatment of congenital cardiac abnormality. At the age of 4 years, she had been hospitalized for ascites and severe congestive failure. At that time the cardiac shadow was found to be enormous. She had been digitalized since that time. There had been retarded physical development and diminished exercise tolerance. Cardiac catheterization had demonstrated conclusive evidence of an interatrial septal defect as well as a normal pulmonary vascular resistance.

Physical examination showed a poorly developed child with prominence of the left precordium. To the left the heart was enlarged to the anterior axillary line. At the apex was a loud systolic murmur and a mid-diastolic rumble; in the pulmonic region was a loud systolic murmur. The pulmonic second sound was duplicated and was much louder than the aortic second sound. The liver edge was palpable 1 centimeter below the costal margin. The neck veins were not distended.

Fluoroscopic examination showed right-sided enlargement of the heart, distinct fullness of the pulmonary artery, and moderate engorgement in the lung fields.

Electrocardiograms showed right bundle branch block and prominent P waves. Fluorescein circulation time was 10 seconds. Venous pressure was 70 millimeters of water.

First operation. On April 3, 1952, right thoracotomy was performed. The chest was opened through a posterolateral incision extending forward beneath the nipple. The pleural space was entered throughout the sixth interspace. The sixth and seventh ribs were divided posteriorly and the fifth and sixth costal cartilages were cut anteriorly; good exposure was obtained. The right auricle was greatly enlarged. There was a faint poorly localized systolic thrill over the heart. A large rubber well was attached to the prominence of the right atrial wall with interrupted No. 0000 Deknatel silk sutures. Although prior to placement of the well, the atrial pressure measured 9.2 centimeters of water by manometer reading, blood rose in the rubber appliance only 5 or 6 centimeters. A defect was found low in the septum, between the posterior atrial wall and the annulus of the tricuspid valve. Not knowing how much of an operative procedure the heart would stand, it was decided to insert a Hufnagel button as quickly as possible. A lucite button 3 centimeters in diameter was positioned. Although the defect had a rather complete rim of septal tissue, this was very thin. The steel prongs of the 3 centimeter button grasped the septal rim only a few millimeters back from the edge of the defect. After closure of the septal defect, the heart diminished greatly in size, and the diffuse thrill disappeared. The well had been open for 12 minutes; it was dismantled and the atrium closed with interrupted figure-of-eight sutures of No. 000 silk. During closure there was evidence of 2:1 atrioventricular blocking, but after closure was completed, the rhythm became normal. The pericardium was closed with interrupted sutures, leaving a defect superiorly for drainage of fluid.

Postoperative course. The initial response was good but within 24 hours there was slight cyanosis of the lips. Cyanosis became worse and was aggravated by exercise. There was progressive evidence of venous congestion, as indicated by distention of the neck veins. Fluorescein circulation time was prolonged to 14 seconds. Arterial oxyhemoglobin saturation was 70 per cent, rising only to 79.4 per cent on inhalation of pure oxygen. The presence of venous congestion and cyanosis, which was not relieved by oxygen inhalation, suggested that the button had become displaced so as to obstruct the tricuspid valve with resultant rise of right atrial pressure and production of a right-to-left shunting of blood through a persistent atrial defect. Fluoroscopic examination confirmed the suspicion that the button had become dislodged from its former position and had migrated to the area of the tricuspid valve. A second intracardiac exploration was carried out in an attempt to retrieve the button and also to attempt closure of the septal defect.

Second operation. On April 28, 1952, in spite of light fibrinous pleural adhesions and a healed suture line on the right atrium, no trouble was encountered in again attaching a large rubber well to the right atrium. Blood rose in the well 4 or 5 centimeters. The button was found to be attached at only one edge of the septal defect, and had flopped over downward and forward to lie within the tricuspid valve orifice. The main portion of the septal defect was open. The button was removed. The 2 centimeter septal defect was then closed by 4 interrupted sutures of No. 000 silk introduced through the well. The well was dismantled and the atrial incision closed with interrupted figure-of-eight sutures of No. 000 silk. As the chest was being repaired, the heart slowed and stopped. After a period of cardiac massage and injection of calcium and adrenalin, ventricular fibrillation was noted. Fibrillation was interrupted by a single electric shock. Synchronized and regular heart beats returned; they gradually increased in vigor. After the chest was closed, the skin color was poor, and peripheral artery pulsations were unobtainable. Within a few minutes a short convulsive seizure occurred, no heart sounds could be heard, and the presence of ventricular fibrillation was proved by electrocardiogram. Shortly thereafter, no electrical tracing could be obtained.

Autopsy. The atrial defect was completely closed by silk sutures. One suture had partially torn through the thin septal edge, but this did not compromise the closure. There were hemorrhages in the myocardium, lungs, subarachnoid space, and subdural space.

CASE 2. M.Z. was a 4 year old female. At the age of 7 months she was known to have a heart murmur. At 2 years, studies revealed right-sided cardiac enlargement and a moderate congestive failure, with basilar rales and a palpable spleen. She was maintained in a satisfactory manner by means of digitalization, a low salt diet, and occasional mercurial diuresis. She grew fairly well during this regimen. Her activity was not limited. There was no history of cyanosis.

Examination showed a slightly underdeveloped child in no distress. There was increased prominence of the left precordium. The apical cardiac impulse was 6 centimeters to the left of the midclavicular line. The apical first sound was accentuated and the pulmonic second sound was split. Prominent systolic murmurs were audible at the apex and in the pulmonic region, and there was an apical mid-diastolic rumble. The neck veins were distended. The spleen and liver were enlarged.

Fluoroscopic examination of the heart showed right ventricular enlargement. The auricles and the pulmonary artery were prominent. There was pulmonary vascular engorgement and a hilar dance.

Cardiac catheterization demonstrated the presence of an atrial left-to-right shunt of 6.7 liters per minute. The systemic flow was 3.3 liters per minute. Pulmonary vascular resistance was normal. Electrocardiograms showed right ventricular hypertrophy and right bundle branch block with prominent P waves. Fluorescein circulation time was 10 seconds.

Operation. Right thoracotomy was performed on April 3, 1952. The right atrium and right ventricle were hypertrophied and dilated. Pulmonary engorgement was pronounced. A large rubber well was attached to the right atrium. Although the atrial pressure prior to placement of the well had measured 20 centimeters of water, after attachment of the well and tilting the body 30 degrees with the legs downward, blood rose in the rubber well only 5 or 6 centimeters. A 2 centimeter defect was found low on the auricular septum. There was an incomplete rim of septal tissue around this. When the defect was partially occluded with two fingers, cardiac irregularity and weakened contractions were noted. It was deemed advisable to terminate the procedure rapidly by insertion of a Hufnagel button. A 3 centimeter lucite button was inserted so that there was no impingement on the coronary sinus or tricuspid annulus, and the atrium was closed after being open for 15 minutes. After closure of the defect, the heart decreased greatly in size. Its activity was markedly reduced as compared to its previous vigorous contractions. Pulmonary engorgement markedly diminished. Immediately after operation, the patient was in rather precarious condition. The radial pulse was only fair. The skin color was satisfactory.

Postoperative course. During the first 24 hours the patient responded but her course was unsatisfactory. The blood pressure remained low and in spite of transfusion and adequate intake of fluid, the urinary output was depressed to less than 400 cubic centimeters per 24 hours. A soft systolic murmur was audible just to the left of the sternum and a gallop rhythm was heard. Electrocardiogram on the second postoperative day showed high peaked T waves. Serum potassium at that time was 6.7 millequivalents per liter and serum sodium was 121 millequivalents per liter. By x-ray film, the button had obviously shifted its position and was apparently lying in the right atrium. Evidence of congestive failure became worse, as manifested by progressive distention of neck veins, hepatic enlargement, and appearance of basilar rales. She expired on the third postoperative day. Permission for autopsy could not be obtained.

CASE 3. D.C. was an 8 year old girl who was known to have congenital heart disease since birth. There had been cyanosis in the neonatal period but none since then. The child had always been considered to be "delicate." Activity was normal although she tired very easily. There was no history suggesting congestive failure.

On examination she was undernourished. The heart was enlarged to the left anterior axillary line. There was a loud systolic murmur in the pulmonic region and a systolic murmur and systolic click at the apex. The pulmonic second sound was split. The spleen was palpable and the liver could be felt 4 centimeters below the costal margin. The neck veins were distended.

Roentgenograms of the chest showed enlargement of the right ventricle and both auricles, dilatation of the pulmonary artery, pulmonary vascular engorgement, and a hilar dance.

Cardiac catheterization showed enormous left-to-right atrial shunting (16.4 liters per minute), a systemic flow of 2.74 liters per minute per square meter body surface area, and normal pulmonary vascular resistance. Electrocardiogram showed right ventricular hypertrophy with right bundle branch block. Fluorescein circulation time was 11 seconds.

Operation. On April 11, 1952, a right thoracotomy showed cardiac enlargement, distention of the vessels of the lung root, and a systolic thrill over the hilum of the lung. A large rubber well was attached to the side of the distended right atrium and blood rose within it to a level of 7 or 8 centimeters. There was an enormous atrial defect measuring 4.5 by 5 centimeters. This lay high in the septum so that there was a margin of septal tissue inferiorly and anteriorly but none superiorly and posteriorly. An attempt was made to pass a 5 centimeter kel-F button in the auricle, but it could not be manipulated into place. A 4.5 centimeter button was positioned and although septal tissue could be grasped at the rim inferiorly and anteriorly, a closure could not be obtained superiorly; this left a crescentic defect where the rim was absent. This was regarded as an unsatisfactory button placement, but it was hoped that at least a baffle would be created which would greatly reduce the size of the shunt. The well had been kept open for 30 minutes.

Postoperative course. Shortly after operation cyanosis appeared. Signs of progressive congestive failure became evident with dyspnea, tachycardia, diffuse crepitant rales, and increasing enlargement of the liver. In spite of rapid digitalization the child's course was progressively downhill. She expired on the third day.

Autopsy. Examination showed complete dislodgement of the button; it lay free within the left atrium. There were 300 cubic centimeters of sanguineous fluid in the right pleural space. There was marked passive congestion of the various viscera.

CASE 4. G.S., a boy of 9, was admitted because of shortness of breath on exertion. At 1½ years of age,

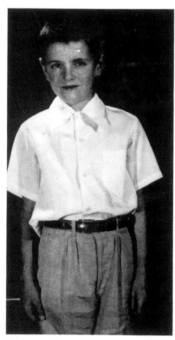

Fig. 19. Patient 4, four months after surgical treatment of interauricular septal defect. Cardiac catheterization shows that the septum is completely closed.

a systolic murmur had been heard. At previous hospital admissions, roentgen examination had shown right ventricular enlargement and pulmonary vascular engorgement. In 1950 cardiac catheterization had demonstrated the presence of an atrial left-to-right shunt flow of 7.1 liters per minute. There was no pulmonary vascular obstruction at that time. Electrocardiogram demonstrated right ventricular hypertrophy and right bundle branch block.

Physical examination showed a rather thin boy. There was prominence of the left precordium. The apex beat was at the anterior axillary line. There was a loud systolic murmur in the pulmonic region and a soft diastolic murmur at the apex. The mitral first sound was split. The liver and spleen were not enlarged.

By T-1824 dye solution the plasma volume was 73 milliliters per kilogram; the blood volume was 129 milliliters per kilogram. Fluorescein circulation time was 10 seconds.

Operation. Findings at right thoracotomy on April 15, 1952, included right atrial and right ventricular enlargement, pulmonary vascular engorgement, and a hilar thrill. A rubber well was attached to the right auricle; blood rose 6 centimeters into it. A septal defect measuring 3 by 2 centimeters was found high and posterior in the septum (Fig. 17). This opening had no rim of tissue at the orifice of the superior vena cava. A disc of nylon sheet, 0.81 millimeter thick, was cut to the dimensions of the

defect and was secured to silk sutures which were to be used for anchoring it into place. Seven of the sutures grasped the rim of septal tissue anteriorly and inferiorly, while 3 of them were passed out from the auricular cavity through the atrial wall in those regions where no septal rim was present. The disc was introduced into the heart, obliterating the defect, and was anchored into place by tying the various sutures. The well had been kept open for 47 minutes. The procedure was well tolerated.

Postoperative course. For a few days after operation there was mild right-sided heart failure, as evidenced by slight elevation of venous pressure, prolongation of circulation time to 13.5 seconds, expansion of the plasma volume to 98 milliliters per kilogram, and tender enlargement of the liver. The patient began to walk on the fourth day. Easy fatigability diminished and he was discharged on the thirteenth postoperative day, showing steady disappearance of the congestive signs.

Subsequent course. The boy was readmitted to the hospital for re-evaluation on June 2, 1952. In the interval he had been able to return to school and ride his bicycle with ease. The left cardiac border remained in the mid-clavicular line. There was a loud third heart sound, and a soft blowing systolic murmur at the apex and at the left sternal border. There was a pericardial friction rub in the second and third left interspaces. The liver had decreased in size and was palpable 1 centimeter below the costal margin. Fluoroscopic examination showed some reduction of pulmonary vascular markings.

Cardiac catheterization showed complete closure of the septal defect. It was possible to pass the catheter from the root of the superior cava into a right pulmonary vein. The finding suggests that the nylon disc has been located in the region of the vein root in such a manner that it lies astride the vein orifice so that a portion of the pulmonary venous drainage is directed into the right auricle. If this explanation is not correct, there must be an anomalous small pulmonary vein entering the right auricle. This small shunt flow of 0.75 liters per minute is in contrast to the preoperative left-right shunt flow value of 7.1 liters per minute. One striking finding of the postoperative catheterization is the fact that rather than the pulmonary artery flow and systemic flow being reduced, the pulmonary artery flow has remained elevated at 10 liters per minute as contrasted to a preoperative value of 9.8 liters per minute, while the systemic flow has shown an elevation from 3.4 liters per square meter per minute to 9.5 liters per square meter per minute. The cause of this elevation of left ventricular output is obscure and cannot be accounted for on the basis of any apparent error in the catheterization technique. There is no evidence of chronic venous congestion in response to high output since the right auricular pressure has fallen following operation from a mean value of 10 millimeters of mercury to 4 millimeters of mercury, and the pulmonary "capillary" pressure has fallen from 13 millimeters of mercury to 7 millimeters of mercury in spite of the threefold increase in left ventricular output. The plasma volume has fallen from a preoperative value of 73 milliliters per kilogram to 59 milliliters per kilogram.

CASE 5. G.C. was a 14 year old girl, on whom a diagnosis of atrial septal defect had been made 3 years previously by cardiac catheterization. When she was 6, a heart murmur had been heard, and after the age of 11 she was noticed to be slightly cyanotic and also short of breath after exertion.

Physical examination showed a pulmonic systolic murmur and an apical mid-diastolic rumble. There was no cyanosis or clubbing.

Roentgen examination revealed enlargement of the right side of the heart and marked pulmonary vascular engorgement.

By electrocardiogram, a right bundle branch block was present.

Cardiac catheterization showed: (1) a left-to-right atrial shunt flow of 14 liters per minute; (2) depression of systemic flow index (2.3 liters); and (3) normal pulmonary vascular resistance. Fluorescein circulation time was 10 seconds. Venous pressure was 80 millimeters of water. By T-1824 dye dilution, the plasma volume was 60 milliliters per kilogram, the blood volume was 103 milliliters per kilogram.

Operation. A right thoracotomy was performed on April 16, 1952. The right auricle and ventricle were greatly enlarged. A systolic thrill could be felt in the dilated vessels at the lung root. A large rubber well was secured to the atrial wall with 20 sutures. The heart action was weak during application of the well and the arterial pressure fell to 60 millimeters systolic. On opening the well, blood rose 11 centimeters into it. Two defects were found in the atrial septum (Fig. 18). A small round orifice 1 centimeter in diameter occupied the central portion of the septum. In the posterior part of the septum there was an elongated opening 5 centimeters long and 1 centimeter wide. This lay just anterior to the orifices of the right pulmonary veins, without any ridge of septal tissue along the posterior margin of the atria. Two sutures of No. 000 Deknatel, placed and tied through the well, were used to close the small central defect, the thinness of the septal tissue raised some doubts whether these would hold. The absence of any ridge of septum along the posterior margin of the larger defect prevented suture being placed entirely within the auricle. Straight needles, carrying No. 000 Deknatel silk, were introduced through the back wall of the right auricle just to the right of the pulmonary veins. With a directing finger immersed in the well, these needles were guided to grasp the edge of the septal margin. The needles were retrieved through the rubber well, and then were passed out of the back wall of the auricle as mattress stitches. Tying up these mattress sutures obliterated the septal opening by pulling the septal rim to the back wall of the atrium, just to the right of the pulmonary veins. The heart action improved during this procedure. Following closure of the second defect, blood in the well became darker and the heart decreased in size. The well was removed and the atrium was closed with interrupted figure-of-eight silk sutures. The well had been open 53 minutes.

Postoperative course. Recovery from anesthesia was prompt and blood pressure stabilized at 115/70 millimeters of mercury 6 hours after operation. Four hours after operation, the blood coagulation time was 5 minutes. Appreciable amounts of sanguineous fluid could be aspirated from the chest during the first 6 days, following which the intercostal catheter was withdrawn. Roentgen examination showed definite reduction in the pulmonary vascular markings. During the first postoperative week, there was evidence suggestive of mild right-sided failure. The liver edge became palpable 3 centimeters below the costal margin; it was tender. The urinary output was low, there was slight elevation of venous pressure, and there was tachycardia. These findings gradually disappeared. The patient walked on the fifth postoperative day and was discharged on the eleventh day.

Subsequent course. The patient was readmitted for study on June 2, 1952. In the interim she had noticed subjective improvement in that she did not "puff" as much as before operation. Activity had been somewhat limited during this period. There was a soft systolic murmur at the apex and under the left clavicle. The liver was palpable 2 centimeters below the costal margin but was not tender. Cardiac catheterization showed some persistence of left-to-right atrial shunting. The volume of shunt flow had decreased from a preoperative value of 14 liters per minute to a volume of 4.7 liters per minute. No conclusions could be drawn concerning which of the two septal defects had the residual opening. The catheter could not be passed into the left auricle, in spite of repeated efforts to do this. Systemic flow showed an elevation from a preoperative figure of 2.3 liters to 2.8 liters per minute per square meter body surface area. The right auricular pressure had fallen from a preoperative mean value of 11 millimeters of mercury to 3 millimeters of mercury. Pulmonary "capillary" pressure had fallen from 17 millimeters of mercury to 8 millimeters of mercury. The plasma volume was 58 milliliters per kilogram

Four months after operation this child appears to be in excellent health. She is most exuberant. She likes to play tennis and engage in other strenuous sports—all of which are entirely new experiences for her.

CASE 6. W.R. was a 16 year old boy who had marked fatigability on exertion. At 12 years a murmur had been detected. At 15 years, roentgenograms had shown enlargement of the heart. At that time an electrocardiogram demonstrated frequent ventricular premature contractions.

Physical examination showed a well nourished and well developed boy without signs of congestive failure. The left precordium was quite prominent. The heart was enlarged to the anterior axillary line and there was a heaving cardiac thrust. There was a harsh apical systolic murmur and a low-pitched systolic murmur along the left sternal border. There was a high-pitched early diastolic murmur along the left side of the sternum. The pulmonic and aortic second sounds were duplicated.

Cardiac fluoroscopy showed a large heart with predominantly right ventricular enlargement, enlarged auricles, prominence of the pulmonary conus, pulmonary vascular engorgement, and a hilar dance.

Cardiac catheterization showed a left-to-right shunt flow through a very large atrial defect (14 liters per minute per square meter body surface), a systemic flow of 3.8 liters per minute per square meter body surface and a reduced pulmonary vascular resistance. Electrocardiogram showed a regular rhythm and right bundle branch block.

Operation. At the time of right thoracotomy on April 26, 1952, the lung substance was found to be greatly engorged and the pulmonary vessels enormously distended. There was a thrill in the hilum of the lung. The heart was enlarged, the right atrium being particularly prominent. A large rubber well was attached to the right auricle; blood rose 8 centimeters into it. Except for a small ridge of septal tissue at the superior caval orifice, the atrial septum was absent. Essentially, there was a common atrium, the opening between the two sides being about 5 centimeters in diameter. An oval sheet of polyethylene, 0.5 millimeter thick, was cut about 5 centimeters wide and 7 centimeters long. Seventeen sutures were introduced through the well into the septal margin of the tricuspid valve ring and the superior septal ridge, or were passed out through the auricular wall in those areas where there was no septal substance to grasp. These various silk stitches were passed through the margins of the polyethylene sheet which was then pushed down into place, and the stitches were tied. Digital palpation of the anchored sheet disclosed that the septal defect was completely closed over, but that the piece of plastic was too long and, therefore, projected down over the annulus of the tricuspid valve. We were loath to remove it or to attempt cutting off its lower end. The heart decreased in size and the pulmonary engorgement diminished after closure of the defect. During the prolonged intracardiac manipulations, the cardiac rhythm was remarkably regular. The well had been kept open 2 hours and 5 minutes.

Postoperative course. Recovery from anesthesia was prompt and the blood pressure stabilized around 110/50 within a few hours. All electrocardiograms taken after operation demonstrated the presence of an auriculoventricular nodal rhythm. The patient was unusually listless. The skin was sallow but there was no scleral icterus. The urinary output was depressed. The venous pressure was elevated to 160 to 170 millimeters of saline. On the morning of the third postoperative day the patient had a sudden spell of gasping respiration and then died.

Autopsy. Examination showed that the septal defect had been effectually closed, but a clot had formed beneath the excess portion of the polyethylene plate. This clot had propagated down into the tricuspid orifice and partially occluded it.

CASE 7. S.W. was an underdeveloped girl of 11 years. She was born prematurely, weighing 2 pounds at birth. There was early retardation of growth and slow mental development. There was marked limitation of tolerance to physical exercise. She could walk only about half a block before tiring. There were no complaints suggestive of congestive failure.

Physical examination showed a thin child appearing about 6 or 7 years of age. There was left-sided prominence of the chest and a heaving cardiac impulse. The apical beat was in the left midclavicular line. There was a high-pitched early systolic murmur in the second left interspace and a questionable early diastolic murmur in the fourth left interspace. The pulmonic second sound was split. The neck veins were slightly distended and the liver was palpable 2.5 centimeters below the costal margin.

Electrocardiograms showed incomplete right bundle branch block and a normal cardiac axis. Fluoroscopy showed that the heart was considerably enlarged with predominance of the right ventricle. The right auricle was moderately enlarged. The pulmonary artery was prominent and the pulmonary vascular markings were distinctly increased.

Catheterization showed left-to-right interatrial shunting (8.3 liters per minute), a systemic flow index of 4.6 liters, normal pulmonary vascular resistance, and a rather wide systemic arterial pulse pressure (femoral arterial pressure 140/80). By the T-1824 dye dilution method, the plasma volume was 67.4 cubic centimeters per kilogram, the blood volume was 109 cubic centimeters per kilogram.

Operation. On June 30, 1952, a right thoracotomy was performed. The right auricle and ventricle were found enlarged. A systolic thrill was palpable over the right pulmonary hilum. A large rubber well was attached to the side of the right atrium and the atrium opened widely. A large, oval defect occupied the central portion of the atrial septum; this measured 3 by 2.5 centimeters. There was a narrow rim of septal tissue around the periphery of the defect. A sheet of polyethylene plastic (0.51 mm. thick) was cut to dimensions similar to the estimated size of the defect and to its approximate contour. With silk sutures around its periphery the disc was then anchored to the septum to lie over and close the defect. All sutures were located in the septal rim by introduction through the well. Nine sutures were employed to hold the polyethylene in place. Digital examination showed the defect to be completely obliterated by this prosthesis. The well had been kept open 40 minutes.

Postoperative course. Immediately following operation the blood pressure was 80 systolic, 50 diastolic, pulse rate 125, and rectal temperature 92 degrees F. The pulse was strong and skin color good. Within a few hours, the temperature rose to normal and the patient's general status was satisfactory. During succeeding days the course was extremely smooth.

The patient walked on the seventh postoperative day. At no time after operation was there evidence of cardiac congestion. The liver has not been enlarged. On the tenth postoperative day, plasma volume was 67.0 cubic centimeters per kilogram and blood volume 108 cubic centimeters per kilogram of body weight. The pulmonic murmur has greatly diminished in intensity. The child was discharged from the hospital in 2 weeks, and at that time appeared to be in very satisfactory condition.

SUMMARY AND CONCLUSIONS

A method has been devised whereby it is possible to attach a rubber well to the right auricle so that the atrium can be opened into this well, thereby providing direct access into the interior of the chamber. This appliance can be left in place for a rather indefinite period of time and intracardiac manipulations can be carried out with precision and great accuracy. With its aid, interauricular septal defects can be felt with the exploring finger and knowledge can be accumulated regarding the size, shape, and position of the opening as well as the nature of the margins which surround the orifice.

With an atrial well approach to the interior of the heart, large interauricular septal defects can be closed by carrying into place a sheet of plastic material which covers the opening and which is securely held in position by sutures which anchor it to remaining rims of septum or to nearby surfaces of the auricular wall. Small defects can be closed by direct suture.

REFERENCES

1. BAILEY, C. P. Material presented at the American College of Physicians, Cleveland, 1952.
2. COHN, R. An experimental method for the closure of interauricular septal defects in dogs. Am. Heart J., 1947, 33: 453.
3. DENNIS, C., SPRENG, D. S., JR., NELSON, G. E., KARLSON, K. E., NELSON, R. M., THOMAS, J. V., EDER, W. P., and VARCO, R. L. Development of a pump-oxygenator to replace the heart and lungs; an apparatus applicable to human patients, and application to one case. Ann. Surg., 1951, 134: 709.
4. DODRILL, F. D. A method for exposure of the cardiac septa. J. Thorac. Surg., 1949, 18: 652.
5. HUFNAGEL, C. A., and GILLESPIE, J. F. Closure of interauricular septal defects. Bull. Georgetown Univ. M. Center, 1951, 4: 137.
6. INGRAHAM, F. D., ALEXANDER, E., JR., and MATSON, D. D. Synthetic plastic materials in surgery. N. England J. M., 1947, 236: 362.
7. MARTIN, W. B., and ESSEX, H. E. Experimental production and closure of atrial septal defects with observations of physiologic effects. Surgery, 1951, 30: 283.
8. MURRAY, G. Closure of defects in cardiac septa. Ann. Surg., 1948, 128: 843.
9. REMINGTON, J. W., HAMILTON, W. F., WHEELER, N. C., and HAMILTON, W. F., JR. Validity of pulse contour method for calculating cardiac output of the dog, with notes on effect of various anesthetics. Am. J. Physiol., 1949, 159: 379.
10. SANTY, P., BRET, J., and MARION, P. Communication interauriculaire traitée par invagination transeptale de l'auricule gauche dans l'auricule droite. Lyon chir., 1950, 45: 359.
11. SWAN, H., MARESH, G., JOHNSON, M. E., and WARNER, G. The experimental creation and closure of auricular septal defects. J. Thorac. Surg., 1950, 20: 542.

CIRCULATORY BYPASS OF THE RIGHT SIDE OF THE HEART*

IV. Shunt between Superior Vena Cava and Distal Right Pulmonary Artery — Report of Clinical Application

WILLIAM W. L. GLENN, M.D.†

NEW HAVEN, CONNECTICUT

IN the first publication of this series of papers attention was called to the need of a method for the direct delivery of venous blood into the pulmonary arterial circulation.[1] The congenital anomalies of the heart that might be remedied from this operation are characterized by malfunction of the right atrium or right ventricle or both. More specifically, the cardiac conditions that would benefit from circulatory bypass of the right side of the heart include stenosis or atresia of the tricuspid and pulmonary outflow tracts, Ebstein's anomaly, single ventricle, bilocular heart and transposition of the great vessels with an associated pulmonary valvular stenosis. Also, in certain cases of pulmonary hypertension in which the changes in the pulmonary arterioles have not become irreversible, the direct delivery of systemic venous blood into the pulmonary arterial circulation may be beneficial at some time after temporary ligation of the right pulmonary artery. Finally, bypass of the right side of the heart may be indicated when there is obstruction of the cavae where they join the heart, or when there is an abnormal insertion of either cava into the left atrium. Other literature pertinent to this problem has been reviewed previously.[1-3]

*From the Department of Surgery, Yale University School of Medicine.

Supported in part by grants from the Victoria Foundation for Cardiovascular Research at Yale and United States Public Health Service (H851-C-7).

†Associate professor of surgery, Yale University School of Medicine.

In the first paper 9 experiments were reported in which the superior vena cava was anastomosed to the distal end of the right pulmonary artery, and observations were made on venous pressure, oxygen saturation of the venous and arterial blood and angiography. It was evident from these early experiments that an anastomosis performed between the superior vena cava and the distal end of the right pulmonary artery usually remained patent postoperatively, and venous-pressure studies in the superior vena cava before and after the anastomosis was opened indicated that at least some of the blood from the superior vena cava passed through the anastomosis into the right pulmonary artery.

appears to be a child or adult with cyanosis due to decreased pulmonary blood flow with normal or diminished pulmonary arteriolar resistance and with a condition that cannot be treated adequately by other methods. Such a patient was recently presented for consideration for surgery, and the shunt was advised on the basis of extensive experimental work carried out in this laboratory over a period of three and a half years.[1-3]

CASE REPORT

The patient (G.–N.H.C.H. 45-77-54), a 7-year-old boy, was first seen in this hospital at the age of 3 months with the chief complaint of "congenital heart disease." The

TABLE 1. *Preoperative Catheterization of the Right Side of the Heart.**

CATHETER POSITION	BLOOD OXYGEN CONTENT	CAPACITY	SATURATION	PRESSURES (CORRECTED)
	vol. %	*vol. %*	*%*	*mm. Hg.*
Right ventricle (mid)	18.7		67	82/10
(?) Right ventricle (mid)	23.4		85	
Right atrium (low)	14.2		51	10/ 4
Right atrium (mid)	16.9	27.56	61	7/ 2
Superior vena cava	17.1		62	9/ 6
Left femoral artery (arterial blood)	20.7		75	88/59

*Performed by Pediatric-Cardiology Staff on 11/9/56.

In the second and third papers in this series[2,3] further studies were carried out to determine longer-term effects of direct anastomosis of the vena cava to the distal pulmonary artery in the laboratory animal. A series of 75 animals was studied in which the anastomosis was made between the superior vena cava and the right pulmonary artery. Studies were also made on a second group of 46 animals, with an anastomosis made between the inferior vena cava, severed from connection with the right atrium, and the distal end of the right pulmonary artery. As a result of these experiments, it is believed that most and possibly all of the blood returning to the heart through the superior vena cava can be made to pass directly into the pulmonary circulation bypassing the right side of the heart. In this limited sense, the right side of the heart is not necessary to propel the venous return through the pulmonary circulation when the pulmonary vascular resistance is normal. Because of the regular occurrence of splanchnic venous congestion and ascites where the shunt between the inferior vena cava and pulmonary artery is made and because no greater flow of blood through the lung is obtained with this shunt than with that between the superior vena cava and right pulmonary artery, it was believed that the former shunt will probably have no practical clinical application except when there is congenital insertion of the inferior vena cava into the left atrium.

The ideal candidate for the shunt between the superior vena cava and right pulmonary artery

present illness revealed that the child's birth was uneventful. In the neonatal period the color was poor, and oxygen was required. His color was described as "blue," and a "murmur" was heard at this time. After discharge from the hospital development appeared to be normal, although his color continued to be blue and this was more evident when he cried. Some difficulty in breathing was observed when he was lying flat.

Over the next 5 years the child developed and gained weight normally. Cyanosis was marked at all times, and exercise tolerance was poor. Between the 5th and 6th years a steadily increasing polycythemia was observed, and on October 19, 1956, the hemoglobin was found to be 25.2 gm. per 100 ml., the red-cell count 7,150,000, and the hematocrit 71 per cent of packed cells. An electrocardiogram, as interpreted by the Pediatric Staff, revealed right-axis deviation, normal sinus rhythm, high-peaked P waves, a vertical heart and right ventricular hypertrophy as evidenced by a high R wave in Lead V_1. One month later cardiac catheterization and angiocardiography were carried out by the Pediatric Staff. The findings of the catheterization are shown in Table 1.

Angiocardiography confirmed the suspicion of the existence of a single ventricle and also demonstrated a transposition of the great vessels, with decreased pulmonary blood flow. It was the consensus of members of the combined service conference that these findings represented a single ventricle, a transposition of the great vessels and a pulmonary stenosis.

Phlebotomy was done about 2 months before operation to reduce the hematocrit from 70 to 63 per cent of packed cells. No vein punctures were permitted in the upper extremities for 5 days before surgery.

At operation on February 25, 1958, an intravenous infusion was started in the long saphenous vein at the ankle. The right side of the chest was entered anteriorly through the bed of the 4th rib. The right pulmonary artery was isolated and found to be large and easily compressible. The superior vena cava was isolated within the pericardium. Cardiac arrest developed during the intrapericardial dissection but responded promptly to massage. Atrial tachycardia was controlled by digitalization. The azygos vein was ligated and divided. The pressure in the right pulmonary artery was found to be 270 mm. of saline solution. The artery was ligated medially and divided. Rubber-shod bulldog clamps were placed on the distal branches. An anastomosis was

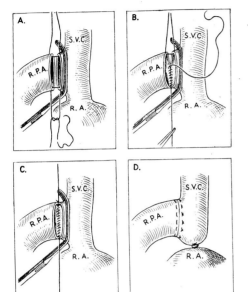

FIGURE 1. *Shunt between the Superior Vena Cava and Right Pulmonary Artery — Technic of Anastomosis.*
R.P.A. = *right pulmonary artery; S.V.C. = superior vena cava; and R.A. = right atrium.*

performed between the distal end of the right pulmonary artery and the side of the superior vena cava at the level of its junction with the azygos vein (Fig. 1). The clamps

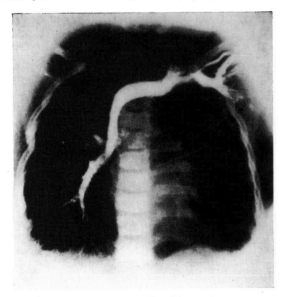

FIGURE 2. *Angiogram Taken Two Months after Operation.*

on the cava and distal branches of the pulmonary artery were removed. The superior vena cava was then ligated at its entrance into the right atrium. Extreme precautions were taken throughout the operation to avoid unnecessary trauma

to the superior vena cava, the pulmonary artery and the right lung.

Immediately after operation there was a marked improvement in the patient's color, and the cyanosis that had been quite evident before operation was now barely discernible. Ambulation was begun on the 6th postoperative day.

The patient returned to the hospital 4 weeks after discharge for a postoperative superior caval angiogram and venous-pressure and oxygen-saturation studies. The angiogram revealed the rapid passage of dye (diatrizoate sodium, 50 per cent) from the left brachial vein and superior vena cava into the distal right pulmonary artery through the anastomosis (Fig. 2). The dye rapidly passed through the lung into the left atrium. There was no evidence of obstruction or venous distention.*

A venous-pressure determination was performed through a 15-gauge needle placed in the left brachial vein with the patient at rest. The pressure varied with each quiet respiration from 118 to 140 mm. of saline solution. Oxygen-saturation studies (Table 2) indicated a marked improvement during rest, with and without 100 per cent oxygen inhalation, and after exercise.†

TABLE 2. *Arterial Oxygen Studies before and after the Shunt.*

PERIOD OF TEST	FEMORAL-ARTERY SATURATION	
	BEFORE OPERATION†	AFTER OPERATION‡
After exercise	42.8	71.6
With rest (20–25 min.)	70.7	86.9
After breathing oxygen for 1 min.	78.4	96.2
Hematocrit (packed red cells)	70.0 (2 mo.)	47.0 (2 mo.)

*Operation, 2/25/58.
†2/14/58.
‡4/23/58.

DISCUSSION

The successful performance of the shunt in this patient is significant, for his complex problems could

*The angiogram was supervised by Dr. Richard Barach.
†Dr. N. K. Ordway made the following calculations on the basis of the catheterization data and studies of femoral-artery oxygen saturation.
In all the calculations the arteriovenous difference of 3.8 vol. per cent observed at the time of catheterization on November 9, 1956, was used. Complete mixing of the blood in the common ventricle is assumed so that the oxygen content of systemic arterial and pulmonary arterial blood is the same at any time. With this as a basis the right-to-left shunt on November 9, 1956, was calculated to have been 58 per cent of the systemic venous return to the heart, and the pulmonary blood flow 73 per cent of the systemic blood flow. On February 14, 1958, the right-to-left shunt calculated out at 63 per cent of the systemic venous return to the heart, and the pulmonary flow at 58 per cent of the systemic blood flow. After operation the net right-to-left shunt is now 28 per cent of the systemic venous return to the heart. The amount of bypass to the right lung brought about by the anastomosis of the superior vena cava to the distal right pulmonary artery is now exactly the difference between the preoperative and postoperative net shunts, or somewhere between 29 per cent and 35 per cent of the systemic blood flow, depending on which of the preoperative figures one uses for net right-to-left shunt. This is in striking concordance with the prediction based on observation on animals.[3] To have produced the same result with a systemic-artery to pulmonary-artery shunting procedure, one would have had to increase the pulmonary flow by a flow through the operative fistula equal to one or one and a quarter times the systemic flow, depending on which of the preoperative figures for right-to-left shunt is used. In either case, this means a pulmonary flow of about one and eight-tenths times the systemic flow, or a pulmonary flow of two and a half to three times the preoperative pulmonary flow, depending again on what figure is used for that. This would amount to a one-and-a-half-fold to twofold increase in output of the common ventricle as opposed to no increase in output from the common ventricle with the superior-vena-cava-pulmonary-artery shunt. A further assumption made is that the flow through the stenotic pulmonary valve to the left lung postoperatively is the same as the total flow to both lungs preoperatively. This is a reasonable assumption since the pressure difference must be about the same because the return to the common ventricle is also the same.
If this operation is applied to a patient with intact ventricular septum such as Epstein's anomaly, the right ventricular output would be reduced by about 29 to 35 per cent whereas the left would not be altered.

not, at least with present knowledge, be corrected by open-heart technics. Also, the use of a shunt between the systemic artery and the pulmonary artery would have had the undesirable effect of increasing the work of the single ventricle. Furthermore, because the shunt could be made as large as the diameter of the vessels would permit, it is likely, if the animal experiments can be used as a guide, that the anastomosis will remain sufficiently wide as the child grows to transmit the total return to the superior vena cava without a further significant increase in venous pressure. The anastomosis performed in this patient was identical to the first one done on a laboratory animal more than three and a half years ago.[1] That first animal is living and well, with a widely patent anastomosis, at the present time.

It is probable that the venous flow through the shunt will not exceed 30 to 40 per cent of the total systemic venous return.[3] But, as is evident from the postoperative clinical and laboratory studies in this patient, this amount of flow will result in marked improvement in arterial oxygenation without increasing the work of the heart. The reduction of 30 to 40 per cent of the venous return to the right side of the heart incident to the creation of the shunt may be beneficial to conditions such as Ebstein's anomaly characterized by right-sided heart failure with normal or hypotensive pulmonary-artery pressure. There was no evidence of increase in the heart size in this patient after operation — if any change took place, the heart appeared slightly smaller.

The most striking change after operation was the increase in exercise tolerance. Cyanosis, which was severe before operation, was barely discernible with the child at rest after operation. Cyanosis increased with exercise, but diminished rapidly on resting. His family noted that he now had no limitation of activity and that only on strenuous exercise was cyanosis marked. When he was asked how the operation helped him, he replied, "Now I can walk up the hill."

The criteria for the selection of patients for the performance of the shunt cannot be too strongly emphasized.[3] The two most important local anatomic features are a pulmonary artery and superior vena cava of large size and a normal or decreased resistance to flow in the pulmonary circulation.

The gratifying result obtained in this first patient encourages me to apply this technic to other patients when there is strict adherence to the criteria for selection and management. Remarkable as this operative procedure is, from the standpoint both of the alteration of the basic circulatory pattern and of the improvement of the arterial oxygen saturation in the cyanotic patient, the possibly fatal consequence of thrombosis of the anastomosis must not be forgotten and no effort spared to avoid this complication.

SUMMARY AND CONCLUSIONS

On the basis of experimental work carried out over a period of three and a half years, the clinical application of anastomosis between the superior vena cava and the distal right pulmonary artery was successfully accomplished. The patient was a seven-year-old boy with a single ventricle, transposition of the great vessels and pulmonary stenosis.

Clinical studies and laboratory tests indicate significant improvement in arterial oxygen saturation and exercise tolerance since operation. Attention is called particularly to the strict criteria for the selection of patients for this operative procedure, and the exceptional precautions taken to prevent thrombosis at the site of anastomosis. For a successful shunt of this type, it is believed to be essential to have a pulmonary artery and superior vena cava of large size and a normal or low resistance to flow through the pulmonary circulation.

A number of congenital malformations of the heart, not previously amenable to adequate treatment, may be benefited by a shunt between the superior vena cava and pulmonary artery.

It is due to the experimental contributions of my surgical colleagues, Drs. J. F. Patiño, S. B. Nuland, P. H. Guilfoil and M. Hume, and Mr. J. E. Fenn that this procedure in the human subject was made possible. I am also indebted to members of the Pediatric Staff, Drs. H. S. Harned, R. Whittemore, R. J. Waters, R. Sunico and N. K. Ordway, for their help in the diagnosis and management of the patient reported herein.

REFERENCES

1. Glenn, W. W. L., and Patiño, J. F. Circulatory by-pass of right heart. I. Preliminary observations on direct delivery of vena caval blood into pulmonary arterial circulation: azygos vein-pulmonary artery shunt. *Yale J. Biol. & Med.* 27:147-151, 1954.
2. Patiño, J. F., Glenn, W. W. L., Guilfoil, P. H., Hume, M., and Fenn, J. E. Circulatory bypass of right heart. II. Further observations on vena caval-pulmonary artery shunts. *S. Forum* 6:189-193, 1955.
3. Nuland, S. B., Glenn, W. W. L., and Guilfoil, P. H. Circulatory bypass of right heart. III. Some observations on long-term survivors. *Surgery* 43:184-201, 1958.

SURGICAL CORRECTION OF TRANSPOSITION OF THE GREAT VESSELS

ÅKE SENNING, M.D., STOCKHOLM, SWEDEN

(From the Thoracic Clinic, Karolinska Sjukhuset, and the Department of Experimental Surgery, Karolinska Institutet)

TRANSPOSITION of the great vessels is a congenital heart malformation which causes cyanosis, with about the same incidence as tetralogy of Fallot. It is one of the most common anomalies which cause death during the first period of life. In complete transposition, the aorta emanates from the right ventricle and receives systemic venous blood. The pulmonary artery emanates from the left ventricle and directs the arterialized blood back to the lungs. The only possibility of survival for children post partum is the presence of associated defects which shunt blood between the systemic and pulmonary circulation. A persistent foramen ovale, an atrial septal defect, a persistent ductus arteriosus, and ventricular septal defect are the most common associated defects and occur in 75 to 100 per cent of the cases reported in the literature.[7, 9]

From a surgical point of view, it can be considered that the pulmonary artery and the aorta have about the same diameter in 60 per cent of the cases. The coronary arteries always leave the aorta and, according to Mustard,[11] they usually extend in front of the pulmonary artery. In 4 of our 6 cases, there were two coronary arteries which originated near each other on the back of the aorta. The right coronary artery was wide and divided into two branches. One right branch corresponded to a normal right coronary artery, and a left branch, extending behind the pulmonary artery, supplied the same region as an ordinary circumflex branch of a left coronary artery. The descending branch of a normal left coronary artery was, in these instances, replaced by a narrow left coronary artery. The right ventricle, maintaining the systemic circulation, is always hypertrophic. The left ventricular myocardium is hypotrophic in cases of intact ventricular septum and closed ductus.

Since the prognosis for these patients is very bad,[4, 7, 9] many attempts have been made to correct transposition of the great vessels. Operative procedures used on the arterial side have been unsuccessful.[2, 3, 8, 11] With operations on the venous side,[4, 6, 9] the survival rate has been improved, but mortality has been high.* Merendino and co-workers[10] have performed interatrial venous transposition with the aid of a plastic prosthesis, with no survivals to the present time. Albert[1] has tried experimentally to use an anterior atrial septal flap for correction.

Two new different surgical methods for complete correction of transposition of the great vessels have been worked out experimentally; one in 1955 on

Received for publication Sept. 29, 1958.

*The best results have been those obtained with Baffes' method.[13]

the arterial side, and one in 1957 on the atrial level.[12]   The methods have been used clinically, with one survival, by the atrial method.   The principle of the experimental work has been to divert the blood flow to or from the ventricles with maintained perfusion pressure in the aorta and the coronary arteries, without using a prosthesis or graft which might result in obstruction of the blood stream later as the children grow.

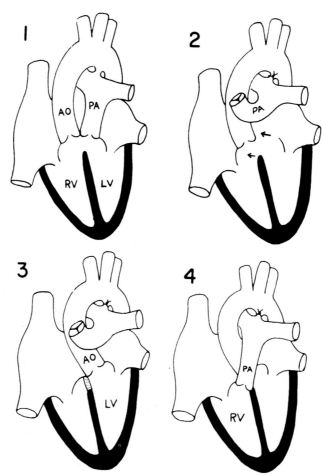

Fig. 1.—Steps in surgical correction on the arterial side of transposition of the great vessels.   *1*, Defect in a case of complete transposition of aorta and pulmonary artery combined with ventricular septal defect and persistent ductus arteriosus.   *2*, First stage of repair: the pulmonary artery with its valves dissected free; the persistent ductus arteriosus ligated.   *3*, Second stage of repair: the root of the aorta sutured to the mitral valve and to the left ventricle; the upper ridge of the ventricular septum sutured to the right of the aortic root.   *4*, Repair completed: the root of the pulmonary artery sutured to the right ventricle.   *AO*—aorta; *PA*—pulmonary artery; *RV*—right ventricle; *LV*—left ventricle.

CORRECTION OF TRANSPOSITION OF THE GREAT VESSELS ON THE ARTERIAL SIDE

With this method, the aorta, including its coronary arteries, is transposed to the left ventricle and the pulmonary artery to the right (Fig. 1).   The pulmonary artery with its valve is dissected from the left ventricle (Fig. 1, *2*).   The resulting hole is limited on the right by the aorta and the interventricular

968   SENNING   Surgery
June, 1959

septum and on the left by the anterior mitral cusp, where this meets the atrial wall in annulus fibrosus. This hole is sutured and thus the anterior mitral cusp is fixed to the aortic root (Fig. 1, 2). A right ventriculotomy is made over the outflow tract. Part of the right aortic border is dissected from the right ventricular wall. An Ivalon sponge prosthesis is sutured into the ventricular septal defect and the upper part of the prosthesis is sutured to the right of the

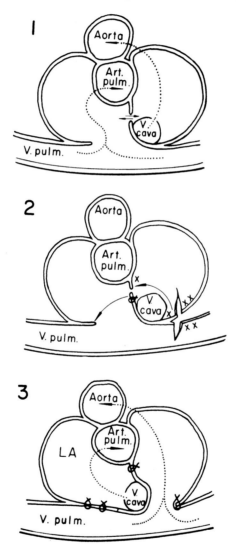

Fig. 2.—Diagram of atrial correction of transposition of the great vessels. *1*, preoperative conditions. *2*, The atrial plastic indicated by arrows. *x* and *xx* indicate incisional edges to be sutured together. *3*, Postoperative condition. Flow pathways indicated.

aorta. Thus, the aorta communicates directly with the left ventricle through the ventricular septal defect (Fig. 1, 3) and then the pulmonary artery root is sutured into the right ventricle (Fig. 1, 4). In this way, complete correction of the transposed vessels is achieved.

This method was used in 3 patients, 2 with and one without ventricular septal defect. The first patient, a 6-month-old child, was operated upon under hypothermia (22° C.), combined with perfusion of oxygenated blood through the carotid arteries and induced ventricular fibrillation. During rewarming, after the cardiac correction had been made, there was good cardiac action and the child was breathing spontaneously, when hemorrhage, caused by fibrinolysis, occurred and the baby died.[5]

In 2 cases, operations were performed under extracorporeal circulation with the AGA heart-lung machine. In both these patients, spontaneous heart action was restored with a good pressure in the pulmonary artery during the extracorporeal circulation. However, the patients could not maintain good arterial blood pressure after the bypass was completed and both died.

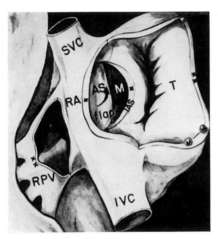

Fig. 3.—Sketch of atrial operation for the correction of transposition of the venous side. Right auricle (*RA*) incised between and in front of venae cavae. Right pulmonary veins (*RPV*) incised at the entrance into the left auricle. Interatrial septum (*IAS*) cut to form a posterior flap (marked with an *arrow*). Tricuspid orifice (*T*), mitral orifice (*M*), superior vena cava (*SVC*), inferior vena cava (*IVC*). The auricularseptal flap will be sutured to the posterior wall of the left auricle in front of the left pulmonary veins, the posterior part of the right auricular wall to the rest of the interauricular septum *x* to *x*, and finally the anterior part of right atrial wall to the right pulmonary veins (*xx* to *xx*).

INTERATRIAL CORRECTION OF TRANSPOSITION

The principle of this operation is illustrated in Figs. 2 and 3.

The operations are performed under extracorporeal circulation with the Crafoord-Senning-AGA heart-lung machine.* A transsternal incision through the fifth costal bed is made. The venous cannulae are introduced into the superior vena cava through the azygos vein, and into the inferior vena cava through the femoral vein. The arterialized blood is returned to the body through the femoral artery. During extracorporeal bypass the aorta is clamped to produce an anoxic cardiac arrest. The clamp is released for a short period every 20 to 25 minutes. If a persistent ductus arteriosus is present, this is ligated. An incision, as long as possible, is made in the right atrium in front of and parallel to the venae cavae. The right pulmonary veins are incised immediately to prevent pulmonary vascular overload; the incision is made as near

*Manufactured by AGA, Lidingö, Sweden.

970   SENNING   Surgery
June, 1959

as possible to the left atrium. The interatrial groove can be slightly dissected to gain some tissue (Fig. 4). By a U-shaped incision, the atrial septum is made into as big a posterior flap as possible. If a large atrial septal defect is present, as in our Case 3, this is widened upward and downward and a posterior flap is formed. The anterior rim of the atrial septum is resected.

When the U-shaped incision is made or the anterior part of the septum is resected, great care must be taken not to damage the A-V bundle and it is therefore safe to leave some tissue intact above and in front of the coronary sinus. In our first 2 patients, the orifice of the coronary sinus was widened into the left atrium by an incision, but in both these patients A-V block occurred.

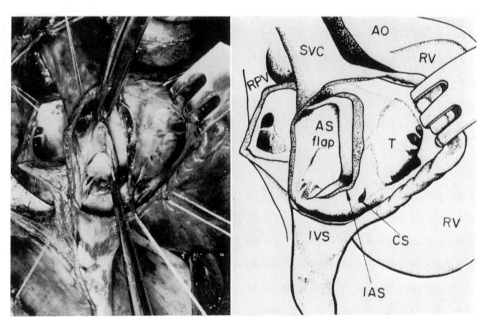

Fig. 4.—Right pulmonary veins (*RPV*) incised along entrance in the left atrium, right atrium incised between, in front of, and parallel to superior vena cava (*SVC*) and inferior venous caval vein (*IVC*). Atrial septum incised creating a posterior flap (*AS* flap, grasped by two forceps). *CS*—Coronary sinus; *T*—tricuspidalis; *RV*—right ventricle; *IAS*—rest of atrial septum. (Postmortem specimen from Case 4.)

Separation of pulmonary veins from the left atrium is achieved by suturing the atrial septal flap to the posterior wall of the left atrium in front of the left pulmonary veins. With three stay sutures placed from the outside of the left atrium, one above, one below, and one between the pulmonary veins and in front of them, the upper corner, the middle part, and the lower corner of the created atrial septal flap are fixed in position. Thereafter, the edge of the atrial septal flap is sutured to the left atrial wall with a continuous over-and-over suture. To get a tight suture line, a finger or an instrument is held behind the flap. In Fig. 5 the suture is completed and Fig. 6 shows the orifices of the left pulmonary veins separated from the anterior part of the left atrium.

Diversion of caval and coronary sinus venous blood to the left and creation of the "venous atrium" are shown in Fig. 7. The anterior edge of the posterior part of the original right atrial wall is fixed to the lower rim of the created atrial septal defect, downward to the anterior and inferior lip of the coronary sinus orifice and then anterior to the entrance of the inferior vena cava. The

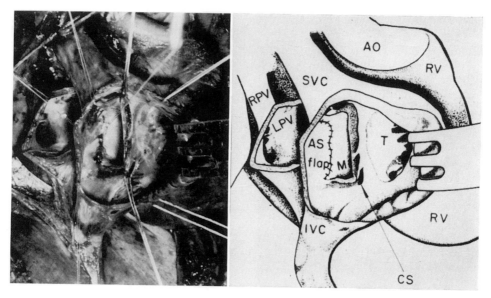

Fig. 5.—Interatrial septal flap sutured to posterior wall of left atrial wall in front of left pulmonary veins. (Postmortem specimen from Case 4.)

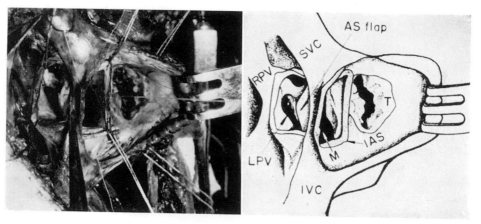

Fig. 6.—The same step as in Fig. 5. Heart rotated forward. The atrial flap is separating the pulmonary veins from the anterior part of the left atrium. (Postmortem specimen from Case 4.)

suture is continued upward over the defect to the posterior wall of the right atrium in front of the superior vena cava. The venous return from the caval veins as well as the coronary sinus blood thus is directed to the left. A "venous atrium'' is created, limited posteriorly by the atrial septal flap, to the right by the posterior part of the right atrial wall, and anteriorly by the remainder of the left atrium.

Creation of an ''arterial atrium'' is shown in Fig. 8. The pulmonary venous return is shut off from the ''venous atrium'' by the atrial septal flap.

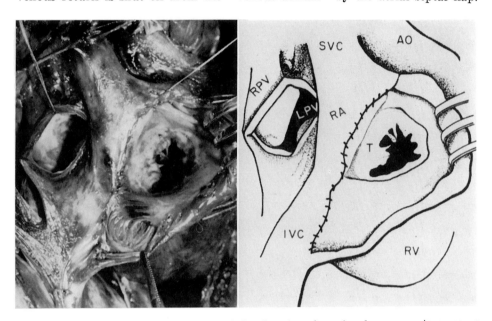

Fig. 7.—Creation of a ''venous atrium'' by diversion of caval and coronary sinus venous blood to the left. The posterior part of the lateral right atrial wall (*RA*) sutured anterior to and to the right of the inferior vena cava and the coronary sinus, further into the created interatrial septal defect and anterior to the superior vena cava. A ''venous atrium'' is created consisting of the anterior part of the left atrium limited posteriorly by the atrial septal flap and to the right by the posterior part of the right atrial wall. Into this venous chamber both caval veins and coronary sinus empty. (Postmortem specimen from Case 4.)

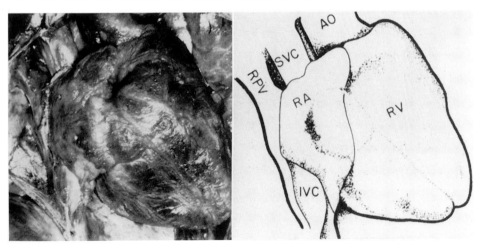

Fig. 8.—The creation of an ''arterial atrium.'' The edge of the anterior rest of the right atrial wall is sutured anteriorly to the wall of both caval veins and to the lateral edge of the incision in the right pulmonary veins. The ''arterial atrium'' consists of the posterior part of left atrium (with the entering pulmonary veins) and the anterior part of the original right atrium. (Postmortem specimen from Case 4.)

Volume 45
Number 6

TRANSPOSITION OF GREAT VESSELS

973

The "arterial atrium" is created by suturing the edge of the anterior part of the right atrial wall, first in front of the entrance of both caval veins into the original right atrium without strangulating the entrance, and then to the lateral incisional edge of the right pulmonary veins. The "arterial atrium" consists of the posterior part of the original left atrium with the entrance of

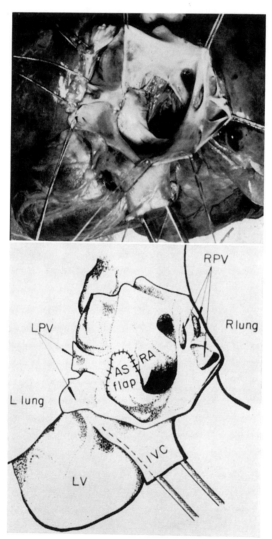

Fig. 9.—"Arterial atrium" opened and seen from behind. Forceps into the "venous atrium" through inferior caval vein. The posterior part of the original left atrium with entering pulmonary veins empty through a wide opening into the anterior remainder of the original right atrium. (Postmortem specimen from Case 4.)

the pulmonary veins, limited anteriorly against the left auricle by the atrial septal flap and communicating widely behind the venae cavae with the anterior remainder of the original right atrium.

Figs. 9 and 10 are shown to clarify the condition of the created atrial chambers. In Fig. 9, the "arterial atrium" with the pulmonary veins is opened from behind with a transverse incision. A pair of forceps is introduced into the "venous atrium" through the inferior vena cava. The atrial septal flap separates the vena cava from the "arterial atrium." The wide communication between the pulmonary veins and the anterior remainder of the original right atrium is seen.

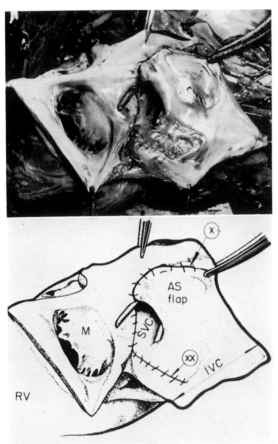

Fig. 10.—"Venous atrium" seen from behind, opened through the inferior vena cava (along incision indicated in diagram of Fig. 9). The posterior wall is folded upward. Forceps in the orifice of the superior vena cava. Suture line between posterior left atrial wall and atrial septal flap is seen above forceps. x—Suture line between posterior part of the right atrial wall and the created atrial septal defect below (xx). Orifice of coronary sinus hidden. (Postmortem specimen from Case 4.)

In Fig. 10 the "venous atrium" is opened along the line indicated in the diagram of Fig. 9. The posterior wall is folded upward and grasped with two clamps. The forceps are inserted from above into the orifice of the superior vena cava. The suture line between the atrial septal flap and the posterior wall of the left atrium is seen above the forceps. The suture line of the posterior part of the lateral wall of the original right atrium, sutured into the created defect to divert venous blood to the left, is seen below the forceps. There is no strangulation of the entrance of the venae cavae into the "venous atrium." (The orifice of the coronary sinus is masked in the photo.)

CASE REPORTS

CASE 1.—A 6-week-old child, severely ill, had a diagnosis of transposition plus persistent ductus arteriosus plus small open foramen ovale. The arterial oxygen saturation was 39 per cent. Ventricular fibrillation occurred before cannulation was finished. Extracorporeal circulation was started. Pulmonary vascular overload with pulmonary edema was caused by flow through a wide typical persistent ductus arteriosus before the ductus could be dissected and clamped. A typical operation was performed. After correction under anoxic cardiac arrest and release of the aortic clamp, spontaneous defibrillation occurred. There was good heart action, but complete A-V block. There was 94 per cent arterial oxygen saturation when the patient was ventilated with 100 per cent oxygen. The child was awake for a few hours. There was increasing respiratory resistance and ventilatory insufficiency developed. The patient died 18 hours postoperatively. Postmortem examination showed complete surgical correction. The lungs were engorged with blood and edematous fluid. Cause of death: pulmonary vascular overload.

CASE 2.—The patient was a boy, 10 years of age, who was cyanotic and underdeveloped. The diagnosis was transposition of great vessels plus ventricular septal defect and valvular pulmonary stenosis. There had been cerebral emboli with hemiplegia at 2 years of age. The arterial oxygen saturation was 62 per cent. The pressures in both ventricles were equilibrated. The operation was a typical atrial correction of transposition of great vessels plus closure of the open foramen ovale plus closure of a ventricular septal defect with insertion of an Ivalon sponge prosthesis and resection of left ventricular subvalvular stenosis plus pulmonary valvular commissurotomy. During the operation, the left ventriculotomy was first sutured directly without resection of the left ventricular outflow tract, but the resistance to the left ventricle was found to be too great. For this reason the ventriculotomy was reopened, the resection made, and the ventriculotomy closed again. Since the ventricular septal defect was closed during this procedure a pulmonary overload with pulmonary edema developed rapidly. The patient died from increasing ventilatory insufficiency 5 hours postoperatively.

CASE 3.—The patient was a 9-year-old boy with cyanosis. The diagnosis was transposition of the great vessels and atrial septal defect. The arterial oxygen saturation was 69 per cent. Selective angiocardiography with injection of dye into the right ventricle showed the aorta originating from an anatomically typical right ventricle with hypertrophic myocardium (Fig. 11, A). The operation was a typical one for atrial correction and ligature of persistent ductus arteriosus under anoxic cardiac arrest. The anterior rim of the atrial septum was resected and the posterior part of the atrial septum used as flap.

After correction and releasing of the aortic clamp, good spontaneous heartbeats with regular auricular and ventricular action were rapidly restored and there was good arterial blood pressure. After the bypass was finished, arterial saturation was 100 per cent on ventilation with 60 per cent oxygen. A tracheostomy was performed and the patient was under artificial ventilation in a respirator for 3 days. There was an uncomplicated postoperative course.

Re-examination 6 weeks postoperatively showed no cyanosis, and catheterization showed no signs of stenosis of the entrance of the venae cavae into the created left "venous atrium," and no shunts on the atrial or ventricluar level. The arterial saturation was 94 per cent (during anesthesia and spontaneous respiration). The patient was in extremely good physical condition.

Angiocardiography with injection into the venous atrium (Fig. 12, A and B) showed normal reflux into both superior and inferior venae cavae and no stenosis. The left ventricle and pulmonary artery were filled from the malformed "venous atrium." During the refilling phase (Fig. 12, C and D), the pulmonary veins are seen separated from the remainder of the left atrium forming together with the remainder of the original right atrium the new "arterial atrium." There were no shunts. These conclusions are confirmed on side views (Fig. 13).

A.

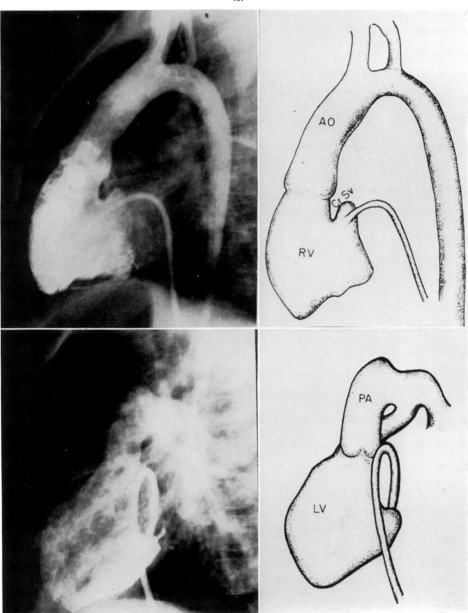

B.

Fig. 11.—Preoperative selective angiocardiograph.

A, Injection in right ventricle. Aorta emanates from an anatomically typical right ventricle. *CrSu*—Crista supraventricularis.

B, Injection in left ventricle. The pulmonary artery emanates from an anatomically typical left ventricle.

(Angiocardiography was performed in the Department of Radiology of the Children's Clinic and Thoracic Clinic, Karolinska Sjukhuset.)

CASE 4.—The patient was a 6-year-old underdeveloped girl with cyanosis. The diagnosis was transposition of the great vessels and ventricular septal defect. The arterial oxygen saturation was 59 per cent. A typical atrial correction was made during 17 minutes of extracorporeal circulation. The aorta was unclamped and there was good regular heart action with regular atrial action and no A-V block. The extracorporeal circulation was interrupted and there was good atrial blood pressure. Extracorporeal circulation was started again and the aorta was clamped. An Ivalon sponge prosthesis was sutured into a 1 by 1.5 cm. wide ventricular septal defect through a left ventriculotomy followed by a complete A-V block with low ventricular frequency and low arterial blood

A. B.

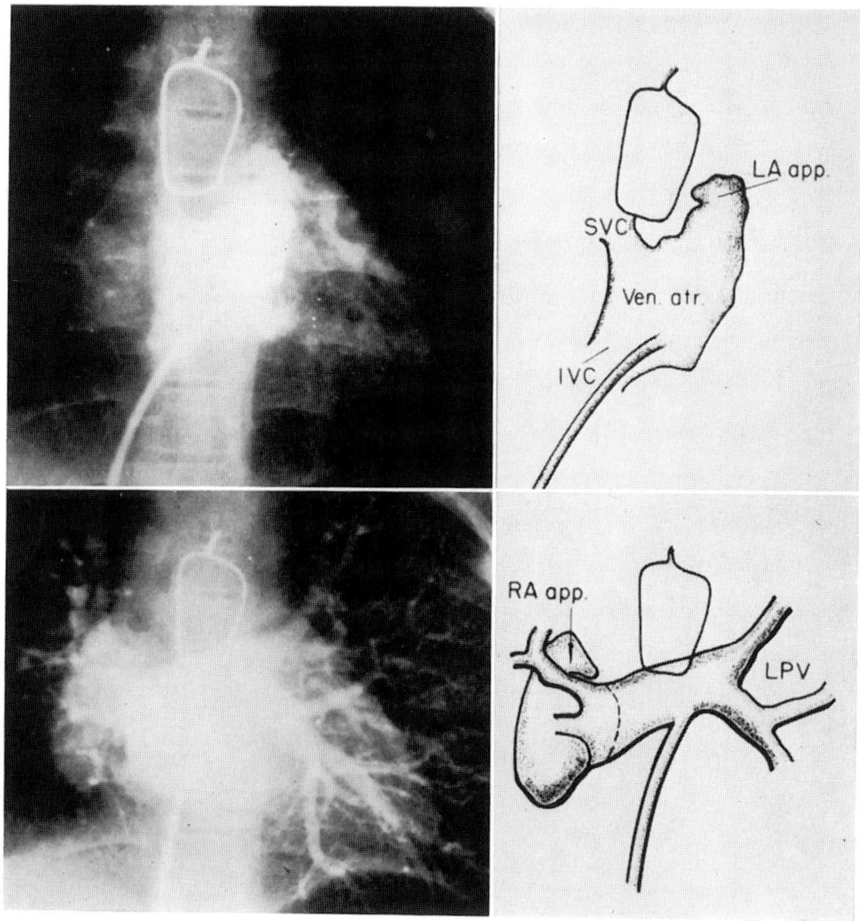

C. D.

Fig. 12.—Postoperative angiocardiography. Injection into "venous atrium." Frontal projection. A and B, "Venous atrium" filled. Reflux into caval veins. LA app.—Left atrial appendage. C and D, "Arterial atrium" in pulmonary refilling phase. RA app.—Right atrial appendage.

pressure. With Adrenalin the A-V block changed to 1:2, with higher frequency and improved blood pressure. It was difficult to maintain good blood pressure. The patient was conscious for 4 hours. The arterial oxygen saturation was 97 per cent. The blood pressure fell and death ensued. On removal of the drainage tubes, about 400 c.c. of blood poured out from the right chest. A postmortem examination showed another 200 c.c. of blood in the chest cavities. The heart showed complete atrial correction (Figs. 4-10). The ventricular septal defect was well closed. The contributing cause of death was intrathoracic bleeding.

DISCUSSION

Transposition of the great vessels is a congenital anomaly with a bad prognosis. Since operations for this anomaly have to be performed in small children, a method for correcting the defect has been developed avoiding the

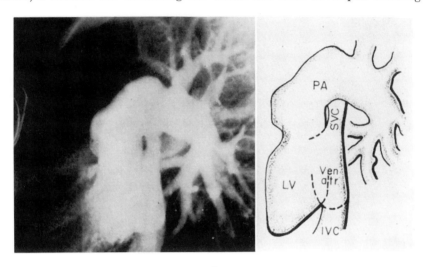

A.

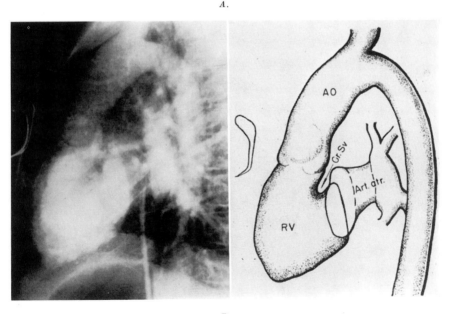

B.

Fig. 13.—Postoperative angiocardiography. Injection into "venous atrium." Side projection.

A, Caval veins, "venous atrium" (*Ven. atr.*), left ventricle, and pulmonary artery visualized.

B, Refilling phase. "Arterial atrium" (*Art. atr.*), right ventricle, and aorta visualized.

use of prosthesis or grafts which later, when the child is growing, may lead to obstruction of the blood stream.

The described method used on the arterial side for correcting transposition was used clinically three times. In all 3 cases there was a good postoperative blood pressure in the pulmonary artery, but in the last 2 cases the pressure in the aorta was very low.

Before the operation, the left ventricle had mainly supplied the pulmonary circulation; however, as in 2 of the cases there was a large ventricular septal defect, the left ventricle should have been sufficiently strong to be able to maintain a good systemic circulation. Possibly there was a mitral or aortic insufficiency due to valvular distortion, resulting from the suture of the hole left after the dissection of the pulmonary artery root. Whether or not there were other causes of death is difficult to judge. This method seemed suitable in cases with large ventricular septal defects but as the surgical technique is rather difficult, no further clinical trials have been made.

Methods for correcting transposition on the atrial level were worked out. Principally, the original atrial chambers are rebuilt to form a "venous atrium" consisting of the anterior part of the original left atrium together with the posterior part of the right atrium. The "arterial atrium" consists of the posterior part of the left atrium with the entrance of pulmonary veins and the anterior part of the right atrium.

There are several procedures to be considered; pulmonary veins can be separated from the left atrium by a duplication of the posterior wall or with the aid of a small prosthesis, or part of the right atrial wall. The venae cavae can be diverted to the left through a created atrial septal defect with the aid of an anterior atrial septal flap or a small prosthesis. The atrial septum can be incised longitudinally, a posterior flap being used to divert pulmonary venous return and an anterior flap to divert systemic venous return.

According to electrocardiographic examination, catheterization, and angiocardiography of the surviving patient, the function of the atrial chambers seems to be good despite this remodeling. In this patient, there are no arrhythmias; the different parts of the atrium seem to contract simultaneously. Catheterization reveals no stenosis between the caval veins and the venous atrium and, on angiocardiography, the reflux to the superior and the inferior venae cavae seems to be normal.

In the first 2 cases, the coronary sinus was incised from the left atrium to facilitate diversion of the coronary sinus blood to the left. This might have been the cause of the A-V block in these 2 patients. In the last patient, the A-V block appeared after closure of the ventricular septal defect.

It is difficult to judge whether or not associated defects should be closed during the same operation. A persistent ductus arteriosus is easily closed and this should be done unless there is a distinct contraindication, for example, excessive pulmonary vascular resistance. An associated ventricular septal defect was closed in Cases 2 and 4. This considerably prolonged the perfusion time and increased operative cardiac trauma and seems to have been the actual cause of death in Case 2, in which a pulmonary vascular overload occurred during closure of the left ventriculotomy. It would evidently have been wise to postpone the final closure of the "arterial atrium." If there is a ventricular septal defect combined with pulmonary stenosis with left-to-right shunt through the ventricular septal defect (as in Case 2), the patient will be cyanotic even if the transposition is corrected on the atrial level. In these cases, it is necessary to make a left ventriculotomy to release the left ventricular outflow stenosis. The ventricular septal defect should be closed at the same time to avoid the risk of pulmonary vascular overload.

In the event of further cases of associated ventricular septal defect we intend not to close the ventricular septal defect during the first operation unless this can be done through the tricuspid orifice without disturbing the septal cusp of the tricuspid valve. If necessary, the ventricular septal defect can be closed during a subsequent operation.

The successful outcome of the atrial correction of transposition in the third case and the findings from re-examinations indicate that the method described here would provide a practical surgical approach to complete transposition of the great vessels.

SUMMARY

1. Two new methods for complete repair of transposition of the great vessels are presented.

2. One method applied on the arterial side has been tried clinically in 3 cases without success.

3. One atrial method for complete transposition without application of prosthesis or grafts was used in 4 patients.

4. One with a successful correction was re-examined. Ideal circulatory conditions were observed.

5. Closure of associated defects is discussed.

REFERENCES

1. Albert, H. M.: Surgical Correction of Transposition of the Great Vessels, S. Forum **5**: 74, 1954.
2. Bailey, C. P., Cookson, B. A., Downing, D. F., and Neptune, W. B.: Cardiac Surgery Under Hypothermia, J. Thoracic Surg. **27**: 73-91, 1954.
3. Björk, V. O., and Bouckaert, L.: Complete Transposition of the Aorta and Pulmonary Artery. An Experimental Study of the Surgical Possibilities for Its Treatment, J. Thoracic Surg. **28**: 632-635, 1954.
4. Blalock, A., and Hanlon, C. R.: The Surgical Treatment of Complete Transposition of the Aorta and the Pulmonary Artery, Surg. Gynec. & Obst. **90**: 1-15, 1950.
5. Blombäck, B., Blombäck, M., Senning, Å., and Wallén, P.: Fibrinolys och fibrinogenolys som orsak till komplikationer inom kirurgi och obstetrik, Nord. med. **53**: 1019, 1955.
6. Graanboom: Quoted by Lillehei, C. W., and Varco, R. L.[9]
7. Hanlon, C. R., and Blalock, A.: Complete Transposition of the Aorta and Pulmonary Arteries. Experimental Observations on Venous Shunts as Corrective Procedures, Ann. Surg. **127**: 385-397, 1948.
8. Kay, E. B., and Cross, F. S.: Surgical Treatment of Transposition of the Great Vessels, SURGERY **38**: 712-716, 1955.
9. Lillehei, C. W., and Varco, R. L.: Certain Physiologic, Pathologic, and Surgical Features of Complete Transposition of the Great Vessels, SURGERY **34**: 376, 399, 1953.
10. Merendino, K. A., Jesseph, J. E., Herron, P. W., Thomas, G. I., and Vetto, R. R.: Interatrial Venous Transposition, SURGERY **42**: 898-909, 1957.
11. Mustard, W. T., Chute, A. L., Keith, J. D., Sirek, A., Rowe, R. D., and Vlad, P.: The Surgical Approach to Transposition of the Great Vessels With Extracorporeal Circuit, SURGERY **36**: 39-51, 1954.
12. Senning, Å.: Transposition av aorta och arteria pulmonalis, Opuscula Medica nr. 2, 1958.
13. Baffes, T. G.: A New Method for Surgical Correction of Transposition of the Aorta and Pulmonary Artery, Surg. Gynec. & Obst. **102**: 227, 1956.

CORRECTION OF PULMONARY ATRESIA WITH A HOMOGRAFT AORTIC VALVE

D. N. Ross

M.B., B.Sc. Cape Town, F.R.C.S.

CONSULTANT THORACIC SURGEON

Jane Somerville

M.D. Lond., M.R.C.P.

SENIOR LECTURER, INSTITUTE OF CARDIOLOGY

NATIONAL HEART HOSPITAL, LONDON W.1

In any large series of patients with Fallot's tetralogy, a few will be found with a complete obstruction of the right ventricle at the pulmonary valve or infundibular level. Lillehei et al. (1955) first described the management of such a case by reimplanting the distal pulmonary artery into the right ventricle, and subsequently the practice has been to reconstruct the outflow tract with plastic material (Lillehei et al. 1964, Sabiston et al. 1964). Although these procedures relieve the obstruction of the right-ventricular outflow tract, significant pulmonary regurgitation inevitably results and imposes a serious volume load on the already hypertrophied right ventricle. In order to correct this, Lillehei has attempted to insert a monocusp valve and others have tried various pericardial reconstructions (Rastelli et al. 1965).

In view of the maintained function of the homograft aortic valve in the descending aorta (Murray 1956) and in the subcoronary position (Ross 1962, 1966), it was decided to use an aortic-valve homograft as a substitute for the absent pulmonary valve.

Case-report

This was an 8-year-old boy. Cyanosis was first noted at the age of 3 months and was constantly present after 1 year. Because of severe intolerance of effort he had to be educated at a school for handicapped children. From the age of 6 years his breathlessness further increased, and he squatted frequently.

Clinical Examination

He was an undersized child, with gross clubbing and central cyanosis at rest. Jugular-venous pulse slightly raised, with small a and v waves. Prominent bulging sternum. Jerky peripheral pulses. Right ventricle moderately enlarged. Auscultation elicited ejection click in aortic area and single second sound; no ejection murmur; continuous murmurs over both sides of the chest, loudest below right clavicle. Hæmoglobin 19·8 g. per 100 ml.

Chest X-ray.—Right arch. Underfilled lung fields.

Electrocardiogram.—P pulmonale, right axis-deviation. R wave in V_1 32 mm. T inversion V_1–V_3.

Cardiac catheterisation.—The findings were as follows:

	Oxygen Saturation (%)	Pressure (mm. Hg)
Femoral artery ..	74	100/40
Superior vena cava	57	..
Right atrium ..	57	a = 4, v = 0
Right ventricle ..	60	100/0

Angiocardiogram showed complete pulmonary-valve atresia. Pulmonary arteries filled from a possible ductus, and collaterals from a large right aortic arch.

Operation

Exploration by D. N. R. on Feb. 14, 1966, through a midsternal incision confirmed the presence of a large aorta, 3 cm. in diameter, and a main pulmonary artery 7 mm. across.

An attempt to find a way through the outflow tract was made by probing, and no connection was found between the right ventricle and main pulmonary artery. After hypothermic bypass was instituted, the right-ventricle outflow tract was opened through a vertical incision, and a blind-ended outflow was seen just beyond the hypertrophied infundibulum. A complete septum was present where the pulmonary valve should have been. A large ventricular septal defect, 2·5 × 1·5 cm., was closed with a 'Teflon' patch and multiple circumferential sutures.

The outflow tract was reconstructed by inserting a small homograft aortic valve with a segment of aorta above, and the anterior cusp of the mitral valve below, which acted as a gusset. A patch of pericardium was inserted between the anterior mitral cusp and a remaining defect in the ventriculotomy.

Postoperative systolic pressures in the main pulmonary artery and right ventricle were 60 mm. Hg when the aortic pressure was 75 mm. Hg.

Postoperative Course

After operation the patient developed features of pulmonary œdema, which was treated with tracheostomy and intermittent positive-pressure respiration as well as anti-failure medication. The clinical and radiological appearances of pulmonary œdema persisted for 8 weeks, and signs of right-heart failure for 3 months, after operation.

Recatheterisation 3 weeks after operation showed a left-to-right shunt into the pulmonary artery, and elevation of the pulmonary capillary venous wedge pressure (P.C.V.):

	Oxygen Saturation (%)	Pressure (mm. Hg)
		P.C.V. mean 27
Right pulmonary artery	82	65/35
Main pulmonary artery	79	65/40
Right ventricle ..	68–67	90/0
Right atrium ..	65, 67	..
Superior vena cava	66	..
Aorta	93	75/50

Aortography demonstrated large bronchial arteries on the anterior aspect of the descending aorta, passing into the hilum; and right pulmonary arteries filled from branches of the right subclavian. In view of the persistent left-heart failure, it was decided to explore the right chest for a ductus. A continuous thrill was felt in the right pulmonary artery, but no duct could be found.

Progress

The patient's heart-failure slowly improved, and he was able to lead a normal active life 6 months later.

Clinical examination.—9 months after operation his weight had increased by 8 lb., and he had grown $1\frac{1}{4}$ in. He was acyanotic at rest and after effort. Jugular-venous pressure normal. Liver normal. Jerky peri-

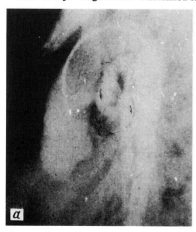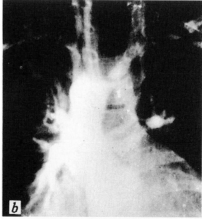

Postoperative aortogram (a, lateral; b, anteroposterior) showing collaterals filling pulmonary arteries.

pheral pulses. Right ventricle unusually pulsatile in 2nd left interspace. Loud ejection click. Loud pulmonary-valve closure, split second sound moving normally. Short grade-3 (out of 4) ejection systolic murmur in pulmonary area. Loud continuous murmurs. No separate immediate diastolic murmur.

Chest radiograph.—Cardiothoracic ratio 52%. Slight increase in lung vascularity.

Electrocardiogram.—Normal P waves. Regression of right-ventricular hypertrophy. R wave in V_1 14 mm. Steep T wave inversion to V_1–V_4.

Discussion

The function of the aortic valve in the pulmonary ring appeared to be excellent, and there was no evidence of pulmonary regurgitation 9 months after operation. The resting gradient (30 mm. Hg) across the right-ventricular outflow tract was at the level of the valve and was probably due to the restricted size of the ring. The main post-operative problem was persistent left-heart failure for 3 months, which required treatment by tracheostomy, digitalis, and daily diuretics. This complication was attributed to the presence of heavy bronchial collaterals, demonstrated by aortography (see figure), which presumably imposed a burden on the left ventricle after closure of the ventricular septum.

The advantage of homograft replacement over other forms of radical surgery for pulmonary atresia is the absence of postoperative pulmonary regurgitation, which may prevent resolution of right-ventricular hypertrophy and lead to persistent right-heart failure despite the disappearance of cyanosis and dyspnœa. Prosthetic valve replacement avoids this complication, but a mechanical valve cannot grow with the patient; and, as most of these patients are children, this may impose serious problems. As yet we have no knowledge of the growth of homograft valves, but they have the advantage that embolic complications, which may occur with prosthetic valves, do not arise, so long-term anticoagulant therapy is not needed.

This technique is suitable for any type of pulmonary atresia, provided there are distal pulmonary-artery branches in continuity; for the trunk of the homograft aorta may be retained and anastomosed to the pulmonary-artery branches or to any main trunk remnant. Homograft aortic valves may also be used in patients with Fallot's tetralogy who have acquired pulmonary atresia, in those with absent or rudimentary valves, or in those with a small valve ring.

Summary

A grossly disabled patient with pulmonary atresia was successfully treated by replacement of the totally obstructed right-ventricular outflow tract by a homograft aortic valve and closure of the ventricular septal defect. It is believed that this technique could be applied to other forms of Fallot's tetralogy with acquired atresia and rudimentary pulmonary valves.

We are grateful to Dr. R. E. Bonham-Carter, who referred the patient to us.

REFERENCES

Lillehei, C. W., Cohen, M., Warden, H. E., Read, R. C., Aust, J. B., De Wall, R. A., Varco, R. L. (1955) *Ann. Surg.* **142**, 418.
— Levy, M. J., Adams, P., Anderson, R. C. (1964) *J. thorac. cardiovasc. Surg.* **48**, 556.
Murray, G. (1956) *Angiology*, **7**, 466.
Rastelli, G. C., Ongley, P. A., Davis, G. D., Kirklin, J. W. (1965) *Proc. Staff Meet. Mayo Clin.* **40**, 521.
Ross, D. N. (1962) *Lancet*, ii, 487.
— (1966) *ibid.* ii, 461.
Sabiston, D. C., Cornell, N. P., Criley, J. M., Neill, C. A. Ross, R. S., Bahnson, H. T. (1964) *J. thorac. cardiovasc. Surg.* **48**, 577.

Addendum

Since this paper was prepared homograft-valve reconstructions of the right-ventricle outflow have been success-

fully carried out in two more patients with Fallot's tetralogy. Also, our attention has been drawn to a report of the use of a homograft replacement in uncomplicated pulmonary-valve stenosis (Marchand, P., Fuller, D. N., Zion, M. M., Zivi, S. *Thorax*, 1966, **21**, 337).

THE LONG-TERM PROGNOSIS OF GENERALISED MILIARY TUBERCULOSIS IN CHILDREN

J. LORBER
M.D. Cantab., F.R.C.P.
READER IN CHILD HEALTH, UNIVERSITY OF SHEFFIELD

GENERALISED miliary tuberculosis, unassociated with tuberculous meningitis, is fortunately a very rare disease now among children in the U.K. No new cases have been admitted to the Children's Hospital, Sheffield, since 1959. In earlier years, however, it was a common disease—between September, 1947, when treatment first became possible, and the end of 1959, 42 children were admitted to the University Department in the Children's Hospital with generalised miliary tuberculosis unassociated with meningitis. In the earliest years 10 children developed caseous tuberculous meningitis while under streptomycin treatment, but no child developed meningitis after the introduction of isoniazid. The 32 children who had no

TABLE I—MILIARY TUBERCULOSIS IN CHILDREN, 1947–59

Age on admission	No. (% of total)
Under 12 mos.	6 (19%)
12–23 mos.	6 (19%)
2–5 yr.	6 (19%)
6–13 yr.	14 (53%)
Total	32

meningitis at any time form the material of this study. There were 16 boys and 16 girls. The age-distribution is shown in table I.

Diagnosis

Miliary tuberculosis was diagnosed on the basis of classical snowstorm appearance of the lung field on chest X-ray in all cases, together with a positive tuberculin test. 19 children (60%) had choroidal tubercles, supporting the diagnosis with this specific physical sign. Tubercle bacilli were recovered from gastric washings, and/or from the urine or caseous glands in 26 cases (81%). Among the 6 children without bacteriological confirmation 4 had choroidal tubercles which helped to strengthen the diagnosis. The large majority of children had fresh primary complexes in their lungs besides the miliary picture, and 2 had pleural effusion. 3 children had tuberculosis of the vertebræ and 1 had tuberculous arthritis of one knee. 1 child had convulsions with a high protein content in the cerebrospinal fluid, without excess of cells or the presence of organisms. This boy was considered to have tuberculomata of the brain. Prolonged anticonvulsant therapy prevented further fits for over fourteen years, but X-rays of his skull some two

TABLE II—INCIDENCE OF EXTRAPULMONARY TUBERCULOSIS

—	Brain	Bones and joint	Lungs*	Pleural effusion
(a) Concurrent with active miliary disease	1	4	1	2
(b) After recovery from miliary disease	..	2	1	..
(c) Postprimary pulmonary T.B. ..	..	..	None	..

* Both had lobectomy for post-tuberculous bronchiectasis.

Volume 55, Number 3   *March* 1968

The Journal of THORACIC AND

CARDIOVASCULAR SURGERY

Surgical repair of the complete form of persistent common atrioventricular canal

G. C. Rastelli, M.D., Patrick A. Ongley, M.D., John W. Kirklin, M.D., and Dwight C. McGoon, M.D., Rochester, Minn.

Repair of the complete form of persistent common atrioventricular (A-V) canal with its severe anatomic derangement is still a formidable task for the cardiovascular surgeon. With the exception of Gerbode and Sabar's[1] report of only one surgical death in 13 cases, the surgical mortality has been 63, 75, and 67 per cent in reported series.[2-4] The technique of repair is far from standardized, and the reports of long-term follow-up have been too scarce to allow appraisal of late results. The whole experience of repair of this lesion at the Mayo Clinic is reviewed herein.* The technical problems of repair are analyzed in the light of new anatomic observations on pathologic material, and a more appropriate repair, used in recent operations, is described.

Material

A total of 38 patients were operated upon between December, 1955, and September, 1967.* There were 21 females and 17 males; the median age was 6 years (range, 10 months to 51 years). Most of the patients had severe symptoms, including heart failure. Clinically mild cyanosis was present in 5 patients; severe cyanosis was present in 2 who had associated pulmonary stenosis. The average preoperative cardiothoracic ratio was 0.62 (range, 0.48 to 0.78). The electrocardiogram showed a negative mean frontal plane QRS axis between –45 degrees and –180 degrees (average, –103 degrees) and a counterclockwise frontal loop[7] in all the cases except 2 in which the mean QRS′ axis was +125 and +130 degrees, respectively. In these 2 cases, the initial frontal

From the Mayo Clinic and Mayo Foundation, Rochester, Minn. 55901: Section of Pediatrics (Dr. Ongley) and of Surgery (Drs. Kirklin and McGoon). Mayo Graduate School of Medicine (University of Minnesota), Rochester, Minn.: Research Associate (Dr. Rastelli).

Received for publication May 29, 1967.

*We appreciate the cooperation of our colleagues, Drs. F. Henry Ellis, Jr., and R. B. Wallace, in allowing us to include patients operated upon by them.

*Eighteen cases have been reported in previous papers.[4-6]

Journal of
Thoracic and Cardiovascular
Surgery

300   *Rastelli et al.*

QRS loop was also counterclockwise. In 1 case, a 12-year-old girl had associated valvular and infundibular pulmonary stenosis; in the other, a 1-year-old girl had associated coarctation, patent ductus arteriosus, left inferior vena cava, and partial anomalous pulmonary venous return.

There were associated cardiovascular anomalies in 16 of the 38 surgically treated patients (Table I). In 18 of the 20 patients catheterized preoperatively, pulmonary flow exceeded systemic flow by a factor of two or more; in the 2 others it was 1.2 and 1.8 times systemic flow. In the absence of pulmonary stenosis, pulmonary artery systolic pressure measured at cardiac catheterization or at operation was mildly increased (< 45 per cent of systolic systemic pressure) in 5 cases, moderately increased (45 to 75 per cent of systolic systemic pressure) in 4 cases, and severely increased (> 75 per cent of systolic systemic pressure) in 26 cases. In 11 patients with severe pulmonary hypertension in whom adequate data were available, the ratio of pulmonary resistance to systemic resistance was 0.31 or less in 5, and 0.4, 0.43, 0.5, 0.5, 0.5 and 0.6, respectively, in the other 6.

A left ventricular angiogram was made in 6 cases. By demonstrating the features characteristic of this malformation,[8] it contributed to the diagnosis of persistent common A-V canal, although it was not useful in the differential diagnosis between the partial and the complete form of the malformation.[9] Left A-V valve incompetence was judged on the basis of apical systolic murmur, size of the left ventricle on thoracic roentgenograms, and assessment of the regurgitant jet by the exploring finger of the surgeon while the heart was beating. It was considered to be present in 33 of the 38 cases (mild or moderate in 26 and severe in 7).

Surgical technique

Operation was performed through a median sternotomy incision, with total cardiopulmonary bypass utilizing a Mayo-Gibbon pump oxygenator. The heart was quieted by one or more short periods (up to 15 minutes each) of aortic cross-clamping (with previous cooling) or by electrically induced and maintained ventricular fibrillation. Various types of repair were performed through a right atriotomy; this was associated with right ventriculotomy in 7 cases. In an attempt to relieve mitral incompetence, the mitral portions of the anterior and posterior common leaflets were usually approximated.

In 31 operations, the interventricular communication was usually obliterated by suturing the anterior and posterior common leaflets to the crest of the muscular septum with interrupted mattress sutures. The interatrial communication was then closed with an Ivalon sponge patch (in early cases) or a pericardial or Teflon patch (more recently). In 5 cases, an additional Teflon patch was used to repair (through a right ventriculotomy) a large interventricular communication existing under the anterior common A-V leaflet. In order to avoid injury to the bundle of His

Table I. *Associated anomalies in 16 patients undergoing surgical repair of persistent common atrioventricular canal*

Anomaly	No.
Patent foramen ovale	11
Ostium secundum	3
Common ventricle	1
Patent ductus arteriosus	4
Left superior vena cava	5*
Pulmonary stenosis (infundibular and valvular)	2
Infundibular pulmonary stenosis with bicuspid pulmonary valve	1
Coronary sinus drained into left atrium	1
Common atrium	2
Stenosis of orifice of right pulmonary veins	1
Accessory mitral orifice	2
Coarctation of aorta	2
Origin of right subclavian artery distal to left subclavian artery	2
Partial anomalous pulmonary venous connection	2
Muscular ventricular septal defect	1

*Drained into left atrium in 1 case.

Volume 55
Number 3
March, 1968

which runs more toward the left side of the interventricular septum, the sutures were carefully placed a few millimeters away from the edge of the septum, toward its right side. For the same reason, in general, fewer sutures were placed in the area of the posterior halves of the A-V valves (which are in close proximity to the bundle) and stitching in the tricuspid leaflet was done without incorporating the septum. It is preferable to achieve a less secure repair in this area than to risk complete A-V block. At this stage of repair, the cardiac action was started to allow immediate detection of any injury to the conduction system and removal of the responsible stitch. Since these precautions have been adopted, the incidence of heart block has greatly diminished. Infundibular resection was carried out in 2 cases through a right ventriculotomy; 1 of these 2 patients had a patch reconstruction of the right ventricular outflow tract.

The type of repair used recently in 7 cases is based on a better understanding of the anatomy of the common A-V valve.[10] Three types of complete A-V canal (Fig. 1) can be recognized on the basis of the anatomy of the anterior common A-V leaflet and the extent and site of interventricular communication:

1. The anterior common A-V leaflet is divided into two portions, one mitral and one tricuspid,* both attached medially to the muscular septum. In this type the membranous septum has formed and the interventricular communication does not extend to the vicinity of the aortic cusps (Fig. 1A). This series had 25 cases of this type.

2. The anterior common A-V leaflet is divided into two portions unattached to the septum but both are attached medially to an anomalous papillary muscle in the right

*This portion is in fact analogous to the normal anterior leaflet of the tricuspid valve.

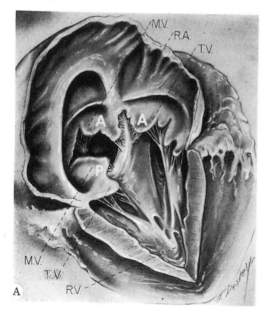

Fig. 1A. Anterior *(A)* common A-V leaflet is divided into two portions, one mitral *(MV)* and one tricuspid *(TV)*, attached medially to interventricular septum with long, nonfused chordae tendineae. In posterior *(P)* common A-V leaflet, mitral *(MV)* and tricuspid *(TV)* portions are not separated. *RV*, right ventricle; *RA*, right atrium.

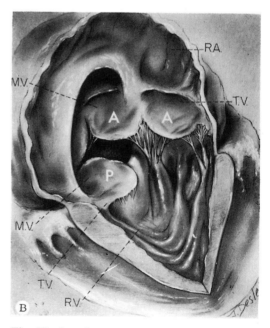

Fig. 1B. Anterior common A-V leaflet is divided but not attached to septum. Mitral and tricuspid components are both attached medially to abnormal papillary muscle arising in right ventricle near septum. Free interventricular communication occurs under anterior common leaflet.

Journal of
Thoracic and Cardiovascular
Surgery

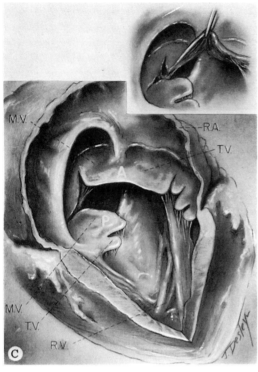

Fig. 1C. Anterior common A-V leaflet is not divided and is not attached to septum *(inset)* so that free interventricular communication, extending to vicinity of aortic cusps, occurs underneath this leaflet. (From Rastelli, G. C., Kirklin, J. W., and Kincaid, O. W.: Angiocardiography in Persistent Common Atrioventricular Canal, Mayo Clin. Proc. 42: 200, 1967.)

ventricle adjacent to the septum (Fig. 1B). There were 3 cases of this type.

3. The anterior common A-V leaflet is undivided and unattached to the septum but freely floats above it (Fig. 1C). Ten cases were of this type. In this and in the preceding type, the interventricular communication is complete under the common anterior leaflet and it extends to the proximity of the aortic cusps.

The posterior common leaflet in all three types is usually rudimentary and shows various anatomic arrangements similar to those described for the anterior common leaflet.

The first type of malformation (Fig. 1A) is the most frequent and usually it has been an isolated finding; the second and the third

types (Figs. 1B and 1C) have been associated with other major cardiac anomalies.

The type of complete A-V canal shown in Fig. 1A in 7 patients was repaired recently, as shown in Fig. 2. The anterior leaflet of the mitral valve was reconstructed by approximating its two components at their base with a few interrupted stitches (Fig. 2, *A*). A single autogenous pericardial or Teflon patch was then used to repair the persistent A-V canal (Fig. 2, *B*). The medial edge of the reconstructed mitral leaflet was attached to the patch with interrupted sutures (Fig. 2, *C*) before closure of the atrial portion of the defect was completed (Fig. 2, *D*). In those cases in which the posterior common leaflet is attached to the interventricular septum by a continuous membrane or by fused chordae (inset, Fig. 2, *A*), between which only insignificant interventricular communication occurs, it may be preferable to suture the patch directly over leaflet tissue so as to incorporate most of it in the mitral valve (Fig. 2, *B*). This technique avoids suturing in the area of the bundle of His. When the posterior common leaflet is not attached to the septum and a significant interventricular communication exists underneath it (inset, Fig. 2, *E*), it is probably best to split the leaflet from the free edge down to the base, slightly to the right of the midline (Fig. 2, *E*), to attach the patch to the right side of the septum (Fig. 2, *F*), and to suture the medial edges of the newly created mitral and tricuspid portions to the patch in a similar fashion as for the anterior common leaflet (Fig. 2, *G*).

Results

There was a total of 19 hospital deaths. None of the 8 patients 2 years of age or less survived. Hospital mortality prior to 1964 was 60 per cent (17 deaths). Hospital mortality in the last 4 years was 20 per cent (10 operated cases, 7 by means of the repair shown in Fig. 2). Complete heart block has occurred in 8 cases (21 per cent), 7 prior to 1959 and only 1 in the last 26 cases. All these cases are included among

Volume 55
Number 3
March, 1968

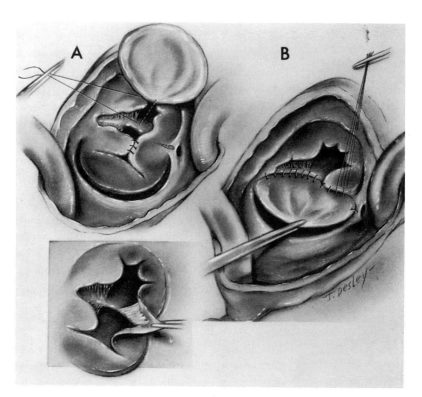

Fig. 2. Method of repair of complete A-V canal of type illustrated in Fig. 1A. *A,* Mitral portions of anterior and posterior common leaflets are approximated; a single patch is used and sutures are started midway in muscular septum to right of crest. *B,* Patch first is sutured between chordal attachment of anterior mitral and tricuspid leaflets. In area of posterior common leaflet, in absence of interventricular communication below this leaflet *(inset),* sutures are placed, while heart is beating, onto leaflet tissue without incorporating underlying muscular septum, thus avoiding stitches in area of bundle of His.

the deaths. In addition, 1 surviving patient has a 2:1 block.

There were two late deaths. One occurred in a 3-year-old boy with severe pulmonary hypertension who had had a transient heart block during operation. Residual mitral valve incompetence was present at the time of dismissal. The boy died 2 months postoperatively during an episode of respiratory infection. Complete heart block had been noted again at that time. The second death occurred in a 19-year-old girl who had an associated partial anomalous pulmonary venous connection which was repaired at the same operation. She died 3 years postoperatively after she had been started on an unknown treatment for rapid heart rate. Progressive mitral valve incompetence had developed since her operation.

The 17 surviving patients have had relief of symptoms for 1 month to 12 years postoperatively. They are leading normal lives with no restriction in activity. The heart has become smaller than its preoperative size in all 17, but it remains slightly enlarged in most of them (Figs. 3, 4, and 5). In most patients the apical systolic murmur noted preoperatively persisted after operation, with unchanged loudness. Sixteen patients are considered to have residual mild or moderate mitral incompetence. One patient who had no incompetence preoperatively is free of incompetence 2 years postoperatively.

Comment

Analysis of the 11 hospital deaths that occurred in the absence of A-V dissociation

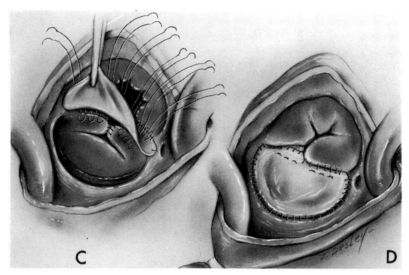

Fig. 2, Cont'd. *C,* After lower edge of patch is sutured in place, upper portion is folded back into right atrium. Medial edge of reconstructed anterior mitral leaflet is then attached with interrupted mattress sutures to patch at height it reaches without tension on underlying chordae tendineae. *D,* Closure of atrial portion of defect is completed with continuous sutures.

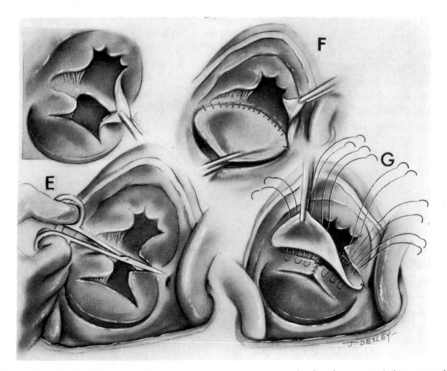

Fig. 2, Cont'd. *E,* When significant interventricular communication is present below posterior common leaflet *(inset),* this structure may be split from free edge down to its base. *F,* Patch is sutured to right side of septum in this area. *G,* Medial edges of both newly created mitral and tricuspid portions of posterior common leaflet are attached to patch before completion or repair of atrial portion of defect.

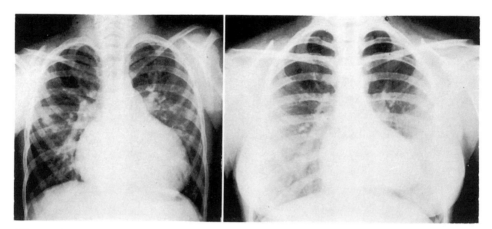

Fig. 3. Thoracic roentgenograms made before *(left)* and 10 years after *(right)* repair of complete form of persistent common A-V canal. Patient was 9 years of age at time of operation.

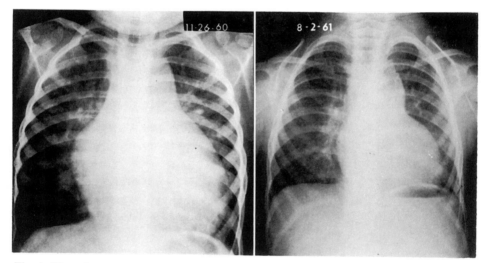

Fig. 4. Thoracic roentgenograms made before *(left)* and 9 months after *(right)* repair of complete form of persistent common A-V canal. Patient was 3 years of age at the time of operation.

shows that the cause of death was related to low cardiac output. Two cyanotic patients had associated severe infundibular pulmonary stenosis. One patient had undergone repair of a common ventricle. In each of the remaining 8 cases, residual mitral incompetence was present or was suspected after the repair. Preoperatively, mitral incompetence was considered to be severe in 3, moderate in 4, and mild or absent in 4 of these 11 cases. The incompleteness of relief of mitral valve incompetence in cases of

partial A-V canal is well recognized.[11] In the successfully treated cases of the complete form also, mitral incompetence existing prior to operation has not been effectively relieved by the operation. The same degree of incompetence may have a more severe effect after the closure of the interatrial communication than it had before. The low cardiac output observed after operation was most likely related to significant residual mitral incompetence. Severe pulmonary hypertension was present in 9 of these 11 pa-

Journal of
Thoracic and Cardiovascular
Surgery

306   *Rastelli et al.*

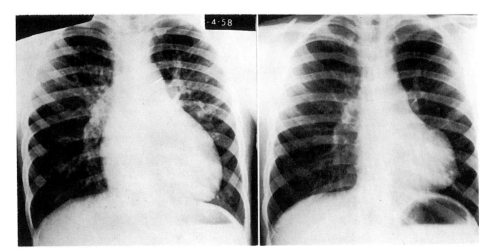

Fig. 5. Thoracic roentgenograms made before *(left)* and 4 years after *(right)* repair of complete form of persistent common A-V canal. Patient was 10 years of age at the time of operation.

tients (excluded are the 2 patients with pulmonary stenosis). Therefore, although pulmonary vascular resistance was generally not severely increased, right ventricular dysfunction probably was a factor in precipitating the low cardiac output syndrome.

An attempt was made to correlate surgical mortality with the three anatomic types of complete A-V canal (see Fig. 1). Prior to the introduction of the surgical repair described herein, hospital mortality has been 47 per cent for repair of the first type and 77 per cent for repairs of the second and the third types combined. This suggests that the latter two types are more difficult to repair and the prognosis is worse in these cases. This is due to the presence of a larger interventricular communication, a smaller total surface area of the anterior common leaflet, and the association of other major cardiac anomalies.

From the postmortem analysis of the available hearts it became apparent that, when the common anterior leaflet was sutured to the interventricular septum to obliterate the interventricular communication in this area, obstruction to left ventricular outflow was created in some cases. This is explainable by the way the left ventricular outflow tract is already characteristically narrowed and elongated in this condition.[8]

Suturing of the anterior common leaflet to the interventricular septum can exaggerate this situation to the point of creating significant obstruction. Also, the attachment of the anterior and posterior common leaflets to the interventricular septum often resulted in loss of mobility of the A-V valves. Mitral stenosis was caused in some cases when the anterior leaflet of the mitral valve was reconstructed by suturing together completely the mitral components of the anterior and posterior common leaflets in the area of the "cleft." In the complete form of A-V canal, this resembles more a wide gap. Elsewhere[10] it has been stressed that the tricuspid valve is not cleft in this condition. In fact, the gap existing between the tricuspid components of the anterior and posterior common leaflets is between an anterior leaflet of the tricuspid valve (see Fig. 1A) or its equivalent (see Figs. 1B and 1C) and a rudimentary tricuspid septal leaflet posteriorly. This gap should therefore be left alone lest its repair cause tricuspid deformity or stenosis.

The type of anatomy illustrated in Fig. 1A, which is fortunately found in most cases, lends itself to the type of repair illustrated in Fig. 2. In these cases the anterior common leaflet has a wider total area and it is divided into two portions, attached

Volume 55
Number 3
March, 1968

medially to the septum; thus, the extent of the interventricular communication underneath the leaflet is reduced. The repair illustrated in Fig. 2 aims at preserving as much as possible the mobility of the A-V valves. The reconstruction of the anterior leaflet of the mitral valve is carried out by approximation of the mitral portions of the anterior and posterior common leaflets starting at their bases but not carried out for the entire length of the "cleft." A better reconstruction of the mitral valve with avoidance of stenosis is thus achieved. Another important feature of this repair is that the attachment of the medial edge of the reconstructed anterior mitral leaflet to the patch avoids obstruction to left ventricular outflow tract.

In the types illustrated in Figs. 1B and 1C, a type of repair similar to that illustrated in Fig. 2 could be carried out, after the anterior common leaflet is split, but it is doubtful that a satisfactory reconstruction of mitral valves may be achieved, because of the scarcity of A-V valvular tissue. In these cases it may be better to incorporate most of the available valvular tissue into the tricuspid valve and to replace the mitral valve with a prosthetic valve. In view of the differences in prognosis and the difficulty in repairing the various types of complete A-V canal, it is important to be able to diagnose preoperatively the exact anatomic variety. This may prove to be possible by left ventricular angiocardiography.[9]

The lack of success in repairing the malformation in infants suggests that it is not advisable to try a complete repair before the patient is 3 years of age. Pulmonary artery banding may be considered for those younger patients with intractable congestive failure due to excessive pulmonary flow. The 2 such infants with the complete form of persistent common A-V canal so treated in our experience have received excellent palliation.

Late results of intracardiac repair are encouraging, although mitral valve incompetence has not been completely relieved by the technique used in the past. It is too early to know whether or not the proposed new surgical technique may result in a more complete relief of mitral incompetence.

Summary

Thirty-eight patients with the complete form of persistent common atrioventricular canal were operated upon at the Mayo Clinic between December, 1955, and September, 1967. The hospital mortality was 60 per cent prior to 1964. It was 20 per cent in the last 4 years (10 cases, including 7 cases in which a new surgical repair was used). The incidence of heart block was 21 per cent; only one instance occurred in the last 26 patients (after 1959). There were two late deaths. The 17 surviving patients have been free of symptoms and are leading normal lives. In most of them there is evidence of persisting mild or moderate mitral valve incompetence. The failures early in the surgical management were mostly associated with heart block, infant age, and associated anomalies. More recently, with better selection of the patients, the failures were more closely related to mitral incompetence which was incompletely relieved by the operation.

The recognition of three anatomic types of complete atrioventricular canal has given a better understanding of the problems involved in surgical repair. A more appropriate type of repair is described and discussed.

REFERENCES

1 Gerbode, F., and Sabar, E. F.: Endocardial Cushion Defects: Diagnosis and Surgical Repair, J. Cardiov. Surg. **5:** 223, 1964.

2 Levy, M. J., Cuello, L., Tuna, N., and Lillehei, C. W.: Atrioventricularis Communis: Clinical Aspects and Surgical Treatment, Am. J. Cardiol. **14:** 587, 1964.

3 Scott, L. P., Hauck, A. J., Nadas, A. S., and Gross, R. E.: Endocardial Cushion Defect: Preoperative and Postoperative Survey, Circulation **26:** 218, 1962.

4 Ellis, F. H., Jr., McGoon, D. C., and Kirklin, J. W.: Surgical Management of Persistent Common Atrioventricular Canal, Am. J. Cardiol. **6:** 598, 1960.

5 Cooley, J. C., Kirklin, J. W., and Harshbarger, H. G.: The Surgical Treatment of Persistent

Journal of
Thoracic and Cardiovascular
Surgery

3 0 8 *Rastelli et al.*

Common Atrioventricular Canal, Surgery **41**: 147, 1957.

6 McGoon, D. C., DuShane, J. W., and Kirklin, J. W.: The Surgical Treatment of Endocardial Cushion Defects, Surgery **46**: 185, 1959.

7 Burchell, H. B., DuShane, J. W., and Brandenburg, R. O.: The Electrocardiogram of Patients With Atrioventricular Cushion Defects (Defects of the Atrioventricular Canal), Am. J. Cardiol. **6**: 575, 1960.

8 Baron, M. G., Wolf, B. S., Steinfeld, L., and Van Mierop, L. H. S.: Endocardial Cushion Defects: Specific Diagnosis by Angiocardiography, Am. J. Cardiol. **13**: 162, 1964.

9 Rastelli, G. C., Kirklin, J. W., and Kincaid, O. W.: Angiocardiography in Persistent Common Atrioventricular Canal, Mayo Clin. Proc. **42**: 200, 1967.

10 Rastelli, G. C., Kirklin, J. W., and Titus, J. L.: Anatomic Observations on Complete Form of Persistent Common Atrioventricular Canal With Special Reference to Atrioventricular Valves, Mayo Clin. Proc. **41**: 296, 1966.

11 Rastelli, G. C., Weidman, W. H., and Kirklin, J. W.: Surgical Repair of the Partial Form of Persistent Common Atrioventricular Canal, With Special Reference to the Problem of Mitral Valve Incompetence, Circulation **31** (Suppl. I): 31, 1965.

Thorax (1971), **26**, 240.

Surgical repair of tricuspid atresia

F. FONTAN and E. BAUDET

Centre de Cardiologie, Université de Bordeaux II, Hôpital du Tondu, Bordeaux, France

Surgical repair of tricuspid atresia has been carried out in three patients ; two of these operations have been successful. A new surgical procedure has been used which transmits the whole vena caval blood to the lungs, while only oxygenated blood returns to the left heart. The right atrium is, in this way, 'ventriclized', to direct the inferior vena caval blood to the left lung, the right pulmonary artery receiving the superior vena caval blood through a cava-pulmonary anastomosis. This technique depends on the size of the pulmonary arteries, which must be large enough and at sufficiently low pressure to allow a cava-pulmonary anastomosis. The indications for this procedure apply only to children sufficiently well developed. Younger children or those whose pulmonary arteries are too small should be treated by palliative surgical procedures.

Only palliative operations (systemic vein to pulmonary artery anastomosis ; systemic artery to pulmonary artery anastomosis) have been performed in tricuspid atresia. Although these procedures are valuable, they result in only a partial clinical improvement, because they do not suppress the mixture of venous and oxygenated blood.

We have initiated a corrective procedure for tricuspid atresia, which completely suppresses blood mixing. The entire vena caval return undergoes arterialization in the lungs and only oxygenated blood comes back to the left heart. This procedure is not an anatomical correction, which would require the creation of a right ventricle, but a procedure of physiological pulmonary blood flow restoration, with suppression of right and

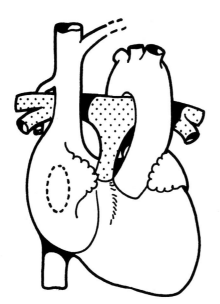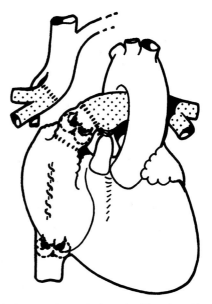

FIG. 1. *Case 2. Tricuspid atresia type II B. Drawing illustrates steps in surgical repair:* (1) *end-to-side anastomosis of distal end of right pulmonary artery to superior vena cava;* (2) *end-to-end anastomosis of right atrial appendage to proximal end of right pulmonary artery by means of an aortic valve homograft;* (3) *closure of atrial septal defect;* (4) *insertion of a pulmonary valve homograft into inferior vena cava; and* (5) *ligation of main pulmonary artery.*

240

Surgical repair of tricuspid atresia 241

left blood mixing. This new surgical procedure has been used in three patients and has been successful in two of them; the first case has been followed satisfactorily for 30 months. The indications for this procedure apply only to children who are sufficiently well developed, without pulmonary arterial hypertension.

Palliative operations remain valuable in other patients and will permit many of them to have a secondary corrective procedure.

SURGICAL TECHNIQUE

The purpose of the operation is to drain the whole vena caval blood to the pulmonary arteries (Fig. 1): the superior vena cava is anastomosed to the distal end of the right pulmonary artery, according to Glenn's procedure; the proximal end of the right pulmonary artery is anastomosed to the right atrium; so, after the atrial septal defect has been closed, the blood of the inferior vena cava is drained towards the left pulmonary artery. The main pulmonary artery is ligated at the point where it leaves the right hypoplastic ventricle, to prevent ventricular blood entering the left lung. In short, the right atrium is used to propel inferior vena caval blood through the left lung. To facilitate this function, the right atrium is provided with two aortic or pulmonary valve homografts: one is inserted into the inferior vena cava at its junction with the right atrium, to prevent blood reflux into the inferior vena cava during atrial systole; the other is used as an anastomosis between the right atrial appendage and the proximal end of the right pulmonary artery, so that, during atrial diastole, there is no reflux from the left pulmonary artery into the right atrium.

The operation is performed through a median sternotomy. After the pericardium has been opened, the heart is examined to confirm the preoperative diagnosis of tricuspid atresia type. The pulmonary arteries also have to be examined carefully to ensure that their size is large enough to permit a cava-pulmonary anastomosis. In addition, it is necessary to measure the pressures in the pulmonary artery, thus making sure that there is no pulmonary arterial hypertension, which would be a contraindication to cavapulmonary anastomosis. This information, suspected from catheterization and angiocardiography, can only be corroborated during operation.

The surgical repair begins with the classic cavapulmonary anastomosis between the distal end of the right pulmonary artery and the right posterolateral aspect of the superior vena cava. End-to-side anastomosis is made, using a Blalock continuous suture (Fig. 2). But the superior vena cava is not yet transected at its entry into the right atrium, because it must be used for superior vena caval cannulation during cardiopulmonary bypass. This transection must be carried out as the last step of the operation.

The proximal end of the right pulmonary artery is then anastomosed to the right atrium by means of an

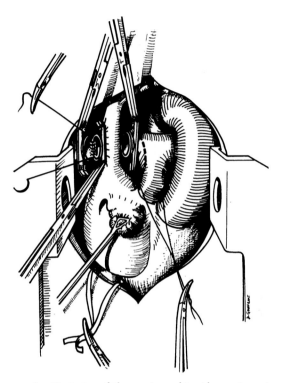

FIG. 2. *First step of the repair: end-to-side anastomosis of distal end of right pulmonary artery to superior vena cava (Glenn, 1958). Drawing illustrates bevelling of proximal end of right pulmonary artery to ensure a correct fit with the aortic valve homograft (see Fig. 3).*

aortic valve homograft (Fig. 3); the aortic wall is tailored to an adequate length; the origin of the right pulmonary artery can also be enlarged by bevelling up to the main pulmonary artery in order to achieve a good fit with the homograft (Fig. 2). End-to-end anastomosis is made using a continuous suture. The homograft (a short segment of the anterior mitral leaflet and septum below the aortic cusps has been kept) is end-to-end anastomosed to the right atrial appendage. There is no problem of fit with the atrial appendage which is, in tricuspid atresia, widely dilated, but fleshy tissues in the atrial appendage should be resected so that they do not hinder blood flow. Such a homograft was used in our second and third cases. In the first case, a younger child, we did not have a small enough homograft. We anastomosed the proximal end of the right pulmonary artery directly to the left lateral side of the upper part of the right atrium (Figs 7 and 8).

The operation then proceeds under cardiopulmonary bypass (Fig. 4), at flow rates of 2 to 2·2 litres/min/m² at normothermia. The duration of cardiopulmonary bypass is about 40 minutes. The ascending

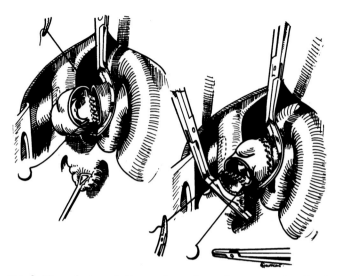

FIG. 3. *Second step of the repair: end-to-end anastomosis of right atrial appendage to proximal end of right pulmonary artery by means of an aortic valve homograft. Drawing illustrates superior vena cava to right pulmonary artery anastomosis, but superior vena cava is not yet transected at its entry into right atrium because it must be used for superior vena caval cannulation during cardiopulmonary bypass.*

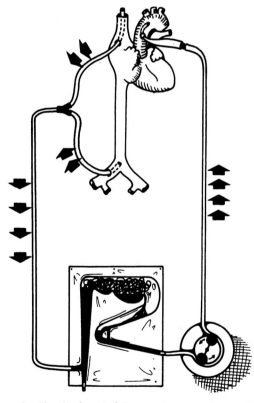

FIG. 4. *Sketch of cardiopulmonary bypass, with cannulation of ascending aorta, superior vena cava, and right iliac vein.*

aorta is cannulated; the superior vena cava is cannulated through a purse-string suture slipped on between the right atrial appendage and the superior vena cava. The inferior vena cava is cannulated by means of the right external iliac vein so that the catheter does not prevent the insertion of the valve homograft into the inferior vena cava level with its junction with the right atrium. When the bypass is started, the superior vena cava is snared by an umbilical tape above the right cava-pulmonary anastomosis and the inferior vena cava is clamped just below its entry into the right atrium. The left ventricle is vented. The aorta is cross-clamped. After the right atrium has been opened (Fig. 5), the atrial septal defect is closed; a pulmonary valve homograft is inserted into the inferior vena caval orifice. This homograft is prepared in the following manner: the whole subvalvular tissue is resected and only 2 to 3 mm of the arterial wall above the cusps is kept to suture the homograft to the atrial wall, using a continuous suture. There is no fear of harm to the bundle of His if the suture is passed sufficiently far behind the coronary sinus.

After the atriotomy has been closed, the air evacuated, and the clamps removed, the main pulmonary artery is ligated or transected. Cardiopulmonary bypass is discontinued as soon as cardiac action is vigorous. When the systemic pressure is above 100 mmHg, the same or slightly higher pressures are looked for in the superior vena cava, the right atrium, and the pulmonary artery as were measured before bypass.

After the cannulae have been removed, the superior vena cava is transected between two clamps at its entry into the right atrium and both ends are sutured (Fig. 6).

Surgical repair of tricuspid atresia 243

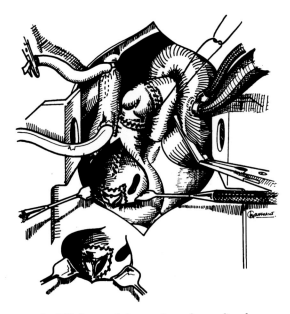

FIG. 5. *Third step of the repair, under cardiopulmonary bypass: closure of atrial septal defect and insertion of a pulmonary valve homograft into inferior vena cava level with right atrium. Superior vena cava is cannulated through a purse-string suture, slipped on between right atrial appendage and superior vena cava, and it is snared by an umbilical tape above cava-pulmonary anastomosis.*

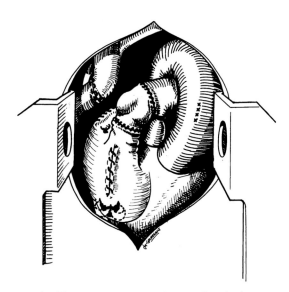

FIG. 6. *The operation at completion, after the last step of the repair: superior vena cava is transected at its entry into right atrium and main pulmonary artery is ligated.*

The pericardium is closed in the upper part without compromising the different anastomoses. The pericardial cavity and the anterior mediastinum are drained ; the sternum is reapproximated with wire sutures and the subcutaneous tissue and skin are closed.

CASE REPORTS

CASE 1   Our first patient, C.F., underwent operation at the age of 12 years.

The face and extremities had been cyanosed from the age of 6 months and the cyanosis had gradually progressed ; at the same time, exertional dyspnoea had appeared when she was admitted to hospital in 1961, at the age of 6 years, for haemodynamic investigations.

Cyanosis was marked. There was clubbing of the fingers and toes. A loud systolic murmur was heard at the apex, radiating along the left of the sternum, with an accentuated second heart sound. Blood pressure was 100/60 mmHg. Manifestations of cardiac failure were not noted. A blood count showed 7,000,000 RBC/mm^3.

Cardiac catheterization and angiocardiography revealed a type I B tricuspid atresia, with pulmonary arteries of good size. The possibility of a cava-pulmonary anastomosis was noted. The child left hospital and was lost sight of.

She was later readmitted to hospital in April 1968. She was very erythrocyanotic and manifested exertional symptoms—dyspnoea and frequent episodes of tachycardia. No signs of cardiac failure were noted. A blood count showed 7,800,000 RBC/mm^3 and the haematocrit was 80%.

Operation (Fig. 7) was performed on 25 April 1968 through a median sternotomy. The findings were tricuspid atresia without transposition of the great vessels (type I B) but with pulmonary arteries of good size and low intra-arterial pressure (15·0 mmHg). A superior vena cava to pulmonary artery anastomosis and an anastomosis between the atrium and the proximal end of the right pulmonary artery were carried out (Fig 8) ; the azygos vein was not ligated. Then, under cardiopulmonary bypass, the atrial septal defect was closed, a pulmonary valve homograft was inserted into the inferior vena cava level with the right atrium, and the main pulmonary artery was ligated. After the cardiopulmonary bypass had been discontinued, the superior vena cava was divided level with the right atrium below the cava-pulmonary anastomosis (Fig. 9).

The initial postoperative course was very satisfactory : cyanosis disappeared. The patient was in sinus rhythm at 90 per minute and the blood pressure was 120/60 mmHg. Ventilation and haematosis were satisfactory. The venous pressure was not raised.

Twenty-four hours postoperatively anuria developed quite suddenly, but metabolic disorders were corrected by one haemodialysis only, while a moderate melaena appeared. The following day urinary

244   *F. Fontan and E. Baudet*

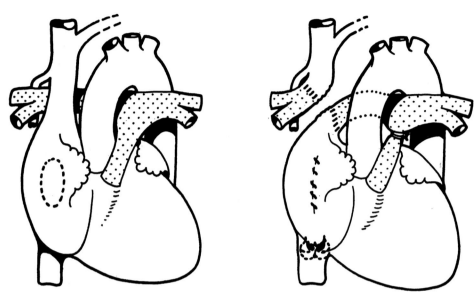

FIG. 7. *Case 1. Tricuspid atresia type I B. Drawing illustrates the repair: anastomosis between right atrium and proximal end of right pulmonary artery was made without interposition of an aortic valve homograft.*

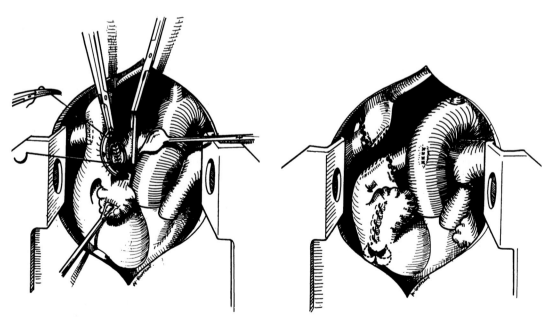

FIG. 8. *End-to-side anastomosis of proximal end of right pulmonary artery to left lateral side of upper part of right atrium.*

FIG. 9. *Case 1. Appearance at completion of operation.*

Surgical repair of tricuspid atresia   245

function returned, after the patient's legs had been raised to improve the stagnant inferior vena caval circulation. From that moment there was no further urinary problem, but intravenous urography revealed a bilateral congenital hydronephrosis.

One month postoperatively a right serofibrinous pleural effusion required suction drainage for a few days.

The child was examined regularly after discharge from hospital and she is quite well after a 30 months' follow-up; she has grown normally and does not show exertional symptoms; she is no longer cyanotic and there is no oedema of the inferior limbs. The liver is just palpable below the costal edge. A chest radiograph shows normal pulmonary vascularity of both lungs. An electrocardiogram indicates a regression of the right atrial hypertrophy. A blood count showed 4,400,000 RBC/mm³ and the haematocrit was 52%. Digitalis and diuretics in standard doses were prescribed. Anticoagulants were not used postoperatively. Physical examination is normal and there is no longer a systolic murmur.

The following postoperative haemodynamic and angiocardiographic investigations were made:

(1) The pressure curve in the superior vena cava fluctuated between 2·0 and 16·0 mmHg with breathing movements. On the other hand, in the inferior vena cava and the right atrium, the pressure was stable, about 15·0 mmHg (Table 1).

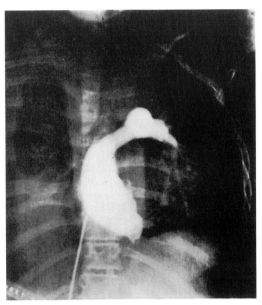

FIG. 10. *Case 1. Postoperative right atrial angiocardiogram, anteroposterior view, showing opacification of right atrium and contrast medium flowing through left pulmonary artery.*

TABLE I

| | | RBC per mm³ | Haematocrit % | Pressure (mmHg) | | |
				SVC	IVC	RA
Preoperative	6 yr	7,000,000	70		8	
	12 yr	7,800,000	80			
Postoperative		4,400,000	52	2 to 16	15	14

(2) Right atrial angiocardiography showed that, except for a slight flow along the catheter (Figs 10 and 11), the contrast medium did not flow back from the right atrium to the inferior vena cava because the valve homograft performed its antireflux function perfectly. The valvular sinus is well seen on the angiocardiogram (lateral view). The contrast medium flowed through the left pulmonary artery and passage though the left lung was unimpeded.

CASE 2 Our second patient, J.B., was a 36-year-old woman, who had been cyanotic since she was a child but was normally developed.

At the age of 18 years she had had a cerebral abscess which was drained without sequelae.

At the age of 30 years she was referred to hospital because of exertional dyspnoea. Marked generalized cyanosis and clubbing of the fingers were noted. A very loud systolic murmur was heard to the left of the sternum, but there were no signs of cardiac failure.

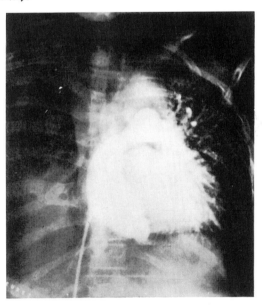

FIG. 11. *Case 1. Postoperative right atrial angiocardiogram, anteroposterior view: passage of contrast medium through left lung is fast, as proved by good opacification of left atrium. Except for a slight flow along catheter, contrast medium does not flow back from right atrium to inferior vena cava, because the pulmonary valve homograft performs its antireflux function perfectly.*

246   *F. Fontan and E. Baudet*

At the age of 33 years exertional dyspnoea, non-productive cough, and headache appeared, but they were improved by symptomatic therapy.

Finally, at the age of 36 years, her exercise tolerance was reduced and dyspnoea became progressively worse. She was admitted to hospital in January 1970.

Cardiac catheterization and angiocardiography confirmed a type IIB tricuspid atresia, with pulmonary arteries which seemed of small size when compared with an enormous transposed aorta, but the right and left branches of the pulmonary artery were, in fact, of nearly normal size.

Operation (Fig. 1) was performed on 20 January, 1970. The pulmonary arterial pressure was 35·0 mmHg. After superior vena cava to right pulmonary artery anastomosis had been carried out (Fig. 2), the superior vena caval pressure was 10·0 mmHg. Anastomosis of the right atrial appendage to the proximal end of the right pulmonary artery was carried out by means of an aortic valve homograft (Fig. 3). Under cardiopulmonary bypass (Fig. 5) the atrial septal defect was closed, the pulmonary valve homograft was inserted into the inferior vena cava, and finally the main pulmonary artery was ligated. After the cardiopulmonary bypass had been discontinued, the superior vena cava was transected below the cava-pulmonary anastomosis (Fig. 6) at its entry into the right atrium.

The initial postoperative course was very satisfactory: cyanosis disappeared; the patient was in sinus rhythm at 80 per minute and ventilation and diuresis were excellent. To maintain an adequate blood pressure it was necessary to produce hypervolaemia by increasing the transfusion rate and tachycardia by isoproterenol.

A superior vena caval syndrome appeared eight days after the operation but disappeared after a few days under treatment with diuretics, while a bilateral serosanguineous pleural effusion required aspiration. On getting up, the patient had no oedema of the inferior limbs and only a moderate hepatomegaly. There was a considerable biological improvement: the blood count was 4,200,000 RBC/mm³ and haematocrit was 50% (Table II).

TABLE II

		RBC per mm³	Haemato-crit %	Pressure (mmHg)		
				SVC	IVC	PA
Preoperative	30 yr	6,750,000	70	5		35
	36 yr	7,200,000	80			
Postoperative		4,200,000	50	10	15	30

It is too soon yet to carry out cardiac catheterization, but these haemodynamic and angiocardiographic investigations will be performed shortly. The clinical course is quite satisfactory 10 months postoperatively: there is no cyanosis and no systolic murmur; cardiac auscultation is normal except for an accentuated second heart sound. There is no venous stasis in the upper half of the body, no pleural effusion, and no oedema of the inferior limbs. There is only a moderate persistent hepatomegaly.

CASE 3   The third patient, N.B., was a 23-year-old woman. Dyspnoea and cyanosis had appeared in childhood. An episode of cardiac failure occurred during pregnancy, in 1969, followed by a premature birth four months before her admission to hospital in December 1969.

Physical examination showed clubbing of the fingers, cyanosis of the extremities, and hepatomegaly. A loud systolic murmur was heard in the whole precordial area. A blood count showed 3,700,000 RBC/mm³ and the haematocrit was 44%.

A diagnosis of tricuspid atresia with dextrocardia, atrial septal defect, and ventricular septal defect was made. There was a low pulmonary arterial pressure of 23·0 mmHg (Table III).

TABLE III

	Pressure (mmHg)			
	RA	PA		
Preoperative				
Maximal		23		
Minimal		13		
Mean	7	16		
	SVC–RPA	IVC	RA	LPA
Postoperative				
Maximal	15		22·5	17·5
Minimal	10		17·5	12·5
Mean		17·5		

Operation was performed in March 1970. First, a superior vena cava to pulmonary artery anastomosis was carried out; then, an anastomosis of the right atrium to the proximal end of the right pulmonary artery, using an aortic valve homograft; finally, under cardiopulmonary bypass, a pulmonary valve homograft was inserted into the inferior vena cava, the atrial septal defect was closed, and the main pulmonary artery was transected and sutured.

The initial postoperative course was satisfactory, with good cardiac action. But, despite blood over-compensation and isoproterenol, her pulse and blood pressure fell slowly 6 hours postoperatively and she died.

At necropsy there was no thrombosis and the anastomoses were patent; but the mitral valve was abnormal, with vegetations and a perforation of 1 cm² in the anterior leaflet. Finally, the right atrium was small and its wall was very thin.

We are of the opinion that failure was due to this mitral insufficiency.

DISCUSSION

A new surgical technique for repair of tricuspid atresia seems worth while. Indeed, in reviewing the literature on the subject, no corrective tech-

Surgical repair of tricuspid atresia   247

nique is mentioned, only palliative procedures.

Some years ago, after the appearance of the first papers on cava-pulmonary anastomosis (Glenn and Patiño, 1954; Glenn, 1958), we conceived the theoretical basis of the operation we report. Experimental research on dogs enabled us to check the technical feasibility of this procedure, but there were no survivals for more than a few hours, perhaps because the haemodynamic status of a normal dog heart does not allow a circulation which involves circulatory bypass of the right side of the heart. We were of the opinion that the right atrium of a normal heart could not provide the required work, whereas a hypertrophied right atrium, as in tricuspid atresia, could supply the additional work represented by a pulmonary arterial pressure higher than the left atrial pressure. However, it seemed to us indispensable to provide the right atrium with valve homografts, one inserted into the inferior vena cava at the level of the right atrium, and the other at the exit from the right atrium to the left lung, to prevent free flow between the inferior vena cava, the right atrium, and the pulmonary artery and, in this way, stasis in the lower half of the body and inadequate cardiac filling.

The pliability and plasticity of the homograft facilitates suturing; but the long-term fate of valve homografts is unknown. Rastelli, Wallace, and Ongley (1969) have reported that calcification of the aortic wall of homografts used to repair truncus arteriosus defects has occurred in each of five patients operated on, without preventing continued function of the leaflets.

Reports from other surgeons (Bigelow *et al.*, 1967; Bigelow, 1968) on the fate of aortic homografts, in place for as long as 13 years in the thoracic aorta, have indicated that the segment of aorta and aortic valves have remained functionally satisfactory with time. Indeed, secondary calcifications seem to occur only in aortic valve homografts; pulmonary valve homografts are rarely affected by these changes and they can be used not only for 'valvation' of the inferior vena cava, but also for an anastomosis between the right atrium and the proximal end of the right pulmonary artery. Barratt-Boyes *et al.* (1969) and Ross (1971) have noted that fresh aortic valve homografts are less likely to become calcified than those that are sterilized and preserved.

A homograft between the right atrium and the proximal end of the right pulmonary artery is not indispensable, because in our first patient we did not use one for want of having one small enough. The result was satisfactory two and a half years

postoperatively. But we are of the opinion that the homograft is probably useful, for the postoperative course was more difficult in this patient and an inferior vena caval syndrome was observed (hepatomegaly, melaena, oligoanuria), though this last syndrome could be explained by the child's congenital bilateral hydronephrosis.

A striking fact in the postoperative course was the need to provide a large amount of fluid infusion (blood and physiological solution) and maintain a tachycardia to ensure a correct haemodynamic balance. During the first three days postoperatively we had to ensure an overcompensation and a tachycardia (about 100 to 120/min) as if the right atrium, 'ventricle-like', could supply a satisfactory left pulmonary blood flow only by ensuring a venous hyperpressure which would help filling and a tachycardia permitting a suitable flow, until a spontaneous balance was obtained. The need for a large volume of fluid infusion is well known in cava-pulmonary anastomosis and is explained by a liquid storage in the upper half of the body. This new technique, which is a double cava-pulmonary anastomosis, could only aggravate this syndrome.

Respiratory assistance should be stopped early because positive pressure prevents central venous return.

Another less explicable feature of the postoperative course was, in both cases, a right or bilateral pleural effusion which required a few pleurocenteses.

The operation is not technically difficult. We have waited for as long as 30 months after operation before reporting this technique. The immediate result is remarkable and remains satisfactory. One element remains unpredictable—the haemodynamic consequences of an eventual atrial rhythm disturbance such as an atrial fibrillation or flutter.

INDICATIONS

The indications for this corrective procedure, though remaining limited, apply to many patients. Our first two patients were anatomically and haemodynamically privileged; they had pulmonary arteries of normal size and low pressure.

The anatomical classification of tricuspid atresia, from Edwards and Burchell (1949) (Fig. 12) and Keith, Rowe, and Vlad (1958), distinguishes two principal types—type I, with normally related great arteries, and type II, with transposition of the great arteries; and three groups in each type—group A, with pulmonary atresia, group B, with

248   *F. Fontan and E. Baudet*

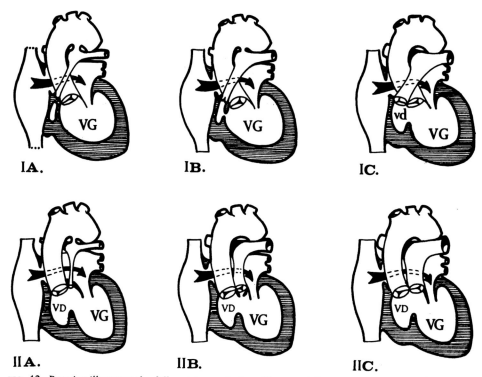

FIG. 12. *Drawing illustrates the different types of tricuspid atresia (from Edwards and Burchell, 1949).*

pulmonary valvular or subvalvular stenosis, and group C, with a normal pulmonary artery and increased pulmonary blood flow.

Most of the children with tricuspid atresia have a poor prognosis and die rather early. In these circumstances, only palliative surgical procedures can be considered (anastomosis in groups A and B and banding of the main pulmonary artery in group C), but we are of the opinion that they could profit from this corrective procedure as soon as they are older and have a bodily development compatible with the anatomical, haemodynamic, and technical necessities of this operation.

REFERENCES

Barratt-Boyes, B. G., Roche, A. H. G., Brandt, P. W. T., Smith, J. C., and Lowe, J. B. (1969). Aortic homograft valve replacement. A long-term follow-up of an initial series of 101 patients. *Circulation*, **40**, 763.

Bigelow, W. G. (1968). Personal communication.

—— Trimble, A. S., Aldridge, H. E., Bedard, P., Spratt, E. H., and Lansdown, E. L. (1967). The problem of insufficiency following homograft replacement of the aortic valve. *J. thorac. cardiovasc. Surg.*, **54**, 478.

Edwards, J. E., and Burchell, H. B. (1949). Congenital tricuspid atresia: a classification. *Med. Clin. N. Amer.*, **33**, 1177.

Glenn, W. W. L. (1958). Circulatory bypass of the right side of the heart. IV. Shunt between superior vena cava and distal right pulmonary artery—Report of clinical application. *New Engl. J. Med.*, **259**, 117.

—— and Patiño, J. F. (1954). Circulatory by-pass of the right heart. *Yale J. Biol. Med.*, **27**, 147.

Keith, J. D., Rowe, R. D., and Vlad, P. (1958). *Heart Disease in Infancy and Childhood*. Macmillan, New York.

Rastelli, G. C., Wallace, R. B., and Ongley, P. A. (1969). Complete repair of transposition of the great arteries with pulmonary stenosis. A review and report of a case corrected by using a new surgical technique. *Circulation*, **39**, 83.

Ross, D. N. (1971). Aortic valvar replacements. In Proceedings VI World Congress of Cardiology, London, September 1970. *Brit. Heart J.*, **33** (Suppl.), 39.

Anatomic correction of transposition of the great vessels

We present a new approach for anatomic correction of transposition of the great arteries. The two coronary arteries, with a piece of the aortic wall attached, are transposed to the posterior artery. The two aortic openings are closed with a patch. The aorta and pulmonary artery are transected, contraposed, and then anastomosed. The interventricular septal defect is closed with a patch, through a right ventriculotomy approach, because the right ventricle is no longer part of the systemic circulation. Two patients, aged 3 months and 40 days and weighing 4,200 and 3,700 grams, respectively, were operated upon with deep hypothermia and total circulatory arrest. There was good recovery from the operation, with normal cardiocirculatory conditions. Renal failure developed in the first patient, and she died on the third postoperative day. During this time the cardiocirculatory conditions were good. The second patient made an uneventful recovery. Hemodynamic studies 20 days after the operation showed complete correction of the malformation. Five and one-half months after the operation, he weighs 7,500 grams, and his development is very good. We believe that this operation will be reproducible by most cardiovascular surgeons and will be an alternative to the Mustard procedure, especially for those patients with interventricular septal defect and pulmonary hypertension.

Adib D. Jatene, M.D. (by invitation), V. F. Fontes, M.D. (by invitation), P. P. Paulista, M.D. (by invitation), L. C. B. Souza, M.D. (by invitation), F. Neger, M.D. (by invitation), M. Galantier, M.D. (by invitation), and J. E. M. R. Sousa, M.D. (by invitation), *São Paulo, Brazil*
Sponsored by E. J. Zerbini, M.D., *São Paulo, Brazil*

The ideal operation for transposition of the great vessels must be one performed at the arterial level. To divide, contrapose, and then reanastomose the great arteries is not a surgical problem. The major technical difficulty in this approach has been the transfer of the coronary arteries. The earliest attempts made more than twenty years ago were uniformly unsuccessful.[1-5] Recently, anatomicopathological and experimental studies have been reported on this subject.[6-8]

This paper presents our initial experience with two infants subjected to anatomic correction of transposition of the great vessels. The case history of one of these patients has been related as a preliminary report.[9]

From the Instituto Dante Pazzanese de Cardiologia do Estado de São Paulo, São Paulo, Brazil.

Read at the Fifty-sixth Annual Meeting of The American Association for Thoracic Surgery, Los Angeles, Calif., April 23, 24, and 25, 1976.

Address for reprints: Dr. Adib D. Jatene, C. Postal 215. São Paulo, SP. Brasil.

Surgical procedure

The patients are operated upon with the use of profound hypothermia (16° C.) and total cardiocirculatory arrest according to the technique described by Mori,[10] Barratt-Boyes,[11] and their colleagues.

The heart is exposed by means of a median sternotomy. The pericardium is opened wide by an inverted T-shaped incision. The ascending aorta and the pulmonary artery are dissected and freed distally to the level of the pericardial reflection and proximally to the level of the anterior and posterior valves. The initial portions of the coronary arteries are dissected free. With the heart beating normally, two sites are selected in the anterior wall of the posterior artery (in this case the pulmonary artery) where the coronary arteries will be located. These two places are identified with a stitch of 6-0 Prolene suture (Fig. 1, *A*). This is important, because when the heart is empty it is possible to open the artery in the wrong place. At the same time an area is selected in the aortic wall, adjacent to the origin of the coronary arteries, which will remain attached to the

364

Volume 72
Number 3
September, 1976

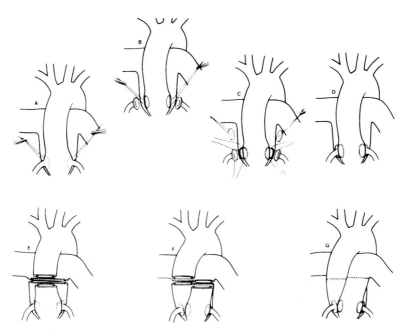

Fig. 1. Schematic drawing of the operative technique (see text).

coronary arteries. The transecting incisions in the aorta (anterior) and pulmonary artery (posterior) must be made at the same level and the sites selected at this time. The differences in diameter between the aorta and the pulmonary artery, instead of being a problem, are helpful when the two vessels are contraposed and reanastomosed. Purse-string sutures are placed in the right atrial appendage and at the apex of the left ventricle (in this case pulmonary ventricle), and cannulas are inserted. Another cannula is inserted in the ascending aorta through a small transverse aortotomy at the point selected for complete transection of the aorta. Perfusion is started and hypothermia to 16° C. is reached in 5 or 6 minutes. The blood is permitted to drain to the heart-lung machine, the aorta is cross-clamped just below the innominate artery, and the cannulas are removed from the aorta and right atrium. The coronary arteries are then excised with the selected piece of the aortic wall attached (Fig. 1, *B*). This maneuver simplifies the subsequent anastomosis. The openings in the aortic wall are closed with a running suture by means of a patch of homologous dura mater preserved in glycerol (Fig. 1, *C*). This is the same material used in the dura mater valve for cardiac valve replacement.[12] It is easier to suture the dura mater than the pericardium. With the two stitches previously placed as a guide, two similar pieces are resected from the posterior artery (in this case the pulmonary artery).

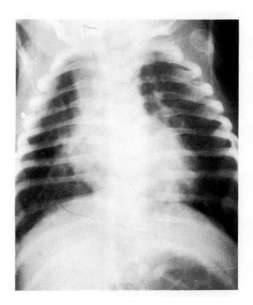

Fig. 2. Case 1. Preoperative roentgenogram.

Two anastomoses are then performed with continuous 6-0 Prolene suture, the coronary arteries being implanted in their new sites (Fig. 1, *D*). The next step is to transect the ascending aorta by using the aortotomy for cannulation. At the same level, the pulmonary artery is transected (Fig. 1, *E*). A continuous running suture is then placed in the distal end of the pulmonary artery starting at the right border. A similar suture is

The Journal of
Thoracic and Cardiovascular
Surgery

366   *Jatene et al.*

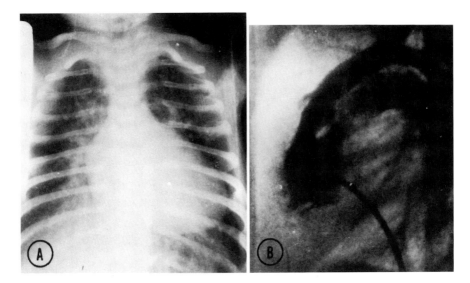

Fig. 3. Case 2. *A,* Preoperative roentgenogram. *B,* Preoperative cineangiogram.

placed at the proximal end of the pulmonary artery starting at the left border (Fig. 1, *F*). These two sutures are intended to equalize the diameters of the vessels which are going to be contraposed and reanastomosed. The distal end of the anterior artery is sutured to the proximal end of the posterior artery, to which the coronary arteries are now attached. The distal end of the posterior artery is sutured to the proximal end of the anterior artery, from which the coronary arteries were removed (Fig. 1, *G*). By this technique we have performed an anatomic and complete correction of the transposed vessels. The interventricular septal defect is closed with a Dacron patch, the approach being through a right ventriculotomy, because the right ventricle is no longer part of the systemic circulation but instead, the pulmonary circulation. After closure of the right ventricle, the cannulas are reinserted, the aortic line being placed in a new aortotomy distal to the suture line. Air is eliminated from the heart, and the patient is rewarmed.

The postoperative care for these infants is the same as that for any subjected to profound hypothermia.

Case reports

Two patients with transposition of the great vessels and interventricular septal defect were operated upon for anatomic correction.

CASE 1. C. P., an 11-day-old white female infant weighing 3,200 grams, was admitted with a history of cyanosis since birth. The clinical diagnosis was transposition of the great vessels. Cardiac catheterization at this time revealed a large interventricular septal defect and transposition of great

arteries. Balloon septostomy was not done because it was not possible to insert the catheter into the left atrium.

At the age of 3 months, her weight was 4,200 grams and she was becoming progressively more cyanotic. A second cardiac catheterization was then performed. Pressures were as follows: right ventricle 100/12 mm. Hg, aorta 100/60 mm. Hg, pulmonary artery 100/58 mm. Hg, and left ventricle 100/12 mm. Hg. The arterial oxygen saturation was 53 per cent. The electrocardiographic tracings showed right ventricular and right atrial hypertrophy. The chest roentgenogram demonstrated that the cardiac shadow was smaller than on the first film made, and there was an increased pulmonary vascularity, but without signs of congestion (Fig. 2).

The operative procedure described was performed on May 4, 1975. The only difference was in the closure of the two openings in the former aorta. The orifice on the left was closed with a pericardial patch and the one on the right with a continuous running suture. The complete correction, including closure of the interventricular septal defect through a right ventriculotomy, was done with the patient under total circulatory arrest. The operation took 75 minutes. After rewarming, the heart recovered completely with no conduction disturbances, and maintained good cardiocirculatory condition. Abnormal bleeding required extra stitches in the sutures of the patched coronary orifices.

The infant had a complete postoperative recovery. The intratracheal tube was removed after 6 hours and the infant was alert. The following day all conditions were good except for the urinary output. On the second day, anuria and elevations of the serum potassium and urea levels were noted. On the third day, before peritoneal dialysis was begun, she had a cardiac arrest and could not be resuscitated despite all attempts at that time. Necropsy showed all the sutures to be in place and the anatomic correction to be good.

CASE 2. P. C. O. B., a 40-day-old white male infant weighing 3,700 grams, was first examined on May 6, 1975. Cyanosis had first been noted 10 days after birth. On

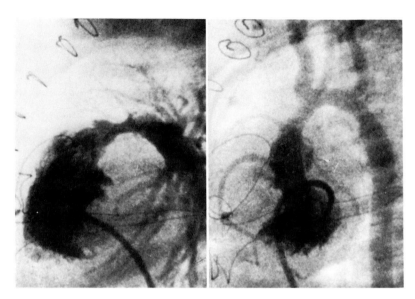

Fig. 4. Case 2. Postoperative cineangiogram.

admission he had a cough, tachypnea, and congestive heart failure with increasing cyanosis. He was treated with digitalis, diuretics, and antibiotics. On physical examination he was cyanotic and the liver was enlarged, the edge being 3 cm. below the right costal margin. There was a Grade 2 systolic murmur at the mesocardium. A roentgenogram revealed an enlarged, egg-shaped heart and a considerable increase in pulmonary vasculature (Fig. 3, *A*). Data obtained from cardiac catheterization showed a pressure of 90/13 mm. Hg in the right ventricle and 90/55 mm. Hg in the aorta. The pressure in the left ventricle was 90/12 mm. Hg and in the pulmonary artery, 75/35 mm. Hg. The arterial oxygen saturation was 88 per cent with the infant under general anesthesia. The cineangiogram confirmed the diagnosis of transposition of the great arteries with a large ventricular septal defect (Fig. 3, *B*).

The patient was operated upon on May 8, 1975, according to the technique described. The postoperative course was uneventful. Twenty days after the operation, right and left heart catheterization studies were performed. The cineangiographic aspect is shown in Fig. 4. We can see the complete correction and the coronary arteries at their new sites. The pressure in the pulmonary artery had dropped to 25/13 mm. Hg and that in the right ventricle to 60/10 mm. Hg. The mean pressures at the left and right atria were 10 and 6 mm. Hg, respectively. The infant was discharged 3 weeks after operation in good condition. He has been re-examined monthly and has had no problems. Ten months after the operation, without medications, he is thriving at normal standards and weighing 8,300 grams.

Comment

The idea of retransposing the great arteries in patients with transposition of the great vessels is not new. The attempts of Bailey and associates[2] and Kay and Cross[3] and the proposal of Björk and Bouckaert[13] leave the coronary arteries in the pulmonary artery. With the technique of Mustard and associates[1] the left coronary artery is taken with the aorta but the right coronary artery remains in the pulmonary artery. Senning[4] was the first who completely corrected the transposition, but his technique is very difficult to use. Idriss and associates[5] in 1961 developed an interesting technique, but the ring of the aorta with the two coronary arteries is difficult to obtain and the anastomoses are all made very near the valve level. At this time all the patients in whom these techniques were tried have died in the operating room or shortly thereafter. Since that time we have not found new attempts in the literature. The papers of Anagnostopoulos,[6, 7] Balderman,[8] and their associates present interesting ideas but no clinical experience.

We based our technique on our experience with aorta-coronary bypasses,[14] and it sounded technically feasible to us. There are two major arguments: First, the coronary arteries are excised with a piece of the aortic wall, so that there are no problems with suture and future stenosis; second, the great vessels are transected far from the valves, so that it is easier to create the anastomoses and to correct any leak that is observed. This technique also permits the adjustment of the sizes of the two vessels. The operation may be technically difficult, but we believe it is reproducible by most of the cardiovascular surgeons. We still believe at the present time that transposition of the great vessels with an intact ventricular septum must be corrected by the Mustard[15] operation. We think in this situation that the left ventricle, having been exposed to a low pressure regimen, perhaps will not be able to

The Journal of
Thoracic and Cardiovascular
Surgery

368   *Jatene et al.*

sustain the load of systemic pressure. The same is true in cases of pulmonary stenosis. The Rastelli[16] operation should be the procedure of choice for this group of patients if the stenosis cannot be relieved properly. However, if the stenosis can be relieved, perhaps relief of stenosis will be adequate for anatomic correction. Our technique will be ideal for transposition of the great vessels with ventricular septal defect or persistent ductus arteriosus and pulmonary hypertension with low arteriolar resistance. We do not know at the present time whether the procedure is adequate for patients who have pulmonary hypertension and high arteriolar resistance.

Some successful similar operations have been performed by Kreutzer,[17] Yacoub,[18] Ross,[19] and Nakamura.[20]

Addendum

After this paper was submitted, we had a disappointing experience. Five infants operated upon died a few hours after the operation or in the operating room. In all these patients there were no technical problems. The first patient, 3 months old, had a severe respiratory infection for which he required assisted ventilation for a week before the operation. At that time he was resuscitated from a cardiac arrest, and the operation was a desperate effort to change the situation. The next 3 patients were between 2 and 3 months old. All of them had patent ductus arteriosus, and 2 of them also had a ventricular septal defect. Evidence of pulmonary hyperresistance was present. The heart size was relatively small. These infants did not have pulmonary vascular congestion or cardiac insufficiency, but they did have severe anoxia. After complete anatomic correction and closure of the patent ductus, the pressure in the pulmonary artery appeared higher than that in the aorta. Output was low. In one of these cases the pressure measured in the left ventricle was 65 mm. Hg and that in the right ventricle 80 mm. Hg. The end-diastolic pressure was high. Opening the ductus decreased both the end-diastolic pressure and the pressure difference between the two ventricles. Despite this maneuver, the patient died.

The fifth patient we considered to be a good subject for this operation. He had signs of low pulmonary resistance with an enlarged heart, congestion of the pulmonary vasculature, and heart failure. After the complete anatomic correction, the aortic pressure was 90/60 mm. Hg and the right ventricular systolic pressure was 40 mm. Hg. This patient had an excellent immediate recovery, with good cardiocirculatory condition and good urinary output. He was completely awake, and the blood gas and electrolyte values were almost normal. Six hours after the operation, he had a sudden cardiac arrest and could not be resuscitated.

Despite this very discouraging experience, we still believe that this technique will be useful, especially if we improve the selection of patients.

On last June 20, we performed another successful anatomic correction on a 9-month-old girl who had transposition of the great vessels and a large ventricular septal defect with signs of low pulmonary resistance. Because the pulmonary artery was to the right, a piece of Dacron tube was used to eliminate tension in the pulmonary flow pathway reconstruction. One month after the operation, the patient is doing remarkably well.

REFERENCES

1 Mustard, W. T., Chute, A. L., Keith, J. D., Sirek, A., Rowe, R. D., and Vlad, P.: A Surgical Approach to Transposition of Great Vessels With Extracorporeal Circuit, Surgery 36: 39, 1954.

2 Bailey, C. P., Cookson, B. A., Downing, D. F., and Neptune, W. B.: Cardiac Surgery Under Hypothermia, J. THORAC. SURG. 27: 73, 1954.

3 Kay, E. B., and Cross, F. S.: Surgical Treatment of Transposition of the Great Vessels, Surgery 38: 712, 1955.

4 Senning, A.: Surgical Correction of Transposition of the Great Vessels, Surgery 45: 966, 1959.

5 Idriss, F. S., Goldstein, I. R., Grana, L., French, D., and Potts, W. J.: A New Technic for Complete Correction of Transposition of the Great Vessels, Circulation 24: 5, 1961.

6 Anagnostopoulos, C. E.: A Proposed New Technique for Correction of Transposition of the Great Arteries, Ann. Thorac. Surg. 15: 565, 1973.

7 Anagnostopoulos, C. E., Athanasuleas, C. L., and Arcilla, R. A.: Toward a Rational Operation for Transposition of the Great Arteries, Ann. Thorac. Surg. 16: 458, 1973.

8 Balderman, S. C., Athanasuleas, C. L., and Anagnostopoulos, C. E.: Coronary Artery in Transposition of the Great Vessels in Relation to Anatomic Surgical Correction, J. THORAC. CARDIOVASC. SURG. 67: 208, 1974.

9 Jatene, A. D., Fontes, V. F., Paulista, P. P., Souza, L. C. B., Neger, F., Galantier, M., and Sousa, J. E. M. R.: Successful Anatomic Correction of Transposition of the Great Vessels: A Preliminary Report, Arq. Bras. Cardiol. 28: 461, 1975.

10 Mori, H., Muraoka, R., Yokota, Y., Okamoti, Y., Ando, F., Fukumasu, H., Oku, H., Ideda, M., Shirotani, H., and Hikasa, Y.: Deep Hypothermia Combined With Cardiopulmonary Bypass for Cardiac Surgery in Neonates and Infants, J. THORAC. CARDIOVASC. SURG. 64: 422, 1972.

11 Barratt-Boyes, B. G., Simpson, M., and Neutze, J. M.: Intracardiac Surgery in Neonates and Infants Using Deep Hypothermia With Surface Cooling and Limited Cardiopulmonary Bypass, Circulation 43, 44: 25, 1971 (Suppl. I).

12 Pigossi, N.: Implantação de dura-máter homógena conservada em glicerina. Estudo experimental em cães, Rev. Hosp. Clin. Fac. Med. São Paulo 22: 204, 1967.

Routine Primary Repair vs Two-stage Repair of Tetralogy of Fallot

JOHN W. KIRKLIN, M.D., EUGENE H. BLACKSTONE, M.D., ALBERT D. PACIFICO, M.D.,
ROBERT N. BROWN, B.S., AND LIONEL M. BARGERON, JR., M.D.

SUMMARY   Fifteen of 194 patients (7.7%) with tetralogy of Fallot operated upon since January 1, 1972 under a protocol of routine primary repair despite young age died in-hospital. Most deaths were from low cardiac output. Young age and smallness of size increased the risk of operation. No deaths occurred among patients older than 4 years. High hematocrit was also a risk factor. Transannular patching has an independent effect in increasing risk. The post-repair ratio of peak pressure in the right ventricle to that in the left did not exert an independent effect. To project current risks of a two-stage approach, we determined that five of 158 patients (3.2%) died in-hospital after secondary intracardiac repair after a previous Blalock-Taussig or Waterston anastomosis between 1967–1978. Using these data and those we have published on the risk of shunting, we project that except in very small babies, the risks of hospital death of a two-stage approach are not less than those of primary repair done without a transannular patch, except when body surface area is less than about 0.35 m². When a transannular patch is used in the primary repair, the two-stage approach is projected to be safer when the child has a body surface area of about 0.48 m² or smaller.

SOME YEARS AGO evidence was presented to support the idea that the basic hospital mortality after intracradiac repair of tetralogy of Fallot is almost zero. However, certain variables (incremental risk factors) were shown in the early years to be associated with increased risk of the operation.[1-3] These included young age, severe cyanosis, and the use of a transannular patch. Complete atrioventricular block and incomplete repair of the ventricular septal defect were incremental risk factors,[1] but have been essentially obviated by the improved surgical techniques introduced about 1959.[4]

This effect of young age persuaded most centers to use a two-stage approach for patients with tetralogy of Fallot who need operation in the first few years of life, consisting of an initial shunting operation and later intracardiac repair. Barratt-Boyes and colleagues began to do routine primary repair even in very young symptomatic infants in 1970, and in 1973 reported that the results from this policy were better than those of two-stage repair.[5-7] Recently, Castaneda also reported excellent results from this policy.[8] The optimal method of managing symptomatic patients in the young age group with tetralogy of Fallot is, however, controversial.[9-11]

We are reporting the results of a protocol, begun in 1972, of routine primary repair even in the very young. In the analysis, we have particularly looked for incremental risk factors. For comparison, we have projected the current risks of the two-stage approach by combining the risks of secondary repair after a previous shunting operation, determined from our experience in 1967–1978, and those currently pertaining to the initial shunting procedure, obtained from our data on the risks of the shunting procedures.[12]

In this evaluation, we have focused on early results because present information indicates that the late results from primary and two-stage repair in comparable subgroups are similar.

Materials and Methods

Between January 1967 and January 1978, 617 patients with tetralogy of Fallot underwent intracardiac repair at the University of Alabama Medical Center (table 1). For this study, we have analyzed in detail the 492 patients with classic tetralogy of Fallot, which is defined by exclusion in table 1. If the pulmonary stenosis was so severe as to result in a pinpoint opening that was not functionally important, the malformation was still called classic tetralogy of Fallot rather than tetralogy of Fallot with pulmonary atresia. If the aorta arose 90% or more from the right ventricle, we considered the malformation to be double outlet right ventricle with pulmonary stenosis rather than tetralogy of Fallot. Twenty-three patients had unusual major associated defects that indicate, in our opinion, that patient management must be on an ad hoc rather than a protocol basis (table 2). These patients are excluded from further analysis, leaving 469 patients. At least 80 patients had other associated anomalies that did not exclude them from the study group (table 3).

Two hundred sixty-five of the 469 patients underwent primary intracardiac repair. One hundred ninety-five of these patients had their operations in the period beginning January 1, 1972, the date on which we began the prospective protocol of routine primary intracardiac repair in infants and small children, and

From the Departments of Surgery and Pediatrics, University of Alabama School of Medicine and Medical Center, Birmingham, Alabama.

Address for reprints: John W. Kirklin, M.D., Department of Surgery, University Station, Birmingham, Alabama 35294.

Received November 9, 1978; revision accepted February 16, 1979.

Circulation 60, No. 2, 1979.

TABLE 1. *Repair of Tetralogy of Fallot (UAB 1967-1978)*

Category	n	Hospital deaths		
		n	%	70% CL
Classic TOF	492*	35	7.1	5.9–8.5%
Classic TOF with p atresia	84†	15	18	13–23%
TOF with subpulm VSD	22	2	9	3–20%
TOF with p incompetence	13‡	3	23	10–41%
TOF with complete AV canal	5	2	40	14–71%
TOF with flap-valve VSD	1	1	100	15–100%
Total	617	58	9.4	8.2–10.8%

*One additional patient, age 25 years, with a previously constructed Potts anastomosis and severe pulmonary vascular disease, had exploratory operation only for confirmation of this complication. She survived.

†Four patients were inadvertently omitted in the report of Alfieri et al. of 80 patients.

‡One additional patient died at sternotomy, preliminary to proposed correction.

Abbreviations: CL = confidence limits; TOF = tetralogy of Fallot; p = pulmonary; subpulm = subpulmonary; VSD = ventricular septal defect; AV = atrioventricular; UAB = University of Alabama, Birmingham.

form the study group for primary repair. Before 1972, three patients younger than 12 months of age underwent primary repair and survived. One who survived underwent repair between 12–24 months of age, and none aged 24–48 months underwent primary repair. During the period 1972–1978, one 3-day-old patient with extreme pulmonary stenosis (who received an emergency Blalock-Taussig shunt in 1975), one 8 days old with extreme pulmonary stenosis and severe hypoplasia of left and right pulmonary arteries (who received open transannular patching as a palliative procedure), and one 5 months old with a re-

TABLE 2. *Repair of Classic Tetralogy of Fallot (UAB 1967-1978) (n = 492)*

Associated condition	n	Hospital deaths		
		n	%	70% CL
Major*	23	6	26	16–39%
Multiple VSDs	12	3	25	11–44%
Anomalous origin LPA or RPA	2	0	0	0–61%
Enormous discrete "bronchial" arteries (like pulmonary atresia)	5	1	20	3–53%
Important subaortic stenosis	2	1	50	7–93%
Isolated dextrocardia	1	0	0	0–85%
Situs inversus totalis	2	1	50	7–93%
Other	80	8	10	7–15%

*One of the 23 patients had two major associated lesions.

Abbreviations: VSD = ventricular septal defect; LPA = left pulmonary artery; RPA = right pulmonary artery; CL = confidence limits; UAB = University of Alabama, Birmingham.

TABLE 3. *Repair of Classic Tetralogy of Fallot (UAB 1967-1978) (n = 492)*

Other associated conditions	n	Hospital deaths		
		n	%	70% CL
Anomalous origin LAD	23	1	4	1–14%
Patent ductus arteriosus	14	1	7	1–22%
Absent RPA or LPA	4	1	25	3–63%
PAPVC	4	0	0	0–38%
PASVC	1	0	0	0–85%
Important TI	3	0	0	0–47%
Important underdeveloped TV	2	0	0	0–61%
Straddling TV	1	0	0	0–85%
Unroofed coronary sinus	1	0	0	0–85%
Important underdeveloped RV	1	0	0	0–85%
Ebstein's anomaly	1	0	0	0–85%
AP Window	1	0	0	0–85%
Stenoses or severe hypoplasia RPA, LPA*	40	7	18	11–26%
Total	80	8	10	7–15%

*This is a minimum number, and we believe these were also present in many additional patients in whom their presence was not specified. Some of the 80 patients had more than one condition; therefore, the individual breakdown will add up to more than the total.

Abbreviations: LAD = left anterior descending coronary artery; RPA = right pulmonary artery; LPA = left pulmonary artery; PAPVC = partial anomalous pulmonary venous connection; PASVC = partial anomalous systemic venous connection; TI = tricuspid incompetence; TV = tricuspid valve; RV = right ventricle; AP = aortopulmonary; CL = confidence limits; UAB = University of Alabama, Birmingham.

cent severe hemiplegia (who received a Blalock-Taussig shunt) failed to undergo primary repair. No patients were considered so ill or had such a severe malformation that operation was not advised.

Between 1967–1978, 204 of the 469 patients un-

TABLE 4. *Repair of Classic Tetralogy of Fallot after Previous Palliative Operations Without Major Associated Lesions (UAB 1967-1978)*

Category	n	Hospital deaths		
		n	%	70% CL
Blalock-Taussig (1)	124	3	2.4	1.1–4.8%
Waterston (1)	34	2	6	2–13%
Potts (1)	16	1	6	1–20%
Blalock-Taussig (2)	5	0	0	0–32%
Waterston + Blalock-Taussig	3	1	33	4–76%
"Closed" Brock	5	1	20	3–53%
Other (single or multiple)	17	2	12	4–26%
Total	204	10	4.9	3.4–7.0%

Abbreviations: CL = confidence limits; UAB = University of Alabama, Birmingham.

derwent intracrdiac repair after a previous palliative operation (table 4). In any planned, two-stage patient management program in the future, the definitive repair would be planned after a single Blalock-Taussig or Waterston shunt. Therefore, the 158 patients who had those procedures formed the study group for secondary repair.

Diagnostic Methods

Each patient was studied preoperatively by cardiac catheterization and angiocardiography. Most, but not all, of the studies were done in our institution. Only in recent years have the details of the bifurcation of the pulmonary artery been studied by special "sitting-up" views, and the internal anatomy by special axial cineradiography.[13, 14]

Surgical Methods

The operations were done with cardiopulmonary bypass, using a rotating disc oxygenator until 1969 and subsequently a disposable bubble oxygenator. In the early years, moderate hypothermia to 28°C and intermittent aortic cross-clamping for 10–20 minutes were used. Beginning in late 1971, profound hypothermia to 20°C was used in nearly all patients. In very small infants younger than 3–4 months of age, the intracardiac operation was done with total circulatory arrest. Otherwise, it was done at a low perfusion flow with the patient at 20°C[15] and one period of cold ischemic cardiac arrest produced by aortic cross-clamping. Cold and cardioplegia were used for myocardial preservation in 1977.[16] Preliminary surface cooling was used in 1972, 1973 and 1974 for infants younger than about 1 year old, but has not been used since.

The right atrium was routinely opened for closure of a patent foramen ovale, if present. Until about 1974 the ventricle was usually opened by a transverse incision; if a transannular patch was needed, a separate vertical incision was made in the infundibulum of the right ventricle and carried across the pulmonary valve ring and out to the bifurcation of the pulmonary artery. Since 1974, a vertical incision has been used and the management of the outflow tract standardized.[17, 18] The ventricular septal defect has been closed with a patch by techniques previously described.[19]

Analytic and Statistical Methods

The records of each of the 617 patients were reviewed, without knowledge of the outcome, to determine the morphology and associated lesions and thus the classification of the patient. The basic data were recorded from the clinical, diagnostic, surgical and hospital records, and all derived values recalculated.

Standard methods were used to obtain medians, means, and standard errors. The *t* tests were calculated under both equal and unequal variance assumptions, selecting the equal variance test if the F statistic for equality of the variances was associated with a *p* value > 0.2.[20] Group data are presented as a mean ± SEM. Proportional data are presented with their 70% confidence limits (CL), roughly corresponding to 1 standard error.[21] Two-tailed *p* values are used throughout.

The significance of the relationship of hospital mortality to categorical (yes-no) risk factors was analyzed using the chi-square test unless the numerator of any proportion had fewer than three events, in which case Fisher's exact test was used. The relationship of mortality to continuous variables (age, body surface area, post-repair ratio of peak pressure in the right ventricle to that in the left ($P_{RV/LV}$), preoperative hematocrit, and date of operation) was explored using the parametric method of logistic regression.[22] The logistic model is:

$$\text{Probability of event} = 1/(1 + \exp[-Z])$$

where exp is the base of the natural logarithms, and Z is the logit[23] expressed as a multivariate regression equation. The equations incorporate both continuous and categorical variables (such as presence of a transannular patch) and their interaction terms. Parameters of the model were estimated by the method of maximum likelihood, using the data from individual patients in an iteratively reweighted, nonlinear regression scheme.[24, 25] Standard deviations of these estimates were rescaled by setting the residual deviance to 1. Models containing multiple risk factors were determined both by an all possible regression scheme — the "best" model being that with the largest explained deviance (also called the log likelihood) — and by stepwise, backward elimination, eliminating sequentially the variable at each separate interaction level having the least significant *p* value > 0.2. In the latter analysis, full and reduced models were compared at each step by taking the difference in deviance and applying the chi-square test with one degree of freedom. An overall chi-square goodness of fit test was used to evaluate the models quantitatively, and all *p* values were greater than 0.2 for lack of fit.* A qualitative tabular analysis by deciles was also made. The logit of grouped data for each continuous variable was examined to determine the appropriate data transformation needed for the analyses.

The projected hospital mortality of two-stage repair is the current hospital mortality for the initial shunting procedure[12] combined with that from secondary repair (obtained from this study) by the equation:

$$P_{hd} \text{ 2-stage} = 1 - (1 - P_{hd} \text{ shunting}) \cdot (1 - P_{hd} \text{ secondary repair})$$

where P_{hd} is the probability of hospital death. The difference in probability of hospital death between primary and two-stage repair was tested after arcsine-square root transformation of each probability.

In comparing primary and two-stage repair,

---

*An exception is noted in the footnote on page 380.

TABLE 5. *Primary Repair of Classic Tetralogy of Fallot Without Major Associated Lesions (UAB 1972-1978)*

Treatment of pulmonary stenosis	n	Hospital deaths		
		n	%	70% CL
Without transannular patch	117	4	3.4*	1.7–6.1%
Transannular patch	74	10	14*	9–19%
Valved external conduit	2	0	0	0–61%
Non-valved external conduit	1	1	100	15–100%
Total	194	15	7.7	5.7–10.2%

*p for difference = 0.01.

Abbreviations: CL = confidence limits; UAB = University of Alabama, Birmingham.

primary repair is considered psychologically, sociologically and economically advantageous and thus advisable, unless two-stage repair is safer. Because many uncertainties are involved in the comparison and because death may be the penalty for a wrong decision, we considered two-stage repair to be safer when its point estimate for the risk of hospital death in the individual patient was less than that of primary repair and the *p* value for the difference 0.2 or less (rather than the more conventional and strict 0.05 or 0.1 or less).

P values greater than 0.2 were considered to indicate that any differences or relations were not true ones. We considered differences or relations to be true when $p \leq 0.05$, probably true when $p = 0.05$–0.1, and possibly true when $p > 0.1$ but ≤ 0.2.

Results

Primary Intracardiac Repair

Fifteen hospital deaths (7.7%, CL 5.7–10.2%) occurred among the 194 patients (table 5). In 11 of the

15 cases, low cardiac output was the cause of death. Permanent complete atrioventricular block has not occurred in this experience.

Young age is still an incremental risk factor in this surgery. The mean age of the surviving patients was 7.3 ± 0.77 years, significantly ($p < 0.0001$) older than that of the nonsurvivors (1.4 ± 0.29 years). Tabular presentation shows the hospital mortality to be the highest in the very young patients (table 6). No patient 4 years of age or older died at the time of repair. Parametric analysis again shows a highly significant relation ($p = 0.0004$) between the probability of hospital death and age at operation; the probability of death increases exponentially as age approaches the neonatal period (fig. 1).

Smallness of size increased the risk of operation. The body surface area of the survivors was 0.75 ± 0.033 m², significantly larger ($p < 0.0001$) than that of the nonsurvivors (0.41 ± 0.029 m²). Parametric analysis confirmed the incremental risk effect of small size ($p = 0.0002$) and showed the risk to rise steeply when body surface area was less than about 0.4 m² (fig. 2). The same relations were evident when size was expressed as weight in kilograms. Multivariate analysis indicates that smallness of size, expressed as body surface area, has an incremental effect ($p = 0.01$) on hospital mortality, independent of age. Indeed, when the effect of size is accounted for, young age contributes no further incremental risk (p for effect of age is 0.21).

The hematocrit of the survivors ($48.3 \pm 0.69\%$) was not significantly different from that of the nonsurvivors ($51 \pm 2.4\%$). By individual parametric analysis, hematocrit was also not significantly related to hospital mortality. Hematocrit, when considered with body surface area in multivariate analysis, does not have an incremental risk effect ($p = 0.3$). However, hematocrit is a sufficiently important risk factor that

TABLE 6. *Classic Tetralogy of Fallot. Primary Repair Without Major Associated Lesions (UAB 1972-1978)*

Age	No transannular patch				Transannular patch				Total			
		Hospital deaths				Hospital deaths				Hospital deaths		
	n	n	%	70% CL	n	n	%	70% CL	n	n	%	70% CL
0 < 3 months	—	—			3	2	67	24–96%	3	2	67	24–96%
≥ 3 < 6 months	6	1	17	2–46%	6	1	17	2–46%	13	3*	23	10–41%
≥ 6 <12 months	13	2	15	5–33%	15	1	7	1–21%	28	3	11	5–20%
≥12 <24 months	13	0	0	0–14%	17	2	12	4–26%	30	2	7	2–15%
≥24 <48 months	22	1	5	1–15%	12	4	33	18–52%	35†	5	14	8–23%
≥48 <60 months	10	0	0	0–17%	7	0	0	0–24%	17	0	0	0–11%
≥ 5 <10 years	29	0	0	0–6%	9	0	0	0–19%	38	0	0	0–5%
≥10 <20 years	8	0	0	0–21%	—	—	—		8	0	0	0–21%
≥20 <30 years	5	0	0	0–32%	3	0	0	0–47%	8	0	0	0–21%
≥30 years	11	0	0	0–16%	2	0	0	0–61%	14‡	0	0	0–13%
Total	117	4	3.4	1.7–6.1%	74	10	14	9–19%	194	15	7.7	5.7–10.2%

*One patient with nonvalved external conduit: 3.98 months—died.
†Patient with valved external conduit alive—25.5 months.
‡Patient with valved external conduit alive—30.3 years.
Abbreviations: CL = confidence limits, UAB = University of Alabama, Birmingham.

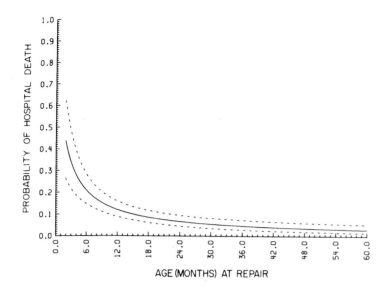

FIGURE 1. *Probability of hospital death as a function of age (shown in months along the horizontal axis) at primary repair (1972–1978). The point estimates are represented by the solid line, and the dashed lines represent the 70% confidence limits. The logistic regression equation is: Z = 0.4 ± 0.73 − 0.94 ± 0.269 · ln (age), where ln (age) is the natural logarithm of age at repair (months). The significance level of coefficients:* p *(age) = 0.0004;* p *(intercept) = 0.6; correlation between coefficients:* r *= −0.92.*

high hematocrit lessens the effect of body surface area on mortality; that is, the hematocrit modifies the body surface area effect ($p = 0.07$ for the interaction).

Transannular patching is an independent incremental risk factor in this experience. Four deaths (3.4%; CL 1.7–6.1%) occurred among the 117 patients in whom no transannular patch was used, compared with 10 deaths (14%; CL 9–19%) among the 74 patients who had transannular patches (p for difference = 0.01). Three patients received valved or unvalved external conduits and are excluded from this portion of the analysis. Among the patients who lived, 36% received transannular patches, compared with 71% of those who died ($p = 0.01$ for the difference). Multivariate analysis indicated that the transannular patch possibly has an effect ($p = 0.12$) independent of age and ($p = 0.13$) body surface area. By parametric

analysis, young age does not appear to have a greater incremental risk effect on patients receiving transannular patches than on those not receiving them, since the interaction of transannular patch and age as regards probability of hospital death is not significant ($p = 0.26$) (fig. 3A). Smallness of size possibly has a greater incremental risk effect on patients receiving transannular patches, in that the interaction of patch and body surface area is possibly significant ($p = 0.19$) (fig. 3B). Both transannular patching ($p = 0.04$) and post-repair $P_{RV/LV}$ ($p = 0.10$) have independent effects, and their interaction is not significant ($p = 0.44$).

Moderately elevated post-repair $P_{RV/LV}$ probably was not an incremental risk factor. However, only nine patients had $P_{RV/LV} \geq 0.85$, and only two had $P_{RV/LV} > 1.0$ (table 7). Post-repair $P_{RV/LV}$ was

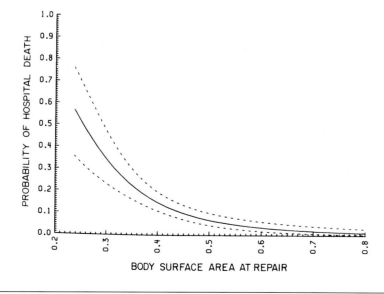

FIGURE 2. *Probability of hospital death as a function of body surface area (BSA) in square meters at primary repair. The presentation is as in figure 1. The logistic regression equation is: Z = −5.3 ± 0.98 − 3.9 ± 1.05 · ln (BSA). Significance level of coefficients:* p *(BSA) = 0.0002,* p *(intercept) <0.0001; correlation between coefficients:* r *= 0.96.*

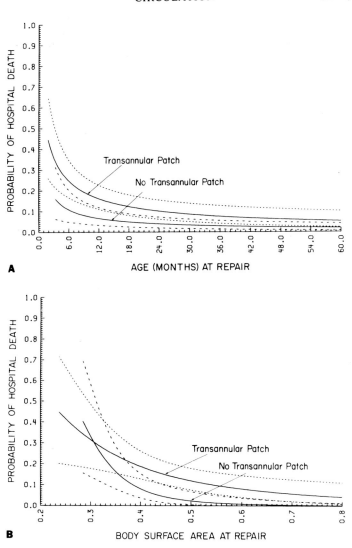

FIGURE 3. *A) Probability of hospital death after primary repair, as a simultaneous function of age at repair and the presence or absence of a transannular patch. The solid lines represent the point estimates, the long-dashed lines the 70% confidence limits for no transannular patch, and the short-dashed lines the 70% confidence limits for transannular patch. The logistic regression equation (in which Patch = 0 for absence of transannular patch and Patch = 1 for presence of transannular patch) is: Z = −0.7 ± 0.96 + 1.0 ± 0.64 · Patch − 0.78 ± 0.280 · ln (age). Significance level of coefficients: p (Patch) = 0.12, p (age) = 0.005, p (intercept) = 0.4; correlation between coefficients: r (intercept, Patch) = −0.60, r (intercept, age) = −0.84, r (Patch, age) = 0.19. The interaction term between patch and age is not significant (p > 0.2), indicating that the slopes of the two curves are not different. B) Probability of hospital death after primary repair as a simultaneous function of body surface area (m²) at repair and the presence or absence of a transannular patch. Presentation is as in 3A. The logistic regression equation is: Z = −8 ± 2.5 − 6 ± 2.5 · ln (BSA) + 4 ± 2.7 · Patch + 4 ± 2.8 · Patch · ln (BSA). Significance level of coefficients: p (Patch) = 0.12, p (BSA) = 0.01, p (Patch · BSA) = 0.19, p (intercept) = 0.002; correlation between coefficients: r (intercept, Patch) = −0.92, r (intercept, BSA) = 0.97, r (intercept, Patch · BSA) = −0.87, r (BSA, Patch) = −0.89, r (BSA, Patch · BSA) = −0.90, r (Patch, Patch · BSA) = 0.97. We consider the interaction term (Patch · BSA) possibly significant (p < 0.2), indicating that the slopes of the curves are different.   The complete logistic regression equation for risk of hospital death after primary repair, including in addition the effect of hematocrit (Hct), is: Z = 4 ± 5.2 + 6 ± 5.6 · ln (BSA) + 0.9 ± 0.69 · Patch − 500 ± 280/Hct − 500 ± 300 · ln (BSA)/Hct. Significance level of coefficients: p (BSA) = 0.31, p (Patch) = 0.20, p (Hct) = 0.08, p (BSA · Hct) = 0.11, p (Intercept) = 0.45; correlation between coefficients: r (intercept, BSA) = 0.93, r (intercept, Patch) = −0.09, r (intercept, Hct) = −0.98, r (intercept, BSA · Hct) = −0.93, r (BSA, Patch) = 0.11, r (BSA, Hct) = −0.91, r (BSA, BSA · Hct) = −0.98, r (Patch, Hct) = 0.00, r (Patch, BSA · Hct) = −0.10, r (Hct, BSA · Hct) = 0.95.*

TABLE 7. *Classic Tetralogy of Fallot. Primary Repair Without Major Associated Lesions (UAB 1972–1978)*

| $P_{RV/LV}$ | No transannular patch | | | | Transannular patch | | | | Total | | | |
| | n | Hospital deaths | | | n | Hospital deaths | | | n | Hospital deaths | | |
		n	%	70% CL		n	%	70% CL		n	%	70% CL
≤ 0.40	58	0	0	0–3%	26	2	8	3–17%	84	2	2	1–6%
$0.40 \leq 0.65$	48	3	6	3–12%	33	7	21	14–31%	81	10	12	9–17%
$0.65 \leq 0.75$	8	1	12	2–36%	8	0	0	0–21%	16	1	6	1–20%
$0.75 \leq 0.85$	2	0	0	0–61%	1	0	0	0–85%	3	0	0	0–47%
$0.85 \leq 1.0$	—	—			5	1	20	3–53%	5	1	20	3–53%
> 1.0	1	0	0	0–85%	1	0	0	0–85%	2	0	0	0–61%
Total	117	4	3.4	1.7–6.1%	74	10	14	9–19%	191*	14	7.3	5.4–9.8%

*Excludes three patients with external conduits.

Abbreviations: $P_{RV/LV}$ = ratio of peak pressure in the right ventricle to that in left; CL = confidence limits; UAB = University of Alabama, Birmingham.

0.457 ± 0.0133 in the hospital survivors, and 0.54 ± 0.044 among those who died (p for difference = 0.08). When patients with transannular patch are analyzed parametrically as a group, $P_{RV/LV}$ does not have a significant effect ($p = 0.3$) on mortality; in the group without a transannular patch, $P_{RV/LV}$ might have a significant effect ($p = 0.14$). By individual parametric analysis of the two groups together, $P_{RV/LV}$ has a significant ($p = 0.04$) effect on hospital mortality, but the rate of increase in risk with higher $P_{RV/LV}$ up to 1.0 is not great (fig. 4). Most important, multivariate analysis shows that $P_{RV/LV}$ was not a significant determinant of hospital mortality ($p > 0.3$) when age, body surface area, hematocrit, and presence or absence of transannular patching are considered.

The results have not improved recently. Thus, the operative date was not related to hospital mortality by either t test or parametric analysis. The total elapsed time of cardiopulmonary bypass (including the time of total circulatory arrest) was 74.9 ± 1.66 minutes in

surviving patients and 88 ± 7.6 minutes in nonsurviving patients ($p = 0.1$). There were no significant differences in the aortic cross-clamp time of those who lived (42.2 ± 0.90 minutes) compared with that of those who died (43 ± 3.6 minutes) when cold ischemic arrest was used, either when analyzed alone or in a multivariate analysis using age, body surface area, hematocrit, and the presence or absence of a transannular patch. The incidence of the use of cold cardioplegia was not significantly different in those who lived vs those who died.

Some interrelations between variables and events are interesting. Transannular patching did not insure a low $P_{RV/LV}$, as patients with high post-repair $P_{RV/LV}$ are more frequently in the group receiving transannular patching. Also, the mean value of $P_{RV/LV}$ for those not receiving transannular patching was 0.434 ± 0.0147, lower than that of 0.51 ± 0.023 among those who did. Post-repair $P_{RV/LV}$ tended to be higher in the younger patients ($r = -0.26$, $p = 0.0003$) and in those with smaller body surface

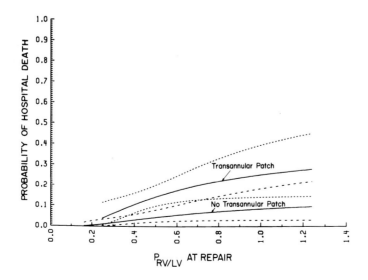

FIGURE 4. *Probability of hospital death after primary repair as a simultaneous function of the post-repair ratio of peak pressure in the right ventricle to that in the right ($P_{RV/LV}$) (in the operating room) and the presence or absence of transannular patch. The presentation is as in figure 3. The logistic regression equation (with notation as in figure 3) is: $Z = -1.7 \pm 1.04 + 1.3 \pm 0.62 \cdot Patch - 0.70 \pm 0.417 / P_{RV/LV}$. Significance level of coefficients: p (patch) = 0.04, p ($P_{RV/LV}$) = 0.095, p (intercept) = 0.10; correlation between coefficients: r (intercept, Patch) = −0.53, r (intercept, $P_{RV/LV}$) = −0.87, r (Patch, $P_{RV/LV}$) = 0.14. Interaction term between patch and $P_{RV/LV}$ is not significant (p > 0.2).*

TABLE 8. *Classic Tetralogy of Fallot. Primary Repair Without Major Associated Lesions (UAB 1972–1978): Proportion of Patients Receiving Transannular Patches*

Age	Total n		With transannular patch		
			n	%	70% CL
< 6	15 ⎫	41/73	9	60	43–75%
6 < 12	28 ⎬	56% (49–63%)	15	54	42–65%
12 < 24	30		17	57	46–67%
24 < 48	34		12	35	26–46%
≥ 48	84		21	25	20–31%
Total	191*		74	39	35–43%

*Excludes three patients with external conduits.
Abbreviations: UAB = University of Alabama, Birmingham; CL = confidence limits.

TABLE 9. *Repair of Classic Tetralogy of Fallot Without Major Associated Lesions after Single Blalock-Taussig or Waterston Shunt (UAB 1967–1978)*

Determinant of hospital mortality	p value
Age*	0.15
Body surface area	0.12
Hematocrit	0.01
Type of shunt	0.9
Date of operation	0.7
Transannular patch	0.6
Post-repair $P_{RV/LV}$	0.4

N = 158 (five deaths).
*Only five patients were younger than 2 years old at intracardiac repair.
Abbreviations: UAB = University of Alabama, Birmingham; $P_{RV/LV}$ = ratio of peak pressure in the right ventricle to that in the left.

area ($r = -0.30$, $p = 0.0001$). Also, the younger the patient, the higher the proportion receiving transannular patches ($p = 0.0004$),* and the smaller the patient's body surface area, the larger the proportion receiving transannular patching ($p < 0.0001$).* The proportion of patients receiving transannular patching at various ages is shown in table 8. The higher the hematocrit, the greater the probability of a transannular patch ($p < 0.0001$).* Transannular patching was used more frequently in the later years of this experience. Thus, transannular patches were used more frequently (p for difference < 0.0001) in the patients undergoing primary repair between 1972–1978 (74 of 191 patients† (39%); CL 35–43%) than in those undergoing primary repair in 1967–1972 (five of 70 patients (7%); CL 4–12%). Multivariate analysis of these 261 patients showed that the date of operation, when corrected for age and the level of preoperative hematocrit, was very significantly and independently related ($p < 0.0001$) to the probability of a transannular patch having been inserted, with more such patches being inserted in the later years of this period.

Secondary Intracardiac Repair after an Initial Anastomotic Operation

Three of 124 patients (2.4%, CL 1.1–4.8%) undergoing intracardiac repair after a single Blalock-Taussig anastomosis between 1967–1978 died in the hospital, a mortality not significantly different ($p = 0.9$) from that of two of 34 patients (6%, CL 2–13%) who had previously undergone a single Waterston anastomosis. Therefore, for purposes of analysis, these two groups were combined. Four of the patients died of low cardiac output, and one died of intractable pulmonary dysfunction. Atrioventricular block did not occur in either group.

Multivariate analysis showed age and body surface

area possibly to be inversely related to the risk of operation (table 9). It showed hematocrit at the time of intracardiac repair to be related to the risk of the operation, and three of the five deaths were in patients with hematocrits >60% at the time of operation. The type of shunt, date of operation (showing that the results have been stable over the study period), presence or absence of transannular patching, and post-repair $P_{RV/LV}$ were not related to mortality in this group of patients. The use of transannular patching increased in the latter part of this experience, as well as in the patients undergoing primary repair.

Multivariate analysis of the combination of the 194 patients who underwent primary repair in 1972–1978 and this group of 158 patients who had previously undergone an anastomotic operation showed that the presence of a shunt had no effect on hospital mortality when the effect of age (p for shunt = 0.6) or body surface area (p for shunt = 0.5) are accounted for.

Comparison of Primary and Two-stage Repair

The projected risk of two-stage repair (see Methods) at age 3–5 years is about 5% (CL 3–7%) (fig. 5). It rises above that when the age at the initial operation (the shunt) is less than 3 months, and when shunting must be done at 1 month of age, the combined risk is 9% (CL 6–12%). No late deaths before age 3 years occurred after the shunting procedures.[12] Six (4%, CL 2–7%, of the hospital survivors of shunting) patients required a second palliative operation before 3 years of age.

For simplicity, we first compared two-stage and primary repair considering only age at initial operation, and whether or not a transannular patch was used at primary repair. With this method, even at the youngest age, the two-stage repair is not safer (see Materials and Methods for definition of "safer") than primary repair without transannular patching (figs. 6A and 6B). When transannular patching is needed in the primary repair, two-stage repair is safer in infants

---

*These p values must be interpreted with caution because p value for lack of fit of model to data was 0.1.
†Excluding the three patients with valved or nonvalved external conduit.

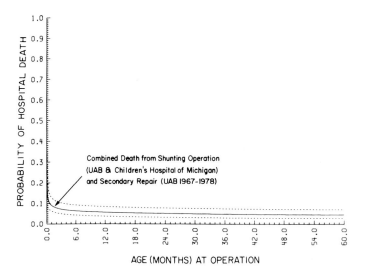

FIGURE 5. *Projected probability of hospital death from two-stage repair of tetralogy of Fallot (initial Blalock-Taussig or Waterston anastomosis and intracardiac repair about 3 years later). This is based upon the combined mortality of the initial shunting procedure, described in detail previously,*[12] *and the mortality of secondary repair (five deaths among 158 patients, mortality 3.2%, confidence limits 1.8–5.3%) from our 1967–1978 experience at the University of Alabama, Birmingham (UAB). The presentation is as in figure 1.*

younger than 24 months old (figs. 6A and 6B).

However, not only age at operation and the presence or absence of transannular patching, but also body surface area and hematocrit are important incremental risk factors in primary repair. Thus, comparison of its risks with those of two-stage repair should take these factors into account. When this is done, the importance of small size and, in patients with transannular patching at primary repair, preoperative hematocrit becomes apparent. For example, two-stage repair is still not safer than primary repair without transannular patch, except in very young patients who are also very small (body surface area less than about 0.35 m²) (fig. 7A). When transannular patching is used, two-stage repair is safer when body surface area is less than about 0.53 m² when hematocrit is not included (fig. 7B). When hematocrit of 52% (the mean hematocrit value of the patients in this subset) is included, two-stage repair is safer only when body surface area is less than about 0.48 m².

Discussion

We have presented data concerning our surgical experience with all types of tetralogy of Fallot so that criteria for inclusion of patients in the study groups are clear. We included data from patients of all ages who underwent primary repair of classic tetralogy of Fallot between January 1972 and January 1978, because statistical analysis of the relation of age at operation and other variables is more reliable when data from the entire experience are included. Policies and practices of intracardiac repair in patients who had previously had a palliative procedure were quite stable between 1967–1978, and the entire period is therefore included in this part of the study.

We used visual examination of tabular data, scattergrams, analysis of mean values, single and multivariant regression analysis, and probability of event

analysis to learn as much as we could from this experience and to present it in usable form.

Primary Intracardiac Repair

In this experience, young age increased the risk of operation, with the effect being strongest as age approached that of the neonatal period. The incremental risk for the effect of age was not evident after about 4 years of age, and no deaths occurred in patients older than 4 years of age at operation. Similarly, smallness of size, expressed as either body surface area or weight, increased the risk of operation, and when this effect was accounted for, young age added no further risk.

The incremental risk effect of young age and small size in primary repair of the tetralogy of Fallot may be unique to our experience. However, data from Barratt-Boyes' recent presentation concerning tetralogy of Fallot suggest a similar effect in his experience.[26] The results of Castaneda et al.[8] in young infants, as a whole, are superior to ours (table 10). The mortality of two deaths among 39 patients in their study is lower ($p = 0.07$) than ours of eight in 44 patients operated in the first year of life. The reasons for this difference should be studied further. However, any possible incremental risk effect of young age and small size in his experience is difficult to assess, because no data from his patients over the age of 1 year are available for trend analysis and the numbers of patients in the various young age groups are small.

If this incremental risk effect of young age and small size is a real one and not limited to our experience, its causes require investigation. We do not believe it is explained by interference with the technical aspects of the operation, for smallness does not prevent accurate intracardiac repair. Since the mechanism of death is low cardiac output in most patients and since high preoperative hematocrit (which is usually associated with severe cyanosis) in-

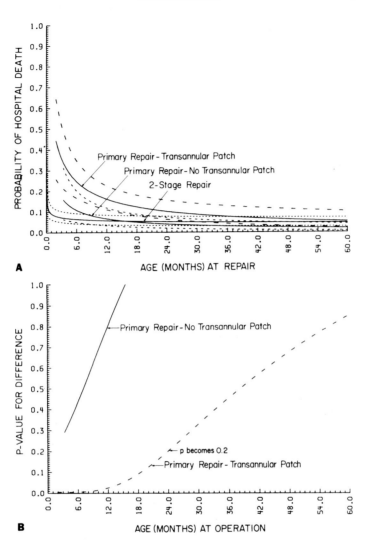

FIGURE 6. *Simplified comparison of the hospital mortality of primary repair (from data used in figure 3A) and that of the two-stage repair (from data used in figure 5), using only age at operation and transannular patch (yes-no) at primary repair. A) Probability of hospital death. When transannular patching is not used, no matter how young the patient, the 70% confidence limits of the two-stage repair overlap those of primary repair (p for difference therefore greater than about 0.1), indicating by one convention of surgical decision-making[36] that primary repair is permitted at any age. B) P value for the difference between the point estimate of the lesser hospital mortality of two-stage repair compared with that of primary repair, according to age at operation and presence or absence of transannular patching. The solid line is the p value for the difference when the primary repair is done with no transannular patch. Since at no age is the p value 0.2 or less, the conclusion would be that at no age in this subset is two-stage repair safer. The dashed line is the p value when a transannular patch is used at primary repair. Two-stage repair is safer when operation is required before 24 months of age.*

creased the incremental risk effect of young age, we believe improved results will require understanding and more appropriate management of the hemodynamics and metabolism of the young, small, and chronically hypoxic heart. The relatively (for the size of the patient) large "dose" of the adverse effects of cardiopulmonary bypass may play a role also, even though total circulatory arrest or a prolonged period of very low flow was used in almost all the infants. This factor is suggested by the fact that we have also shown an incremental risk effect of very young age and small size in a different setting — repair of the complete form of common atrioventricular canal.[27]

Transannular patching appears to be an incremen-

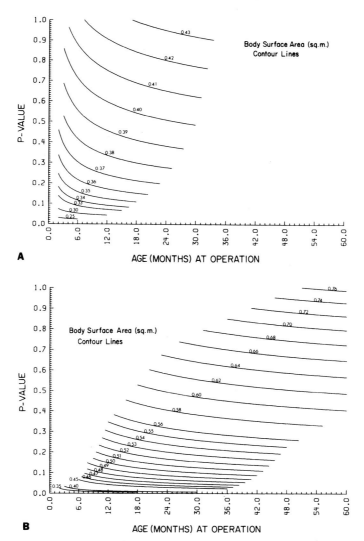

FIGURE 7. *Plots similar to those in figure 6B, but representing more completely (the small hematocrit effect is not included) the calculations for deciding in a given patient whether two-stage repair is safer (see Materials and Methods) than primary repair. A) Effect of age and body surface area in patients in whom no transannular patch was used at primary repair. Along the vertical axis is the p value for the difference between the lower point estimate of the combined risk of two-stage repair and that of primary repair. In patients younger than 6 months of age, for example, primary repair is as safe as two-stage repair (p > 0.2) only when body surface area is greater than about 0.36 m². The spread of each contour line is related to the actual spreads of age for a given body surface area in the primary repair study group. For example, by linear regression analysis we find the standard deviation of body surface area to be ±0.07 m² at age 60 months (5 years). B) Effect in patients in whom transannular patch is used at primary repair. Two-stage repair is safer whenever body surface area is less than 0.53 m², when hematocrit is not considered.*

tal risk factor, as in our earlier experience at the Mayo Clinic.[1, 3] The effect of transannular patching in increasing the risk of operation is not evident in this experience in patients older than about 4 years of age, because, as already noted, no deaths occurred in that subset. This probably explains why we could not show an incremental risk effect of transannular patching in our patients undergoing secondary repair, most of whom were older at the time of repair. It may also explain the weak effect of transannular patching in the cases reported by Poirier, McGoon, and colleagues, as their data indicate that most of these patients were older than 4 years.[28] In contrast, no statistically significant adverse effect of transannular patching in infants can be shown in Castaneda's data.[8] The two deaths in his experience were both in patients receiving

TABLE 10. *Results of Primary Intracardiac Repair for Classic Tetralogy of Fallot* (Castaneda)[8]*

Age (months)	No transannular patch				Transannular patch				Total			
		Hospital death				Hospital death				Hospital death		
	n	n	%	70% CL	n	n	%	70% CL	n	n	%	70% CL
0 < 3	1	—	0	0–86%	8	1	12	2–36%	9	1	11	1–33%
≥ 3 < 6	5	—	0	0–32%	8	1	12	2–36%	13	1	8	1–24%
≥ 6 < 12	6	—	0	0–27%	11	—	0	0–16%	17	—	0	0–11%
Total	12	—	0	0–15%	27	2	7	2–17%	39	2	5	2–12%

*Omits one patient aged 0.2 months with absent pulmonary valve who died, and one aged 10.2 months with pulmonary atresia and small right and left pulmonary arteries who had palliative transannular patching and lived. Recalculated from Castaneda et al.[8]

Abbreviation: CL = confidence limits.

transannular patching. If transannular patching truly has an incremental risk effect on hospital mortality, we believe it may be related in part to the volume overload of the right ventricle resulting from the severe pulmonary valve incompetence and in part to the mechanical (or hemodynamic) effect of the patch itself in the ventricular wall.

In this regard, it seems clear that the proportion of patients in all categories receiving transannular patching has increased in the recent years of our experience. In the latter part of our earlier period of experience with the tetralogy of Fallot at the Mayo Clinic (up to 1967), and in the early part of this present experience in Alabama, the proportion of patients receiving transannular patches was low, about 15%. In recent years in all categories it has risen to 30–50%. We believe this has resulted from a nondeliberate lowering of the acceptable post-repair $P_{RV/LV}$ without a patch, and an almost unconsciously accepted idea that patients receiving transannular patches "did as well" as those without them. Therefore, the proportion of patients receiving transannular patches in series reported by others probably results as much from the bias of the surgeons as from the case material. The present analysis indicates that we should return to a policy of using transannular patches only when it is reasonably certain they are necessary.

While a low post-repair $P_{RV/LV}$ after repair is highly desirable, we have not been able to show that post-repair $P_{RV/LV}$ is an independent determinant of the risk of primary repair unless it is inordinately elevated (above 0.85 in the operating room after repair). This is similar to our earlier findings.[3] Furthermore, no matter how well the $P_{RV/LV}$ is reduced by inserting a transannular patch, the 70% CL of the probability of hospital death do not fall below those of primary repair without transannular patching when the post-repair $P_{RV/LV}$ is below 1 (fig. 4). We have neither seen nor read of functionally poor late results or the need for reoperation as long as late postoperative $P_{RV/LV}$ is below about 0.75, the ventricular septal defect well closed and the pulmonary valve ring intact. Furthermore, Calder and colleagues,[29] as well as Muraoka and colleagues,[30] have shown that the intact ring and the main pulmonary artery grow nicely after primary repair without transannular patching in infancy.

Secondary Intracardiac Repair

The analysis indicates that secondary repair after a single Blalock-Taussig or Waterston anastomosis is a safe procedure, particularly in patients whose hematocrit is not above 60%. Since, as in our previous Mayo Clinic experience,[2, 3] the presence or absence of a shunt did not affect hospital mortality in any age group, we conclude that shunting exerts its favorable effect primarily by allowing the intracardiac repair to be done at a later age, rather than by enlarging the left ventricle, or "preparing the lungs." Possibly, a part of its effect is in bringing the patient to operation less hypoxic than he or she would have been otherwise.

Primary vs Two-stage Repair

This analysis indicates that with the methods we have used, only when the very young patient is also very small is a two-stage approach safer than primary repair when a transannular patch is not required. When a transannular patch is required, the two-stage approach is in general safer than primary repair up to 24 months of age.

We have altered our patient management program to a selective one, based upon age, body surface area, hematocrit, and the probable need for a transannular patch. Data from the preoperative cineangiogram are used to determine whether a transannular patch will probably be required.[31] Then, based on whether the patient probably will or will not receive a transannular patch, as well as age, body surface area, and hematocrit, we calculate the risks of primary repair and two-stage repair (figs. 7A and 7B).* We do primary repair unless the two-stage repair is considered to be safer. If the calculations show the two-stage repair to be safer, we do a Blalock-Taussig shunt, and intracardiac repair is deferred until 3–5 years of age. We believe these criteria should be

---

*An appendix is available on request, providing the equations, parameter estimates, and variance-covariance components necessary for calculating the risks of primary vs two-stage repair, according to the data drom this study. These functions can be used to program any of the currently available hand-held programmable calculators (we have used the Hewlett-Packard models HP-67 and HP-97).

generally applicable, although they are not needed by those obtaining uniformly good results from routine primary repair in infants. Prospective testing over the next 3–5 years will be required to prove the usefulness of these criteria. Dobell and colleagues,[32] Starr and colleagues,[33] and Bender and colleagues[34] have reported excellent results from their somewhat different selective policies in the past.

Our recommendation may be temporary, for further research, we hope, will more clearly identify the factors in the myocardial damage that must underlie most of the deaths from low cardiac output, and will develop ways of preventing these. Further research may identify the causes and thus allow prevention of the other two causes of death, hemorrhagic pulmonary edema without elevated left atrial pressure, and the syndrome of severe hyperpyrexia, agitation, peripheral constriction and progressing hemoconcentration that we believe is a reaction to the complex situation of cardiopulmonary bypass as now practiced. However, if it is shown that a preliminary anastomotic operation allows later repair with preservation of the pulmonary valve in an appreciable number of patients who would have required a transannular patch had the repair been done primarily in infancy, the policy may have merit for a considerable period of time.

Acknowledgment

We are pleased to acknowledge the contribution of the skillful work of Sandy O'Brien in the graphics and in manuscript preparation.

References

1. Kirklin JW, Payne WS, Theye RA, DuShane JW: Factors affecting survival after open operation for tetralogy of Fallot. Ann Surg 152: 485, 1960
2. Kirklin JW, Ellis FH Jr, McGoon DC, DuShane JW, Swan HJC: Surgical treatment for the tetralogy of Fallot by open intracardiac repair. J Thorac Surg 37: 22, 1959
3. Kirklin JW, Wallace RB, McGoon DC, DuShane JW: Early and late results after intracardiac repair of tetralogy of Fallot. Ann Surg 162: 578, 1965
4. Kirklin JW, McGoon DC, DuShane JW: Surgical treatment of ventricular septal defect. J Thorac Cardiovasc Surg 40: 763, 1960
5. Kerr AR, Barratt-Boyes BG: Surgery of tetralogy of Fallot in infancy: comparison of shunt palliation and primary intracardiac repair. *In* Heart Disease in Infancy, edited by Barratt-Boyes BG, Neutze JM. London, Churchill Livingstone, 1973, pp 197–210
6. Barratt-Boyes BG, Neutze JM: Primary repair of tetralogy of Fallot in infancy using profound hypothermia with circulatory arrest and limited cardiopulmonary bypass: a comparison with conventional two-stage management. Ann Surg 178: 406, 1973
7. Barratt-Boyes BG: Primary definitive intracardiac operations in infants: tetralogy of Fallot. *In* Advances in Cardiovascular Surgery, edited by Kirklin JW. New York, Grune & Stratton, 1973, pp 155–172
8. Castaneda AR, Freed MD, Williams RG, Norwood WI: Repair of tetralogy of Fallot in infancy. Early and late results. J Thorac Cardiovasc Surg 74: 372, 1977
9. Arciniegas E: Discussion of paper by Castaneda et al.: Repair of tetralogy of Fallot in infancy. Early and late results. J Thorac Cardiovasc Surg 74: 380, 1977
10. Chopra PS, Levy JM, Dacumos GC Jr, Berkoff HA, Loring LL, Kahn DR: The Blalock-Taussig operation: the procedure of choice in the hypoxic infant with tetralogy of Fallot. Ann Thorac Surg 22: 235, 1976
11. Daily PO, Stinson EB, Griepp RB, Shumway NE: Tetralogy of Fallot. Choice of surgical procedure. J Thorac Cardiovasc Surg 75: 338, 1978
12. Arciniegas E, Blackstone EH, Pacifico AD, Kirklin JW: Classical shunting operations as part of 2-stage repair for the tetralogy of Fallot. Ann Thorac Surg. In press
13. Bargeron LM Jr, Elliott LP, Soto B, Bream PR, Curry GC: Axial cineangiography in congenital heart disease. Section 1. Concept, technical and anatomic considerations. Circulation 56: 1075, 1977
14. Elliott LP, Bargeron LM Jr, Bream PR, Soto B, Curry GC: Axial cineangiography in congenital heart disease. Section II. Specific Lesions. Circulation 56: 1084, 1977
15. Kirklin JW, Pacifico AD, Hannah H III, Allarde RR: Primary definitive intracardiac operations in infants: intraoperative support techniques. *In* Advances in Cardiovascular Surgery, edited by Kirklin JW. New York, Grune & Stratton, 1973, pp 85–99
16. Conti VR, Bertranou EG, Blackstone EH, Kirklin JW, Digerness SB: Cold cardioplegia vs hypothermia as myocardial protection: a randomized clinical study. J Thorac Cardiovasc Surg 76: 577, 1978
17. Pacifico AD, Kirklin JW, Blackstone EH: Surgical management of pulmonary stenosis in tetralogy of Fallot. J Thorac Cardiovasc Surg 74: 382, 1977
18. Blackstone EH, Kirklin JW, Pacifico AD: Decision-making in the repair of tetralogy of Fallot based on intraoperative measurements of the pulmonary arterial outflow tract. J Thorac Cardiovasc Surg. In press
19. Kirklin JW, Karp RB: The Tetralogy of Fallot from a Surgical Viewpoint. Philadelphia, WB Saunders Company, 1970
20. Barr AJ, Goodnight JH, Sall JP, Helwig JT: A User's Guide to SAS-76. Raleigh, North Carolina, SAS Institute, Inc, 1976, pp 275–277
21. Wallis WA, Roberts HV: Statistics: A New Approach. New York, The Free Press, 1965, pp 467, 468
22. Walker SH, Duncan DB: Estimation of the probability of an event as a function of several independent variables. Biometrika 54: 167, 1967
23. Berkson J: A statistically precise and relatively simple method of estimating the bioassay with quantile response, based on the logistic function. Am Stat Assn J 48: 565, 1953
24. Bradley EL: The equivalence of maximum likelihood and weighted test squares estimates in the exponential family. J Am Stat Assn 68: 199, 1973
25. Nelder JA, Wedderburn RWN: Generalized linear models. J R Stat Soc, Series A 135: 370, 1972
26. Barratt-Boyes BG: Primary repair of tetralogy of Fallot in infants. Presented at Postgraduate Course on Cardiac Surgery, American College of Surgeons, Dallas, Texas, October 19, 1977
27. Berger TJ, Blackstone EH, Kirklin JW, Bargeron LM Jr, Hazelrig JB, Turner ME Jr: Survival and probability of cure without and with surgery in complete atrioventricular canal. Ann Thorac Surg 27: 104, 1979
28. Poirier RA, McGoon DC, Danielson GK, Wallace RB, Ritter DG, Moodie DS, Wiltse CG: Late results after repair of tetralogy of Fallot. J Thorac Cardiovasc Surg 73: 900, 1977
29. Calder AL, Barratt-Boyes BG, Brandt PWT, Neutze JM: Postoperative evaluation of patients with tetralogy of Fallot repaired in infancy: including criteria for the use of outflow patching and a radiological assessment of pulmonary regurgitation. J Thorac Cardiovasc Surg. In press
30. Muraoka R, Yokota M, Matsuda K, Tabata R, Hikasa Y: Long-term hemodynamic evaluation of primary total correction of tetralogy of Fallot during the first two years of life. Arch Jpn Chir 42: 315, 1973
31. Blackstone EH, Kirklin JW, Bertranou EG, Labrosse CJ, Soto B, Bargeron LM Jr: Preoperative prediction from cineangiograms of post-repair right ventricular pressure in tetralogy of Fallot. J Thorac Cardiovasc Surg. In press
32. Dobell ARC, Charrettee EP, Chughtai MS: Correction of tetralogy of Fallot in the young child. J Thorac Cardiovasc Surg 55: 70, 1968

Special Article

Open-Heart Surgery at the Mayo Clinic
The 25th Anniversary

JOHN W. KIRKLIN, M.D.
Department of Surgery, Division of Cardio-Thoracic Surgery, University of Alabama School of Medicine and Medical Center, Birmingham, Alabama

In about 1952, a patient at the Mayo Clinic with pulmonary stenosis and intact ventricular septum died 2 days after an operation that I had performed. Severe secondary subvalvular obstruction thwarted the surgical attempt to relieve the right ventricular outflow obstruction by a closed pulmonary valvotomy, a phenomenon and a case described, among others, in a subsequent publication by a group of us at the Mayo Clinic.[1] Dr. J. E. Edwards, in pathology, Dr. E. H. Wood, in physiology, and I concluded, after study of the autopsy specimen from this case, that an open technique was necessary for successful management of such cases, and that since the cardiac septa were intact, a technique of right heart bypass should provide this opportunity. (Discussions about this in Earl Wood's small office in the Medical Sciences Building were hampered by the noise from the overhead ventilator, as a protection against which he often wore large "noise reducers" such as are worn around jet aircraft!) We were concerned that an oxygenator, which would be necessary for total cardiopulmonary bypass, would introduce extreme complexities. Drs. David Donald, in experimental surgery, Earl Wood, Mr. R. E. Jones, head of the engineering section, and I then visited three institutions where pump-oxygenators had been developed but were not being used clinically. After these visits, we revised our opinion that we should develop right heart bypass as a clinical tool and decided that we could, after further research and development, probably adapt the Gibbon-IBM pump-oxygenator[2] for successful clinical application.

No successful operations had been done in man with the use of cardiopulmonary bypass at the time our small group made our decision. Gibbon,[3] in 1939, had shown the feasibility of total cardiopulmonary bypass in the experimental animal. Dennis and colleagues[4] at the University of Minnesota had done extensive laboratory studies with pump-oxygenators and had one unsuccessful clinical case in 1951. A number of investigators in various parts of the world had reported experimental studies with various kinds and sizes of pump-oxygenators, including Björk[5] and Senning[6] in Stockholm. Their work led ultimately to a successful human application for removal of a left atrial myxoma, by Crafoord and associates.[7] As we were reflecting about all this in 1952, we wondered why successful clinical application of pump-oxygenators to cardiac surgery had not been accomplished.

We, along with Drs. H. B. Burchell in cardiology, J. W. DuShane in pediatric cardiology, H. J. C. Swan in physiology, and Robert Patrick in anesthesiology, requested and received permission to proceed with (1) the design and building of a "Mayo-Gibbon" pump-oxygenator in the engineering shops of the Mayo Clinic (none was produced commercially at that time), (2) a laboratory program of research and development, and (3) ultimate clinical application if successful. Two and a half years of intense work followed, in which we were joined by Drs. Peter Hetzel and Harry Harshbarger. By 1955, we were in a position to proceed with clinical application, as indicated by two brief publications early that year.[8,9]

Meantime, Gibbon,[10] in 1953, had successfully repaired an atrial septal defect in a 17-year-old girl, but four subsequent patients died.[11] Lillehei and colleagues at the University of Minnesota, ably supported by Varco, had begun their pioneering work in open-heart surgery in the spring of 1954,[12] using the "azygos-flow principle"[13,14] and another human being as the oxygenator during "controlled cross-circulation." A number of spectacularly successful operations were performed at the University of Minnesota with this technique. Indeed, as an outgrowth of this experience there was some discussion to the effect that artificial oxygenators could never be successful because of their damaging effect on blood. It is not difficult to imagine the pressures we were subjected to from inside and outside our institution to abort our efforts in favor of "controlled cross-circulation."

Early in 1955, five patients were identified for the initial use at the Mayo Clinic of a pump-oxygenator for cardiac surgery. They were selected after careful review of a large number of patients who needed open operations for their otherwise ultimately fatal heart disease, for which no other kind of surgical treatment would be possible. Each family was told that we would use a new and hitherto unproven method, with which we had extensive laboratory but no clinical experience. We explained the risks, imponderables, and possible benefits of the operations. The first operation, repair of a large ventricular septal defect in a 5½-year-old child, was performed on Mar. 22, 1955. Our plan was to proceed with the other four operations even if the first patient died, so great was our confidence in the methods we had developed in the laboratory work. In spite of temporary dislodgement of the arterial line during bypass, the first operation was successfully done, and the patient's postoperative course was uneventful. These five patients and three more formed the basis of the world's first publication concerning a group of patients operated on with use of cardiopulmonary bypass and a pump-oxygenator.[15] Of the eight patients, four died postoperatively—one with a complete atrioventricular canal defect, one with tetralogy of Fallot and a Blalock-Taussig anastomosis, one 4-month-old infant with ventricular septal defect, and one 11-year-old girl with a large ventricular septal defect, pulmonary vascular disease, and scoliosis. Now, 25 years later, as a result of the intense efforts of clinicians and investigators all over the world, the

method is used quite safely and many times a day in hospitals in almost every country in the world.

The Mayo Clinic has reason for pride in the 25th anniversary of those early events. In the interim, the entire field of cardiac surgery has developed. Its techniques have become beautifully refined, so that technically complex operations can be done inside the hearts of small babies, artificial valves can be inserted at very low risk, and anastomoses can be made to coronary arteries, only a millimeter or two in diameter. The intensive care unit developed in response to the needs of cardiac surgical patients (the very first intensive care unit of any kind may have been the cardiac surgery intensive care unit developed by St. Marys Hospital and the Mayo Clinic in 1957). Interestingly, many cardiac surgical patients now convalesce simply and uneventfully as a result of the many advances that have been made, particularly in myocardial preservation during operation.[16] The need for intensive care is minimal today in this subset of cardiac patients. Therefore, cardiac surgeons may now be able to make a contribution to increasing cost-effectiveness by decreasing the intensity of the postoperative care given many of their patients, although this is made difficult by the large operational and intellectual superstructure presently concerned with intensive care.

Some of the basic problems associated with the clinical use of pump-oxygenators are as real and unsolved today as they were in 1955. They are not necessarily apparent, since the knowledge and skills that have been developed by all those concerned with cardiac surgery have reduced the risks of many kinds of heart surgery nearly to zero.[17,18] But when we repair very complex kinds of heart disease, particularly in the very young, the very sick, and the very old, important risks are still imposed by the unsolved problems of cardiopulmonary bypass with pump-oxygenators. These include the physicochemical changes produced in the formed and unformed elements of blood by exposure to nonbiologic surfaces, which produce profound and widespread structural and functional abnormalities in the patients. They include the physiologic sequelae of 1 or 2 hours of the nonpulsatile flow associated with clinical cardiopulmonary bypass. Although effects are for the most part transient, they do increase the risks of the operations and the intensity of care needed by some patients intraoperatively and early postoperatively. Solutions to these complex problems would not be only intellectually rewarding, and save lives, but would also considerably increase the cost-effectiveness of cardiac surgery. These residual problems require the com-

Mayo Clin Proc, May 1980, Vol 55

bined efforts of basic scientists (particularly, probably, immunochemists and protein chemists and physiologists) and clinicians for their solutions; unfortunately, they are being studied in only a few centers.

We could, of course, set aside these problems, rejoice in our accomplishments, and accept the idea that nature sets certain limits to everything, including cardiac surgery. Billroth[19] expressed such a view in 1897 when he said that cardiac surgery had reached the limits set by nature. Those in 1954 who urged aborting the pump-oxygenator effort must have had a similar notion. Not the passage of time but the efforts of many people have proven the idea to be wrong at both points in time. I believe acceptance of such an idea today would also be wrong.

REFERENCES

1. Kirklin JW, Connolly DC, Ellis FH Jr, Burchell HB, Edwards JE, Wood EH: Problems in the diagnosis and surgical treatment of pulmonic stenosis with intact ventricular septum. Circulation 8:849-863, 1953
2. Miller BJ, Gibbon JH Jr, Fineberg C: An improved mechanical heart and lung apparatus: its use during open cardiotomy in experimental animals. Med Clin North Am, 1953, pp 1603-1624
3. Gibbon JH Jr: The maintenance of life during experimental occlusion of the pulmonary artery followed by survival. Surg Gynecol Obstet 69:602-614, 1939
4. Dennis C, Spreng DS Jr, Nelson GE, Karlson KE, Nelson RM, Thomas JV, Eder WP, Varco RL: Development of a pump-oxygenator to replace the heart and lungs; an apparatus applicable to human patients, and application to one case. Ann Surg 134:709-721, 1951
5. Björk VO: Brain perfusions in dogs with artificially oxygenated blood. Acta Chir Scand 96 [Suppl] 137:1-122, 1948
6. Senning Å: Ventricular fibrillation during extracorporeal circulation: used as a method to prevent air-embolisms and to facilitate intracardiac operations. Acta Chir Scand [Suppl] 171:1-79, 1952
7. Crafoord C, Norberg B, Senning Å: Clinical studies in extracorporeal circulation with a heart-lung machine. Acta Chir Scand 112:220-245, 1957
8. Jones RE, Donald DE, Swan HJC, Harshbarger HG, Kirklin JW, Wood EH: Apparatus of the Gibbon type for mechanical bypass of the heart and lungs: preliminary report. Proc Staff Meet Mayo Clin 30:105-113, 1955
9. Donald DE, Harshbarger HG, Hetzel PS, Patrick RT, Wood EH, Kirklin JW: Experiences with a heart-lung bypass (Gibbon type) in the experimental laboratory: preliminary report. Proc Staff Meet Mayo Clin 30:113-115, 1955
10. Gibbon JH Jr: Application of a mechanical heart and lung apparatus to cardiac surgery. In Recent Advances in Cardiovascular Physiology and Surgery. Minneapolis, University of Minnesota, 1953, pp 107-113
11. Gibbon JH Jr: Personal communication
12. Warden HE, Cohen M, Read RC, Lillehei CW: Controlled cross circulation for open intracardiac surgery. J Thorac Surg 28:331-341, 1954
13. Andreasen AT, Watson F: Experimental cardiovascular surgery: discussion of results so far obtained and report on experiments concerning a donor circulation. Br J Surg 41:195-206, 1953
14. Cohen M, Warden HE, Lillehei CW: Physiologic and metabolic changes during autogenous lobe oxygenation with total cardiac by-pass employing the azygos flow principle. Surg Gynecol Obstet 98:523-529, 1954
15. Kirklin JW, DuShane JW, Patrick RT, Donald DE, Hetzel PS, Harshbarger HG, Wood EH: Intracardiac surgery with the aid of a mechanical pump-oxygenator system (Gibbon type): report of eight cases. Proc Staff Meet Mayo Clin 30:201-206, 1955
16. Kirklin JW, Conti VR, Blackstone EH: Prevention of myocardial damage during cardiac operations. N Engl J Med 301:135-141, 1979
17. Barnhorst DA, Oxman HA, Connolly DC, Pluth JR, Danielson GK, Wallace RB, McGoon DC: Isolated replacement of the aortic valve with the Starr-Edwards prosthesis: a 9 year review. J Thorac Cardiovasc Surg 70:113-118, 1975
18. Rizzoli G, Blackstone EH, Kirklin JW, Pacifico AD, Bargeron LM Jr: Incremental risk factors in hospital mortality after repair of ventricular septal defect. J Thorac Cardiovasc Surg (in press)
19. Billroth T: Cited by Löwenbach G: Beitrag zur Kenntniss der Geschwülste der Submaxillar-Speicheldrüse. Virchows Arch [Pathol Anat] 150:73-111, 1897

25 Years Ago in *Proceedings*

"In a series of operations upon eight patients who had severe congenital heart disease, each with symptoms of advanced severity indicating a poor prognosis, the mechanical pump-oxygenator system adequately maintained the patients during the period of perfusion. Use of this system established excellent conditions for precise, unhurried intracardiac surgery. The foregoing facts demonstrate the usefulness of this technic in the surgical treatment of certain abnormalities of the heart and great vessels."

Kirklin JW, DuShane JW, Patrick RT, Donald DE, Hetzel PS, Harshbarger HG, Wood EH: Intracardiac surgery with the aid of a mechanical pump-oxygenator system (Gibbon type): report of eight cases. Mayo Clin Proc 30:201-206 (May 18), 1955

The Boston Medical and Surgical Journal

TABLE OF CONTENTS

June 28, 1923

Original Articles.

CARDIOTOMY AND VALVULOTOMY FOR MITRAL STENOSIS. EXPERIMENTAL OBSERVATIONS AND CLINICAL NOTES CONCERNING AN OPERATED CASE WITH RECOVERY.

BY ELLIOTT C. CUTLER, M.D., BOSTON,

AND

S. A. LEVINE, M.D., BOSTON.

[From the Surgical Clinic of the Peter Bent Brigham Hospital and the Laboratory of Surgical Research of the Harvard Medical School.]

DURING the recent decennial celebration of the former and present members of the nursing and professional staff of the Peter Bent Brigham Hospital, we presented (May 24, 1923) a case of mitral stenosis upon which we had operated four days previously in an attempt to alleviate the condition by diminishing the degree of stenosis of the valve.

It so happened that Professor Wenckebach of Vienna was visiting our clinic just at this time. The great enthusiasm and approval of the method of attack of the problem that he manifested, and the considerable discussion and general in-terest that the presentation of the case aroused, made it appear advisable to us to detail as exact a preliminary report as is possible at the present time. So far as we can determine, this is the only case on record of such a surgical attack upon a mitral stenosis being completed. Doyen[1] previously attempted a similar case, but his patient did not survive the operation.

Ever since Sir Lauder Brunton[2] in 1902 suggested the possibility of the surgical treatment of valvular disease of the heart, investigators have studied the experimental creation of valvular lesions. Papers by McCallum,[3] Cushing and Branch,[4] Bernheim,[5] Schepelmann,[6] and Carrel and Tuffier[7] from 1906 to 1914 describe fully the experimental methods in use. All of these methods were only successful in creating defective valves resulting in regurgitation. The most successful methods consisted in inserting a knife-hook (valvulotome) into the apex or down the aorta and cutting or tearing out valve cusps. Carrel and Tuffier added a new method of creating an insufficiency by the use of an endothelial transplant over the region of valves, the ring at the base of the valve then being cut, thus permitting a bulging at that point. In 1922 Allen and Graham[8] reported investigations of a similar nature with the addition that they used a cardioscope in which a small knife was carried, and by inserting the instrument *via* the left auricular appendage they were able to cut the mitral valve under direct vision.

For over two years we have sought to clear up by experimentation some of the points still left unanswered by all this work. The chief difficulty has always been to create a stenosis. Obviously until this can be produced further animal investigation will not tell us what benefits accrue when such a lesion is converted into an insufficiency. Temporary, but purely temporary, stenoses can be made by placing a thread in the ring about the base of the valves and tying it snugly. We attempted to improve on this by various methods of partial ventriculectomy, by plicating, and by plastic operations at the region of the valves. None of these methods proved successful in our hands. The experience gained, however, proved of great value, chiefly educating us in the ability of the heart muscle to stand trauma, in the methods of restoring an injured heart to renewed function, and in our ability to locate and "feel" valves in a writhing, pulsating organ.

We had reached a point where it appeared to us that further knowledge could only be gained by an attempt in an actual case, and much as we feared the difficulties, our experimental work gave us the courage to carry out what must appear as a hazardous trial. Our experimental work with the cardioscope left us with the impression that the greater intricacy of the operation and the greater amount of time consumed with this method was such that it seemed wiser to use the simpler and more speedy route through the ventricular wall with the valvulotome in the first human case.

The opportunity arrived through the interest and vision of Dr. Maurice Fremont-Smith, who asked us to see in consultation with him a child in the Good Samaritan Hospital. The history is as follows:

The patient is a girl 12 years old, whose chief complaints are dyspnea and bloody sputum. The family history is unimportant except that the father has cirrhosis of the liver. The patient had measles, mumps, chicken-pox, and whooping cough as a child, and until the age of six had frequent colds and sore throat, after which her tonsils and adenoids were removed. Also as a child she had growing pains with fever, although the mother states that she never had rheumatic fever or chorea.

Since having influenza in 1918 there has been a slight cough at intervals and some dyspnea on exertion for two years. After dancing at a festival in June, 1921, she became very dyspneic. For several months after that she was in and out of bed, but the dyspnea continued. During the following winter she went to school part of the time. She was in various hospitals for a few weeks at a time but would always develop marked dyspnea on slight effort. Severe pain in the upper back developed during September, 1922, and the dyspnea became worse.

Later the cough became troublesome and then there was a severe cough with bloody expectoration. From November, 1922, to May, 1923, she was in bed at the Good Samaritan Hospital under the care of Dr. Maurice Fremont-Smith, with whom we had the opportunity of seeing her.

During the past six months repeated attempts were made to get the patient out of bed, but each time the pulse would become rapid—120 to 140—and the dyspnea would increase. During this time there were frequent pulmonary hemorrhages. She would raise from 20 to 300 c.c. of pure bright blood at a time and would seem desperately sick, so that for a while she was on the danger list.

On May 15, when we saw her, the patient presented the following picture: She was sitting up comfortably in bed, but could not lie flat. There was slight cyanosis of the lips and no clubbing of the fingers. The general examination was not remarkable except for the chest. The pulse was small, regular, and slightly rapid. The precordial region bulged forward considerably. At the apex a distinct diastolic thrill could be felt in the fourth and fifth spaces. The apex impulse was diffuse and could be felt a finger's breadth outside the nipple line. There was definite enlargement of the heart, measuring 4.5 cm. to the right and 8.5 cm. to the left of the midsternal line. In the pulmonary area a shock could be felt synchronous with the closure of the pulmonary valve. On auscultation the heart was found to be regular—126 to the minute. There was a moderate systolic murmur at the apex and a louder rumbling diastolic murmur, filling the entire diastole and ending with a presystolic accentuation and a somewhat snapping first heart sound. Along the left sternal border and at the base a diastolic murmur was heard, but this was considered the same one as the apical murmur. The pulmonary sound was markedly accentuated. There were no signs of adherent pericardium. The cervical veins were not distended and the liver was neither tender nor palpable. There was no edema of the legs. The lungs showed a fair number of moist râles at both bases, but otherwise were not remarkable. The blood pressure was systolic 98 and diastolic 64.

The laboratory findings were as follows: the urine was slightly cloudy, acid, specific gravity 1020, no albumen, and no sugar. The sediment was negative. The hemoglobin was 85 per cent., the erythrocyte count was 4,160,000, and the white count was 8200. The stained smear was normal except for a slight achromia. Stool examination was negative.

A seven-foot x-ray plate of the heart showed a prominent left auricle and a somewhat enlarged heart. The lung findings suggested congestion. The vital capacity of the lungs was 1100 c.c. (52 per cent. of normal according to the surface area standards). The electrocardiograms showed evidence of right ventricular preponderance and exaggerated auricular waves. The ventricular complexes were otherwise normal.

In general, the picture presented was one of mitral stenosis in a child who had no cardiac reserve. She could be fairly comfortable in bed except for the repeated attacks of severe hemoptysis. It proved to be impossible to get her out of bed. Our studies indicated that the heart muscle was still in fair condition and that the stenosis was sufficient to be an important factor from a purely mechanical point of view.

Operation May 20, 1923. Morphine .008 gm. and atropin .00045 gm. were given subcutaneously at 7 A.M. At 8 A.M. the patient was brought to the operating room and another control roentgenogram taken in the cardiac bed.* At 8.25 A.M. ether was begun by the open mask method and the first stage of anesthesia quickly passed through. The child was then placed on the operating table in a semi-upright position, a catheter passed into the nasopharynx through the nose, and anesthesia continued from this time on without any difficulties by using the Connell machine. The electrocardiograph leads and blood pressure apparatus were connected up and the anterior thorax and upper abdomen prepared with alcohol and bichlorid. After a preliminary incision line had been scratched on the skin, towels, frame-cover, and sterile sheets were arranged.

At 8.45 A.M. the operation was commenced, the exposure elected being the elaboration of Milton's median sternotomy known as the Duval-Barasty median thoraco-abdominal-pericardiotomy.[9] A median incision was made over the sternum from opposite the first interspace to within two inches of the umbilicus. The ensiform was freed of muscular attachments (recti and diaphragm) and removed. Fingers of the right hand were then passed beneath the sternum and the pericardium and pleurae dissected away from it. The sternum was then split in the mid-line up to a point opposite the second intercostal space, where the gladiolus was cut across. Using slow and gentle retraction, the thorax was then opened outwards, the pleurae being swept back from the chest wall as it opened outwards by wet gauze dissection. The two halves of the sternum were held open by a Tuffier rib spreader and a perfect exposure of the pericardium obtained. The pericardium was then split up its anterior surface almost to the very base of the heart, taking care to avoid the pleurae, which nearly meet in this area. Next, the posterior pericardium and diaphragm were divided together towards the suspensory ligament, thus permitting the bottom of the

wound to open widely and exposing the entire heart to view and manipulation.

The pulse, which was 180 during the early stages of anesthesia, had dropped to 120, and the pressure had dropped from 110/50 to a systolic of 50. At times it was difficult to get any blood pressure reading whatever, and during such times the pulse was practically imperceptible. Realizing that heart muscle will stand severe trauma better if gradually initiated to its task, the heart was several times rolled out of its position with the left hand, allowing us to see more perfectly the left ventricle, which was almost completely hidden by the dilated right ventricle and huge auricles. At this point about $\frac{1}{2}$ c.c. of 1 to 1000 adrenalin solution was allowed to drip over the heart, followed by some hot salt solution. At once the heart responded by vigorous and full contractions. This moment was seized as our most propitious one, and rolling the heart out and to the right by the left hand, the valvulotome, an instrument somewhat similar to a tenotome or a slightly curved tonsil knife, and the one with which we were most familiar in our experimental work, was taken in the right hand and plunged into the left ventricle at a point about one inch from the apex and away from the branches of the descended coronary artery, where two mattress sutures had already been placed. The knife was pushed upwards about $2\frac{1}{2}$ inches, until it encountered what seemed to us must be the mitral orifice. It was then turned mesially, and a cut made in what we thought was the aortic leaflet, the resistance encountered being very considerable. The knife was quickly turned and a cut made in the opposite side of the opening. The knife was then withdrawn and the mattress sutures already in place were tied over the point at which the knife had been inserted. There was absolutely no bleeding. Hot saline was dripped onto the heart, whose action continued good. A sterile stethoscope placed on the heart yielded such a confusion of sounds that no reliance could be placed on the information obtained. We would have liked to repeat our manipulation, but felt the risk too great.

The closure was simple. The posterior pericardium and diaphragm were closed by a continuous suture of silk, next the small opening in the abdomen in a similar fashion, and the anterior pericardium likewise. No opening had been made in the pleurae and there had been no respiratory disturbance throughout the procedure. The divided sternum was allowed to come together, and after being held tightly by an encircling silver wire suture, the periosteum on either side of the divided bone, both at the horizontal and vertical divisions, was approximated by multiple interrupted sutures of fine silk. Fine silk sutures were used to close the subcutaneous tissue and skin. A simple gauze dressing with fairly tight towel swathe was then applied.

*A bed was devised by Dr. Burgess Gordon, of the Peter Bent Brigham Hospital, having a canvas back in which a patient could be radiographed and x-ray plates could be taken at a distance of six feet without moving the patient. This permits of frequent observations in sick patients without disturbing them.

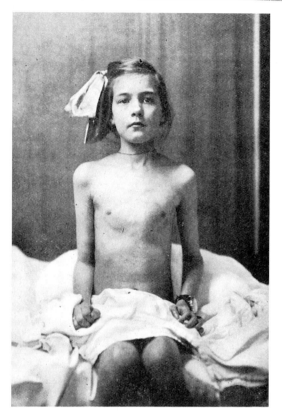

Photograph May 19, 1923.
(Operation May 20, 1923.)

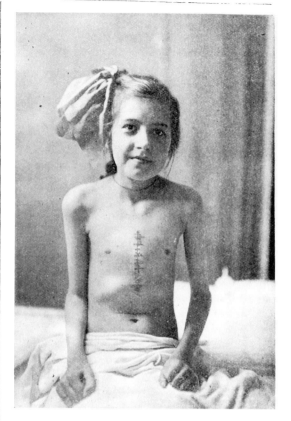

Photograph May 21, 1923.
(Eleven days after operation.)

The operation was over by 10 A.M. At this time the pulse was 140, respiration 40, and blood pressure, 80 systolic, 40 diastolic. The general condition seemed good. Immediate x-ray studies were made and the patient placed in bed.

The patient became conscious in less than an hour, and at once began to complain of severe sternal pain with respiration. It was necessary to control this by the liberal use of morphin for 48 hours. The pulse ranged around 130, the respirations around 25 for the first 24 hours, and the systolic pressure remained close to 90 most of the time. The day following operation the temperature rose to 101, the pulse to 140, and respirations to 45, and the patient showed all the signs of a postoperative pulmonary complication of the right upper lobe of a type repeatedly described by one of us.[10] In view of the severity of this complication, the outlook at this stage looked very dubious, but the child responded well to digitalis and oxygen therapy, and was greatly helped and comforted by her faith in and affection for her nurses, on whom the chief burden fell. Towards the end of her third postoperative day, the temperature and pulse and respiratory rates fell, the signs in the right apex rapidly cleared except for some sticky râles, and after a comfortable night the patient seemed in as good general condition as before operation.

Indeed, we felt so sanguine of her ultimate recovery that she was brought down to the large amphitheater and presented before the reunion group of doctors and nurses the fourth day after operation (May 24, 1923). From this time on her recovery was rapid, as it is in most children once the period of convalescence becomes well established. Her appetite, spirits, strength, and general condition responded marvelously. Seven days after operation the sutures and all dressings were removed. The wound was perfectly healed, but there remained an extraordinary bulging of the precordia and the region underlying the sternum. (See photographs before and after operation.)

Accurate observations on the heart sounds were not possible during the first four or five days because of the dressings, and because the critical condition of the patient did not seem to justify any prolonged examination. Later on, however, careful study of the heart findings was made. The diastolic thrill and diastolic murmur were distinctly diminished in intensity at the apex, and the apical systolic murmur was increased. A pericardial to and fro friction developed, which was best heard at the third right interspace near the sternum. This has gradually grown fainter. It is not at all unlikely that a pericardial effusion was also present. It did not seem wise to tap the pericar-

Volume 188
Number 26 MITRAL STENOSIS—CUTLER AND LEVINE 1027

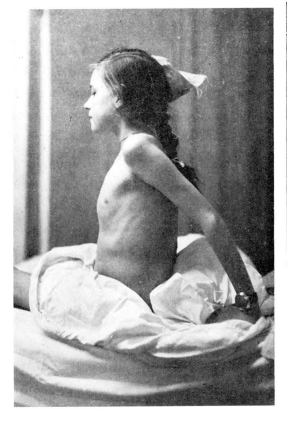

Photograph May 19, 1923.
(Operation May 20, 1923.)

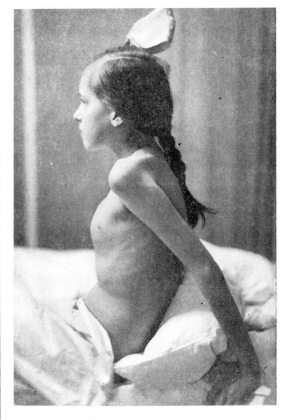

Photograph May 31, 1923.
(Eleven days after operation.)

dium for diagnosis as the patient was doing so well. The diminution of the diastolic murmur and thrill might be accounted for by the pericardial effusion, but then the increased intensity of the systolic murmur would have to be due to greater insufficiency of the mitral valve resulting from the operation.

At this stage of our observations we cannot with accuracy define just what has occurred nor what benefits may have accrued, if any. It is true that we do not feel very sanguine about the latter, although, should any improvement occur in the patient's vital capacity, that might be taken as a definite indication that some alleviation of the stenosis had resulted. The experience with this case, however, is of importance in that it does show that surgical intervention in cases of mitral stenosis bears no special risk, and should give us further courage and support in our desire to attempt to alleviate a chronic condition, for which there is now not only no treatment, but one which carries a terrible prognosis. Unquestionably further attempts will be made, and our own experience in this instance has shown us technical improvements that should render a subsequent attempt both less hazardous as well as more hopeful for success.

Summary.—A human case of mitral stenosis was operated upon with recovery. The method of attack used was one evolved after years of laboratory investigation concerning the surgery of the heart.

REFERENCES.

1 Tuffier, T.: La Chirurgie du Coeur. Cinquieme Congres de la Soc. Int. de Chirurgie, Paris, 19-23 juillet, 1920, Rapports, Proces-verbaux et Discussions publies par le Docteur L. Mayer, Brussels, M. Hayez, 1921, 5-75.

2 Brunton, Sir Lauder: Preliminary Note on the Possibility of Treating Mitral Stenosis by Surgical Methods. The Lancet, 1902, 1, 352.

3 MacCallum, W. G.: On the Teaching of Pathological Physiology. Johns Hopkins Hosp. Bull., 1906, xvii, 251-254.

4 Cushing, H., and Branch, J. R. B.: Experimental and Clinical Notes on Chronic Valvular Lesions in the Dog and Their Possible Relation to a Future Surgery of the Cardiac Valves. Jour. Med. Res., 1907-8, xii, 471-486.

5 Bernheim, B. M.: Experimental Surgery of the Mitral Valve. Johns Hopkins Hosp. Bull., 1909, xx, April, No. 217.

6 Schepelmann, E.: Herz Klappen Chirurgie. Experimentelle Untersuchungen. Deutsche Ztschr. f. Chir., Leipz., 1912-13, cxx, 502-579.
—Zur Chirurgie des Segel Klappenstenose des Herzens. Munchen. med. Wchnschr., 1913, lx, 47.
—Versuche zur Herz-chirurgie. Archiv. f. klin. Chir., Berlin, 1912, xcvii, 739-751.

7 Tuffier, T., and Carrel, A.: Patching and Section of the Pulmonary Orifice of the Heart. Jour. Exp. Med., 1914, xx, No. 1, 3-8.
Etude Anatomopathologique et Experimentale sur la Chirurgie des Orifices du Coeur. Presse Méd., Paris, 1914, xxii, 173-177.

8 Allen, D. S., and Graham, E. A.: Intracardiac Surgery. A New Method. Jour. Am. Med. Assn., 1922, 79, 1028-1030.

9 Keen, W. W.: Surgery. Philadelphia and London, W. B. Saunders Co., 1921, vii, 725-728.

10 Cutler, E. C., and Hunt, A. M.: Postoperative Pulmonary Complications. Arch. Surg., 1920, 1, 114.
Cutler, E. C., and Hunt, A. M.: Postoperative Pulmonary Complications. Arch. Int. Med., 1922, xxix, 449.
Cutler, E. C.: The Etiology of Postoperative Pulmonary Complications. Surgical Clinics of North America, 1922, 11, 935.

THE SURGICAL TREATMENT OF MITRAL STENOSIS.

BY

H. S. SOUTTAR, C.B.E., M.CH., F.R.C.S.,

SURGEON (WITH CARE OF OUT-PATIENTS), LONDON HOSPITAL.

THERE can be no more fascinating problem in surgery than the relief of pathological conditions of the valves of the heart. Despite the consecutive changes to which these lesions may have given rise in the cardiac muscle, the relief of the lesions themselves would undoubtedly be of immense service to the patient and must be followed by marked improvement in his general condition. Expressed in these terms, the problem is to a large extent mechanical, and as such should already be within the scope of surgery, were it not for the extraordinary nature of the conditions under which the problem must be attacked. We are, however, of opinion that these conditions again are purely mechanical, and that apart from them the heart is as amenable to surgical treatment as any other organ. Incisions can be made into its chambers, portions of its structure can be excised, and internal manipulations can be carried out, without the slightest interference with its action, and there is ample evidence that wounds of the heart heal as readily as those in any other region.

The conditions which appear as fundamental are, first, that the operations have to be carried out on a structure in rapid movement; and secondly, that no interference whatever with the circulation must take place. The first is not quite so difficult as it sounds, for it is possible to fix the actual portion of the heart which is under operation, but it must obviously limit the possibilities of repair. In animals the second condition may sometimes be ignored, and the circulation has been clamped for as much as two minutes. This, however, would never be justifiable in a human being, in view of the extreme danger to the brain from even the shortest check to its blood supply. Any manipulations which are carried out must therefore be executed in the full flow of the blood stream, and they must not perceptibly interfere with the contractions of the heart.

The simplest valvular lesion for surgical interference is stenosis of one of the valves, and of these the mitral valve is perhaps the most accessible. I have been interested for some time in the development of a suitable technique for reaching this valve, and I owe to Dr. Otto Leyton the opportunity presented by the following case for putting my ideas to the test. A description of the case itself will give the clearest indication of the method of approach I adopted and of the technique which I devised.

Description of Case.

L. H., aged 15, was admitted to the London Hospital in January, 1921, suffering from chorea and mitral stenosis. Her subsequent history was one of many relapses, with steadily increasing failure of compensation. In September, 1924, she was admitted with haemoptysis, vomiting, and severe dyspnoea. She was cyanosed, her feet were swollen, and her liver was enlarged and tender. After three weeks in hospital she had greatly improved and was sent to a convalescent home, whence three weeks later she was discharged.

Early in March, 1925, she appeared at the London Hospital with cough, dyspnoea, and pain in the limbs. She was sent home to bed and given digitalis and aspirin, but she did not improve. After a severe attack of epistaxis and precordial pain she was again admitted as an in-patient.

She was a thin girl with a bright malar flush. Her pulse rate was 128, and respirations 32. Cardiac pulsation was visible over a large area of the left chest, and the rib cartilages in this area were very soft and had a forward bulge. The apex beat was in the fifth space, outside the mid-clavicular line, and the area of cardiac dullness extended to the second space above. In the mitral area there was a long rumbling diastolic murmur, followed by a soft blowing systolic murmur, the latter being conducted out into the axilla. A presystolic murmur was present, but was not very marked. The liver was not obviously enlarged, but was slightly tender on palpation.

After a week's rest in bed her pulse fell to 80 and her respirations to 24, while her general condition greatly improved. Her pulse was now small but perfectly regular, with a systolic pressure of 95 mm. There was no presystolic murmur or thrill, but a long diastolic murmur of low pitch was followed by a soft blowing systolic murmur.

In view of her many relapses it appeared that her heart was unable to establish compensation for the combined stenosis and regurgitation from which she suffered, and it was therefore decided to attempt to relieve the stenosis by surgical means.

Operation.

On May 6th, 1925, under intratracheal anaesthesia, a curved incision was made along the fourth left intercostal space, up along the middle of the sternum, and outwards along the first left intercostal space. The skin and subcutaneous tissues, with the left breast, were turned outwards, exposing an area of the chest wall about five inches square. On the outer side of this area a short horizontal incision was made along each of the three ribs exposed (Fig. 1), and through these incisions the ribs

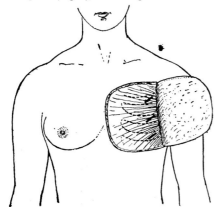

Fig. 1.—Skin and subcutaneous tissue reflected, with ribs exposed prior to division.

were in turn divided. The chest wall was now divided a little within the line of the original incision by cutting through the muscles and costal cartilages, and the flap so formed was turned outwards, the pleura being included in the flap (Fig. 2).

A very full exposure of the left side of the pericardium was thus obtained, while with an intratracheal pressure of 15 mm. Hg there was only moderate collapse of the left lung. The action of the heart now became extremely hurried, the pulse rising to 150, and it was evident that until it settled down nothing further could be attempted. After five minutes' delay the beats became slower and steadier, and it was decided that we could safely proceed. The pericardium was opened by a vertical incision three inches long, in the centre of which the left auricular appendage came prominently forward (Fig. 3). Two sutures were passed through the upper and lower margins of the appendage, so that it could be readily drawn forward. As the heart was still beating very rapidly the wound was covered with hot saline pads and a subcutaneous injection of 1/100 grain of strophanthin was given. After a delay of ten minutes the heart had steadied down to a rate of 120, and the blood pressure, which had fallen to 60 mm., had returned to 80 mm.

The auricular appendage was now drawn forward, a soft curved clamp (Fig. 4) was applied to its base, and it was

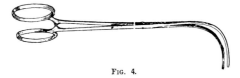

Fig. 4.

incised in an antero-posterior direction with scissors (Fig. 5). Into this opening the left forefinger was inserted (Fig. 6), the

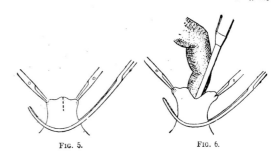

Fig. 5.   Fig. 6.

clamp was withdrawn, and the appendage was drawn over the finger like a glove by means of the sutures. The whole of the inside of the left auricle could now be explored with facility. It was immediately evident from the rush of blood against the finger that gross regurgitation was taking place, but there was not so much thickening of the valves as had been expected. The finger was passed into the ventricle through the orifice of the mitral valve without encountering resistance, and the cusps of the valve could be easily felt and their condition estimated.

The finger was kept in the auricle for perhaps two minutes, and during that time, so long as it remained in the auricle, it appeared to produce no effect upon the heart beat or the pulse. The moment, however, that it passed into the orifice of the mitral valve the blood pressure fell to zero, although even then no change in the cardiac rhythm could be detected. The blood stream was simply cut off by the finger, which presumably just fitted the stenosed orifice. As, however, the stenosis was of such moderate degree, and was accompanied by so little thickening of the valves, it was decided not to carry out the valve section which had been arranged, but to limit intervention to such dilatation as could be carried out by the finger. It was felt that an actual section of the valve might only make matters worse by increasing the degree of regurgitation, while the breaking down of adhesions by the finger might improve the condition as regards both regurgitation and stenosis.

It was now decided to withdraw the finger and close the appendage. Unfortunately, at the critical moment of withdrawal the lower retaining suture cut through, the appendage slipped back into the pericardium, and there was a sudden gush of blood, which, however, was instantly checked by pressing the appendage against the heart. With a little manipulation the tip of the appendage was now grasped between the finger and thumb, which held it securely closed while an assistant passed a silk ligature round it and tied it off. The pericardium was closed, and a certain amount of blood, which in this *contretemps* had escaped into the pleural cavity, was removed with moist gauze pads. The intratracheal pressure was raised so as to cause the left lung to expand, and the wound was closed in layers, the ribs being accurately sutured in position. Before the flap was actually closed a small quantity of 60 per cent. alcohol was injected into the intercostal nerves just outside the point at which the ribs had been divided.

Immediately the chest was closed the heart's action returned to normal, and on the conclusion of the operation the general condition of the patient was indistinguishable from that at the beginning. She had a bright colour and an excellent pulse. Except at the moment when the suture cut out her condition had never caused the slightest anxiety, and even then there was only a momentary drop in the blood pressure. The whole operation took precisely sixty minutes.

She made an uninterrupted recovery, the freedom from pain or any disturbance which might have been expected to result from the operation being remarkable. Her general condition appeared to be greatly improved, but the physical signs showed little or no change. She was sent to the country and kept in bed for six weeks, but as at the end of that time her pulse rate had remained constant at about 90 she was gradually

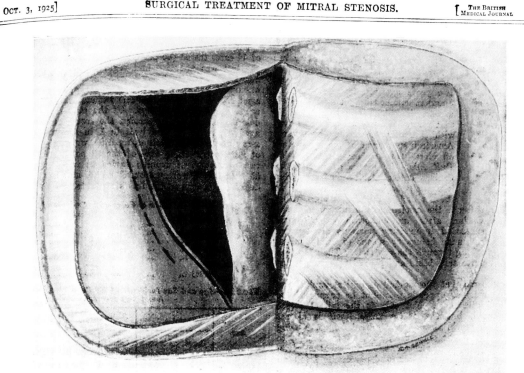

FIG. 2.—Ribs divided, and flap, formed by cutting through muscles and costal cartilages, turned back; left side of pericardium exposed.

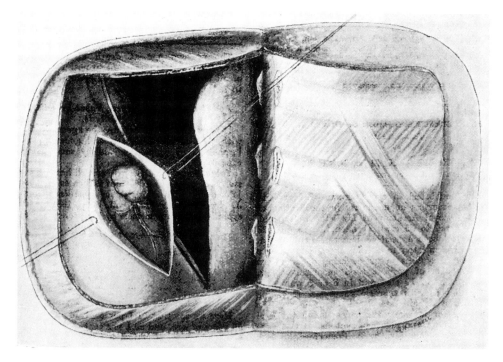

FIG. 3.—Vertical incision in pericardium, exposing left auricular appendage.

allowed to get up. At the end of three months she declared that she felt perfectly well, although she still became somewhat breathless on exertion.

REMARKS.

I believe that this is the first occasion upon which an attempt has been made to reach the mitral valve by this route in the human being, or to subject the interior of the heart to digital examination. The value of the method cannot possibly be judged on a single case, but I think that I may claim to have shown that the method is practicable and that it is reasonably safe. Indeed, the features which most struck all who were present at the operation were the facility and the absolute safety of the whole procedure, while even on a first attempt the amount and precision of the information to be gained by digital exploration were very remarkable. I had intended to divide the aortic cusp by passing a thin hernia bistoury along my finger (Fig. **7**) and thus to relieve the stenosis, and this could have been done with perfect facility had it been considered advisable.

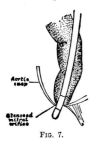

FIG. 7.

The problem of cardiac surgery has frequently attracted the attention of both physicians and surgeons, and two years ago the BRITISH MEDICAL JOURNAL summed up, in an admirable article, its history and position at that time. It is now being attacked with characteristic energy by several American surgeons from various points of view. On the experimental side Duff Allen, by means of a most ingenious optical device, has succeeded in actually seeing the mitral valve in the cat and in dividing a cusp, using the approach through the auricular appendage. On the clinical side Cutler, after an elaborate experimental investigation, succeeded in excising portions of stenosed mitral valves in human beings by means of an ingenious valvulotome, working through the ventricle. The operation was, however, necessarily blind and proved to be somewhat dangerous.

It appears to me that the method of digital exploration through the auricular appendage cannot be surpassed for simplicity and directness. Not only is the mitral orifice directly to hand, but the aortic valve itself is almost certainly within reach, through the mitral orifice. Owing to the simplicity of the structures, and, oddly enough, to their constant and regular movement, the information given by the finger is exceedingly clear, and personally I felt an appreciation of the mechanical reality of stenosis and regurgitation which I never before possessed. To hear a murmur is a very different matter from feeling the blood itself pouring back over one's finger. I could not help being impressed by the mechanical nature of these lesions and by the practicability of their surgical relief.

BIBLIOGRAPHY.

Allen, D. S.: Intracardiac Surgery, *Arch. Surg.*, 1924, viii, 317.

Cutler, E. C., Levine, S. A., and Beck, C. S.: The Surgical Treatment of Mitral Stenosis, *Arch. Surg.*, 1924, ix, 689.

BRITISH MEDICAL JOURNAL (leading article), September 22nd, 1923, p. 530.

Mitral Replacement: *

Clinical Experience with a Ball-Valve Prosthesis

ALBERT STARR, M.D., M. LOWELL EDWARDS, B.S.

*From the Department of Surgery and Division of Thoracic Surgery,
University of Oregon Medical School, Portland, Oregon*

THE MORBID ANATOMY of rheumatic mitral disease is such that in many instances nothing short of excision and replacement will allow adequate relief of the hemodynamic abnormality. Experience with eight such patients in whom mitral replacement has been performed with a ball-valve prosthesis forms the basis of this report.

Considerable work has been performed by other investigators in the development of a total mitral prosthesis for the dog and experience with human mitral replacement prior to our own attempts have been recorded. In the animal laboratory these studies have included the testing of flap valves of various materials,[3, 6, 9] ball valves,[3] sleeve valves without chordae,[11] flexible sleeve or leaflet valve with chordae,[1, 5, 7, 8] homologous aortic valve,[7] and autogenous pulmonary valves.[12] Problems of fixation, valve function and thrombotic occlusion of the prosthesis have prevented long-term survival in most instances. Human mitral resection and replacement has been reported by Kay,[8] Braunwald,[2] Lillehei,[10] Ellis.[4] While early satisfactory results were obtained in some patients, survival beyond three months has not been reported to now.

Prosthesis

The experience of this laboratory with mitral replacement in the dog reported elsewhere [14, 15] led to the development of the ball valve prosthesis shown in Figure 1 from which all subsequent valves in this

series have evolved. Firm and lasting fixation has been achieved by the use of interrupted sutures placed through the mitral annulus and through a knitted Teflon cloth ring to which the prosthesis is attached as shown in Figure 2. Satisfactory hydraulic function in the dog was demonstrated by left atrial pressure tracings immediately following implantation (Fig. 3) and by postoperative cardiac catheterization, angiocardiography, and cine-angiocardiography performed from two to 12 months following implantation. Some of the valves in the long-term survivor group have radio-opaque balls or steel pins inserted into the balls so that valve function and ball spin have been observed with fluoroscopy.

The prosthesis currently employed in the human and the relative dimensions of the two sizes are pictured in Figure 4. A cutaway drawing of the construction is depicted in Figure 5. The case is cast in one piece stainless steel or Stellite 21 and the final dimensions are achieved from the crude castings by machining or grinding. A mirror finish is produced by buffing and electro-polishing. The surface is then silicone coated and carefully inspected. Unless flawless with regard to minor imperfections or irregularities of surface the valve is rejected from further assembly. The knitted Teflon cloth fixation ring is attached by Teflon spreader rings and braided Teflon thread. The ball is of Dow-Corning medical grade heat-cured silastic.

Prior to insertion the valve is cleaned in detergent and autoclaved. Since the initiation of clinical use of the valve minor changes in material and geometry have

* Presented before the American Surgical Association, Boca Raton, Florida, March 21–23, 1961.

This work is supported in part by a grant-in-aid from the Oregon Heart Association.

726

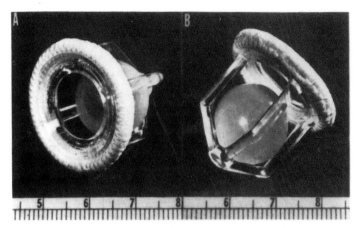

FIG. 1. The Lucite caged ball valve used in the first long-term dog survivor in this laboratory. A. View of inlet side; B. View of outlet side.

been made. The cages used for Patients 1 and 2 were of Lucite. A change to a metallic cage in subsequent cases allowed a reduction in the external dimensions of the valve with no loss of internal dimension or sacrifice of strength. The fixation device binding the Teflon cloth to the valve in Patients 1–7 consisted of stainless steel spreader rings and stainless steel wire. While all metals used were of the same formulation it was believed prudent to avoid the use of multiple metallic parts for fear of electrolytic corrosion. Subsequent valves have therefore been made with Teflon spreader rings and Teflon thread. The struts of the cage angulated in cases 1–7 was changed to a gentle curve in the current valve. This increases the surface area of contact between the ball and cage in the open position and reduces wear.

While the laboratory demonstration of firm and lasting fixation, satisfactory hydraulic function, and long-term survival is important in the evaluation of a proposed valve substitute there will remain uncertainty regarding the long-term wearing ability of a prosthesis. Extracorporeal accelerated fatigue testing is therefore mandatory prior to clinical use. The mitral ball valve lends itself well to such study since the end point of the test is not the demonstration of total disruption of the valve but easily detectable changes of the size, shape and weight of the silastic ball. Using the

accelerated fatigue test pump developed in this laboratory the valve has been opened and closed at 6,000 cycles per minute at a closing pressure of 150 mm. Hg with the ball so restrained that closure is not a random event in regard to ball surface but is

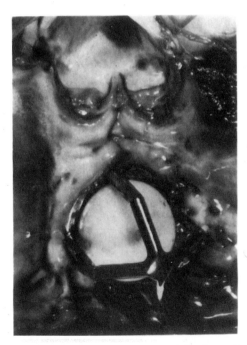

FIG. 2. Left ventricular aspect of dog heart 39 days following mitral replacement with the stainless steel cage barium impregnated silastic ball valve. The Teflon cloth margins are endothelialized and are firmly anchored to the annulas by fibrous ingrowth. The aortic root is demonstrated and the aortic valve remains undistorted.

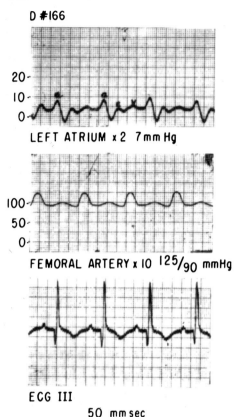

D #166

20-
10-
0-

LEFT ATRIUM x 2 7mm Hg

100-
50-
0-

FEMORAL ARTERY x 10 125/90 mmHg

ECG III

50 mm sec

Fig. 3. Operating room pressures following mitral replacement in the dog with the Lucite valve shown in Figure 1. Left atrial pressure tracing is normal both in magnitude and configuration as shown above.

confined to the same area with each cycle. Three weeks of testing in this manner revealed no change in ball dimension, shape, or weight. The proper interpretation of the extracorporeal test must be tentative and cautious. However, assuming a normal pulse of 80 per minute and similar closing pressures *in vivo* the acceleration is 75-fold. Since the area taking part in the closure is one-tenth of the ball surface area the prevention of ball spin and random closure accelerates the test an additional 10-fold. The total minimal acceleration is therefore 750-fold and at this rate the ball has received the mechanical equivalent of approximately 43 years *in vivo*.

Clinical Material

The mitral ball valve prosthesis was considered available for initial trial in July 1960, and by February 1961, eight patients had undergone resection and replacement therapy for rheumatic mitral disease. Pertinent data concerning this group are presented in Table 1. All patients were seriously incapacitated and were taking digitalis and diuretics. Five patients were in chronic congestive failure despite strict medical therapy in the hospital and were functional Class IV. Most of the patients had severe cachexia with marked weight loss and muscle wasting. Patients 1 and 2 had a history of previously closed commissurotomy and in Patient 1 this was followed by an unsuccessful open procedure for mixed stenosis and insufficiency. Atrial fibrillation was present in all cases.

The usual murmurs of mitral disease were present at the apex and five patients had early diastolic murmurs at the base

TABLE I. *Human Mitral Replacement*

Pt. No.	Age	Sex	Classification Anat.	Funct.	Date Surgery	Perfusion Time (min.)	Assoc. AI	Results	Comment
1	33	F	Pure MI	IV	8/25/60	108	None	Died	Air embolism 10 hrs. postop.
2	52	M	MS, MI	IV	9/21/60	112	None	Alive	At work as truck dispatcher
3	28	F	Pure MI	IV	10/27/60	89	None	Alive	At work—graduate student
4	45	M	Pure MS	IV	11/ 2/60	151	None	Died	Renal shutdown—11th day
5	32	F	Pure MI	III	1/12/61	58	Slight	Alive	Discharged 4th wk.
6	42	F	Pure MI	III	1/19/61	60	None	Alive	Discharged 3rd wk.
7	41	F	MS, MI	IV	1/26/61	61	None	Alive	Staph. endocarditis—under treatment
8	44	M	MS, MI	III	2/22/61	71	Slight	Alive	No complications

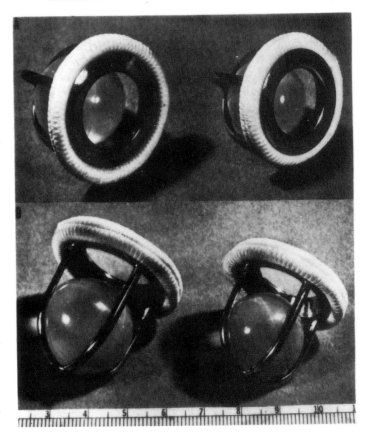

FIG. 4. The mitral ball valve prosthesis for human implantation. A. View of inlet side; B. View of outlet side.

suggesting aortic or pulmonic insufficiency. Left heart visualization by percutaneous retrograde femoral artery catheterization with injection of contrast agent above and below the aortic valve was performed on all potential candidates for open mitral surgery. Slight regurgitation of contrast agent into the left ventricle following supravalvular injection was demonstrated in one patient and this was correctly considered preoperatively to be injection artifact. Two patients with no evidence of aortic insufficiency on x-ray had slight regurgitation at operation. However, angiocardiography of this type was effective in screening patients preoperatively for subclinical aortic insufficiency of sufficient severity to require aortic cross clamping to maintain operative exposure.

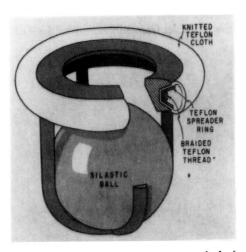

FIG. 5. Cut-away drawing showing method of fixation of Teflon cloth to the metallic cage by spreader ring and Teflon thread.

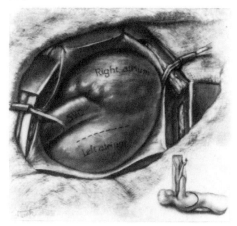

FIG. 6. Operative exposure employed in mitral valve replacement.

All patients had preoperative right heart catheterization demonstrating low cardiac output, pulmonary hypertension, and left atrial hypertension. The data obtained from studies in Patients 2 and 3 whose postoperative catheterization results are available for comparison are presented in Table 2.

Operative Technics

With the patient in the full lateral position exposure is obtained through the entire right fifth intercostal space (Fig. 6). The pericardium is opened anterior to the phrenic nerve. No attempt is made to free the ventricles from adhesions resulting from

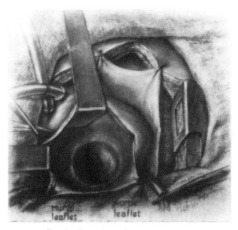

FIG. 7. After total cardiopulmonary bypass has been established the valve is exposed as shown.

previous surgery or pericarditis. The margins of the pericardial incisions are sutured to the drapes to produce a stable operative field and pressures are recorded by needle puncture of the left atrium and pulmonary artery. The cavae are surrounded by tapes. Cannulation is performed in the usual manner using the right common femoral artery or external iliac artery for inflow.

Cardiopulmonary bypass is performed as previously described at a flow of 2.5 l./meter^2/body surface/min. which in most instances is reduced to 1.8 l./meter^2/body surface/min. as mild hypothermia to 32° C. is produced.[13] A direct approach via the left atrial wall is preferred and was performed in all instances except Patients 2 and 4, in whom the left atrium was considerably smaller and less accessible than the right atrium. Under these circumstances the transseptal approach provides satisfactory exposure. The left atrium is opened as shown in Figure 7 and the mitral valve exposed. Once the atrium is emptied of blood care is taken to keep the mitral valve incompetent so that foam is not expelled into the aorta. Further protection against air embolus is achieved by flooding the operative field with carbon dioxide. The valvular pathology may be so extensive that resection consists of piecemeal debridement of the mitral annulus.

If the pathology permits, removal of the valve *in toto* saves considerable time. The shorter perfusion time shown in Table 1 in the later cases resulted from adherence to this principle when possible. The attached margin of the aortic leaflet is usually sufficiently flexible so that its junction with the aortic root is clearly discernible. Under these circumstances resection is started by incising this leaflet near the attached margin with no fear of aortic injury, and this incision is continued around the annulus leaving a margin of 3.0 to 4.0 mm. of valve tissue in place (Fig. 8A). On the aortic side this allows the placement of sutures without aortic valve injury and around the remainder of the annulus the residual margin of valve leaflet serves as a marker for he placement of sutures and provides ough fibrous material that will facilitate irm anchoring of the prosthesis without too leep a bite into the myocardium. With traction upward on the divided valve the papillary muscles are cut and the valve removed. Removal of papillary muscle is not necessary to provide room for the prosthesis so that if adhesions of the papillary muscles to the ventricular wall are present the chordae are divided individually.

In the extensively calcified valve the junction of leaflet with annulus is not clear and it is therefore safer to achieve mobility of the valve prior to resection by dividing the chordae tendineae first (Fig. 8B). The motion of the leaflet thereby achieved allows clear definition of the junction of the valve with annulus and division of the attached margins can follow with safety.

Following resection and inspection of the left ventricle for loose debris one of the two sizes of prostheses is selected and placed in the annulus for a direct fitting. The margins of the Teflon cloth ring must fit easily into the valve orifice and it is best to err on the side of the smaller prosthesis when in doubt. The selected valve is then removed from the heart and 0-silk sutures are placed through the mitral annulus and the cloth margin of the prosthesis. To avoid confusion these are placed through the anterior and posterior commissure first and the remaining sutures inserted one quadrant at a time, using three to four sutures within each quadrant (Fig. 9). The sutures are kept from entangling by placement on a flexible spring. Sixteen to 20 sutures are required for firm fixation and when all are in place the prosthesis is slid down into the annulus and these are tied and cut. The valve is kept incompetent to avoid air embolism by passing a blunt forceps through the prosthesis. The left atrium is then allowed to fill with blood and the atriotomy partially closed. The rewarmed patient is removed from cardiopulmonary bypass, the forceps producing valvular incompetence removed and the remaining atriotomy closed with a partially occluding clamp. This clamp is

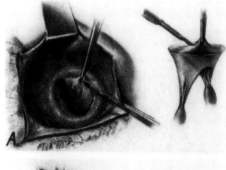

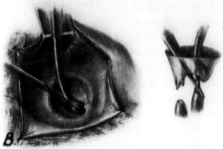

FIG. 8. A. Method of excision initiated by incising aortic leaflet near attached margin. B. Alternate method of excision initiated by dividing chordae tendineae.

opened once or twice to flush the atrium of air after bypass has been completed. The right superior pulmonary vein is checked for air by needle aspiration and decannulation is effected in the usual manner.

Operative Findings

There was considerable variation in the extent of calcification, loss of surface area, subvalvular contractures, and commissural fusion of the mitral valve found in surgery. The specimens shown in Figures 10–12 were amenable to total removal rather than piece-meal debridement and hence represent the least damaged valves resected. The operative findings are described below for each patient.

Patient 1. The pathology at the time of mitral commissurotomy in 1953 is not known. At the time of open mitral surgery in March 1960 the mitral annulus was found to be small and the anterior commissure fused for a distance of 3–4 mm. The mural leaflet was rolled under and functionless. The aortic leaflet was flexible and free of calcification and seemed adequate in surface area. The fused commissure was divided and a single

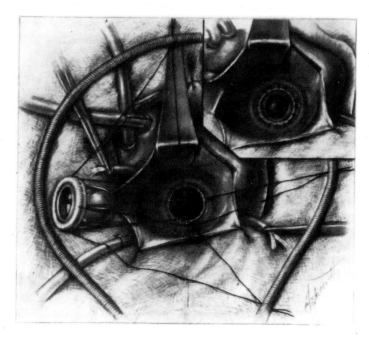

FIG. 9. Method of placement of silk sutures. Insert shows valve in place.

leaflet replacement with a roll of compressed Ivalon sponge was sutured into place. Mitral replacement was performed on August 25, 1960, because of persistent congestive failure with repeated bouts of pulmonary edema due to overwhelming mitral insufficiency. The Ivalon leaflet had not undergone any change in size and was free of thrombus material. The sutures anchoring this leaflet were divided and the leaflet easily removed. During the resection of the mitral valve the extent of subvalvular shortening was greater

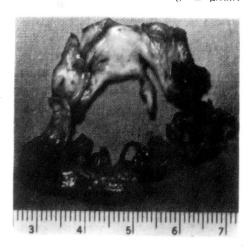

FIG. 10. Operative specimen from Patient 5 with pure mitral insufficiency. There is marked loss of surface area and chordal shortening.

than was anticipated at the time of previous surgery. The posterior papillary muscle was adherent to the left ventricular wall and the posterior aspect of the aortic leaflet was pulled down to this by shortened chordae.

Patient 2. At the time of mitral commissurotomy in 1956 complete calcification of the mitral valve was found and fracture of the posterior medial commissure was not possible. Mitral replacement was performed on September 21, 1960 with a preoperative diagnosis of predominant stenosis with insufficiency. The mural leaflet was completely destroyed by fibrosis and calcification. The aortic leaflet was massively calcified, and thickened to 1.0 cm. at its free margin. The posterior papillary muscle was adherent to the ventricular wall and the chordal support of the aortic leaflet was shortened and thickened. A fixed orifice of 3–4 mm. was present.

Patient 3. Mitral replacement was performed on October 27, 1960 with a preoperative diagnosis of pure mitral insufficiency. The mitral valve ring was slightly dilated to about three fingers. The mural leaflet was completely rolled under and functionless. The anterior leaflet was free of calcification, flexible, and decreased in surface area posteriorly. The free margin of the aortic leaflet was thickened to 3–4 mm. and pulled downward by chordal shortening especially posteriorly. Annuloplasty was performed narrowing the orifice to two finger breadths but persistent severe regurgitation required that a resection procedure be done.

Patient 4. Mitral resection and replacement vas performed on November 2, 1960, with a preperative diagnosis of calcification of the atrial vall, mural thrombus, and severe mitral stenosis. soft thrombus material was present over the entire atrium and extended into the orifices of the pulmonary veins. The entire left atrial wall with the exception of the septum was calcified. The valve orifice was 3–4 mm. in diameter and regurgitation was not evident. The mural leaflet was markedly retracted and thickened. The aortic leaflet was flexible along its attached margins but calcified and thickened to 5.0 mm. along the free margin. Leaflets were contracted to about half normal surface area; severe subvalvular contracture was evident.

Patient 5. Mitral valve replacement was performed on January 12, 1961 with a preoperative diagnosis of pure mitral insufficiency. The mitral annulus was of normal size and there was no fusion of the commissures. Calcification was not present.

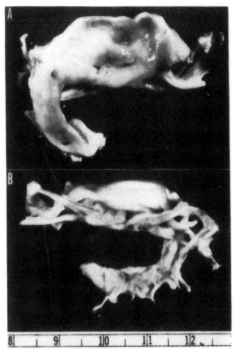

FIG. 12. Operative specimen from Patient 8 with predominant mitral insufficiency. A. View from atrial aspect; B. View from ventricular aspect.

Flexibility was maintained but there was marked loss of substance of both leaflets. The anterior leaflet was rolled under, especially posteriorly and pulled downward into the left ventricle by extreme chordal shortening (Fig. 10).

Patient 6. Mitral replacement was performed on January 19, 1961 with a preoperative diagnosis of pure mitral insufficiency. The mitral annulus was of normal size and the mural cusp was deficient in surface area and held tightly against the ventricular wall. The aortic leaflet was flexible and there was no evidence of fusion of the commissures. Posteriorly the aortic leaflet was markedly deficient in surface area; in addition, chordae attaching to the free margin of this leaflet were shortened resulting in marked limitation of mobility.

Patient 7. Mitral replacement was performed on January 26, 1961 with a preoperative diagnosis of calcific mitral stenosis and insufficiency. There was no dilatation of the mitral annulus. The valve orifice was 10–12 mm. in diameter and there was fusion of both commissures. Severe calcification was present in both leaflets and this was especially heavy posteriorly where blocks of calcium crossed the zone of commissural fusion. There was marked loss of surface area of the leaflet and extreme shortening of the chordae tendineae (Fig. 11).

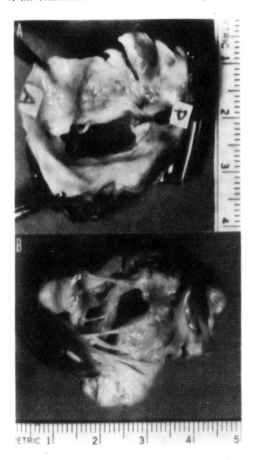

FIG. 11. Operative specimen from Patient 7 with calcific stenosis and insufficiency. A. View from atrial aspect; B. View from ventricular aspect.

TABLE 2. *Right Heart Catheterization Before and After Human Mitral Valve Replacement*

Pt. No.	Time of Study		RA	PA			Wedge		Index c/Meter²/ min.	O₂ Cons. cc./min.
				S	D	M	M	V		
2	Pre-op	Rest*	7	60	36	42	28	3	2.6	300
	Post-op (15 wks)	Rest	5	36	17	22	12	—	1.9	236
		Exercise	—	54	20	36	14	—	2.1	420
3	Pre-op	Rest	2	50	16	35	20	45	1.9	176
	Post-op (14 wks)	Rest	1	29	10	17	7.5	—	2.5	150
		Exercise	—	46	13	26	12	—	3.6	342

* Pre-op. study performed by Henry T. Lang, Jr., M.D. and Ralph Berg, Jr., M.D., Spokane, Washington.

Patient 8. Mitral resection and replacement was performed on February 22, 1961 with a preoperative diagnosis of predominant mitral insufficiency. At operation there was no mitral annulus dilatation. There was slight fusion of both commissures and marked loss of leaflet surface area (Fig. 12).

Results

The two deaths and two serious complications following mitral replacement are noted in Table 1. Patient 1 was returned to the recovery room following an uneventful operation and was awake with normal signs. She was able to sit up for a postoperative chest film which revealed an air fluid level in the right chest that was mistakenly interpreted as partial hemopneumothorax. Ten hours postoperatively as she turned to lie on her right side she expired of massive air embolism. Postmortem x-rays confirmed the air fluid level represented sequestered air in her left atrium.

The prophylactic measures agains air embolism described in the previous section were taken in this patient with the exception of flushing out the left atrium after bypass was discontinued. This maneuver performed by momentarily opening the partially occluding clamp on the atriotomy incision would most likely have avoided this death.

The second fatality occurred in Patient 4 and resulted from renal shutdown on the eleventh postoperative day. Bypass was prolonged in this patient because of poor exposure related to the small size of the calcified left atrium and the need to recover dislodged muralthrombus at frequent intervals during the procedure. The patient was returned to the recovery room with normal vital signs but failed to awaken. Left hemiplegia, coma, and anuria persisted to his death. His cardiac status remained good with no evidence of congestive failure or hypotension until shortly before death. Autopsy examination revealed right cerebral infarction and lower nephron nephrosis. Examination of the heart revealed firm fixation of the prosthesis. There were small adherent clots on the suture line and over the teflon cloth but no thrombus material on the valve itself.

One patient (No. 5) required reoperation for massive hemorrhage from a laceration of the left ventricle produced by the rod used in this case to maintain mitral incompetence while the left atriotomy was being closed. Upon reopening the right thoracotomy massive bleeding was noted from the left side of the heart. The right chest was closed and the ventricular tear repaired through a left anterior thoracotomy. The patient subsequently made an uneventful recovery and was discharged from the hospital four weeks postoperatively in excellent condition.

Patient 7 developed an acute staphylococcal endocarditis on the third postoperative day which responded to appropriate antibiotic therapy. All subsequent blood cultures were negative and she is at present in the hospital still under treatment.

The remaining patients (No. 2, 3, 5, 6) are at home and doing well. Patient 8 has had an uncomplicated course but has not yet been discharged from the hospital. The first survivor (Patient 2) is back at work as a truck dispatcher and the second survivor (Patient 3) is a graduate student.

Postoperative Cardiac Status

All patients undergoing resection and replacement of the mitral valve in this clinic had a satisfactory hemodynamic result as reported in Table 3. There was no difficulty in discontinuing cardiopulmonary bypass and left atrial pressures fell to normal in the operating room except in Patient 8 in whom the mean left atrial pressure fell from 20 to 18 mm. Hg. There was complete freedom from extra-systoles of ventricular origin that might imply impingement of the valve on the left ventricular endocardium. Transient supraventricular tachycardia or rapid atrial fibrillation with rates up to 160/min. were well tolerated in the immediate postoperative period without hypotension or evidence of pulmonary congestion. While all patients had normal venous pressures during the first few postoperative days congestive failure as manifest by moderate hepatic enlargement and tenderness was not unusual beginning from the fifth day to the second week after surgery and responding to increased doses of digitalis and diuretics. All patients showed a dramatic change in heart size and configuration by the time of discharge (Fig. 13, 14).

Phonocardiography was performed on the surviving patients and confirmed the absence of murmurs due to mitral disease. A typical phonocardiogram before and after replacement is shown in Figure 15. The mean interval in this series between the onset of the Q-wave in the electrocardiogram and the closing sound of the valve was 0.06 seconds and falls within the normal limits for the intact mitral valve. The mean interval between the semilunar valve closure and the "opening snap" of the prosthesis was 0.10 seconds. The patients were pleased by the diminution in cardiac noise and activity noted early in their recovery period but there was occasional awareness of the valve sound in the very thin patient when at bedrest or disrobed. The closure sound in such patient is audible without a stethoscope if the ear is within a few inches of the naked chest. The wearing of a hospital gown or clothing renders the valve inaudible at this range.

Two patients have thus far had postoperative cardiac catheterization and the results are shown in Table 2. The mean pulmonary artery pressure and wedge pressures were normal at rest and only slightly elevated in Patient 2 with exercise. The cardiac index rose in both instances with exercise with a normal response evident in Patient 3.

Red cell survival studies are planned in all patients and were completed in Patient 2, five months following valve implantation. The results are shown in Figure 16.

Anticoagulant Therapy

All patients were given oral anticoagulant therapy beginning on the seventh post-

TABLE 3. *Operating Room Pressures Before and After Human Mitral Replacement*

Pt. No.	Left Atrium						Pulmonary Artery						Femoral Artery	
	Before			After			Before			After			Before	After
	V	ED	M	V	ED	M	S	D	M	S	D	M	Before	After
1	22	12	17	14	9	11	—	—	—	—	—	—	75/55	90/70
2	40	25	32	15	10	13	50	37	45	35	20	25	100/60	75/45
3	50	17	37	10	7	9	50	25	37	35	20	25	100/65	90/50
4	25	15	20	12	5	9	60	35	45	50	35	40	130/80	100/75
5	27	13	17	12	7	10	35	25	30	35	25	30	150/95	115/75
6	25	15	20	15	8	10	30	25	28	—	—	—	115/80	95/60
7	55	32	42	18	14	15	60	50	52	35	25	30	100/70	75/50
8	35	20	25	22	15	18	40	27	35	—	—	—	130/75	100/60

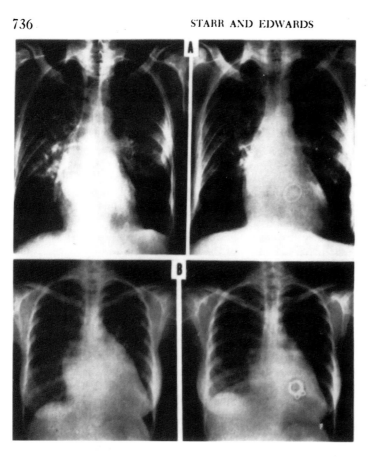

FIG. 13. A. Pre- and postoperative chest x-ray of Patient 2 in whom a Lucite cage valve with steel spreader ring was used. B. Chest X-ray of patient 3 immediately before and one month after mitral replacement.

operative day. There have been no thromboembolic difficulties in the six surviving patients. Patients 2 and 3 were given heparin beginning on the third postoperative day but the subsequent late right hemothorax developing in both patients resulted in reliance upon oral medication alone with a prothrombin depressing drug. It is of interest that because of this complication anticoagulant drugs were discontinued during the second postoperative week in patients 2 and 3 without embolic phenomena. Patient 3 also underwent excision of a left inguinal encapsulated hematoma two months following valve replacement and was again maintained with a normal clotting mechanism for one week without complications. The need for postoperative anticoagulant therapy following human mitral replacement still remains in doubt. However, experience with thromboembolic difficulties in the dog following implantation with a similar prosthesis and the occasional occur-

rence of this complication with the Hufnagel valve in the descending aorta of the human suggests the possible vulnerability of an intracardiac ball valve in this regard. Chronic atrial fibrillation was present in all patients and in itself increases the risk of embolism. Until further experience with human mitral replacement is obtained it seems prudent to maintain a state of diminished blood coagulability in these patients indefinitely.

Discussion

Considerably more information is required before the search for the ideal mitral prosthesis may be discontinued. In the interim, however, the results presented in this report, in terms of extracorporeal accelerated fatigue testing and animal and human implantation, suggest that under certain circumstances the use of the ball-valve mitral prosthesis is justified. The indications for mitral replacement with this prosthesis are lated to the operative findings and the comparative risks and advantages of replacement versus more conservative surgical management. The immediate risks of mitral valve implantation in terms of mortality and morbidity are acceptable when consideration is given to the poor functional status of the patient prior to operation and to the present developmental nature of the procedure. Satisfactory hemodynamic results can be expected with some regularity following the valve replacement procedure since the hydraulics of the valve varies only with the size of the prosthesis. However, the advantages of the prosthesis over plastic procedures on the mitral valve in terms of predictability of hemodynamic result must be balanced by the unknown long-term hazards involved in total dependence upon an intracardiac appliance. For this reason the only indication for mitral replacement in this series has been the opera-

tive findings of a hopelessly diseased valve not amendable to any reasonable plastic procedure in a patient with severe symptomotology (functional Class III or IV) from whom prior permission for the use of the prosthesis has been obtained.

Evaluation of the pathology in terms of the need for replacement is not difficult in those cases of complete bone-like calcification of the valve with marked loss of valve substance and chordal contracture. Pure stenosis or a combined lesion with predominant stenosis is usually present in this group of cases and these findings may be predicted by preoperative cardiac fluoroscopy. Even in the presence of pure stenosis primary replacement is indicated in this group. Considerably more judgement is required in the evaluation of the insufficiency group. In the patient with marked dilatation of the annulus, flexible aortic leaflet with adequate surface area, and rolling un-

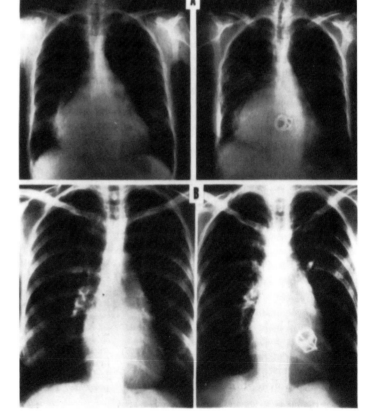

FIG. 14. A. Chest x-ray of Patient 5 immediately before and one month following mitral replacement. B. Chest x-ray of Patient 7 immediately before and one month following mitral replacement.

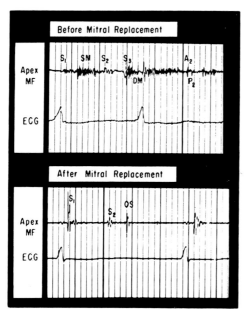

FIG. 15. Phonocardiogram of Patient 3 measured immediately prior and three months following mitral replacement. O.S. represents "opening snap" of prosthesis.

der of the mural leaflet annuloplasty with or without mural leaflet replacement may give excellent results. Ruptured chordae tendineae with annular dilatation also represents a prime indication for conservative operative management. In the absence of annular dilatation or ruptured chordae severe mitral insufficiency is usually the product of marked loss of surface area of one or both leaflets and extensive contracture of the subvalvular mechanism. It is in this group with serious involvement of both leaflets and their chordal support that mitral replacement is considered. It is possible to underestimate the contribution of subvalvular patholgy to regurgitation since decompression of the heart during cardiopulmonary bypass takes some of the tension off the chordae. The poor result following single leaflet replacement for destroyed mural leaflet in patient number one in this series was clearly related at the time subsequent mitral resection to a failure to appreciate the degree of chordal shortening involving this leaflet. This error

was not repeated in the subsequent cases of pure mitral insufficiency (Patients 3, 5, 6).

There are marginal instances in which the results of annuloplasty or leaflet extending procedures are difficult to predict unless these procedures are actually performed. It is reasonable under these circumstances to attempt to conserve the patient's valve and then assess the results either visually or by palpation and pressure studies immediately after bypass. Should there be dissatisfaction with the results obtained, the repair can be taken down and the valve replacement performed at the same sitting.

Summary and Conclusion

Mitral replacement with a ball-valve prosthesis has been performed on eight patients. The prosthesis prior to this experience was demonstrated to provide firm and lasting fixation to the mitral annulus, satisfactory hydraulic function and long-term survival in the dog. All patients had a satisfactory hemodynamic result documented by pressure studies in the operating room. There were two postoperative deaths that were unrelated to the prosthesis and the remaining patients are convalescing satsifactorily. The first two surviving patients, operated upon in September and October 1960, are free of cardiac symptoms and back at work.

The results obtained thus far in terms of cardiac catheterization, phonocardiography, red cell survival, and the need for anticoagulant therapy are presented.

Mitral valve replacement at present is indicated only in severely incapacitated patients with operative findings of a hopelessly damaged valve not amenable to any plastic procedure and in whom operation cannot reasonably be postponed.

Acknowledgments

The authors express their appreciation to Silas Braley, of Dow-Corning, for his help in supplying silicone rubber and other silicone products used in the fabrication of the prosthesis, to Norman Jeckel, of U. S. Catheter and Instrument Company, for making available various Teflon cloth

Volume 154
Number 4
MITRAL REPLACEMENT
739

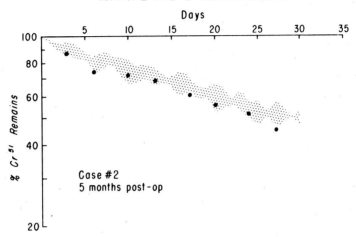

FIG. 16. Radioactive chromium tagged red cell study of Patient 2. Shaded area represents the normal limits in this laboratory.

products used in the fixation ring, and to R. R. Miller, of Precision Metalsmiths Incorporated, Cleveland, Ohio, for his help with metallurgical problems involving casting technics. The prostheses used in this study were obtained from the Edwards Laboratories Inc., 603-H Alton Street, Santa Ana, Calif.

Addendum

Since submission of this paper, four more patients have had mitral replacement with no operative deaths and one late death due to staphylococcal endocarditis. This patient and Patients 7 and 8, who also died of endocarditis two months after replacement, was operated upon during an epidemic of staphylococcal infections involving other cardiac surgical patients and requiring temporary closure of the operating suite. All seven survivors continue to maintain dramatic initial functional response.

Bibliography

1. Braunwald, N. S., T. Cooper and A. G. Morrow: Experimental Replacement of the Mitral Valve with a Flexible Polyurethane Foam Prosthesis. Conference on Prosthetic Valves for Heart Surgery. U.S.P.H.S. Edited by K. Alvin Merendino, C Thomas, 1960.

2. Braunwald, N. S., T. Cooper and A. G. Morrow: Complete Replacement of the Mitral Valve. J. Thoracic Surg., 40:1, 1960.

3. Ellis, F. H., Jr. and A. H. Bulbullian: A Prosthetic Replacement Mitral Valve: Preliminary Experimental Observations. Proc. Staff. Meet., 33:532, 1958.

4. Ellis, F. H., Jr.: Discussion of Frater, R. W., Ellis, F. H., Jr.: Problems in the Development of an Artificial Mitral Valve. Confer-

ence no Prosthetic Valves for Heart Surgery. U.S.P.H.S. Edited by K. Alvin Merendino, C. C Thomas, 1960.

5. Esmond, W. G., S. Attar, R. A. Cowley, S. Braley and R. R. McGregor: Design and Implantation Trials of Silastic, Dacron, Ivalon Prosthetic Mitral Valves. Conference on Prosthetic Valves for Heart Surgery. U.S.P.H.S. Edited by K. Alvin Merendino, C. C Thomas, 1960.

6. Frater, R. W. and F. H. Ellis, Jr.: Problems in the Development of an Artificial Mitral Valve. Conference on Prosthetic Valves for Heart Surgery, U.S.P.H.S. Edited by K. Alvin Merendino, C. C Thomas, 1960.

7. Howard, H. S., V. L. Willman and C. R. Hanlon: Mitral Valve Replacement. Amer. Coll. Surg. Cong. (46th) Proc. Surg. Forum IX, 256, 1960.

8. Kay, E. B., C. Nogueira and H. A. Zimmerman: Correction of Mitral Insufficiency under Direct Vision. Circulation, 21:568, 1960.

9. Kernan, M. C., M. M. Newman, B. S. Levowitz, J. H. Stuckey and C. Dennis: A Prosthesis to Replace the Mitral Valve. J. Th. Surg., 33:698, 1957.

10. Lillehei, C. W.: Discussion of Long, David, M., Jr., Sterns, L. P., Finsterbusch, W. Meyne, N., Varco, R. L., Lillehei, C. W.: Reconstruction and Replacement of the Mitral Valve with Plastic Prostheses. Conference on Prosthetic Valves for Heart Surgery. U.S.P.H.S. Edited by K. Alvin Merendino, C. C Thomas, 1960.

11. Long, David M., Jr., L. P. Sterns, W. Finsterbusch, N. Meyne, R. L. Varco and C. W. Lillehei: Reconstruction and Replacement of the Mitral Valve with Plastic Prostheses.

STARR AND EDWARDS Annals of Surgery
October 1961

Conference on Prosthetic Valves for Heart Surgery. U.S.P.H.S. Edited by K. Alvin Merendino, C. C Thomas, 1960.

12. Shumway, Norman: Personal communication.

13. Starr, A.: Oxygen Consumption during Cardiopulmonary Bypass, J. Thoracic Surg., 38: 46, 1959.

14. Starr, A.: Total Mitral Replacement: Fixation and Thrombosis. Am. Coll. of Surgeons, Clin. Cong. (46th) Proc. Surg. Forum XI, 258, 1960.

15. Starr, A. and M. L. Edwards: Mitral Replacement: The Shielded Ball Valve Prosthesis. J. Thoracic Surg. 1961 (in press).

DISCUSSION

DR. MICHAEL E. DEBAKEY: I must say that this paper persuades me to re-evaluate my attitude toward ball valves. I have been somewhat prejudiced against them because of my very early experience with their use in changing the directional flow in blood pumps. Our more recent experience with the use of such ball valves, as in the Hufnagel valve in aortic insufficiency, also tended to make me somewhat prejudiced.

Perhaps today with much better materials, materials that obviously have less effect upon the cellular and other components of the blood, these valves may be less harmful and therefore more useful.

Nonetheless, it seems to me that this is very impressive work on the part of Drs. Starr and Edwards. Everyone who is familiar with this area of pathology and with the problems relating to correction of this type of lesion knows the difficulties involved in attempting to replace the mitral valve. Although these results are yet too early for final evaluation, they are most encouraging.

DR. GEORGE H. A. CLOWES, JR.: As one who has heard the story on this business of artificial valves practically since its beginning in connection with the Artificial Internal Organ Society, I am equally impressed with Dr. DeBakey.

This is a most remarkable piece of work, to have had six out of eight patients survive. I simply want to outline briefly some of the problems that have confronted workers in this field that Dr. Starr was a little too modest to talk about.

Now I know that from his excellent paper on oxygen consumption, and so on, he did a very careful job of work before he did this thing. But lots of competent people like Drs. Koll, Kay, Muller and others have worked on it. They found that the great problem was not that they could not put in valves that would work, but that they always produced thrombi in dogs. This was true particularly at the junction between the myocardium or endocardium and the prosthetic substance. On the left side if these thrombi dropped off, the animal died of a cerebral embolism, and this inevitably took place within three or four weeks.

For that reason, many of us have been very reticent about putting in these artificial protheses. We have been waiting for the time when we thought we had to do it; but Dr. Starr has succeeded in doing it, and he has proved the point that was brought out at the NIH meeting in Chicago last fall concerning artificial heart valves, that probably man does not react as violently as the animal does in producing a clot at the interference between myocardium and the artificial prosthesis. It may be that man is a better candidate for this type of thing than the animal.

DR. ALBERT STARR: (Closing) We were prejudiced against the ball valve for use as an intracardiac prosthesis, and it was difficult to state in the short presentation the various steps that led to the choice of this "repugnant" intracardiac appliance.

Numerous other types of valves were tried, and as Dr. Clowes has mentioned, the problem of thrombosis in the dog made evaluation impossible. However, with the ball-valve prosthesis it was possible to obtain long-term dog survivors without anticoagulant treatment. I believe the reason for this is that the valvular mechanism is not attached to the body of the prosthesis itself. The clot in the dog grows by direct extension like an infiltrating tumor rather than by multicentric origin, so that the clot which forms on the margin of the valve at its point of attachment is less likely to interfere with valve function with the ball valve as compared with other types of prosthesis in which leaflets are anchored to the mitral annulus itself. I think this explains our ability to obtain long-term survival with the dog with the ball valve.

Some of the dogs who were not on anticoagulant treatment have had embolic problems requiring on one occasion reoperation for saddle emboli. For this reason, the patients in this series are receiving anticoagulant therapy. All had atrial fibrillation. Many of them have had anticoagulants before operation. The price we pay for adequate hydraulic function in terms of anticoagulant treatment is really not great.

The valve that we currently use in the dog is somewhat different from the ball valve in the human. We have found that if we shield the suture line with some bland material such as silastic so that the zone of injury of the endocardium is separated from the circulation, that the tendency to thrombotic occlusion is completely overcome and embolic complications even without anticoagulant therapy following implantation in the dog are markedly reduced.

Biological factors affecting long-term results of valvular heterografts

Alain Carpentier, M.D. (by invitation), Guy Lemaigre, M.D. (by invitation),

Ladislas Robert, M.D. (by invitation), Sophie Carpentier, M.S. (by invitation), and

Charles Dubost, M.D. (by invitation), Paris, France

Sponsored by Frank Gerbode, M.D., San Francisco, Calif.

The use of biological tissue in surgery springs from a natural tendency of man to consider with affection all natural material and with suspicion any artificial substitute. This more sentimental than scientific attitude is, however, still justified at the present time in cardiac surgery because of the real advantages of valvular graft replacement, such as excellent hemodynamic function, absence of hemolysis, thrombosis, and embolism, and avoidance of postoperative anticoagulant therapy.

Heterografts in comparison with homografts provide more practical conditions for obtaining an unlimited number of samples, removed under sterile conditions, from selected donors. In addition, by the use of different animal species (lamb, pig, or calf), it is possible to obtain a great variety of sizes to supply the needs of all valvular replacement, both in adults and children. Despite these advantages, heterografts have their own disavantages, which must be em-

phasized to show this method of valvular replacement in its true aspect.

Having been the subject of a great deal of study in this laboratory[10, 11, 14] as well as in others,[16, 21, 30] the technical problems seem to be solved whereas the biological problems still remain relatively unknown, although they play a great part in the long-term results of such grafts.

Thus, despite continuous investigations, several questions still remained unanswered, such as: What is the host reaction to differently treated tissue? Is the effect of host cell ingrowth into the valve beneficial or harmful? What is the long-term fate of collagen and elastin? And, finally, what is the adequate method for preservation of such grafts?

Continuous analysis of data accruing from our clinical experience and from immunological and biochemical research have helped provide answers to some of these questions.

Normal and pathological evolution of grafts

Since September, 1965, the date of the first successful heterograft replacement of the aortic valve in a human,[7] we have made extensive use of this valve substitute. Some patients who died or were reoperated upon for reasons listed in Table I, made it possible to examine the graft at various time

From the Laboratoire d'Etude des greffes et prothèses valvulaires, Institut de Progenèse, Faculté de Médicine, 15, rue de l'Ecole de Médicine, Paris, France, and the Clinique de Chirurgie Cardiaque Hôpital Broussais, Paris, France.

Supported by the Délégation Génerale á la Recherche Scientifique et Technique.

Read at the Forty-ninth Annual Meeting of The American Association for Thoracic Surgery, San Francisco, Calif., Mar. 31, April 1 and 2, 1969.

467

Journal of
Thoracic and Cardiovascular
Surgery

Table I. *Treatment and fate of grafts examined at and after 3 months of implantation**

Patient, age (yr.)	Date of operation	Valvular replacement	Duration (mo.)
KIR. 23	Nov. 1965	Aortic, direct suture	3
KUR. 26	Dec. 1965	Aortic, direct suture	4
BUS. 42	Dec. 1965	Aortic, direct suture	34
St OY. 50	Dec. 1965	Aortic, direct suture	37
PAS. 31	May 1967	Mitral, frame-mounted	9
ASS. 28	June 1967	Mitral, frame-mounted	11
QUE. 23	June 1967	Mitral, frame-mounted	5
PON. 47	June 1967	Mitral, frame-mounted	3
SCAR. 19	Jan. 1968	Mitral, frame-mounted Aortic, direct suture Tricuspid, frame-mounted	10

*All patients were successfully reoperated upon, except for 2 who died postoperatively.
†M.S.: Mercurial solution 1 (1/100,000), 2 (1/300,000).
‡D.R.C.C.: Distention and prolapse of the right coronary cusp.

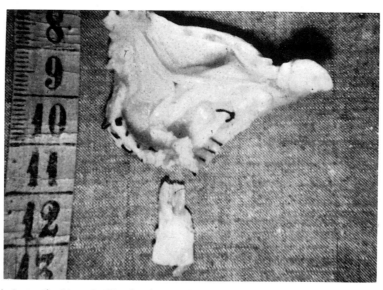

Fig. 1. A 3-month-old graft. The fixation stitch tied across one commissure cut through, and the commissure, displaced upward, produced regurgitation. (Graft was preserved in a mercurial solution and directly implanted in the aortic position. The patient was successfully reoperated upon.)

intervals after operation. From gross and histologic study it is possible to derive a general description of the normal evolution as well as the complications of the grafts.

1. Material

Sixty-one grafts were implanted in 53 patients suffering from pulmonary, tricuspid, aortic and/or mitral disease. Eleven grafts removed from 9 patients were checked at periods ranging from 3 months to 3 years. Four grafts were in place 3 to 6 months, five for 6 to 12 months, and two for 1 to 3 years.

Mechanical failures due to technical fault were found in 5 cases: one valve had a section of one commissure by a stitch (Fig. 1), one valve had folding of the aortic sleeve be-

Volume 58
Number 4
October, 1969

Valvular heterografts 4 6 9

Method of preservation	Cause of failure	Cellular ingrowth	Collagen
M. S. 1†	Rupture of commissure	Immunolog. competent cells	Normal
M. S. 1	Folding	O	Denaturation
Freeze-dried	Infection	Inflammatory	Necrotic
M. S. 1	Biological failure	Fibroblasts	Denaturation
M. S. 2†	DRCC‡	Immunolog. competent cells	Necrotic
M. S. 2	Infection	O	Normal
Formalin	Biological	Immunolog. competent cells	Necrotic
M. S. 2	DRCC‡	O	Normal
Conditioned (not protected)	DRCC‡	Inflammatory	Normal
Formalin	Biological	Inflammatory	Necrotic
M. S. 2	Biological	O	Denaturation

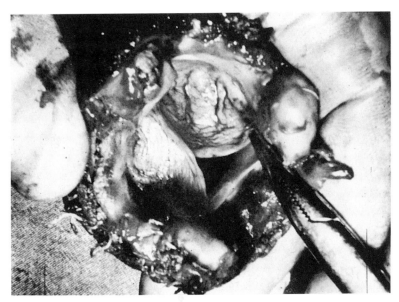

Fig. 2. A 3-month-old graft. Photograph shows prolapse of the right coronary cusp, made fragile by previous trimming. (Graft was preserved in a mercurial solution, frame-mounted, and placed in the mitral position. The patient was successfully reoperated upon.)

cause of inadequate fixation of the lower rim, three valves placed in the mitral position had a prolapse of the right coronary cusp which had been made fragile by trimming (Fig. 2.)

Biological failures were found in 4 cases. The valves were satisfactorily inserted but tears occurred because of histologic alterations.

The method of preservation used in 7 cases was a chemical sterilization, in 1 case freeze drying, in 2 cases formalin, and in 1 case our current method was used.

2. Normal evolution

Specimens, removed either during the postoperative period or later because of mechanical failure, made possible the description of the stages of the normal evolution of heterografts preserved by usual methods.

For some months after insertion, valves maintained their preoperative aspect and thickness. A thin filmy covering was apparent at both suture lines and on the surface of the graft (see Fig. 1). After 6 months, definition of suture lines became increasingly difficult and, because of a high degree of incorporation of the grafted tissue it was, on occasion, impossible to remove all the aortic sleeve of the valve.

Microscopic examination revealed that the graft retained its original architecture but with slight alterations in detailed structure: during the first months occasional thin

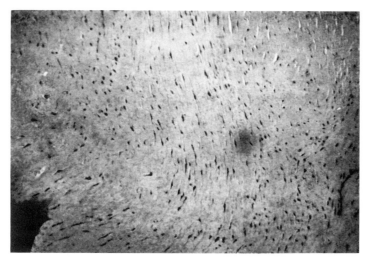

Fig. 3. A 3-year-old graft. The histologic section shows focus of fibroblasts in the aortic sleeve (hematoxylin and eosin; orig. mag. × 60). (Graft was preserved in a mercurial solution and directly implanted in the aortic position. The patient was successfully reoperated upon.)

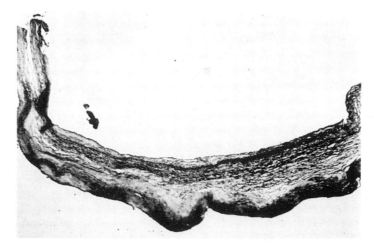

Fig. 4. An 11-month-old graft. Histologic section shows well-preserved structure, acellular. There is a slight modification of collagen (hyalinization) and elastic fibers. (Elastic stain with van Gieson counterstain; orig. mag. × 20.) (Graft was preserved in a mercurial solution, frame-mounted, and implanted in the mitral position. The patient was successfully reoperated upon for septicemia.)

Volume 58
Number 4
October, 1969

Valvular heterografts 4 7 1

discrete deposits of fibrin were seen on cusp surfaces and on the sleeves. In some specimens, on the surfaces and within the superficial layers of both sides of the cusps, were found small linear groups of pyroninophilic mononuclear cells which presumably represented the only evidence of an immunological response to the foreign tissue. Grafts between 6 and 12 months old showed little increase in the extent of the intimal fibrin sheaths but, contrary to fresh homografts, these fibrin sheaths were very thin. In one graft no fibrin was observed. Scattered cells, mainly histiocytes, were present in grafts at this stage, but there were no inflammatory cells or evidence of immunological reaction.

In a 3-year-old graft, a focus of fibroblasts with stained new collagen was observed in the sleeve and in the sheaths covering the base of the cusps, but did not extend to the cusps. (Fig. 3). Collagen showed an aspect of hyalinization and elastic fibers were fragmented in some areas, but the general architecture remained identical (Fig. 4).

It is important to point out that these architectural modifications were generally slight, except in cusps affected by mechanical dysfunction related to the technique of insertion. In these cases fragmentation and necrosis of collagen fibers were common. This fact demonstrates the interactions between technical and biological factors and emphasizes the necessity of a perfect reconstruction of the normal valve position.

3. Graft pathology

Three types of biological failures have been observed on four specimens between 5 months and 3 years in age.

a. Immunological reactions. In 2 cases, immunological reaction was the cause of the valve failure. One valve had a tear of a commissure. The other had a tear of the marginal border of the noncoronary cusp. The ruptured areas had a watery appearance resembling edema fluid.

Histologically, a large focus of pyroninophilic cells that is, lymphocytes, plasma cells and macrophages, were observed at the site of ruptures. In the same site, collagen was necrotic (Fig. 5).

Despite these pathological changes, the host serum showed no antibodies to heart muscle by the tanned-cell technique or to valve tissue by a fluorescent technique.

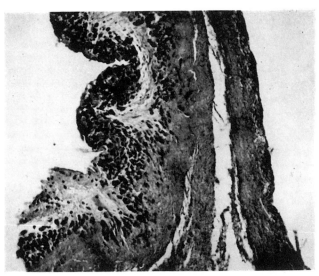

Fig. 5. A 5-month-old graft. Histologic section of the posterior leaflet shows focus of pyroninophilic cells extending from the aortic sleeve (hematoxylin and eosin; orig. mag. × 60). (The patient was successfully reoperated upon.)

Journal of
Thoracic and Cardiovascular
Surgery

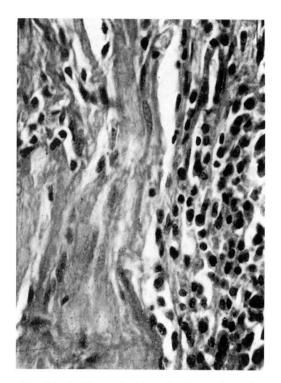

Fig. 6A. A 10-month-old graft. Histologic section shows inflammatory cell infiltration at the base of the cusp. (The valve was preserved in formalin and implanted in the aortic position. The patient was reoperated upon 10 months later and died postoperatively because of acute cardiac failure [triple valve replacement].) (Hematoxylin and eosin; orig. mag. × 100.)

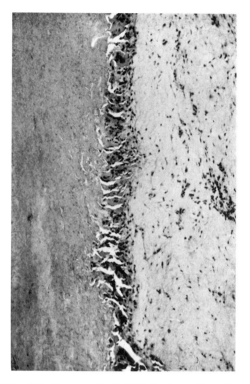

Fig. 6B. Same patient. Histologic section shows inflammatory cells at the graft/host interface (hematoxylin and eosin; orig. mag. × 40).

b. Inflammatory reactions. In 3 other cases, areas of nonspecific inflammatory cells were observed with plasmodial cells, macrophages, histiocytes, and relatively numerous eosinophils. (Fig. 6A). Degenerative change appeared in the adjacent collagen and elastic fibers, showing fragmentation of the fibers and areas of necrosis.

No bacteria were seen on the gram-stained specimen except in 1 patient.

Both immunologically competent cells, and inflammatory cells were mainly observed in the graft sleeve, either in the region of graft host interface (Fig. 6B) or along the threads used to secure the graft. The holes created by these sutures seemed to facilitate the cell ingrowth (Fig. 7).

c. Denaturation of collagen and elastin.

Denaturation of collagen and elastin without any cellular infiltration was observed in 3 cases. Macroscopically the graft appeared fragile, thin, and transparent. Histologic appearance showed extensive and pronounced fibrous tissue changes involving all three cusps. Generally, cusps appeared eosinophilic and amorphous, with fibrinoid aspect (Fig. 8). Another specimen showed areas of complete necrosis (Fig. 9). In all cases, the general architecture of the graft was modified and the elastic fibers were disintegrated. No calcification was observed in any specimen.

4. Discussion

Studies of the morphologic evolution of the grafted valve have not yet been reported by other authors who are now using this method of valvular replacement,[17, 23, 30] but doubtless they will be reported in due course. Ionescu[24] recently reported, in Ma-

Volume 58
Number 4
October, 1969

Valvular heterografts 4 7 3

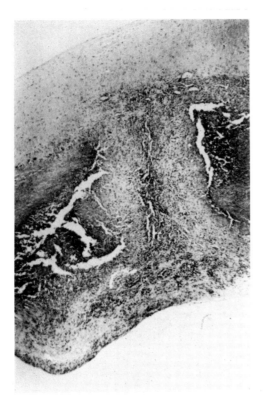

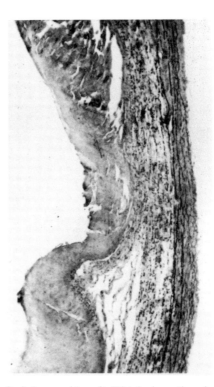

Fig. 7. A 34-month-old graft. Histologic section shows inflammatory cell penetration along a thread used to secure the graft (hematoxylin and eosin; orig. mag. × 40). (The valve was preserved by freeze-drying and then placed in the aortic position. The patient was successfully reoperated upon.)

Fig. 8. A 3-year-old graft. Histologic section shows denaturation of collagen and fragmentation of elastic fibers (elastic stain with van Gieson counterstain; orig. mag. × 40). (The valve was preserved in a mercurial solution and then placed in the aortic position. The patient was successfully reoperated upon.)

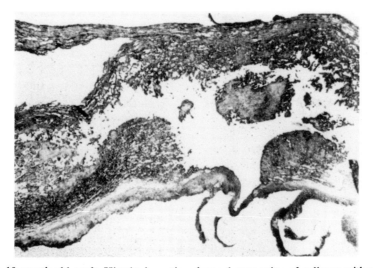

Fig. 9. A 10-month-old graft. Histologic section shows denaturation of collagen with necrosis—acellular (hematoxylin and eosin; orig. mag. × 40). (The valve was preserved in mercurial solution, frame-mounted, and implanted in the tricuspid position.)

Journal of
Thoracic and Cardiovascular
Surgery

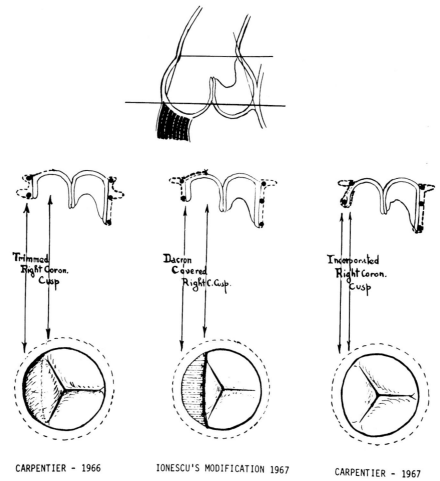

CARPENTIER - 1966   IONESCU'S MODIFICATION 1967   CARPENTIER - 1967

Fig. 10. Techniques of mounting the grafts into a frame, the muscular part of the right coronary cusp becomes fragile after trimming (*left*) and therefore must be reinforced either by a fabric pledget (*center*) or by a slight asymmetry of the frame (*right*), allowing greater flow areas.

drid, 6 cases of such valve failure in valves prepared with formalin.

We believe the following conclusions can be derived from this study.

An aortic valve heterograft will give dependable physiologic function both in the aortic and mitral positions, if the valve configuration is retained by careful reconstruction of the normal valve position. This may be accomplished with a direct suture technique,[10] or preferably with the use of a support ring which will allow the aortic heterograft to be adapted for use in any intracardiac position.[11] This support, described in 1966,[10] was subsequently modi-

fied in order to prevent the mechanical distention of the muscular part of the right coronary cusp[14] (Figs. 10 and 11).

These technical considerations look very important, even from a biological point of view, because, as we have seen above, an early valve dysfunction can create severe secondary histologic alteration of the valve.

In regard to the long-term fate of the valves, contrary to accepted opinions, it seems that the host cell ingrowth is more often harmful than beneficial. Fibroblasts and new collagen were rarely observed and were limited to very small portions of the valves.

Volume 58
Number 4
October, 1969

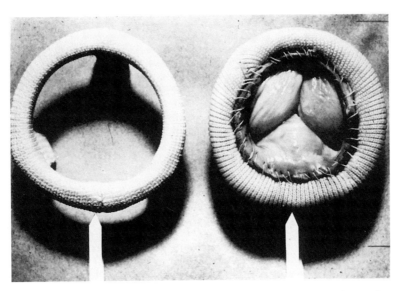

Fig. 11. Asymmetric frame provides support for the right coronary cusp *(arrows).*

An early reaction with mild infiltration of immunocompetent or inflammatory cells was frequently observed but generally disappeared after several months. In some instances this cellular reaction became extensive and destroyed a part of the graft. For this reason, we believe it is more useful to prevent cellular ingrowth than to hope for a hypothetical regeneration of the graft.

Immunological reactions observed point out the persistent antigenicity of some heterografts, and led to our search for antigenic factors implicated in these reactions. Denaturation of collagen and elastin after several years appears to be a major problem. Even in the absence of inflammatory reaction, collagen denaturation can occur, although this molecule usually has a very high degree of stability.

Criteria for evaluation of a method of preservation

These considerations suggest that the method of preservation of the valve plays a determinant role in the long-term fate of the graft. They also permit stating the criteria of efficiency for a method of preservation of the grafts: (1) guaranteed sterilization, (2) preservation of the mechanical properties (strength and flexibility), (3)

protection against cellular ingrowth, (4) prevention of immunological reaction by elimination of the antigenic components, and (5) prevention of long-term denaturation of collagen.

Among these factors we would like to study particularly the three last factors because they are the most important for the long-term fate of such grafts.

1. Protection against cellular ingrowth. As we said above, cellular ingrowth into the valve generally appeared harmful. Fibroblast penetration was very rare and limited to the sleeve or to the sheaths covering the cusps, whereas inflammatory cell penetration frequently occurred and was more extensive. Contrary to our previous thinking,[10] prevention of host cell penetration seems desirable.

Cellular ingrowth can be prevented by employing an appropriate method of preservation which reduces the antigenicity of the valve as well as by mechanical protection. This mechanical protection can be achieved by interposition of a thin silicone-impregnated cloth between the host and the graft and by covering the aortic sleeve with the same material (Figs. 12 and 13).

2. Prevention of immunological reaction. The histologic studies related above suggest

Journal of
Thoracic and Cardiovascular
Surgery

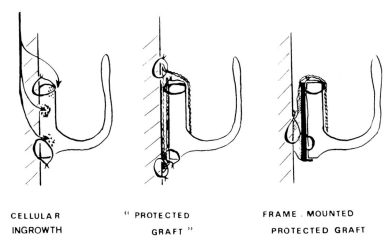

CELLULAR   " PROTECTED   FRAME . MOUNTED
INGROWTH   GRAFT "   PROTECTED GRAFT

Fig. 12. Techniques for the prevention of cellular ingrowth.

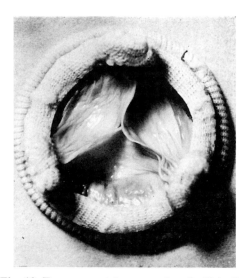

Fig. 13. Frame-mounted, protected graft. Note the cloth extended at the base of the cusp, hiding the aortic sleeve and sutures.

that persistent antigenic factors in the graft can induce an immunogenic cellular response.

To investigate this problem the different macromolecular fractions of fresh valves and valves treated by different methods of preservation were extracted and studied in this laboratory by the method of extraction, described by Robert,[35] then the antigenicity of the different valvular extracts was tested by several methods including: hemagglutination tests using antisera of rabbits immunized with the different fractions extracted from valves, intradermal tests in immunized guinea pigs, and immunofluorescent and histologic studies of differently treated valves subcutaneously implanted in rats.[14]

The components of a valve could be divided into two parts with respect to their degree of antigenicity: First, cells, soluble proteins, mucopolysaccharides, and structural glycoproteins which had a high degree of antigenicity. Second, collagen and elastin which appeared less antigenic. In some instances, collagen could induce an immunological response. The specificity of this molecule is probably due to its spatial arrangement and to peptides of low molecular weight, termed telopeptides,[34] extending from the triple helix body of the molecule. That is probably why enzymatic treatment or some tanning agents were able to reduce collagen antigenicity.

Comparative extractions from fresh valves and from valves treated by different methods of preservation showed significant differences. But none of the methods showed complete elimination of antigenic components, especially the structural glycoproteins (Table II).

3. Denaturation of collagen. Despite its high stability, collagen, when placed in an homologous or heterologous recipient, can

Volume 58
Number 4
October, 1969

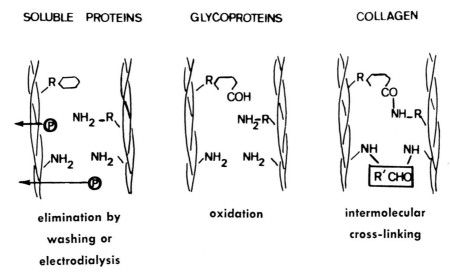

SOLUBLE PROTEINS   GLYCOPROTEINS   COLLAGEN

elimination by   oxidation   intermolecular
washing or   cross-linking
electrodialysis

Fig. 14. Diagrammatic representation of the different stages of the method for conditioning heterografts. (Figures represent the triple helix at the molecule of collagen with telopeptides extending from the body of the molecules.)

Table II. *Evaluation of the different techniques for preservation in relation to the criteria stated*

	Antigenic components			Nonantigenic component		Sterility	Tensile strength
	Cells	Soluble protein	Glyco-protein	Collagen	Elastin		
Hanks solution	–	+	–	0	0	0	0
Deep frozen	–	–	–	0	0	0	0
Freeze-dried	+	–	–	0	–	–	–
Irradiation	+	–	–	0	0	+	0
Propiolactone	+	+	–	–	–	+	+
Formaldehyde	+	–	–	+	0	+	+
Mercurial solution 1	+	+	....	–	–	+	–
Mercurial soution 2	+	+	–	0	–	+	0
Electrodialysis, oxidation and cross-linkage*	+	+	+	+	0	+	+

Legend: . . . . = Action. + = Favorable. 0 = Nul (or no action). – = Unfavorable.
*Our current technique.

be destroyed by the means of enzymatic actions. Telopeptides, which are largely responsible for the antigenicity of the molecule, are probably the sites of enzymatic action.

On the other hand, intermolecular cross-links are able to play an important role in determining the resistance to reabsorption of the graft.[39]

Various tanning agents, such as formalin, chromic acid, and polyacrolein have been used as cross-linking inducing factors by several authors.[25, 30, 37] These agents are not able to assure a correct and definitive protection of the graft because the intermolecular cross-links are reversible and because all glycoproteins and telopeptides are not eliminated.[37]

4. Method for conditioning heterografts.
A method for preservation of heterografts

478 *Carpentier et al.*

Journal of
Thoracic and Cardiovascular
Surgery

based upon these data and considerations has been developed in this laboratory.[14] According to the criteria of efficiency stated above, this method assures: sterilization of the graft, preservation of its mechanical properties, elimination or denaturation of the antigenic components, and prevention of denaturation of collagen (Fig. 14).

The basic principles of this method are as follows: Soluble proteins are eliminated by washing or electrodialysis. Mucopolysaccharides and structural glycoproteins are denatured by oxidation, according to the works of Moczar and Robert. The sodium periodate used for this purpose creates free aldehyde groups which spontaneously cross-link with free amino groups of other molecules. After 24 hours this oxidation must be neutralized by the use of ethyleneglycol. Then the valve is placed in glutaraldehyde buffered solution which reacts to cross-link with other free amino groups of lysine or other amino acids.

Practically speaking the method used is as follows: After removal from the heart, the valve is placed for at least 2 hours in Hanks solution with constant stirring (magnetic stirrer). During the trimming and measuring operations the valve must be dipped in sterile Hanks solution to prevent dehydration. The valve is then placed in a solution of sodium metaperiodate for 24 hours at 40° C. in the dark. (One part sodium metaperiodate solution 3 per cent to 2 parts of Hanks solution filtered through a Millipore filter GS and stored at 40° C. in the absence of light.)

The valve is then placed in a solution of ethyleneglycol for 1 hour with constant stirring (magnetic stirrer): ethyleneglycol (1 ml.) and Hanks solution (99 ml.), filtered through a Millipore filter and stored at 4° C. The valve is finally placed in a solution of glutaraldehyde in which it can be stored for several months at 4° C. (Twenty-five per cent glutaraldehyde solution, 2.6 ml., and phosphate buffer, 97.4 ml. To obtain the buffer mix: *Disodium phosphate solution,* 80 ml. [disodium phosphate 23.87 Gm., add distilled water to make 1,000 ml.] *Mono-*

potassium phosphate solution, 20 ml. [monopotassium phosphate, 9.07 Gm., add distilled water to make 1,000 ml.]).

Clinical results

The clinical results will be discussed with particular reference to the different techniques of preservation used.

Clinical material (Table III, see also Table I). Since November, 1965, sixty-one grafts were implanted in 53 patients. These patients were divided into 3 series in relation to the techniques of insertion and preservation of the graft used.

In a first series of 12 patients, operated upon between November, 1965, and June, 1966, the aortic valve was replaced by an aortic heterograft with a direct suture technique previously reported.[10] One valve was preserved by freeze drying, the other eleven were sterilized by the means of a mercurial solution (1/100,000 concentration).

In a second series of 11 patients operated upon between April, 1967, and June, 1967, frame-mounted grafts were used for replacement of the mitral valve in 9 patients and of

Table III. *Material (61 grafts: 53 patients)*

First series, 1965-1966 (Directly inserted grafts, sterilized with a mercurial solution or freeze dried)		12
Aortic valve replacement	12	
Second series, 1967 (Frame-mounted grafts, sterilized by mercurial solution, or formalin)		11
Mitral valve replacement	9	
Mitral and tricuspid valve replacement	2	
Third series, 1967-1968 (Frame-mounted conditioned and protected grafts)		30
Mitral replacement	14	
Aortic replacement	7	
Pulmonary replacement	2	
Tricuspid replacement (Ebstein's disease)	3	
Double aortic and mitral replacement	2	
Triple aortic mitral tricuspid replacement		2

Volume 58
Number 4
October, 1969

Valvular heterografts 479

both mitral and tricuspid valves in 2. The graft, inserted into a frame especially designed for this purpose[10-11] were implanted with a double suture line technique previously reported.[11] The valves were sterilized by mercurial solution (1/30,000 concentration) in 9 patients and by formalin in 2.

In a third series of 30 patients operated upon between November, 1967, and January, 1969 frame-mounted grafts were used for different types of replacement: of the mitral valve in 14 patients, of the aortic valve in 7 patients, of the pulmonary valve in 2 patients suffering from a pulmonary valvular agenesia, of the tricuspid valve in 3 patients suffering from Ebstein's disease, of both aortic and mitral valves in 2 patients, of aortic, mitral, and tricuspid valves in 2 patients.

The grafts were protected against cell penetration, adhering to the principles stated above, and the muscular part of the right coronary cusp was incorporated into the frame according to a method previously described.[14] The grafts were preserved or, precisely speaking, "conditioned for implantation" by the means of the method described above, except in 4 patients in whom formalin was used.

Results (Tables I and IV). In the first series of patients, there was no operative death as a result of valvular insufficiency. Two patients died in the postoperative period because of a low cardiac output. One patient died of septicemia, 10 months postoperatively. In 4 patients, a severe aortic insufficiency occurred from 3 months to 3 years later. The cause of this failure was mechanical in 2 patients and biological in the 2 others (Table I). These 4 patients were successfully reoperated upon using a prosthetic valve for replacement and their subsequent courses have been uncomplicated. Five patients remain well, but 2 of them have a soft Grade 2/6 diastolic murmur which has been unchanged. No anticoagulants were used at any time postoperatively.

In the second series, 1 patient died during operation. Another patient died 9 months postoperatively because of subacute bac-

Table IV. *Complications*

First series, 1965-1966 (Sterilized, directly implanted grafts)		12
Operative mortality	2	
Late mortality (infection)	1	
Mechanical failure	2	
Biological failure	2	
Second series, 1967 (Sterilized frame-mounted grafts)		11
Operative mortality	1	
Late mortality (infection)	1	
Mechanical failure	2	
Biological failure	2	
Third series, 1967-1968 (Conditioned protected frame-mounted grafts)		30
Operative mortality	4	
Late mortality (triple repl.)	1	
Complications	0	

terial endocarditis. In 4 patients, a severe valvular insufficiency occurred at periods of time ranging from 3 to 11 months. All of these patients were also successfully reoperated upon and the cause of failure was a prolapse of the right coronary cusp in 2 patients and histologic alterations of the tissue in the 2 others (see Table I). Five patients remain perfectly well (follow-up: 20 to 24 months).

In the third series of 30 patients, there were 4 operative deaths. One patient with a triple valve replacement died 10 months after operation because of persistent cardiac failure and cachexia. Twenty-five patients are alive and much improved. Only 2 patients have a soft and stable Grade 1/6 murmur. Among these 25 patients, 16 have had a follow-up of 10 months or more.

Discussion (Table V)

Comparative evaluation of the 3 series of patients operated upon with different techniques of graft implantation and preservation emphasizes the importance of these two factors, particularly the method of preparation used. Comparison between the second and the third series for the same period of

Table V. *Durability of valves*

	Per cent of well functioning valves at different periods of time				
	2 mo.	*6 mo.*	*1 yr.*	*2 yr.*	*3 yr.*
First Series: 12 (sterilized grafts directly implanted)	83%	58%	50%	50%	33%
Second series: 11 (frame-mounted sterilized grafts)	87%	54%	45%	37%	
Third Series: 30 (frame-mounted conditioned and protected grafts)	87%	82%	82%		

follow-up suggests that the use of the "conditioned and protected frame-mounted grafts" may be considered a real improvement.

There have been no emboli in any of the patients. Patients who were operated upon for aortic or pulmonary valve replacement did not have anticoagulant therapy at any time. Patients who were operated upon for a mitral or tricuspid replacement were treated with anticoagulants for at least 1 month postoperatively. Then the treatment was discontinued except in patients who had persistent auricular fibrillation.

Summary and conclusions

Analysis of the data accruing from the present series of histologic, biochemical, and clinical investigations provides answers to some of the questions raised in the introduction of this paper.

1. The host reaction to the grafted tissue is in relation to the degree of antigenicity of this tissue, so that the method of preservation of the graft must eliminate the principal antigenic components of the tissue, that is, soluble proteins, cells, glycoproteins, mucopolysaccharides.

2. Host cell ingrowth is generally harmful because the cells are usually immunologically competent or inflammatory and not fibroblasts. Thus, it appeared desirable to prevent cell ingrowth by appropriate methods of preservation of the graft as well as by mechanical protection.

3. Denaturation of the implanted collagen

with time is one of the chief biological problems. It may be preventable by intermolecular cross-linkage.

4. Finally, there is increasing evidence that the method of preservation of the graft is the main factor which affects the long-term fate of such grafts.

The method of preservation that we propose, although it appears to be a real improvement, is only another step in the research and investigation that this method of valvular replacement must have to achieve dependability.

REFERENCES

1 Angel, W. W., Wuerflein, R. D., and Shumway, N. E.: Mitral Valve Replacement With the Fresh Aortic Valve Homograft, Surgery **62:** 807-813, 1967.
2 Angel, W. W., Iben, A. B., Stinson, E. B., and Shumway, N. E.: Multiple Valve Replacement With the Fresh Aortic Homograft, J. THORACIC & CARDIOVAS. SURG. **56:** 323, 1968.
3 Barratt-Boyes, B. G., Lowe, J., Cole, D., and Kelly, D.: Homograft Replacement for Valve Disease, Thorax **20:** 495, 1965.
4 Berghuis, J., Rastelli, G. C., van Vliet, P. D., Titus, J. L., Swan, H. J. C., and Hellis, F. H., Jr.: Homotransplantation of the Canine Mitral Valve, Circulation **29:** 47-53, 1964 (Suppl. 1).
5 Bernhard, A., Ringdal, R., Babotai, I., Linder, H. P., Krayenbuhl, H. P., and Senning, Å.: Zur homotransplantation der mitralklappe, Thoraxchirurg. **13:** 89-95, 1965.
6 Bigelow, W. G., Trimble, A. S., Auger, P., and Wigle, E. D.: Aortic Homograft Valve Replacement of the Mitral Valve. Long-term Success, J. THORACIC & CARDIOVAS. SURG. **54:** 438, 1967.
7 Binet, J. P., Carpentier, A., Langlois, J., Duran,

ANNALS OF SURGERY

VOL. 102   NOVEMBER, 1935   No. 5

TRANSACTIONS of the AMERICAN SURGICAL ASSOCIATION

MEETING HELD IN BOSTON, MASS.

THE DEVELOPMENT OF A NEW BLOOD SUPPLY TO THE HEART BY OPERATION*

CLAUDE S. BECK, M.D.

CLEVELAND, OHIO

FROM THE DEPARTMENT OF SURGERY OF THE WESTERN RESERVE UNIVERSITY SCHOOL OF MEDICINE AND THE LAKESIDE HOSPITAL, CLEVELAND, OHIO

Two relatively small arteries supply the most vital muscular structure of the body. This muscular organ is in constant motion, and to make its movements free and frictionless it is enclosed in a moist envelope of mesothelium. In providing man with this anatomic pattern Nature so frequently has deprived him of an important compensatory mechanism, namely, the ability to develop an adequate collateral blood supply to this organ. The heart is anchored in the body by the great vessels at its base, and while the entire surface of the heart is in direct contact with adjacent structures it has a minimum of direct continuity with the rest of the body. The only continuity that the heart has with the rest of the body is through the walls of the great vessels, some fat, a few nerves and lymphatics that constitute its anchorage, and these structures are relatively avascular tissues. This anatomic arrangement has made the heart a defenseless organ when its normal blood supply is interrupted. The appalling incidence of sudden death from heart failure attests to the destructive nature of coronary closure. Under normal conditions the myocardium receives practically all its blood through the left and right coronary arteries. The thebesian channels opening directly from the left ventricular cavity offer a second possible source of blood supply.[1] The importance of these channels has been the subject of argument. It has been claimed by some that the flow through the thebesian vessels is of little importance. This statement is based on the assumption that the thebesian channels are compressed, perhaps completely collapsed, by the tension of contracting muscle fibers during systole when the pressure in the ventricular cavity is being built up, and as these channels open during diastole the

---

* Some of the experimental data were presented in an address to the Caduceus Honorary Society of the Emory University Medical School on May 17, 1934.

801

pressure in the ventricular cavity synchronously falls. The third possible source of blood supply to the heart is through the extracardiac anastomoses that are present in the tissues at the base of the heart.[2] When the blood flow through the coronary arteries is reduced gradually, compensatory mechanisms are established. Complete closure of a major coronary artery is compatible with life, if the closure takes place sufficiently slowly. Indeed, complete closure of both major coronary arteries may be compatible with life,[3] but the number of times that the process of occlusion has gone on to completion in each of the two major coronary arteries is excessively small. The occlusion must occur at such a rate as to permit the other sources of blood supply to develop. Usually while this substitution is being made, life is snuffed out like a candle flame.

I have been interested in the heart as a surgical organ since 1923, and during this period of time a rather extensive background of surgical experimentation on the heart has been accumulated, as the result of over 1200 experimental operations which have been done by my assistants and myself. I made the observation several years ago that blood vessels extended between the heart and an adherent scar. At that time Dr. R. A. Griswold[4] and I were interested in studying chronic compression of the heart produced experimentally and we were trying to resect an adherent scar from the surface of the heart. In so far as these small vascular connections between the heart and adherent tissues were concerned, we simply noted their presence. At that time they had no other significance for us. Last November, while a compressing scar was being resected from a human heart, a broad band of scar extending from the base of the left ventricle to the parietal pericardium was transected. Brisk bleeding occurred from the cut ends of the scar and the bleeding was more brisk from the cardiac end than from the pericardial end. This was the first direct observation made at the operating table that blood actually flowed between myocardium and adherent tissues. This observation had now assumed new and additional significance because in the meantime we had been attempting to produce a collateral vascular bed to the heart experimentally. This observation confirmed our belief that vascular connections between heart and adherent tissues could be produced in the human being. I desire to give credit to Dr. Alan R. Moritz for directing my attention to the subject of vascularization of cardiopericardial adhesions. Moritz, Hudson and Orgain[5] not only demonstrated anatomically the presence of blood vessels in cardiac adhesions by the injection of carbon particles into the coronary arteries but also Doctor Moritz believed that under certain conditions these blood vessels might function and become an important source of blood supply to the heart. He directed my attention to a case reported by Thorel in 1903. This patient had complete obliteration of both major coronary arteries, and Thorel suggested the possibility of the heart receiving a supply of blood through adhesions that were present.

Could the heart be given a new source of blood supply by operation? I carried out the first experiments in an attempt to study this problem in

Volume 102
Number 5
CARDIAC SURGERY

February, 1932, and shortly thereafter Dr. V. L. Tichy collaborated with me, not only in the technical surgery that was involved but also in the solution of many problems.[6] Doctor Moritz followed the work with interest and gave us valuable suggestions concerning the injection and study of the specimens.[7, 8] In these experiments the collateral vascular bed consisted of parietal pericardium and pericardial fat. The epicardium and the lining of the parietal pericardium were removed with a burr because it was our belief that these structures acted as a barrier to the growth of blood vessels into the heart. The results of these experiments were as follows: (1) Almost total occlusion of right and left coronary arteries near the aorta was compatible with life if the heart had been provided with a collateral vascular bed. The occlusion of arteries was produced by silver bands which were compressed in stages at repeated operation. (2) Dye penetrated the myocardium through the collateral bed, and we assumed that if particles of dye entered the myocardium as freely as they did, that blood also flowed into the myocardium through these vascular channels. We believe that we succeeded in giving the heart a new source of blood supply and that this was sufficient to maintain cardiac function. (3) A pressure-differential was necessary to promote anastomosis between the cardiac and extracardiac vascular beds. In other words, a physiologic need for blood in the myocardium was necessary for such anastomoses to develop. The physiologic need for blood was produced by occlusion of the major coronary arteries by silver bands which were placed around the arteries and which were compressed in stages at successive operations. (4) The development of anastomoses between the myocardium and the collateral bed was demonstrable three weeks after operation. More recently we have succeeded in demonstrating anastomoses between extracardiac and cardiac beds two weeks after the bed was applied to the myocardium.

During the past eight months additional experimental operations have been carried out with the assistance of Dr. Ernest Bright and Miss Alice B. Maltby. In these experiments pedicle grafts of muscle were used together with the pericardial and mediastinal fat for the vascular bed. Omentum was also brought up through an opening in the diaphragm and sutured to the heart. These experiments have not yet been published but I shall refer briefly to some of the results:

(1) Anastomoses readily develop between skeletal muscle and cardiac muscle provided the normal blood supply to the heart has been reduced. If the coronary arteries were not partially occluded the anastomoses between omentum or skeletal muscle and myocardium, although present to some extent, did not become well developed.

(2) A collateral vascular bed gives the heart partial, but not complete, protection when the right coronary artery is occluded in one stage. When the descending ramus of the left coronary artery is ligated in one stage, the degree of protection afforded by a collateral vascular bed is slight. The conclusion that can be drawn is that a collateral vascular bed protects the heart when the right coronary artery is occluded in one stage. The larger

CLAUDE S. BECK

Annals of Surgery
November, 1935

the coronary artery occluded, the less is the protective effect. The evidence, however, was definite that the presence of a collateral vascular bed protected the heart from the ravages of sudden occlusion of a major coronary artery. In this respect the operation becomes a prophylactic measure, and if the experimental data can be applied to patients with coronary sclerosis it would seem that this operation should be done early in the course of the disease, before replacement of myocardium by scar tissue and fat has taken place or before the heart has been brought to a standstill by occlusion.

(3) The right coronary artery, the ramus descendens of the left coronary artery, or the ramus circumflexus of the left coronary artery, can be ligated successfully almost as a routine if the ligation is carried out in two stages.

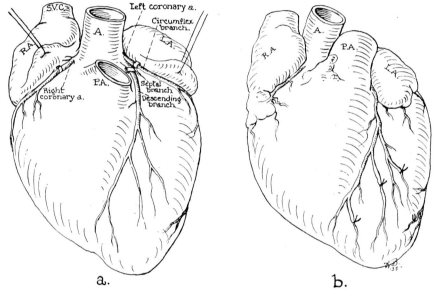

FIG. 1.—Two types of operations are shown: (a) shows the usual sites where silver bands were applied to the coronary arteries. A reduction of 30 to 50 per cent in the cross sectional area of these three arteries was compatible with life. (b) shows another type of experiment. Four or five peripheral branches of the coronary arteries over the apex of the heart were ligated. This experiment was always fatal. In (a) the reduction in total coronary blood flow was considerably greater than in (b). The heart cannot tolerate ischemia of a severe degree even though the area of ischemia is small. The collateral bed produced by operation can transport blood to such ischemic areas.

The explanation for this is that the reduction in blood flow brought about by the partial constriction of this vessel—and as little as 20 per cent of the cross section is efficacious—is compensated for by the development of collateral vessels. After this compensatory mechanism has been established, complete occlusion of the artery does not produce complete ischemia of the muscle. The myocardium remains viable after complete occlusion and additional channels become established.

(4) Distribution of blood to every part of the myocardium is of vital importance. If one relatively small portion of the myocardium is rendered ischemic by the peripheral ligation of four or five arterial branches, ventricular fibrillation develops and this is routinely fatal (Fig. 1). An equal

804

distribution of blood to the myocardium is essential for maintenance of function.

(5) The collateral vascular bed is functional not only in making a new source of blood supply available to the heart but it also helps to distribute blood to various portions of the myocardium. In this respect the collateral vascular bed produced by operation acts as an anastomotic bridge that transports blood from the bed of one coronary vessel to the bed of another coronary vessel where the blood flow is deficient.

The question naturally arises as to whether or not the presence of the new vascular bed might interfere with the movement of the heart. The importance of adhesions to the heart has been greatly overemphasized in the past. Cardiopericardial adhesions usually are silent lesions of little or no clinical significance. In none of our experiments did we find that the circulation was in any way embarrassed by these adhesions. Adhesions to the heart can embarrass the circulation in several ways: (1) A constricting bed of scar tissue may produce chronic cardiac compression. Adhesions in this clinical syndrome are entirely incidental and of no significance. (2) Adhesions between the heart and chest wall may act as a harness through which the heart pulls and expends energy. In our experiments the heart was not so extensively and intimately bound to the chest wall as to produce embarrassment. (3) The heart may be sharply angulated from its normal axis by such adhesions so that it cannot effectively function.

With this experimental work as a background it was decided to attempt to apply the data to a patient suffering from coronary sclerosis. To select a satisfactory case was not without difficulty and then to have the selected patient give his consent to have an operation performed on his heart (an operation that had never been done before on a human being) required something of the heroic spirit. For this reason I wish to mention the name of the patient, Joseph Krchmar, of Chardon, Ohio. I believe he has made a contribution to surgery. I also want to give credit to his physician, Dr. Walter Corey of Chardon. Doctor Corey had the imagination to see the possibilities of the experiments and he made a serious attempt to secure a patient for the operation. I also want to thank the internists, Dr. Joseph T. Wearn and Dr. Harold Feil. Doctor Feil is collaborating in the clinical aspects of this work.

CASE REPORT

J. K. was admitted to the Lakeside Hospital February 3, 1935. He was 48 years old, a white male, married, formerly a coal miner, more recently a farmer. His complaint was pain in the chest, over the heart, to the left of the sternum. He remembers the onset of the pain distinctly. A sharp pain appeared suddenly over the heart while he was at work nine years ago. It was accompanied by dyspnea and dizziness. After this initial attack he went back to fairly heavy labor until five years ago. Then, because of repeated attacks of substernal oppression, he moved to a farm. The precordial oppression was accentuated after meals. The patient claims that he had not done heavy work for the past five years, but he has done such things as plowing. During the last year or two he suffered from attacks of sharp, knife-like pains over the heart. These radiated to the left shoulder and down the left arm to the elbow. During these attacks of pain

CLAUDE S. BECK

Annals of Surgery
November, 1935

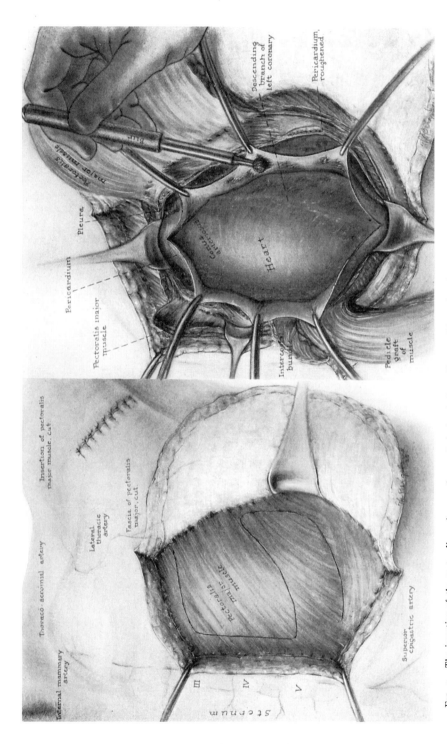

Fig. 3.—The pericardium was opened. The inner surface of the pericardium is roughened with a burr.

Fig. 2.—The insertion of the pectoralis major muscle was incised. A flap of skin and pectoral fascia was turned laterally. The pectoral muscle was incised as shown. This provided a pedicle graft of muscle with its attachment lateral to the sternum.

806

530

531

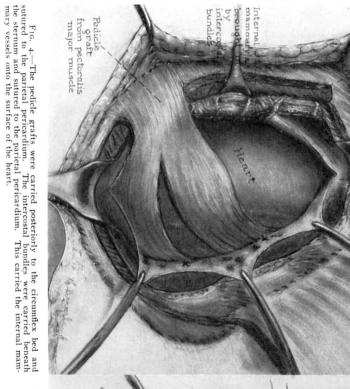

FIG. 4.—The pedicle grafts were carried posteriorly to the circumflex bed and sutured to the parietal pericardium. The intercostal bundles were carried beneath the sternum and sutured to the parietal pericardium. This carried the internal mammary vessels onto the surface of the heart.

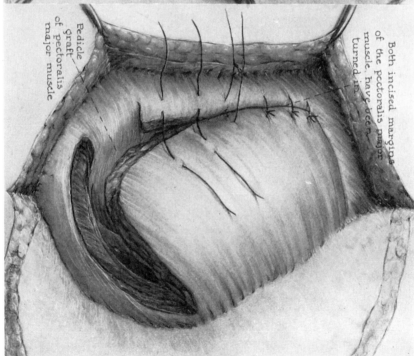

FIG. 5.—The parietal pericardium was left open and the incised margins of the pectoral muscles were inverted so that they came into contact with the heart.

807

he felt suffocated, was dyspneic and the heart palpitated. Epigastric distress after meals was also a prominent symptom. Numbness and tingling of the left hand and fingers frequently accompanied the pain. Ten days before admission to the hospital the patient, while carrying some wood into his house, was seized with violent, sharp, precordial pain, dyspnea and dizziness. He went to bed where he remained until he came to the hospital.

The patient was well developed, well nourished and of a phlegmatic temperament. His expression was worried. Examination of the precordium was negative. The heart was slightly enlarged to the left. On admission to the hospital the systolic pressure was 155 and the diastolic pressure was 95 Mm. Hg. The peripheral arteries were moderately thickened and tortuous. Exercise produced substernal oppression but no sharp pain. The electrocardiogram after exercise showed no significant change. While in the hospital the

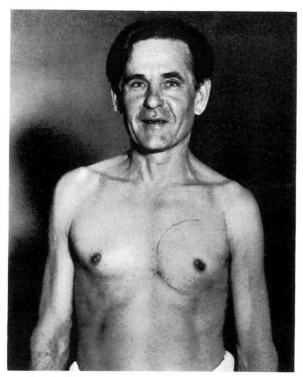

FIG. 6.—Patient three and one-half months after operation.

patient suffered a sudden, severe, knife-like attack of pain after taking a bath. The pain was precordial, to the left of the sternum, and did not radiate. At the same time he became cyanotic, very dyspneic and extremely apprehensive. Amyl nitrite gave him relief. A diagnosis of coronary sclerosis and angina pectoris was made. The electrocardiographic findings would indicate that there was no bundle damage thus far. He also had generalized arteriosclerosis and a mild degree of hypertension.

The patient consented to operation. He desired to go home to visit with his family but he returned to the hospital at midnight because of pain and a fear of impending death.

Operation.—February 13, 1935. Gas-oxygen anesthesia was used. The insertion of the left pectoral muscle was incised at the suggestion of Dr. W. C. McCally, for the purpose of mobilizing this muscle. This wound was closed. A curved incision was then made to the left of the sternum. (Fig. 2). The fascia was dissected from the left

CARDIAC SURGERY

pectoral muscle. The inferior portion of the pectoral muscle was incised for the purpose of making a pedicle graft. An incision was then made through the pectoral muscle parallel to the sternum exposing the third, fourth, and fifth costal cartilages. The muscle was freed from the chest wall. These cartilages were removed. The inter-costal bundles were cut laterally leaving them attached to the region of the internal mammary vessels. The pericardium was incised from base to apex (Fig. 3). The lining of the pericardium everywhere was roughened by means of a burr. The epicardium was removed in shreds by means of a burr. This produced a great many extra systoles and some dilatation of the heart. Rest periods were given. At the suggestion of Doctor Wearn I tried to palpate the coronary vessels but with the heart moving I could not be sure that I could feel them. The pedicle graft was then divided longitudinally and both pedicles were swung around to the circumflex area of the heart. These grafts were sutured laterally and posteriorly to the parietal pericardium (Fig. 4). The intercostal bundles and the medial margin of the pectoral muscle were carried beneath the sternum and attached to the parietal pericardium. These structures carried the internal mammary artery onto the surface of the heart. The lateral margin of the pectoral muscle was then inverted so that the incised surfaces were in contact with the heart (Fig. 5). The fascia of the pectoral muscle was sutured; the skin was closed. The wound was not drained.

Three and one-half months have elapsed since the operation (Fig. 6). The patient has been kept in the hospital during this period but during the last six weeks he has been doing light work, such as serving trays, moving beds. *etc.* For several weeks after operation he had indigestion after meals. This has disappeared. He claims that he has no precordial pain; that the feeling of oppression over the heart has disappeared, that he has no sharp radiating pains to the shoulder and arm. He claims that he is well. He can exercise without pain, although up to the present time he has done no hard physical work. I have emphasized the importance of describing accurately what symptoms he has, but to me and to everyone else who talks with him he claims that he is better. Objectively I can say that he appears to be better. The worried expression has left him, and he has a fine spirit.

SUMMARY

The heart can be given a new blood supply experimentally. On the basis of this work a collateral vascular bed to the heart should offer some benefit to patients suffering from coronary sclerosis. A collateral vascular bed was given to a patient with coronary sclerosis on February 13, 1935. Three and one-half months after operation the patient claims that he has been greatly benefited. However, it will be necessary to have a number of such results before we can attach any clinical significance to this operation. I want to emphasize the point that the work is still in the experimental stage and I do not recommend the performance of this operation until it is established by operation upon a number of patients.

ADDENDUM: September, 1935. Seven months have now elapsed since the operation on the first patient. He continues to work as a gardener; he has no pain and he claims that he is cured. I have carried out the operation on five additional patients, making the total number seven. The third patient had an extremely marked degree of arteriosclerosis. At the operating table I could palpate the ramus descendens. It was hard, tortuous and several millimeters in diameter. The patient had been incapacitated sine 1942. One and one-half years ago a total thyroidectomy was done. He has kept his basal metabolic rate at about minus 20 by taking thyroid extract. His life had been of a vegetative nature, spending as he did 20 hours a day in bed. Two and one-half months have elapsed since we did the cardiac anastomosis. He states that he is completely free from all pain and discomfort. He is able to take twice the dose of thyroid extract that he took before the operation and his basal metabolic rate is plus 2. He is up and about six to eight hours a day and his interest in life has returned. He is still an invalid and he is still weak, but the complete absence of pain, his normal basal metabolic rate, his increased activities and interests, are facts that may be of real significance in establishing the operation as a beneficial procedure. The fourth patient is a well known surgeon from Ashland, Kentucky, who came to me because he believed in the soundness of my operation. He had suffered a myocardial infarct with dilatation and failure. He also had diabetes mellitus. He believes that he has shown some improvement but the pulse rate on occasions becomes rapid and he has had several attacks of anginal pain since operation. A sufficiently long interval has not elapsed to comment on the other cases. These cases will be reported by Dr. Harold Feil and myself.

REFERENCES

[1] Wearn, Joseph T.: The Rôle of the Thebesian Vessels in the Circulation of the Heart. Jour. Exper. Med., vol. 47, pp. 293–316, February, 1928.

[2] Hudson, Charles L., Moritz, Alan R., and Wearn, Joseph T.: The Extracardiac Anastomoses of the Coronary Arteries. Jour. Exper. Med., vol. 56, pp. 919–925, December, 1932.

[3] Leary, Timothy, and Wearn, Joseph T.: Two Cases of Complete Occlusion of Both Coronary Orifices. Am. Heart Jour., vol. 5, p. 412, April, 1930.

[4] Beck, Claude S., and Griswold, R. A.: Pericardiectomy in the Treatment of the Pick Syndrome; Experimental and Clinical Observations. Arch. Surg., vol. 21, pp. 1064–1111, December, 1930.

[5] Moritz, A. R., Hudson, C. L., and Orgain, E. S.: Augmentation of the Extracardiac Anastomoses of the Coronary Arteries Through Pericardial Adhesions. Jour. Exper. Med., vol. 56, p. 927, 1932.

[6] Beck, C. S., and Tichy, V. L.: The Production of a Collateral Circulation to the Heart. Am. Heart Jour., in press.

[7] Beck, C. S., Tichy, V. L. and Moritz, A. R.: Production of a Collateral Circulation to the Heart. Proc. Soc. Exper. Biol. & Med., vol. 32, pp. 759–761, 1935.

[8] Moritz, A. R. and Beck, C. S.: The Production of a Collateral Circulation to the Heart. II. Pathological-Anatomical Study. Am. Heart Jour. (in press).

DISCUSSION.—DR. JOHN B. FLICK (Philadelphia, Pa.).—The experimental work of Claude Beck, in establishing a collateral vascular bed in the myocardium of animals and thus protecting the myocardium from anoxemia due to coronary occlusion, furnishes an entirely new avenue of approach in combating cardiac ischemia due to coronary artery disease in human beings.

Sir Thomas Lewis says, "The malady originally described by Heberden under the term angina pectoris is one in which pain of characteristic type occurs during effort. It is by far the commonest form of malady in which angina pain occurs. The pain may be interpreted as resulting when the blood supply to the heart, or part of the heart, is limited and consequently inadequate when the heart is called upon to do work at a certain increased rate—a condition of relative ischemia."

The operative treatment of angina pectoris first proposed by Francois Frank in 1899 and first practiced by Jonnesco in 1916 was purely symptomatic and was not intended to eradicate the disease. The surgical act aimed at division of the nervous arc thus preventing the patient from recognizing the symptom pain (Elliott C. Cutler). Since then various neurosurgical procedures along similar lines have been devised for the relief of cardiac

810

CARDIAC SURGERY

pain and practiced with more or less success, but they have not gained greatly in popularity, possibly because of technical difficulties and possibly because of the uncertainty of the results.

Removal of the normal thyroid gland in the treatment of heart disease was proposed by Blumgart, Lavine and Berlin and was practiced for the first time on December 14, 1932, at the Peter Bent Brigham Hospital in Boston. Strikingly beneficial results from this operation have since been obtained in the group of patients suffering from angina pectoris. The rationale of this procedure for the treatment of heart disease has its basis in the reduction of the metabolic demand on the heart by the total ablation of the thyroid gland.

Beck's operation strikes directly at the myocardial ischemia and theoretically should be beneficial where the ischemia is due to organic changes in the walls of the cardiac vessels. Experience alone can determine the place in surgery of Beck's ingenious and logical operation and he is to be congratulated upon a fine piece of work which at least has proved that a collateral circulation can be established experimentally in the myocardium of animals.

DR. ELLIOTT C. CUTLER (Boston, Mass.).—I should like to be among those who congratulate Doctor Beck upon what I know to be the end-result of a vast amount of work and a most ingenious investigation.

This morning our President spoke of our job as one of keeping Nature from taking us away before our time, but I wonder whether we should apply our energies to people as young as forty, as suggested by Doctor Cheever. I had the opportunity to see Doctor Beck's first patient as he was recovering from the operation and the ordeal did not seem unusual.

It is certain that the attack proposed by Doctor Beck and the physiologic background for this procedure are much more admirable, much better suited and far more certain to hold hope for ultimate good than any procedure yet proposed for those cardiac disorders that have as beginnings and cause ischemia of the myocardium.

Whether one is to turn in muscle flaps which many of us have tried in other conditions without much success, whether one is to use the fat about the pericardium, or whatever the actual method of establishing the collateral circulation is to be, it is certain that the understanding of what seems necessary and which Doctor Beck has attempted to carry out in these experiments constitute the most logical attempt that has ever been suggested.

The difficulty, of course, is going to be the same as we all have found in other conditions, now that ingenuity of the surgeon has brought us so far apace, *i.e.*, to convince our medical colleagues that our undertakings are desirable, or perhaps educate them to help us choose which case is desirable for the definite procedure.

Knowing how in this country surgery of the pericardium has lagged behind such surgery elsewhere, partly because of the attitude of our internists, one can imagine the difficulties in this field of choosing the proper case of arteriosclerotic heart disease, angina or hypertensive heart disease, as the one best suited for such procedure. I have no doubt if Doctor Beck keeps at it, and he fortunately has a group of medical colleagues who are interested and will help him, he will be able to tell us in a few years which form of heart disease is best suited and most likely to be relieved by this procedure.

I think we should all congratulate him sincerely for an admirable piece of work.

DR. W. F. RIENHOFF, JR. (Baltimore, Md.).—Independently and without any knowledge of Doctor Beck's experiments, or interest in this problem, we

811

Annals of Surgery
November, 1935

began in October, 1934, investigating different methods of supporting an interrupted coronary circulation. We have used a series of old dogs for the reason that the independent development of a collateral circulation in younger animals is so readily achieved that recovery from ligation of the right or left anterior descending coronary artery may be clinically uneventful and easily survived by the animal. Doctor Beck did not state whether his series of dogs were young or old. In the older dogs, in our experience, ligation of the left anterior descending branch of the left coronary artery almost always resulted in either ventricular fibrillation or a marked arrhythmia. Ligation of the left coronary artery before departure of the circumflex resulted invariably in ventricular fibrillation. In a small series of nine dogs, Dr. E. Cowles Andrus, Dr. August Jonas and myself obtained electrocardiographic studies before beginning the experiment, and used only those animals in whom the electrocardiograms were normal. Under ether anesthesia, an incision was made in the fifth interspace on the left side exposing the pericardial sac which latter was opened. The central tendon of the diaphragm was then incised and the omentum drawn up into the left thoracic cavity. The epicardium was then moistened with half strength iodine and the omentum wrapped, so to speak, completely about the heart, entirely covering the anterior surface. To insure maintaining this position the omentum was fastened to the epicardium by two interrupted fine silk sutures. The pericardial sac was not closed but the hiatus in the central tendon of the diaphragm was pulled snug about the omentum. After this cardio-omentopexy had been performed, Doctor Andrus found the type of electrocardiographic curve present, suggested a coronary occlusion. Whether this alteration in the electrical reaction of the dog's heart was due to the small amount of iodine painted on the epicardium or whether it was due to the two stitches placed in the heart wall, away from the coronary vessels, was not determined. Three to six weeks later, ligation of the entire left coronary artery just below its origin from the aorta and above the division into the left anterior descending and circumflex arteries was accomplished by taking a deep bite with a French No. 2 needle in the ventricular wall in the region of the left coronary artery just beneath the tip of the left auricle. The distension of the coronary veins distal to the ligature proved its location. No disturbance in cardiac rhythm followed these ligations after previously performed cardio-omentopexy, either clinically or in the electrocardiogram. The dogs were not at all ill and were up and around their cages the next day. Whereas before similar ligation was invariably fatal, not one animal succumbed after adhesion of the omentum to the heart had been produced. At the second operation extensive adhesions were revealed to have occurred between the omentum and the heart wall. These bled profusely when slightly separated. The electrocardiograph remained the same following the first and second operative procedures. In other words, ligation of the entire left coronary vessel in this series of old dogs was relatively inconsequential when the coronary circulation was properly supported by an outside source of blood supply. We are in the process of sacrificing and injecting our specimens. Carmine gelatin was used for the coronary circulation, being injected in the aorta. This solution will not go beyond the arterioles and thus will not fill the capillary bed in the myocardium. No injection mass entered the cavities of the heart and therefore the thebesian vessels were not injected. Prussian blue mass was injected into the celiac axis, thus filling the omental vessels. This mass will fill the capillary bed and in the as yet incompletely cleared specimens, seems to have penetrated the capillary branches of the coronary system.

Volume 102
Number 5 CARDIAC SURGERY

These specimens will be reported on later. We have not entertained the hope that this procedure of cardio-omentopexy will be clinically applicable except possibly in such cases of coronary thrombosis that might be seen at an early stage of the interruption of the coronary circulation.

Dr. J. Shelton Horsley (Richmond, Va.).—Is there not some difference between the circulation of the blood from the omentum and that from the pectoral muscle? According to the procedure described by Doctor Beck the pectoral muscles were severed near their insertion, and a portion of the muscle turned onto the heart. This would, of course, involve destroying the nerve supply to the pectoral muscles, with consequent atrophy of the muscle and diminution of its blood supply, even if no vessels had been actually injured when the muscle was divided. The omentum, however, when brought up to the heart would suffer no trophic changes, and consequently circulation would not be impaired by such conditions as beset the pectoral muscles when they are divided near their insertion.

Doctor Beck.—The second patient upon whom we carried out our operation died one week later. A thrombus developed at the bifurcation of the aorta and occluded the left common iliac artery. The ischemia of the leg was very painful and the patient died within several hours. The thrombus developed at the site of an atheromatous ulcer of the abdominal aorta. The coronary arteries showed extensive and marked sclerosis. The right coronary artery was completely occluded about 14 Mm. from its ostium. The lumina of the ramus descendens and of the ramus circumflexus of the left coronary artery were markedly constricted but not completely occluded. The myocardium of the right ventricle showed extensive replacement by fat. There was no evidence of infarction in the left ventricle. The pedicle grafts of skeletal muscle and the adjacent fat and pericardium were adherent to the myocardium and for the present at least I am satisfied with this part of the operation.

In our experience ligation of the ramus circumflexus of the left coronary artery in one stage had a high mortality, even though a collateral vascular bed had been provided for the heart. Ligation in two stages is usually successful. This statement applies to the right and to either major branch of the left coronary artery.

The pedicle grafts of skeletal muscle brought in from the chest wall are deprived of some of their normal blood supply. We know, however, that the body has a great capacity to develop blood vessels and in our experiments we obtained excellent anastomoses between the vessels of cardiac muscle and of skeletal muscle. We used omentum in a number of experiments. Anastomoses between the coronary bed and the vessels of the omentum can be obtained. I am doubtful whether omentum could be used on a human patient because the opening in the diaphragm complicates the operative procedure. Experience may alter this point of view.

The Bristol
Medico-Chirurgical Journal

" Scire est nescire, nisi id me
Scire alius sciret."

SUMMER, 1937.

THE CAREY COOMBS MEMORIAL LECTURE

DELIVERED AT A MEETING OF THE SOCIETY
ON WEDNESDAY, MAY 5th, 1937.

THE PRESIDENT (Dr. R. C. CLARKE)
in the Chair.

BY

LAURENCE O'SHAUGHNESSY, F.R.C.S.,

Consultant Surgeon to the Lambeth Cardiovascular Clinic
(L.C.C.), London.

ON

THE PATHOLOGY AND SURGICAL TREATMENT
OF CARDIAC ISCHÆMIA.

IN the first place I should like to express my gratitude for the opportunity of delivering this lecture. It is quite clearly a lecture which could better be delivered by many more competent authorities than myself; for it is a lecture in memory of a great physician who

I

---

spent his active life in the study of cardiovascular disease, while I have merely laboured on the fringes of the subject, and that only of recent years.

I was already familiar with some of Coombs's writings, and it has been a most welcome task during the last few weeks to review in closer detail those which I had not previously read. It soon became apparent to me that many of the more significant aspects of his work could not be dealt with in this lecture. There was his discovery of the " submiliary nodule " in rheumatic carditis, his important contributions to the pathology and treatment of rheumatism, and his valuable work on its social and economic importance. There was also his very beautiful and detailed description of some of the rarer manifestations of cardiovascular disease — I refer especially to his important paper on abnormalities of the pulmonary artery. However, on reading his Lumleian Lecture for 1930 I was struck by the accuracy with which the pathology of cardiac ischæmia was described, and in some of his other papers I have looked for further evidence of his views on coronary disease, a subject which is relevant to our work in the Lambeth Cardiovascular Clinic. I mean to show very briefly how his views have been confirmed and amplified by subsequent clinical and experimental work.

Anginal pain is common to all types of cardiac ischæmia, and in 1930 the " aortic " theory of cardiac pain, of which Sir Clifford Allbutt had been so able an exponent, had still its strong adherents. Coombs however asserted that anginal pain originated in the heart itself, for he had observed that the anginal pain

---

of syphilitic aortitis differed in no way from the angina associated with generalized atheroma of the coronary tree ; and while it might well be that the aortic plexus could be involved in aortitis, this was clearly not the case in coronary sclerosis. The one factor common to all types of coronary insufficiency was a defective supply of oxygen to the myocardial cells, and Coombs therefore considered that interference with cell metabolism caused cardiac pain. There is much recent work to support this view—the clinical researches of Sir Thomas Lewis may be cited.

In syphilitic coronary insufficiency there is a normal peripheral coronary tree—a very beautiful injection specimen prepared by Dr. Bruce Perry illustrates this particular point in the lecture; but as Coombs himself expressed it, the coronary blood supply is strangled at its source, for the orifices of the vessels are obstructed, and in addition loss of the normal elasticity of the wall of the aorta, together with deformity in varying degree of the aortic valves, disturbs the normal mechanism by which blood is fed to the coronary tree. In coronary atheroma Coombs believed that it was loss of the elasticity of the coronary vessels which rendered them incapable of those subtle variations which adequate function of this vital segment of the vascular tree demands. Loss of elasticity in its most extreme form is, of course, seen in calcification of the coronary vessels. It was from this type of cardiac ischæmia that John Hunter died. Coombs had seen coronary thrombosis occur as a complication of coronary atheroma, and he appreciated to the full the part which some incidental infection, especially of the respiratory tract, may play in

---

determining the moment at which an actual deposit of clot on some roughened area of the vessel wall may cause complete obstruction of its lumen.

The anginal pain of severe anæmia Coombs explained on the grounds that here, although distribution of the blood supply to the heart could proceed normally, the fluid supplied was incapable of providing the myocardium with that rich oxygen supply which under all conditions normal cardiac action requires.

The most striking evidence of the importance of cardiac ischæmia as a common factor in a variety of heart affections has been provided by Büchner, Weber and Haager. Their monograph contains a careful record of forty-three fatal cases of cardiac ischæmia and correlation of the clinical findings, including, of course, electrocardiographic studies, with the post-mortem appearances both macroscopic and microscopic. Although in many of their cases anginal pain was a prominent symptom this was not invariable, and in some cases dyspnœa on attempted exertion, recurrent attacks of pulmonary œdema or attacks of congestive heart failure provided the evidence for impaired cardiac function. The problem of the ischæmic heart, which may progress even to the point of perforation of an infarct without pain, is one of the most fascinating in cardio-vascular pathology, and it may be that its solution lies in more systematic examination of the autonomic nervous system in such cases. Their series includes obvious cases of coronary thrombosis in an otherwise normal coronary tree, thrombosis complicating atheroma of the coronary arteries, cases of hypertensive heart failure with gross atheroma of the tree but no actual obstruction, fatal cases of syphilitic aortitis when only the orifices of the coronary vessels were affected, and even one or two cases of heart failure following chronic bronchitis and emphysema in the presence of coronary atheroma. In all this group of cases there were characteristic electrocardiograms, and at autopsy careful examination of the heart revealed pathological changes in the myocardium. After obstruction of a main coronary artery gross evidence of an old or recent infarct was invariably present, and in other cases, where no actual block of the circuit was present but merely a general impairment of its lumen, scattered areas of recent necrosis or old fibrosis could invariably be detected by serial sections.

As Coombs pointed out, there is one condition in which angina may be a prominent symptom despite normal coronary arteries, and this is severe anæmia. Büchner in his ingenious experiments provided a rational explanation of this apparent inconsistency. He produced an intense anæmia in his rabbits by hæmorrhage and then set them to work on a treadmill. His animals died, and at autopsy multiple areas of necrosis were found scattered throughout the myocardium—a familiar finding in coronary obstruction in man. He obtained similar results if he reduced the oxygen-carrying capacity of the blood by inducing a state of carbon-monoxide poisoning, and thus the obvious fact that anoxæmia of the cardiac muscle is the determining cause of death in cardiac ischæmia received experimental confirmation.

Under some conditions coronary occlusion is a fatal event, but the organism is often in a position to

effect a remarkable degree of natural compensation, so that even successive attacks of coronary thrombosis may be survived and sometimes an astonishing degree of normal activity may be regained in the interval, sometimes years in extent, between the initial and the second attack. Natural compensation is especially favoured, as Sir Clifford Allbutt long ago pointed out, if the process of coronary obliteration is one of slow onset; but even in Chiari's famous case of embolus of the right coronary artery (one of the few *clear* records in the literature of coronary embolism as distinct from thrombosis) his patient survived this insult for two days, when a second embolism of the left coronary artery abruptly terminated his life.

Natural compensation for occlusion of the coronary tree may be effected in several ways. Although it seems quite possible that there may be subtle compensatory mechanisms of which we know nothing, the mechanism of at least some of them is clear, and the following possibilities for the provision of an alternative blood supply exist :—

1. Anastomoses between the right and left coronary arteries may come into action when one or other main trunk is occluded.

2. The Thebesian vessels may act as an additional source of cardiac nutrition.

3. The natural collateral channels which connect the coronary tree with the vasa vasorum of the great vessels may become more pronounced.

4. The heart may acquire a new and additional blood supply if it adheres to the parietal pericardium.

1. *Inter-coronary Anastomoses.*

The free communications between the branches of the right and left coronary arteries, which were first effectively demonstrated in the exquisite preparations of Spalteholz, probably constitute the most important compensatory mechanism in cardiac ischæmia. That mechanism is effective in diffuse obstruction of the tree (athero-sclerosis and arterio-sclerosis), and it must play an essential part when actual occlusion of one of the main trunks (right coronary, descending branch of the left coronary, or circumflex) occurs. At the same time occlusion of a main trunk, whether it is sudden or gradual, is followed by an infarct of the heart wall. An explanation of the apparent inconsistency between the anatomical researches of Spalteholz and the effect of coronary occlusion as seen in the experimental animal or the living patient is provided by the ingenious experiments of Crainicianu. Crainicianu perfused the coronary trees of human hearts shortly after death under carefully-controlled conditions of pressure and temperature. He was able to show that the total volume of fluid perfused in a given time could be modified by experimental ligature of various branches of the tree, and also that the volume flow in a given time was less in hearts that were the seat of coronary disease. As he very reasonably points out, this method of examination will reveal what may be termed " physiological " obstruction in the capillary bed which histological examination may fail to demonstrate.

The degree of natural compensation by this means in an acute case of coronary occlusion probably depends, as in cases of peripheral vascular occlusion,

on the restoration of an optimum blood-pressure, relaxation of any spasm in those portions of the coronary circuit still patent, and localization rather than extension of the thrombus ; for an extending thrombosis will occlude side branches of the affected vessel and militate against the formation of a collateral circulation.

2. *The Thebesian Vessels.*

The Thebesian vessels are small channels which connect all four chambers of the heart with the venous and capillary bed of the coronary tree. Their morphology has been demonstrated in injection studies by Grant and Viko and by Wearn. The exact part played by these vessels in compensation for cardiac ischæmia is unknown, but there is some recent work which suggests that it may be an important one. Slater and Kornblum record a remarkable case of mitral stenosis complicated by bilateral coronary occlusion, in which good compensation was maintained at least for a time, and they suggest that the altered pressure relationship within the heart owing to the mitral lesion may have made the Thebesian circulation abnormally efficient. Leary and Wearn report two cases of syphilitic aortitis with bilateral coronary occlusion which seemed to have had good compensation, and suggest that in these patients the Thebesian vessels must have been of service. Nevertheless, these patients died of heart failure, and there is no pathological evidence to suggest that the Thebesian vessels can in any way replace the normal coronary circulation, although the possibility remains that they may assist in compensation for a defective circulation.

3. *The Natural Collateral Channels of the Coronary Tree.*

Minute arteries which connect the coronary arterial tree with the vasa vasorum of the aorta and the pulmonary artery were first demonstrated by Langer. He also found that material injected into the coronary tree could be recognized in the vessels of the mediastinum and the diaphragm, and even lying far out in the lung under the bronchial mucosa. An occasional and very interesting finding was the presence of a minute artery taking origin in the aorta some distance above the sinus of Valsalva and pursuing an independent course to ramify on the basal region of the heart. Langer's findings have been confirmed by more recent work, but few observations appear in the literature as to the state of these vessels in persons dead of cardiac ischæmia. Von Redwitz, however, noted in some of his exhaustive post-mortems the presence of a network of small vessels at the root of the aorta and pulmonary artery.

4. *The Formation of New Extra-Cardial Anastomoses.*

The heart can only acquire a new collateral blood supply if partial or complete destruction of the epicardium takes place, so that an adhesion may form between the heart and the parietal pericardium. This important mechanism is only available in those rare cases when the victim of coronary occlusion has previously suffered obliteration of his pericardial space as a result of an old pericarditis, or when following a coronary occlusion an actual infarct is produced with its base on the epicardial surface of the heart.

Examples of this extreme degree of natural

compensation are very rare, but since Sternberg first recorded the syndrome of pericarditis epistenocardica there have been other reports of angina complicated by pericarditis with a favourable immediate outcome. Sternberg's patient was a man of 48 who suffered a coronary thrombosis, and in whom a clinical diagnosis of pericarditis was made by auscultation. He made a good recovery, and returned to active life for two years before dying of heart failure. At autopsy a large cardiac aneurysm was found adherent to the parietal pericardium. Mönckeberg cites other similar instances. One of these, a case published by Fujinami, is very striking. Sir Clifford Allbutt recorded the case of a doctor who suffered a severe attack of angina pectoris, after which he was bedridden for some time, and during his illness pericardial friction was detected. He recovered and returned to active practice. The opposite picture was presented by two cases of cardiac aneurysm of which I had personal experience. So far as can be determined the site of vascular obstruction was the same as in the cases cited, but in neither case had pericardial adhesions formed. One patient died from progressive heart failure and the other from hæmo-pericardium following perforation of the aneurysm into the pericardial sac a few months after the initial attack.

It is true that this type of compensation is available only to a small number of cases of coronary thrombosis. White only found it present eight times in 62 cases, and in Parkinson's and Bedford's 83 autopsies on coronary occlusion there were 11 cases of pericarditis, and in 100 cases examined clinically pericardial friction was only heard in 7. On the other hand, in Coombs's

series of 148 cases of coronary thrombosis he detected pericardial friction on forty-two occasions; and although it was his opinion that the immediate mortality was higher in these cases, it would appear from his figures that the subsequent course of those patients who did survive was rather more favourable than in the other group. Of course, his period of observation had been short, and in view of the importance which this question has now assumed it would be of extreme interest to know the course run by his group of patients during the last five years.

Despite their comparative rarity, there is every indication of the practical importance of these adhesions when they are present. Wearn and his associates carried out injection studies on the human cadaver, and could demonstrate a vascular connection between the coronary tree and the parietal pericardium when adhesions were present. I was concerned in a case in which pericardectomy was carried out for *concretio cordis.* The patient died some three months later, and in the interval, although the mechanical relief afforded by the operation was demonstrated in a reduction of her ascites and venous pressure, an unusual type of cardiac irregularity had developed. After death histological examination showed scattered areas of necrosis and fibrosis in part of the auricular wall, from which the adherent pericardium had been stripped.

It is interesting to speculate on the relation of these natural reparative processes to the prognosis of the various types of cardiac ischæmia.

An established case of syphilitic aortitis should theoretically be of the greatest disadvantage, for here

intercoronary anastomoses can be of little service if the orifices of both vessels are occluded, endarteritis of the vasa vasorum of the aorta and pulmonary artery is likely to render them less efficient as collateral channels, the heart remains free in the pericardium, and therefore additional collaterals cannot reach it, and so the only mode of compensation remaining is a rather doubtful Thebesian supply.

The gradual development of diffuse atheroma of the coronary tree should enable compensation to be established through the natural collateral channels, but unless a frank coronary thrombosis occurs late in the disease an infarct cannot form, and there is no chance of the natural acquisition of a new blood supply.

THE TECHNIQUE OF CARDIO-OMENTOPEXY.

The following description illustrates one of the methods we have worked out at the Buckston Browne Farm Laboratory of the Royal College of Surgeons of England and in the Lambeth Cardio-vascular Clinic, by which the processes of natural compensation may be initiated and supplemented by operation.

After suitable premedication general anæsthesia is induced and maintained with the Tiegel-Henle apparatus, which supplies oxygen under positive pressure together with vaporized ether. With the patient on his back, the chest is entered through an incision along the fifth intercostal space extending from the midline to the anterior axillary line. The fifth and sixth costal cartilages are divided near the sternum after the manner of Kirschner and by

THE CAREY COOMBS MEMORIAL LECTURE   121

the use of a large Sauerbruch intercostal retractor the pericardium is exposed. The phrenic nerve is identified and crushed with a hæmostat, and once this has been done the pressure in the anæsthetic apparatus is reduced (from 10 to 6 cm. of water) and the table is tilted to the right. As a result of these manœuvres the left leaf of the diaphragm appears in the operation field, and after the insertion of two sutures the muscle is incised. The abdomen is then explored through the diaphragmatic incision ; a suitable portion of the omentum is obtained and brought through into the chest. The wound in the diaphragm is then closed by suture. The table is brought back to its original position, the degree of inflation of the lung is again increased, and the heart, covered by the pericardium, is once more in view. With caution the pericardium is incised and the graft is attached to the surface of the heart and to the edges of the pericardium by suture with fine linen thread. Finally the chest wound is closed in layers in the usual way.

CASE HISTORY.

A missionary's widow, aged 65, had led a strenuous life for many years in high altitudes. Angina pectoris for twelve years : attacks had become more frequent and more severe, and she had been almost confined to bed for over eighteen months, being finally unable even to wash herself. (A sister had angina.) She was referred to the clinic by Dr. L. Lyne, of Hove, and was admitted on 1st October. Examination : very obese ; heart enlarged to anterior axillary line ; soft aortic systolic murmur and very short diastolic whiff ; radiogram confirmed cardiac enlargement ; B.P. 247/117 ; no œdema ; electrocardiogram showed complete bundle-branch block with large amplitude of Q R S complexes in leads I and III.

122   MR. LAURENCE O'SHAUGHNESSY

After ten days' treatment with general massage, starch free diet, and administration of theamine and amytal, cardio-omentopexy was performed at Lambeth Hospital on 16th October, 1936, with the assistance of Dr. Mansell and Dr. Berry under general anæsthesia by Dr. Hasler. Aleuronat was injected into the pericardial sac and at the site of graft. At the end of operation the pulse-rate was 69, the B.P. 170/90, and the electrocardiogram showed no change. Recovery was interrupted by a paroxysm of auricular fibrillation, which began 30 hours after operation and ceased spontaneously 9½ hours later. There were two anginal attacks during the first fortnight and none subsequently. General massage was begun after five weeks, and she was allowed to wash herself. In six weeks the blood-pressure had returned to 240/112 and was causing symptoms. She is now getting up daily for one to two hours and has kept free of angina. On a balanced diet the blood-pressure has fallen to 210/120. Physical signs of pulmonary collapse have been present at the left base since operation. The electrocardiogram shows no change.

She was allowed gradually to increase her activities, and was eventually discharged to St. Benedict's Hospital on 3rd February, 1937. From the time that she was treated with five grains of quinidine sulphate daily there was only one more brief paroxysm of auricular fibrillation. Her progress at St. Benedict's Hospital was uninterrupted, and she was discharged from there on 18th March. When last seen on 23rd April she was complaining of no symptoms except painful feet. She was able to climb stairs and to go out to church, shopping, etc., and was quite free from anginal pain. She proposed to go home to Hove on 26th April. Her systolic blood-pressure was 220.

In the course of our operations we have made some incidental observations which may be of interest. It is, of course, no new thing for the surgeon to expose and operate on the human heart. Since Rehn demonstrated the possibility of operation for cardiac wounds in 1897

THE CAREY COOMBS MEMORIAL LECTURE   123

such interventions have become almost commonplace. Before the operation of cardio-omentopexy was devised, although I had exposed and operated on a very large number of animal hearts, my experience of cardiac surgery (as distinct from the surgery of the pericardium) in man had been limited to one or two interventions for stab-wounds, and the dramatic attendant circumstances left me little time for deliberate inspection. In any event the victims of cardiac wounds do not as a rule have diseased hearts.

During our operations we have had occasion to recognize one essential difference between hypertrophy and dilatation of the heart, for in dilatation the coronary vessels are unduly prominent, being forced out from the interventricular sulcus, and we now know that it is necessary to treat such a heart with special care. We have also seen the various types of pericardium—the tense sac over a true hypertrophy which is difficult to incise lest the heart itself be wounded, the slack pericardium over a heart of normal size, and the rather delicate pericardium enclosing a serous effusion. We have also had what is perhaps the unique experience of exposing the heart in a patient suffering from heart block, when we observed cardiac contractions proceed at the rate of 36.

We have also been struck by the greater vascularity of the structures which surround the heart in man as contrasted with the lower animals. The pericardium itself is often highly vascular, and the inferior sternopericardial ligament, insignificant both in the cadaver and in the experimental animal, has been a prominent and richly vascular structure in most of our patients. It is reasonable to suppose that man is under

124   MR. LAURENCE O'SHAUGHNESSY

a greater necessity to develop his defences against cardiac ischæmia than are the lower animals, and I have previously pointed out that cardio-omentopexy, as well as bringing a new blood supply into direct relationship with the ischæmic area and the coronary tree, serves to reinforce the normal collaterals in the mediastinum and to give them access to the heart.

CONCLUSION.

In the present state of knowledge it is impossible to lay down any rigid indications for surgical intervention in cardiac ischæmia. From a consideration of the pathology of the various cardiac disorders it is clear that ischæmia plays an important rôle in many and a dominant rôle in some, and in the Lambeth Clinic we have demonstrated that surgical intervention is practicable and relatively safe, even under rather unfavourable circumstances. Our patients have included a man of 72 and a bed-ridden woman of 65. We are not neglecting the obvious factor of arterial spasm in angina pectoris, but we maintain that spasm is only significant when coronary disease is present. In the laboratory we have paid considerable attention to the nervous factor in coronary obstruction—I am most grateful to Professor Leriche, of Strasbourg, for the personal explanation of his views—and in certain cases we are prepared for operative intervention on the autonomic nervous system.

The selection of patients for operation is in the hands of the medical staff of the Lambeth Cardio-vascular Clinic—Lord Dawson of Penn, Dr. Dan T. Davies, and Dr. H. E. Mansell. We have only operated on a relatively small proportion of the cases sent to us,

THE CAREY COOMBS MEMORIAL LECTURE   125

and in the present stage of the work we have felt it advisable to restrict our interventions to the most severe cases.

In one of his papers Coombs pleaded for the exact correlation of anatomical examination with the clinical findings. At Lambeth we are for the first time able to correlate our clinical findings with what the late Lord Moynihan so well described as the " pathology of the living," and while our researches are only at their beginning, and are in no sense comparable in volume or importance to the vast output which was Coombs's own contribution to cardiology, it may be that in some measure we shall reap where he and other of the great cardiologists have sown.

REFERENCES.

Allbutt, Sir Clifford, *Diseases of the Arteries*, vol. 2. London: Macmillan, 1915.

Büchner, Franz und Walter v. Lucadou, *Beitr. z. Path. Anat.*, 1934, 93, 165.

Büchner, F., Weber, B., Haager, B., *Koronarinfarkt und Koronarinsuffizienz*. Leipzig: Georg Thieme, 1935.

Chiari, H., *Prag. Med. Wochsch.*, 1897, 22, 61.

Coombs, C. F., *Rheumatic Heart Disease*. Bristol: John Wright, 1924; *Lancet*, 1927, i. 579, 634; Clarke, R. C. et. al., *Quart. J. Med.*, 1927, 21, 51; *Bristol Med.-Chir. J.*, 1927, 144, 249; *Proc. Royal Soc. Med.*, 1928, 21, 727; *Quart. J. Med.*, 1930, 23, 233; *Lancet*, 1930, ii. 227, 281, 333, Aug. 2, 9, 16 (Lumleian Lecture); *Brit. J. Surg.*, 1930, 18, 326; *Bristol Med.-Chir. J.*, 1931, 48, 179; *Quart. J. Med.*, 1932, i. (New Series) 179.

Crainicianu, A., *Virchow's Arch. für Path. Anat.*, 1922, 238, 1.

Fujinami, A., *Virchow's Arch. für Path. Anat.*, 1906, 159, 447.

Grant, P. T., and Viko, L. E., *Heart*, 1929, 15, 103.

Langer, *Bericht d. K. Akad. d. Wissensch.*, Wien, 1880.

Leary, T., and Wearn, J. T., *Amer. Heart J.*, 1930, 5, 412.

Leriche, R., Macewen Memorial Lecture for 1934, Glasgow University, No. 35.

Lewis, Sir Thomas, *Arch. of Int. Med.*, 1932, 49, 713–727.

Mönckeberg, J. G., *Die Erkrankungen des Myocardiums und des spezifischen Muskelsystems, im Handbuch der speziellen Pathologischen Anatomie und Histologie*, F. Henke and O. Lubarsch, Springer, Berlin, 1934.

Moritz, A. R., Hudson, C. L., and Orgren, E. C., *Jour. Expt. Med.*, 1932, 56, 919.

Parkinson, J., and Bedford, D. E., *Heart*, 1928, 14, 194.

von Redwitz, E., *Virchow's Arch. für Path. Anat.*, 1909, 197, 433.

Rehn, L., *Verhand. d. Gesellsch. d. Naturforscher, und Aerzte.*, 1896.

Slater, R., and Kornblum, D., *Jour. Amer. Med. Assoc.*, January, 1934.

Spalteholz, Werner, *Die Arterien der Herzwand*. Leipzig: S. Hirzel, 1924.

Sternberg, M., *Wiener Med. Wchschr.*, 1910, 60, 14.

INTERNAL MAMMARY CORONARY ANASTOMOSIS IN THE SURGICAL TREATMENT OF CORONARY ARTERY INSUFFICIENCY*

Arthur Vineberg, M.D. and Gavin Miller, M.D.

Montreal, Que.

THIS paper constitutes a preliminary report of clinical cases which have undergone transplantation of the left internal mammary artery into the left ventricle as a treatment for coronary artery insufficiency. The theoretical and experimental basis on which this procedure is based will be briefly described.

Experimental Data

Many attempts have been made experimentally to improve ventricular myocardial circulation such as, the application of fat or muscle grafts to the heart, the use of irritating foreign bodies such as talc, or asbestos fibres to produce adhesions between pericardium and myocardium. Fauteux[1] attempted to improve the myocardial circulation by cardiac vein ligation and Beck[2] by means of arterialization of the coronary sinus. One of us (A.V.) has attempted to obtain this improvement by the direct implantation of a living artery, namely the left internal mammary artery into the left ventricular myocardium. The artery is placed within a tunnel in the myocardium and in over 200 experiments the degree and frequency of new anastomoses have been experimentally proved by injection studies, radio-graphs, plastic casts and serial sections.[3, 4] Anastomosis occurred in 50 to 75% of these animals, depending on the technique of implantation used. No animal developed infarction or died following anterior descending branch ligation when a large anastomosis had developed. All these experiments have been controlled and the control group, without implantation of a living vessel into the heart muscle, showed a mortality of 90%, and in 10% a large infarction developed following the same ligation of the anterior descending branch.[5, 6] (It is recognized that thrombosis of the anterior descending branch of the left coronary artery is the most common cause of death in human coronary artery disease.)

The anastomoses which developed have been shown both by injection and by histological serial section to be true arterial branches. It has been reported by Glenn[7] that these branches only live for 8 weeks. Our observations have definitely shown that they last at least 58 weeks which is the longest observation made before the animal was sacrificed to confirm the persistence of these vessels.[8] The direction of blood flow through the implanted internal mammary artery was studied in order to determine whether or not blood was being brought to the ventricular myocardium through the internal mammary artery. Direct determination of blood flow in the internal mammary artery was difficult, so the indirect method was used. Animals which survived anterior descending branch ligation of the left coronary artery were subjected after 4 weeks to complete and sudden occlusion of the implanted internal mammary artery. If the internal mammary artery was maintaining the circulation of the left ventricle then, following its ligation, either death or infarction should result. This is exactly what happened. In three animals with an internal mammary implant that had survived anterior descending branch ligation, the internal mammary artery was ligated. One animal died within 24

* From the Department of Surgery, Royal Victoria Hospital and the Department of Experimental Surgery, McGill University, Montreal, P.Q.

Canad. M. A. J.
Mar. 1951, vol. 64 VINEBERG AND MILLER: CORONARY DISEASE 205

hours and displayed an œdematous cyanotic area of the anterior wall of the left ventricle. One survived for 3 days before dying from a large infarct in the same location. The 3rd animal survived, but examination of the sacrificed specimen revealed that multiple intercoronary anastomoses were present.

The experimental results just described were obtained by implanting the internal mammary artery into normal dogs' hearts. It was suggested that in human coronary insufficiency such a procedure would be of little value because of the presence of occluded coronary vessels and associated myocardial ischæmia. It was, therefore, decided to experimentally produce coronary artery insufficiency in the dog. This was done by wrapping the origin of the anterior descending branch of the left coronary artery with a sclerosing type of cellophane.[9] The cellophane surrounding the origin of the anterior descending branch of the left coronary artery set up a periarterial fibroplasia which resulted in a gradual contraction through scar tissue of the coronary artery with narrowing of its lumen. This caused a reduction in blood flow through the narrowed vessel, and resulted in ischæmia of the left ventricular muscle supplied by the anterior descending branch of the left coronary artery. The degree of myocardial ischæmia was evaluated by estimating the exercise tolerance of the animal on a motorized treadmill. Before the cellophane wrap was placed around the coronary artery the animals would run 9 to 12 minutes at 8½ miles per hour on the treadmill. With this amount of exercise the animals became tired, began to lag on the mill and would break alternatively from a gallop to a run. Eventually they would become anxious to escape the mill. When the exercise was discontinued these animals would pant, but would drink water and appear similar to any other normal dog after exercise. Five months after these animals had had a piece of cellophane wrapped around their anterior descending branch of the left coronary artery they would run for 1 6/10 minutes on the treadmill before becoming extremely anxious, begin to whine and salivate profusely. If the exercise was not terminated they would attempt to lie down or drag their feet on the revolving platform. When the mill was stopped they would drop where they stood and resist all coaxing to move for some minutes and would not drink water. Animals that had reached this stage were then subjected to a left internal mammary artery implant. Four months after the implant those animals which had definitely developed an internal mammary coronary anastomosis had a return of exercise tolerance to 7 minutes or more. This occurred in spite of a completely occluded anterior descending branch of the left coronary artery. When an internal mammary coronary anastomosis failed to develop there was no improvement in exercise tolerance in such animals after implantation.

Because of these experimental results it was thought that implantation of the internal mammary artery into the left ventricular myocardium might be of value in the treatment of human cases of coronary artery insufficiency.

HUMAN CASES OF CORONARY ARTERY INSUFFICIENCY TREATED BY INTERNAL MAMMARY ARTERY TRANSPLANT

Selection of cases.—The estimation of clinical results is always difficult and the results of any given surgical procedure may vary according to the severity of the disease process at the time of operation. There are certain well-known pathological facts concerning coronary artery sclerosis and thrombosis which greatly influence the selection of cases for internal mammary artery implant. Perhaps the most important is the fact that coronary artery sclerosis in general is confined to the first 3 or 4 cm. of the coronary artery. It has been stated that arteries beyond the first 3 or 4 cm. of the coronary vessels show lesser degrees of sclerosis and rarely is sclerosis seen after the 3rd or 4th order of branching. Sections have shown that in cases of severe coronary artery sclerosis the vessels lying within the heart muscle are generally free of arterial disease. Thus, an internal mammary artery placed in the ventricular muscle is placed in an area where the arteries are comparatively healthy. In this way fresh blood can be brought to the network of non-sclerosed arteries and arteries which exist beyond the points of coronary artery obstructions.

In cases of coronary artery thrombosis with myocardial infarct,[10] the picture is entirely different. In these cases, if the patient survives, an area of myocardial infarction the muscle undergoes degeneration and eventually heals by scar formation. In most cases there will be healthy muscle surrounding the area of the healed infarct. It is also stated that during the process of healing new blood vessels grow into the infarcted area; thus the history of a left coronary artery thrombosis with recovery does not constitute a contraindication to internal mammary artery implantation. The new living arteries can be placed in healthy muscle which is present at the edge of the healed infarct and, if necessary, into the intraventricular septum itself. With this in mind, it is clear that patients who have recovered from coronary artery thrombosis and infarction may be considered as candidates for an internal mammary artery transplant. Our last patient was known to have had two attacks of coronary artery thrombosis with a posterior wall infarct. At operation there was still what appeared to be good muscle posteriorly. There was, however, evidence of scarring on the posterior surface towards the apex which extended for a half inch or more to the anterior surface of the left ventricle. The internal mammary artery was placed into healthy muscle which was present just proximal to this scarred area. We have been reluctant to operate upon patients who are able to carry on their normal daily activities. We have to date only operated upon those patients who are unable to carry on because of the severity of their anginal pain. Patients with an enlarged left ventricle and myocardial decompensation have been considered poor risks and have not been accepted. Every attempt has been made to exclude other sources

206   VINEBERG AND MILLER: CORONARY DISEASE   [Canad. M. A. J.
[Mar. 1951, vol. 64

of anginal pain and to make certain that the pain from which the patient is suffering is due to coronary insufficiency. Where there is a doubt and particularly when other organic disease such as cholelithiasis exists, the associated disease has been treated first.*

Preoperative investigation.—Each patient has undergone extensive investigation in order to establish a diagnosis of coronary insufficiency and to determine its extent. A careful clinical history has been supplemented by detailed electrocardiographic studies made at rest and after exercise. In order to correlate the anginal pain with myocardial ischæmia electrocardiograms have been taken after exercise at the height of the anginal pain. A record was made on each patient as to the extent of his exercise tolerance prior to operation as indicated by the number of stairs he could climb in a given time before experiencing the onset of anginal pain.

In each patient a careful survey has been made to exclude sources of pain which were not cardiac in origin. Complete radiographic studies have been made of the œsophagus, stomach, duodenum and gallbladder, as well as of the thorax and lungs. In each case a Mosenthal test, nonprotein nitrogen, basal metabolic rate, blood cholesterol, blood sugar and hæmograms were also recorded.

CASE 1

Mr. J.P., (referred by Dr. L. I. Frohlich of Montreal) age 53, occupation, tailor. Admitted to the Royal Victoria Hospital, April 24, 1950. On admission the patient's chief complaint was that of substernal pain which radiated to the left jaw and down the left arm to the wrist. Occasionally the pain radiated to the back in the interscapular region. The pain was brought on by exertion and emotion. It was an aching, pressure type of pain, and was not very sharp. It was first noticed 14 years ago, gradually becoming more severe. The patient had been unable to work for three years prior to admission and had suffered pain day and night. Some, but not complete, relief was obtained by nitroglycerin. Exercise tolerance was limited to one city bock; walked very slowly before onset of anginal pain occurred. There was a history of 40 pounds loss of weight in the past 10 years. There was also a history of intolerance to fatty foods with eructations of gas and inability to eat a large meal.

General physical examination revealed a well nourished white male of good colour. Temperature was 98, pulse 80, respiration 20, blood pressure 120/90. There was a right, direct inguinal hernia. There were bilateral varicose veins.

Exercise tolerance test.—The patient developed pain after going up 22 steps in a 10 minute period. The electro-cardiograms, taken before and after exercise, are shown in Figs. 1 and 2 respectively. Blood and spinal fluid serology were negative. The lungs, œsophagus, stomach, duodenum and gallbladder were radio-

logically normal. Blood analysis for sugar and cholesterol were found to be within normal limits. There was no increase in white blood count or the sedimentation rate.

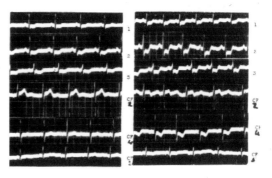

Fig. 1   **Fig. 2**

Fig. 1.—Electrocardiogram taken after 3 hours' rest in bed. A slurring of QRS complexes. Depression of S-T interval in leads 1, 2 and 3. Lead CF_2 normal. CF_4 shows a low T-wave as does CF_5. Myocardial changes with coronary insufficiency. Rate 60 per minute. **Fig. 2.**—Electrocardiogram taken at height of pain after 22 steps climbed in 10 minutes. The standard leads show a marked depression of the S-T intervals after exercise. A marked coronary insufficiency. The CF leads show a diphasic T-wave. CF_4 a negative T and a shallow negative T in CF_5. Evidence of marked coronary insufficiency. Rate 90.

Operation.—On April 28, 1950, implantation of the left internal mammary artery into the left ventricular myocardium was carried out. Prior to the commencement of the anæsthetic, the patient experienced severe substernal pain which was not relieved by two tablets of nitroglycerin. An electrocardiogram taken at this time did not show any changes indicative of coronary thrombosis. The blood pressure was unaltered so it was decided to proceed with the operation. The left thorax was entered through the 5th intercostal space by an anterolateral approach. The 4th and 5th ribs were resected subperiostally 10 cm. lateral to the sternum, including part of their cartilages. Approximately 1.5 cm. of cartilage was left in position. Procaine 1% was injected into the pericardium and was also given intravenously as a continuous drip. At this time the blood pressure, which had slowly been dropping, was recorded at 70/50. Patient was placed in the Trendelenberg position and the blood pressure returned to 90/70. The internal mammary artery was freed from the chest wall between the 4th and 6th intercostal spaces. The intercostal arteries 4th and 5th were doubly ligated with 000 catgut. The internal mammary artery was tied with cotton and severed between ligatures. The pericardium was opened. The left ventricular muscle was firm and was covered by a layer of fat. A traction

Canad. M. A. J.
Mar. 1951, vol. 64]   Vineberg and Miller: Coronary Disease   207

suture was placed in the apex of the heart. The 6th intercostal artery was cut and bled freely and was pulled with the internal mammary artery into a tunnel in the myocardium. The internal mammary artery was held in position by a traction suture which was tied about it. The entire procedure of implantation took about 3 minutes. There was little evidence of ventricular irritability or arrhythmia. The blood pressure at the time of implantation was 70/60 which quickly returned to 110/80 after the thorax was closed. The pulse rate throughout the operation was comparatively slow at about 100 per minute. The left thorax was drained. The total blood loss during operation was 260 c.c., as measured by the gravimetric method.

Postoperative course.—For the first 12 hours after operation the blood pressure remained steady at 110/72 with a pulse rate of 108 per minute. The patient was conscious and appeared clinically quite well. Gradually the blood pressure sank until 24 hours after operation it was 86/62. The pulse rate, however, had dropped to 96 per minute and the patient's general condition was excellent. He was removed from the oxygen tent and given a liquid diet. An electrocardiogram taken approximately 24 hours after operation showed anterior myocardial changes and coronary insufficiency, but the rhythm was regular, and the a-v conduction time was normal. In spite of the low blood pressure the patient's general condition remained excellent throughout the succeeding two days. At 5.54 p.m., April 30 he attempted to use the bed pan. This was followed by a rapid drop in blood pressure and elevation of pulse rate to 160 per minute. On May 1, at 12.30 a.m., chest pain developed and there was an increase of the respiration rate to 22. At 1.25 a.m. the chest pain became more severe and the condition of the patient rapidly deteriorated. He expired at 1.45 p.m.

The interval between completion of operation and death was a little over 2½ days.

Pathological Findings

The three main coronary arteries were pipe-stem in character for their first 3 or 4 cm. All the coronary arteries showed multiple areas of marked stenosis due to arteriosclerotic plaquing. The right coronary artery was completely blocked by an old, firm, greyish thrombosis. The left anterior descending branch was completely occluded for a distance of 1 cm. by a recent, soft,

dark-brown thrombosis. The anterior wall of the left ventricle and intraventricular septum showed evidence of recent infarction.

The internal mammary artery which had been implanted was patent throughout. There was no hæmatoma at the site of implant (see Fig. 3).

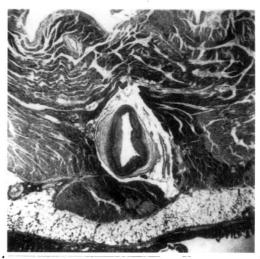

Fig. 3.—Shows the internal mammary artery lying in the human myocardium 62 hours after implantation.

Death was due to a recent thrombosis of the anterior descending branch of the left coronary artery with ventricular infarction. There was an associated atelectasis of the left lower lobe.

Case 2

Mr. D.M., age 54. Admitted to the Royal Victoria Hospital, October 22, 1950. Discharged December 5, 1950. This patient, 7 months prior to admission, developed severe precordial pains which radiated down the left arm. Pain was initiated by exercise and was associated with shortness of breath. Pain frequently followed the ingestion of solid food. This was so pronounced that for a few months prior to admission patient lived on a liquid diet. His exercise tolerance was limited to about one city block. There was a bad family history. His father and two paternal uncles died of heart disease. One brother had had coronary artery thrombosis.

Physical examination revealed a well nourished slightly obese adult male with sallow complexion and a somewhat myxœdematous appearance to his face. The abdomen was pendulous due to excessive fat. Pulse 68 to 74, temperature 98, respiration 18, blood pressure ranged between 140/100 to 106/60.

Exercise tolerance.—Fifty-six steps with 7″ elevation were climbed in 2½ minutes before pain in the precordium and left arm occurred. A control electrocardiogram taken at rest is shown in Fig. 4, and an electrocardiogram exercise taken at the height of pain is shown in Fig. 5.

Blood serology and chemistry for sugar and nonprotein nitrogen were normal. Radiographic studies of the lungs, œsophagus, stomach, duodenum and gallbladder were normal. There was no elevation of the white count or sedimentation rate. The Mosenthal test showed excellent concentration and output. The basal metabolic rate was normal.

208 VINEBERG AND MILLER: CORONARY DISEASE [Canad. M. A. J.
[Mar. 1951, vol. 64

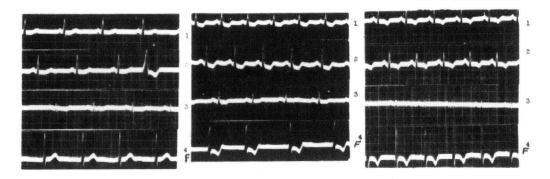

Fig. 4   Fig. 5   Fig. 6

Fig. 4.—Sinus rhythm. Normal auriculo-ventricular conduction time. QRS complexes slurred. Right ventricular extra systoles in lead II. Low voltage T-waves in all leads. Diphasic P-waves in lead III. Ventricular rate 60 per minute. Lead 4F adds nothing more. **Fig. 5.**—Regular rhythm. Normal auriculo-ventricular conduction time. QRS complexes slurred. R-T intervals depressed in leads I and II. Diphasic T-waves in lead III. Ventricular rate 90 per minute. Lead 4F shows a depressed S-T and negative T-waves. Coronary insufficiency. **Fig. 6.**—Regular rhythm. Normal auriculo-ventricular conduction time. Negative T-waves in leads I and II. QRS complexes slurred. Ventricular rate 90 per minute. Lead 4F shows an acutely inverted T-wave. The picture is that of recent anterior infarction.

Operation.—In this patient and in the subsequent case, the blood pressure was maintained throughout the operation by means of a continuous intravenous drip of neosynephrin. The blood pressure was 130/60 at the commencement of the anæsthetic and was never permitted to drop below 120/70 throughout the entire operation which lasted approximately 2½ hours. It was necessary to increase the rate of flow of neosynephrin at various times during the operation in order to prevent the blood pressure from dropping. The technique followed was approximately the same as that described in the first case, except for the approach which was made through the 5th intercostal space with severance of the 4th and 5th ribs just distal to the costal cartilages. The heart at the time of implant showed little disturbance. The blood pressure was maintained throughout. There was no fall in blood pressure during the operation such as occurred in the first patient. The anæsthetic used was cyclopropane and ether.

Postoperative convalescence.—The immediate postoperative blood pressure was well maintained and varied from 142/106 to 100/70. At the time of discharge, the blood pressure varied from 140/80 to 100/74. The pulse rate 48 hours after operation reached 120 per minute. This slowly diminished, and at time of discharge was between 80 and 90. The postoperative convalescence was essentially uneventful except for the complication of a paralytic ileus which was easily controlled by Wangensteen drainage.

There was also a diffuse pleuritis of the left thorax which gradually improved.

The patient was allowed to sit on the side of the bed on the 10th postoperative day, and was permitted to sit in a chair on the 23rd day. He was discharged to his home five weeks after operation. At the time of his discharge he was able to eat solid food and walk slowly. There was no anginal pain after eating or during walking. An electrocardiogram taken the day before discharge is shown in Fig. 6. Recent communication from this patient states that he is completely free of pain and working.

CASE 3

Mr. E.S., age 49. Admitted to the Royal Victoria Hospital, November 9, 1950. Discharged December 18, 1950. This patient, in December, 1947, developed uræmia and was extremely ill. In 1948 after playing 27 holes of golf, he experienced severe pain in his left arm which radiated to the chest. A diagnosis of left posterior branch coronary occlusion was made. Since that time he has suffered from anginal pain which radiated up his left arm to the precordial region and sternum. Occasionally, the pain went into the throat and jaw. The anginal-like pain was initiated by any change of pace. It was particularly severe on getting out of bed in the morning or on walking rapidly. It was relieved by nitroglycerin. Sometimes it was so severe that patient was forced to take demerol.

Temperature was 97.2, pulse rate varied from 112 to 90, respirations 18, blood pressure varied from 174/120 to 120/90. Physical examination was essentially normal.

Exercise tolerance.—Ninety steps were taken in 1½ minutes without increasing the pain. The pain, however, was present before starting the exercise. Control and exercise electrocardiograms are shown in Figs. 7 and 8. Blood chemistry for serum cholesterol, sugar and non-protein nitrogen were within normal limits. The basal metabolic rate, hæmogram and Mosenthal test were normal. Radiographic examination of the lungs, œsophagus, stomach, duodenum and gallbladder were normal.

Canad. M. A. J.
Mar. 1951, vol. 64] VINEBERG AND MILLER: CORONARY DISEASE

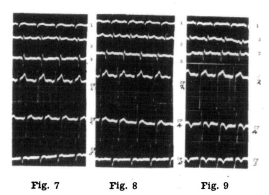

Fig. 7   Fig. 8   Fig. 9

Fig. 7.—Regular rhythm. Normal auriculo-ventricular conduction time. Left-sided preponderance. QRS complexes slurred. Q-wave in leads II and III. T-wave flattened in all standard leads. Ventricular rate 90 per minute. Leads CF₂ and 4 add nothing. CF₅ shows negative T-waves. Myocardial changes. Coronary insufficiency. **Fig. 8.**—Regular rhythm. Normal auriculo-ventricular conduction time. QRS complexes slurred; Q-waves in leads II and III. T-waves of greater voltage. Ventricular rate 90 per minute. Leads CF₂, CF₄ and CF₅ are unchanged. **Fig. 9.**—Regular rhythm. Normal A-V conduction time. Left-sided preponderance. QRS complexes slurred. Q waves in leads 2, 3. Negative T-waves with elevated S-T in lead 1. R-T elevated in lead 3. Ventricular rate 90/min. Leads CF₄ and CF₅ show an acutely negative T-wave. Anterior myocardial infarction.

Operation.—On November 20, 1950, under cyclopropane and ether, an internal mammary artery implant was carried out. The blood pressure at the commencement of the anæsthetic was 130/80, and was quite difficult to maintain before and during operation. Large amounts of neosynephrin were given in order to keep the blood pressure at approximately 130/80. A total of 4 c.c. of 1% neosynephrin was used in this case from the time the anæsthetic was commenced to the conclusion of the anæsthetic. The pulse rate at the beginning of the operation was 110 per minute. It climbed to 140 and 150 per minute and then settled down to approximately 130 per minute for the duration of the procedure. The operative technique followed was essentially the same as in the second case, except for the fact that the 5th rib and costal cartilage were removed, which facilitated exposure. The implantation of the left internal mammary artery into the myocardium of the left ventricle caused little cardiac disturbance. It should be noted here that in this case and in the second case the 6th intercostal arteries were not bleeding at the time of implant.

Postoperative convalescence.—The pulse rate reached 130 at the end of 48 hours. This slowly settled down to vary between 80 and 100 where it was at the time of his discharge. The immediate postoperative blood pressure varied between 142/100 to 100/72. This patient developed a paralytic ileus and a patch of pneumonia in the right lower lobe. Paralytic ileus was treated by means of gastric and duodenal decompression and the pneumonia with streptomycin and aureomycin. The patient was given 3 grains of quinidine before and after operation. He was permitted out of bed at the end of three weeks and returned to his home four weeks after the operation. At the time of his discharge he showed marked improvement of his anginal pectoris. There remained only a slight pain in the left wrist upon getting out of bed in the morning. This did not require nitroglycerin or demerol. The discharge electrocardiogram is shown in Fig. 9.

DISCUSSION

In our experimental work it has been shown that when the internal mammary artery is placed in the ventricular myocardium it forms new arterial branches which anastomose with the left coronary circulation. When this occurs, the heart is protected against death by infarction following the occlusion of the anterior descending branch of the left coronary artery. It has also been shown that those animals which have survived a ligation of the anterior descending branch of the left coronary artery die or develop infarction when the implanted internal mammary artery is occluded. An internal mammary coronary artery anastomosis has been shown to be of functional value. It has relieved artificially produced coronary artery insufficiency. It is reasonable to assume on the basis of our experimental work and the pathological facts of coronary artery sclerosis that an internal mammary artery implant may be of value in the treatment of human coronary artery insufficiency.

Cases have to be carefully selected and treated by a medical-surgical team, and it is our opinion that the use of quinidine pre- and post-operatively with procaine during the operation is important in preventing ventricular fibrillation. Our first patient, we believe, develped his coronary thrombosis because of the continuous low blood pressure which was present throughout the operation. In order to bring these patients through an intra-thoracic operation without further damaging their coronary artery system, we believe it is necessary to maintain their blood pressures above 100 mm. Hg. throughout the entire operative procedure.

The postoperative care of these cases is fundamentally a medical problem. Unlike other thoracic cases, these patients should not be moved frequently in the first few postoperative days. It would seem best to treat them postoperatively much in the same manner as a case of coronary artery thrombosis. Interpretation of postoperative electrocardiographs is difficult because of the disturbances created by the implantation of a pulsating artery into the anterior wall of the left myocardium. Clinically there has been no evidence of coronary artery thrombosis developing after operation in the two cases which have survived. It is too early to estimate results.

Summary

1. The internal mammary artery can be implanted in the ventricular myocardium in man with recovery.

2. There appears to be no disturbance in cardiac function resulting from the implant procedure.

3. The internal mammary artery in man, as in the animal, was found to be completely patent 62 hours after implantation in the one fatality that occurred.

4. In spite of the burying of an open vessel in the myocardium, there was no evidence of hæmorrhage or intramural hæmatoma.

5. The last two cases appear to have been improved at the time of discharge.

We wish to express our appreciation for the counsel, criticism and continued support which have been given by Drs. Lyman Duff, Donald Webster and C. A. MacIntosh. In particular do we wish to thank Dr. G. R. Brow for his careful selection of cases for operation and for his help in their postoperative care.

References

1. Fauteux, M.: *Surg., Gynec. & Obst.,* 71: 151, 1940.
2. Beck, C. S. and Tichy, V. L.: *Am. Heart J.,* 10: 849, 1935.
3. Vineberg, A. M.: *Canad. M. A. J.,* 55: 117, 1946.
4. Vineberg, A. M. and Jewett, B. L.: *Canad. M. A. J.,* 56: 609, 1947.
5. Vineberg, A. M.: *J. Thorac. Surg.,* 6: 839, 1949.
6. Vineberg, A. M. and Niloff, P. H.: *Surg., Gynec. & Obst.,* 91: 551, 1950.
7. Glenn, F. and Beal, J. M.: *Surgery,* 27: 841, 1950.
8. Vineberg, A. M., Niloff, P. H. and Miller, D.: Proc. Royal Coll. Physicians and Surgeons of Canada, Montreal, December, 1950. In Press.
9. Miller, D. and Vineberg, A. M.: Proc. of Surgical Forum, American College of Surgeons, Boston, October, 1950. In Press.

Books on Art for War-damaged Libraries.—In response to a Unesco appeal for art books and prints to war-damaged libraries, the San Francisco Museum of Art has sent material of this kind to Austria, Czechoslovakia, Germany, the Netherlands and Poland. Subscriptions to various American art periodicals have also been donated.—(UNESCO.)

The New England
Journal of Medicine

Copyright, 1958, by the Massachusetts Medical Society

Volume 259   NOVEMBER 20, 1958   Number 21

DIRECT-VISION CORONARY ENDARTERECTOMY FOR ANGINA PECTORIS*

WILLIAM P. LONGMIRE, JR., M.D.,† JACK A. CANNON, M.D.,‡ AND ALBERT A. KATTUS, M.D.§

LOS ANGELES, CALIFORNIA

OF the numerous surgical procedures[1-7] so far designed to increase blood flow to the myocardium in patients with angina pectoris, none have won wide acceptance since conclusive evidence of their therapeutic benefit has been lacking. It seemed to us that the most effective means of increasing myocardial blood flow would be to remove the obstructing atheromatous plugs from the coronary arteries themselves. Experience with peripheral arterial endarterectomy suggested the possibility of a direct surgical approach by this method to occluded coronary arteries. The feasibility of such an operation was supported by both pathologic and experimental observations of one of us (J.A.C.). This report presents in detail the case histories of 5 patients treated for incapacitating angina pectoris by direct-vision coronary endarterectomy.

The operation was devised on the basis of the following four premises: that the patient with severe angina pectoris is likely to have complete occlusion of at least one of the three major coronary branches (the right coronary, the left anterior descending and the left circumflex artery); that the occlusive process is likely to be located near the aortic origins of these vessels; that the distal coronary tree beyond the occlusion is likely to be patent and supplied with blood through collateral anastomotic channels that would be expected to have attained a maximum state of development; and that it is technically possible to perform definitive endarterectomy on vessels the size of the human coronary arteries.

The first two of these premises are derived from the classic pathological studies of Blumgart, Schlesinger and Davis.[8] The third is based in part on the same studies and in part on the physiologic studies of Gregg, Thornton and Mautz,[9] as well as on the coronary angiographic experiments of one of us

(J.A.C.).[10] The fourth premise is based upon the extensive experience of one of us (J.A.C.) in working out the surgical technic of coronary endarterectomy in dogs and in human hearts obtained at autopsy.

In the course of the animal experiments, suitable instruments were designed and fabricated for carrying out the procedure. These consist of modified intimal stripping loops, of the same basic design as those used in human femoropopliteal endarterectomy, and a small elevator with an adjustable blade for the initial dissection (Fig. 1).

The patients selected for coronary endarterectomy were those who had incapacitating angina pectoris of such severity that they were incapable of gainful employment. The diagnosis of coronary insufficiency was beyond question, since they had typical histories of angina on effort and marked changes in electrocardiograms taken during exercise. None of the patients had definite evidence of recent or remote myocardial infarction. All were in the relatively young age group (thirty-eight to fifty-three years).

To obtain objective evidence of the efficacy of the operation, a treadmill exercise test was devised that we hoped would provide a semiquantitative index of the severity of the disease preoperatively and an indication of the degree of improvement postoperatively. The patient walks up a 10 per cent grade on a motor-driven treadmill at the rate of 1.5 miles per hour with a bipolar, transthoracic, electrocardiographic lead strapped securely to the chest. The electrode of the right arm is placed in the right posterior axillary line at a level of the angle of the scapula, whereas the left-arm electrode is placed in the V_4 position. The electrocardiogram is run during exercise at the Lead-1 position. The times at which ST-segment displacement or anginal pain or both occur are noted, and the time required for return to normal of the electrocardiogram is observed.

CASE REPORTS

CASE 1. E.J.M., a 38-year-old cabinetmaker, entered the University of California Hospital on December 16, 1957, with the chief complaint of chest pain for several years.

Two and a half years previously he had noted for the 1st time a pressing pain in the anterior aspect of the chest

*From the departments of Surgery and Medicine, University of California Medical Center.
Aided by a grant-in-aid (H-1787) of the United States Public Health Service.
†Professor of surgery and Chairman of the Department of Surgery, University of California School of Medicine.
‡Associate professor of surgery, University of California School of Medicine.
§Associate professor of medicine (cardiology), University of California School of Medicine.

during sexual intercourse. In the next few months, the same chest pain came on while he was walking. On walking the block and a half from his car to work, he had to stop 2 to 3 times because of chest pain, which he described as a weight pressing on the chest. Subsequently, the chest pain was associated with aching in the left arm and hand. In addition to the aching pain, there was a tingling and numbness in the hand so severe that on 1 occasion he dropped his lunch pail while walking to work. Sometimes, nitroglycerin relieved the pain promptly. On other occasions, he found it necessary to take several nitroglycerin

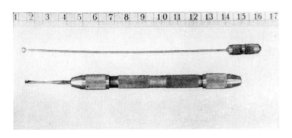

FIGURE 1. *Special Instruments Designed for Coronary Endarterectomy, Showing, Below, an Elevator to Dissect the Thickened Intimal Core from the Media and Adventitia and, Above, a Loop Stripper to Dissect the Core Proximally and Distally from the Incision in the Coronary Artery.*

tablets. Often, 1½ hours elapsed before relief was obtained. On at least 2 occasions he became unconscious during an attack. Owing to the increasing frequency and severity of the attacks of chest pain on exertion, he was forced to stop work in September, 1957. There were 2 8-week periods of complete bed rest.

On physical examination the heart was not enlarged. The precordium was quiet, and there was no palpable apical impulse. The rhythm was regular, sounds were of good quality, and there were no murmurs. The lungs were clear to auscultation. The blood pressure was 140/85. The liver and spleen were not palpable. There was no peripheral edema.

A roentgenogram of the chest showed a normal-sized heart. An electrocardiogram with the patient resting was normal. Master's 2-step test was positive. The treadmill exercise test resulted in ST-segment depression after 1 minute of walking. Exercise was stopped at 1½ minutes because of chest pain. Two minutes later the ST segments had become isoelectric, but the T waves had become markedly inverted. The tracing required 10 minutes to return to normal (Fig. 2).

On December 20 a bilateral anterior thoracotomy was performed. The chest was entered through the 4th interspace, and the sternum was transected. The myocardium was diffusely streaked with white fibrous tissue, but there was no evidence of a gross infarct. The right coronary artery was first exposed from its origin for a distance of 3 cm. by dissection of the densely adherent epicardial fat. This portion of the vessel was firm and rigid, and the lumen seemed to be completely occluded. The left circumflex artery was soft, pliable and patent. The proximal portion of the left anterior descending vessel was rigid and nodular. Clamping of the right coronary artery and the anterior descending artery for 4 minutes each failed to produce any change in the electrocardiogram or in the heart action. The blood supply for the entire myocardium seemed to be conducted largely by the circumflex artery. Occlusion of this artery for a brief period produced slight but definite diffuse cyanosis of the myocardium and depression of the ST segments in the electrocardiogram. It was striking that the sclerosis was confined to the main coronary vessels and their primary branches. The smaller arteries appeared grossly normal.

Both the right main coronary and the left anterior descending coronary artery were resected, with removal of a thrombus, and a satisfactory pulsation was re-established

in both vessels (Fig. 3 and 4). The rate and rhythm of the heart and the blood pressure were unchanged throughout the procedure. The patient's condition was excellent at the conclusion of the operation.

During the final stages of the procedure, heparin was administered systemically in an attempt to maintain a clotting time of between 10 and 15 minutes. During the next 8 hours, however, there was evidence of continued bleeding into the right pleural space. A massive hemothorax developed on the right and was evacuated at re-exploration of the right side of the chest. Despite a tracheotomy performed on the 2d postoperative day, a staphylococcal pneumonitis developed in the left lower lobe. This responded to vigorous antibiotic therapy. Fluid and air, which accumulated in the right hemithorax, were removed by repeated thoracentesis. A persistent wound infection that developed over the middle portion of the chest incision slowly healed.

There has been no recurrence of anginal pain in the 9-month period since operation. The treadmill exercise test was repeated 3 weeks after operation. Walking for 7 minutes did not produce any symptoms of chest pain or any significant change in the electrocardiographic pattern. There was no depression of the ST segment or inversion of the T wave (Fig. 2). Four months after operation a repeat treadmill test produced no symptoms or electrocardiographic changes during or after a 20-minute exercise period. The patient has been permitted to return to part-time work.

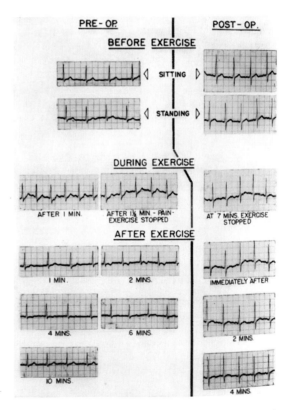

FIGURE 2. *Treadmill Exercise Test in Case 1, Showing the Tracing Made Three Weeks after Operation.*
During the second test there was no anginal pain and no depression of the ST segment or inversion of the T wave.

CASE 2. G.L., a 53-year-old ex-machinist, was admitted to the University of California Hospital with the complaint of severe chest pain of 4 years' duration. The pain, which was described as cramping, was located beneath the sternum, but at times it spread diffusely over the anterior aspect of the chest. It did not radiate to the neck or arms and was brought on by exertion, emotion and eating. Occasionally, the pain awakened the patient early in the morning. Attacks occurred from one to many times a day, depending upon the amount of activity. Each attack lasted for 5 minutes to 1 hour. Relief was obtained by rest and nitroglycerin, although this drug caused headaches.

Four years previously the patient had been forced to stop his usual work because of pain. After trying 3 or 4 other types of less active work, he was forced to stop work altogether. There was no history suggestive of an acute coronary occlusion with infarction of the myocardium.

Physical examination showed a moderately obese man. The heart was not enlarged. The sounds were somewhat faint but otherwise normal. Rhythm was regular. The pulse rate was 60, and the blood pressure 142/84. Peripheral pulses were present, equal and regular. The lungs were clear. The liver and spleen were not palpable. There was no peripheral edema.

A roentgenogram of the chest showed slight enlargement of the left ventricle and elongation of the aorta. An electrocardiogram with the patient resting was normal. The treadmill exercise test produced severe pain after 8 minutes of walking. At that time there was a 1-mm. depression of the ST segment followed by inversion of the T wave. The electrocardiogram reverted to normal after 12 minutes of rest. This test was considered to have confirmed the diagnosis of coronary insufficiency with angina pectoris.

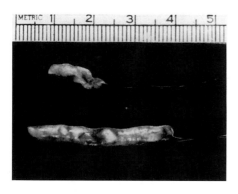

FIGURE 3. *Occluding Intimal Core Removed from the Right Coronary Artery in Case 1.*

A bilateral, anterior thoracotomy was performed on January 28, 1958, through the 4th interspace, with division of the sternum. Cyclopropane anesthesia was used. The right coronary artery was first visualized by dissection of the epicardial fat. The main segment of the vessel was thickened and firm, with numerous hard plaques palpable. The distal branches of the vessel, however, appeared and felt normal. An occluding clamp was placed on the main right artery for a period of 4 minutes without any change in the color of the myocardium, in the electrocardiographic tracing or in the heart action. A 1-cm. longitudinal incision was made in the wall of the vessel. The lumen was almost completely occluded; there was only a slight ooze of blood from the opened unclamped vessel. The thickened intimal core was dissected from the media of the vessel and divided and stripped proximally into the aorta and distally into the smaller branches. There was then a free flow of blood from both the proximal and distal lumen of the artery; 2 ml. of 1:100 heparin solution was instilled into the artery as the incision was closed.

A similar procedure was performed on the left anterior descending coronary artery, with the removal of a 2-cm. segment of thickened obstructing intimal core. Intermittent irregularities of cardiac action were produced by the rotation of the heart required to expose the left anterior descending coronary artery. During closure of the arteriotomy the heart suddenly dilated, and irreversible asystole occurred despite the vigorous application of all usual resuscitative measures.

CASE 3. J.E.B., a 47-year-old former plasterer, entered the University of California Hospital on February 25, 1958, with the complaint of chest pain of 4 years' duration. Although he had been told that he had a moderately high blood pressure, he had been in good health until approximately 4 years before, when he began to have substernal pain. He associated this pain with the smoking of 2½ packages of cigarettes per day. At first, he relieved the pain by reducing the number of cigarettes smoked. However, the pain slowly increased with such frequency and severity that he had been forced to stop work 2 years previously. At the time of admission, he had pain occasionally at rest. It was

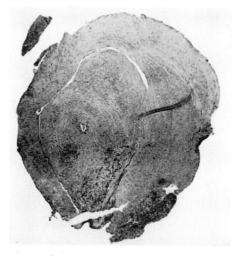

FIGURE 4. *Cross-section of the Intimal Core Removed from the Right Coronary Artery in Case 1, Demonstrating a Tiny Patent Lumen before Stripping.*

usually precipitated by eating, smoking, exercise or emotional excitement. The pain, which was located over the middle anterior aspect of the chest, usually started as a dull ache and progressed to a severe crushing pain, which radiated to the medial surface of the left arm and neck. It lasted "minutes" to "several hours" and was relieved by 10 to 20 nitroglycerin tablets per day. There had been no episodes suggestive of myocardial infarction or heart failure. Three months of rest and anticoagulant therapy and the loss of 13.6 kg. (30 pounds) in weight resulted in only slight improvement in symptoms.

Physical examination showed a well nourished man. The heart was not enlarged, the sounds were well heard, and there were no murmurs. The rhythm was regular, and the pulses equal. The blood pressure was 160/100. The pulse was 82, and the respirations 20. The lungs were clear. The liver edge was palpable 1 cm. below the right costal margin. The spleen was not felt. There was no peripheral edema.

Roentgenograms of the chest showed enlargement of the left ventricle, with slight dilatation of the ascending aorta. An electrocardiogram with the patient resting showed slight sagging of the ST segment in leads V₄ and V₅. During the treadmill exercise test the ST segments gradually became depressed to a maximum of 1.5 mm. in 2½ minutes. At this time a dull precordial pain, which reached moderate severity and was associated with a heavy aching sensation in the left arm, developed. Exercise was terminated after 3 minutes, and the tracing returned to normal in 6 minutes. The pain disappeared in 4 minutes. These findings were considered to have confirmed the diagnosis of coronary insufficiency with angina pectoris.

On February 28 the chest was entered through a bilateral anterior thoracotomy incision in the 4th interspace, with division of the sternum. The heart was moderately enlarged. No gross scar was visible in the myocardium. The right main coronary artery was exposed from its origin at the aorta out to its terminal branches. The main vessel felt solid and could not be compressed. Scattered, small, opaque plaques could be seen in some of the smaller branches of the left anterior descending coronary artery. The 1st branch from the main right coronary vessel seemed to pulsate slightly and was considered to be at least partially patent. Occlusion for 6 minutes of the right main coronary artery distal to this point produced no change in the color of the myocardium, in the electrocardiographic tracing or in the action of the heart.

With the aid of a binocular loupe the vessel was opened distally through a 1-cm. longitudinal incision. There was no bleeding from the opened, unclamped artery. The thickened intimal core was dissected from the media, and it was then divided and stripped proximally to the aorta and distally down into the main branches. Removal of the core proximally was followed by vigorous arterial bleeding. Good back bleeding was obtained after removal of the core from the distal portion of the artery. A small amount of powdered heparin was placed in the lumen of the vessel, and the incision was closed. A vigorous pulsation was palpable in the vessel. The left coronary artery was palpated. The circumflex artery felt soft and pliable. The anterior descending coronary branch felt firm, and it was isolated. Segmental cyanosis of the myocardium and depression of the ST segment in the electrocardiographic tracing occurred when the vessel was temporarily occluded. We concluded, therefore, that the vessel was at least partially patent and elected not to perform an endarterectomy. The patient's condition was excellent at the conclusion of operation.

One week later he was ambulatory and free of anginal pain.

In the three months since operation he has been markedly improved. He has occasionally had mild attacks of pain in the left arm but never severe enough to require medication. He convalesced uneventfully from repair of an inguinal hernia carried out to qualify him for return to work. On treadmill tests performed 18, 21 and 54 days after operation, he was able to walk 10, 15 and 15 minutes respectively. He complained of a mild, vague ache in the left shoulder or in the anterior aspect of the chest on each occasion, but there was no increase with continued exercise and no response to nitroglycerin. On each occasion the electrocardiogram in the resting position revealed T-wave abnormalities attributed to postoperative pericardial changes, but there was no significant ST-segment or T-wave change during or after exercise.

CASE 4. H.F., a 53-year-old osteopathic physician, entered the University of California Hospital on March 14, 1958, with the chief complaint of severe chest pain on exercise. He had first noted the onset of sudden chest pain while walking up a hill 2 years before. The pain lasted for 10 minutes and was described as severe and crushing over the precordium. Similar attacks had been precipitated by exercise since that time. Since November, 1957, he had been awakened during the night by severe precordial pain on a number of occasions. Walking for ½ block on level ground caused attacks of pain. The frequency of attacks varied, but it was not unusual for him to have as many as 10 attacks of pain per day. Attacks were also precipitated by heavy meals, cigarettes and emotional stress. He had been taking pentaerythritol tetranitrate for 3 months, without any appreciable improvement in his condition. The pain was usually promptly relieved by nitroglycerin, and if precipitated by exercise it was relieved by rest. The frequency of these attacks had forced him to retire from his profession 3 months before admission.

On physical examination the heart was not enlarged. The rhythm was regular, and the sounds were of good quality. The aortic 2d sound was louder than the pulmonic. There were no murmurs. The blood pressure was 120/80. The pulse was 80. The lungs were clear to auscultation. The liver and spleen were not palpable. There was no peripheral edema.

Roentgenograms of the chest showed the cardiac silhouette to be within normal limits. There was emphysema of both lungs, with evidence of pleural thickening at the bases. An electrocardiogram taken at rest was interpreted as normal. On Master's 2-step exercise test the patient made 20 ascents in 1½ minutes. Immediately after exercise the record showed a 2-mm. ST-segment depression in Lead V₄. Two minutes after exercise there was still sagging of the ST segments. Again, at 6 minutes after exercise, a 1-mm. depression of the ST segments remained, although the T waves were becoming taller. Wolff–Parkinson–White complexes appeared intermittently in tracings taken immediately after exercise. Treadmill tests were performed on 3 occasions before operation, and on 2 of these, the electrocardiogram became abnormal after the patient climbed 3 steps to the treadmill. Tests were terminated after 3½, 3½ and 5½ minutes because of chest pain and ST-segment depression of 2 mm. or greater. The electrocardiographic changes were considered typical of subendocardial injury, and they required 7, 5 and 10 minutes, respectively, after exercise to return to normal. The test was considered strongly positive and confirmatory of the clinical impression of coronary-artery insufficiency with angina pectoris.

On March 17 a bilateral anterior thoracotomy was performed through the 4th interspace, and the sternum was transected. The left anterior descending coronary artery was completely occluded by a thickened atheromatous intima. A pulsatile blood flow was re-established in the vessel by thromboendarterectomy. The obstructing core was removed from the origin of the vessel peripherally into the major branches. A 1-cm. core was also removed from the septal branch. The wall of the right coronary artery was thickened, but the vessel was not occluded. The vessel was exposed throughout its length but not opened.

The course after operation was uneventful. The patient has had no further attacks of anginal pain during the 6 months since operation. He did complain of paresthesia of the skin over the anterior chest wall above the operative scar, these sensations being precipitated by anything touching the area. Treadmill tests were performed on March 31 and May 25. Exercise was continued for 10 minutes and 15 minutes respectively without chest pain or any electrocardiographic changes on either occasion.

CASE 5. M.N., a 54-year-old salesman, was admitted to the University of California Hospital on March 25, 1958, with the complaint of intractable anginal pain unrelieved by coronary vasodilator drugs. The pain, which had gradually increased in frequency and intensity over the past 10 years, was described as a deep, squeezing, pressurelike sensation over the left aspect of the chest, with radiation to the top of the shoulder, down the inner aspect of the left arm and into the fingers. This pain was brought on by exercise, eating and cold weather. It was relieved only partially by nitroglycerin. A 2d type of pain, which had been present for approximately 1½ years, was described as a sharp, stabbing pain starting in the left upper portion of the chest, radiating up into the neck and jaws and the left postauricular region, and behind the left eye. This pain was not affected by nitroglycerin but was diminished with codeine and relieved by meperidine. There were also increasing symptoms of dyspnea on exertion, shortness of breath, paroxysmal nocturnal dyspnea, night sweats, palpitation and intermittent ankle edema.

Two years previously the patient had been admitted to a hospital with what was diagnosed as myocardial infarct. For 4 months he had practically been bed-ridden except for sitting in a chair occasionally. Anginal pains were frequently precipitated by as little effort as turning over in bed. One week before admission he "blacked out" while eating breakfast and was resuscitated with oxygen administered by members of the local fire department. There was a strong family history of xanthelasma.

Physical examination showed a well developed, well nourished man in no acute distress. He was alert and cooperative, but generally quite apprehensive about his condition. Large xanthelasmas were present on the eyelids. The heart was enlarged. The sounds were of good quality, and there were no murmurs. The blood pressure was 144/88, and the pulse 87 and regular. Fine, moist rales were present in the mid-lung fields posteriorly. Inspiratory and expiratory rales were heard at both bases posteriorly at the time of admission. These rales cleared during the hospital course before operation. No ankle edema was present.

Roentgenograms of the chest demonstrated moderate hypertrophy of the left ventricle and dilatation of the aorta. There was a questionable area of calcification in the region of the left anterior descending coronary artery. The lung fields were clear. The serum cholesterol was 407 mg. per 100 ml. An electrocardiogram taken at rest showed digitalis effect, but there was no evidence of old or recent myocardial infarction.

The 1st attempt to perform a treadmill test was postponed because of an attack of severe anginal pain, with marked depression of the ST segments, while the patient was sitting in a chair. A 2d test was performed on the following day. Exercise was discontinued after 3 minutes because of chest pain and ST-segment depression of 3 mm. on the electrocardiogram. This was interpreted as a strongly positive exercise test.

On April 7 a bilateral anterior thoracotomy incision was made through the 4th interspaces. A thrombus was removed from the completely occluded left anterior descending coronary, and good pulsation established in the vessel. The right coronary branch was at least partially patent and was not opened.

Several large emphysematous blebs were noted in both lungs at the time of operation.

The immediate postoperative course was complicated by a moderately severe subcutaneous emphysema and a subcutaneous wound infection in the right axillary portion of the incision. Both conditions cleared satisfactorily.

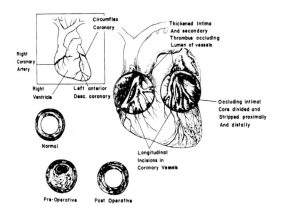

FIGURE 5. *Technic of Operation, Showing Exposure of the Right Main Coronary and Left Anterior Descending Coronary Arteries, with Longitudinal Incisions into the Vessels, and Also Diagrammatic Cross-sections of a Normal Coronary Artery, an Artery Occluded by Atheromatous Intima and the Vessel after Intimal Stripping.*

Warfarin therapy was instituted 10 days after operation and has been continued.

On a treadmill test performed 2 weeks after operation the patient was able to exercise for 7 minutes, with a 2-mm. depression of the ST segment. He continued to have occasional mild attacks of substernal pain on exercise. The left postocular pain has been entirely relieved.

He was seen in the outpatient clinic on May 28, when the following note was made:

Since operation he has had 4 or 5 episodes of retrosternal pain radiating to the left arm. He is, however, able to walk 6 to 10 blocks on level ground and to walk up 15 to 20 steps without stopping. On one occasion (May 22) chest pain developed while he was carrying groceries upstairs. After a heavy meal on the following

day anginal pain developed. He was seen in the emergency room, where it was noted that he had gained 4.1 kg. (9 pounds). After an induced diuresis, he had felt well and had been spending 2 hours daily in his office. Physical examination was unchanged.

Treadmill tests were performed on 4 occasions between 2 and 8 weeks after operation. On 3 occasions exercise was terminated after 3, 7 and 7 minutes because of precordial pain and an aching sensation in the left forearm. During and immediately after exercise there was 1-mm. to 2-mm. ST-segment depression on the electrocardiogram. On 1 test, 18 days after operation, the patient tolerated 10 minutes of

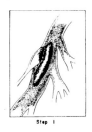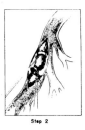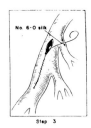

FIGURE 6. *Stripping of the Intimal Core.*

Step 1 shows the longitudinal incision in the vessel and elevation of the intimal core.

Step 2 shows the intimal core divided, its end ligated and the loop stripper ready to be advanced into the vessel.

Step 3 shows the core removed, powdered heparin inserted into the lumen and the incision closed with continuous No. 000000 arterial silk suture.

exercise without pain or electrocardiographic changes. The electrocardiogram at rest is now normal except for digitalis effect.

DISCUSSION

A bilateral anterior thoracotomy was utilized in all cases. The sternum was transected, and the pleural spaces were entered through the fourth interspaces. Exposure of the right main coronary artery was excellent. Rotation of the heart to the right was required to expose the left anterior descending coronary vessel. This approach is not satisfactory for adequate exposure of the left circumflex artery (Fig. 5). The first step of the procedure is palpation and inspection of the main coronary vessels and their smaller branches. If all the smaller peripheral vessels of a coronary artery are occluded, there is obviously little reason to proceed with endarterectomy of the major vessel. On the other hand, if the peripheral vessels are soft, pliable and translucent, the epicardial fat is dissected away from the right main coronary and left anterior descending coronary arteries. In segments where atheroma is most severe, the epicardial fat is scarred and densely adherent to the vessel. In more normal areas the fat strips with ease from the surface of the coronary artery. This finding provides a useful landmark to indicate areas of occlusion in the vessel. Further inspection and palpation indicate the extent of atheromatous changes. The vessel is gently occluded for a period of three to six minutes, while the color of the myocardium supplied by the vessel, the electrocardiographic tracing and the heart action are closely observed. If no changes are noted, the vessel is not supplying blood to the myocardium and may be assumed to be completely occluded.

A 1-cm. incision is then made over the middle portion of the vessel (Fig. 6). A binocular loupe is helpful in the remaining dissection. It is possible to develop a plane of cleavage between the thickened intimal core and the media of the vessel. The core is divided, and the ends tied with No. 0000 silk suture. The ends of the ligature are left long, passed through the special coronary loop stripper and used to effect countertraction on the core. With the stripper, the core is freed proximally into the aorta and distally down into the major branches. At times, it may be necessary to make additional small arteriotomies at the origins of major branches to remove portions of the intimal core that extend into these branches and obstruct the progress of the stripper. Adequate removal of the core proximally will be followed by vigorous spurting of blood from the proximal lumen. A steady flow of back bleeding from the distal end will indicate an adequate clearing of the distal segment of the vessel and a patent run-off bed.

The vessel is gently occluded, a small amount of sterile, powdered heparin is placed inside the lumen of the vessel, and the incision is closed with a running No. 000000 silk arterial suture.

The right main coronary artery and the left anterior descending coronary artery were both resected in 2 of our cases. It is possible that rotation of the heart necessary to exposure of the left descending coronary artery in Case 2 was responsible for the irreversible asystole that occurred. The right coronary artery alone was resected in the third and fourth cases, for the anterior descending arteries gave evidence of being partially patent. In Case 5 the left anterior descending coronary artery alone was resected. It seems probable that re-establishing a good blood flow in any one of these vessels would result in marked improvement in total coronary blood flow and probably in symptomatic improvement, since it is to be expected that the maximally dilated collateral channels would be capable of distributing the additional blood flow to all ischemic areas of the myocardium.

A general principle in the treatment of occlusive vascular disease elsewhere in the body, — in the iliac or femoral arteries, for instance, — by either endarterectomy or bypass graft, is that there must be a patent peripheral arterial system, a patent "run-off" bed. The same principle is essential, of course, in coronary endarterectomy. Opening the occluded main coronary vessels can only be of value if the branches and more peripheral vessels are patent.

Preoperative coronary angiography was considered a possible method for evaluating the patency of the peripheral coronary tree, as well as for identifying the sites of occlusion. In these cases it was not used, however, because one of us (J.A.C.) had found a high prevalence of ventricular fibrillation when coronary angiography was attempted on a series of dogs with coronary-artery ligations.[11] Operative experience has shown that the limits of atheromatous change can be estimated during surgery by palpation and inspection of the vessels. Furthermore, it has been found that adequate coring out of the occluded coronary artery distal to the incision in the vessel will result in a brisk retrograde flow of arterial blood from the coronary collateral anastomoses, thereby attesting to the patency of the peripheral coronary vascular bed at the time of surgery. At present, we are making no attempt to assess preoperatively the pathologic anatomy of the coronary tree.

It should be emphasized that the surgical attack is made on virtually occluded arteries, so that there is no time limit on the duration of the clamping and manipulation of the vessels involved. The longest time required to complete endarterectomy in any one of the vessels of this series was forty minutes from the original clamping to the establishment of free flow through the vessels.

A crucial question has been whether or not the vessels repaired will remain patent. Because of the bleeding problem encountered in Case 1, we have not used systemic anticoagulant therapy subsequently* but have resorted to heparin applied locally in the vessels after endarterectomy and 25-mg. doses of heparin intravenously every six hours during the early postoperative period. Low-fat diets have, of course, been employed postoperatively in the hypercholesterolemic patients. Thus far, we have purposely selected for treatment patients who did not have definite evidence of infarction, thereby hoping that the intact myocardium would tolerate the stress of operation better than an extensively damaged one and that maximal symptomatic improvement might be expected by an increase in the flow of blood to the undamaged myocardium. If the method continues to show promise, the indications for operation will probably be extended to include patients with myocardial infarction.

Although the brief period of observation since operation is inadequate to assess the ultimate value of this procedure, the subjective improvement, with marked reduction or disappearance of the characteristic anginal pain in the 4 surviving patients, and the striking improvement in the electrocardiographic tracings taken postoperatively during the treadmill exercise are encouraging.

*Heparin was not used in sufficient amount to produce the usually recommended prolongation of clotting time.

SUMMARY AND CONCLUSIONS

Direct-vision coronary endarterectomy has been employed for the first time in the treatment of 5 patients with coronary atherosclerosis and typical symptoms of angina pectoris without definite evidence of myocardial infarction.

In all cases it has been possible to remove an almost totally occluding, thickened intimal core from one or more of the main coronary vessels and to reestablish blood flow through the vessel at the time of operation.

Asystole occurred near the completion of the operation in 1 patient. In the brief period since operation, 2 patients have been completely relieved of their pain, and the frequency and intensity of anginal attacks have been greatly reduced in the other 2 patients. Marked improvement in the electrocardiographic tracings taken during exercise has been noted in all cases.

These results indicate that it is technically feasible by this procedure to re-establish blood flow in previously obstructed major coronary arteries. Experience with additional cases and longer periods of observation after operation will be necessary to make a final assessment of the value of the procedure.

REFERENCES

1. O'Shaughnessy, L. Experimental method of providing collateral circulation to heart. *Brit. J. Surg.* **23**:665-670, 1936.
2. Thompson, S. A., and Raisbeck, M. J. Cardio-pericardiopexy: surgical treatment of coronary arterial disease by establishment of adhesive pericarditis. *Ann. Int. Med.* **16**:495-520, 1942.
3. Carter, B. N. Discussion of Beck, C. S. Revascularization of heart. *Ann. Surg.* **128**:854-864, 1948.
4. Schildt, P., Stanton, E., and Beck, C. S. Communications between coronary arteries produced by application of inflammatory agents to surface of heart. *Ann. Surg.* **118**:34-45, 1943.
5. Vineberg, A. M. Development of anastomosis between coronary vessels and transplanted internal mammary artery. *Canad. M. A. J.* **55**:117-119, 1946.
6. Beck, C. S., Stanton, E., Batiuchok, W., and Leiter, E. Revascularization of heart by graft of systemic artery into coronary sinus. *J.A.M.A.* **137**:436-442, 1948.
7. Bailey, C. P., May, A., and Lemmon, W. M. Survival after coronary endarterectomy in man. *J.A.M.A.* **164**:641-646, 1957.
8. Blumgart, H. L., Schlesinger, M. J., and Davis, D. Studies on relation of clinical manifestations of angina pectoris, coronary thrombosis, and myocardial infarction to pathologic findings, with particular reference to significance of collateral circulation. *Am. Heart J.* **19**:1-91, 1940.
9. Gregg, D. E., Thornton, J. J., and Mautz, F. R. Magnitude, adequacy and source of collateral blood flow and pressure in chronically occluded coronary arteries. *Am. J. Physiol.* **127**:161-175, 1939.
10. Cannon, J. A., Clifford, C. A., Diesh, G., and Barker, W. F. Accurate diagnostic coronary arteriography in dog. *S. Forum* **6**:197-199, 1956.
11. Cannon, J. A. Unpublished data.

Saphenous Vein Autograft Replacement of Severe Segmental Coronary Artery Occlusion

Operative Technique

Rene G. Favaloro, M.D.

Direct operation on the coronary artery has been performed in 180 patients at the Cleveland Clinic up to October, 1967. Recently, a new operative technique has been applied in 15 patients with extensive and severe obstruction of the right dominant coronary artery, specifically to overcome some of the unfavorable results that occurred when pericardial patch reconstruction was performed.

OPERATIVE TECHNIQUE

The operation is performed while the patient's circulation is maintained by total cardiopulmonary bypass at normal temperature. The left femoral artery is utilized for insertion of the arterial line, except in those patients with severe peripheral arteriosclerosis and in these the ascending aorta is cannulated. At the time the left femoral artery is exposed, using the same incision, the left saphenous vein is dissected free at the point where it joins the femoral vein. A segment of the saphenous vein is resected; a ligature is applied to the proximal end of the isolated segment, as an indicator of the direction of the flow, whereas the distal stump is left open. With this identification, it is easy to place the graft in the appropriate position (inverted), thus preventing impairment of the flow by the valves within the vein. The venous return is via individual cannulation of the superior and inferior venae cavae. A vent is obtained by inserting a catheter into the left atrium through the right superior pulmonary vein.

With the heart beating and the aorta unclamped, the right coronary artery is dissected, and sutures of 2-0 silk are placed above and below the obstruction, held by modified "baby gallbladder" clamps, the curves of which easily surround the vessel. After the artery is exposed, bulldog clamps (with rubber covers, to prevent tissue damage) are applied distal and proximal to the obstruction.

The uppermost surface of the obstruction is incised longitudinally until the lumen is reached. The proximal bulldog clamp can be released intermittently in order to facilitate the procedure. As soon as the lumen is entered, blood flow is evident. With a long, sharp, right-angled scissors, the incision is elongated distally and proximally until a good patent lumen is obtained (Fig. 1). Dilators are gently

From the Department of Thoracic and Cardiovascular Surgery, The Cleveland Clinic Foundation, Cleveland, Ohio.

Accepted for publication Dec. 11, 1967.

Vein Autograft for Coronary Occlusion

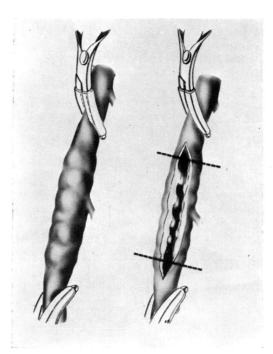

FIG. 1. *On the left, the coronary artery is shown dissected and clamped. On the right side, a longitudinal incision is made on top of the obstruction and is elongated until a patent lumen is found. Dotted lines show the place of transection in order to obtain an enlarged stump.*

introduced to ascertain whether or not further obstruction is present in either direction; this is the only reason for using a dilator. Enforced dilatation may tear the endothelium, and local thrombosis may ensue. The amount of backflow can be assessed by releasing the distal bulldog clamp. Significant backflow eliminates the need for distal perfusion; hence, the artery is clamped, and the surgical procedure continues without interruption. Inadequate return of blood necessitates perfusion of the distal segments through a small plastic cannula with blood at normal temperature.

The coronary artery is then transected about 2 or 3 mm. below the beginning of the longitudinal incision. This point of transection is an important landmark, as it is possible from there to enlarge the lumen of the stump and prevent narrowing of the coronary artery. The anastomosis is done with interrupted sutures of 6-0 silk. The first suture is placed posteriorly (Fig. 2); the saphenous vein is approximated, and the suture is tied. The rest of the sutures are placed alternately from one side to the other side of the first suture (Fig. 3). Approximately ten sutures are usually required; they should be placed close together to prevent leakage.

After the anastomosis is completed, the proximal bulldog clamp is released and the patency of the anastomosis is ascertained. Seldom must extra sutures be used when suturing has been meticulous. The bulldog clamp is next applied on the saphenous vein, and the distal portion of the stump is prepared in the same fashion. If distal perfusion is being used, it is discontinued at this moment. The distal anastomosis is performed in the same manner. The last three sutures are placed without tying them, to be sure that they are properly located. At this time the distal bulldog clamp is also released, and then two of the sutures are tied.

FAVALORO

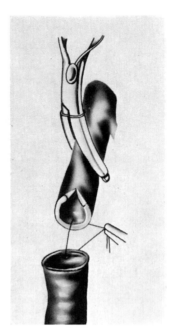

FIG. 2. The first suture is being placed posteriorly; the saphenous vein is approximated and the suture is tied.

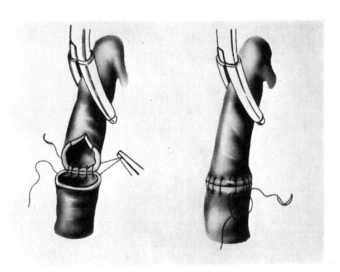

FIG. 3. The proximal anastomosis. On the left side, the sutures have been placed alternately from one side to the other side of the first suture. On the right, the completed anastomosis.

Before the last suture is tied, the proximal bulldog clamp is released so as to fill the lumen with blood and exclude any air trapped inside the coronary arteries (Fig. 4).

The anastomoses are performed with the aorta partially clamped; the heart continues to beat during the entire procedure. The coronary circuit receives blood of normal temperature. When the motion of the heart interferes with

Vein Autograft for Coronary Occlusion

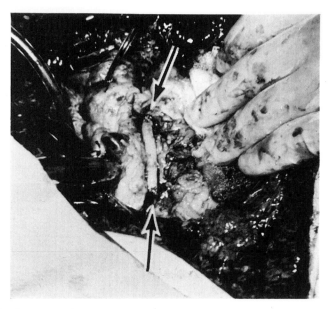

FIG. 4. *Saphenous vein autograft at the end of the procedure.*

proper placing of sutures, the aorta is totally clamped for no longer than 10 minutes, slowing the heart action and thus facilitating the surgical maneuvers.

RESULTS

This operation has been performed in 15 patients, all of whom are alive. Each of them had severe segmental occlusion of the right dominant coronary artery. One patient had previously undergone a right coronary endarterotomy. Three patients also benefited by simultaneously undergoing left internal mammary artery implantation, since severe obstruction of the left coronary artery system was present. The last patient had a 95% occlusion in the upper third of the right coronary artery, starting at the ostium. The saphenous vein graft was placed in the lower portion of the ascending aorta; there, a small opening was made and a side-to-end anastomosis was accomplished. The distal anastomosis was effected with the routine end-to-end anastomosis in the middle third of the right coronary artery. Six of these patients had undergone postoperative cine-coronary angiography studies showing excellent function of the graft (Figs. 5, 6).

COMMENT

A complete follow-up on the 180 patients who had had direct coronary artery surgery (coronary endarterotomy with pericardial patch graft) including selective coronary angiography (Sones' technique) showed that 13% exhibited significant narrowing, and 29% had total occlusion at the site of the patch. This occurred most often in patients with long segmental occlusions.

The indications for endarterotomy rather than endarterectomy have been discussed in previous reports [1–3], and obviously, at present,

FAVALORO

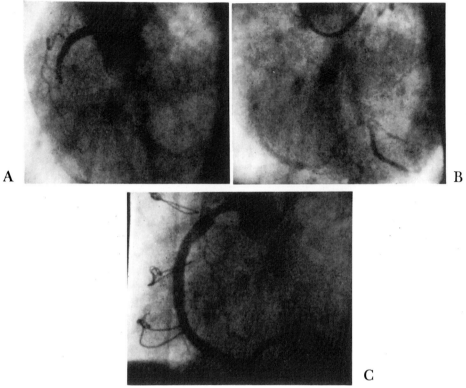

FIG. 5. *Coronary angiogram of a 55-year-old Caucasian woman with total occlusion of the right coronary artery (A). Perfusion of distal right coronary artery by collateral branches from the left coronary artery (B). Total reconstruction of right coronary artery by a saphenous vein autograft (C).*

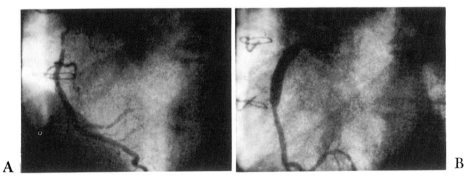

FIG. 6. *Coronary arteriogram of a 42-year-old Caucasian man who underwent a right coronary endarterotomy with pericardial patch graft in April, 1967. Postoperative catheterization shows severe segmental occlusion (A). A saphenous autograft replacement was performed in Sept., 1967. Catheterization on tenth postoperative day shows the vessel to be patent (B).*

true endarterectomy cannot be performed upon the coronary circulation. Placement of the pericardial patch graft on top of an irregular wall that usually has many crevices provides an ideal stratum for

Vein Autograft for Coronary Occlusion

further thromboses and occlusion. Saphenous vein interposition requires only two end-to-end anastomoses, thereby shortening the time of the operation, and the segment can be replaced by a smooth wall that will prevent occlusion. The concept that the coronary artery should be transected after a longitudinal incision is made is a fundamental and important step for two reasons: the transection can be done a few millimeters farther down, enlarging the lumen of the coronary artery stump; and crushing of the endothelium is prevented. In 1 patient in whom the transection was done before the artery was opened it was difficult to find the lumen. To facilitate placing of the sutures when the coronary artery is small, two sutures can be inserted in opposite sides, and by gentle traction the lumen can be kept open.

It is believed that performing the operation while the patient is being perfused with blood of normal temperature has significantly reduced the operative mortality and morbidity. We no longer use hypothermia and selective cooling of the heart on patients who undergo cardiac operations.

SUMMARY AND CONCLUSION

A new operative technique is described to correct severe segmental occlusion of the right dominant coronary artery. A saphenous vein autograft replaces the occluded arterial segment. Fifteen patients were operated upon without mortality. Postoperative angiographic catheterization has demonstrated excellent function of the grafts. Further application of the technique will help to determine the possibilities of its use on the left coronary artery in selected patients who have severe localized obstruction.

ADDENDUM

Since this paper was written, the total number of patients with whom this new operative technique has been applied has grown. The total number of cases is now 55. Fifty-two cases involved segmental occlusion of the right coronary artery; the other 3 involved the circumflex branch of the left coronary artery. Of the total, there were only 2 hospital deaths.

REFERENCES

1. Effler, D. B., Groves, L. K., Sones, F. M., Jr., and Shirey, E. K. Endarterectomy in the treatment of coronary artery disease. *J. Thorac. Cardiov. Surg.* 47:98, 1964.
2. Effler, D. B., Groves, L. K., Suarez, E. L., and Favaloro, R. G. Direct coronary artery surgery with endarterotomy and patch-graft reconstruction: Clinical application and technical considerations. *J. Thorac. Cardiov. Surg.* 53:93, 1967.
3. Effler, D. B., Sones, F. M., Jr., Favaloro, R. G., and Groves, L. K. Coronary endarterotomy with patch-graft reconstruction: Clinical experience with 34 cases. *Ann. Surg.* 162:590, 1965.

The New England
Journal of Medicine

©Copyright, 1979, by the Massachusetts Medical Society

| Volume 301 | JULY 12, 1979 | Number 2 |

NONOPERATIVE DILATATION OF CORONARY-ARTERY STENOSIS

Percutaneous Transluminal Coronary Angioplasty

ANDREAS R. GRÜNTZIG, M.D., ÅKE SENNING, M.D., AND WALTER E. SIEGENTHALER, M.D.

Abstract In percutaneous transluminal coronary angioplasty, a catheter system is introduced through a systemic artery under local anesthesia to dilate a stenotic artery by controlled inflation of a distensible balloon.

Over the past 18 months, we have used this technic in 50 patients. The technic was successful in 32 patients, reducing the stenosis from a mean of 84 to 34 per cent (P<0.001) and the coronary-pressure gradient from a mean of 58 to 19 mm Hg (P<0.001). Twenty-nine patients showed improvement in cardiac function during follow-up examination. Because of acute deterioration in clinical status, emergen-cy bypass was later necessary in five patients; three showed electrocardiograpic evidence of infarcts.

Patients with single-vessel disease appear to be most suitable for the procedure, and a short history of pain indicates the presence of a soft (distensible) atheroma likely to respond to dilatation. We estimate that only about 10 to 15 per cent of candidates for bypass surgery have lesions suitable for this procedure. A prospective randomized trial will be necessary to evaluate its usefulness in comparison with surgical and medical management. (N Engl J Med 301:61-68, 1979)

IN 1964, Dotter and Judkins[1] introduced the tech-nic of transluminal angioplasty for the treatment of atherosclerotic obstruction of the femoral artery. Despite their enthusiasm, the technic has been largely ignored in the United States. In Europe, however, several physicians have used this technic to treat large numbers of patients.[2]

Because of the technical difficulties, complications and limited usefulness of transluminal angioplasty in the treatment of obstruction of the peripheral arte-ries, we sought to modify the original technic of Dotter and Judkins. A double-lumen dilatation catheter with a nonelastic balloon was developed.[3] Such catheters have been used since February, 1974, in patients with obstructions of the femoropopliteal and iliac arteries and have yielded low complication rates and no mor-tality.[4]

Recently, we modified this catheter to allow us to develop a technic for percutaneous dilatation of renal-artery[5] and coronary-artery stenosis.[6] This technic was used in human beings[7] after preliminary trials in dogs and cadavers.[8-10] We present here preliminary results obtained with the technic in the past 18 months.

From the Section of Cardiology, Medical Policlinic, Department of Medicine, and Surgical Clinic A, University Hospital, Zurich, Switzerland (address reprint requests to Dr. Grüntzig at Medical Policlinic, Department of Medicine, University Hospital, Rämistrasse 100, CH-8091 Zurich, Switzerland).

Supported by a grant from the Swiss National Science Foundation.

MATERIALS AND METHODS

Technic

The basic equipment consists of two catheters (Firma H. Schneider, Zurich), the guiding catheter, which has an outer diameter of French 8-9, and the dilating catheter. The guiding cath-eter is inserted into the femoral artery according to the method of Seldinger or through a brachial arteriotomy under local anesthe-sia. The guiding catheter is advanced in a retrograde manner into the ascending aorta and positioned in the orifice of the coronary artery requiring dilatation. This catheter guides the dilating cathe-ter into the stenotic arterial branch. The dilating catheter contains a double lumen to permit pressure measurements, contrast injec-tion and inflation of the balloon. At the tip of this catheter, a short soft wire, 5 mm long, projects beyond the balloon (Fig. 1) and directs the catheter into the artery, thus avoiding injury to the arte-rial wall. By means of a fluoroscopic-image intensifier, the dilating catheter is advanced into the stenotic area. The balloon is filled with a liquid mixture of contrast medium and is inflated for three to four seconds at a pressure of 4 to 5 bar (400 to 500 kPa); the balloon is then deflated, blocking the artery for about 15 to 20 seconds (Fig. 2). Inflation and deflation of the balloon are controlled by a calibrated pressure pump (Firma H. Schneider).

To estimate the extent of coronary-artery disease and the effect of dilatation, coronary angiography is peformed immediately before and after transluminal angioplasty. It is important to obtain views laterally, from both oblique angles and hemiaxially.[11] The degree of stenosis is calculated from the mean stenosis seen in all projections and was determined by one of us (A. R. G.). In all cases, pressure was monitored, and pressure gradients across the lesions were recorded. A pacemaker was readily available during the procedure.

Drug Treatment

The patient is given aspirin (1.0 g per day) for three days, starting the day before the procedure. Heparin and low-molecular-weight dextran are administered during dilatation; warfarin is started after the procedure and is continued until the follow-up study six to nine months later. To prevent coronary spasms, nitroglycerin and nifedipine are given before and during the procedure. The patient is discharged two days after angioplasty.

Patient Selection and Evaluation

Patients with an accessible stenosis less than 1 cm in length, as judged from coronary arteriograms, and a short history of pain (less than one year) are most suitable for the procedure. The patients should also be likely candidates for operation as a result of disabling symptoms and their clinical status.

Results of previous catheterization studies and coronary angiograms of potential candidates for the procedure are shown to and discussed with the cardiac surgeons. The possible benefits and risks of the procedure and alternative treatments are explained to the patients. After informed written consent is obtained, the procedure is performed when the surgeon, anesthesiologist and operating room with cardiopulmonary bypass equipment are available.

Before transluminal angioplasty, the patient undergoes a baseline, quantitative, submaximal, bicycle ergometric examination in the upright position,[12-14] which is repeated two days after dilatation. We classified the patients, according to the results of the stress tests, as follows: no pain or electrocardiographic changes with marked exertion (Class I); pain with marked exertion (≥50 per cent of the predicted age, sex and height-adjusted working capacity consistent with steady state) (Class II); pain with minimal exertion (<50 per cent of the predicted working capacity) (Class III); or pain at rest (Class IV). A ^{201}Tl myocardial-perfusion scintigram can also be performed during the ergometric examination[15-17] to evaluate perfusion after dilatation.

A 12-lead electrocardiogram and cardiac-enzyme estimation are performed before treatment and repeated every eight hours for the first 24 hours. Stress tests are given every three months for the first year, and coronary angiography is performed six to nine months after dilatation.

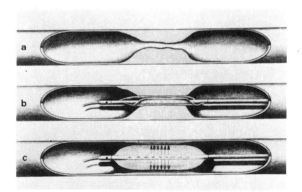

Figure 1. Percutaneous Transluminal Coronary Angioplasty and Catheters Used in the Procedure.

(a) Stenosis of the coronary artery is shown. (b) The double-lumen balloon catheter is introduced by use of a guiding catheter positioned at the orifice of the left or right coronary artery; at the tip of the dilating catheter is a short soft wire, which guides the catheter through the vessel. Proximal to the wire is a side hole connected to the main lumen of the dilating catheter. This lumen is used for pressure recording and contrast-material ejection. The dilating catheter is advanced through the coronary artery with the balloon deflated. (c) The balloon is inflated across the stenosis to its predetermined maximal outer diameter of 3.0 to 3.7 mm at a fluid pressure of 4 to 5 bar (400 to 500 kPa), thereby enlarging the lumen. After balloon deflation, the catheter is withdrawn.

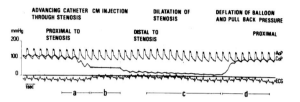

Figure 2. Original Tracing with Recording of Mean Pressure and Electrocardiogram during Dilatation, September 16, 1977, in a 39-Year-Old Man with Severe Angina and 85 Per Cent Stenosis of the Left Coronary Artery.

CoP denotes coronary pressure, and AoP aortic pressure. The left-hand tracing (a) was the proximal pressure (114/96/105 mm Hg); the initial reduction in pressure occurred as the dilating catheter was passed across the lesion (24/16/20 mm Hg), occluding the artery. The position of the catheter was then checked by ejection of contrast medium (CM) distal to the stenosis through the main lumen of the dilating catheter (b). The balloon was inflated across the lesion (c), thereby enlarging the lumen. For 25 seconds, the coronary artery was totally occluded. No pain or change in the S-T segment occurred on the electrocardiogram. Dilatation reduced the stenosis from 85 to 29 per cent and the pressure rose (100/90/95 mm Hg) above the initial distal pressure. There was no substantial further rise in pressure in the pullback pressure curve (106/91/97 mm Hg) (d). This observation indicated a good hemodynamic result, which was confirmed by the second arteriogram taken after coronary angioplasty.

Angiograms of this patient are shown in Figure 5.

Patients

From September, 1977, to January, 1979, 50 patients underwent coronary angioplasty (Table 1). The patients were 31 to 67 years of age, with a mean of 49. Forty-six patients were men, and four were women. The mean duration of angina pectoris since the patient first experienced pain had been 13±30 months (mean ± S.D.). Twenty-six patients (52 per cent) showed electrocardiographic evidence of mural or nontransmural infarction.

Thirty patients (60 per cent) had single-artery disease (no other artery involved, with 50 per cent or greater reduction in luminal diameter) of the left anterior descending coronary artery, left circumflex artery or the right coronary artery. The remaining patients had two or three affected arteries. Eight patients (16 per cent) had previously received coronary-artery-bypass grafts and showed recurrent stenosis and symptoms.

Despite adequate medical therapy (beta-blocking agents and long-acting nitrates), exercise-induced angina pectoris (functional Classes II and III) or angina at rest (functional Class IV) was present in 36 (72 per cent) and 14 patients (28 per cent), respectively.

Detailed histories on all patients have been deposited with the National Auxiliary Publication Service.*

RESULTS

We attempted to dilate 53 vessels in 50 patients; 42 patients had severe stenoses of various coronary arteries, and eight other patients were studied after coronary-artery-bypass grafting (Table 2). As judged by a

A four-page table is available. Order NAPS Document 03466 from ASIS/NAPS c/o Microfiche Publications, P.O. Box 3513, Grand Central Station, New York, NY 10017. Remit in advance, $3 for each microfiche-copy reproduction or $5 for each photocopy. Outside the United States and Canada, postage is $3 for a photocopy or $1 for a microfiche. Make checks payable to Microfiche Publications.

10 per cent or greater reduction of stenosis and pressure gradient, we successfully treated 34 vessels in 32 patients (66 per cent), namely, 29 of the 46 (63 per cent) coronary arteries and five of the seven (71 per cent) graft stenoses. The mean duration of angina pectoris had been nine months (range, one to 108) in the successfully treated patients.

The coronary stenosis was reduced on average from 84 ± 9 to 34 ± 16 per cent (paired Student's t-test; $P<0.001$). The mean coronary-artery pressure distal to the stenosis increased from 27 ± 10 to 66 ± 15 mm Hg ($P<0.001$), after dilatation, with a mean systemic pressure of 85 mm Hg. The pressure gradient was therefore reduced from 58 ± 14 to 19 ± 13 mm Hg ($P<0.001$). The decrease of the mean pressure gradient correlated well with the decrease of the stenosis after treatment (Fig. 3).

We were unable to dilate 19 vessels in 18 patients. In these subjects, the mean duration of angina pectoris had been 20 months (range, one to 192). Thirteen stenotic arteries could not be repaired because of anatomic factors, such as tortuosity of the right coronary artery, a sharp angle at the point where the left

Table 1. Patient Description and Results of Dilatation.

No. of Patients	50
Age (yr)	
Mean	49
Range	31–67
Sex	
Male	46
Female	4
Duration of angina (mo) mean ± SD	13±30
Functional classification (no. of patients)	
Class I	0
Class II	18
Class III	18
Class IV	14
Coronary disease (no. of patients)	
One vessel	30
Two vessels	7
Three vessels	5
Status after coronary-artery-bypass grafting	8
Failure	18
Medical therapy (no. of patients)	1
Elective coronary-artery bypass (no. of patients)	10
Emergency coronary-artery bypass (no. of patients)	7
Primary success (no. of patients)	32
Follow-up period	
Mean (mo)	9
Range (mo)	3–18
Success (no. of patients)	24
Death (no. of patients)	2
Recurrence	6
Repeated dilatation (no. of patients)	*3*
Coronary-artery bypass (no. of patients)	*1*
Medical therapy (no. of patients)	*2*
Complications of 60 procedures, including 50 attempts, 3 repetitions & 7 emergency coronary-artery-bypass grafts	
Elevation of creatine phosphokinase (MB fraction) (≥10 U/liter)	6 (10%)
Mean of peak values (U/liter)	35
Range of peak values (U/liter)	12–74
Myocardial infarction (elevation of creatine phosphokinase [MB fraction] & positive electrocardiogram)	3 (5%)
Pulsating hematoma at puncture site (groin)	1

Table 2. Results of Coronary Angioplasty.

Artery	No. of Patients	Dilatation Completed Successfully	Recurrence in Follow-up Period
		no. of patients	*no. of patients*
Left coronary	2	2	0
Left anterior descending coronary	33	21	3
First diagonal branch of left anterior descending coronary	1	0	0
Left circumflex	1	1	0
Right coronary	8	4	0
Status after grafting	8	6	3
Venous graft	5	3	2
Native vessel	1	1	0
Both	2	2	1
Total	53	34	6
No. of patients	50	32	6

anterior descending coronary artery branches off or tightness and eccentricity of the stenosis. In four patients, the stenotic area was passed and the balloon inflated, but the situation deteriorated; in two subjects, no reduction of stenosis or pressure gradient was possible. Seventeen of these 18 patients required surgical intervention, seven within 24 hours and 10 within four weeks. There were no surgical complications from the procedure.

Clinical success was classified as either primary (by the time of discharge) or late (any time thereafter). The 32 patients treated successfully showed improvement in clinical symptoms and stress tests leading to functional reclassification of 29 patients in the primary period (Fig. 4). Three patients were not functionally reclassified in this period; one improved after discharge, and two had recurrences in the follow-up period.

Fifteen of the 20 patients with single-vessel disease showed marked improvement (into Class I); however, only three of six with multiple-vessel disease could be so reclassified. Of the six other patients who were dilated successfully, one remained in Class II, one improved from Class II to I, two from Class IV to II and two from Class IV to III. Therefore, most patients who failed to reach Class I had many stenoses, but only some of the lesions could be dilated.

The mean working capacity at steady state rose from 86 ± 48 to 128 ± 42 W (32 patients; $P<0.001$). This change represented an increase from 53 to 80 per cent of the predicted age, sex and height-adjusted working capacity. In patients with single-vessel disease, the working capacity increased from 90 ± 45 to 143 ± 31 per cent (20 patients; $P<0.001$), which was within the normal range.

Thallium scintigrams performed during exercise were taken before and after the dilatation in 18 of 32 patients; they showed improvement of perfusion in 15 but revealed no change after dilatation in three patients who had normal scintigrams before the operation.

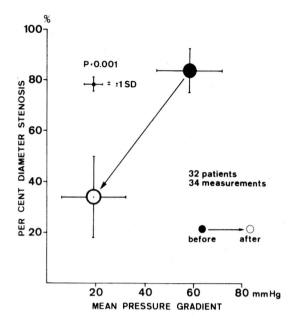

Figure 3. Pressure Recordings across Coronary Stenoses in 32 Patients (34 Vessels Dilated) with Primary Success.

The relation of the resting mean pressure gradient across the stenosis to the percentage of reduction in vessel diameter due to stenosis is shown before and after coronary dilatation. Significant decreases in pressure gradient and percentage diameter of stenosis were observed, with a correlation coefficient of r = 0.79; P<0.001.

By April, 1979, six recurrences had been observed (Tables 1 and 2); all occurred within three months after dilatation. Angiograms were obtained in all six patients. Three recurrences occurred after dilatation of stenotic saphenous-vein bypass grafts. One of these patients underwent repeated angioplasty, and the others were treated medically. The fourth recurrence was recorded in a patient with pseudoxanthoma elasticum and widespread progression of the disease. Coronary-artery bypass grafting was necessary. The fifth and sixth recurrences were observed after successful dilatation of severe stenosis of the left anterior descending coronary artery; in those cases, coronary angioplasty was repeated, again with at least initial success.

In the 50 attempts and three repeated dilatations, there were no deaths, no evidence of embolization, no central-nervous-system deficits and one femoral hematoma requiring evacuation (Table 1).

Of the 32 patients who underwent successful dilatation and the three who had repeated dilatations in the follow-up period, only one showed elevation of creatine phosphokinase (MB, or heart, fraction). This patient had renal failure, previous myocardial infarction and pain at rest owing to multiple-vessel disease and a lesion of the left main coronary artery. The ejection fraction was normal. He was the only patient who was denied an operation at the surgical conference because of the poor condition of the distal coronary arteries. The main-stem lesion was dilated, reducing

Two patients have died. One death was unrelated to the procedure and occurred nine months later. The second death occurred unexpectedly in a 45-year-old man (Patient 36) who had extensive hypertrophy of the medial smooth-muscle cells of the left main stem; the extent of hypertrophy had been underestimated on the basis of several angiograms, and the vessel was therefore incompletely dilated. The patient died two months after the procedure. Autopsy showed no occlusion or dissection of the left main coronary artery and no infarction. The cause of death was not clear.

Thirty-one patients had at least one follow-up examination, with a mean follow-up time of nine months (range, three to 18). Improvement of functional class was maintained in 20 patients; five patients showed further improvement, whereas six showed deterioration to a lower functional class (Fig. 4).

Follow-up angiograms were obtained six to nine months after dilatation for 16 of 25 patients showing consistent clinical improvement. The vessels remained widely patent. There was improvement in caliber and vessel smoothness in 13 of these 16 patients. Recurrence of stenosis (30 to 40 per cent) occurred in two patients, although they remained in Class I. Figure 5 shows dilatation of one stenotic left anterior descending coronary artery; the same procedure is shown in Figure 6 for a right coronary artery and in Figure 7 for a bypass-graft circumflex lesion.

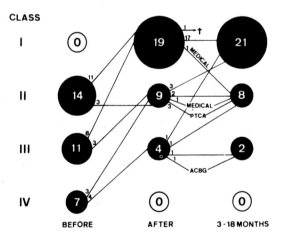

Figure 4. Analysis of Functional Status before and after Dilatation in 32 Patients Treated Successfully.

Before dilatation, 14 patients were in Class II, 11 in Class III and seven in Class IV. After dilatation, only three did not improve to a better functional class. All except one patient had at least one follow-up examination three months after the procedure. This patient died (†) two months after the procedure. Most patients retained higher functional status or showed further improvement (five patients), whereas six had recurrences, which were treated with a second dilatation (PTCA) in three patients, coronary bypass in one (ACBG) and medical therapy in two. The size of each circle is proportional to the number of patients.

Vol. 301 No. 2 THE NEW ENGLAND JOURNAL OF MEDICINE 65

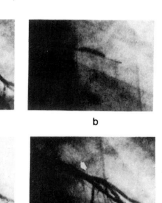

a   b

c   d

Figure 5. A 38-Year-Old Man with Typical Angina Pectoris since August, 1977 (75 W, Three Minutes, Pain, Elevation of S–T Segment, Left-Bundle-Branch Block, 49 Per Cent of Predicted Working Capacity).

(a) Coronary angiography showed 85 per cent stenosis of the left anterior descending coronary artery (right-anterior oblique view, 30°). A ^{201}Tl scan showed a severe anteroseptal defect after stress testing on September 15. (b and c) Dilatation was performed on September 16. An angiogram taken after dilatation showed a patent vessel with a 29 per cent residual stenosis. The mean coronary-pressure gradient across the lesion had decreased from 85 to 2 mm Hg. After dilatation, marked improvement of the thallium scan and normalization of the stress test occurred (200 W, three minutes, S–T segment normal, no bundle-branch block, 121 per cent working capacity, Class I). (d) A coronary angiogram on October 20, four weeks after coronary angioplasty, showed further improvement of vessel patency and wall smoothness. The ^{201}Tl myocardial-perfusion scintigram after exercise was normal on March 6, 1978, six months after coronary angioplasty. Stress testing in July gave the following results: 175 W, three minutes, no pain, S–T segment normal, 115 per cent working capacity, Class I.

the stenosis from 80 to 65 per cent and the mean pressure gradient from 47 to 8 mm Hg, but the balloon blockage of coronary blood flow (already severely impaired) over several 20-second intervals may have caused myocardial necrosis, producing a maximum creatine phosphokinase (MB fraction) level of 50 U per liter. The electrocardiogram remained unchanged. However, the patient improved for eight months after dilatation and progressed into Class III. The patient then experienced a myocardial infarction resulting from reocclusion of the stenotic left anterior descending coronary artery. Angiograms at autopsy and pathological examination revealed a patent left main coronary artery.

The procedure failed in 18 patients. One patient with severe stenosis of the first diagonal branch of the left anterior descending coronary artery, exercise induced angina pectoris, pain at rest and nontransmural myocardial infarction showed improvement but presented with recurrent spasms after dilatation — a likely explanation of the myocardial necrosis

(peak value of creatine phosphokinase [MB fraction], 20 U per liter) and the electrocardiographic evidence of lateral-wall infarction. The remaining 17 patients underwent coronary-artery-bypass grafting, seven of them within 24 hours. Of the 10 elective cases, none showed deterioration of symptoms, elevations of the MB fraction of creatine phosphokinase or electrocardiographic evidence of infarction after attempted dilatation. Six of the seven patients treated surgically within 24 hours were considered to require operations because of complications resulting from the procedure. The seventh patient had been scheduled for an emergency operation, and we were not able to dilate the stenotic area. In five of the six patients showing complications, a critical stenosis became a total stenosis, suggesting imminent infarction. Creatine phosphokinase (MB fraction) was measured after bypass grafting and showed elevations to maximum values of 12 to 74 U per liter (normal, <10) in four patients, two of whom demonstrated definite evidence of infarct on electrocardiograms. In the sixth patient, severe spasms occurred in the stenotic area after dilatation, resulting in elevations of the S–T segment that resolved within a few minutes. Re-examination showed that the stenosis had not been reduced, so we decided to operate on the patient on the same day, even though there was no elevation of creatine phosphokinase. Five of the seven patients who underwent emergency operations had clinical re-evaluations six to eight months later. Four patients reached functional Class I, and one improved from Class IV to II.

DISCUSSION

The successful application of the balloon-dilatation technic to peripheral arteries[4] in the past five years encouraged us to try the method on coronary arteries. The technic is comparatively simple and has the advantage of providing instantaneous revascularization without the need for open-heart surgery.

At present, the technic is limited by anatomic factors, such as vessel tortuosity, sharply angled arteries, cul-de-sac-like lesions and fibrotic or calcified stenoses. Most of our 18 failures can be attributed to these factors. Careful evaluation of the angiogram may reduce failures due to anatomic factors, and attention to the patient's history, in which a short duration of symptoms seems to correlate well with the distensibility of atheroma (mean duration of angina, nine months in primary successes versus 20 months in failures), may eliminate unsuitable hard lesions from consideration. These circumstances will limit this therapy to a small number of patients with coronary-artery disease. We estimate that 10 to 15 per cent of our surgically treated patients are suitable for the procedure at present.

Coronary angioplasty was successful in 32 of 50 patients, reducing stenosis from 84 to 34 per cent and decreasing the mean pressure gradient from 58 to 19

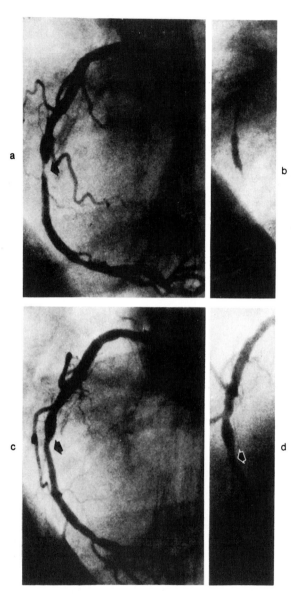

Figure 6. A 43-Year-Old Man with Typical Angina Pectoris since July, 1977 (150 W, Three Minutes, Pain, Depression of the S-T Segment, 75 Per Cent of Predicted Working Capacity, Class II).

(a) Coronary angiography (left-anterior oblique view, 60°) showed 82 per cent stenosis of the right coronary artery, 64 per cent stenosis of the left anterior descending coronary artery and 50 per cent stenosis of the left circumflex artery (not shown). A thallium scan showed an inferior perfusion defect after a stress test. (b and c) Dilatation was performed on November 21, 1977. The stenosis was reduced to 31 per cent. At the same time, stenosis of the left anterior descending coronary artery was reduced from 64 to 33 per cent. The mean coronary-pressure gradient decreased from 51 to 8 mm Hg and from 56 to 27 mm Hg, respectively. Myocardial perfusion, measured on November 28, improved after angioplasty. (d) Restudy eight months after coronary angioplasty, on July 10, 1978, had shown a patent right coronary artery, with further improvement of vessel patency. A thallium scan on April 18 showed normal myocardial perfusion after exercise. January, 1979: 200 W, three minutes, no pain, S-T segment normal, 102 per cent of predicted working capacity, Class I.

mm Hg. However, the pressure gradient across the stenosis provides only an index of the severity of the lesion since insertion of the dilatation catheter (Figs. 3 and 4) contributes to the stenosis. However, if there is no change in heart rate or blood pressure, a decline in the mean pressure gradient after dilatation must represent a reduction in stenosis since the size of the catheter remains the same. The increase in distal coronary pressure after dilatation of the balloon can therefore be used to determine whether the balloon should be inflated again to achieve optimal results.

Restoration of the original lumen, although ideal, is not necessary, since improvement in working capacity from 86 to 128 W was especially clear-cut in patients with single-vessel disease. The improvement of ^{201}Tl myocardial perfusion after dilatation underlines this observation.[18]

The question that now arises is whether the beneficial effect can be substantiated in follow-up studies. Although our experience with the procedure is limited, the first 16 patients restudied six months after dilatation did show results similar to the experience with peripheral vessels[4] and are thus encouraging. Moreover, in 13 patients, further improvement of vessel patency and wall smoothness was observed. This observation may reflect a self-healing process that took place after the controlled injury caused by balloon inflation, resulting in compression of the atheroma, with intimal tearing and enlargement of the outer diameter of the vessel. Similar changes have been described in histologic studies after dilatation of peripheral arteries.[4,9,19] The restoration of good blood flow through the dilated segment of the vessel seems to have a major role in this process.

On the other hand, six recurrences occurred in the follow-up period, namely, three of 27 patients who underwent coronary-artery dilatation and three of five undergoing dilatation of saphenous-vein-graft stenosis. Two of the former and one of the latter were subjected to repeated angioplasty, with anatomic and clinical primary success. The different kind of disease may explain the high incidence of recurrence in graft stenosis. Further experience will show whether we should eliminate this lesion from consideration.

Two points must be made. We have not been too successful in dilating stenotic main stems of left coronary arteries. It has been difficult to estimate the extent of disease in this area and the presence of concomitant spasm. We feel that these factors contributed to the death of one patient two months after dilatation. Secondly, although the procedure is relatively simple, it requires special experience. Moreover, the potential complications are both serious and sudden, so that it is mandatory that a competent surgeon be available for emergency coronary-artery bypass should it become necessary. The procedure should not be performed in hospitals lacking this facility. We believe that early surgical inter-

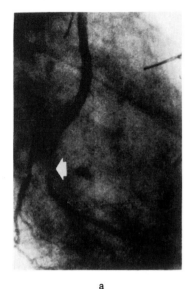 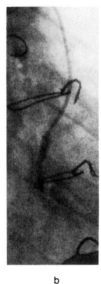 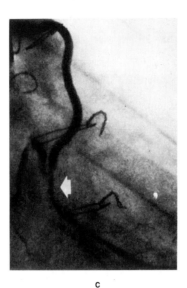 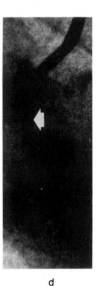

a   b   c   d

Figure 7.

A 43-Year-Old Man Who Received Grafts Bypassing the Right Coronary, Left Anterior Descending Coronary and Left Circumflex Arteries in July, 1977, and Showed Recurrence of Symptoms since July, 1977 (50 W, Three Minutes, Pain, Depression of
S–T Segment, 32 Per Cent of Predicted Working Capacity; January, 1978: Pain at Rest, Class IV).

(a) Arteriography (right-anterior oblique view, 30°) showed stenosis of the graft bypassing the left circumflex artery at the distal implantation site and progression of the disease to the recipient vessel (92 per cent stenosis). Occlusion of the bypass graft
across the right coronary artery was demonstrated, as was 30 per cent stenosis of the graft bypassing the left anterior
descending coronary artery, 64 per cent stenosis of the left anterior descending and 100 per cent of the right coronary arteries. A ^{201}Tl scintigram showed an inferoposterior-perfusion defect after stress testing. (b and c) Dilatation was performed on
January 23, 1978. This patient was the first for whom we know the status after coronary-artery bypass. Stenosis of the left circumflex artery decreased from 92 to 20 per cent, and the native vessel of the left anterior descending coronary artery
decreased from 64 to 23 per cent. Myocardial imaging returned to normal. Stress-test results improved (100 W, three minutes,
pain, depression of the S–T segment, 64 per cent of predicted working capacity, Class II). (d) Re-evaluation on August 25, eight
months after coronary angioplasty, showed a patent graft and recipient vessel with improved anatomic structure. Myocardial
scintiscanning on May 8 had revealed no perfusion defect after exercise, and stress-test results improved (125 W, three
minutes, pain, depression of the S–T segment, 80 per cent of predicted working capacity, Class II).

vention prevented major infarction in five patients. In
two of them, forceful manipulation of the dilatation
catheter caused an intimal dissection at the stenosis,
whereas in the others, complete occlusion of the stenosis occurred after uneventful dilatation. The precise
mechanism of the occlusion is not clear. Inspection of
the artery at operation revealed neither vessel damage
and extravasation nor peripheral embolization. It is
possible that the fibrous "cap" of the atheroma ruptured and that a partial dissection occurred in the diseased intima, creating a flap that occluded the stenotic area.

We emphasize that our results are preliminary.
More information and follow-up data are needed
before coronary angioplasty can be accepted as one
form of treatment for coronary-artery disease. However, the results in patients with single-vessel disease
are sufficiently good to make the procedure acceptable
for prospective randomized trials. Such trials are
clearly needed if we are to evaluate the efficacy of
this new technic as compared with current medical
and surgical treatments.

We are indebted to Drs. M. Turina and Ch. Krayenbuehl for performing the emergency operations, Dr. R. Gattiker of the Department of Cardiac Anesthesiology, M. Schlumpf for preparation of
the follow-up data and Dr. R. Pyle for help with the manuscript.

REFERENCES

1. Dotter CT, Judkins MP: Transluminal treatment of arteriosclerotic
   obstruction: description of a new technic and a preliminary report of its
   application. Circulation 30:654-670, 1964
2. Percutaneous Vascular Recanalization. Edited by E Zeitler, AR Grüntzig, W Schoop. Heidelberg, Springer, 1978
3. Grüntzig A: Die perkutane Rekanalisation chronischer arterieller
   Verschlüsse (Dotter-Prinzip) mit einem doppellumigen Dilatations-
   katheter. Fortschr Röntgenstr 124:80-86, 1976
4. Idem: Die perkutane transluminale Rekanalisation chronischer
   Arterienverschlüsse mit einer neuen Dilatationstechnik. Baden-Baden,
   G Witzstrock Verlag, 1977
5. Grüntzig AR, Kuhlmann U, Vetter W, et al: Treatment of renovascular
   hypertension with percutaneous transluminal dilatation of a renal-
   artery stenosis. Lancet 1:801-802, 1978
6. Grüntzig AR: Perkutane Dilatation von Coronarstenosen — Be-
   schreibung eines neuen Kathetersystems. Klin Wochenschr 54:543-545,
   1976
7. Idem: Transluminal dilatation of coronary-artery stenosis. Lancet
   1:263, 1978

The Lancet · Saturday 27 November 1982

LONG-TERM RESULTS OF PROSPECTIVE RANDOMISED STUDY OF CORONARY ARTERY BYPASS SURGERY IN STABLE ANGINA PECTORIS

European Coronary Surgery Study Group*

Summary   This report presents the final results (follow-up 5–8 years) of a prospective study in 768 men aged under 65 with mild to moderate angina, 50% or greater stenosis in at least two major coronary arteries, and good left ventricular function. 395 were randomised to coronary artery bypass surgery, 373 to no treatment; 1 patient in the surgery group was lost to follow-up. These original groups were compared, whatever subsequently happened to the patients. Survival was improved significantly by surgery in the total population, in patients with three-vessel disease, and in patients with stenosis in the proximal third of the left anterior descending artery constituting a component of either two or three vessel disease, and non-significantly in patients with left main coronary disease. An abnormal electrocardiogram at rest, ST-segment depression $\geqslant 1 \cdot 5$ mm during exercise, peripheral arterial disease, and increasing age independently point to a better chance of survival with surgery. In the absence of these prognostic variables in patients with either two or three vessel disease the outlook is so good that early surgery is unlikely to increase the prospect of survival. In terms of anginal attacks, use of beta-adrenergic blockers and nitrates, and exercise performance the surgical group did significantly better than the medical group throughout the 5 years of follow-up, but the difference between the two treatments tended to decrease.

*Past and present participants:
Coordinating centre, Göteborg.—E. VARNAUSKAS (director of study), S. B. OLSSON, the late E. CARLSTRÖM, THOMAS KARLSSON.
Participating centres.—Edinburgh: D. G. JULIAN, H. C. MILLER, M. F. OLIVER. Glasgow: A. R. LORIMER, I. HUTTON, R. G. MURRAY, A. TWEDDEL, T. LAWRIE, W. BAIN, the late P. CAVES, D. WHEATLEY. Helsinki: M. H. FRICK, P. T. HARJOLA, M. VALLE. Leiden: B. BUIS, J. DRAULANS, A. G. BROM, H. A. HUYSMANS. London: C. M. OAKLEY, J. F. GOODWIN, W. MCKENNA, H. H. BENTALL, W. P. CLELAND, K. S. C. WONG (Hammersmith Hospital); R. BALCON, M. HONEY, J. E. C. WRIGHT (London Chest Hospital); E. SOWTON, P. ROY, A. C. EDWARDS, J. CRICK, A. YATES (Guy's Hospital). Harefield Hospital, Harefield, Middlesex: M. TOWERS, R. THOMSON, S. A. QURESHI, R. PRIDIE, M. YACOUB. Oslo: S. SIMONSEN, O. STORSTEIN, L. EFSKIND, T. FRÖJSAKER (Rikshospitalet); E. SIVERTSEN, L. MELDAHL, G. SEMB (Ulleväl Hospital). Prague: J. FABIAN, the late L. HEJHAL, F. FIRT. Zürich: M. ROTHLINE, A. SENNING: W. MEIER.

Introduction

PREVIOUS reports of this prospective randomised study revealed a gradually increasing difference in survival between the medically and surgically treated groups.[1-3] The projected minimum follow-up time of 5 years for all patients is now completed. Some patients have been followed up for as long as 8 years. This report compares final results of survival and symptomatic changes in the two treatment groups. In addition, prognostic factors other than treatment are examined with respect to survival.

Patients and Methods

Previous reports have given a comprehensive description of patients, methods, and procedure.[1-4] In summary, 768 men, aged under 65, with angina pectoris of three months or longer duration, 50% or greater obstruction in at least two major coronary arteries, and a left ventricular ejection fraction of $0 \cdot 5$ or more were randomised to medical or surgical treatment between September, 1973, and March, 1976. Patients with severe anginal pain which could not be controlled by medical therapy were not included. In terms of prognostically important variables, the medical group of 373 patients did not differ from the surgical group of 395 patients.

Both groups had high-level medical care from the beginning of the study. Coronary artery bypass grafting was done as soon as possible after randomisation—mean delay $3 \cdot 9 \pm 3 \cdot 5$ SD months. If at any time a patient in the medical group had unacceptable symptoms despite adequate medical therapy, he was eligible for surgery.

An average of $1 \cdot 9$ grafts per patient were inserted in the two-vessel-disease subgroup and $2 \cdot 4$ grafts per patient in the three-vessel-disease subgroup. The graft patency rate was 90% within 9 months and 77% between 9 and 18 months after surgery.

All patients were to be followed up to their death or to the closing date of the study—the date of 5-year follow-up for the last included patient—March 24, 1981. In addition to 5-year follow-up, about 60% of the patients were followed for 6 years, 25% for 7 years, and 10% for 8 years.

For statistical analysis the group of patients randomised to medical treatment was compared with the group randomised to coronary bypass surgery. "Medical" patients who subsequently received surgery, having deteriorated despite medical therapy, and "surgical" patients who either refused surgery or died before operation were retained in their randomly allocated treatment groups. This approach compares two *policies* of treatment.[5] Some workers have suggested that "medical" patients who eventually receive surgery should be regarded as lost to follow-up at the time of surgery and "surgical" patients who are not operated on should be excluded from the statistical analysis. Although incompatible with the logic of trial design, such "censored" results have been compared in other randomised and non-randomised studies.[6,7] In

1174

THE LANCET, NOVEMBER 27, 1982

the present study censored survival figures and symptomatic changes were compared merely to demonstrate the extent of deviation of censored results from those obtained by the proper method of comparison. We have refrained from comparing all patients actually operated on with all not operated on: this does not provide a valid measure of the value or otherwise of elective bypass surgery, since the two categories were not separated from each other at random.[5]

An incidence test based on Edgeworth expansion was used to identify variables predictive of 5-year survival and to test survival differences between the two treatment policies at 5 and 8 years. The test is a generalisation of the log rank test such that not only zero-one variables (e.g., belonging to medical or surgical group) but also continuous variables (e.g., age) can be studied. Furthermore, the test makes it possible to eliminate the influence of a background variable such as age when testing the correlation to survival of a factor such as duration of symptoms (Odén A, unpublished).

Cox's proportional hazards regression analysis was performed to estimate the effect of mode of therapy (medical versus surgical) on 5-year survival with correction for variables predictive of survival. χ^2 and t tests were used to compare the two treatment policies with respect to other variables, and correlations between variables were tested with Pitman's non-parametric permutation test.

Results

Lost to Follow-up

In the medical group 3 patients were lost to follow-up, at $2 \cdot 5$, 3, and 4 years. In the surgical group 1 patient was lost immediately after randomisation and 2 others at $2 \cdot 5$ and $3 \cdot 5$ years. The "surgical" patient who was lost to follow-up immediately after randomisation (before surgery) is completely excluded from the follow-up analysis, reducing the number of patients in the surgical group to 394, and the total to 767.

Compliance with Randomised Treatment

100 (27%) of the 373 patients randomised to medical treatment had a coronary bypass operation because of disabling angina pectoris despite full medical therapy. At 5 years the number of these medical deviants was 90 (24%). 26 (7%) of the 394 patients randomised to surgical treatment were not operated on: 6 died, 29–82 days after randomisation, before the operation could be done; 19 refused surgery; and 1 had intercurrent liver disease contraindicating surgery.

Deaths (table I)

Numbers in parentheses represent 5-year results. 69 (61) of the 373 patients randomised to the medical group died: there were 60 (56) deaths among the 273 (283) patients who were treated medically throughout the whole observation period

and 9 (5) among the 100 (90) patients who subsequently received surgery.

41 (30) of the 394 patients randomised to surgical treatment died—33 (23) among the 368 patients who were operated on and 8 (7) among the 26 patients who were not operated on.

Operative (in-hospital) mortality was $3 \cdot 6\%$ for a total of 494 operations. It was $3 \cdot 3\%$ for 368 "surgical" patients and 4% for 100 "medical" patients who were operated on for the first time. 23 patients required a second operation and 3 of them a third. Operative mortality for the 26 reoperations was $7 \cdot 7\%$.

The most frequent cause of death was cardiac; it was entirely responsible for the mortality difference between the two treatments.

Factors Related to Survival

27 variables recorded at the time of randomisation were considered potentially relevant to prognosis on the basis of previous studies and clinical judgment. They were analysed by incidence test in order to identify those which independently predicted survival in the total patient population. Seven of them were found to be independent predictors—(i) extent of disease; (ii) location of lesion(s) in the proximal third of the left anterior descending artery (proximal LAD); (iii) resting electrocardiogram (ECG) suggestive of previous possible or probable myocardial infarction and/or with specified abnormalities according to the criteria of the HIP study;[8] (iv) ischaemic ST-segment response predominantly in lead V_5 during maximum level of a multistage symptom/sign-limited bicycle exercise; (v) peripheral arterial disease diagnosed from history and physical examination; (vi) age; and (vii) mode of treatment. Mode of treatment was highly predictive of survival. Six other independent predictors were used to refine the comparison of the two treatments. Variables such as smoking, history of myocardial infarction, serum cholesterol, arrhythmias, and conduction defects found at single physical examination, severity of angina pectoris, blood-pressure, and variables related to left ventricular function were not independently predictive of survival in this selected patient population.

Survival

Survival curves and p values for the differences between the two treatment policies are shown in figs 1–5.

Total group.—The advantage in "survival" rate for patients randomised to surgery was highly significant (fig. 1, left). The policy of surgery conferred a 53% decrease in 5-year mortality.

TABLE I—DEATHS

Cause	Medical group (n = 373)			Surgical group (n = 394)*		
	Medically treated (n = 273)	Operated on (n = 100)†		Not operated on (n = 26)	Operated on (n = 368)‡	
		In-hosp.	Late		In-hosp.	Late
Cardiac, sudden	26	0	2	4	2	3
Cardiac, not sudden	26	3	0	3	4¶	4
Related to surgical procedures	0	1	0	0	5	0
Cerebrovascular	1	0	0	0	2¶	3
Non-cardiovascular	1	0	2	0	0	5
Insufficient data	6	0	1	1	1	4
Total	60	4	5	8	14	19

*1 lost patient excluded; †103 operations; ‡391 operations; ¶1 reoperation.

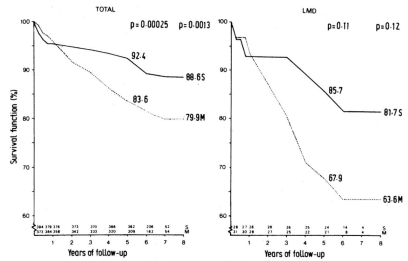

Fig. 1—Survival curves for randomised medical (M) and surgical (S) groups in the total population, and in the subset of patients with left main disease (LMD).

Numbers along the bottom represent patients at risk at the beginning of each period.

There was a large survival difference between the two treatments in patients with *left main disease* (LMD): at 5 years the mortality rate in the surgical subgroup was 56% lower than that in the medical group; the numbers were, however, small (28 and 31) and the difference was not statistically significant (fig. 1, right). None of the patients had isolated LMD; it was combined with lesions in at least two major branches.

In the surgical subgroup of patients with *three-vessel disease* the 5-year mortality rate was significantly lowered, by 66% (fig. 2, left). In patients with two-vessel disease, however, there was no significant survival difference (fig. 2, right).

In the subgroup of patients with $\geqslant 50\%$ *stenosis in the proximal third of the LAD* constituting a component of either two or three vessel disease there was a highly significant difference between the two survival curves (fig. 3, right), with mortality at 5 years lowered by 60%.

There was no significant survival difference between the two treatments for the patients *without proximal LAD*

stenosis, although all of them had either two or three vessel disease (fig. 3, left).

Of the patients with two-vessel disease, 40% had no obstruction in the proximal third of the LAD. In the medical subset of these patients the survival at 5 years (95·0%) was higher than that in the surgical subset (91·1%), largely owing to early mortality after surgery. The difference between the two survival curves was not significant (p>0·20). In 60% of the patients with two-vessel disease one of the two diseased vessels was the proximal segment of the LAD. 5-year survival for the medical subset of these patients was 83·7%. The policy of surgery improved survival (91·2%) but not to the level of statistical significance (p=0·15).

Although the presence of proximal LAD stenosis in the subgroup with three-vessel disease was also prognostically important, the influence of this stenosis on survival seemed less than in the subgroup with two-vessel disease. The number of three-vessel-disease patients without coexistent proximal LAD disease was small.

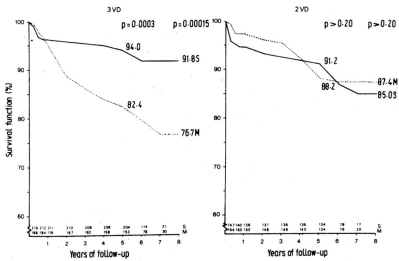

Fig. 2—Survival curves for the subsets of patients with three-vessel disease (3VD) and two-vessel disease (2VD).

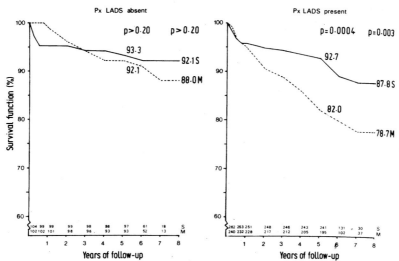

Fig. 3—Survival curves for the two subsets of patients defined by the absence or presence of stenosis in the proximal segment of the left anterior descending artery (Px LADS) as component of two or three vessel disease.

In patients with an *abnormal resting electrocardiogram* the policy of surgery improved survival more than it did in those with normal resting electrocardiogram (p values at 5 and 8 years 0·0052 and 0·0196, respectively).

In patients with *ischaemic ST-segment depression* of >1·5 mm during a symptom/sign-limited multistage exercise test the prognosis was significantly improved with the policy of surgery—mortality rate at 5 years decreased by 60% (fig. 4, right). Among the patients with 0–1 mm ST depression mortality in the two groups did not differ significantly (fig. 4, left). In 65 "medical" and 46 "surgical" patients exercise tests were not performed mainly because one centre refrained from doing the test. Some patients could not perform bicycle exercise for technical/medical reasons.

The presence of *peripheral arterial disease* was associated with greatly decreased survival, and in this group the surgical policy lowered mortality rate by 68%, but the difference was significant also in patients without peripheral arterial disease

(fig. 5). The number of patients with peripheral arterial disease was small—30 in the medical group and 28 in the surgical. In 26 "medical" and 19 "surgical" patients information regarding peripheral arterial disease was not available.

There was an association between age and survival. Although the policy of surgery significantly improved survival for the younger as well as for the older patients, the survival difference between the treatments was more striking in the older patients.

When *8-year survival* was examined all but one of these significant and non-significant differences persisted. The exception was the subgroup of patients with normal resting ECG, among whom there was no longer a significant difference in survival between the two groups.

Analysis of *censored survival* data—"medical" patients eventually operated on counted as lost to follow-up at the time of surgery, and "surgical" patients not operated on

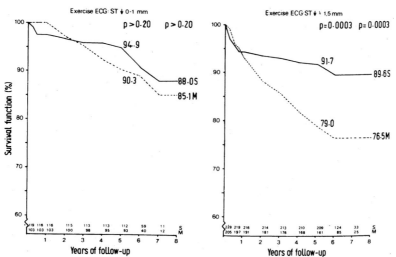

Fig. 4—Survival curves for subset of patients with exertional ST-segment depression by 0–1 mm and the subset with ≥1·5 mm ST depression.

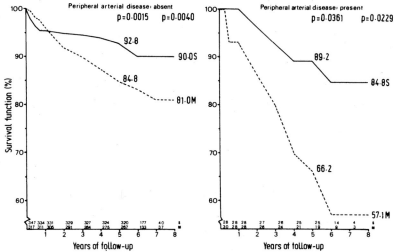

Fig. 5—Survival curves for the subsets of patients with and without peripheral arterial disease.

excluded—showed a 2–9% general increase of 5-year survival difference between the two treatments. The medical survival curves became depressed because of a gradually increasing number of censored deviants while the surgical curves frequently improved owing to relatively high mortality among the censored non-operated patients. Although the level of significance for censored survival differences between the two treatments was in most instances higher than that for uncensored survival differences, a decrease of p value from a non-significant level (0·15) to a significant level (0·02229) was found only in the subgroup of patients with two-vessel disease and coexistent proximal LAD stenosis.

Probability of surviving 5 years with either of the two modes of treatment was estimated by Cox's regression analysis with a proportional hazards model adjusting for independent predictors of survival. There were six variables independently predictive of survival in the total population and in the medical group; they were not of significant importance in the surgical group. In table II estimated survival for "medical" patients with selected sets of predictors can be compared with estimated survival for the "surgical" patients. It is clear that the probability of beneficial effect of surgery increases with increasing number of preoperative prognostic predictors. No improvement or even shortening of 5-year survival with surgery seems to be probable in two or three vessel disease without the presence of additional prognostic indicators.

Smoking, Drugs, and Angina Pectoris

Individual follow-up data of variables other than mortality were not obtained in all patients. Check-up information at 1, 2, 3, 4, and 5 years of follow-up was available in 70–80% of patients. Changes in smoking habits, drug treatment, and angina pectoris were analysed by comparison of data for each year of follow-up with data obtained at the time of randomisation for the respective patients.

At the time of randomisation each treatment group had 43% smokers. The proportions of smokers at the follow-up of 1, 2, 3, 4, and 5 years were 33%, 30%, 32%, 32%, and 35% in the medical group and 26%, 27%, 33%, 30%, and 31% in the surgical group. There were no significant differences in the overall changes of smoking habits between the two groups at any time of follow-up. Only

the proportion of patients who stopped smoking at 1 year was significantly greater in the surgical than in the medical group (22% vs 14% p>0·05).

The proportion of patients receiving a *beta-blocker* at the time of randomisation was 74% in the medical group and 75% in the surgical. At follow-up of 1–5 years the proportions of patients receiving beta-blocker treatment were 76%, 72%, 69%, 68%, and 71% in the medical group and 22%, 25%, 34%, 32%, and 34% in the surgical. The difference in overall changes of beta-blocker treatment between the two groups was highly significant. A much larger proportion of patients in the medical group than in the surgical group were receiving a beta-blocker on all five occasions (p<0·001) (fig. 6).

The proportion of patients on *nitrate* treatment at the time of randomisation was 78% in the medical group and 82% in the surgical group. Changes in nitrate treatment throughout the follow-up of 5 years were very similar to those in the beta-blocker treatment—a significant decrease of nitrate medication was seen in the surgical group (p<0·001).

TABLE II—ESTIMATED 5-YEAR SURVIVAL POLICY OF NO SURGERY: COX'S REGRESSION ANALYSIS*

	Predictors of survival†			
Diseased vessels	Prox. LAD stenosis	Periph. arterial disease	ST depression on exercise	Survival (%)
2	No	No	0–1	98
3	No	No	0–1	96
2	Yes	No	0–1	94
3	Yes	No	0–1	92
LMD	—	No	0–1	89
2	Yes	No	≥1·5	88
	Unadjusted survival			85
3	Yes	No	≥1·5	83
LMD	—	No	≥1·5	78
2	Yes	Yes	≥1·5	69
3	Yes	Yes	≥1·5	60
LMD	—	Yes	≥1·5	50
3	Yes	Yes	≥1·5	40‡
LMD	—	Yes	≥1·5	29‡

*For policy of surgery the above predictors had no influence on survival, and the unadjusted survival rate was 93%.

†Resting ECG normal and age 50 in all instances except ‡, where resting ECG is abnormal.

1178

THE LANCET, NOVEMBER 27, 1982

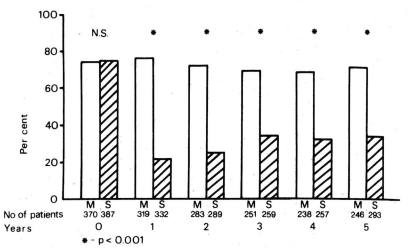

Fig. 6—Proportions of patients receiving beta blocker treatment at the time of randomisation (0) and annual follow-up of 1–5 years.

M = medical group; S = surgical group.

At the time of randomisation 9% of patients were on *digitalis* in the medical group and 13% in the surgical group. At the annual follow-up of 1–5 years the proportions of patients receiving digitalis were 13%, 17%, 17%, 15%, and 15% in the medical group and 21%, 23%, 20%, 23%, and 21% in the surgical group. Although all figures of the surgical group were slightly higher than those of the medical, the differences between the two groups were significant (p<0·05) only at 1 and 4 years.

At the time of randomisation 11% of the "medical" and 10% of the "surgical" patients were on *diuretics*. Changes after randomisation were small and there were no significant differences between the groups.

Angina pectoris was mild in 60% and moderately severe in 40% of patients in the medical group at the time of randomisation. The corresponding figures for the surgical group were 56% and 44%. Angina pectoris improved throughout the whole observation period in a significantly (p<0·001) larger proportion of patients in the surgical group (83%, 79%, 78%, 77%, and 75%) than in the medical group

(45%, 48%, 51%, 53%, and 60%) (fig. 7). The greatest difference between the two groups was in the proportion of angina-free patients—58%, 55%, 50%, 48%, and 46% in the surgical group, and 14%, 16%, 21%, 22%, and 28% in the medical group (p<0·001). The improvement in the medical group was largely due to operations.

Exercise Performance (fig. 8)

At the time of randomisation the average maximum exercise level achieved was 100 W (range 21–225 W) for the medical group and 98 W (25–200 W) for the surgical group. As judged by mean values of paired differences in the "maximum" exercise level between the five occasions of follow-up and randomisation, exercise performance increased in both groups. The increase in the medical group was 9, 7, 12, 5, and 14 W, and in the surgical group 28, 24, 22, 19, and 20 W. The difference between the groups favouring surgery was significant up to 4-year follow-up (p<0·001, <0·001, <0·01, <0·001). At 5 years the difference was not significant (p=0·14).

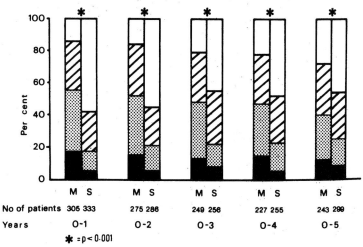

Fig. 7—Changes in angina pectoris at 1–5 years in relation to time of randomisation (0).

M = medical group; S = surgical group.

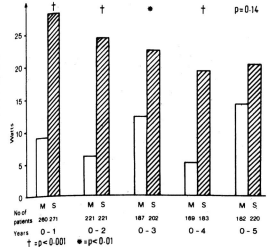

Fig. 8—**Improvement of exercise performance at 1–5 years in relation to time of randomisation (0).**

Discussion

The present study was designed primarily to answer the question whether coronary bypass surgery prolongs life in patients with chronic angina pectoris who do not require surgery for relief of symptoms. To achieve this objective it was necessary to limit the study to relatively high risk patients in whom surgery would be expected to yield greatest survival benefit. According to the experience available at the start of the study (1973) the following categories of patients were therefore not included in the study: patients who constituted an unreasonable surgical risk because of poor left ventricular function or other complicating conditions, such as uncontrolled arterial hypertension; patients with diseases independently predictive of greatly shortened life; and patients with one-vessel disease, because their prognosis was considered to be so good that vast numbers of patients would have to be recruited to show a significant survival difference within 5 years. Since the antianginal effect of bypass operation was known at the time of the start of the study, patients with severe intractable angina were likewise not included. Consequently, the results and conclusions cannot be readily applied to categories of patients other than those included.

This study compares policies of treatments rather than strictly the medical treatment with the surgical. The policy of no immediate surgery in patients randomised to the medical group actually corresponds to what many clinicians advise—that is, high-level medical care, with surgery offered only to patients whose symptoms deteriorate to an unacceptable level. Our results in the patients randomised to the surgical group indicate that coronary bypass grafting is the treatment of choice even when angina pectoris responds adequately to medical management. The difference between the two survival curves is highly significant at the projected 5-year follow-up of all patients and also at 8-year follow-up completed by a gradually decreasing proportion of patients. Retrospective stratification of patients by independent prognostic variables and comparison of survival within each prognostic stratum shows that the greatest benefit of the policy of surgery is obtained in high risk patients. Coronary obstructions pointing to high risk patients in the total population and in the medical group are: (a) left main disease with concomitant narrowing in three or two of the main

branches; and (b) proximal LAD stenosis in the presence of either three or two vessel disease. Expectation of life is further diminished by one or more of the following independent predictors (in order of importance): peripheral arterial disease; ST-segment depression in exercise ECG; ischaemic changes in resting ECG; and increasing age.

Absence of the expected prognostic influence of variables related to left ventricular function, including history of previous myocardial infarction, is most probably explained by the chosen criteria for patient selection: patients with congestive heart failure and those with a left ventricular ejection fraction less than 0·5 were not included in the study. Likewise, patients with uncontrolled arterial hypertension were not admitted.

Estimated 5-year survival and the effect of surgical treatment on survival (Cox's regression analysis) varies considerably with different combinations of predictors (table II). Although the extent and location of coronary artery disease seem to be the major determinants, estimated survival and effect of surgery is greatly influenced by other variables, especially those reflecting generalised arteriosclerotic disease and/or severe myocardial ischaemia—e.g., peripheral arterial disease and exertional ST-segment depression of 1·5 mm or more, respectively.

Was the beneficial effect of the policy of surgery on long-term survival really due to coronary bypass grafting? Although departures from the randomised treatment seem to have influenced the results, analysis of censored data pointed to bigger differences between the two treatments; in some instances, the statistical significance of the differences was even increased. We can only speculate about the possible survival effect of a small transient decrease in smoking and a permanent decrease in treatment with beta-blockers and nitrates after operation.

Our results cannot be directly compared with those of the Veterans Administration study.[6,9] In the VA study many of the patients had a left ventricular ejection fraction less than 0·5, operative mortality was higher, and graft patency was lower. Nevertheless, when these factors are taken into consideration the survival results seem in general agreement; surgery is favoured in patients with left main disease and three-vessel disease respectively. A non-randomised study, in which survival in medically and surgically treated patients was compared by Cox's regression model with adjustment for important survival-related baseline characteristics, demonstrated improved survival with surgical therapy similar to that in the present study.[7]

By comparison with medical and surgical series reported between 1975 and 1981, our 5-year survival rates for left main disease, three-vessel disease, and two-vessel disease are in the upper range,[10] indicating that the observed differences between the treatment groups are due not to poor survival with medical management but to improved survival with bypass surgery.

In the surgical group, symptomatic improvement in terms of postoperative angina, use of beta-adrenergic blockers and nitrates, and exercise performance was of the same magnitude as generally reported by experienced centres and significantly superior to that of the medical group. Although the symptomatic improvement with surgery was maintained throughout 5 years the difference between the two treatments tended to decrease with time, a finding reported by others.[11,12]

On the evidence of this study, coronary bypass grafting should be seriously considered as the treatment of choice in certain patient categories even when angina pectoris responds

1180

adequately to medical management. The selection of patients should be based not only on the extent and location of operable stenoses but also on survival-related characteristics determined by non-invasive investigation. The greatest survival benefit of surgery is obtained in patients at high risk. Surgery is unlikely to improve 5-year survival in patients with good left ventricular function whose ST segment is depressed less than 1·5 mm on exertion, whose resting ECG is normal, and who are free from peripheral arterial disease.

We thank A. Odén for statistical advice.

Correspondence should be addressed to Prof. E. Varnauskas, Sahlgrenska Hospital, s-413 45 Göteborg, Sweden.

REFERENCES

1. European Coronary Surgery Study Group. Coronary bypass surgery in stable angina pectoris: survival at two years. *Lancet* 1979; i: 889–93.
2. European Coronary Surgery Study Group. Prospective randomized study of coronary artery bypass surgery in stable angina pectoris. Second interim report. *Lancet* 1980; ii: 491–95.
3. European Coronary Study Group. Prospective randomized study of coronary artery bypass surgery in stable angina pectoris: a progress report on survival. *Circulation* 1982; **65** (suppl. II): 67–71.
4. Varnauskas E, Olsson B. The European Multicenter CAB trial. In: Yu PN, Goodwin JF, eds. Progress in cardiology. Philadelphia: W. B. Saunders, 1977: 83–89.
5. Peto R, Pike MC, Armitage P, et al. Design and analysis of randomised clinical trials requiring prolonged observation of each patient: I. Introduction and design. *Br J Cancer* 1976; **34:** 585–612.
6. Takaro T, Hultgren HN, Detre KM, Peduzzi P. The Veterans Administration Cooperative Study of Stable Angina: current status. *Circulation* 1982; **65** (suppl. II): 60–67.
7. Hammermeister KE, DeRouen TA, Dodge HT. Comparison of survival of medically and surgically treated coronary disease patients in Seattle Heart Watch: a non-randomised study. *Circulation* 1982; **65** (suppl. II): 53–59.
8. Weinblatt E, Frank CW, Shapiro S, Sager RV. Prognostic factors in angina pectoris—a prospective study. *J Chron Dis* 1968; **21:** 231–45.
9. Takaro T, Peduzzi P, Detre KM, Hultgren HN, et al. Survival in subgroups of patients with left main coronary artery disease. Veterans Administration cooperative study of surgery for coronary arterial occlusive disease. *Circulation* 1982; **66:** 14–22.
10. Varnauskas E. Coronary bypass surgery in prevention of premature mortality. *Adv Cardiol* (in press).
11. Tecklenberg PL, Alderman EL, Miller DC, et al. Changes in survival and symptom relief in a longitudinal study of patients after bypass surgery. *Circulation* 1975; **51/52** (suppl. I): 98–104.
12. Campeau L, Lespérance J, Hermann J, et al. Loss of the improvement of angina between 1 and 7 years after aorto-coronary bypass surgery. *Circulation* 1979; **60** (suppl. I): 1–5.

Aneurysm of Thoracoabdominal Aorta Involving the Celiac, Superior Mesenteric, and Renal Arteries. Report of Four Cases Treated by Resection and Homograft Replacement [*]

MICHAEL E. DeBAKEY, M.D., OSCAR CREECH, JR., M.D., GEORGE C. MORRIS, JR., M.D.[**]

Houston, Texas

MOST aneurysms of the abdominal aorta fortunately arise below the origin of the renal arteries, so that resection is not associated with serious ischemic damage to vital structures.[10] In the small proportion of cases, however, in which the aneurysm is located in the upper segment of the abdominal aorta including its major visceral branches, this problem assumes grave significance. In such cases there is considerable danger of producing fatal ischemic damage to such vital structures as the liver, kidneys, and gastro-intestinal tract, as a consequence of temporary arrest of blood flow to these organs during the period required to excise the aneurysm and replace it with an aortic homograft.

This report is concerned with our experiences with resection of aneurysms of this latter type and replacement by homografts in four cases. The aneurysms in all of these cases extended from the lower descending thoracic aorta to the lower abdominal aorta and involved the celiac, superior mesenteric, and one or both renal arteries. So far as we have been able to determine from a

review of the literature, there have been no records of similar cases in which all these vessels were involved, although two cases with involvement of some of these vessels were recently reported. In one of these the aneurysm arose below the origin of the normally placed left renal artery but involved the renal artery of an ectopic right kidney, and it was successfully resected and arterial continuity to the right kidney restored after replacement with a homograft.[21] In the other case the aneurysm, involving the celiac, superior mesenteric, and left renal arteries, was successfully resected and the segment replaced with a homograft so that continuity to the celiac and superior mesenteric arteries was restored but the left kidney was excised.[22]

In the four cases to be reported the operative procedure consisted in excision of the aneurysm and replacement with an aortic homograft with restoration of continuity to the celiac axis and superior mesenteric arteries in all, as well as to both renal arteries in two and to one of the renal arteries in the other two cases. Because of the extensive nature of this operative procedure and the problems it poses in terms of technical management as well as functional disturbances of vital organs, it seems desirable to record these cases and to consider certain observations derived from this experience, relating particularly to surgical management and to significant studies on renal and hepatic function.

[*] Presented before the American Surgical Association, White Sulphur Springs, West Virginia, April 11–13, 1956.

Supported in part by the Houston Heart Association.

[**] From the Cora and Webb Mading Department of Surgery, Baylor University College of Medicine, and the surgical services of the Veterans Administration, Methodist, and Jefferson Davis Hospitals, Houston, Texas.

550　　　　　　　　　　DeBAKEY, CREECH AND MORRIS　　　　　　Annals of Surgery
October 1956

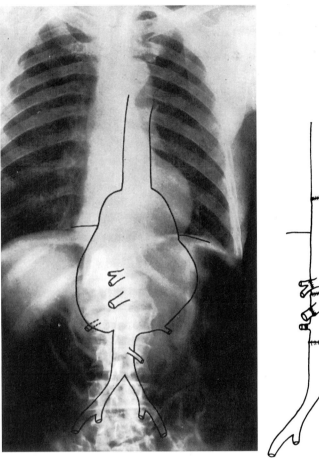

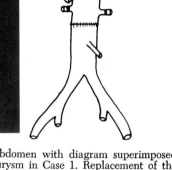

Fig. 1. Composite roentgenogram of the chest and abdomen with diagram superimposed to show location and extent of the thoracoabdominal aneurysm in Case 1. Replacement of the excised segment of aorta and aneurysm by homograft with restoration of continuity of the aorta, celiac, superior mesenteric, and renal arteries is shown in the diagram on the right.

CASE REPORTS

Case 1. J. H., a Negro farmer 66-years-old, was admitted to the Houston Veterans Administration Hospital Aug. 10, 1955, because of pain in the abdomen, left flank and back, of 2 years' duration. The pain initially was felt only in the upper portion of the abdomen but gradually extended to the back and left flank. The patient had lost about 30 pounds in weight during his illness and had had to discontinue farming because of failing strength.

The patient had had gonorrhea and probably a penile lesion, the nature of which could not be accurately ascertained.

On admission the blood pressure was 158 mm. Hg systolic and 100 mm. Hg diastolic. The heart was not enlarged and no murmurs were detected. The abdomen was somewhat protuberant, particu-

larly in the epigastrium, where vigorous pulsations were visible. Palpation disclosed a firm mass in the upper part of the abdomen extending from the xiphoid process almost to the umbilicus. It was somewhat irregular in outline, with an expansile pulsation. A systolic murmur was audible over the entire mass.

Roentgenographic examination of the chest and abdomen revealed a large soft-tissue shadow extending from the level of the eleventh thoracic to the third lumbar vertebra (Fig. 1). The bodies of the twelfth thoracic and first and second lumbar vertebrae were extensively eroded (Fig. 2). An aortogram disclosed a large dumbbell-shaped aneurysm extending from the ninth thoracic vertebra to the second lumbar vertebra. The waist of the dumbbell appeared to be at the level of the aortic hiatus of the diaphragm. Intravenous pye-

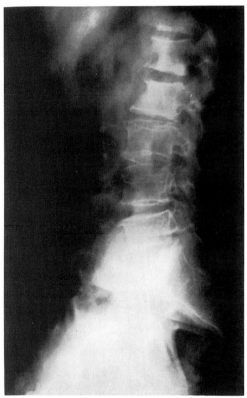

Fig. 2. Lateral roentgenogram of the abdomen in Case 1 showing erosion of the bodies of the twelfth thoracic, first and second lumbar vertebrae.

lography outlined the collecting systems of both kidneys but failed to disclose their relationship to the aneurysm. An electrocardiogram showed normal sinus rhythm with slight evidence of left ventricular hypertrophy. Laboratory studies disclosed slight increase in the globulin fraction of the serum proteins and moderate reduction in platelet count.

On Aug. 31, 1955, operation was performed under general body hypothermia. Surface cooling was accomplished with a Thermo-O-Rite® blanket, the temperature having been reduced to 32.8° C. (91° F.). A left thoracolumbar approach was employed with entrance into the pleural cavity through the bed of the eighth rib. The pleural space was obliterated by dense fibrous adhesions, and posteriorly in the paravertebral gutter and adjacent mediastinum there was evidence of old and recent hemorrhage. The lower lobe of the lung was mobilized and retracted upward. The descending thoracic aorta was isolated about 6 cm. above the diaphragm and encircled with tape. The aneurysm was found to arise about 4 cm. above the diaphragmatic hiatus and extended well below the

renal arteries. The posterior parietal peritoneum over the abdominal aorta and the ligament of Treitz were divided. The aorta below the aneurysm was encircled with umbilical tape. In order to expose the anterior surface of the aneurysm, it was necessary to remove the spleen and divide the attachments of the tail of the pancreas. The splenic flexure of the colon was mobilized, and retraction of the stomach and pancreas to the right and the colon downward exposed the aneurysm. The left kidney lay on the left anterior lateral wall of the sac, its vein passing laterally across the aneurysm to the inferior vena cava. The left kidney was dissected from Gerota's fascia and turned medially to expose the artery at the hilum. This vessel was then dissected medially and found to arise from the left lateral wall of the aneurysm about 5 cm. from its distal end. Mobilization of the left renal vein exposed the right renal artery which also arose from the aneurysm. Superior mesenteric and celiac arterial trunks were next isolated and encircled with tapes.

Occluding clamps were applied to the aorta above and below the aneurysm and to the renal, superior mesenteric, and celiac arteries. The sac was then opened widely and excised except for the portion adherent to the eroded vertebral bodies. The major branches were divided at their origin from the aneurysm to preserve maximum length. A segment of abdominal aortic homograft containing stumps of the renal, superior mesenteric, and celiac arteries was then used to bridge the defect and to restore continuity to all of these major vessels (Fig. 1). Following completion of these anastomoses the occluding clamps were released and normal circulation through the aorta was reestablished. The respective periods of arrest of circulation are shown in Chart III. The remnant of aneurysmal sac at the site of vertebral erosion was sutured along its margin for hemostasis. The omentum was then brought posteriorly and placed around the graft and into the vertebral defect. Penrose drains were placed into the vertebral bed of the aneurysm and brought out through a stab wound in the left flank. The diaphragm was repaired, an intercostal catheter was inserted into the left pleural space for underwater drainage, and the thoracic and abdominal wounds were closed.

During operation the rectal temperature drifted to 32.2° C. (90° F.). Rewarming was begun about one hour prior to completion of the operation, and the temperature returned to normal 4½ hours later. During the operation raw surfaces bled excessively. At that time the prothrombin time was 15 per cent, clotting time 45 seconds, and platelet count 100,000. Intravenous administration of 50 mg. of vitamin K-1 oxide caused prompt re-

CHART I. *Data Relating to Renal Function in Case 2*

CHART I

Determination	Before Operation	After Operation (days)			
		2	7	11	23
Urine Volume ml./24 hrs.	1000	162	1175	1150	1140
Urine Specific Gravity	1.023	1.024	1.014		1.013
Blood Urea Nitrogen mg. %	14	78	42	20	22
Urea Clearance	(1) 27%—normal max. clearance (2) 29%—normal standard clearance				
Renal Blood Flow ml./min.		29			644
Renal Plasma Flow ml./min.		16			389
Glomerular Filtration Rate ml./min.		1			69
Plasma Sodium meq./l.		141	133	138	144
Plasma Potassium meq./l.		5.9	4.3	4.0	2.6
Sodium Excretion meq./l.		8			8
Potassium Excretion meq./l.		12			30

duction in oozing and improvement in prothrombin and clotting times.

On the first postoperative day the patient was fully conscious, moved the extremities well, and appeared to be in good condition. The urinary output averaged about 7 ml. an hour.

On the second postoperative day urinary output remained about 7 ml. an hour and the blood urea nitrogen rose to 50 mg./100 ml. During the evening the patient developed severe acute pulmonary edema and was treated by venesection with removal of 500 ml. of blood and administration of aminophyline, norepinephrine, and oxygen under positive pressure. The patient's condition gradually improved, but it was necessary to continue intravenous administration of norepinephrine.

At 3 a.m. on the third postoperative day, severe pulmonary edema again developed and the patient became unconscious. Tourniquets were applied to the extremities, tracheostomy was performed, and oxygen was administered under pressure with a Halliburton positive pressure, demand-assist valve. The blood urea nitrogen had risen to 70 mg./100 ml. The urinary output was increased, however, to a total of 440 ml. in 24 hours.

On the fourth postoperative day the patient's general condition remained about the same. There was, however, a significant rise in the total urine volume for the 24 hour period, the amount being 1,183 ml. Urinary steroid excretion studies showed a significant reduction in adrenal cortical activity; therefore, an infusion of 100 mg. of cortisone was given.

Bronchopulmonary secretions remained a problem throughout the next day although there appeared to be slight improvement. The blood urea nitrogen had risen to 96 mg./100 ml. Throughout the day the urinary output remained at a high level, 1,066 ml. having been excreted during the 24 hour period. However, renal blood flow, renal plasma flow, and glomerular filtration rate were reduced to negligible levels, the actual figures being 22 ml. per minute, 12 ml. per minute, and 4 ml. per minute, respectively. Serum bilirubin had increased to 4.4 mg. and cephalin flocculation to 2 +.

Six days after operation the patient was still stuporous although he responded somewhat to painful stimuli. The blood urea nitrogen had risen to 124 mg./100 ml. and the hourly urinary volume gradually declined. A total of 500 mg. of cortisone was given intravenously. Although the total urinary volume for the 24 hour period was 522 ml., during the last 2 or 3 hours the urinary output was zero.

The patient's condition rapidly deteriorated on the seventh postoperative day, manifested by pro-

CHART II. *Studies of Hepatic Function Before and After Operation in the Cases Reported Herein*

CHART II. *Studies of Liver Function*

Determination	Case 1 (105 min.)*			Case 2 (36 min.)*		Case 3 (47 min.)*		Case 4 (102 min.)*		
	Con-trol	P.O. 1	P.O. 5	Con-trol	P.O. 19	Con-trol	P.O. 5	Con-trol	P.O. 7	P.O. 9
Bilirubin	0.5	1.1	4.4	0.7	0.3	0.7	1.3	0.4	2.2	2.0
Ceph. Flocc.	Neg.	1+	2+	Neg.	2+	Neg.	2+	Neg.	2+	2+
Thymol Turbidity	2	1	1	2	1	4.3		1	1	1
Alk. Phosphatase	3.5		4.3	4	3	3.5		3.1		11.0
Serum Protein	8.5			6.5	6.0	6.6	5.3	5.5	4.5	4.2
Prothrombin	85%	80%	80%	100%	75%	55%	100%	95%	45%	50%

* Period of simultaneous occlusion of aorta, celiac and superior mesenteric arteries.

gressive fall in blood pressure despite vasopressor agents and by complete anuria. Pulmonary edema became overwhelming and the patient died at 3:50 a.m. on Sept. 7, 1955.

At necropsy there were bilateral pulmonary edema and pneumonitis. With the exception of multiple small hemangiomas the liver was normal. The kidneys were swollen and pale, and on microscopic examination there was hyalinization of glomeruli and necrosis of tubules. The homograft was intact and patent.

Case 2. C. B. M., a man 65-years-old, was admitted to the Houston Veterans Administration Hospital on Oct. 13, 1955, for treatment of an aneurysm involving the lower thoracic and upper abdominal aorta. About 18 months previously, severe pain had developed in the left subcostal area, which seemed to be precipitated by sitting or standing. At first the pain was relieved by lying on the right side, but in recent months it had been unaffected by change in position and had increased in severity, involving also the left flank and upper lumbar region. About 6 weeks previously, the patient had been admitted to another hospital, where roentgenograms revealed an aortic aneurysm.

The patient had no knowledge of previous syphilitic infection.

The blood pressure on admission was 120 mm. Hg systolic and 80 mm. Hg diastolic. His chest was emphysematous and slightly asymmetric owing to prominence of the left anterior costal margin. However, expansion was equal bilaterally. In the epigastrium, and particularly beneath the left costal margin, vigorous aortic pulsations were evident, although a definite mass was not felt.

Laboratory studies revealed slight albuminuria and hematuria. The erythrocyte count was 4,000,-000, hemoglobin 13.7 grams, and leukocyte count

5,250, with a normal differential count. Blood urea nitrogen was 14 mg./100 ml., and urea clearance was normal (Chart I). Hepatic function studies were also normal (Chart II). Results of the serologic test for syphilis were positive. Postero-anterior and lateral roentgenograms of the chest and abdomen revealed a large fusiform aneurysm of the lower thoracic and upper abdominal aorta, the walls of which were outlined by calcium (Fig. 3). At its origin the thoracic aorta was sharply angulated to the left, and distally the aneurysm appeared to extend as far as the third lumbar intervertebral space, displacing the esophagus and stomach anteriorly (Fig. 3). The vertebral bodies were not eroded. Intravenous pyelograms showed normal excretory renal function and suggested that the renal arteries arose from the lower portion of the aneurysm.

On Oct. 19, 1955, operation was performed under general anesthesia. A left thoracolumbar approach was used with the pleural cavity being entered through the bed of the resected seventh rib. Preliminary exploration disclosed a large fusiform aneurysm arising in the lower third of the thoracic aorta and extending into the left hemithorax. There was sharp angulation of the thoracic aorta just proximal to the origin of the aneurysm. The greatest diameter of the aneurysm was at the level of the diaphragm, where it measured approximately 16 cm. The mediastinal pleura over the lower thoracic aorta was incised, the aorta was mobilized above the aneurysm, and a tape was passed about it. The aneurysm extended below the diaphragm for a distance of about 15 cm., its total length approximating 24 cm. The posterior peritoneum overlying the lower abdominal aorta was next incised together with the ligament of Treitz, the aorta in the region of the inferior mes-

554   DeBAKEY, CREECH AND MORRIS   Annals of Surgery
October 1956

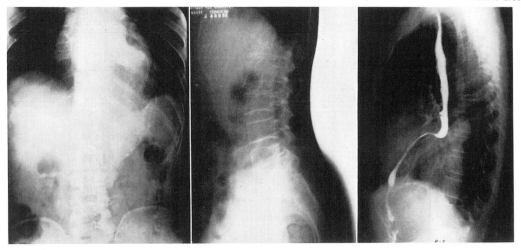

Fig. 3. Posteroanterior and lateral roentgenograms in Case 2 reveal a large fusiform aneurysm involving the lower thoracic and upper abdominal portions of the aorta. The walls of the aneurysm are outlined by calcium. The thoracic aorta is sharply angulated to the left at the upper end of the aneurysm. An esophogram with barium shows the esophagus to be displaced anteriorly by the aneurysm.

enteric artery was exposed, and a tape was passed about it. The parietal peritoneum was incised from the aortic hiatus, beneath the diaphragm to the left, behind the spleen, and downward in the left colic gutter. The spleen, splenic flexure of the colon, pancreas and stomach were then mobilized and retracted to the right, thus exposing the perirenal fat about the left kidney and the left retroperitoneal portion of the aneurysm. The left kidney was dissected from Gerota's fascia, its vein and artery were identified, and tapes were passed about them. From above the diaphragm the mediastinal pleural attachments to the aneurysm were incised and reflected, and the dissection was continued inferiorly to free the diaphragm and its crura from the aneurysm. The celiac, superior mesenteric, and right renal arteries were then isolated. With the exception of the inferior mesenteric artery, all major visceral branches of the aorta arose from the aneurysm (Fig. 4).

In order to minimize the period of arrest of visceral blood flow during resection of the aneurysm, a temporary shunt made of polyvinyl sponge, with an internal diameter of 14 mm. and approximately 40 cm. in length, was utilized. The shunt was attached to the descending thoracic aorta above the origin of the aneurysm by an end-to-side anastomosis and then similarly implanted into the abdominal aorta just above the level of the inferior mesenteric artery (Fig. 11c). The aorta proximal to the aneurysm was then doubly clamped and divided. Blood flow to the aneurysm and the branches arising from it now occurred by way of

the shunt. Removal of the aneurysm was begun at its proximal end, but because of the thin necrotic posterior wall and the danger of hemorrhage from perforation, an occluding clamp was applied just proximal to the superior mesenteric artery and above the origin of the renal arteries and another occluding clamp applied to the celiac axis. Blood flow to the kidneys and superior mesenteric artery was thus maintained by the shunt, but blood flow to the celiac artery was interrupted. The proximal portion of the aneurysm between the occluding clamps was then removed, and the intercostal vessels arising from the posterior wall of its thoracic portion were secured by suture ligature. A portion of the posterior wall could not be completely excised, but the intimal layer with the attached laminated thrombi was removed. Occluding clamps were placed on the left renal artery, and it was divided. The left renal branch of the homograft was then anastomosed to this vessel (Fig. 12a). Occluding clamps were then placed on the abdominal aorta distal to the aneurysm and on the superior mesenteric and right renal arteries, and the remainder of the aneurysm was removed. The distal end of the homograft was anastomosed to the abdominal aorta, following which a noncrushing clamp was placed across the graft just above the left renal artery and just below its right renal branch and the occluding clamp on the abdominal aorta released to restore blood flow to the left kidney by way of the shunt (Fig. 12c). The graft was then anastomosed to the right renal artery, and the occluding clamp was moved above that vessel on the homograft to permit blood flow to the right

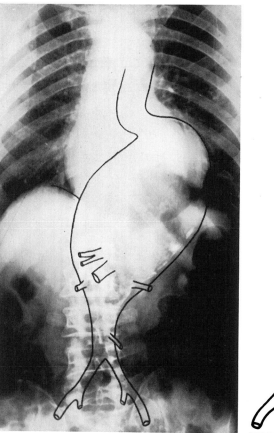
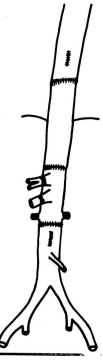

FIG. 4. Composite roentgenogram of the chest and abdomen with diagram superimposed to show location and extent of the thoracoabdominal aneurysm in Case 2. Replacement of the excised segment of aorta and aneurysm by homograft with restoration of continuity of the aorta, celiac, superior mesenteric, and renal arteries is shown in the diagram on the right.

kidney. This maneuver was repeated as the anastomoses to the superior mesenteric and celiac arteries were performed. The respective periods of arrest of circulation through these vessels are shown in Chart III. Anastomosis of the upper end of the graft to the thoracic aorta completed insertion of

CHART III. *Periods of Occlusion of the Celiac, Superior Mesenteric, and Renal Arteries in the Cases Reported Herein in Minutes*

CHART III. *Period of Occlusion in Minutes*

Case No.	Celiac Artery	Superior Mesenteric	Right Renal	Left Renal
1	120	105	105	105
2	44	36	27	23
3	114	47	15	43
4	116	102	46	0

the graft. Occluding clamps were then removed to allow blood to flow in a normal fashion through the thoracic and abdominal portions of the aorta and into its major branches (Fig. 4). Exclusion clamps were reapplied, the shunt was removed, and the openings were closed with interrupted silk sutures (Fig. 5). Incisions in the posterior peritoneum over the abdominal aorta and beneath the diaphragm and in the left colic gutter were closed with continuous catgut sutures. The spleen was removed because of laceration. The aortic hiatus was then reconstructed, and the diaphragm was repaired. A catheter was inserted into the left pleural space through the eighth intercostal space for underwater drainage, and the thoracic and abdominal wounds were closed. A tracheostomy was then performed.

Operation lasted 8½ hours. During the procedure 4,500 ml. of whole blood was administered,

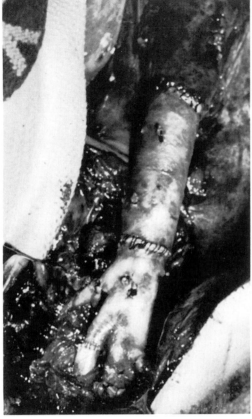

FIG. 5. Photograph made at operation in Case 2 showing the homograft in place. The celiac, superior mesenteric, and left renal arteries are visible, but the right renal artery lies behind the superior mesenteric artery. The proximal site of implantation of the shunt is just above the proximal aortic anastomosis.

and at the end of operation the patient's general condition appeared satisfactory.

During the first postoperative day, the urinary output was 15 ml. By the end of the second postoperative day, however, urinary output had increased to 162 ml. and renal function studies showed severe depression (Chart I). There was progressive increase in urinary volume during the next few days and by the fifth day the 24 hour urinary volume was 1,240 ml. The blood urea nitrogen reached a maximal level of 79 mg./100 ml. on the 3rd postoperative day and subsequently declined to a normal level by the 11th postoperative day. Renal function studies showed a return to normal on the 23rd day (Chart I) and liver function studies were essentially normal on the 19th day (Chart II).

Good peristalsis was evident on about the 4th postoperative day, and the patient was eating nor-

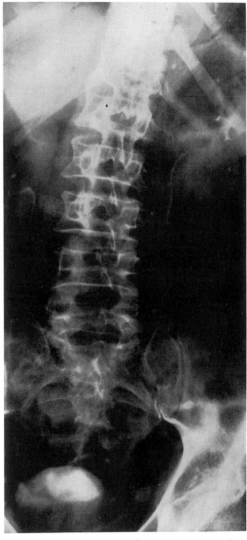

FIG. 6. Intravenous pyelogram in Case 2 four months after operation reveals normal function of both kidneys.

mally by the end of the 1st week. A necrotic area in the left groin resulting from extravasation of norepinephrine on the first postoperative day was debrided on the 26th postoperative day, and 15 days later the area was covered with a split thickness skin graft. The patient was discharged on Jan. 4, 1956, fully recovered and in good condition.

He returned for examination on Feb. 19, 1956. Intravenous pyelograms disclosed normal function of both kidneys (Fig. 6). Discrete renal function studies at this time were found to be normal, the actual figures for renal blood flow, renal plasma flow and glomerular filtration rate being respectively 792, 475 and 68 ml./minute. An aortogram

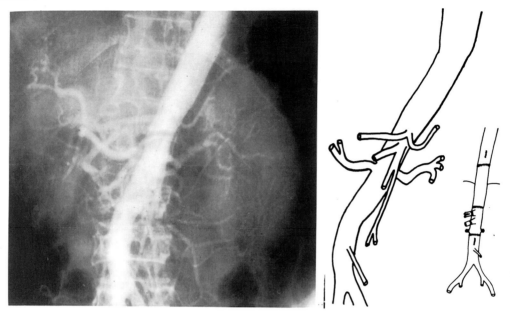

FIG. 7. Aortogram made five months after operation in Case 2 reveals normal patency of the aorta, celiac, superior mesenteric and renal arteries.

on March 23, 1956 demonstrated patency and normal filling of the renal, superior mesenteric, and celiac arteries (Fig. 7).

Case 3. P. T., a man 42-years-old, was admitted to the Methodist Hospital on Nov. 5, 1955, complaining of a sense of fulness and increasing pain in the upper part of the abdomen of one year's duration. During the preceding 4 months, the pain had become so severe that large doses of narcotics were necessary for relief. The pain, which was most severe in the epigastrium and left upper abdominal quadrant, was not related to eating and was not relieved by antacids. An aortogram made at another hospital 3 months previously had disclosed an aneurysm of the lower thoracic and upper abdominal portions of the aorta. Operation was performed at that time, but because the aneurysm involved the renal arteries, it was not resected.

The patient had had brucellosis many years previously and was known to have had hypertension for one year prior to admission. There was no history of venereal disease.

On admission, the blood pressure was 180 mm. Hg systolic and 130 mm. Hg diastolic. An operative scar extended in an oblique direction from the umbilicus to the left costal margin. Examination of the abdomen was difficult because of extreme tenderness in the epigastrium, although a pulsating mass was palpable.

The only significant laboratory findings were a few granular casts and a trace of albumin in the urine. Roentgenograms of the chest showed a soft tissue mass in the posterior mediastinum protruding to both the right and left of the spine (Fig. 8). Abdominal films showed the mass to protrude to the left of the lumbar spine at the level of the third and fourth lumbar vertebrae. Calcification was present in the peripheral portions of the mass. Intravenous pyelograms revealed a normal kidney and ureter on the right but poor concentration on the left. An electrocardiogram disclosed normal sinus rhythm with slight left ventricular hypertrophy and slightly prolonged P–R interval.

On Nov. 10, 1955, operation was performed through a left throacoabdominal approach with excision of the previous scar. Upon retracting the lung anteriorly, the mid-descending thoracic aorta was found to be sharply angulated in a horseshoe fashion. At the lower end of this angulation was a large aneurysm, which extended distally through the diaphragm.

The descending thoracic aorta above the aneurysm was mobilized, and a tape was placed about it. The spleen was resected, and an incision was made in the left lateral posterior peritoneum; this detached the splenic flexure of the colon and permitted retraction of the stomach, colon, and pancreas to the right. Gerota's fascia was incised, and the left kidney was mobilized from its bed and retracted to the right and inferiorly. The left renal artery was isolated and was found to arise from the lower portion of the aneurysm. The ligament of Treitz and the posterior peritoneum overlying the abdominal aorta in the region of the inferior

558   DeBAKEY, CREECH AND MORRIS   Annals of Surgery
                                                                    October 1956

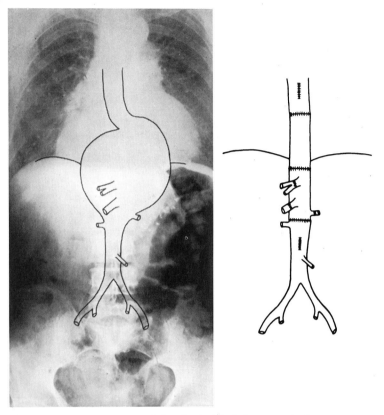

Fig. 8. Composite roentgenogram of the chest and abdomen with diagram superimposed to show location and extent of the thoracoabdominal aneurysm in Case 3. Replacement of the excised segment of aorta and aneurysm by the homograft with restoration of continuity of the aorta, celiac, superior mesenteric and left renal arteries is shown in the diagram on the right.

mesenteric artery were incised. The lower abdominal aorta was mobilized, and a tape was placed about it distal to the aneurysm. The aneurysm was then mobilized by removal of the diaphragmatic attachments to its surface, and the superior mesenteric and celiac arteries were isolated. The aneurysm extended distally to a point just beyond the origin of the left renal artery but above the origin of the right renal artery (Fig. 8). A shunt of compressed polyvinyl sponge was then anastomosed to the side of the descending thoracic aorta above the aneurysm and to the anterior aspect of the abdominal aorta below the aneurysm. The left renal artery was then divided at its origin from the aneurysm, and the left renal branch of a lyophilized homograft was anastomosed to it. Occluding clamps were placed on the descending thoracic aorta above the aneurysm, on the abdominal aorta just proximal to the right renal artery and on the celiac and superior mesenteric arteries, and the aneurysm was excised. The distal portion of the **abdominal aortic homograft was anastomosed to**

the abdominal aorta. The homograft was then occluded above the renal arteries. Upon removal of the abdominal aortic clamp, blood flow to the kidneys was restored through the shunt.

The superior mesenteric and then the celiac arteries were next anastomosed to the graft, following which the homograft was anastomosed to the lower end of the descending thoracic aorta, and the occluding clamp on the aorta removed with resultant restoration of normal blood flow (Fig. 8). The periods of occlusion for the left renal, superior mesenteric, and celiac arteries are shown in Chart III. The shunt was removed and the aortotomy wounds were closed. The posterior remnant of the wall of the aneurysm was oversewn with a continuous suture for hemostasis, a pedicled omental graft was wrapped about the homograft, and the posterior peritoneum over the abdominal aorta was closed with a continuous suture. The left kidney was replaced in its bed and the peritoneum in the left gutter was reapproximated. Appendectomy was then performed.

CHART IV. *Data Relating to Renal Function in Case 3*

CHART IV

Determination	Before Operation	After Operation (days)			
		2	7	11	22
Urine Volume ml./24 hrs.	1000	306	3595	5560	1800
Urine Specific Gravity	1.026	1.013	1.010		1.014
Blood Urea Nitrogen mg. %	20	60	80	27	
Renal Blood Flow ml./min.	461	212	396		596
Renal Plasma Flow ml./min.	277	121	226		358
Glomerular Filtration Rate ml./min.	67	19	44		59
Plasma Sodium meq./l.	122	128	132	132	128
Plasma Potassium meq./l.	5.2	3.8	4.3	4.3	3.5
Sodium Excretion meq./l.	63	61	280		101
Potassium Excretion meq./l.	40	62	52		38

The diaphragm was repaired, and an intercostal drainage tube was inserted through the ninth intercostal space and connected to water sealed drainage. The wound was then closed. A catheter was placed in the right side of the chest through the fifth intercostal space, since the right hemithorax had been entered through the mediastinum during the procedure. The patient received 6,500 ml. of whole blood during the procedure, which lasted about 7 hours. At the conclusion of the operation the blood pressure was 150 mm. Hg systolic and 90 mm. Hg. diastolic.

Within the first 90 minutes after operation, 250 ml. of urine was excreted, and urinary output continued at a rate of 5 to 20 ml. per hour during the first 48 hours (Chart IV). By the 4th day, the urinary volume had reached 1,820 ml. with maximal diuresis on the ninth day, when 5,950 ml. of urine was excreted. Subsequently, the output declined to normal levels. The blood urea nitrogen level had risen to 100 mg. on the 5th day but returned to normal by the tenth day. Glomerular filtration rate was severely reduced on the day after operation but returned to normal by the 22nd day. Peristaltic activity became normal by the 4th postoperative day, when the nasogastric tube was removed. Hepatic function studies revealed a slight increase in serum bilirubin and a cephalin flocculation of 2 + (Chart II).

After the first postoperative week the patient required only occasional small doses of codeine

and by the 10th postoperative day he was completely ambulatory, asymptomatic and taking a normal diet. He was discharged on Dec. 4, 1955, in good condition. On Mar. 31, 1956, excretory pyelograms were normal.

Case 4. A. G., a white man 65-years-old, was admitted to the Houston Veterans Administration Hospital Oct. 25, 1955, for treatment of a thoracoabdominal aneurysm, diagnosed about 2 months previously at the time of subtotal gastric resection for peptic ulcer.

On admission, the blood pressure was 130 mm. Hg systolic and 90 mm. Hg diastolic. Examination revealed a well healed upper abdominal midline incision and a palpable pulsating mass in the left upper abdominal quadrant. Laboratory findings were essentially normal. Roentgenograms of the chest revealed no abnormalities, but an anteroposterior roentgenogram of the abdomen disclosed calcification of the wall of the aneurysm (Fig. 9). Aortography, performed through a catheter passed through the left brachial artery into the thoracic aorta, revealed aneurysmal involvement of both the lower thoracic and upper abdominal portions of the aorta. Intravenous pyelograms were normal, although discrete renal function studies disclosed slight reduction in glomerular filtration rate. No abnormalities were detected in the electrocardiogram.

On Nov. 12, 1955, operation was performed through a left thoracoabdominal approach. Exploration revealed a fusiform aneurysm involving

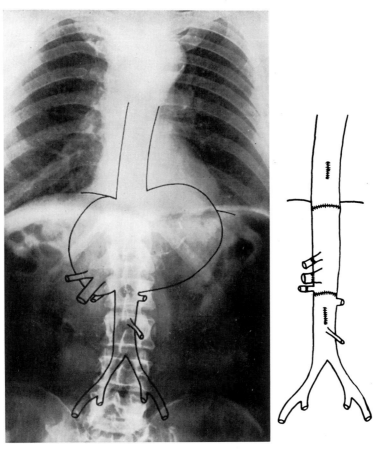

Fig. 9. Composite roentgenogram of the chest and abdomen with diagram superimposed to show location and extent of the thoracoabdominal aneurysm in Case 4. Replacement of the excised segment of aorta and aneurysm by the homograft with restoration of continuity to the aorta, celiac, superior mesenteric and right renal arteries is shown in the diagram on the right.

the distal third of the descending thoracic aorta and extending through the diaphragm to include the upper abdominal aorta. The thoracic aorta above the aneurysm was mobilized, and a tape was passed about it. The diaphragm was then incised to the surface of the aneurysm. The posterior peritoneum beneath the left leaf of the diaphragm was incised laterally, the incision continuing behind the spleen and down the paracolic gutter as far as the sigmoid colon. The stomach, spleen, pancreas and colon were then mobilized and retracted to the right to expose the left anterolateral surface of the aneurysm and distal abdominal aorta below. The posterior peritoneum over the lower abdominal aorta was incised just above the inferior mesenteric artery, the aorta below the aneurysm was mobilized, and a tape was passed about it. The left renal vein was then isolated and mobilized. The left renal artery was exposed and found to arise just distal to the aneurysm. The

right renal artery, however, had its origin from the aneurysmal sac about 4 cm. from its distal end. The superior mesenteric and celiac arteries arising from the aneurysm were likewise exposed and mobilized, and tapes were passed about them. With exclusion clamps, a temporary by-pass shunt of compressed polyvinyl sponge was then implanted into the aorta above and below the aneurysm (Fig. 10). With blood flow established through the shunt, occluding clamps were applied to the aorta above the aneurysm just distal to the shunt and below to the aneurysm at a level above the origin of the left renal but below the origin of the right renal artery. After occlusion of the superior mesenteric and celiac arteries, the aneurysm was opened widely and excised. A lyophilized abdominal aortic homograft containing the right renal, celiac, and superior mesenteric arteries was utilized to replace the excised segment of aorta. The right renal branch of the homograft was first

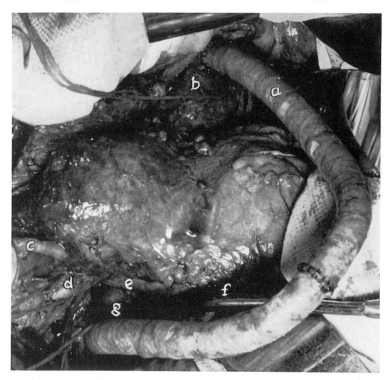

Fɪɢ. 10. Photograph made at operation in Case 4. The shunt (a) has been implanted into the thoracic aorta above (b) and into the abdominal aorta below (g). The celiac (c) and superior mesenteric (d) arteries have been isolated and tapes passed about them. The left renal vein (e) crosses the lower portion of the aneurysm. The left renal artery has been identified and a tape (f) passed about it.

anastomosed to the right renal artery, after which the distal end of the aortic homograft was anastomosed to the distal segment of aorta. By removal of the occluding clamp above the origin of the right renal vessel, blood flow was restored to the right kidney, flow to the left kidney not having been interrupted during the procedure. Anastomosis of the superior mesenteric artery to the graft was completed, and following this the celiac artery was anastomosed to the graft. The proximal anastomosis between the homograft and the thoracic aorta was next completed (Fig. 9). The shunt was removed, the abdominal viscera were replaced, and the posterior peritoneum was approximated. Several rubber drains were placed into the bed of the aneurysm along the eroded surface of the vertebral bodies and brought out in the left flank. The diaphragm was then repaired, an intercostal catheter was inserted into the left pleural space for underwater drainage, and the wound was closed. The periods of occlusion for the celiac, superior mesenteric, and right renal arteries are shown in Chart III.

Following operation, the blood pressure remained at preoperative levels. The urinary volume

for the first postoperative day was 199 ml. and the blood urea nitrogen was 33 mg./100 ml. Subsequently, the daily urinary volume progressively increased to 2,020 ml. by the 8th postoperative day. Blood urea nitrogen increased to 136 mg. per 100 ml. on the 8th day and began to decline thereafter. Hepatic function studies showed some deviations from normal, but his general condition was satisfactory (Chart II). By the 8th postoperative day the patient was ambulatory, taking a soft diet, and asymptomatic. During the following week his condition seemed to be daily improving, and arrangements for his discharge were being made.

On the 13th postoperative day, the patient began to have bloody diarrheal stools and on the following day vomited a large quantity of bright red blood and became hypotensive. At abdominal exploration, the site of bleeding was found to be a marginal ulcer at the gastrojejunostomy. The ulcer was resected, but the patient became hypoxic and died after cardiac arrest developed. At necropsy, all the anastomoses were patent, and both kidneys appeared relatively normal.

DISCUSSION

There are two important considerations in extirpation of aneurysms of this type, stemming primarily from the location and extent of the lesion. The first of these is concerned with the technical performance of the procedure and the second with the potential ischemic damage to such vital abdominal organs as the kidneys, liver, and gastrointestinal tract as a result of temporary arrest of circulation to them during performance of the procedure. The former has an important bearing upon the latter, since ischemic damage to tissues is largely dependent upon the period of circulatory arrest. To be sure, there is considerable variation in the tolerance of different tissues to ischemia, but in all of them limits exist as to the duration of circulatory arrest that will permit subsequent survival. Although these limits may be affected by a number of factors, including particularly development of collateral circulation as a result of the lesion itself, this cannot always be determined with sufficient reliability prior to operation. Accordingly, this aspect of the problem, namely, prevention of fatal ischemic damage to tissues during performance of the procedure, assumes major significance.

Two methods are available to overcome this problem. The first consists in the use of hypothermia to reduce oxygen demand by the tissues and the second in the use of a temporary shunt to conduct blood around the occluded segment with performance of the procedure in a manner to minimize the period of circulatory arrest. The former method was employed in the first case, but because it did not prove successful, the latter method was used in the subsequent three cases. The gratifying results obtained in these cases suggest that it is the preferable method, and for this reason its more detailed consideration seems desirable.

TECHNICAL CONSIDERATIONS

Because of the extensive nature of these aneurysms, involving both the lower thoracic and upper abdominal aorta, adequate exposure is essential. This may be satisfactorily obtained by a left thoracoabdominal approach. The patient is placed in the supine position with the left side of the chest slightly elevated and the left arm suspended from an overhead support (Fig. 11a). The incision is made over the left seventh or eighth rib, extending from the midaxillary line anteriorly and obliquely across the costal margin to the midabdominal line and then curving inferiorly as a midabdominal incision to a point well below the umbilicus (Fig. 11a). The left pleural and peritoneal cavities are entered, and after division of the costal cartilages, the diaphragm is incised radially from its peripheral attachment to the aortic hiatus, and the rib-spreader is inserted. This provides satisfactory exposure of the entire extent of the aneurysm as well as the aorta immediately above and below the lesion.

After adequate exploration to determine more precisely the extent and nature of the lesion, it is desirable to expose, by careful sharp and blunt dissection, the aorta immediately above and below the aneurysm and to encircle these segments of the aorta with umbilical tape as a safety measure for control of hemorrhage. The major visceral branches, such as the celiac, superior mesenteric and renal arteries arising from the aneurysm, are then similarly treated (Fig. 11b). In order to expose these vessels satisfactorily, as well as to permit subsequent excision of the aneurysm, a left retroperitoneal approach is employed. This is done by dividing the posterolateral parietal peritoneal attachment along its left border with mobilization of the visceral organs to the right side.

The shunt, which has previously been prepared, is then sutured into place by end-to-side anastomosis, with the use of partial tangential occlusion clamps, to the descending thoracic aorta immediately above the aneurysm and to the abdominal aorta just above the bifurcation (Fig. 11c). For this

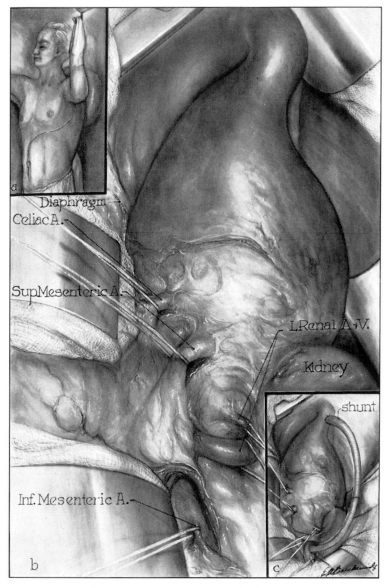

FIG. 11. Drawings made at operation in Case 2. (*a*) The patient is placed in the supine position with left shoulder slightly elevated and left arm supported overhead. Left thoracolumbar incision is employed. (*b*) The aorta above and below the aneurysm has been exposed and the celiac, superior mesenteric, and left renal arteries and the left renal vein have been isolated and tapes passed about them. The right renal artery lies behind the superior mesenteric artery and is not seen. (*c*) A shunt made of compressed polyvinyl sponge has been attached as an end-to-side anastomosis to the descending thoracic aorta above the aneurysm and to the abdominal aorta below the aneurysm.

purpose, it has been found desirable to use a shunt made of compressed polyvinyl sponge (Ivalon®) with a lumen 14 mm. in diameter [7, 8] (Fig. 10).

Once these steps have been completed and the shunt is functioning satisfactorily and conducting blood into the abdominal aorta below the aneurysm, attention may be directed toward mobilization and resection of the aneurysm. By careful sharp and blunt dissection, the aneurysm is freed from surrounding structures as well as possible,

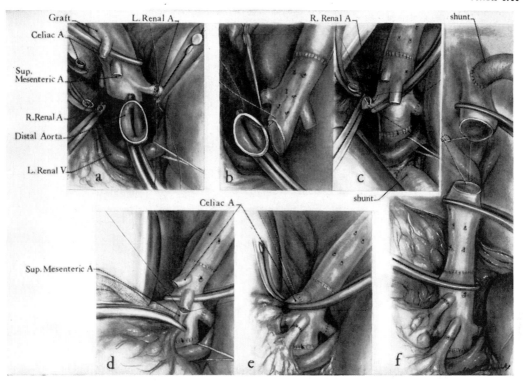

FIG. 12. (*a*) Anastomosis of the left renal artery to its comparable segment on the aortic homograft. The technic of anastomosis here as elsewhere consists in a continuous through-and-through suture of arterial silk. (*b*) Anastomosis of the distal end of the aortic homograft to the abdominal aorta. (*c*) With the anastomosis of the homograft to the left renal artery and to the abdominal aorta completed, an occluding clamp is applied to the graft in an oblique manner so that it lies below the origin of the right renal artery and above the origin of the left renal artery. The previously applied occluding clamp on the abdominal aorta has now been released, permitting restoration of blood flow to the left kidney through the shunt. The anastomosis to the right renal artery is then performed. (*d*) Anastomosis of the graft to the superior mesenteric artery. It may now be observed that the occluding clamp lies between the origin of the superior mesenteric and both renal arteries, thus permitting blood flow to be restored to both kidneys during the anastomosis of the superior mesenteric artery. (*e*) Anastomosis of the celiac artery. It may be noted again that the previously applied occluding clamp below the superior mesenteric artery has been moved up so as to lie immediately above it in order to permit restoration of blood flow through this vessel during the anastomosis of the celiac artery. (*f*) With the celiac artery anastomosis completed and the occluding clamp reapplied above it, blood flow has been restored to all the major visceral branches of the homograft during the completion of the final anastomosis to the descending thoracic aorta above.

following which special noncrushing arterial occlusion clamps are applied to the aorta immediately below the upper attachment of the shunt and immediately above its lower attachment, as well as to the celiac, superior mesenteric, and renal arteries. By this means circulation through the aneurysm is completely arrested, and it may be excised with minimal blood loss. In some instances it has not been feasible to free the aneurysm satisfactorily because of its intimate adherence to surrounding structures. Under these circumstances, as for example in Cases 1, 3, and 4, it may be preferable to apply the occluding clamps as already described and, after complete arrest of circulation through the aneurysm, it may be safely entered and removed by intramural dissection of the aneurysmal sac.

When the aneurysm has thus been excised, aortic continuity may be restored by means of a properly fitting abdominal aortic homograft, including the branches of the celiac, superior mesenteric, and renal

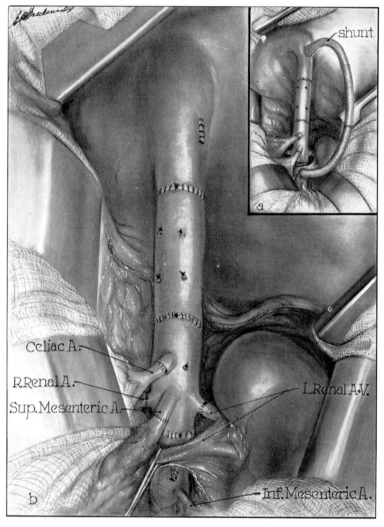

FIG. 13. Drawing showing completion of the homograft replacement in Case 2. (*a*) All anastomoses have been completed and blood flow through the aorta has been restored although the shunt is still in place. (*b*) The shunt has been removed and the openings in the aorta repaired.

arteries. In order to minimize the period of circulatory arrest to the abdominal organs, particularly the kidneys, which are considered more susceptible to ischemia, the anastomoses are performed in the following order. The left renal artery is attached first to its counterpart on the graft by end-to-end anastomosis, with the use of continuous through-and-through suture of 00000 arterial silk (Fig. 12a). Similar anastomosis is performed to unite the graft to the opening in the abdominal aorta (Fig. 12b). An oc-

clusion clamp is applied to the graft somewhat obliquely so that it lies above the origin of the left renal artery but below the origin of the right renal artery, and the occluding clamp on the abdominal aorta immediately above the lower attachment of the shunt is released (Fig. 12c). This permits restoration of circulation into the left renal artery through the shunt. The anastomosis to the right renal artery is performed as previously described (Fig. 12c). Upon completion of this anastomosis, an occluding clamp is applied to the graft above the origin of both renal arteries but below the origin of the superior mesenteric artery, and the previously applied occluding clamp is released to permit blood flow into both renal arteries (Fig. 12d). In a similar manner, after the anastomosis to the superior mesenteric artery has been performed, the occluding clamp is moved above it while the anastomosis is performed to the celiac axis (Fig. 12e). After completing the latter anastomosis this maneuver with the occluding clamp is repeated, following which the final anastomosis is made between the graft and the opening in the lower thoracic aorta (Fig. 12f). In this manner circulation by way of the shunt is restored successively into each major visceral artery as rapidly as its anastomosis is performed. Following completion of the final anastomosis of the graft to the thoracic aorta, the occluding clamps at this level are removed and blood flow is restored in a normal manner through the graft (Fig. 13a). The shunt is then removed and the openings in the aorta are closed by a continuous suture of arterial silk (Fig. 13b). In cases in which the aneurysm has produced erosion of the vertebral bodies and a large excavated area, it is desirable to wrap the graft with a pedicled flap of omentum in order to provide it with a protecting bed of vascular tissue. The abdominal viscera are then replaced in their normal positions, and the posterolateral peritoneal attachments on the left side are approximated. The opening in the diaphragm is closed, and after a catheter has been placed in the left pleural space for underwater drainage, the wound is closed in layers.

PHYSIOLOGIC CONSIDERATIONS

The ischemic effects of temporary interruption of circulation to the major abdominal organs in man have not been clearly defined owing to the paucity of such observations. Moreover, studies directed toward this problem in animals have not yielded entirely satisfactory information. Thus, although the effects of ischemia on the kidney have been extensively investigated experimentally, variable results have been obtained depending to a large extent on the methods employed to produce renal ischemia as well as the type of animal used for this purpose. It has been demonstrated, for example, that occlusion of the renal artery for two hours in unilaterally nephrectomized rabbits uniformly produced death from renal damage.[1] On the other hand, in rats this procedure is apparently well tolerated, since most of the animals will survive this period of occlusion, but extension of this period beyond three hours reduces survival by about 50 per cent.[27, 28] In dogs longer periods of renal artery occlusion may also be tolerated with progressive increase in mortality after two hours.[16, 17, 25, 40, 44] Although renal function is temporarily reduced during the early period, it gradually returns to normal over a period of two to three weeks. Similarly, autotransplantation of the kidney into the groin or neck, with complete interruption of its blood supply for periods up to two and one-half hours, results in severe temporary depression of renal function.[34] Renal homotransplants apparently behave in a similar fashion.[13, 14, 26] Dempster described a type of anuria that developed in 5 to 16 per cent of animals following autotransplantation and homotransplantation of kidneys. This anuria, which differs from the early depression of function customarily encountered, consists in complete failure to excrete urine after re-establishment of blood flow. It probably results from ischemia and arteriolar spasm incident to transplantation, since increased speed in removing and transplanting the kidney apparently decreases the incidence of this type of anuria.

The significance of the method of producing renal ischemia is well illustrated by experiments carried out in our laboratory.

Thus, two-hour occlusion of the aorta immediately above the renal arteries has a negligible effect on renal function in the dog.[31, 32] Similarly, unilateral renal artery occlusion for two hours is well tolerated, although it results in moderate depression of renal function in the occluded kidney but not in the contralateral kidney.[23, 31, 32, 39] On the other hand, simultaneous occlusion of the aorta and one renal artery for two hours results in severe depression of renal blood flow and glomerular filtration rate in the occluded kidney.[31, 32] Particularly significant is the fact that in this latter group of animals renal function in the kidney whose renal artery was not occluded remains unaffected, despite the fact that the aorta was occluded immediately above this point. It is also significant that the pressure in the aorta distal to the level of occlusion was found to be approximately 25 mm. Hg. These observations would suggest that this degree of subfiltration arterial pressure resulting from collateral blood flow provides a high degree of protection from ischemic damage to the kidney. These experiments were repeated utilizing hypothermia, and it was found that this afforded moderate protection to the kidney subjected to complete ischemia.[33]

Much less precise information is available on the ischemic effects of temporary arrest of circulation to the kidney in man.[9] Semb,[41] in performing segmental resection of the kidneys for tuberculosis, clamped the entire renal pedicle for one and one-half hours without significant alteration of renal function. Similarly, Bahnson[2, 3] reported survival of a patient following occlusion of both renal arteries for 37 minutes, although another of his patients died from renal failure after occlusion of the aorta above the renal arteries for 110 minutes. In the case recently reported by Ellis and associates,[21] occlusion of the aorta and one renal artery for 95 minutes produced no significant reduction in renal function.

In describing the results of renal homotransplantation in nine patients, Hume and co-workers[26] reported resumption of function in kidneys that had been totally ischemic for 200 minutes. Similarly, Merrill and associates,[30] in performing homotransplantation of a healthy kidney from one identical twin to another, observed that total anoxia of the kidney for a period of 90 minutes does not mitigate against resumption of adequate function.

Thus, it is apparent from these experimental and clinical observations that considerable variations exist in the safe period of tolerance of the kidney to anoxia, ranging from less than one hour to over three hours. Obviously, there are a number of variables that influence this problem, including age, pre-existing renal disease, collateral blood supply, individual variations, and the like. In this connection it may be significant that three of the four patients reported herein were in the seventh decade. In these cases arrest of circulation to the kidneys for periods of less than one hour was well tolerated, but prolongation of this period for more than one and one-half hours, despite the use of hypothermia, resulted in fatal ischemic damage to the kidneys.

In the first case in which operation was performed under hypothermia complete renal ischemia bilaterally for 105 minutes resulted in acute, severe oliguria of 48 hours' duration, followed by gradual increase in urinary volume. However, in spite of the fact that urinary output had increased to 1,183 ml. on the fourth day after operation, glomerular filtration rate and renal blood flow were minimal and death from uremia occurred on the seventh postoperative day. Microscopically, there were extensive hyalin changes in the glomeruli and tubular necrosis. These events suggest that the fatal renal failure was a direct result of prolonged renal ischemia. If the patient could have survived the first week, perhaps renal recovery would have taken place, a possibility that is suggested by the experience with renal autotransplants.[13, 14, 34]

In the second case blood flow to the right and left kidneys was interrupted for 27 and 23 minutes, respectively (Chart III). The pattern of recovery was similar to that observed in acute renal failure from other causes and consisted of early oliguria followed by diuresis with return to normal function about the third week. Discrete renal function studies in this case point to ischemic involvement of the entire nephron initially with glomerular recovery preceding tubular recovery (Chart I).

Renal response in the third case was strikingly similar to that in the second case although the right kidney was ischemic for only 15 minutes, while the left was ischemic for 43 minutes. In this instance the occurrence of pronounced diuresis suggested more extensive tubular involvement. Nonetheless, recovery was practically complete by the end of the third week. The response in the fourth case was somewhat similar, although as might be anticipated from the unilateral ischemia, depression of renal function was only moderate and recovery was more rapid than in the other cases.

These limited observations do not permit definite conclusions to be drawn regarding the maximum safe period of complete renal ischemia. They do, however, point to the importance of minimizing this period. It seems reasonable to state that in cases of this kind periods up to 45 minutes may be safely tolerated, but extension beyond this time is increasingly hazardous. It would also appear that hypothermia of moderate degree, i.e., with reduction of body temperature to 32.2° C. (90° F.), cannot be relied upon to provide adequate protection against fatal ischemic damage to the kidneys when the period of ischemia extends over 100 minutes.

Whereas observations on the effects of renal ischemia in man are relatively few, there are even fewer data pertaining to the effects of ischemia on the liver and gastro-intestinal tract. There are a number of older reports of ligation of the thoracic aorta for aneurysm and considerable recent experience with temporary occlusion for resection of aneurysms,[10-12] but these are not pertinent since only partial ischemia of these structures is produced in this way. Nor are the observations following celiac or hepatic artery ligation for bleeding esophageal varices relevant, since an extensive collateral network is still functioning.

The tolerance of the liver to ischemia has been extensively investigated in experimental animals, but the results of these studies have been quite variable.[4-6, 15, 18-20, 24, 29, 35, 36, 38, 43] According to these experiments, for example, the maximum safe period of arrest of circulation to the liver varies from somewhat less than one half hour to a little more than one hour. These variations in results are apparently due to a number of factors, including particularly the different species of experimental animals used, the different methods of producing arrest of hepatic circulation with consequent differences in the degree of completeness of occluding the afferent hepatic circulation, the presence of anomalous or accessory arteries to the liver, and the administration of antimicrobial agents. For these reasons it is difficult to evaluate these experimental observations in determining more precisely the critical period of hepatic anoxia. The weight of evidence would suggest, however, that this period closely approaches one half hour. There is also some experimental evidence to suggest that this period may be prolonged to one hour by the use of hypothermia.[5, 37, 42]

This problem in man is even less well defined owing to the paucity of such observations. Wangensteen[45] reported performance of left hepatic lobectomy in three cases with simultaneous occlusion of the hepatic, gastroduodenal, and superior mesenteric arteries and the portal vein. In the two patients who survived operation the periods of ischemia were 33 and 24 minutes respectively, whereas in the patient who died there were two periods of ischemia of 12 and 15 minutes each interrupted by a 20-minute period of release of ischemia. Two somewhat similar cases of left hepatic lobectomy for metastatic carcinoma have also been reported by Burch, Traphagen, and Folkman.[4] In their first patient who recovered, the aorta above the celiac axis and the portal vein were occluded for 10 minutes with no apparent disturbance in liver function. Similar occlusion for the same period of time was done in the second case, but the patient developed extensive mesenteric thrombosis which subsequently caused his death. More recently, Shumway and Lewis [42] reported four cases of right hepatic lobectomy performed under hypothermia in which temporary arrest of hepatic circulation was produced by occlusion of the thoracic aorta at the level of the tenth intercostal space, the inferior vena cava above and below the liver, the hepatic artery, and the portal vein. In the two patients who survived operation the period of ischemia was 45 minutes, while in the other two patients who died it was 33 and 40 minutes, respectively.

The four cases reported herein afforded a unique opportunity to observe the effects of relatively complete interruption of arterial blood supply to the liver and gastro-intestinal tract. Thus, with the aorta occluded above the diaphragm and below the renal arteries, and with celiac and superior mesenteric arteries interrupted, the liver was nourished only by the portal venous flow. The effectiveness of this afferent nutrient vessel to the liver was also greatly diminished through reduction of arterial blood flow to the portal bed since this was derived primarily from the inferior mesenteric artery. In the three successful cases the periods of hepatic ischemia ranged from 44 to 116 minutes. Yet in no instance

was hepatic function seriously deranged (Chart II). It cannot be stated with certainty that hypothermia was responsible for the apparent tolerance of the liver to ischemia of two hours in the first case, since the patient survived only one week. There was no evidence, however, during this time nor at autopsy of significant liver derangement. The most consistent changes were noted in serum bilirubin levels and in the cephalin flocculation. In view of the large amount of whole blood administered during operation, however, the slight increase in serum bilirubin does not appear to be significant. Accordingly, these observations would suggest that in man the liver can tolerate occlusion of its major arterial blood supply for relatively long periods, almost two hours, without significant alteration in function.

In the first case arterial blood flow to the entire gastro-intestinal tract was interrupted for 105 minutes. Postoperatively, there were moderately severe intestinal distention and diarrhea suggesting some disturbances but otherwise no evidence of serious ischemic damage to these organs. In the remaining cases the superior mesenteric artery was occluded for periods ranging from 36 to 102 minutes, but a temporary aortic shunt maintained blood flow through the inferior mesenteric artery so that the gastro-intestinal tract was not completely ischemic. In none of these cases was intestinal distention or diarrhea a problem, and resumption of gastro-intestinal function took place in a normal manner following operation.

SUMMARY

1. Four cases of extensive thoracoabdominal aneurysm of the aorta treated by resection and homograft replacement are reported. In all of these cases the aneurysm extended from the lower descending thoracic aorta to the lower abdominal aorta and involved the celiac, superior mesenteric, and one or both renal arteries. The

operative procedure consisted in excision of the aneurysm and replacement with an aortic homograft with restoration of continuity to the celiac axis and superior mesenteric arteries in all as well as to both renal arteries in two and to one of the renal arteries in the other two cases.

2. The most important consideration in extirpation of aneurysms of this type arises from the potential ischemic damage to such vital organs as the kidneys, liver, and gastro-intestinal tract as a consequence of temporary arrest of circulation to them during performance of the procedure. Two methods are available to overcome this problem, namely hypothermia and the use of a temporary shunt to conduct blood around the occluded segment with the performance of the procedure in a manner to minimize the period of circulatory arrest.

3. Hypothermia was used in the first case, but the patient died of renal failure one week after operation. The superior mesenteric and both renal arteries were occluded for 105 minutes and the celiac artery for 120 minutes.

4. In the other three cases temporary shunts were employed permitting significant reduction in the period of temporary arrest of circulation to the abdominal viscera. The successful results obtained in these cases emphasize the importance of performing the procedure in such a manner as to minimize the period of ischemia to these vital structures.

5. In the three successful cases the period of occlusion of the renal arteries ranged from 15 to 46 minutes. Serial renal function studies in these cases revealed a characteristic pattern of depression of function, as reflected by increase in the blood urea nitrogen level and significant reduction in renal blood flow and glomerular filtration rate, during the first four or five days after operation with progressive return to normal during the subsequent ten days to two weeks.

6. The period of occlusion of the celiac artery in these cases ranged from 44 to 116 minutes. Studies of hepatic function revealed no significant alterations.

7. The period of arrest of circulation through the superior mesenteric artery varied from 36 to 102 minutes and no significant disturbances in gastro-intestinal function were observed.

BIBLIOGRAPHY

1. Badenoch, A. W. and E. M. Darmady: The Effects of Temporary Occlusion of the Renal Artery in Rabbits and its Relationship to Traumatic Uraemia. J. Path. and Bact., 59: 79, 1947.

2. Bahnson, H. T.: Definitive Treatment of Saccular Aneurysms of the Aorta with Excision of Sac and Aortic Suture. Surg., Gynec. and Obst., 96: 383, 1953.

3. Bahnson, H. T.: Treatment of Abdominal Aortic Aneurysm by Excision and Replacement by Homograft. Circulation, 9: 494, 1954.

4. Burch, B. H., D. W. Traphagen and M. J. Folkman: The Use of Aortic Occlusion in Abdominal Surgery with a Report of Two Human Cases. Surgery, 34: 672, Oct. 1953.

5. Burch, B. H., D. W. Traphagen, M. J. Folkman, D. A. Rosenbaum and E. C. Mueller: Temporary Aortic Occlusion in Abdominal Surgery. Surgery, 35: 684, May 1954.

6. Child, C. G., III, R. D. McClure, Jr. and D. M. Hays: Studies on Hepatic Circulation in Macaca Mulatta Monkey and in Man. Surg. Forum, American College of Surgeons, p. 140, 1952.

7. Cooley, D. A., D. E. Mahaffey and M. E. DeBakey: Total Excision of the Aortic Arch for Aneurysm. Surg., Gynec., & Obst., 101: 667, Dec. 1955.

8. Creech, O., Jr., M. E. DeBakey and D. E. Mahaffey: Total Resection of the Aortic Arch. Surgery (In press).

9. Creech, O., Jr., M. E. DeBakey, G. C. Morris, Jr. and J. H. Moyer: Experimental and Clinical Observations on the Effects of Renal Ischemia. Surgery, 40: 129, July 1956.

10. DeBakey, M. E., D. A. Cooley and O. Creech, Jr.: Resection of the Aorta for Aneurysms and Occlusive Disease with Particular Reference to the Use of Hypothermia. Analysis of 240 Cases. Trans. Amer. Coll. Cardiology, 5: 153, 1955.

CLINICAL APPLICATION OF A NEW FLEXIBLE KNITTED DACRON ARTERIAL SUBSTITUTE*

MICHAEL E. DE BAKEY, M.D., DENTON A. COOLEY, M.D., E. STANLEY CRAWFORD, M.D., AND GEORGE C. MORRIS, JR., M.D.†

Houston, Texas

The direct surgical treatment of various forms of aortic and arterial disease often requires a vascular replacement. Homografts were first employed successfully for this purpose and both technically and functionally have provided highly gratifying results. Their major disadvantage, however, lies in the inconvenience associated with their procurement and preparation and the fact that they are not available in sufficient quantities to meet the increasing demands for their use. For these reasons attention has been directed toward development of a satisfactory arterial substitute for homografts which would be free of these disadvantages. Various materials such as Ivalon, nylon, Orlon, Dacron, and Teflon have been used for this purpose and fashioned into tubes by different methods including heat-sealing, sewing, braiding, knitting, and weaving. In a previous publication we reviewed our experience with these various types of synthetic arterial substitutes based upon observations derived from an analysis of 317 cases in which they were employed.[1] The functional results in this series of cases were generally satisfactory and provided additional evidence that tubular fabrics of these synthetic materials could be used as substitutes for homografts. There were, however, certain disadvantages associated with most of them, particularly in their technical application. For these reasons and with the hope of overcoming some of these objections, efforts were continued toward the development of a more satisfactory arterial substitute.

As a result of these efforts and in cooperation with Professor Thomas Edman of the Philadelphia Textile Institute, a new knitting machine was designed with particular specifications to produce seamless knitted Dacron tubes in different sizes and in the form of bifurcations as well as multi-branch tubes.[2] Various types of synthetic filament yarns were tested from nylon to Teflon, but the most suitable was found to be Dacron texturized on the Flufon process. To achieve greater flexibility a process of cross-crimping the tubular knitted fabric by heat-setting was used. Various means of coating and chemically treating the fabric were tried but were discarded after

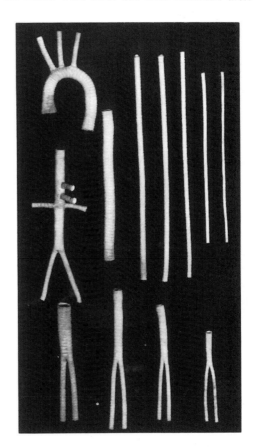

FIG. 1. Photograph showing various types and sizes of Dacron grafts for replacement of different anatomic segments of the aorta and peripheral arteries.

* Supported in part by the United States Public Health Service under Grant H-3137, the American Heart Association, the Houston Heart Association, and Mr. Arthur Hanisch.

† From the Cora and Webb Mading Department of Surgery, Baylor University College of Medicine, Houston, Texas.

862

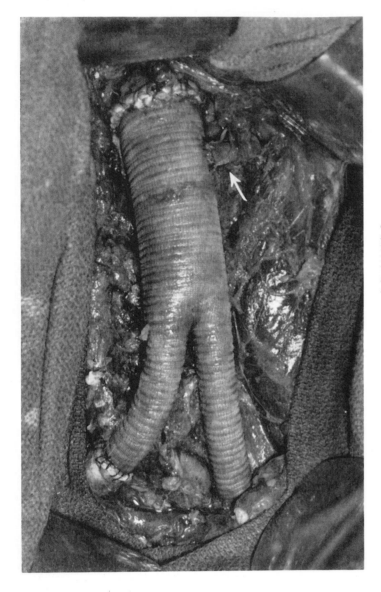

FIG. 2. Photograph made at operation following resection of aneurysm of abdominal aorta involving left renal artery and replacement by Dacron bifurcation graft with end-to-side anastomosis to left renal artery as indicated by arrow.

tests showed that the thoroughly cleansed but untreated Dacron fabric was more satisfactory.

Investigations of this knitted Dacron arterial substitute in the laboratory have demonstrated that it meets certain requirements of strength, durability, and flexibility. Among its desirable characteristics are the following: (1) It may be repeatedly sterilized by autoclaving in the usual manner without weakening of the fabric. (2) It is available in tubes of various sizes and shapes including secondary branches for ready adaptability to all segments of the major arterial system (fig. 1). (3) Because of its knitted construction it is nonfraying and may be cut with the scissors or scalpel at an angle or holes may be cut in its side for anastomosis of branches (fig. 2). (4) It may be clamped with arterial clamps without harm to the fabric. (5) Its flexibility and elasticity greatly facilitate its anatomic and technical application under a wide variety of circumstances.

An important consideration in the use of this knitted Dacron graft is the fact that like any untreated fabric material it is porous and will allow

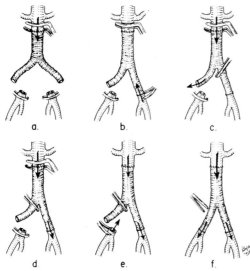

FIG. 3. Drawings illustrating technical application of bifurcation Dacron graft for replacement following resection of aneurysm or occlusive disease of abdominal aorta. (a) Following completion of aortic anastomosis proximal occluding clamp on aorta is released for a few seconds to permit flushing of atheromatous debris or accumulated clot formation. (b) Following completion of the left iliac anastomosis, occluding clamp on this vessel is released permitting retrograde blood flow into graft and thus flushing it of accumulated clot. (c) An occluding clamp is applied to left iliac limb of graft just distal to bifurcation and the occluding clamp on aorta is momentarily released to flush out thoroughly any accumulated clots. (d) The occluding clamp on left iliac limb of graft is removed and applied to right iliac limb, and the aortic occluding clamp is slowly and intermittently released over a period of several minutes permitting restoration of circulation through graft and into left iliac artery. (e) Distal occluding clamp on right iliac artery is temporarily released to permit retrograde flushing of any accumulated clots before performing anastomosis. (f) After completing anastomosis to right iliac artery, distal occluding clamp is removed first and proximal clamp is then slowly and intermittently released permitting restoration of circulation to right iliac artery.

blood to seep through its wall until sufficient clotting has taken place in the interstices of the fabric. In our early experience this was considered an objectionable feature and various methods of treating the fabric were tried in an effort to make it "water-proof" and eliminate this porosity. Experimental studies, however, indicated that this porosity may be considered a desirable feature since it permits subsequent ingrowth of fibrous tissue to produce firm attachment of the new intima lining the inner surface. Accordingly,

certain technical maneuvers were developed which would minimize blood loss from seepage through the graft. This may be illustrated by describing the technical application of a bifurcation Dacron graft for replacement following resection of aneurysms or occlusive disease of the abdominal aorta or as a bypass in accordance with our experience.

At the outset of the operation pre-clotting of the graft is done by thoroughly immersing it in a small quantity of the patient's own blood. After the aortic anastomosis has been completed, the proximal occluding clamp on the aorta is released for a few seconds (fig. 3a). This is done for two reasons: first, it permits the blind segment of the aorta proximal to the occluding clamp to be flushed of atheromatous debris or clot formation, and second, it permits further sealing of the interstices of the graft by fibrin formation.

Attention is then directed toward anastomosis of one of the iliac limbs of the graft, and after this has been completed the following maneuvers are performed. The distal occluding clamp on the iliac artery is released first permitting retrograde blood flow into the graft and thus flushing it of any accumulated clots (fig. 3b). An occluding clamp is then applied to the iliac limb of the graft just distal to the bifurcation and the occluding clamp on the aorta is momentarily released to permit thorough flushing and to wash out any accumulated clots in the graft (fig. 3c). Further assurance of removal of all clots from within the graft may be provided by insertion of the suction tip into the lumen of the graft through the other open iliac limb of the graft. The occluding clamp on the anastomosed iliac limb is then removed and applied to the other iliac limb of the graft just distal to the bifurcation (fig. 3d). The aortic occluding clamp is then slowly and intermittently released over a period of several minutes permitting restoration of circulation through the graft and into the anastomosed iliac artery (fig. 3d). Before performing the anastomosis to the remaining iliac artery, it is desirable to release momentarily the distal occluding clamp to permit retrograde flushing of its blind segment in order to remove any clots or atheromatous debris that may have accumulated in the meantime (fig. 3e). Following completion of this anastomosis, the distal occluding clamp is released first and then the proximal clamp is slowly and intermittently released (fig. 3f). The application of warm moist

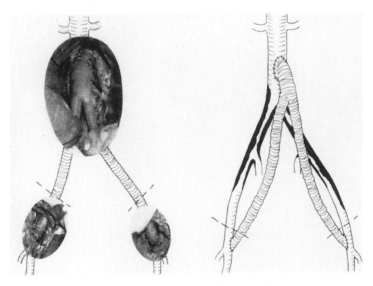

FIG. 4. Photographs made at operation showing use of bypass bifurcation Dacron graft in treatment of occlusive disease of abdominal aorta and iliac arteries. As indicated in diagram on right, trunk of bifurcation Dacron graft is attached as end-to-side anastomosis to abdominal aorta just below origin of renal arteries, and bifurcation limbs of graft are similarly attached to common femoral artery below occlusion permitting restoration of normal circulation to lower extremities.

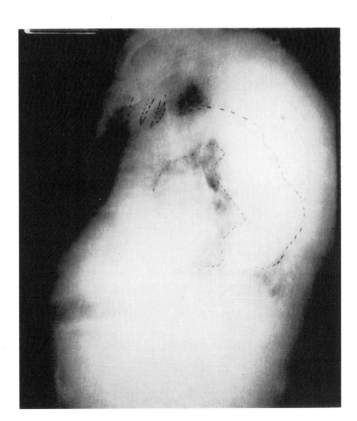

FIG. 5a. Angioaortogram in patient with extensive fusiform aneurysm of descending thoracic aorta arising just distal to left subclavian artery.

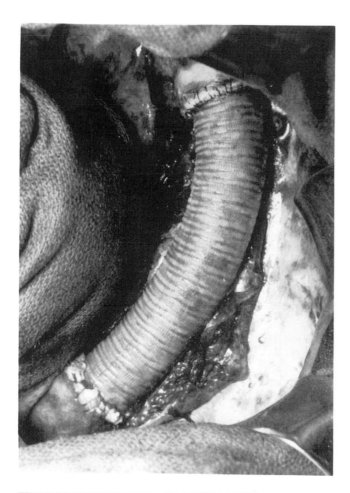

FIG. 5b. Photograph made at operation in same patient showing successful replacement of resected aneurysm with Dacron graft.

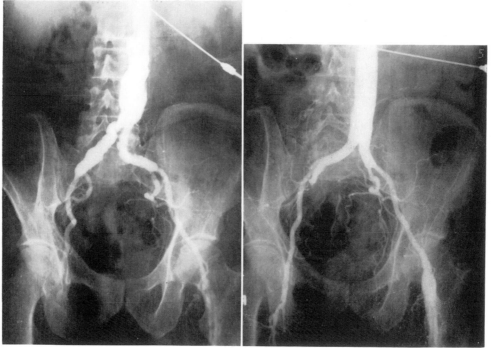

FIG. 6. (a, left) Preoperative aortogram in patient with extensive arteriosclerotic aneurysm of abdominal aorta involving bifurcation and common iliac arteries. (b, right) Aortogram in same patient made approximately one year after operation showing excellent function of bifurcation Dacron graft used to replace excised aortic aneurysm.

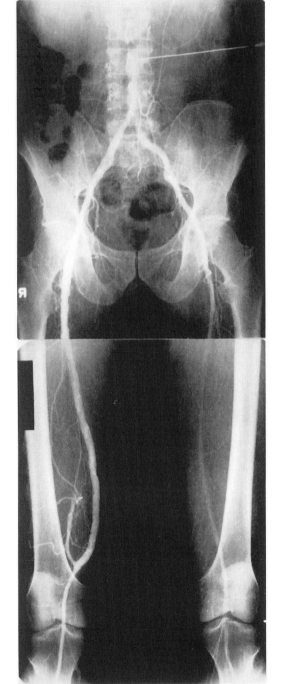

Fig. 7. Aortogram made almost 14 months after operation showing restoration of circulation in right lower extremity by means of bypass Dacron graft attached by end-to-side anastomoses to common femoral artery above and to popliteal artery below.

pads under slight pressure further enhances sealing of the graft and the anastomoses.

Similar technical maneuvers may be employed in the application of this graft under variable circumstances either as a single straight tube for bypass operations or in the performance of multibranched anastomoses. A particular advantage lies in the fact that it may be converted from a temporary shunt into the permanent graft under certain circumstances in which it is desirable to minimize or avoid temporary arrest of circulation such as in the region of the aortic arch or the upper segment of the abdominal aorta from which arise the major vessels to the abdominal viscera.

In an aneurysm involving the aortic arch, for example, and in which the proximal segment of the ascending aorta is involved, the Dacron graft may be attached with end-to-side anastomoses to the uninvolved segment of the ascending aorta and to the descending limb of the aortic arch distal to the aneurysm. With the use of similar end-to-side anastomoses the trunk of a bifurcation Dacron graft is attached to the previously inserted Dacron graft and its three limbs to the innominate and left common carotid arteries. By this means occluding clamps may be applied to the intervening segment of the aortic arch to permit its resection while aortic and cerebral circulation is maintained through the Dacron grafts. Another Dacron graft may be used to replace the excised segment of the aortic arch with anastomosis to the left subclavian artery to complete the procedure. The Dacron grafts which served the purpose of a temporary shunt to maintain aortic and cerebral circulation during the resection are allowed to remain as permanent grafts, thus minimizing the extent of the operative procedure.

This advantage of conversion of the Dacron graft used first as a temporary shunt into the subsequent permanent graft is further illustrated in cases of extensive aneurysms involving the thoracoabdominal segment of aorta including the celiac, superior mesenteric, and renal arteries. Under these circumstances a Dacron graft with appropriate branches is first attached by end-to-side anastomoses to the descending thoracic aorta above the aneurysm and to the uninvolved segment of the abdominal aorta below the aneurysm. The left renal artery is then attached by end-to-end anastomosis to its corresponding branch on the graft and circulation through the

TABLE 1

Tabulation of results obtained following use of Dacron grafts, other synthetic grafts, and homografts derived from analysis of our clinical experience

Dacron Grafts	No. Cases	Deaths	Graft Failures	Successful
Thoracic aorta				
Aneurysms	51	13 (25%)	0	38 (75%)
Occlusions	18	1 (5.5%)	0	17 (94%)
Abdominal aorta				
Aneurysms	235	6 (2.6%)	1 (0.4%)	228 (97%)
Occlusions	163	1 (0.6%)	3 (2%)	159 (98%)
Peripheral arteries				
Aneurysms	27	2 (7%)	1 (4%)	24 (89%)
Occlusions	243	2 (0.8%)	17 (7%)	224 (92%)
Total Dacron grafts	737	25 (3.4%)	22 (3%)	690 (94%)
Total other synthetic grafts	341	29 (8%)	27 (8%)	285 (84%)
Total homografts	593	62 (10%)	24 (4%)	507 (85%)
Total all grafts	1,671	116 (7%)	73 (4%)	1,482 (89%)

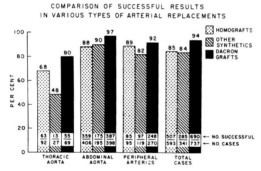

FIG. 8. Graphic representation showing higher incidence of successful results following use of Dacron grafts than other synthetic grafts as well as homografts in various vascular segments.

Dacron graft is permitted. The graft is now functioning as a temporary shunt and in this manner the total period of arrest of circulation to the left renal artery should not exceed more than 10 to 15 minutes, which is well within the critical period. Occluding clamps may then be applied to the aorta above and below the aneurysm and to the celiac, superior mesenteric, and right renal artery and the aneurysm resected. The right renal artery is then attached to its corresponding branch on the Dacron graft by end-to-end anastomosis and circulation restored to the right kidney by releasing the occluding clamps on these vessels. In this manner, arrest of circulation to the right kidney should not exceed about 20 minutes. The superior mesenteric and celiac

arteries are then consecutively anastomosed to their corresponding branches on the Dacron graft and circulation to these vessels restored by releasing the occluding clamps. The procedure may then be completed by suture closure of the aortic ends above and below the end-to-side attachments of the Dacron graft. In this manner the Dacron graft which has served as a temporary shunt is converted into the permanent graft thus greatly facilitating the operative procedure and minimizing the period of arrest of circulation to these critical vessels.

Since early in 1957 we have employed this Dacron graft almost exclusively in the treatment of a wide variety of aortic and arterial diseases (figs. 4 and 5). Analysis of this experience, which now includes a total of 737 cases, reveals results that are in general most satisfactory. Although insufficient time has elapsed to provide long-term evaluation of the functional efficacy of these grafts, follow-up observations extending for periods ranging from a year to a year and a half have been most gratifying and within this period of time have revealed no failures which could be attributable to the graft (figs. 6 and 7). Moreover, a comparison of these results with those obtained in our previous experience with the use of other types of synthetic vascular replacements and with homografts indicates the Dacron graft to be superior in all respects (table 1; fig. 8). Particularly noteworthy is the fact that the incidence of failures attributable to the graft was significantly less in the Dacron series than in other synthetic grafts. To be sure, an important factor contributing to the reduction in mortality in the more recent Dacron series is improvement in surgical management resulting from increased experience. The fact remains, however, that the mortality in the Dacron series is significantly lower than in the other series and this fact along with the distinctly higher incidence of over-all successful results provides good evidence of its clinical value and efficacy.

Michael E. De Bakey, M.D.
Baylor University College of Medicine
Houston, Texas

REFERENCES

1. CRAWFORD, E. S., DE BAKEY, M. E., AND COOLEY, D. A.: The clinical use of synthetic arterial substitutes in 317 patients. A.M.A. Arch. Surg., *76:* 261, 1958.
2. EDMAN, T.: Tubing for arterial surgery knit on V-bed flat unit. Knitted Outwear Times, *26:* 7, 1958.

RESECTION OF ENTIRE ASCENDING AORTA IN FUSIFORM ANEURYSM USING CARDIAC BYPASS

Denton A. Cooley, M.D.

and

Michael E. De Bakey, M.D., Houston, Texas

Fusiform aneurysm of the ascending aorta is a common form of aortic disease and is associated with a grave prognosis. Although excisional therapy is now established as the method of choice for aneurysms of the aorta, this form of treatment for aneurysms of the ascending aorta has been limited until the present time to sacciform lesions in which the neck is relatively small. In such instances tangential excision of the aneurysm with lateral aortorrhaphy may be curative if the adjacent aortic wall is not also involved by the degenerative process. In fusiform aneurysms and in most extensive sacciform lesions this method of treatment cannot be utilized and segmental resection of the ascending aorta with homograft replacement is necessary. Because of the fatal consequences from even brief occlusion of the ascending aorta, no aneurysm in this anatomic location has been treated successfully by segmental aortic resection. This report is concerned with a case of successful resection of the ascending

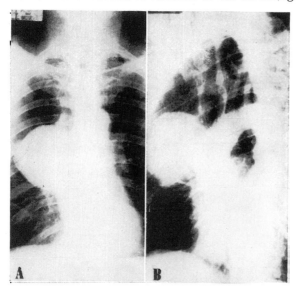

Fig. 1.—Roentgenograms of chest, showing, A, mass about 9 cm. in diameter in right superior mediastinum and, B, an oblique view of the aortogram confirming the diagnosis of aneurysm of the ascending aorta partially filled with thrombus.

aorta for an aneurysm with homograft replacement and with use of temporary cardiac bypass and a mechanical pump oxygenator.

Report of a Case

A 50-year-old male was admitted to Jefferson Davis Hospital on Aug. 18, 1956, complaining of increasing chest pain of several years' duration. About 25 years previously he had been

From the Cora and Webb Mading Department of Surgery, Baylor University College of Medicine, and the Surgical Service, Jefferson Davis Hospital.

kicked in the chest by a horse, but the first diagnosis of aortic aneurysm was made seven years later on routine roentgenography. No history of syphilis was obtained. Physical examination revealed an abnormal pulsation that was maximum in the right second intercostal space adjacent to the sternum and moderate venous distention in the right supraclavicular region. Blood pressure was 110/70 mm. Hg. There were no cardiac murmurs and there was no enlargement. Neurological examina-

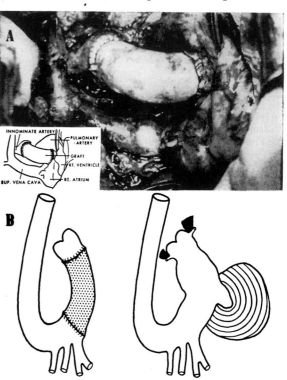

Fig. 2.—A, photograph made at operation, showing the homograft replacing the ascending aorta from just above the coronary ostia proximally to base of innominate artery distally. B, Drawing made from aortograms, showing location of lesion in ascending aorta and the method of surgical correction with aortic homograft.

tion was normal. Laboratory studies revealed a normal hemogram and urinalysis. Serologic tests for syphilis were negative. The electrocardiogram was also normal. Roentgenography and fluoroscopy of the chest revealed a pulsatile mass approximately 9 cm. in diameter in the right superior mediastinum projecting anteriorly, and aortography confirmed the diagnosis of aneurysm (fig. 1).

Bilateral thoracotomy was performed on Aug. 24 through the right fourth and left third intercostal spaces, and the sternum was divided in the midline upward to the suprasternal notch. The aneurysm was extensive, originating just above the coronary ostiums within the pericardium, and involved the entire ascending aorta to the origin of the innominate artery. The aorta was encircled with traction tapes proximal and distal to the lesion. A temporary cardiac bypass with a modified DeWall-Lillehei pump oxygenator was used, with a blood flow rate of 35 cc. per kilogram body weight per minute, or approximately 2,800 cc. per minute total. Most of the oxygenated blood was returned to the arterial system via a catheter threaded into the abdominal aorta through the right femoral artery. A small catheter was placed in the right common carotid artery for cerebral perfusion at 200 cc. per minute during occlusion of the innominate and carotid artery.

The cardiac bypass was begun with total inflow occlusion, and the ascending aorta at the coronary ostia was cross-clamped. Distally the aortic arch and innominate artery were occluded proximal to the left common carotid artery. The ascending aorta was resected and a sterile frozen aortic homograft was inserted into the defect using continuous sutures of 000 arterial silk (fig. 2). About 10 minutes after the bypass was commenced, cardiac standstill occurred, and no attempt at cardiac resuscitation was made until the clamps on the aorta were released after 31 minutes of total perfusion. Cardiac massage was then instituted, restoring myocardial tone while the pump oxygenator still functioned. Ventricular fibrillation ensued but was promptly corrected with two electric shocks of 110 volts, 1.5 amp. Vigorous cardiac action resumed with a sinus rhythm. Bleeding from the graft was not severe and the

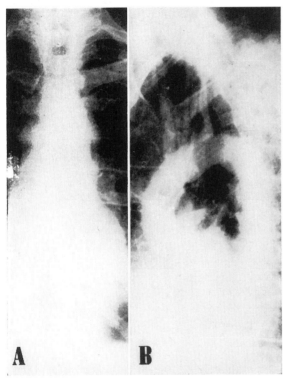

Fig. 3.—Roentgenograms of chest made three weeks after operation, showing, A, absence of mediastinal mass and, B, satisfactory function of the graft.

heparin sodium given prior to the bypass was counteracted with a similar quantity of protamine sulfate injection. The incision was closed, and bilateral subaqueous drainage was used.

Postoperative recovery was uneventful, and the patient was discharged from the hospital on Sept. 13, approximately three weeks after operation. Roentgenograms and aortograms revealed satisfactory healing and function of the graft (fig. 3).

Comment

This case demonstrates the feasibility of temporary cross-clamping of the ascending aorta during 30 minutes of cardiac bypass without artificial perfusion of the coronary vessels. Although cardiac standstill occurred, resuscitation was easily accomplished, and, because the same procedure may be tolerated for even longer periods in the experimental animal, it appears that the method is practical and relatively safe in terms of myocardial circulation. Presumably the coronary ori-

fices were temporarily occluded in this patient by the proximal clamp, but, in instances in which the clamp is applied distal to the coronary ostiums, blood remaining in the left ventricle will perfuse the coronary system during the period of aortic occlusion and cardiac bypass. Another important feature in the recovery of this patient was the success of temporary carotid perfusion, which indicates that this method may be modified slightly and used in resection of the entire aortic arch for aneurysm.

Summary and Conclusions

Excisional treatment of aneurysms of the aorta is widely accepted as the best method for such lesions, but application of this method to certain anatomic regions of the aorta is technically difficult. Segmental resection and homograft replacement for extensive aneurysms of the ascending aorta presents a complicated technical problem, because temporary cross-clamping of the aorta at this level is rapidly fatal. In a 50-year-old man, the entire ascending aorta was successfully resected with homograft replacement with use of temporary cardiac bypass.

1200 M. D. Anderson Blvd. (25) (Dr. Cooley).

Protein Needs in Surgical Patients.—Following World War II. . . . hundreds of wounded soldiers, sailors, and marines, [who] returned to our country from the far-flung theaters of war for final treatment. . . . showed . . . evidence of protein deficiency, such as anemia, hypoproteinemia, cachexia, indolent looking wounds, nutritional edema, and so on. . . . Beattie found the same thing in England, and then clearly demonstrated how protein added to the diet improved the healing process. . . . Many American surgeons . . . have emphasized the prevalence of protein and other nutritional deficiencies and the importance of preventing or correcting them before and after operation or injury. . . . In regard to the . . . protein-deficient patient there is an advantage in considering two protein compartments, i. e., the fixed tissue proteins which are large, and the circulating proteins (plasma protein and hemoglobin, which are relatively small. . . . Plasma and hemoglobin deficits are relatively easy to correct, thanks to the ready availability of blood banks. Tissue protein deficiencies are best corrected by oral feeding, yet many patients have such profound anorexia that they will not ingest anything but simple liquids which usually contain no protein. . . . It is often necessary to resort to tube feedings. . . . In a few patients the gastrointestinal tract cannot be used; here parenteral feeding is the only way to prevent inevitable starvation. Protein alimentation in this way is now possible by the infusion of adequate mixtures of amino acids and polypeptides (hydrolyzed protein). . . . This method closely imitates the natural method by which protein is absorbed from the gastrointestinal tract as amino acids and polypeptides. . . . This relatively new method of protein feeding equals and may in some cases excel the benefits of a smaller protein intake by mouth. But let me emphasize that intravenous feeding does not and cannot compete with oral feeding. Intravenous feeding competes only with starvation. In fact, in successfully combating starvation during periods when the gastrointestinal tract cannot be used, it restores or maintains the patient . . . that oral feeding can be started and increased much sooner. Intravenous protein feeding, when properly used, not only does not compete with oral feeding, it actually encourages and facilitates resumption of the normal method of eating temporarily interrupted by surgical or other disease.—R. Elman, M.D., Protein Needs in Surgical Patients, *Journal of the American Dietetic Association,* June, 1956.

SURGERY
Gynecology & Obstetrics

DECEMBER 1957

VOLUME 105
NUMBER 6

SUCCESSFUL RESECTION OF FUSIFORM ANEURYSM OF AORTIC ARCH WITH REPLACEMENT BY HOMOGRAFT

MICHAEL E. DE BAKEY, M.D., F.A.C.S., E. STANLEY CRAWFORD, M.D.,

DENTON A. COOLEY, M.D., F.A.C.S., and GEORGE C. MORRIS, JR., M.D.,

Houston, Texas

TREATMENT OF AORTIC ANEURYSMS by resection with restoration of continuity by aortorrhaphy or graft replacement has now become well established. Limiting factors to successful application of this method have been concerned primarily with the nature and location of the lesion and with the necessity for temporary arrest of aortic circulation during performance of the procedure. For aneurysms located distal to the left common carotid artery these factors have been satisfactorily overcome by use of hypothermia and the temporary shunt. For aneurysms proximal to this level, however, they have constituted much more difficult and hazardous problems. For one thing, arrest of circulation at this level interrupts cerebral blood flow which, even after a few minutes, can result in fatal ischemic damage to the central nervous system. Also, occlusion of the ascending aorta rapidly imposes such a serious strain upon the left ventricle that acute cardiac failure may ensue.

From the Cora and Webb Mading Department of Surgery, Baylor University College of Medicine, and the surgical services of the Jefferson Davis, Methodist, and Veterans Administration Hospitals, Houston, Texas.

Efforts to solve these problems were directed first toward use of temporary shunts which would permit maintenance of circulation during exclusion of the aortic arch. On the basis of their experimental studies in which multiple, small-bore, polyethylene tubes were employed for this purpose, Schafer and Hardin used this method on a patient whose aortic arch was resected, but the patient died in the operating room. A somewhat similar attempt was made by Stranahan and associates, who utilized a larger bore shunt 10 millimeters in diameter from ascending to descending aorta with one limb of the shunt to the innominate artery. Although the patient survived the operation, he died shortly after completion of the procedure. Significantly, there were manifestations of right hemiplegia, suggesting cerebral damage from failure to provide circulation through the left common carotid artery.

We previously reported the use of the temporary shunt principle for resection of aneurysms of the aortic arch in 3 patients (1, 3). The shunts, made of polyvinyl sponge

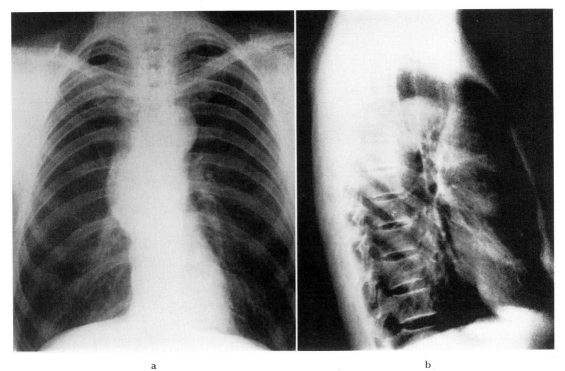

a   b

FIG. 1. a, Posterior anterior roentgenogram of chest showing aneurysm arising in ascending aorta, the right lateral margin of which is outlined by flecks of calcium; b, lateral projection suggests involvement of transverse arch.

(ivalon) with an internal diameter of 14 millimeters in the first 2 cases and 20 millimeters in the third case, were anastomosed end-to-side to the ascending and descending aorta and to both the innominate and left common carotid arteries. Despite use of hypothermia and the shunt, the first patient died on the sixth postoperative day of cerebral damage from temporary ischemia resulting from thrombosis of the right carotid shunt. Both hypothermia and the shunt procedure were also employed in the second case. Although this patient regained consciousness within 30 minutes after completion of the operation and appeared to be progressing satisfactorily, respiratory difficulties subsequently developed which presumably led to his death 6 hours later. In the third case only the shunt was employed. The immediate postoperative course seemed satisfactory, as evidenced by the fact that by the ninth postoperative day he was ambulatory and taking a regular diet. Un-

fortunately, a mediastinal infection developed which led to his death 2 days later. Despite the fact that none of these patients ultimately survived, owing to development of tragic complications, this experience demonstrated the technical feasibility of the procedure. The method has, however, certain disadvantages. For one thing, the necessity of performing and later removing the 4 end-to-side anastomoses of the shunt prolongs operative time, which in some of these patients may increase the operative risk. For another, it may not be possible to apply the shunt in cases in which the aneurysm arises quite proximally on the ascending aorta. Under these circumstances, the length of ascending aorta proximal to the aneurysm is insufficient to permit attachment of the shunt.

For these reasons consideration was given to the use of temporary cardiac bypass with the artificial heart-lung apparatus. After the feasibility of this method had been demon-

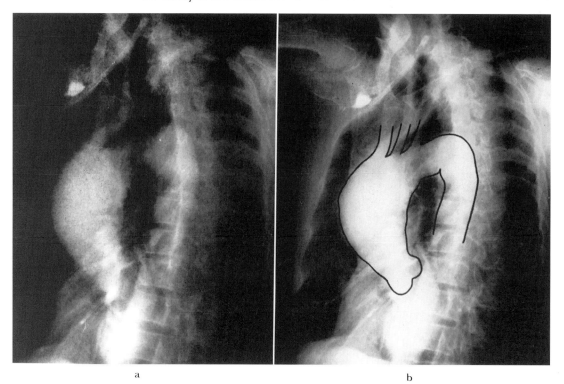

a   b

FIG. 2. a, Angiocardiogram with, b, superimposed outline showing fusiform aneurysm involving ascending aorta and transverse arch.

strated experimentally, temporary cardiac bypass was employed successfully in a patient with an aneurysm involving the entire ascending aorta, which was resected and replaced with a homograft (2). It is now a little over 1 year since this operation was performed, and the patient is well and has resumed normal activities. The successful application of this procedure led us to the belief that it provides a better method of resecting aneurysms of the aortic arch. This conviction has been strengthened by its successful application for this purpose in another patient whose aneurysm involved both the ascending aorta and transverse arch as illustrated in the following case report.

CASE REPORT

B. M., a 56 year old white man, was admitted to the Methodist Hospital, Houston, Texas, March 12, 1957, because of pain in the left side of the chest of 1 year's duration. Nine years previously the patient received multiple injections of penicillin because of a positive reaction to the serologic test for syphilis. Fol-

lowing this therapy the patient remained well and worked as a carpenter until 1 year before admission when he developed pain in the left side of the chest. Roentgenographic examination of the chest then revealed the presence of an aneurysm in the thoracic aorta, and since subsequent examinations showed progressive enlargement of the aneurysm, the patient was referred for surgical therapy.

Physical examination on admission to the hospital was essentially normal. Blood pressure was 122 millimeters of mercury systolic and 70 millimeters of mercury diastolic, and the pulse was regular. Results of electrocardiography and routine examinations of the blood and urine, including serologic tests for syphilis, were normal. Roentgenographic examination of the chest revealed an aneurysm in the region of the aortic arch (Fig. 1). A thoracic aortogram performed March 14, 1957 showed a moderate sized fusiform aneurysm involving the ascending and transverse segments of the aortic arch including the origins of the innominate and left common carotid arteries (Fig. 2).

On March 21, 1957, operation was performed under general anesthesia. With the patient in the supine position, both thoracic cavities were opened through an anterior incision made across the sternum and into both third intercostal spaces (Fig. 3). After the

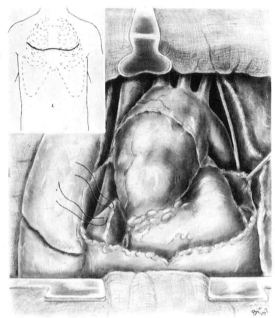

Fig. 3.

Fig. 3. Drawing made at operation showing technique employed in resection of aneurysm. Inset shows incision used through anterior third intercostal spaces with transection of sternum. After opening pericardium and freeing mediastinal structures from aortic arch and its branches, the fusiform aneurysm is visualized arising from base of ascending aorta to origin of left subclavian artery.

Fig. 4. Diagram showing method of exclusion of aortic arch using extracorporeal circulation.

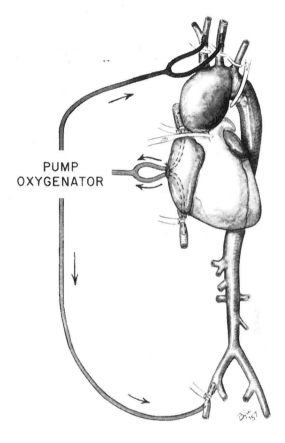

PUMP OXYGENATOR

Fig. 4.

mediastinum was separated from the anterior chest wall, the base of the heart and upper mediastinum were well exposed by retraction of the chest wall on each side with rib spreaders. The aneurysm was fusiform and involved a segment of the aorta that began 4 centimeters beyond the base of the heart and extended to the origin of the left subclavian artery (Fig. 3). Although the descending segment of the aortic arch was elongated and kinked, the diameter of the lumen in this region was essentially normal. The entire aortic arch and its branches were completely exposed by opening the pericardium and dissecting this structure, together with other mediastinal tissues including the pulmonary artery, from these vessels. After completely mobilizing the aortic arch, the aorta, both proximal and distal to the aneurysm, and the major aortic branches were encircled with umbilical tapes for traction during application of clamps.

An artificial heart-lung apparatus using a modified DeWall-Lillehei oxygenator was primed with 6 units of heparinized blood. The superior and inferior venae cavae were mobilized within the pericardial cavity and

encircled with umbilical tapes to be used later as temporary tourniquets. After the patient had been given 100 milligrams of heparin, a No. 16 tygon catheter was inserted into each vena cava through a small incision made in the right auricular appendage and secured in place by pursestring sutures. A similar catheter was inserted into the common iliac artery through an arteriotomy made in the right common femoral artery, and 2 smaller catheters were inserted into the innominate and left common carotid arteries, respectively, through small arteriotomies made distal to the aneurysm in the thoracic segments of these vessels. These 2 catheters only partially filled the lumen of these arteries and were held in place by small pursestring sutures surrounding the arteriotomies. Cerebral circulation was thus maintained at all times.

The venae cavae were occluded around the catheters in these vessels, and the total cardiac inflow was diverted into the oxygenator, from which oxygenated blood was pumped into the right common iliac, innominate, and left common carotid arteries. The rate of blood flow into the iliac artery was 2,100 cubic centimeters per minute, and into each of the in-

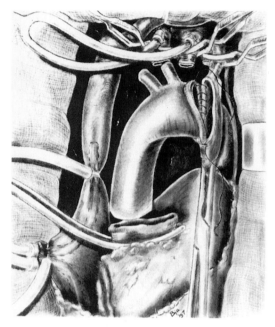

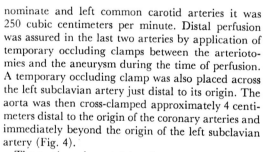

FIG. 5. Drawing showing replacement of aortic arch following its excision with anastomosis of homograft to distal aortic opening using continuous suture of No. 000 arterial silk.

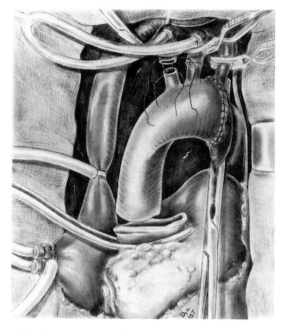

FIG. 6. Anastomoses of homograft to distal aortic opening and to left common carotid artery have been completed, and the next anastomosis to innominate artery is being performed.

nominate and left common carotid arteries it was 250 cubic centimeters per minute. Distal perfusion was assured in the last two arteries by application of temporary occluding clamps between the arteriotomies and the aneurysm during the time of perfusion. A temporary occluding clamp was also placed across the left subclavian artery just distal to its origin. The aorta was then cross-clamped approximately 4 centimeters distal to the origin of the coronary arteries and immediately beyond the origin of the left subclavian artery (Fig. 4).

The aortic arch containing the aneurysm was then excised and replaced by a reconstituted lyophilized aortic arch homograft, care having been taken to preserve the vagus, recurrent laryngeal, and phrenic nerves. The graft was inserted by anastomosis of the distal aorta and then the left common carotid, innominate, and proximal aorta in that order, using continuous over-and-over through-and-through sutures of No. 000 silk (Figs. 5 to 8). At the completion of the anastomoses 150 milligrams of protamine sulfate was given, and the bulldog clamps, which had previously been placed on the innominate, left common carotid and subclavian arteries, were removed after which the distal and proximal aortic clamps were removed in that order. The tourniquets occluding the venae cavae were immediately released, the pump discontinued, and normal circulation was restored through the heart and lungs. The entire perfusion

time was 43 minutes. The operation was completed by removing the perfusion catheters, repairing the mediastinum, and closing the chest wall. Catheters were inserted into each thoracic cavity for drainage. Pathologic examination of the specimen removed at operation showed the characteristic findings of a fusiform aneurysm of the ascending aorta and transverse arch, probably of syphilitic origin (Fig. 9).

Immediately after the operation, the patient responded to questions and moved all extremities. Recovery was essentially uneventful, and the patient was discharged from the hospital 16 days after the operation. He has since been observed several times and at this writing, 5 months postoperatively, his condition continues to be satisfactory and he has resumed working full time as a carpenter. Roentgenograms of the chest made at his last follow-up examination approximately 5 months after operation revealed essentially normal findings (Fig. 10).

DISCUSSION

The limiting factors to the successful application of resection of aneurysms of the proximal portion of the aortic arch suggested the need for a better method to solve the problem and led to consideration of the concept of extracorporeal circulation for

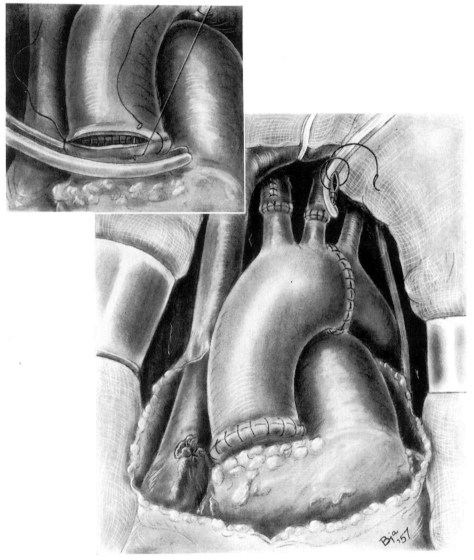

Fig. 7. Drawing showing in inset final anastomosis of homograft to base of ascending aorta. After completion of all anastomoses to homograft, all occluding clamps are released restoring normal circulation. Perfusion catheters are removed, and the arteriotomies for this purpose in innominate and carotid arteries are repaired by lateral arteriorrhaphy.

Successful Resection of Fusiform Aneurysm of Aortic Arch with Replacement by Homograft.—
Michael E. De Bakey, E. Stanley Crawford, Denton A. Cooley, and George C. Morris, Jr.

662   *Surgery, Gynecology & Obstetrics · December 1957*

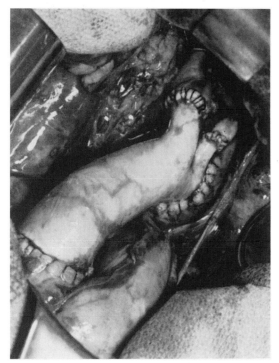

Fig. 8. Photograph at operation showing homograft replacing ascending aorta and transverse arch including branches to innominate and carotid arteries.

this purpose, particularly in light of increasing experience demonstrating its successful employment in the treatment of intracardiac lesions. Accordingly, experiments were conducted in which an artificial heart-lung apparatus with a modified DeWall-Lillehei bubble diffusion oxygenator was used. With total cardiopulmonary bypass being provided by this means and use of flow rates of approximately 35 cubic centimeters per kilogram of body weight, it was found that circulation through the aortic arch could be arrested for periods up to 1 hour without serious cardiac or neurologic disturbances. Of particular importance was the fact that cardiac function was maintained in a relatively normal manner but obviously with reduced cardiac output during the period of occlusion of the aortic arch. With pulmonary ventilation also being maintained during this time, presumably the blood that remains in the cardiopulmonary system after total inflow occlusion provides adequate circulation to maintain myocardial viability. In this connection it is

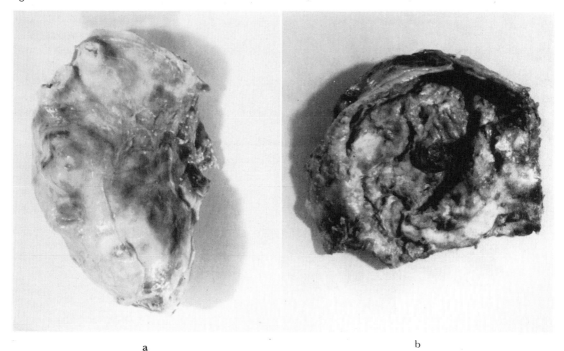

a

b

Fig. 9. Photographs of: a, intact excised specimen showing fusiform aneurysm of ascending aorta and transverse arch, and, b, opened specimen showing degenerative changes in wall.

of interest to observe that in our first patient on whom this method was employed for resection of an aneurysm of the ascending aorta, cardiac arrest occurred about 10 minutes after occlusion of the aorta and persisted during the remaining 21 minutes required to complete the graft replacement. It was possible, however, to resuscitate the heart after release of the occluding clamp. It is believed that cardiac arrest occurred in this patient because it was necessary to apply the occluding clamp so far proximally on the ascending aorta that it obstructed the ostia of one or both coronary arteries. In the case herein reported the clamp could be applied above this level and cardiac function was maintained throughout the procedure.

In the clinical application of this method certain technical aspects of the procedure deserve consideration. In our early experience the approach employed consisted of anterior thoracotomy through the third interspace on both sides, with transection of the sternum and median extension of the incision cephalad to the supraclavicular notch and median sternotomy. In our more recent experience it has been found preferable to avoid the addition of the median sternotomy since adequate exposure can be obtained by bilateral thoracotomy through the third interspaces and this permits more stable closure of the chest wall. If the aneurysm extends so far into the superior mediastinal space as to interfere with proper exposure of the great vessels, it is preferable to expose the common carotid arteries by separate small incisions in the neck. In the dissection to free the aortic arch and aneurysm from surrounding structures, considerable care should be exercised to avoid injury to the innominate vein and pulmonary artery, which are often intimately adherent to the aneurysm. Under these circumstances, it may be preferable to abandon efforts to free these structures completely until after circulation through the aortic arch has been arrested. The aneurysm may then be safely entered, its contents evacuated, and its wall removed from surrounding structures by in-

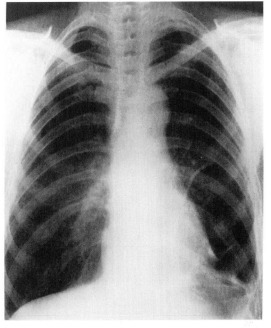

FIG. 10. Roentgenogram of chest made approximately 2 weeks after operation revealing absence of right mediastinal shadow representing aneurysm which was present in preoperative film shown in Figure 1.

tramural dissection. The important step at this stage of the operation is to obtain complete circumferential mobilization of sufficient segments of the aortic arch proximal and distal to the aneurysm and of the great vessels arising from the arch to permit application of the occluding clamps.

Extracorporeal circulation is provided in the standard manner, with $\frac{3}{16}$ inch plastic catheters inserted into the venae cavae to divert venous cardiac inflow into the artificial heart-lung apparatus from which oxygenated blood is returned to the patient through catheters inserted in the common femoral and both common carotid arteries (Fig. 4). Relatively small cannulas (No. 10 or 12 French polyvinyl plastic catheters) are used for the latter vessels in order to avoid obstruction to carotid circulation before perfusion with the pump-oxygenator is begun. By this means carotid circulation is maintained throughout the procedure. Relatively low flow rates of approximately 35 cubic centimeters per kilogram of body

664 *Surgery, Gynecology & Obstetrics · December 1957*

weight per minute were employed in accordance with our experience with this method for intracardiac lesions. Somewhat higher flow rates were used for carotid perfusion, since there is reason to believe that the central nervous system is less tolerant of anoxia than other tissues of the body. For this reason efforts were made to approximate normal cerebral blood flow which has been found by Kety and Schmidt to be 54 cubic centimeters per 100 grams of tissue. Accordingly, optimum flow rates for carotid perfusion should range between 500 and 800 cubic centimeters per minute divided equally between both carotid arteries. Further experience, however, may indicate that even higher flow rates may be desirable.

After excision of the aortic arch lesion the graft replacement is performed by using continuous through-and-through sutures of No. 000 arterial silk for the anastomoses. It is preferable to perform the anastomosis of the graft to the distal end of the aortic arch first and then to the left common carotid and innominate arteries in that order with the final anastomosis to the ascending aorta since this method facilitates their technical performance. Under some circumstances, however, it may be desirable to perform the distal and proximal aortic anastomoses first after which the aortic clamps along with the vena caval occlusion could be released in order to restore normal cardiopulmonary function as rapidly as possible. The flow through the pump-oxygenator would then be reduced to the amount required to maintain carotid perfusion during the time required to complete the anastomoses to these vessels.

SUMMARY

The two major problems associated with resection of aneurysms of the proximal portion of the aortic arch are concerned with the rapidly fatal consequences of arrest of circulation through this vital segment of the aorta upon the heart and central nervous system. Earlier efforts to solve these problems were directed toward use of temporary shunts to provide circulation during excision and replacement of the diseased segment and use of hypothermia to reduce cardiac output and oxygen requirement by the tissue. Although these methods proved to be feasible and to some extent effective in overcoming these problems, they have certain disadvantages that impose additional risks to the operation. Moreover, in some cases in which, for example, the aneurysm arises quite proximally on the ascending aorta, it is not technically possible to make use of the shunt.

These disadvantages have been circumvented by use of temporary cardiopulmonary bypass with the artificial heart-lung apparatus. This method was first successfully employed about 1 year ago in a patient with an aneurysm involving the ascending aorta, which was resected and replaced with a homograft. Its successful application in a second patient reported herein with a fusiform aneurysm involving both the ascending aorta and transverse arch, treated by excision and homograft replacement including restoration of continuity to both the innominate and left common carotid arteries, would suggest that it provides a better method for the resection of fusiform aneurysms of the aortic arch.

REFERENCES

1. COOLEY, DENTON A., MAHAFFEY, DANIEL E., and DE BAKEY, MICHAEL E. Total excision of the aortic arch for aneurysm. Surg. Gyn. Obst., 1955, 101: 667.
2. COOLEY, DENTON A., and DE BAKEY, MICHAEL E. Resection of entire ascending aorta in fusiform aneurysm using cardiac bypass. J. Am. M. Ass., 1956, 162: 1158.
3. CREECH, OSCAR, JR., DE BAKEY, MICHAEL E., and MAHAFFEY, DANIEL E. Total resection of the aortic arch. Surgery, 1956, 40: 817.
4. KETY, S. S., and SCHMIDT, C. F. The nitrous oxide method for the quantitative determination of cerebral blood flow in man: theory, procedure, and normal values. J. Clin. Invest., 1948, 27: 476.
5. SCHAFER, P. W., and HARDIN, C. A. The use of temporary polythene shunts to permit occlusion, resection, and frozen homologous graft replacement of vital vessel segments. Surgery, 1952, 31: 186.
6. STRANAHAN, ALLAN, ALLEY, ROLF D., SEWELL, WILLIAM H., and KAUSEL, HARVEY W. Aortic arch resection and grafting for aneurysm employing an external shunt. J. Thorac. Surg., 1955, 29: 54.

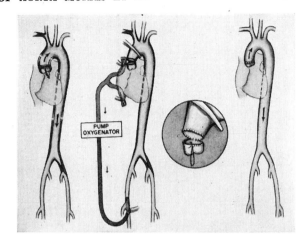

Fig 1.—Operative design for surgical repair and restoration of normal hemodynamics.

Correction of Acute Dissecting Aneurysm of Aorta with Valvular Insufficiency

George C. Morris, Jr., MD, Walter S. Henly, MD, and Michael E. DeBakey, MD, Houston

DISSECTING ANEURYSM is a serious condition proving fatal in more than 75% of cases. The more common subacute or chronic types beginning in the descending thoracic aorta have been managed satisfactorily by resection and graft replacement for nearly a decade.[1] Recent reports have described elective repair for the more extensive type of dissecting aneurysm beginning just above the aortic valve in a few fortunate patients surviving weeks or months after the onset of the dissecting process.[1-6] The purpose of this report is to describe complete correction of this condition in its acute form and to illustrate the problem and its successful emergency treatment by a case report.

The process begins with a transverse tear, often circumferential, in the intimal and medial layers of the aorta just above the aortic valve (Fig 1). Through this tear the force of blood dissects the aortic wall, creating a false lumen. The process

From the Cora and Webb Mading Department of Surgery, Baylor University College of Medicine.

often extends along the entire length of the aorta and out along its great branches. Proximal progression of the dissection may dislocate the aortic valve leaflets, creating aortic insufficiency. The false lumen encroaches on the coronary arteries, often narrowing both and creating coronary arterial insufficiency. Death from this more lethal and rapidly fatal type of dissecting aneurysm often occurs within hours or several days following one of the complications, such as rupture of the dissecting process into the pericardium, myocardial ischemia, or the acute effects of aortic valvular insufficiency.

Operative design for surgical repair and restoration of normal hemodynamics is straightforward and effective (Fig 1). Using cardiopulmonary bypass with an aortic clamp proximal to the innominate artery, the ascending thoracic aorta is transected just above the aortic valve. At this level, the characteristic circumferential intimal tear giving rise to the dissecting process is exposed for direct repair. The double lumen can be visualized, as well as the disrupted and incompetent aortic valve. Obliteration of the false lumen proximally by continuous suture through all layers of the aorta restores the aortic valve leaflets to a normal position re-establishing competency of the valve. Similarly, the false lumen is obliterated distally by continuous suture. End-to-end anastomosis of the divided aorta completes the essential features of the operation. The cleavage in the aortic wall which was formerly a false lumen is subsequently allowed to heal by refusion of the aortic wall layers. An illustrative case demonstrates the effectiveness of this form of emergency surgical management in a patient with classical manifestations of this most grave and formidable type of acute dissecting aneurysm.

Report of a Case

A 32-yr-old physician had been in excellent health until Aug 15, 1962. While reading, he was suddenly seized by excruciating anterior and posterior chest pain. He was able to telephone a physician, but then collapsed. Within an hour, there was obvious aortic valvular insufficiency, absence of the right radial and left femoral pulses, and a loud bruit over the right carotid artery. Six hours after onset, the patient was admitted to the Methodist Hospital in Houston. Physical examination revealed a blood pressure of 110/10 mm Hg in the left arm and 70/10 mm Hg in the right arm. The left femoral pulse was absent and the right femoral pulse had a collapsing quality. On cardiac examination, the most striking finding was an exceedingly loud regurgitant murmur of aortic incompetence. A short systolic murmur over the base of the heart was transmitted to the cervical area. The patient did not have the Marfan syndrome. An electrocardiogram showed only right axis deviation and a portable chest x-ray suggested slight broadening of the thoracic aorta. No other significant clinical studies were carried out and operation was begun 7 hr after onset of the condition. Rapid preparation for cardiopulmonary bypass was facilitated by the use of a disposable plastic oxygenator primed with 5% glucose in water. A midline sternotomy was used for exposure with the patient in the supine position. During the period of total cardiopulmonary bypass, intermittent coronary artery perfusion by cannula was employed. Immediately after the repair aortic valvular competency was apparent on pulse pressure tracings, and normal peripheral pulses were restored. Pleural effusion requiring several aspirations and atelectasis complicated an otherwise uneventful recovery. Subsequent to these problems the patient was restored to normal health with no abnormal clinical findings. Three weeks after operation, an angio-aortogram was performed which showed a normal aortic valve and thoracic aorta (Fig 2). The patient returned for follow-up examination 4 mo after operation. He had been working for 2 mo and was asymptomatic. Physical examination was unremarkable and arterial pulse pressure and electrocardiographic tracings were normal.

Comment

Direct repair of acute dissecting aneurysm arising in the supravalvular position not only provides for restoration of normal hemodynamics and prevention of death but probably mitigates against future recurrence. The latter should be made possible by increased cohesion in the medial layers of the aortic wall as the obliterated false lumen heals by fibrosis. Present availability of oxygenators requiring only a small amount of glucose in water or dextran priming facilitates emergency preparations for cardiopulmonary bypass for this grave and urgent problem.[7] Clinical manifestations of this condition are so characteristic that an immediate diagnosis can be made with confidence usually on the basis of simple history and physical examination, thus expediting an early emergency operation before death and before development of secondary degenerative changes in the aorta and aortic valve.

Summary

Repair of dissecting aneurysm of the aorta beginning below the left subclavian artery by excision and graft replacement has been successfully applied for nearly a decade. More recently elective repair of the more formidable supravalvular type of aortic dissection has been successfully performed. Immediate availability of cardiopulmonary bypass has made possible emergency repair of the supravalvular type of acute dissecting aneurysm.

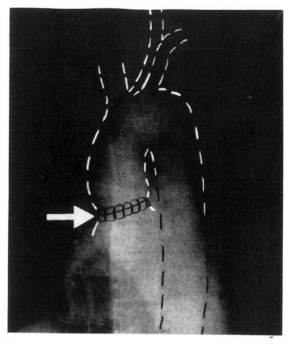

Fig 2.—Normal aortic valve and thoracic aorta in patient 3 weeks after operation for correction of acute dissecting aneurysm.

Such an approach provides the opportunity to save the lives of patients who might otherwise die soon after the process begins, and facilitates technical correction before development of secondary degenerative changes in the aorta and aortic valve.

Baylor University College of Medicine, Texas Medical Center, Houston (Dr. Morris).

This study was supported in part by grants from the American Heart Association, the Texas Heart Association, and the US Public Health Service.

Generic and Trade Names of Drug

Dextran—*Dextran, Expandex, Gentran.*

References

1. DeBakey, M.E., et al: Surgical Treatment of Dissecting Aneurysm of Aorta, Analysis of Seventy-Two Cases, *Circulation* 24:290, 1961.
2. Bahnson, H.T., and Spencer, F.C.: Excision of Aneurysm of Ascending Aorta with Prosthetic Replacement During Cardiopulmonary Bypass, *Ann Surg* 151:879, 1960.
3. Hufnagel, C.A., and Conrad, P.W.: Dissecting Aneurysms of Ascending Aorta: Direct Approach Repair, *Surgery* 51:84, 1962.
4. Hufnagel, C.A., and Conrad, P.W.: Intimo-Intimal Intussusception in Dissecting Aneurysms, *Amer J Surg* 103:727, 1962.
5. Muller, W.H., Jr.; Dammann, J.F., Jr.; and Warren, W.D.: Surgical Correction of Cardiovascular Deformities in Marfan's Syndrome, *Ann Surg* 152:506, 1960.
6. Spencer, F.C., and Blake, H.: Report of Successful Surgical Treatment of Aortic Regurgitation from Dissecting Aortic Aneurysm in Patient with Marfan Syndrome, *J Thorac Cardiov Surg* 44:238, 1962.
7. Cooley, D.A.; Beall, A.C., Jr.; and Grondin, P.: Open-Heart Operations with Disposable Oxygenators, 5 Per Cent Dextrose Prime, and Normothermia, *Surgery* 52:713, 1962.

Thorax (1968), **23**, 338.

A technique for complete replacement of the ascending aorta

HUGH BENTALL AND ANTONY DE BONO

From the Royal Postgraduate Medical School, London, and Hammersmith Hospital

A technique for complete replacement of the aortic valve and ascending aorta in cases of aneurysm of the ascending aorta with aortic valve ectasia is described. The proximal aortic root was too attenuated to afford anchorage to the aortic prosthesis, so this was sutured to the ring of a Starr valve and the prostheses were inserted *en bloc*. The ostia of the coronary arteries were anastomosed to the side of the aortic prosthesis.

Aneurysmal dilatation of the ascending aorta is often associated with ectasia of the aortic valve ring and presents clinically as aortic incompetence. In Marfan's syndrome or cystic medial necrosis this may develop with dramatic suddenness in an ostensibly healthy individual.

The dilatation of the valve ring makes repair or replacement with other than a prosthetic valve difficult. The aneurysm, which is either a true dilatation or dissection, is best treated by excision and replacement with a tubular prosthesis, as the wall is invariably attenuated. This is not difficult provided that the aorta distal to the aneurysm and proximal to the arch is suitable for anastomosis.

Proximally, in most cases, the aortic prosthesis can be sutured to a rim of aorta, leaving the coronary ostia undisturbed, while a valve prosthesis is placed in the usual sub-coronary position (Cooley, Bloodwell, Beall, Hallman, and De Bakey, 1966).

However, it sometimes happens that the root of the aorta is so involved in the disease process that the wall is too attenuated to be sutured to the proximal end of the aortic prosthesis. In this situation the management of the coronaries is the main concern of the surgeon.

CASE REPORT

A man aged 33 years had been in excellent health until a few months before admission, when his wife had noticed a loud cardiac murmur and he developed signs and symptoms of gross aortic regurgitation. Angiocardiography showed a large aneurysmal dilatation of the ascending aorta, not involving the vessels of the arch but associated with free aortic regurgita-

tion. He was in incipient cardiac failure with an effective cardiac output of 1.8 l./min./m.²

OPERATION   A mid-sternal thoracotomy revealed a large globular dilatation of the ascending aorta. Its bulging inelastic wall was so thin that blood could be seen eddying within. Figure 1 gives an idea of the attenuation of the wall.

Total cardiopulmonary bypass was established, and, after cross-clamping the aorta distal to the aneurysm, the aorta was opened, and the coronaries were cannulated and perfused in the usual way. The aortic valve ring was much dilated and the wall was extremely thinned down to the ring.

It was clear that it would not be possible to join the aortic wall above the coronaries to an aortic prosthesis. It was therefore decided to suture the tube prosthesis directly to the ring of a Starr valve. A No. 13 Starr valve was sutured to one end of a crimped Teflon aortic prosthesis, as shown in Figure 2. The aortic cusps having been excised, sutures were placed in the aortic ring and through the Starr valve ring. These were tied, fixing the Starr valve and the attached Teflon tube.

At this stage the coronary cannulae were outside the lumen of the aortic replacement. Holes were cut in the aortic prosthesis at the site of the coronary ostia, which were then re-cannulated, this time through the lumen of the tube (Fig. 3). The aortic wall was sutured to the perimeter of the holes in the Teflon tube, thus reincorporating the coronary ostia within the new aorta.

The distal anastomosis was then completed, leaving a vertical slit (Fig. 3 (5)) through which the coronary cannulae were removed and air was evacuated. This was then closed with a clamp while the aortic clamp was released and retrograde coronary perfusion was started again without any delay. The wall of the aneurysm was closed over the prosthesis.

The patient made an uneventful recovery and remains well after nine months.

A technique for complete replacement of the ascending aorta 339

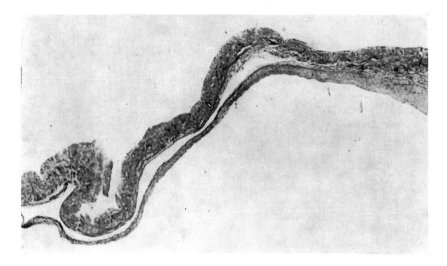

FIG. 1. *Section of aortic aneurysm just above aortic valve, showing extreme thinning. Wall about one-tenth normal thickness. (L.E.H.V.G. ×40.)*

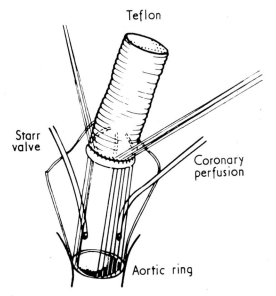

FIG. 2. *Starr valve has been sutured to aortic prosthesis: sutures have been placed in aortic ring before fixing the combined prostheses.*

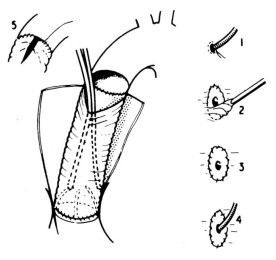

FIG. 3. *Combined prostheses in situ. Insets 1 to 4 show details of holes fashioned in the side wall of the Teflon tube to reincorporate the coronary ostia within the lumen of the new ascending aorta. Inset 5 shows the vertical slit in the prosthesis.*

The technique used is reported as it offers an alternative method of dealing with this type of aortic disease when the whole of the ascending aorta has to be replaced.

REFERENCE

Cooley, D. A., Bloodwell, R. D., Beall, A. C., Hallman, G. L., and De Bakey, M. E. (1966). Surgical management of aneurysms of the ascending aorta. *Surg. Clin. N. Amer.*, **46**, 1033.

30 December 1967   S.A. Medical Journal   1271

THE OPERATION

A HUMAN CARDIAC TRANSPLANT: AN INTERIM REPORT OF A SUCCESSFUL OPERATION PERFORMED AT GROOTE SCHUUR HOSPITAL, CAPE TOWN

C. N. Barnard, M.D., M.Med., M.S., Ph.D., D.Sc. (Hon. Causa), F.A.C.S., F.A.C.C., *Department of Surgery, University of Cape Town and Groote Schuur Hospital, Cape Town*

On 3 December 1967, a heart from a cadaver was successfully transplanted into a 54-year-old man to replace a heart irreparably damaged by repeated myocardial infarction.

This achievement did not come as a surprise to the medical world. Steady progress towards this goal has been made by immunologists, biochemists, surgeons and specialists in other branches of medical science all over the world during the past decades to ensure that this, the ultimate in cardiac surgery, would be a success.

The dream of the ancients from time immemorial has been the junction of portions of different individuals, not only to counteract disease but also to combine the potentials of different species. This desire inspired the birth of many mythical creatures which were purported to have capabilities normally beyond the power of a single species. The modern world has inherited these dreams in the form of the sphinx, the mermaid and the chimerical forms of many heraldic beasts. Modern scientists have a more realistic approach and explored the possibility of treating certain diseases affecting specific organs by replacement of these organs with grafts.

The recent history of transplantation of the heart began with the experiments of Carrel and Guthrie in the early years of this century.[1,2] Gradually our knowledge increased and progress towards this goal continued through the years with the work of many other brilliant men[3-10] and, in particular, through the invaluable contributions of Shumway and his associates.[11-15]

Against the background of this research and with our own experience in the experimental laboratories, backed by the knowledge of the surgical management and post-operative care of patients undergoing major cardiac surgery, the time arrived when a cardiac transplant could be contemplated with hope of success.

PREPARATIONS FOR THE OPERATION

A patient was selected who was considered to have heart disease of such severity that no method of treatment short of cardiac transplantation could succeed. A suitable donor was obtained who had compatible red cell antigens and a similar leucocyte antigen pattern.

The donor was taken to the operating theatre on supportive therapy and the recipient was taken to the adjoining operating theatre. The donor was prepared for total cardio-pulmonary bypass and a disposable oxygenator primed with Ringer's lactate solution was kept in readiness in this theatre. In the adjoining theatre, where the recipient had been placed, the DeWall-Lillehei pump oxygenator[16-19] was prepared and primed with fresh, citrated blood using haemodilution (2 parts blood : 1 part diluent consisting of 1,200 ml. 10% invert sugar in Ringer's lactate with 335 ml. THAM,* calcium 5 ml. of a 10% solution per pint of diluent and 15 ml. heparin).

*Trishydroxymethylaminomethane.

THE OPERATION

As soon as it had become obvious that, despite therapy, death was imminent in the donor, the recipient was anaesthetized and the saphenous vein and common femoral artery were exposed through a right groin incision. The saphenous vein was cannulated and this cannula was used for intravenous fluid administration and venous monitoring. The heart of the recipient was exposed through a median sternotomy incision. The pericardium was opened and the superior and inferior venae cavae and ascending aorta were isolated and encircled with cotton tapes. A careful examination of the recipient's heart showed that no treatment other than transplantation could benefit the patient.

As soon as the donor had been certified dead (when the electrocardiogram had shown no activity for 5 minutes and there was absence of any spontaneous respiratory movements and absence of reflexes), a dose of 2 mg. heparin/kg. body-weight was injected intravenously. The donor's chest was then opened rapidly, using a median sternotomy, and the pericardium was split vertically. A catheter was connected to the arterial line of the oxygenator and was then inserted and secured in the ascending aorta. A single 5/16-in. cannula was inserted into the right atrium via the right atrial appendage for venous return to the oxygenator. Bypass and cooling were commenced in the donor. A vent was placed in the left ventricle, via its apex, and put onto slow suction to prevent distension of the atonic left ventricle. The flow rate was adjusted to 3.5 l./min. This general body cooling was continued until the mid-oesophageal temperature had dropped to 26°C, as the kidneys were also to be protected for use in a transplantation procedure in another hospital.

When the mid-oesophageal temperature had reached 26°C the aortic cannula was adjusted so that it pointed towards the aortic valve. The flow was reduced to 0.5 l./min. and the aorta was then cross-clamped so that only the myocardium of the donor's heart was perfused. The heart was cooled down to 16°C. Perfusion was discontinued and the heart was excised by dividing the aorta distal to the innominate artery, the inferior vena cava being transected on the diaphragm and the superior vena cava at the level of the azygos vein. The right and left pulmonary arteries were divided and the main pulmonary artery was freed. The left atrium was mobilized by dividing the 4 pulmonary veins. The heart was now free. The excision had taken 2 minutes.

The venous catheter in the donor heart was removed from the right atrium. The arterial cannula and left ventricular vent were disconnected from the heart-lung machine but were left in place as positioned in the heart. The heart was placed in a bowl containing Ringer's lactate solution at 10°C and was transferred to the adjacent theatre where, in the meantime, the recipient had been connected to the heart-lung machine.

Perfusion of the donor heart was recommenced immediately (0·4 l./min.) by connecting the arterial cannula to a coronary perfusion line, and as soon as the aorta had filled to displace the air, it was clamped distal to the perfusion cannula so that the coronary arteries would be perfused. The heart was vented continuously during this procedure, and a period of 4 min. had elapsed between cessation of perfusion in the first theatre and the resumption of cardiac perfusion in the second operating theatre.

After systemic heparinization of the recipient the cardiopulmonary bypass was commenced. The flow rate was 3 l./min. (1·8 l./sq.m. body-surface area/min.). Arterial return was through a 5·4-mm. ID metal cannula inserted into the right common femoral artery and venous return to the pump was performed by means of two 5/16-in. diameter cannulae inserted through the right atrial appendage into the superior and inferior venae cavae. During insertion of the cannula into the right common femoral artery, it was noticed that this vessel was atherosclerotic. After 7 min. of bypass it was noticed that the arterial line pressure had risen to over 300 mm.Hg. Accordingly, a 5·6-mm. ID cannula was inserted into the ascending aorta through a stab incision, controlled with a purse-string suture, and bypass was discontinued momentarily while the arterial line was disconnected and re-connected to the cannula in the ascending aorta.

Bypass was recommenced after 3 min., the flow now being increased to 4·2 l./min. (2·5 l./sq.m. body-surface area/min.) and cooling was continued until the patient's mid-oesophageal temperature had reached 30°C. The arterial line pressure was now 120 mm.Hg.

The patient's heart was excised after cross-clamping the aorta proximal to the aortic cannula. The aorta was transected immediately above the coronary ostia and the pulmonary artery divided immediately above the pulmonary valve ring. The ventricles were detached from the atria as near as possible to the atrioventricular groove. The atrial septum was divided as close to the ventricles as possible. The excision was performed in order to leave a cuff of left atrial wall surrounding the ostia of the pulmonary veins and to preserve the part of the right atrium carrying the venae cavae.

Transplantation of the Graft

The donor's heart was placed in the pericardial cavity; the coronary sinus blood was allowed to drip from the donor heart into the pericardial sac and was aspirated from here back to the pump. The bases of the left and right atria were prepared. The base of the left atrial wall around the 4 pulmonary veins was excised and the base of the right atrium was incised, an incision being made posteriorly from the orifice of the inferior vena cava to the orifice of the superior vena cava. It was evident that the portion of the left atrium of the patient's heart to which the donor heart would have to be anastomosed was too large. This area was thus plicated, tucking in the wall of the patient's left atrium both superiorly and inferiorly next to its junction with the interatrial septum.

The left atrium of the donor heart was first attached to the patient's left atrium by anastomosing the opening in the posterior wall of the donor's left atrium to the left atrial wall and septum of the patient's heart. This was done using double layers of 4-0 continuous silk. The right atrium was then anastomosed; the posterior opening in the donor's right atrium to the remaining right atrial wall and septum of the patient's heart. Throughout this period the vena-caval catheters were left in place as introduced, in the patient's right atrial appendage, and did not interfere with the anastomoses.

The donor's pulmonary artery was trimmed down to the required length and was anastomosed to the recipient's pulmonary artery using continuous 5-0 silk sutures, doubly sewn. Perfusion of the donor heart was discontinued. The aorta was cut to fit the patient's aorta and the anastomosis was completed with continuous 4-0 silk sutures, doubly sewn. The donor's left ventricle was vented throughout this procedure. The aortic clamp was released, permitting perfusion of the myocardium from the patient's aorta. The left ventricular apex was tilted up to allow air to escape from the left heart, and the right heart was needled in order to exclude all air from this chamber.

A pint of citrated blood was added to the perfusate after 50 min. of bypass and subsequently 2 further pints were added to the bypass machine, being reconstituted in the usual way by the addition of THAM, calcium and heparin. After completion of the aortic anastomosis, rewarming was commenced after 165 min. of total cardiopulmonary bypass and the flow was increased to 4·5 l./min. (2·7 l./sq.m./min.). After 184 min., partial bypass was commenced by withdrawing the caval cannulae into the atrium and removing the superior vena-caval catheter. With a mid-oesophageal temperature of 36°C and a rectal temperature of 31°C, after a total perfusion duration of 196 minutes, 35 joules of energy were applied to the heart from a DC defibrillator. The first shock was successful in restoring good coordinated ventricular contraction. The heart was beating at a rate of 120/min. in nodal rhythm. At this stage it had been without coronary perfusion for 7 min., at normothermia, and for 14 min. at 22°C, and it had been perfused artificially with the heart-lung machine for a total period of 117 min.

Rewarming was continued for a further 15 min., when an intravenous drip of isoprenaline hydrochloride was commenced, preparatory to discontinuing bypass. The left ventricular apex was tilted up again and the left ventricle was aspirated to remove all air. The left ventricular vent was removed and the opening in the apex was closed with purse-string silk sutures. One minute later bypass was discontinued.

The arterial line pressure was 65/50 mm.Hg and the venous pressure 6 cm. saline at this stage. The heart beat was not forcible and bypass was recommenced after a ½ min., being continued for a further 2 min. When the pump was stopped, the systemic pressure was 85/55 mm. Hg and the venous pressure was 8 cm. saline. One minute later the pump was again started and perfusion resumed for another 3 min. to further improve the heart beat. On discontinuing bypass, the systemic pressure was 95/70 mm.Hg, venous pressure 5 cm. saline, and cardiac contractions were satisfactory. Bypass was finally stopped 221 min. after commencement, with interruptions totalling 4½ min. The lowest mid-oesophageal temperature reached during the operation was 21·5°C.

Protamine sulphate was now administered by slow intravenous infusion, the dosage being calculated at 1·25 times the dosage of heparin administered before bypass. Haemostasis was excellent and no further sutures were required in any of the suture lines. The cannula in the ascending aorta was removed and the aorta repaired with 3-0 silk purse-string sutures. The recipient's atrial appendage was excised and the edges of the wound were closed with silk sutures.

After lavage of the pericardial sac with a warm, normal saline solution, the pericardium was closed with a continuous suture of chromic catgut around a size 20 F plastic catheter. A further chromic catgut suture re-united the 2 lobes of the thymus and a size 24 F plastic mediastinal drainage tube was inserted. Haemostasis of the divided sternum was achieved, and the sternum was approximated with interrupted stainless-steel wire binding, passed through the sternum with an awl. The divided linea alba was closed with interrupted sutures of monofilament nylon and the soft tissues anterior to the sternum were coapted with a running chromic catgut suture. A subcutaneous suture of plain catgut and a continuous skin suture of monofilament nylon completed the thoracotomy closure. The groin wound was closed with interrupted chromic catgut and monofilament nylon, without drainage.

A nasotracheal tube was inserted for maintenance of postoperative mechanical ventilation. The chest X-ray, electrocardiogram, arterial and venous pressures, urinary output and peripheral circulation were assessed and all were satisfactory. The patient was returned to the postoperative room.

POSTOPERATIVE CARE

The postoperative care of the patient was concentrated on:

1. Maintaining a satisfactory cardiac output.
2. Suppressing the immunologic reaction to the transplanted organ.
3. The prevention of infection.

Cardiac Output

The adequacy of the cardiac output was judged by monitoring the following parameters:

1. The systolic blood pressure, measured $\frac{1}{4}$-hourly by palpation distal to an arm-pressure cuff.
2. The venous pressure, measured by inferior vena caval cannulation, established at surgery and connected to a disposable venous-pressure set.
3. The rate and rhythm of the heart, by recording the peripheral pulse rate and by electrocardiographic monitoring. This apparatus displays a continuous trace of standard lead II and gives visual and audible signals of each R wave, and incorporates a heart-rate meter.
4. The volume of the peripheral pulses and the peripheral circulation, by palpation and inspection.
5. Renal function, by measuring the urinary output every 2 hours and by performing daily creatinine clearance studies.
6. The temperature is recorded $\frac{1}{4}$-hourly by means of an indwelling rectal probe.

7. Acid-base balance studies are performed by the Astrup method.
8. Serum electrolyte investigations performed twice daily in the first few days and subsequently once daily.

Any evidence of deterioration in the cardiac output is treated vigorously by correcting abnormalities in the acid-base balance or serum electrolytes. Maintenance of adequate cardiac function was ensured initially by intravenous administration of isoprenaline hydrochloride in accurately regulated dosage of a 1 : 400,000 solution in 5% dextrose in water. Tachycardia was treated by slow digitalization with digoxin.

Suppression of the Immunologic Reaction to the Transplanted Organ

The following parameters were studied to detect any evidence of threatened rejection of the heart:

(a) the leucocyte response in the blood stream,
(b) deterioration in cardiac output,
(c) change in the serum enzyme levels which could indicate myocardial damage,
(d) changes in the voltage of the R wave of the electrocardiograph.

Anticipated rejection was treated by the use of steroids, commencing on the day of operation with intravenous hydrocortisone 500 mg. administered over 24 hours, and in addition 60 mg. prednisone administered orally. The hydrocortisone dosage was gradually reduced by 100 mg. daily while the prednisone dosage was maintained at 60 mg./day. The heart was irradiated locally, using a 1 curie source of cobalt, starting with a dose of 100 rads. on day 3, then 85 rads. on day 4 and 200 rads. on days 5, 7 and 9, given in the Radiotherapy Department.

Initially, 150 mg. azathioprine was administered daily through a nasogastric tube; as soon as urinary function improved, this was increased to 200 mg.

Threatened rejection was treated by administration of 200 mg. prednisone and 200 μg. actinomycin C daily for 3 days. The dosage of prednisone was gradually reduced.

Prevention of Infection

As absolute sterility of the patient's environment is not possible, the following preventive measures were adopted.

1. Pre-operative Period

(a) *Patient.* The patient is washed daily with hexachlorophene soap. Swabs are taken from the skin, nose, throat, mouth and rectum and are examined for the possible presence of potential pathogens, especially yeasts, *Pseudomonas aeruginosa,* Klebsiella species, beta-haemolytic streptococci and staphylococci. Antibiotic sensitivities of these organisms are determined where possible. Any obvious septic lesion is treated vigorously.

(b) *Staff.* Nurses and medical staff who are to handle the patient postoperatively have swabs taken from the nose, mouth, throat and rectum for bacteriological examination to determine if they are carriers of any potential pathogens.

(c) *Room.* A room is set aside in the unit, which is then thoroughly cleaned in the following manner:
(i) gaseous disinfection under bacteriological control,
(ii) thorough washing of all walls and floor with a

phenolic disinfectant, using boiled cleaning utensils,

(*iii*) thorough washing of the bed with liberal amounts of the correctly diluted phenolic disinfectant,

(*iv*) autoclaving of the mattress which is then covered in plastic, and autoclaving of the pillows, and

(*v*) flushing of the wash-basin 3 times daily with a suitably diluted phenolic disinfectant.

(*d*) *Apparatus.* Any apparatus to be used near or on the patient is carefully checked for cleanliness. This applies particularly to the oxygen tent, the suction apparatus and the Bird respirator.

This apparatus is dismantled as completely as possible and thoroughly cleansed mechanically, then all parts which can be autoclaved or boiled are so treated. Parts which cannot be boiled or autoclaved are treated by gaseous disinfection, or a phenolic disinfectant. Particular attention is given to any humidifying unit. The water in this unit is changed daily and the water container is boiled at the end of each day, pre- and postoperatively.

2. *Postoperative Period*

The patient is transferred to the specially prepared room. All staff attending the patient wear caps, masks, canvas overshoes and sterile gown and gloves, as for any sterile procedure. After any form of attention to the patient, the gloved hands are rinsed in the iodopher disinfectant and dried on disposable paper towels.

The patient's sheets and cotton blanket are changed twice daily, taking due care not to disturb the air excessively while doing this. The floors are mopped twice daily with a phenolic disinfectant. The bedpan and urinal are stored in a phenolic disinfectant. They are rinsed in hot water and dried before use.

In addition the following measures are taken:

(*a*) *Patient.* Every second day, swabs for bacteriological examination are taken from the nose, throat, mouth and anus to assess the presence of potential pathogens, or a change in bacterial flora.

All venepunctures, intravenous therapy sites and injection sites are treated as for a sterile surgical procedure. Daily blood cultures are performed. Careful attention is given to the perineum and scrotal region. These areas are dusted daily with hexachlorophene and Mycostatin powder.

The minimal number of personnel attend the patient.

(*b*) *Staff.* Nose, throat, mouth and rectal swabs are taken for bacteriological investigations every week to assess the presence of any potential pathogens. Antibiotic treatment was introduced as required.

The diabetes was controlled as for any patient with diabetes who has undergone major surgery, by means of frequent testing of urine for sugar and ketone bodies, and regulating a dosage of soluble insulin accordingly. This aspect did not present any particular problems.

SUMMARY

The first human heart transplant is described. The steps leading up to this event are outlined briefly and the operative technique is detailed. The postoperative care of the patient following this successful operation is described.

REFERENCES

1. Carrel, A. (1937): Bull. Johns Hopk. Hosp., **18**, 18.
2. Carrel, A. and Guthrie, C. C. (1905): Amer. Med. (Philad.), **10**, 1101.
3. Mann, F. C. (1933): Arch. Surg., **26**, 219.
4. Marcus, E., Wong, S. N. T. and Luisada, A. A. (1951): Surg. Forum, **2**, 212.
5. Neptune, W. B., Cookson, B. A., Bailey, C. P., Appler, R. and Rajkowski, F. (1953): Arch. Surg., **66**, 174.
6. Blanco, G., Adam, A., Rodriguez-Perez, D. and Fernandez, A. (1958): *Ibid.*, **76**, 20.
7. Uebermuth, H. (1959): München med. Wschr., **101**, 529.
8. Webb, W. R., Howard, H. S. and Neely, W. A. (1959): J. Thorac. Surg., **37**, 361.
9. Reetsma, K., Delgado, J. P. and Creech, O. (1960): Surgery, **47**, 292.
10. Bing, R. J., Chiba, C., Chrysolou, A., Wolf, P. L. and Gudbjarnason, B. (1962): Circulation, **25**, 273.
11. Shumway, N. E., Lower, R. R. and Stofar, R. C. (1959): Surg. Gynec. Obstet., **109**, 750.
12. Lower, R. R. and Shumway, N. E. (1960): Surg. Forum, **11**, 18.
13. Lower, R. R., Stofar, R. C. and Shumway, N. E. (1961): J. Thorac. Cardiovasc. Surg., **41**, 196.
14. Lower, R. R., Stofar, R. C., Hurley, E. J., Dong, E. J., Cohn, R. B. and Shumway, N. E. (1962): Amer. J. Surg., **104**, 302.
15. Lower, R. R., Dong, E. J. and Shumway, N. E. (1965): Paper presented at meeting of Society of Thoracic Surgeons, 12 February.
16. Barnard, C. N., Phillips, W. L., De Villiers, D. R., Casserley, R. D., Hewitson, R. P., Van der Riet, R. L. and McKenzie, M. B. (1959): S. Afr. Med. J., **33**, 789.
17. McKenzie, M. B. and Barnard, C. N. (1958): *Ibid.*, **32**, 1145.
18. Barnard, C. N., Terblanche, J. and Ozinsky, J. (1961): *Ibid.*, **35**, 107.
19. Barnard, C. N., McKenzie, M. B. and De Villiers, D. R. (1960): Thorax, **15**, 268.

Diagnosis of human cardiac allograft rejection by serial cardiac biopsy

Philip K. Caves, F.R.C.S., Edward B. Stinson, M.D., Margaret E. Billingham, M.D.,

Alan K. Rider, M.D., and Norman E. Shumway, M.D., Stanford, Calif.

The diagnosis of acute rejection episodes following cardiac transplantation in man has been dependent principally on electrocardiographic changes and clinical examination.[1, 2] Such diagnostic indices have permitted the recognition and successful treatment of most acute rejection episodes.[2] It is recognized, however, that these methods represent indirect assessment of the host immune response and depend upon established impairment of graft function due to immunological injury.

Recent studies in dogs after orthotopic cardiac transplantation have indicated that the electrocardiographic changes characteristic of acute graft rejection develop 24 to 48 hours after histologic evidence of rejection can be demonstrated in graft biopsies.[3] The technique employed to biopsy canine hearts has been adapted to clinical use, and a simple, safe method now exists for obtaining endomyocardial biopsies from the human heart via a percutaneous approach.[4] In this report we describe the use of this new technique for obtaining serial endomyocardial biopsies in the management of 2 patients following cardiac transplantation.

Methods

The operative methods for cardiac transplantation and protocols for postoperative immunosuppression have been described in detail.[2, 5, 6] Biopsies were performed with a Konno-Sakakibara bioptome which had been modified as previously described.[7] On most occasions two biopsy specimens were obtained during each procedure.

Technique. Full details of the biopsy technique have been presented.[4] Under local anesthesia a catheter sheath is introduced into the right internal jugular vein by means of standard techniques. The bioptome is then passed through the sheath into the internal jugular vein and advanced to the right atrium. Under fluoroscopic control, the biopsy forceps are guided into the apex of the right ventricle where the biopsy specimen is obtained from the endomyocardium. After removal of the first specimen from the forceps, the instrument is reintroduced and a second specimen obtained in similar fashion. The sheath is then removed from the vein, and pressure is applied over the puncture site for 5 minutes. With this technique, the internal jugular vein remains patent and available for use in subsequent biopsy procedures. The entire procedure is completed in 5 to 10 minutes. Each specimen is divided

From the Division of Cardiovascular Surgery (Drs. Caves, Stinson, and Shumway), Department of Surgery, Department of Pathology (Dr. Billingham), and Division of Cardiology (Dr. Rider), Department of Medicine, Stanford University School of Medicine, Stanford, Calif. 94305.

This investigation was supported by National Institutes of Health Research Grant No. HL 13108, from the National Heart and Lung Institute, and Research Grant No. RR 70, from the General Clinical Research Centers, Division of Research Resources.

Received for publication June 11, 1973.

Address for reprints: Philip K. Caves, M.B., F.R.C.S., Cardiovascular Surgery Division, A246, Stanford University Medical Center, Stanford, Calif. 94305.

461

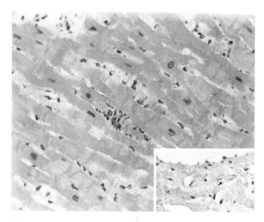

Fig. 1. Case 46. First biopsy 12 days post-transplantation. Signs of early rejection are present, with interstitial edema and an inflammatory cell infiltrate. *Inset* shows edema of the endocardium. (Hematoxylin and eosin; original magnification ×320.)

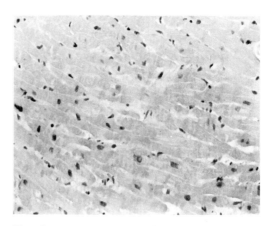

Fig. 2. Case 46. Third biopsy 28 days post-transplantation. The previous histologic changes of acute rejection have been almost completely reversed with treatment. (Hematoxylin and eosin; original magnification ×320.)

and prepared for light and electron microscopy and for immunofluorescence studies.

Case reports

CASE 46.* A 26-year-old man with the diagnosis of idiopathic nonobstructive cardiomyopathy was admitted to Stanford University Medical Center in August, 1972, for evaluation for cardiac transplantation. He had first developed congestive heart failure in 1967 and at that time had undergone cardiac catheterization, which showed depressed left ventricular function without valvular dysfunction or coronary artery disease. Under medical treatment he remained in New York Heart Association Functional Class II until July, 1972, when increasingly severe congestive heart failure required rehospitalization. Because of further clinical deterioration, including cardiogenic shock, cardiac transplantation was recommended.

Upon admission to Stanford Medical Center the patient was diaphoretic and dyspneic at rest. The arterial blood pressure was 110/70 mm. Hg with an infusion of isoproterenol at 4 μg per minute. The apical beat was diffuse and heaving in quality, and there was a systolic thrill palpable in the midaxillary line. A Grade 2/6 holosystolic murmur and summation gallop were heard at the apex. Severe hepatic enlargement was present. Chest roentgenograms showed gross cardiomegaly and pulmonary vascular congestion.

Bedside cardiac catheterization showed a mean pulmonary artery pressure of 45 mm. Hg and a wedge pressure of 40 mm. Hg. The cardiac out-

put was 2.8 L. per minute and the calculated pulmonary vascular resistance 1.8 units.

Cardiac transplantation was performed on Aug. 17, 1972 when a donor of compatible ABO blood type became available. At operation the excised portion of the recipient heart weighed 500 grams, and the left ventricle was enormously dilated and hypertrophied. Microscopic examination showed hypertrophy of muscle bundles with increased interstitial fibrosis, findings compatible with the diagnosis of idiopathic cardiomyopathy.

The patient's initial postoperative convalescence was satisfactory, and bedside determinations of cardiac output by the Fick technique showed a progressive rise to normal levels by the fourth postoperative day. His Σ electrocardiographic voltage (algebraic sum of the QRS voltages in Leads I, II, III, and V_1) rose to approximately 8 mv. and stabilized at this level. On postoperative Day 12 the first percutaneous transvenous endomyocardial biopsy was taken, although there were no clinical signs of rejection. The biopsy (Fig. 1) showed interstitial edema with a mononuclear infiltrate. Scattered "immunoblasts" stained positively with methyl green-pyronine. The endocardium was edematous. These changes were interpreted as indicative of moderately severe acute rejection. Two days after this biopsy the Σ electrocardiographic voltage showed a progressive, sharp fall which continued over the next 2 days. An early diastolic gallop rhythm became audible at the cardiac apex. Increased immunosuppressive treatment for acute rejection was given, including methylprednisolone (1 Gm. intravenously) daily for 3 days, actinomycin D (200 μg intravenously) daily for 2 days, heparin (given systemically) and antithymocyte globulin.

*Case numbers refer to number held in current Stanford cardiac transplantation series.

Volume 66
Number 3
September, 1973

Diagnosis of cardiac allograft rejection 4 6 3

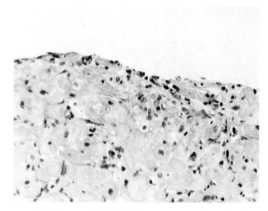

Fig. 3. Case 46. Fifth biopsy illustrating the histologic changes during the second acute rejection episode 39 days post-transplantation. Edema and a focal inflammatory cell infiltrate are present in the endocardium and myocardium. (Hematoxylin and eosin; original magnification ×320.)

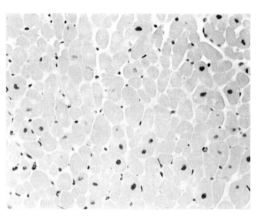

Fig. 4. Case 46. Sixth biopsy 46 days post-transplantation. A second course of increased immunosuppression has reversed the previous histologic changes with the restoration of a normal myocardium. (Hematoxylin and eosin; original magnification ×320.)

A second biopsy was performed on postoperative Day 20, 4 days after initiation of treatment for acute rejection; by this time the Σ electrocardiographic voltage had returned to approximately 8 mv. The specimen showed no interstitial edema and only a sparse lymphocytic infiltrate, indicating reversal of the rejection process. A third biopsy was performed 8 days later (postoperative Day 28) at a time when clinical and electrocardiographic parameters of graft function were completely stable. This specimen showed only mild thickening of the endocardium due to edema, with entrapment of a few mononuclear cells. The myocardium showed an interstitial fibrinous exudate with minimal mononuclear cellular infiltration (Fig. 2). Over the ensuing 8 days the Σ electrocardiographic voltage decreased progressively, and atrial premature contractions developed. A fourth biopsy specimen (postoperative Day 36) showed a more pronounced infiltrate of large mononuclear cells and lymphocytes. The Σ electrocardiographic voltage continued to decrease, and a fifth biopsy, performed on Postoperative Day 39, showed a markedly thickened endocardium with fibrinous exudate and inflammatory cells (Fig. 3). Interstitial edema was present throughout the myocardium, and there was widespread infiltration with mononuclear and polymorphonuclear cells. In addition, extravasated red blood cells were present, and the myocytes were swollen and vacuolated.

A second course of increased immunosuppressive treatment for acute rejection was then given. The Σ electrocardiographic voltage improved but did not return to prerejection levels. A sixth biopsy on postoperative Day 46, however, showed a normal myocardium (Fig. 4). The patient's clinical condition remained stable, but over the next week the Σ electrocardiographic voltage varied significantly on daily recordings. A seventh biopsy, performed on postoperative Day 53, again showed nearly normal myocardium.

An eighth biopsy was performed on postoperative Day 63 before discharge from hospital. The patient's clinical condition was stable and the Σ electrocardiographic voltage, though variable on a daily basis, was near base-line prerejection values. This biopsy was again indicative of acute rejection with interstitial myocardial mononuclear and polymorphonuclear cellular infiltration, endothelial cell swelling of small vessels, and areas of myocytolysis. Many lymphocytes stained positively with methyl green–pyronine. Over the following week the Σ electrocardiographic voltage fell sharply and the patient developed atrial flutter, an arrhythmia nearly always associated with acute rejection. A ninth biopsy on postoperative Day 70 showed widening of the endocardium with a fibrinous exudate and inflammatory cells. The myocardium showed marked interstitial edema and polymorphous interstitial infiltrate of red blood cells, polymorphonuclear leukocytes, and lymphocytes, many of which stained positively with methyl green–pyronine. Small blood vessels showed endothelial cell swelling. A third course of increased immunosuppression for acute graft rejection was given, and 1 week later a tenth endomyocardial biopsy showed considerable histological improvement with only mild interstitial edema and cellular infiltration. Mononuclear cells positive for methyl green–pyronine were no longer present. The Σ electrocardiographic voltage increased again to approximately 8 mv., and the cardiac rhythm reverted to sinus rhythm.

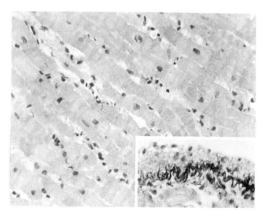
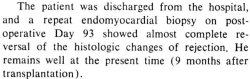

Fig. 5. Case 47. Sixteen days post-transplantation. Early acute rejection is seen with interstitial edema, fibrinous exudate, and an inflammatory cell infiltrate. (Hematoxylin and eosin; original magnification ×320.) *Inset* shows endocardial edema but no infiltrate. (Trichrome stain; original magnification ×340.)

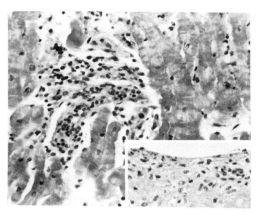

Fig. 6. Case 47. Nineteen days post-transplantation. This second biopsy shows moderately severe, acute rejection with an increased inflammatory cell infiltrate extending to the endocardium *(inset).* (Hematoxylin and eosin; original magnification ×320.)

The patient was discharged from the hospital, and a repeat endomyocardial biopsy on postoperative Day 93 showed almost complete reversal of the histologic changes of rejection. He remains well at the present time (9 months after transplantation).

CASE 47. A 47-year-old man presented for evaluation for cardiac transplantation with a history of myocardial infarction 6 months prior to admission. Following myocardial infarction, the patient suffered intractable congestive heart failure and had New York Heart Association Class IV disability. Cardiac catheterization and left ventricular cineangiography in June, 1972, had shown a left ventricular end-diastolic pressure of 40 mm. Hg, a cardiac index of 1.6 L. per minute per square meter, and an ejection fraction of 16 per cent. Cardiac transplantation was performed on Aug. 20, 1972, when a suitable donor became available. At operation a control endomyocardial biopsy was taken from the right ventricle of the donor heart and showed normal myocardium.

The patient's early postoperative convalescence was satisfactory, and his clinical status and Σ electrocardiographic voltage were stable when he first underwent transvenous endomyocardial biopsy on postoperative Day 8. This biopsy specimen showed normal heart muscle. His clinical status and Σ electrocardiographic voltage remained stable, and endomyocardial biopsy was repeated on postoperative Day 16. This specimen showed changes typical of early acute graft rejection, with edematous thickening of the endocardium and an interstitial infiltrate of polymorphonuclear and mononuclear cells. Many of the latter stained positively with methyl green-pyronine. The myo-

cytes appeared swollen, and interstitial edema was present (Fig. 5). During the next 3 days the patient remained clinically well, but the Σ electrocardiographic voltage decreased progressively, and a third biopsy on postoperative Day 19 revealed an increase of interstitial infiltration with mononuclear cells, which were now also distributed within the endocardium (Fig. 6). In addition, endothelial swelling was noted in small blood vessels.

Increased immunosuppressive treatment for acute graft rejection was given, and the Σ electrocardiographic voltage promptly improved. A fourth endomyocardial biopsy on postoperative Day 26 showed reduction of interstitial mononuclear cellular infiltration. Repeat biopsy 1 week later (postoperative Day 33), at which time the Σ electrocardiographic voltage was stable at its prerejection level, showed normal myocardium and endocardium, with complete disappearance of the previously observed histologic changes (Fig. 7).

Maintenance immunosuppression was then reduced. However, the Σ electrocardiographic voltage decreased, and another biopsy on postoperative Day 36 showed recurrence of changes indicative of acute rejection. Accordingly, a second course of increased immunosuppression was given and continued for 7 days. Throughout this period his clinical condition remained excellent. Three subsequent biopsies on postoperative Days 46, 50, and 60 showed progressive resolution of rejection injury, and at the time of discharge on postoperative Day 65 almost normal endomyocardium was present.

At the present time, the patient remains well 9 months after transplantation.

Volume 66
Number 3
September, 1973

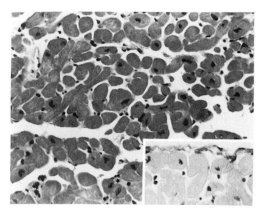

Fig. 7. Case 47. Thirty-three days post-transplantation. Following increased immunosuppression, this fourth biopsy shows normal myocardium with normal endocardium *(inset)*. (Hematoxylin and eosin; original magnification ×320.)

Discussion

The early diagnosis of acute graft rejection and its complete reversal with immediate augmentation of immunosuppressive therapy are essential to long-term survival following cardiac transplantation. It is recognized that the parameters utilized clinically for the detection of acute cardiac rejection episodes—electrocardiographic voltage changes and arrhythmias, diastolic gallop rhythms, and changes on the echocardiogram—represent only indirect indices of rejection since they reflect impairment of graft function at some time after the initiation of immunological injury by host defense mechanisms. Thus the desirability of additional methods for early and acurate diagnosis of cardiac allograft rejection is obvious.

Transvenous endomyocardial biopsy was introduced in this laboratory in 1972 as a means of directly assessing the accuracy of new aids for the diagnosis of acute rejection of cardiac allografts in dogs.[3, 7] Experience with this new technique proved that repeated cardiac biopsies could be safely accomplished and that histologic examination of biopsy material provides an accurate means for early diagnosis of acute rejection. Study of serial biopsies from transplanted hearts in control and immunosuppressed dogs demonstrated that the development of histologic changes of acute rejection is progressive and takes place over several days. Cardiac biopsies obtained at the beginning of a rejection episode showed histologic changes 2 to 4 days before alterations in clinical or electrocardiographic parameters appeared. Biopsies taken after apparently successful treatment of a rejection episode showed complete reversal of the histologic changes of rejection.[3, 8] This experience suggested that serial endomyocardial biopsies in human heart recipients would provide valuable information regarding the onset and severity of graft rejection and that they might permit more accurate immunosuppressive treatment. Routine application of serial cardiac biopsy in man, however, was dependent upon the development of a simple technique for repeated introduction of the biopsy forceps into the donor heart. The adaptation of percutaneous cannulation of the right internal jugular vein for this purpose[4] provided a safe method for serial cardiac biopsy, as described in these 2 patients.

The 2 patients reported here are the first in whom serial endomyocardial biopsy was used in the diagnosis and management of early acute graft rejection after cardiac transplantation. This experience has established serial endomyocardial biopsy as an important new aid in the management of cardiac transplant recipients.

The absence of either false negative or false positive biopsies in these 2 patients suggests that the biopsy technique is both specific and reliable in the diagnosis of acute graft rejection. On each occasion that the biopsy histology appeared normal, the patients were clinically well without evidence of rejection. Conversely, histologic evidence of advancing rejection was invariably followed by confirmatory clinical signs which prompted initiation of increased immunosuppressive treatment.

Importantly, the first postoperative rejection episode was histologically evident in each patient 2 to 4 days before rejection could be established clinically on the basis of significant changes in the electrocardiogram or physical examination. Even more striking was the third rejection episode in Patient 46 at the time of his discharge from hospital. Serial electrocardiograms during this interval were quite stable, but his eighth biopsy specimen suggested an ongoing, moderately severe rejection process. This was confirmed by a progressive decrease in electrocardiographic voltage over the next 7 days and the onset of atrial flutter. Thus it would appear that the biopsy technique provides an early and sensitive index of cardiac graft rejection.

Serial endomyocardial biopsy in these patients also allowed an accurate assessment of the response to immunosuppressive treatment. The regression of histologic changes in biopsies repeated after increased immunosuppressive treatment for rejection correlated well with normalization of clinical parameters.

The pathological changes associated with acute cardiac graft rejection are usually diffusely distributed throughout the myocardium and should, therefore, be detectable by biopsy technique. Because of the potentially focal nature of some lesions, however, two biopsy specimens were removed during each procedure. Excellent correlation between the two specimens was present on all but one occasion. In this one exception one of two specimens in Case 47 showed a relatively large area of fibrous tissue. A subsequent biopsy also showed fibrosis, and this was finally considered to be the result of healing in previous biopsy sites. Such fibrosis was not taken into consideration in the histologic assessment of rejection.

Summary

Our initial experience with serial percutaneous transvenous endomyocardial biopsy in 2 heart transplant recipients has established this procedure as a valuable new aid in the diagnosis and management of acute rejection episodes after cardiac transplantation. Transvenous cardiac biopsy is rapid and safe, and it is readily accepted as part of the early postoperative routine.

REFERENCES

1 Stinson, E. B., Dong, E., Jr., Bieber, C. P., Schroeder, J. S., and Shumway, N. E.: Cardiac Transplantation in Man. I. Early Rejection, J. A. M. A. **207:** 2233, 1969.

2 Griepp, R. B., Stinson, E. B., Dong, E., Jr., Clark, D. A., and Shumway, N. E.: Acute Rejection of the Allografted Human Heart: Diagnosis and Treatment, Ann. Thorac. Surg. **12:** 113, 1971.

3 Billingham, M. E., Caves, P. K., Dong, E., Jr., and Shumway, N. E.: The Diagnosis of Canine Orthotopic Cardiac Allograft Rejection by Transvenous Endomyocardial Biopsy, Transplant. Proc. **5:** 741, 1973.

4 Caves, P. K., Stinson, E. B., Graham, A. F., Billingham, M. E., Grehl, T. M., and Shumway, N. E.: Percutaneous Transvenous Endomyocardial Biopsy, J. A. M. A. In press.

5 Stinson, E. B., Dong, E., Jr., Iben, A. B., and Shumway, N. E.: Cardiac Transplantation in Man. III. Surgical Aspects, Am. J. Surg. **118:** 182, 1969.

6 Caves, P. K., Stinson, E. B., Griepp, R. B., Rider, A., Dong, E., Jr., and Shumway, N. E.: Experience With Fifty-four Cardiac Transplants at Stanford University, Surgery **74:** 307, 1973.

7 Caves, P. K., Billingham, M. E., Schulz, W. P., Dong, E., Jr., and Shumway, N. E.: Transvenous Biopsy of Canine Orthotopic Heart Allografts, Am. Heart J. **85:** 525, 1973.

8 Caves, P. K., Billingham, M. E., Dong, E., Jr., and Shumway, N. E.: The Serial Histological Changes of Cardiac Allograft Rejection in Dogs. Transplantation. In press.

Hemodynamic observations in the early period after human heart transplantation

Serial hemodynamic measurements, including determination of cardiac output by the Fick technique, were obtained in 10 human cardiac recipients for intervals up to 38 days after transplantation. Immediately postoperatively, donor cardiac output was severely depressed because of limitation of stroke volume. Spontaneous recovery of cardiac output and stroke volume then occurred gradually over the first 4 postoperative days to normal or nearly normal levels. Rate augmentation by atrial and/or ventricular pacing early after transplantation had little effect on donor heart performance, but isoproterenol caused significant enhancement of graft function and is now used routinely in postoperative management. Serial hemodynamic monitoring proved to be of little use in the predicion or confirmation of acute graft rejection episodes.

Edward B. Stinson, M.D.,* Philip K. Caves, M.D., F.R.C.S.,
Randall B. Griepp, M.D., Philip E. Oyer, M.D., Alan K. Rider, M.D.,
and Norman E. Shumway, M.D., *Stanford, Calif.*

I n the canine model of orthotopic cardiac transplantation, previous studies have shown that hemodynamic and mechanical performance of the donor left ventricle is significantly depressed immediately after operation.[1, 2] Improvement in donor ventricular function to normal or nearly normal levels then occurs gradually over the first 2 to 4 days after transplantation. Clinical observations have suggested that similar depression of graft function is present after transplantation of the human heart, but the magnitude and time course of such functional alterations have not been defined. We therefore measured cardiac output daily

in 10 recipients for intervals up to 38 days after transplantation. The effects of atrial and ventricular pacing and isoproterenol on graft hemodynamics in the immediate postoperative period were also studied. In addition, serial base-line hemodynamic measurements were obtained during episodes of acute graft rejection.

Patients and methods

The operative techniques for heart transplantation in man and methods for the diagnosis of graft rejection and immunosuppression have previously been described in detail.[3-5] In the 10 patients included in this study, an indwelling polyethylene catheter, placed percutaneously through the chest wall, was inserted into the recipient pulmonary artery at the time of transplantation. Mixed venous blood samples and measurements of mean pulmonary artery pressure (saline manometer) were obtained with this catheter. Cardiac output was derived by the

From the Department of Cardiovascular Surgery, Stanford University Medical Center, Stanford, Calif. 94305.

Supported by grants from the National Heart and Lung Institute, HL 13108 and RR70, General Clinical Research Centers, Division of Research Resources.

Received for publication Aug. 2, 1974.

Address for reprints: Edward B. Stinson, M.D., Department of Cardiovascular Surgery, Stanford University Medical Center, Stanford, Calif. 94305.

*Established Investigatorship, American Heart Association.

264

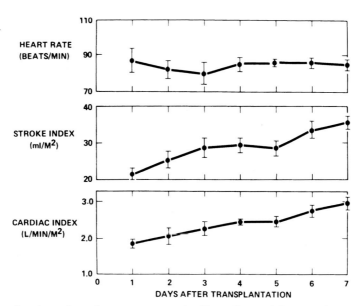

Fig. 1. Base-line hemodynamic measurements in 10 cardiac recipients during the first week after transplantation. *Vertical bars* indicate ± SEM.

standard Fick technique. Gas collections for measurement of oxygen consumption were obtained for a 5 minute period; the exhalation manifold of the mechanical respirator was used immediately postoperatively and subsequently a standard mouthpiece. After tracheal extubation, the daily studies were performed in late morning, 3 to 4 hours after breakfast, and after a 30 minute period of bed rest. Arterial blood samples for analysis of oxygen content were obtained daily for the first 5 postoperative days and then every 2 to 3 days, or more frequently if indicated by apparent instability of pulmonary function. When direct measurements were not obtained, values for arterial blood oxygen saturation were assumed on the basis of the most recent determination. Pulmonary artery catheters were maintained for 11 to 38 days postoperatively (average 22 days); no complications caused by the catheters were detected.

Within the first 24 hours (average 14 hours) after transplantation, the effects of isoproterenol at varying infusion rates on cardiac output and mean arterial blood pressure (measured in radial artery with calibrated aneroid manometer), as well as

pulmonary arterial and central venous pressures, were determined in 6 patients. A stabilization period of 15 to 30 minutes was allowed after institution or change in dose of isoproterenol before repeat measurements of oxygen consumption, arterial and venous blood oxygen content, and pressures. The hemodynamic effects of donor heart pacing at rates 35 to 79 per cent above control, with temporary right atrial (3 patients) or right ventricular (4 patients) pacing wires implanted at the time of operation, were also studied. A 5 minute interval for stabilization was allowed after each change in heart rate induced by pacing.

Stroke index was calculated in a standard manner. Acute hemodynamic changes associated with pacing or administration of isoproterenol were compared to control measurements by means of Student's t test for paired observations, a two-tailed significance level being assigned to the p value.

Results

Base-line hemodynamic measurements. Average cardiac index without myocardial inotropic support, measured within 24 hours of transplantation in all 10 subjects, was initially depressed at 1.83 ± 0.16 (SEM)

The Journal of
Thoracic and Cardiovascular
Surgery

266 *Stinson et al.*

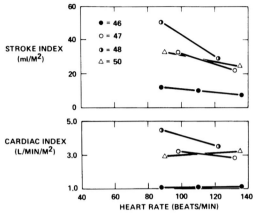

Fig. 2. Effects of right ventricular pacing on stroke index and cardiac index in 4 recipients.

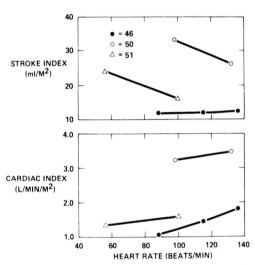

Fig. 3. Effects of donor atrial pacing on stroke index and cardiac index in 3 recipients.

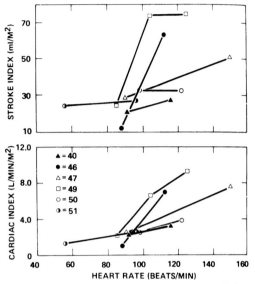

Fig. 4. Effects of isoproterenol (average infusion rate 2.2 μg per minute) on stroke index and cardiac index in 6 recipients.

L. per minute per square meter (range 1.34 to 2.61). It subsequently rose progressively to nearly normal levels by the fourth postoperative day (2.44 ± 0.11 L. per minute per square meter, p < 0.01). A slight additional increase to 2.97 ± 0.19 L. per minute per square meter (p < 0.05) occurred over the next 3 days, but thereafter average cardiac index at rest showed no significant changes, except during episodes of acute graft rejection in some cases (see below). The gradual and progressive improvement in average cardiac index during the first week after transplantation was due entirely to parallel increases in stroke index, which

initially was depressed at 21.4 ± 1.7 ml. per square meter and subsequently rose to 29.5 ± 2.0 (p < 0.05) and 35.2 ± 2.5 ml. per square meter on the fourth and seventh postoperative days, respectively. No significant variation in mean group values for heart rate occurred during this interval. These data are summarized in Fig. 1.

Mean pulmonary artery pressure, which at preoperative cardiac catheterization averaged 36.1 ± 3.3 mm. Hg in the 10 patients studied, was 26.4 ± 1.6 mm. Hg (p < 0.05) immediately after transplantation and then decreased gradually to 22.2 ± 1.4 mm. Hg by the end of the first postoperative week. Average central venous pressure was 11.6 ± 0.9 mm. Hg at the time of initial postoperative study and then subsequently rose to a high value of 16.5 ± 1.6 on the second postoperative day (p < 0.05). It then declined gradually to 7.6 ± 0.7 mm. Hg by the end of the first week.

Ventricular pacing (Fig. 2). Augmentation in donor heart rate from an average 91 beats per minute (sinus rhythm) to 131 beats per minute by electrical pacing via a right ventricular epicardial wire in 4 patients within 24 hours of transplantation was as-

Volume 69
Number 2
February, 1975

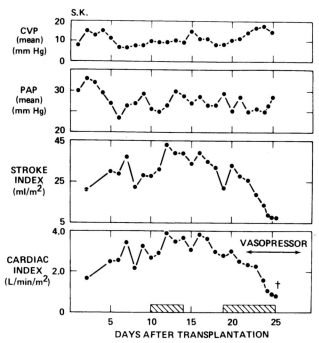

Fig. 5. Serial hemodynamic values in Case 45. Death due to intractable graft rejection occurred on postoperative Day 25. *Hatched areas* at bottom of figure indicate periods of high-dose immunosuppressive treatment for acute rejection. *CVP,* Central venous pressure, *PAP,* Pulmonary artery pressure.

sociated with no significant change in average cardiac index (decreased in 2 patients, increased in 1, and unchanged in 1). However, there was a decline in stroke index from 32.3 ± 7.9 to 21.0 ± 4.6 ml. per square meter ($p < 0.10$). Mean arterial, pulmonary arterial, and central venous pressures showed no significant changes from control with ventricular pacing at the above heart rates.

Atrial pacing (Fig. 3). In contrast to the effects of right ventricular pacing, an increase in donor heart rate induced by right atrial pacing from an average control rate of 81 beats per minute to 123 beats per minute in 3 patients was associated with a modest and consistent rise in average cardiac index from 1.87 ± 0.7 to 2.28 ± 0.6 L. per minute per square meter; this increase was of borderline statistical significance because of the small number of subjects studied ($p < 0.10$). Average stroke index declined from 23.0 ± 6 to 18.3 ± 4 ml. per square meter ($p > 0.10$); however, in 1 patient (Case 46) it remained constant at a low level

(12.0 ml. per square meter) as donor heart rate was increased from a control value of 88 sequentially to 115 and then 136 beats per minute by atrial pacing. Although mean arterial and pumonary arterial pressures tended to rise and central venous pressure to decline with atrial pacing, these changes were not statistically significant.

Isoproterenol (Fig. 4). Infusions of isoproterenol in 6 patients (average dose 2.2 μg per minute), sufficient to raise donor heart rates to levels achieved by atrial or ventricular pacing, increased cardiac index significantly in all. Average cardiac index rose from a control value of 2.04 ± 0.3 to 5.62 ± 1.1 L. per minute per square meter ($p < 0.01$). The augmentation of cardiac index with isoproterenol was associated with marked increases in stroke index from a mean value of 23.8 ± 2.9 to 46 ± 8.2 ml. per square meter ($p < 0.01$), as well as heart rate (control 85 ± 6 versus 120 ± 7 beats per minute during isoproterenol, $p < 0.01$).

Mean arterial blood pressure changed inconsistently during isoproterenol infusions; average mean arterial pressure rose slightly from 91.5 ± 7.2 to 95.8 ± 8.3 mm. Hg (p > 0.05). Mean pulmonary arterial pressure, in contrast, increased during isoproterenol infusions in every case, from an average value of 22.4 ± 3.2 mm. Hg to 25.6 ± 3.6 mm. Hg (p < 0.01). Average central venous pressure declined significantly from 11.9 ± to 9.7 ± mm. Hg (p < 0.01).

Hemodynamics during rejection. Eight episodes of acute graft rejection in 6 patients were diagnosed and managed during the period of daily hemodynamic measurements (six episodes were histologically confirmed by graft endomyocardial biopsy).[5] In only three of these instances did measured cardiac index decrease to subnormal values (< 2.5 L. per minute per square meter). In each case the decline of cardiac index was due entirely to reduction of stroke volume, unaccompanied by significant changes in heart rate. Furthermore, the duration of subnormal cardiac index was limited to 1 and 2 days in the 2 patients in whom graft rejection was reversible with increased immunosuppressive treatment. The third patient (Case 45) died of intractable graft rejection that was associated with progressive deterioration of cardiac output despite support with high doses of catecholamines; terminally, stroke volume in this case decreased to 12.0 ml. per beat (stroke index 7.8 ml. per square meter) (Fig. 5).

The detection of subnormal cardiac index in these three instances occurred at the same time or after the diagnosis of rejection had been established on the basis of standard criteria,[6] although in two a downward trend had developed 1 to 3 days before cardiac index decreased below the lower limit of normal. The significance of such trends, however, could be substantiated only in retrospect because of the limitations of methodologic error. In other words, daily measurement of cardiac output by the methods employed provided no useful predictive index of graft rejection in comparison to the usual clinical methods for rejec-

tion diagnosis. Similarly, analysis of mean pulmonary arterial and central venous pressures in patients sustaining episodes of acute cardiac rejection during periods of daily hemodynamic monitoring showed no significant correlations between these variables and the onset of diagnosed rejection.

Discussion

Previous studies in dogs undergoing orthotopic cardiac transplantation have shown that hemodynamic and mechanical indices of left ventricular performance are significantly depressed immediately after operation.[1, 2] Spontaneous recovery in donor heart performance then occurs gradually over the first 2 to 4 postoperative days. Of the principal determinants of cardiac output (i.e., ventricular preload, afterload, heart rate, and contractile state), contractile state has been shown to be the critically limiting factor in dysfunction of the donor left ventricle immediately after transplantation. The most likely cause of the observed impairment in myocardial contractility is anoxic injury sustained during transfer of the graft from donor to recipient, although an additive or synergistic effect of acute withdrawal of sympathetic myocardial support (denervation) cannot be excluded. Similar, reversible depression of myocardial performance has been shown to result from acute short-term (20 to 30 minutes) anoxia imposed on the normal canine heart.[6]

The present studies offer direct confirmation of functional depression of the transplanted human heart immediately postoperatively, comparable in magnitude and time course to that documented in canine studies. Limitations of the Fick technique for bedside estimation of cardiac output in our patients are recognized, inasmuch as a methodological standard error of 5 to 10 per cent, even under well-controlled conditions, is generally accepted.[7] The homogeneity of our data, however, both in individual patients and in trends between patients, suggests that errors incurred were not remarkably disparate from those noted above.

The present studies do not provide differentiation of right versus left ventricular dysfunction as predominant in the observed pattern of hemodynamic depression and recovery after transplantation. Indeed, prior observations indicate that right ventricular failure may dominate the recipient's immediate postoperative cardiovascular status, as assessed clinically; in patients with excessive elevation of pulmonary vascular resistance, it may cause death intraoperatively or within hours after transplantation.[8] Available evidence, then, suggests that the recipient's hemodynamic status early after transplantation is determined primarily by a variable degree of generalized but reversible impairment of myocardial function that may also be modulated importantly by the external workload imposed acutely on the donor right ventricle.

Heart rate augmentation by ventricular pacing in those recipients studied early postoperatively produced no detectable improvement in cardiac output because of proportional decreases in stroke volume. Donor atrial pacing at rates higher than control, however, was accompanied by consistent though modest improvement in cardiac output. This suggests preservation of donor atrial transport function, despite the altered morphology of these chambers after transplantation. These data are consistent with previous observations in human recipients late postoperatively.[9] In the canine cardiac recipients, atrial pacing early postoperatively has been shown to markedly increase cardiac output because of a relative invariance of stroke volume despite wide ranges in heart rate.[10, 11] Our limited clinical measurements do not illustrate a quantitatively comparable relationship between donor rate and output. The reason for the discrepancy is unknown but may relate to maintenance of lower effective ventricular filling pressures in human cardiac recipients or to the effects of pulmonary vascular changes, as noted previously.

The positive myocardial inotropic and chronotropic effects of isoproterenol in doses commonly used clinically resulted in substantial increases in cardiac output in all the recipients studied. Because of its salutory hemodynamic effects and the predictability of depressed graft performance early after transplantation, isoproterenol is now used routinely in the management of recipients for 1 to 4 days, beginning intraoperatively.

A further intent of the present study was to document in man the time course and degree of hemodynamic deterioration associated with acute graft rejection. It has been recognized clinically for several years that donor heart performance may be significantly depressed during advanced stages of acute rejection; however, the pattern and magnitude of such functional deterioration have not been sufficiently defined to permit evaluation of hemodynamic measurements as a clinically useful tool for diagnosis of rejection or establishment of prognosis. The results of our studies indicate that hemodynamic monitoring (including determination of cardiac output) does not constitute a sensitive diagnostic technique. In only three of eight diagnosed episodes of acute cardiac rejection in our patients did cardiac output decline to levels that could be considered definitely below the limits of error. Furthermore, the duration of subnormal cardiac output was limited to 1 to 2 days in two of these three instances. In the one exception (Fig. 5), deterioration of stroke volume and cardiac output was progressive and was associated with irreversible immunologic injury. It is also noteworthy that in this case prognosis was readily apparent on the basis of established clinical criteria for the severity of rejection.[4] These findings, however, do not exclude the potential usefulness of more reliable and sensitive techniques for characterization of donor heart performance. For example, the analysis of instantaneous left ventricular dynamics by means of implanted tantalum coil intramyocardial markers visualized cineradiographically has allowed precise quantitation of the functional state of orthotopically transplanted canine hearts.[11] Preliminary studies in man have been undertaken.

The Journal of
Thoracic and Cardiovascular
Surgery

270 Stinson et al.

REFERENCES

1 Stinson, E. B., Griepp, R. B., Bieber, C. P., and Shumway, N. E.: Hemodynamic Observations After Orthotopic Transplantation of the Canine Heart, J. THORAC. CARDIOVASC. SURG. **63:** 344, 1972.

2 Stinson, E. B., Tecklenberg, P. L., Hollingsworth, J. F., Jones, K. W., Sloane, R., and Rahmoeller, G.: Changes in Left Ventricular Mechanical and Hemodynamic Function During Acute Rejection of Orthotopically Transplanted Hearts in Dogs, J. THORAC. CARDIOVASC. SURG. **68:** 783, 1974.

3 Stinson, E. B., Dong, E., Jr., Iben, A. B., and Shumway, N. E.: Cardiac Transplantation in Man. III. Surgical Aspects, Am. J. Surg. **118:** 182, 1969.

4 Griepp, R. B., Stinson, E. B., Dong, E., Jr., Clark, D. A., and Shumway, N. E.: Acute Rejection of the Allografted Human Heart, Ann. Thorac. Surg. **12:** 113, 1971.

5 Caves, P. K., Stinson, E. B., Billingham, M. E., Rider, A. K., and Shumway, N. E.: Diagnosis of Human Cardiac Allograft Rejection by Serial Cardiac Biopsy, J. THORAC. CARDIOVASC. SURG. **66:** 461, 1973.

6 Levine, F. H., Copeland, J. G., Melvin, M. B., and Stinson, E. B.: Extended Evaluation of Anoxia on Ventricular Performance and Compliance, Circulation **46:** 184, 1972 (Suppl II).

7 Wade, O. L., and Bishop, J. M.: Cardiac Output and Regional Blood Flow, Philadelphia, 1962, F. A. Davis Company.

8 Stinson, E. B., Griepp, R. B., Dong, E., Jr., and Shumway, N. E.: Results of Human Heart Transplantation at Stanford University, Transplant. Proc. **3:** 337, 1971.

9 Stinson, E. B., Schroeder, J. S., Griepp, R. B., Shumway, N. E., and Dong, E., Jr.: Observations on the Behavior of Recipient Atria Following Cardiac Transplantation in Man, Am. J. Cardiol. **30:** 615, 1972.

10 Chartrand, C., Angell, W. W., Dong, E., Jr., and Shumway, N. E.: Atrial Pacing in the Postoperative Management of Cardiac Homotransplantation, Ann. Thorac. Surg. **8:** 152, 1969.

11 Mattila, S., Ingels, N. B., Daughters, G. T., Adler, S. C., Wexler, L., and Dong, E., Jr.: The Effects of Atrial Pacing on the Synergy and Hemodynamics of the Orthotopically Transplanted Canine Heart, Circulation **48:** 386, 1973.

The New England
Journal of Medicine

Volume 306   MARCH 11, 1982   Number 10

HEART-LUNG TRANSPLANTATION

Successful Therapy for Patients with Pulmonary Vascular Disease

Bruce A. Reitz, M.D., John L. Wallwork, M.B., Ch.B., Sharon A. Hunt, M.D., John L. Pennock, M.D., Margaret E. Billingham, M.B., Philip E. Oyer, M.D., Ph.D., Edward B. Stinson, M.D., and Norman E. Shumway, M.D., Ph.D.

Abstract We report our initial experience with three patients who received heart-lung transplants. The primary immunosuppressive agent used was cyclosporin A, although conventional drugs were also administered.

In the first patient, a 45-year-old woman with primary pulmonary hypertension, acute rejection of the transplant was diagnosed 10 and 25 days after surgery but was treated successfully; this patient still had normal exercise tolerance 10 months later. The second patient, a 30-year-old man, underwent transplantation for Eisenmenger's syndrome due to atrial and ventricular septal defects. His graft was not rejected, and his condition was markedly improved

eight months after surgery. The third patient, a 29-year-old woman with transposition of the great vessels and associated defects, died four days postoperatively of renal, hepatic, and pulmonary complications.

We attribute our success to experience with heart-lung transplantation in primates, to the use of cyclosporin A, and to the anatomic and physiologic advantages of combined heart-lung replacement. We hope that such transplants may ultimately provide an improved outlook for selected terminally ill patients with pulmonary vascular disease and certain other intractable cardiopulmonary disorders. (N Eng J Med. 1982; 306:557-64.)

PULMONARY vascular disease is a discouraging illness in its terminal stage, whether the disorder is idiopathic or due to congenital heart disease (Eisenmenger's syndrome); vasodilators are unsuccessful, and care is only supportive. It has been appreciated for many years that lung or combined heart-lung transplantation may be the only treatment for these entities. However, neither type of transplantation has been successful, because of the complications from immunosuppression in transplants of lung tissue,[1] ventilation-perfusion imbalance in single-lung transplants,[2] and failure of bronchial healing.[3] Recent experimental work from our laboratory has demonstrated the technical ease of performing combined heart-lung transplantation,[4,5] as well as the long-term survival of primates treated with cyclosporin A after undergoing the procedure.[6] This laboratory work, together with extensive clinical experience with cardiac transplantation[7] (including the use of cyclosporin A), preceded a clinical trial of combined heart-lung trans-

plantation for end-stage pulmonary vascular disease at our center. This report summarizes our experience with three patients who received heart-lung transplants between March 9 and July 28, 1981.

METHODS

Patients considered for heart-lung transplantation had pulmonary vascular disease and severe symptoms; their clinical deterioration was such that they were thought to have a poor prognosis for six-month survival. The design and protocol of the trial were approved by the Committee for Human Subjects in Research at Stanford University Medical Center. The cyclosporin A for clinical use was provided by Sandoz (Basel). The first patient had idiopathic pulmonary vascular-disease, and the subsequent two patients had pulmonary vascular disease that was secondary to congenital heart disease.

CASE REPORTS

Patient 1

This 45-year-old woman had primary pulmonary hypertension. Approximately five years before, orthopnea and dyspnea on exertion had developed. As these symptoms progressively worsened, pedal edema and chest pain occurred. Pulmonary arterial hypertension was confirmed by cardiac catheterization in March 1980. The pulmonary-artery pressure was 72/38 mm Hg (mean, 50), and the cardiac index was 1.9 liters per minute per square meter of body-surface area. There was no evidence of any other cardiac disease. The pulmonary-artery pressure was not appreciably affected by 100 per cent oxygen, sodium nitroprusside infusion, or hydrala-

From the departments of Cardiovascular Surgery, Medicine (Division of Cardiology), and Pathology, Stanford University School of Medicine, Stanford, Calif. Address reprint requests to Dr. Reitz at the Department of Cardiovascular Surgery, Stanford University School of Medicine, Stanford, CA 94305.

Supported in part by a grant (HL-13108) from the National Heart, Lung, and Blood Institute.

558   THE NEW ENGLAND JOURNAL OF MEDICINE   March 11, 1982

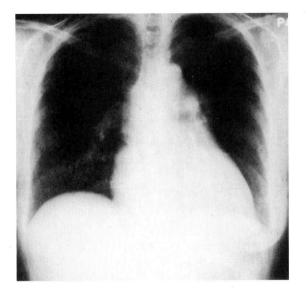

Figure 1. Pretransplantation Chest Roentgenogram of Patient 1.

The heart, right ventricle, and central pulmonary artery are enlarged.

zine. The possibility of collagen vascular disease or silent pulmonary embolism was considered but was ruled out by negative studies. A chest roentgenogram is shown in Figure 1. Over the next year the patient had marked symptomatic deterioration. Various pulmonary vasodilators were administered but then discontinued because of systemic hypotension. Exercise tolerance was minimal, and signs of right heart failure progressed. She became more dependent on continuous oxygen therapy and had several episodes of hemoptysis, syncope, and worsening chest pain. Her progressive disability and poor life expectancy led to consideration of transplantation.

After giving written informed consent, the patient underwent combined heart and lung transplantation on March 9, 1981. The donor was a 15-year-old boy with the same blood type and approximately the same size. He had sustained severe head trauma and was declared brain dead after he had been maintained on a respirator for 48 hours. The recipient and donor were in adjoining operating rooms during transplantation.

The operative technique consisted of median sternotomy and anterior pericardiectomy; both phrenic nerves were preserved on pedicles of pericardium. Cannulation for cardiopulmonary bypass was performed through the right atrium into the superior and inferior venae cavae. The arterial return from the pump-oxygenator was directed into the high ascending aorta. After institution of cardiopulmonary bypass, the ascending aorta was clamped and the heart and lungs of the recipient were excised at the aorta just above the aortic valve, the arterioventricular groove of the right atrium, and across the trachea at a point just above the carina. A similar dissection was performed simultaneously in the donor, except that the superior vena cava was ligated and the superior and inferior venae cavae were cut separately. The donor's heart and lungs were flushed with cold cardioplegic solution (4°C) to remove all donor blood from the graft.[8] Before implantation the graft was cooled further with topical cold saline. With the recipient's heart and lungs removed, small bleeding points in the posterior mediastinum were controlled with electrocautery. Care was taken to preserve the recurrent laryngeal nerve around the arch of the aorta, as well as the vagus nerves on the esophagus. Implantation began with anastomosis of the trachea (running 4-0 Prolene suture), which was followed by aortic anastomosis (4-0 Prolene). The right atrium of the graft was opened from the inferior vena cava toward the right atrial

appendage; this cuff was anastomosed to the recipient's right atrial cuff (3-0 Prolene continuous suture). At this point the aorta was unclamped, and the heart and lungs were resuscitated. After a short period on cardiopulmonary bypass, the transplanted heart and lungs maintained the patient's circulation without difficulty.

In the immediate postoperative period arterial blood gases were satisfactory, and the patient was extubated within 36 hours. Immunosuppression consisted of cyclosporin A, rabbit antihuman thymocyte globulin, methylprednisolone, and azathioprine (Fig. 2). The patient remained weak, with slow recovery from the operation. Seven days after transplantation the results of a cardiac biopsy were normal and the chest roentgenogram was relatively clear. Over the next week, a marked increase in interstitial edema on roentgenography was accompanied by deteriorating arterial blood gases. Ten days after operation a cardiac biopsy showed changes consistent with early acute rejection. Intravenous hyperalimentation, started about one week postoperatively, contributed to the fluid overload. Because of decreasing lung compliance, hypoxemia, and increased work of breathing, it was necessary to insert an endotracheal tube and provide ventilatory support. Intravenous methylprednisolone together with rabbit antihuman thymocyte globulin was given in order to reverse the rejection (Fig. 2). Fiberoptic bronchoscopy showed normal mucosa in the trachea of the graft and no abnormality at the suture line. After 48 hours of ventilation and anti-rejection therapy, pulmonary function improved dramatically and extubation proceeded without difficulty. A second episode of acute cardiac allograft rejection, 25 days after operation, was documented by endomyocardial biopsy; it was accompanied by mild changes of increased interstitial edema on roentgenography. This rejection

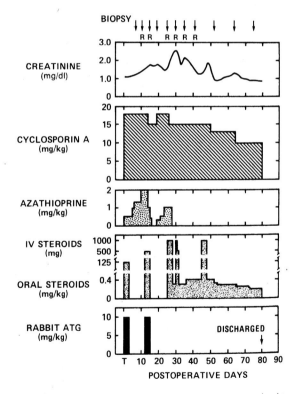

Figure 2. Transplantation Course and Immunosuppression in Patient 1.

The times of transvenous endomyocardial biopsy are indicated by arrows at the top panel; biopsies that revealed acute rejection are marked by R. ATG denotes antihuman thymocyte globulin.

To convert creatinine values to micromoles per liter, multiply by 88.4.

Vol. 306   No. 10   THE NEW ENGLAND JOURNAL OF MEDICINE   559

was treated again by pulse therapy with methylprednisolone (Fig. 2). Thirty days after transplantation the maintenance dose of azathioprine was discontinued, and prednisone therapy was initiated in a dose of 0.2 mg per kilogram of body weight per day. Since resolution of this second rejection episode, the results of frequent cardiac biopsies have continued to be normal and chest roentgenograms have shown continued improvement without evidence of rejection or infection.

The patient was discharged from the hospital on the 85th postoperative day and has been followed as an outpatient on a weekly basis. During this time systemic arterial hypertension of about 150/110 mm Hg has been treated with methyldopa and hydrochlorothiazide. The dose of cyclosporin A has been gradually tapered to 8 mg per kilogram per day, and the prednisone dose has remained 5 mg twice a day. Monthly biopsies have continued to show no evidence of rejection. Cardiac catheterization, performed four months postoperatively, revealed completely normal pressures on the right and normal cardiac output. Pulmonary-function tests demonstrated decreased lung volumes (total capacity and vital capacity), normal flows (peak and at one second), and minimal obstruction of airflow (Table 1) and showed that pulmonary gas exchange was well maintained during moderately severe exercise (Table 2). A recent chest roentgenogram is shown in Figure 3. The side effects of cyclosporin A therapy have been a mild resting tremor, moderate hirsutism, intermittent nausea, vomiting, and diarrhea. At 10 months after transplantation the patient is able to perform all household activities as well as she did before her symptoms of pulmonary hypertension developed. The only infectious complication has been transient cutaneous herpes simplex.

Patient 2

A 30-year-old man had congenital heart disease associated with the Holt–Oram syndrome. The cardiac defects included large atrial and ventricular septal defects. The diagnosis of congenital heart disease was not made until the patient was 12, at which time the pulmonary vascular resistance was elevated. A pulmonary-artery banding procedure was performed; thereafter, serial cardiac catheterization showed progression of pulmonary vascular disease. In 1980 the pulmonary vascular resistance was greater than the systemic, and the ratio of the pulmonary to the systemic shunt (Q_p:Q_s) was 0.24. The patient noticed progressive shortness of breath, fatigability, exertional chest pain, and cyanosis. These symptoms continually worsened, and about three years before transplantation phlebotomies were required for polycythemia and transient cerebral ischemia. Immediately before transplantation, phlebotomy was performed on a weekly basis in order to keep the

Table 2. Post-transplant Pulmonary Function during Exercise.*

PULMONARY FUNCTION	PATIENT 1 (AT 6 MO)		PATIENT 2 (AT 4 MO)	
	AT REST	HIGHEST EXERCISE LEVEL †	AT REST	HIGHEST EXERCISE LEVEL †
Treadmill slope (per cent)	—	7.5	—	12.5
Treadmill velocity (km/hr)	—	4	—	5.5
Ventilation (liters/min)	5.40	22.52	9.35	66.72
Tidal volume (ml)	186	375	312	1516
Frequency (breaths/min)	29	60	30	44
Oxygen consumption (ml/min)	168	605	289	1784
Heart rate (beats/min)	110	120	103	150

*Partial data from a study of graded treadmill exercise.

†Measured at the end of five minutes of exercise.

hematocrit below 70 per cent. Numerous episodes of hemoptysis and anterior chest pain occurred both at rest and with exertion.

Because of the severity of the symptoms and the estimated poor outlook for six-month survival, this patient was accepted as a candidate for heart-lung transplantation and underwent operation on May 1, 1981. The donor was a 25-year-old man who had suffered brain death as the result of an automobile accident; he had been given assisted ventilation for 60 hours before the transplantation. The operative technique was similar to that described for Patient 1.

The immediate postoperative course was complicated by excessive mediastinal bleeding, which required reexploration on two occasions within the first 12 hours. This bleeding proved to be from bronchial and esophageal collateral vessels in the posterior mediastinum. The remainder of the postoperative course was uncomplicated. The patient was extubated 24 hours later; excellent pulmonary function was maintained. Over the first 10 postoperative days an increasingly severe interstitial pulmonary edema developed (Fig. 4). Biopsy of the endomyocardium (Fig. 5), conducted seven days after surgery, ruled out graft rejection as the cause of this edema. The patient was treated with diuretics, and chest roentgenograms showed gradual improvement. As in Patient 1, immunosuppression consisted of cyclosporin A, rabbit antihuman thymocyte globulin, azathioprine, and prednisone (Fig. 6). Azathioprine was given for two weeks and then replaced by prednisone. Serial endomyocardial biopsies (Fig. 6) were all interpreted as showing no evidence of rejection. Creatinine levels rose for a short period, presumably because of the cyclosporin A; they returned to normal as the dose was decreased. The patient had excellent symptomatic improvement and was discharged on the 45th postoperative day.

Three additional cardiac biopsies, taken at monthly intervals during outpatient-clinic visits, were normal. Right heart catheterization revealed normal pressures, and pulmonary-function tests showed decreased lung volumes and good airflow (Table 1). During exercise, ventilation increased from 9.35 liters per minute (at rest) to 66.7 liters per minute (on a treadmill with a slope of 12.5 per cent and a speed of 5.5 km per hour); other findings are given in Table 2. A recent chest roentgenogram is shown in Figure 7. At present the patient takes cyclosporin A (7 mg per kilogram per day) and prednisone (6 mg twice a day), walks 6.5 km, and rides a stationary bicycle for 6.5 to 10 km a day without difficulty. The side effects of cyclosporin A have been minimal, and no appreciable complications have appeared.

Patient 3

A 29-year-old woman was recognized in infancy as having transposition of the great vessels and ventricular and atrial septal defects. When she was 2½ a Baffes procedure was performed.[9] Her condition improved until her teen-age years, when cardiopulmonary function became progessively limited. Serial cardiac catheterizations documented the development of pulmonary vascular disease. A palliative Mustard procedure, performed when the patient was 25, brought only temporary benefit. Dyspnea on exertion,

Table 1. Patient and Donor Characteristics and Post-transplant Pulmonary Function at Rest.

CHARACTERISTIC	PATIENT 1	PATIENT 2
Patient		
Height (cm)	152	175
Weight (kg)	48	57
Donor		
Height (cm)	Not available	180
Weight (kg)	65	77

PULMONARY FUNCTION	PATIENT 1		PATIENT 2	
	OBSERVED (AT 6 MO)	PREDICTED*	OBSERVED (AT 4 MO)	PREDICTED*
Total lung capacity (liters)	1.86	3.55	3.63	6.35
Residual volume (liters)	0.94	0.93	0.90	1.43
Ratio of residual volume to total lung capacity	0.50	0.26	0.25	0.23
Vital capacity (liters)	0.93	2.62	2.73	4.84
Forced expiratory volume (per cent)				
At one second	82	>72	89	>72
At three seconds	100	>95	98	>95

*Based on patient's height and weight.

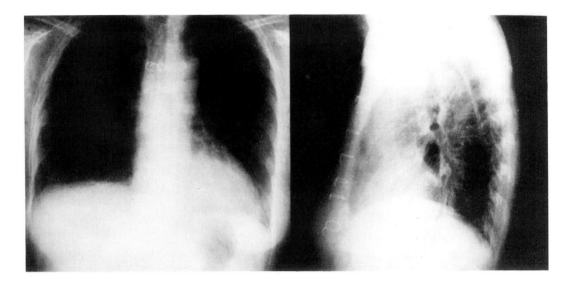

Figure 3. Recent Posterior-Anterior and Lateral Chest Roentgenograms of Patient 1.
This is a representative film obtained six months after transplantation.

fatigue, mild edema, and multiple supraventricular and ventricular arrhythmias occurred. Six months before transplantation the patient had an episode of ventricular fibrillation, from which she was resuscitated without sequelae. The arrhythmias continued despite treatment.

Heart and lung transplantation was performed on July 28, 1981. At the time of operation dense adhesions from the previous cardiac surgery were encountered. Because the pericardium had been removed for the Mustard procedure, it was difficult to separate the phrenic nerves from the heart. A previously unsuspected, calcified patent ductus arteriosus was encountered. Reimplantation of the graft proceeded as described in Patient 1, leaving intact the homograft replacement of the inferior vena cava from the Baffes procedure. However, when cardiopulmonary bypass was first discontinued, there was extensive bleeding from the old calcified homograft where it had fractured. Repair stitches narrowed this conduit further. It was necessary to resume cardiopulmonary bypass and replace the inferior vena cava homograft with a separate portion of new donor aorta. Coagulopathy resulted after this long period of cardiopulmonary bypass (total, six hours, 50 minutes), and the diffuse bleeding was difficult to control. Several coagulation factors were administered, and finally the chest could be closed.

Renal, hepatic, and then pulmonary failure developed postoperatively. Despite maximal therapy, the patient succumbed to these complications four days later. At autopsy, ischemic changes were seen in the kidneys and liver. The pulmonary graft was quite edematous, and there were patchy areas of pneumonia. There was no evidence of graft rejection or tracheal necrosis. The donor heart had focal areas of ischemia that were compatible with vasopressor therapy; the recipient's heart and lungs had very advanced pulmonary vascular disease and the expected congenital cardiac abnormalities.

DISCUSSION

Survival and marked symptomatic improvement has occurred in patients undergoing combined heart-lung transplantation for end-stage pulmonary vascular disease. We believe that three factors are responsible for this success: (1) preliminary laboratory experience with the procedure in primates; (2) the use of cyclosporin A as a primary agent for immunosuppression; and (3) the anatomic and physiologic ad-

vantage of combined heart-lung transplantation with its technical simplicity, matched ventilation and perfusion, and ability to manage immunosuppressive treatment by monitoring the cardiac allograft.

Laboratory experience was critical to the early success of heart-lung transplantation in these patients. A technique for performing the operation was developed that resulted in consistent survival in primates,[4,5] the ability of primates to withstand complete cardiopulmonary denervation was confirmed, and cyclosporin A was shown to significantly prolong allograft survival.[4] The early development of intersti-

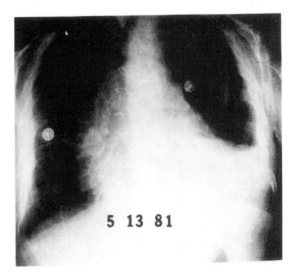

Figure 4. Posterior-Anterior Chest Roentgenogram of Patient 2, 12 Days after Surgery.
A diffuse interstitial infiltrate is present in both lung fields, and the left hemidiaphragm is elevated.

tial pulmonary edema was seen in both autotransplants and allotransplants.[4] This is probably the same process that occurs in the transplanted lung of dogs receiving unilateral transplants and is called the "reimplantation response."[10] The phenomenon is transient and may be due in part to ischemic injury during transplantation or disruption of pulmonary lymphatics. It is best treated by fluid restriction and diuretics and resolves about three weeks after transplantation.[4] Both Patients 1 and 2 had this complication between the first and third weeks after operation.

Cyclosporin A is a unique cyclic polypeptide that was first shown by Borel et al. to have dramatic antilymphocytic properties.[11] Its action appears to be directed toward the inhibition of T-cell growth factor,[12] affecting T-lymphocyte killer cells more than T-lymphocyte helper cells.[13] The retention of polymorphonuclear-cell function and the apparent lack of detrimental effects on healing mechanisms has made cyclosporin A especially suitable for lung transplantation, in which infection and bronchial anastomotic rupture have been responsible for failure in most patients.[4,6,14] In our laboratory, rhesus monkeys undergoing combined heart and lung transplantation have lived for two years while under continuous treatment with cyclosporin A. In other experimental work, Norin et al. have demonstrated prolongation of allograft survival in unilateral lung transplants in dogs.[15]

Cyclosporin A has been used in cardiac transplantation at our center since December 1980; at present 19 of 21 patients with primary cardiac transplants treated with this drug are alive one month to 10 months after transplantation. Previous clinical reports of kidney and liver transplantation[16,17] and our own experience with heart transplantation in animals and patients[6,18,19] have shown the need for additional immunosuppression either with antithymocyte glob-

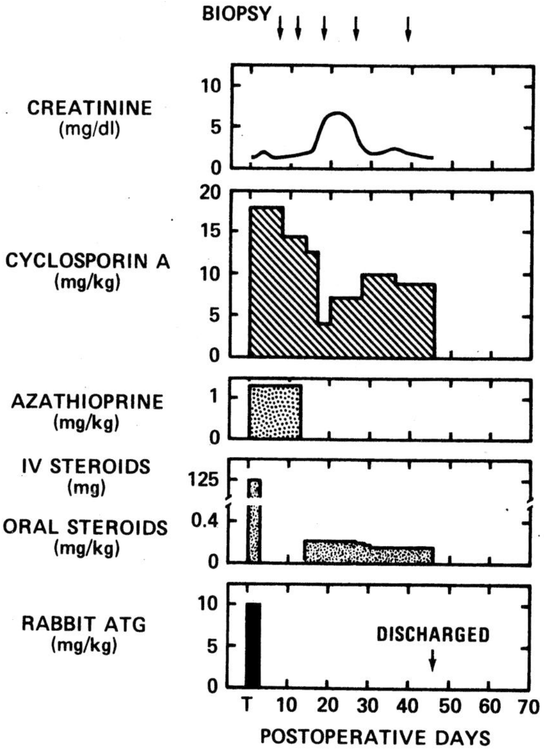

Figure 6. Transplantation Course and Immunosuppression in Patient 2.

For explanation of symbols and abbreviations, see Figure 2 legend.

ulin or prednisone. However, these medications can be used in considerably smaller doses than those used in conventional immunosuppressive regimens.

In reports of previous attempts at heart-lung transplantation in human beings, survival ranged from 12 hours to 23 days. The first of these patients was an infant with a complete atrioventricular canal and pulmonary edema; pulmonary insufficiency was the cause of death just 12 hours postoperatively.[20] The second patient underwent transplantation for chronic lung disease and did well initially but died at eight days from pneumonia.[21] A third patient, also undergoing transplantation for chronic lung disease, had a leak from the right bronchus 12 days postoperatively, required pneumonectomy, and died 23 days postoperatively.[22] At the time that these procedures were done, no animal receiving a combined heart-lung transplant had survived for more than 10 days.[23] The complications encountered in the second and third patients were similar to those following unilateral lung transplant, and were in part due to conventional immunosuppression by corticosteroids and azathioprine.

The results of lung transplantation alone have also been very disappointing. There have been 36 reported cases of lung transplantation in human beings,[1,3] with survival beyond two months occurring in only

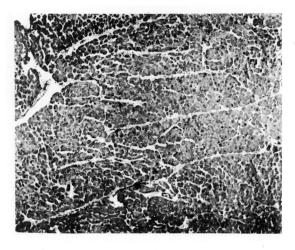

Figure 5. Tissue from Endomyocardial Biopsy of Patient 2, 12 Days after Surgery.
The specimen is normal, showing no evidence of rejection (hematoxylin and eosin).

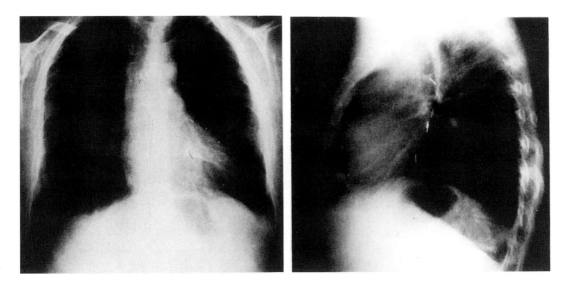

Figure 7. Recent Posterior-Anterior and Lateral Chest Roentgenograms of Patient 2.
This film is representative and was obtained eight months after operation.

two patients (six months and 10 months). Death has been caused by graft rejection, pneumonia, pulmonary insufficiency, and bronchial anastomotic rupture.

Much experience in lung transplantation in animals (mostly in dogs) has been reported. This work has elucidated the problems associated with disruption of pulmonary lymphatics,[10] the pattern of histologic appearance of allograft rejection,[24] bronchial anastomotic healing,[25] lung preservation before transplantation,[26] and the differences in prolonging allograft survival by various protocols of immunosuppression.[27] Achieving long-term survival of unilateral lung transplants in animals by means of conventional immunosuppression has been difficult because of many of the same factors responsible for failure in patients. Unlike animals, many patients who have received a lung transplant have chronic pulmonary infection in the contralateral lung, which quickly contaminates the transplant.

A group with a relatively favorable outlook for unilateral lung transplantation may be patients with primary pulmonary vascular disease, since they rarely have chronic lung infection. This group would acquire ventilation-perfusion abnormalities; however, animals that have undergone unilateral transplantation and contralateral pulmonary-artery ligation have had long survival periods.[28] It has not been shown, however, that single-lung transplantation carries less morbidity than combined heart-lung transplantation. Speculation concerning the type of lung transplant that may be appropriate for pulmonary vascular disease will continue until further experience with each procedure is obtained.[29]

We believe that in heart-lung transplantation, the adjustment of immunosuppression is notably im-

proved by histologically evaluating the cardiac allograft. There has been substantial experience with cardiac transplantation to document the efficacy of such monitoring. In our program, survival has improved from 20 per cent at one year in 1968 to 67 per cent at one year over the past five years.[7] Also, further improvement in survival may result from the introduction of cyclosporin A. The advances in cardiac transplantation that have improved survival, other than serial endomyocardial biopsy, include refinements in selecting patients, measures to prevent graft atherosclerosis, the development of a potent rabbit antihuman thymocyte globulin preparation, the use of immunologic monitoring, and the increased availability of donor hearts through procuring them from distant donors.

In nonhuman primates receiving combined heart-lung grafts in our laboratory, a close concordance has been documented between rejection of the heart and rejection of the lung, in regard to both onset and severity. This concordance has been substantiated by our early experience with the heart-lung recipients described above, in whom both acute allograft rejection was diagnosed and successful treatment followed by serial endomyocardial biopsies. Cardiac (and presumably pulmonary) allograft rejection was detected and treated 10 and 25 days postoperatively in Patient 1, with resolution of the changes evident on pulmonary roentgenography and cardiac biopsy. The possibility that roentgenographic evidence of interstitial pulmonary edema compatible with either rejection or "reimplantation response" was due to rejection was ruled out by a negative cardiac biopsy in Patient 2 on the seventh postoperative day. Previously, transbronchial lung biopsy has not been helpful in experimental lung transplantation,[30] and open-lung biopsy poses unacceptable morbidity for patients with lung transplants. Immunologic monitoring may prove useful in following isolated lung transplants, allowing differentiation between roentgenographic and functional pulmonary changes as due to rejection or infection. Cardiac-allograft monitoring seems to be most helpful in combined heart-lung transplantation.

Although transplantation of the cardiopulmonary axis is conceptually simple, requiring only three relatively easy anastomoses, great care must be taken during dissection in both recipient and donor. Of particular importance is careful preservation of both right and left phrenic nerves, the vagus nerves on the esophagus, and the left recurrent laryngeal nerve passing around the aorta at the ductus arteriosus or ligamentum arteriosum. Patient 1 had evidence of delayed gastric emptying, probably reflecting some damage to the intrathoracic vagal innervation of the stomach; Patient 2 had partial paresis of the left hemidiaphragm that was due to trauma of the left phrenic nerve. The preservation of these nerves is more difficult when previous operations have caused the formation of adhesions.

The death of Patient 3 from operative complications suggests that extensive previous cardiac surgery is a relative contraindication to this procedure. In this patient, the entire pericardial and pleural spaces were obliterated with adhesions, leaving an extensive raw surface with resulting hemorrhage that was difficult to control. Moreover, in a patient who has had a Baffes procedure, the previous homograft replacement of the inferior vena cava should be removed and a separate anastomosis of the vena cava performed.

In addition to patients with pulmonary vascular disease, a number of patients with other diseases may be treated by heart-lung transplantation. Among these are cardiac and pulmonary developmental abnormalities such as severe pulmonary atresia or diffuse pulmonary arteriovenous fistulas. Patients with diffuse pulmonary disease, including interstitial fibrosis, cystic fibrosis, or advanced chronic obstructive pulmonary disease, may be treated in this way. Changes in thoracic volumes acquired in the course of some of these latter diseases (e.g., advanced emphysema) may present a problem in regard to transplantation of organs with relatively normal volumes.

A major concern in lung transplantation has been the availability of suitable donors. Donors for the recipients reported here were found within a reasonable waiting period — 28 to 36 days. The donors had satisfactory lung function and no serious infection, despite neurologic death and ventilatory support for 48 to 60 hours before transplantation. The number of potential organ donors will increase when distant procurement and preservation of heart-lung grafts are possible.

Our results are encouraging, in that combined heart-lung transplantation was of benefit to patients with terminal pulmonary vascular disease. The patients' hemodynamics returned to normal, function

markedly improved, and allograft rejection was diagnosed and treated on the basis of cardiac biopsy. In the two surviving patients there has been no pulmonary infection or complications of tracheal healing. We hope that heart-lung transplantation will provide an improved outlook for terminally ill patients with pulmonary vascular disease or with cardiac and pulmonary disease with other causes.

Addendum: Since the submission of the manuscript, two more patients have undergone heart-lung transplantation at our center: a 40-year-old man with Eisenmenger's syndrome secondary to a ventricular septal defect (October 10, 1981) and a 37-year-old woman with primary pulmonary hypertension (December 1, 1981). Both patients have had satisfactory recoveries to date and are improved.

We are indebted to Mary Burge, M.S.W., Lois Christopherson, M.S.W., Patricia Gamberg, R.N., and Joan Miller, R.N., for their help in managing these patients, and to the physicians who provided medical information and follow-up care.

REFERENCES

1. Veith FJ. Lung transplantation. Surg Clin North Am. 1978; 58:357-64.
2. Stevens PM, Johnson PC, Bell RL, Beall AC Jr, Jenkins DE. Regional ventilation and perfusion after lung transplantation in patients with emphysema. N Engl J Med. 1970; 282:245-9.
3. Nelems JMB, Rebuck AS, Cooper JD, Goldberg M, Halloran PF, Vellend H. Human lung transplantation. Chest. 1980; 78:569-73.
4. Reitz BA, Burton NA, Jamieson SW, et al. Heart and lung transplantation: autotransplantation and allotransplantation in primates with extended survival. J Thorac Cardiovasc Surg. 1980; 80:360-72.
5. Reitz BA, Pennock JL, Shumway NE. Simplified operative method for heart and lung transplantation. J Surg Res. 1981; 31:1-5.
6. Reitz BA, Bieber CP, Raney AA, et al. Orthotopic heart and combined heart and lung transplantation with cyclosporin A immune suppression. Transplant Proc. 1981; 13:393-6.
7. Baumgartner WA, Reitz BA, Oyer PE, Stinson EB, Shumway NE. Cardiac homotransplantation. Curr Probl Surg. 1979; 16(9):1-61.
8. Watson DC, Reitz BA, Baumgartner WA, et al. Distant heart procurement for transplantation. Surgery. 1979; 86:56-9.
9. Baffes TG. A new method for surgical correction of transposition of the aorta and pulmonary artery. Surg Gynecol Obstet. 1956; 102:227-33.
10. Siegelman SS, Sinha SBP, Veith FJ. Pulmonary reimplantation response. Ann Surg. 1973; 177:30-6.
11. Borel JF, Feurer C, Magnée C, Stähelin H. Effects of the new antilymphocytic peptide cyclosporin A in animals. Immunology. 1977; 32:1017-25.
12. Larsson E-L. Cyclosporin A and dexamethasone suppress T cell responses by selectively acting at distinct sites of the triggering process. J Immunol. 1980; 124:2828-33.
13. Hess AD, Tutschka PJ. Effect of cyclosporin A on human lymphocyte responses *in vitro*. I. CsA allows for the expression of alloantigen-activated suppressor cells while preferentially inhibiting the induction of cytologic effector lymphocytes in MLR. J Immunol. 1980; 124:2601-8.
14. Calne RY. Immunosuppression for organ grafting: observations on cyclosporin A. Immunol Rev. 1979; 46:113-24.
15. Norin AJ, Veith FJ, Emeson EE, Montefusco CM, Pinsker KL, Kamholz SL. Improved survival of transplanted lungs in mongrel dogs treated with cyclosporin A. Transplantation. 1981; 32:259-60.
16. Calne RY, Rolles K, White DJG, et al. Cyclosporin A initially as the only immunosuppressant in 34 recipients of cadaveric organs: 32 kidneys, 2 pancreases, and 2 livers. Lancet. 1979; 2:1033-6.
17. Starzl TE, Klintmalm GBG, Porter KA, Iwatsuki S, Schröter GPJ. Liver transplantation with use of cyclosporin A and prednisone. N Engl J Med. 1981; 305:266-9.
18. Jamieson SW, Burton NA, Bieber CP, et al. Cardiac allograft survival in primates treated with cyclosporin A. Lancet. 1979; 1:545.
19. Pennock JL, Oyer PE, Reitz BA, et al. Cardiac transplantation in perspective for the future: survival, complications, rehabilitation, and cost. J Thorac Cardiovasc Surg. (in press).
20. Cooley DA, Bloodwell RD, Hallman GL, Nora JJ, Harrison GM, Leachman RD. Organ transplantation for advanced cardiopulmonary disease. Ann Thorac Surg. 1969; 8:30-42.
21. Wildevuur CRH, Benfield JR. A review of 23 human lung transplantations by 20 surgeons. Ann Thorac Surg. 1970; 9:489-515.

Appendix B: Pioneers in cardiac surgery

Aird, Iain, FRCS

London, England

1. Professor of Surgery at the Hammersmith Hospital who stimulated the developments in cardiac surgery by Cleland, Bentall and Melrose.
2. Performed early separation of Siamese twins.

Alley, Ralph D, MD

Albany, New York

1. Performed the first successful resection traumatic aortic arch aneurysm using external shunts (1953).
2. Exemplary teacher and clinician who built a strong national and international bridge of professional and social exchange.

Austen, W Gerald, MD

Boston, Massachusetts

1. Collaborator with Kantrowitz and Buckley in intra-aortic balloon circulatory assistance.
2. Performed the first repair in a patient in shock from acute ruptured papillary muscle after myocardial infarction (1963). This was a forerunner of emergency coronary surgery in early infarction or unstable angina.
3. With Buckley, Daggett, Mundth, Laver and the MGH Group combined metabolic, pharmacological, mechanical and technical support for critically ill heart surgery patients.
4. Past President American Heart Association and Society of Thoracic Surgeons.

Bahnson, Henry T, MD

Pittsburgh, Pennsylvania

1. Developed operations for aortic aneurysms.
2. Collaborator with Blalock in surgery of congenital and acquired heart disease.
3. Introduced monocusp aortic valve repair to palliate rheumatic heart disease.

Bailey, Charles P, MD

New York, New York

1. Co-founder of modern cardiac surgery.
2. Developed 'commissurotomy' for mitral stenosis.
3. Creator of many closed operations for congenital and acquired heart disease.
4. Clarified and applied many physiologic principles for clinical use collaborating with Zimmerman, Hirose and others.
5. Edited massive textbook on cardiac surgery; the state-of-the-art at that time.
7. Innovator in valve reconstruction and coronary artery surgery.
8. Helped demonstrate heart surgery as a practical therapy to an unwilling world.

Barnard, Christiaan N, MD

Cape Town, South Africa

1. Performed the first heart transplant (1967).
2. Developed heterotopic transplantation.
3. Worked with new heart valves and was first to replace the valve in Ebstein's anomaly.

Barratt-Boyes, Sir Brian G, FRCS, KBE

Auckland, New Zealand

1. Brilliant innovator in aortic valve homograft techniques.
2. Promulgator/developer of deep hypothermic circulatory arrest techniques.
3. Innovator in surgical correction of congenital heart defects.

Beall, Arthus C, Jr, MD

Houston, Texas

1. Performed the first successful emergency pulmonary embolectomy using total cardiopulmonary bypass.
2. Performed the first successful emergency operation for traumatic aortic valve insufficiency.
3. Prosthetic valve designer.
4. Fostered medical, engineering, industrial and government communication via The Association for the Advancement of Medical Instrumentation of which he is a past President.
5. Past President of the American College of Chest Physicians.
6. Advisor to the government and private sectors regarding device safety legislation.

Beck, Claude S, MD

Cleveland, Ohio

1. Proponent of collateralisation of coronary circulation by vascular adhesions similar in principle to the procedures of O'Shaughnessy, Lezius and Harken.
2. He reversed coronary venous flow with an arterial shunt as a method of myocardial revascularisation.
3. Pioneer in open-chest cardiac resuscitation.
4. Co-worker in Cutler and Levine's mitral valvulectomy operation (1923).
5. Articulated Beck's Triad (the physiological signs of constrictive pericarditis and cardiac tamponade).

Bentall, Hugh, FRCS

London, England

1. Developed aortic root replacement with Anthony De Bono.
2. Professor of Cardiac Surgery at the Hammersmith Hospital and helped to develop cardiac surgical programmes in many European countries.

Berkovits, Barouh, FACC

Wellesley, Massachusetts

1. Developer of direct-current defibrillator, tested by Lefemine.
2. Engineered the cardioverter, tested and used by Lown.
3. Engineer-designer of the demand pacemaker with Zarouff and Harken.
4. Designer of the atrioventricular sequential pacemaker.

Bigelow, William G, MD

Toronto, Canada

1. Studied and applied extensive observations of the microcirculation, deriving source material from the anatomist Knisely.

2. Developer of biological valves.
3. Pioneer investigator of hypothermia for cardiac operations.
4. Collaborated with Callaghan and Hopps in early pacemaker work with two-point focal electrode to excite SA node. The selfless sharing of information with Zoll is a tribute to them and a model to the scientific world.

Billroth, Professor Christian Albert Theodor
Zurich and Vienna
1. Great abdominal and general surgeon, but also classical obstructionist and nihilist who is best characterised by his own words: 'Any surgeon who would attempt an operation on the heart should lose the respect of his colleagues.' (Circa 1875)

Björk, Viking O, MD
Stockholm, Sweden
1. Developed direct percutaneous left-heart catheterisation and angiography.
2. Investigator of biomaterials and artificial intima.
3. Developer of a disc oxygenator (1947) with Crafoord and engineer Andersson.
4. Pioneer in patient monitoring and intensive care, and innovator in the field of mechanical devices.
5. Inventor of the Björk–Shiley prosthetic heart valve.

Blalock, Alfred, MD
Baltimore, Maryland
1. Physiologist/surgeon, innovator and teacher.
2. With Burwell, studied and corrected constrictive pericarditis.
3. Studied the thymus and its effect on circulation, including myasthenia gravis and shock.
4. With the paediatric cardiologist Helen Taussig, developed the subclavian-to-pulmonary artery shunt for congenital cyanotic heart disease.
5. Conducted fundamental studies on the nature and treatment of shock.
6. To name a few of those surgeons whose lives he influenced leaves him without peer: Bahnson, Cooley, Gott, Hanlon, Longmire, Maloney, McGoon, Morrow, Muller, Sabiston, Scott, Spencer.

Borst, Hans, MD
Hanover, Germany
1. Pre-eminent German Professor and teacher.
2. Leader in thoracic aortic surgery. Devised the elephant trunk technique for two-stage thoracic aortic replacement.
3. Past President of the European Society of Cardiothoracic Surgery.

Braunwald, Eugene, MD
Boston, Massachusetts
1. Professor of Cardiology at Harvard Medical School, and the world's foremost expert in the aetiology and management of heart failure. Editor of the leading textbook of cardiology.
2. The only physician to be admitted to the American Academy of Science.

Braunwald, Nina, MD
Bethesda, Maryland
1. 'First lady' of cardiac surgery and wife of the great cardiologist Eugene Braunwald.
2. Developed the Braunwald–Cutter prosthetic heart valve and innovator in many ofther areas of cardiac surgery.

Brewer, Lyman, MD

Los Angeles, California

1. World War II pioneer in 'Wet Lung in War Casualties' (1944).
2. Introduced elective cardiac arrest to control haemorrhage of heart wounds (1965).
3. Explored the nature of spinal cord injuries following correction of coarctation of the aorta. This had clinical and medico-legal significance.
4. Chairman of National Thoracic Surgery Manpower Study (1970–74).

Brock, Lord Russell, PRCS

London, England

1. Performed closed mitral valvulotomy, closed pulmonary valvulotomy and closed pulmonic infundibular resection (1948).
2. Pioneered percutaneous left ventricular puncture to assess aortic obstruction.
3. Described functional obstruction of left ventricular outflow tract (1955).
4. Past President of the Royal College of Surgeons of England.

Brom, Gerard, MD

Leiden, Netherlands

1. Leading surgeon of complex congenital heart defects in the Netherlands.

Brunton, Sir Thomas Lauder

London, England

1. Experimental pharmacologist and surgeon who in 1902 drew attention to the English cardiologist Samway's suggestion that notching of the stenotic mitral valve should provide a palliative compromise through mitral insufficiency. He suggested extensive experimental preparation, which he had too little time to conduct himself but suggested that others carry on the project. For 'suggesting that others carry on with a dangerous operation,' he was ruthlessly criticised for both his concept and principles.

Cabrol, Christian, MD

Paris, France

1. Pioneer of techniques in aortic root replacement.
2. Leading French transplant surgeon and proponent of artificial heart technology. Had the largest series of Jarvik 7 total artificial hearts in the bridge-to-transplant setting.

Carpentier, Alain J, MD

Paris, France

1. Assessed behaviour of biological valves with various methods of preparation and use.
2. Developed and evaluated techniques of mitral and tricuspid valve repair.
3. Pioneered the technique of cardiomyoplasty.

Carrel, Alexis, MD

Lyon, France

1. Devised practical techniques for arterial anastomoses (1905).
2. Conceived of artificial hearts and created perfusion pumps with the aviator Lindberg.
3. Suggested open-heart surgery by caval occlusion.
4. Planned (experimentally) heart valve surgery and correction of localised coronary artery disease (1910).
5. Described methods for future resections of aortic aneurysms.

6. Predicted and experimentally practised organ transplantation and was aware of problems of 'biological relationship between tissues'.
7. First American Nobel Laureate in Medicine and Physiology (1912).

Castaneda, Aldo R, MD

Boston, Massachusetts

1. Performed extensive laboratory work (with the Minneapolis group) on the effect of cardiopulmonary bypass on formed blood elements and the use of cardiopulmonary bypass for combined heart–lung autotransplantation in primates. This lead to long term survival of animals after heart–lung transplantation.
2. Applied this laboratory work to the correction of complicated congenital lesions in the first few months of life, using deep hypothermia and circulatory arrest.
3. Past President of the American Association for Thoracic Surgery.

Cooley, Denton A, MD

Houston, Texas

1. One of heart surgery's most brilliant technical surgeons.
2. Aggressive developer of improved techniques for relieving congenital and acquired heart disease.
3. Early proponent of ischaemic arrest for open heart surgery.
4. Extended the use/availability of the bubble oxgyenator in the disposable plastic form as developed by Gott.
5. Proponent of thoracic aortic surgery and artificial hearts.
6. Past President of the Society of Thoracic Surgeons, USA.

Crafoord, Clarence, MD

Stockholm, Sweden

1. Developed respirator equipment and life support techniques predicated on the early work of Sauerbruch, Giertz and others.
2. Student of thromboembolic diseases.
3. Colleague and friend of Erik Jorps, who determined the chemical formula of heparin and introduced it in its pure form. With the physiologist Howell, he was the first to point out the anticoagulant effect of the substance he called 'heparing'.
4. Co-developed heart–lung machines with Björk, Senning and engineer Andersson.
5. Performed the second successful open heart operation, removal of myxoma of the left atrium.
6. Pioneer thoracic surgeon in the areas of coarctation of the aorta, lobectomy, pneumonectomy etc.

Cutler, Elliott Carr, MD

Boston, Massachusetts

1. Initiated valvotomy for mitral stenosis with Samuel A Levine as collaborating cardiologist. This was a brave but disappointing adventure.
2. One of the last to believe that the great surgeons should be competent in all areas (a standard he very nearly attained).
3. Gave Harken his valve instruments. Made Harken Consultant in Thoracic Surgery during World War II, and stimulated the development of modern heart surgery by supporting Harken's removal of shell fragments from the heart.

David, Tirone, MD

Toronto, Canada

1. Innovator in both aortic and mitral valve repair techniques.
2. Developer of the Toronto Stentless Bioprosthesis.

Davila, Julio C, MD

Warsaw, Wisconsin

1. Performed first operation which corrected mitral regurgitation by annular constriction.
2. Built first mechanical pulse duplicator in America for study of cardiac valve mechanics.
3. Made various original observations on valvular function and on the role of the left ventricle in valvular disease.
4. Elucidated mechanisms of thrombosis in valvular prosthesis in relation to altered flow patterns.
5. Experimented in early refinements of cardiopulmonary bypass (with cooling and plasma dilution). Developed thermodilution for measurement of cardiac output in one clinical setting, and applied various instrumental methods for physiological measurements in valvular disease (first to directly measure transmitral valve flow).

Day, Hughes, MD

Kansas City, Kansas

1. Founder and developer of Coronary Care Units.

DeBakey, Michael E, MD

Houston, Texas

1. Developed the roller pump used in John Gibbon's machine and other heart–lung machines.
2. Developed Dacron artificial arteries and biomaterials for cardiac implantation.
3. Developed effective surgical methods for treatment of a wide spectrum of aneurysms of the aorta and major arteries (1952 and later).
4. Performed the first successful carotid endarterectomy (1953).
5. Developed left ventricular bypass for circulatory assistance.
6. The first aortocoronary saphenous vein bypass with long term survival performed on his service by Edward Garrett in 1964.
7. Pioneer developer of mechanical hearts.
8. Champion of cardiovascular causes *pro bono publico*, and the most influential surgical politician in the United States. Still powerful and active in his late 80's.

Dennis, Clarence, MD

Setauket, New York

1. First to use a pump oxygenator to provide circulation during open heart operations (two patients, April 1951 — neither survived).
2. Studied reduction of oxygen utilisation by left heart bypass (1963).
3. First to use mechanical pump support for chronic heart failure (1955) and myocardial infarction with shock (1958).
4. Experimented with caged-ball heart valves (1957).
5. Developed external counterpulsation with Senning and Wesolowski (1963).
6. Performed physiological and metabolic investigations of cerebral ischaemia, embolism and bleeding.

DeVega, Manuel, MD

Malaga, Spain

1. Developed the DeVega tricuspid annuloplasty.

DeWall, Richard A, MD

Dayton, Ohio

1. Pioneer developer of first clinically useful bubble oxygenator, subsequently modified to the Bentley disposable oxygenator.

Dodrill, F Dewey, MD
Detroit, Michigan
1. Performed first open heart surgery using right and left heart bypass successfully with the patient's lung as the oxygenator. First used left heart bypass for mitral stenosis.
2. Characterised the damaging effects of extracorporeal circulation on the lung.

DuBost, Charles, MD
Paris, France
1. Performed first resection and restoration of continuity in abdominal aortic aneurysm (1951).
2. Innovator of instruments and techniques.
3. Co-developer with Carpentier of glutaraldehyde-preserved heterografts for mitral and aortic replacement.
4. Performed endocardiectomy for endocardial fibroelastosis.
5. Developer of the pacemaker.

Duran, Carlos, MD
Missoula, Montana
1. Pioneer of homograft and heterograft techniques with Gunning in Oxford.
2. Proponent of aortic and mitral valve repair techniques.

Edwards, Jesse F, MD
St Paul, Minnesota
1. Made correlations of morbid pathology and physiology to give a new understanding of the heart as a surgical goal.

Effler, Donald B, MD
Syracuse, New York
1. Pioneer in the treatment of ischaemic heart disease.
2. His own epitaph: 'The SOB had enough talent to do a given operation well and was smart enough to reduce it to its simplest form.'

Elkin, Daniel C, MD
Atlanta, Georgia
1. Pioneer in repairing wounds of the heart (1941 and later).

Elkins, Ronald, MD
Oklahoma City, Oklahoma
1. Leading proponent of the pulmonary autograft (Ross) procedure.

Favaloro, René G, MD
Buenos Aires, Argentina
1. Developed bilateral internal mammary artery implant as an extension of the Vineberg operation through midline incision (1966). Combined this form of revascularisation with aneurysmectomy.
2. Used saphenous vein grafts first as interposition and bypass, then aortocoronary saphenous vein bypass (1967).
3. Developed saphenous vein bypass in acute coronary insufficiency and impending myocardial infarction (1968).

Ferguson, Thomas, MD
St Louis, Missouri
1. Esteemed Editor of *The Annals of Thoracic Surgery*.

2. Past President of the American Association for Thoracic Surgery.

Fontan, François, MD
Bordeaux, France
1. Developed bypass of the right ventricle in tricuspid atresia which formed the basis for the treatment of univentricular hearts.
2. Pre-eminent French Professor with his own vineyard.

Frazier, OH (Bud), MD
Houston, Texas
1. Leading protagonist of mechanical circulatory support in the bridge-to-transplant setting.
2. Co-worker with Cooley in the development of permanent artificial hearts.

Gerbode, Frank L, MD
San Francisco, California
1. With Bramson and Osborn, developed clinically successful membrane oxygenator.
2. Developed operations for complicated endocardial cushion effects.
3. With Osborn and IBM, developed computerised monitoring for critically ill patients.
4. With Osborn, established a very important private research institute, The Institute of Medical Science.

Gibbon, John H, Jr, MD
Philadelphia, Pennsylvania
1. Developer of IBM heart–lung machine in collaboration with his wife, Mary.
2. Performed the first successful open heart operation using complete cardiopulmonary bypass (atrial septal defect, 1953).

Glenn, William WL, MD
New Haven, Connecticut
1. Developed techniques for correcting congenital and acquired heart disease, including patent ductus arteriosus and mitral stenosis.
2. Introduced the use of elective electrical ventricular fibrillation.
3. Developed operations to bypass the right ventricle and carry out pulmonary valvulotomy.
4. Developed artificial cardiac pacemakers.
5. Past President of the American Heart Association.

Glover, Robert P, MD
Philadelphia, Pennsylvania
1. Collaborator with CP Bailey in performance of first modern mitral valve operation (commissurotomy). The patient was admitted, and operated on, on his service at Episcopal Hospital in Philadelphia.
2. He had the gift of simplifying scientific and medical information which made him one of the most effective proponents and popularisers of cardiac surgery (mitral commissurotomy), in particular among the general medical public and the laity.
3. He performed the first resection of a postinfarction aneurysm of the left ventricle (1953). His patient died 10 days after from massive GI bleeding secondary to stress gastric ulcer. The ventricular incision was healing well.
4. He was among the most active founders of the American College of Cardiology and one of its first Presidents.
5. He died at the peak of his career, of cancer of the colon. His studies of the lymphatic spread of this tumour (while a trainee at the Mayo clinic) are recognised as a landmark report.

Gorlin, Richard, MD
New York, New York

1. Cardiac physiologist and clinician. Promulgator and innovator of many physiological measurements and their clinical application.
2. With his engineer father, developed the formula for calculating effective valve orifices. The constant in the formula derived from the assumption that Harken's digital estimate was correct. Subsequent prospective estimates in hundreds of patients confirmed the validity of 'the Gorlin formula'.

Gott, Vincent L, MD
Baltimore, Maryland

1. Developed thrombus-resistant heparinised surfaces for use in heart valves (1963).
2. Collaborated with Weirich and Lillehei in developing transthoracic myocardial pacing systems (1957).
3. With Dewall, developed a bubble oxygenator (1957), and modified it to disposable oxygenator as used by Cooley.
4. Developed biomaterials as vessels and shunts.
5. Leading surgeon in the treatment of the Marfan aorta.
6. Past President of the Society for Thoracic Surgeons, USA.

Griepp, Randall, MD
New York, New York

1. Pioneer in the field of thoracic aortic surgery, particularly in the areas of hypothermia, cerebral protection and aortic arch replacement.

Gross, Robert E, MD
Boston, Massachusetts

1. Performed closure of patent ductus arteriosus (1938) as suggested by John Munro (1907).
2. Performed resection of coarctation of aorta in collaboration with Hufnagel (1945).
3. Developed numerous techniques in the field of congenital cardiovascular anomalies.
4. Early leader in developing field of general paediatric surgery, as well as paediatric cardiac surgery.

Harken, Dwight E, MD
Cambridge, Massachusetts

1. Performed the first consistently successful elective intracardiac surgery (removal of shell fragments from the heart, 1944–45).
2. Shared in the development of mitral valvuloplasty for mitral stenosis (1948).
3. Developed technique for closed aortic valvuloplasty. Developed heart valves, heart–lung machines, instruments and surgical techniques for acquired and congenital heart disease.
4. Performed the first successful human implantation of caged-ball valve in normal anatomical site (1960).
5. With Clauss and Birtwell, developed aortic counterpulsation as a mechanism of reducing left ventricular work and increasing coronary perfusion.
6. Placed first totally implantable demand pacemaker (1966), developed by Berkovits and tested with Zaroff, Zuckerman and Matloff.
7. Tested with Lefemine the efficacy and safety of Berkovits' direct current defibrillator in the laboratory, and applied its first clinical use.
8. Collaborator with Beall and others in developing The Association for the Advancement of Medical Instrumentation as a forum for medicine, engineering, industry and government.
9. Established the first designated Intensive Care Unit with Edith Heideman at Peter Bent Brigham Hospital (1951). Nurse Heideman became a director of nursing at the Henry Ford Hospital in Detroit.

10. Past President of the American College of Cardiology, and Chairman of the Heart House campaign.

Heimbecker, Raymond O, MD
London, Canada

1. Performed *in vivo* microcirculation research in collaboration with Bigelow from 1949, with special emphasis on microaggregation in shock.
2. Performed homograft valve placement in thoracic aorta with Murray in 1955 and the first clinical homograft mitral valve replacement in March 1962, following laboratory studies of their function and fate (from 1959).
3. Involved in the early development of extracorporeal circulation with special emphasis on hypothermia and temperature control by heat-exchanger devices.
4. Performed experimental studies of acute myocardial ischaemia and the effects of acute and chronic resection.

Holmes-Sellors, Sir Thomas, PRCS
London, England

1. Pioneer of closed cardiac operations, particularly pulmonary valvotomy and closure of atrial septal defect.
2. Distinguished 'gentleman' of thoracic surgery and President of the Royal College of Surgeons.

Hufnagel, Charles A, MD
Washington, DC

1. Developed plastics for blood contact implants, blood vessels, heart valves, extracorporeal instrumentation and artificial kidneys.
2. Designed and used the ball valve in the descending aorta for aortic insufficiency.
3. Pioneer in low profile mitral valves.
4. First used a cloth-type prosthesis for vascular replacement.
5. Introduced external shunts for the correction of coarctation of the aorta.
6. Developed vessel preservation by rapid freezing.
7. Developed ethylene oxide tissue sterilisation.
8. Pioneered local hypothermia for myocardial protection.

Jude, James R, MD
Miami, Florida

1. With Knickerbocker and Kouwenhoven developed external cardiac massage. This was of extreme importance in itself, but also because it stopped the epidemic of open thoracotomy and manual systole. External cardiac massage was important particularly in the Intensive Care Unit, and it led to the development of Coronary Care Units by Hughes Day.

Kantrowitz, Adrian, MD
Detroit, Michigan

1. Demonstrated that augmentation of diastolic aortic pressure could increase coronary blood flow (1953).
2. Performed the first human implantation of a permanent left ventricular assist device (1967).
3. Early developer of cardiac pacemakers.
4. Performed second human heart transplant after extensive laboratory procedures.
5. First to use the balloon counterpulsation pump in humans (1967).

Kay, Earle B, MD
Cleveland, Ohio

1. Developer of numerous closed heart operations (1946–56).

2. Developed operation for transposition of great vessels (1955).
3. With Cross, developed the rotating disc pump oxygenator (1955).
4. Pioneer in myocardial protection by metabolic and perfusion techniques.
5. Developed heart valves simultaneously and independently of the work of Harken and Muller (1960).
6. Developed tricuspid stent annuloplasty for tricuspid and mitral valve insufficiency subsequently applied by Blondeau, DuBost and Carpentier.
7. Worked with biological heart valves. Developed with Suzuki an early low profile mitral valve with essentially physiological function.
8. One of the most versatile clinical surgeons in myocardial revascularisation. Worked with retroperfusion of the coronary sinus.

Kay, Jerome Harold, MD

Los Angeles, California

1. Student of cardiac arrest and its management by 'external' massage and external defibrillation.
2. Developed instruments, heart–lung machines and heart valves.
3. Strong advocate of valve repair rather than replacement.

Kirklin, John W, MD

Birmingham, Alabama

1. Improved Gibbon's screen oxygenator for wide and practical use.
2. Leader in computerisation of monitoring and treatment of critically ill patients.
3. Pioneer in all areas of cardiac surgery but particularly congenital heart disease and biological valve replacement.
4. Possessed of a unique ability to simplify and apply new surgical techniques.
5. Master of harvesting, distilling and presenting multi-faceted experimental and clinical material in usable form.
6. Past President of The American Association for Thoracic Surgery, and Editor of *The Journal of Thoracic and Cardiovascular Surgery*.

Kolff, Willem J, PhD, MD

Salt Lake City, Utah

1. Pioneer in development of artificial organs, particularly the renal dialysis apparatus during World War II and the artificial heart (1957) with Robert Jarvik.
2. With Moulopoulos and Topaz, developed the intra-aortic balloon for counterpulsation (1961).
3. Pace setter in the field of artificial organs.

Kouchoukos, Nicholas MD

St Louis, Missouri

1. Leader in the fields of myocardial revascularisation and thoracic aortic surgery.

Lam, Conrad R, MD

Detroit, Michigan

1. Pioneer of surgical techniques for correcting congenital and acquired heart disease, including induced cardiac (potassium chloride or acetylcholine) arrest.
2. Performed physiological studies involving the mechanism of death from intracardiac air and its reversibility, with T Gahagan.
3. Pioneered the use of newly purified heparin (1939).

Landsteiner, K, MD

Vienna, Austria

1. Discovered that 'human blood contained isoagglutinins capable of agglutinating other human blood'.
2. Divided human blood into groups (1900).

Lev, Maurice, MD

Chicago, Illinois

1. Evolved the morbid pathology of congenital heart disease into a sound foundation for corrective surgery.
2. His own epitaph: 'The guy who saved a few kids from heart block.'

Lillehei, C Walton, MD

St Paul, Minnesota

1. Creator and innovator of perhaps more techniques and concepts than any other living heart surgeon.
2. Developed open heart surgery by cross circulation of a father to his infant (1954).
3. Collaborated with DeWall in development and use of the bubble oxygenator (1955).
4. Developed plastic disposable bag bubble oxygenator.
5. Introduced haemodilution and moderate hypothermia techniques for open heart surgery.
6. With Lande, developed simple disposable membrane oxygenator (1967).
7. Invented heart valves.
8. Extended the opportunities afforded him by Wangensteen to his own illustrious disciples, including Shumway, Gott, Barnard and others.

Litwak, Robert S, MD

New York, New York

1. Early investigator of intracardiac homografts.
2. With Gadboys, evolved the concept and understanding of homologous transfusion reactions. This and subsequent work supported haemodilution techniques for open heart surgery.
3. Developed a left ventricular circulatory assist system to support critically ill patients which could be discontinued without reopening the chest.

Loop, Floyd, MD

Cleveland, Ohio

1. Pursued developments in coronary artery surgery after the beginnings by Favoloro and Sones.
2. Developed the cardiac surgery programme at the Cleveland Clinic and was one of the first cardiac surgeons to become Chief Executive of a leading institution.

Lower, Richard R, MD

Richmond, Virginia

1. Pioneer in cardiac transplantation and investigator of rejection modes.

McGoon, Dwight C, MD

Rochester, Minnesota

1. Pace setter for surgical procedures to correct complex congenital heart disease.
2. Sponsor of professional bridges of communication, national and international.
3. Editor of *The Journal of Thoracic and Cardiovascular Surgery*.

Magill, Sir Ivan Whiteside

London, England

1. Opened opportunities for thoracic and heart surgery with intratracheal anaesthesia.

Magovern, George J, MD

Pittsburgh, Pennsylvania

1. Early advocate of central venous pressure monitoring in the postoperative patient as a guide to blood volume replacement.
2. Developed a sutureless technique of fixation for aortic and mitral ball valve prostheses (1961). His collaboration with engineer and instrument designer Harry Cromie was central to this success.
3. Past President of the Society of Thoracic Surgeons, USA.

Malm, James R, MD

New York, New York

1. Demonstrated reproducibility and low mortality in the correction of tetralogy of Fallot and developed infant cardiac surgery in several areas.
2. With others including Kirklin, evaluated homografts and their potential, and the limitations of some sterilisation and preservation techniques.

Meredino, K Alvin, MD

Riyadh, Saudi Arabia

1. Investigator in laboratory and clinical use of behaviour of biological valves.
2. Ingenious developer of plastic techniques for acquired valvular insufficiency and atrioplastic procedures to correct congenital transposition of the great vessels.

Morrow, A Glenn, MD

Bethesda, Maryland

1. Pioneered left heart catheterisation by the transbronchial technique based on Allison's concept.
2. Performed the first direct vision valvotomy under general hypothermia for congenital aortic stenosis.
3. Performed the first successful complete mitral valve replacement with synthetic material simulating a normal mitral valve (in collaboration with Nina Braunwald), one day after Harken's first successful caged-ball aortic valve replacement (1960).
4. Investigated biomaterials for patches and valve leaflets.
5. Performed basic studies in hypertrophic subaortic stenosis, its mechanism, diagnosis and surgical correction.
6. Contributed to the concept of porcine heterografts on a flexible stent (first implantation, 1970).
7. Contributed to the unique climate in the National Heart and Lung Institute that has improved diagnostic and surgical techniques for correcting congenital and acquired heart disease.

Muller, W Harry, Jr, MD

Charlottesville, Virginia

1. Developed pulmonary vascular changes in experimental animals secondary to pulmonary hypertension.
2. With F Damman, developed the pulmonary banding operation.
3. Performed the first operation for total anomalous venous return.
4. Performed definitive repair of Marfan's syndrome by resecting the ascending aortic aneurysm and repairing the aortic valve.
5. Performed early definitive repair of a dissecting aneurysm with the pump oxygenator.

Murray, DW Gordon, MD, FRCS(C.), FRCS(E)

Toronto, Canada

1. Innovative and technical genius who made enormous contributions in the development of cardiovascular surgery.
2. Early pioneer of the use of heparin to prevent pulmonary emboli.
3. First used human homograft valves (inserted in descending aorta). Used homograft veins and showed that they arterialised.
4. Tried subclavian coronary artery anastomosis in dogs (1940s).
5. Tried fascia lata for valve replacement.
6. Produced the first artificial kidney in America (second in the world).

Mustard, WT, FRCS

Toronto, Canada

1. Ingenious and courageous pioneer in the surgical correction of transposition of the great vessels.

Nadas, Alexander S, MD

Boston, Massachusetts

1. Made clinical and physiological correlation leading to the establishment of the speciality of paediatric cardiology; published the first comprehensive textbook of paediatric cardiology.
2. Medical collaborator with surgeon Robert E Gross in developmental phases of open and closed cardiac and great vessel operations.

O'Shaughnessy, Laurence, FRCS

Newcastle-Upon-Tyne, England

1. Used omentum and irritant paste to cause revascularisation via vascular adhesions (1933). Was aware of Thorel's case (1903) of patient who died of carcinoma of the lung, but who had 'adhesive pericarditis' and complete obliteration of the main coronary arteries.
2. Suggested valvotomy for congenital pulmonary valve stenosis.
3. Died in his own casualty-clearing hospital of tension pneumothorax in the Dunkirk retreat, World War II.

Paget, Sir Stephen

London, England

1. Leading surgeon of his time. His classical dour prediction of 1896 was: 'The heart alone of all viscera has reached the limits set by nature to surgery. No new method and no new technique can overcome the natural obstacles surrounding a wound of the heart.' (Ludwig Rehn of Frankfurt succeeded in 1896.)

Piwnica, Armand, MD

Paris, France

1. Proponent of aortic homograft and stentless valve techniques in France.
2. Past President of the European Society of Cardiothoracic Surgery.

Potts, Willis J, MD

Chicago, Illinois

1. Brilliant paediatric surgeon.
2. Developed pulmonary artery/aortic shunt for cyanotic congenital heart disease.

Rehn, Ludwig, MD
Frankfurt, Germany
1. Successfully sutured a stab wound of the heart in 1896. A great victory of a 'doer' over the 'doubter' Paget. (The doubters always have a statistical advantage.)

Roe, Benson B, MD
San Francisco, California
1. Pioneered the use of elective ventricular fibrillation.
2. Utilised left atrial pressure measurement after open heart surgery to reduce the mortality of low output syndrome.
3. Promulgator of the disposable bubble oxygenator.
4. Developed and refined techniques for congenital anomalies, including Ebstein's anomaly.

Ross, Donald N, FRCS
London, England
1. Described the sinus venosus congenital defect.
2. Introduced aortic homograft valves into clinical use.
3. Performed the 'Rastelli operation,' right ventricular outflow tract reconstruction with valve conduit before Rastelli (1966).
4. Developed the pulmonary autograft operation for aortic replacement.

Sabiston, David C, Jr, MD
Durham, North Carolina
1. Extended understanding of physiology of the myocardium and coronary circulation as it relates to myocardial contraction and revascularisation.
2. Studied the diagnosis and nature of pulmonary embolism.
3. Explored fluid fluorocarbon for oxygen transport in experimental extracorporeal circulation.
4. Added clarity to the physiopathology of myocardial infarction.
5. Performed early aortocoronary artery bypass (probably first in a human patient, who lived 3 days) (1962). Published with beautiful illustrations (1974).
6. Structured the management of dissecting aneursyms.

Sakakibara, Shigeru, MD
Tokyo, Japan
1. With Konno, developed a cardiac biotome for use before open heart surgery and developed the first transvenous myocardial biopsy technique.
2. Devised oxygenators, and combined them with hypothermia (1956 and later, originally with Konno).
3. With Arai, developed many ingenious operations in the laboratory, then clinically, for congenital heart disease. Performed the first cardiovascular operation in Japan (1956).
4. Founded the Heart Institute of Japan at Tokyo Women's Medical College.

Sealy, Will C, MD
Durham, North Carolina
1. Explained postoperative arteritis and paradoxical hypertension related to coarctation of the aorta and the nature of hypertension in coarctation.
2. Pioneered surface cooling with extracorporeal circulation; used deep hypothermia and circulatory arrest controlled by the first heat exchanger (with Ivan Brown and Glenn Young).
3. Mapped atrial internodal conduction paths.

4. Explained shunt flow pathophysiology.
5. Performed the first correction of WPW dysrrhythmia.
6. Developed bundle of His and AV node exclusion in dysrrhythmias.
7. Performed studies on hypercapnea, alkalosis and acid–base balance.

Senning, Åke, MD
Zurich, Switzerland
1. Introduced elective fibrillation in heart surgery.
2. Combined efforts to develop a heart–lung machine with Crafoord and Björk (1954).
3. Corrected total anomalous venous return (1956).
4. Developed circulatory assist techniques by left heart bypass (some with Dennis).
5. Developed atrial repair of TGA (1958) — Senning's operation.
6. Performed the first pacemaker implantation (1958).

Shumway, Norman E, MD
Stanford, California
1. The prime investigator in the field of cardiac transplantation. He has forged the multidisciplinary effort and persisted when others abandoned the operation.
2. Developed the unit at Stanford and refined many techniques in adult and congenital cardiac surgery.

Sones, Mason, MD
Cleveland, Ohio
1. Developed the equipment and techniques for coronary angiography. Investigated the diagnosis, prognosis and results of both medical and surgical treatment of heart disease. His work added the essential precision to open the field of coronary artery surgery.

Souttar, Sir Henry, FRCS
London, England
1. Successfully explored mitral valve digitally via the left atrial appendage (1925). When asked by Harken why he did not repeat the magnificent operation, he replied, 'Because I could not get another case ... the physicians declared it was all nonsense ... it is of no use to be ahead of one's time.'

Spencer, Frank C, MD
New York, New York
1. Deemed 'the Larrey of the Korean War' for his excellent management of arterial injuries in battle casualties.
2. Pioneer in monitoring of patients after open heart surgery and circulatory assistance guided by appropriate blood gas and electrolyte measurements.
3. Technical innovator and designer of instruments, including silastic coronary perfusion cannulae.

Stark, Jarda, FRCS
London, England
1. Pioneer of congenital heart surgery with David Waterston and Marc DeLeval at the Hospital for Sick Children, Great Ormond Street.
2. Past President of the European Society of Cardiothoracic Surgery.

Starr, Albert, MD

Portland, Oregon

1. The most meticulous investigator, innovator and clinical user of caged-ball valves. His standards of quality control in valve development and follow-up of patients set the standards for others.
2. Innovator of surgical techniques for congenital and acquired heart defects.

Streider, John W, MD

Boston, Massachusetts

1. Made the first attempt to close a patent ductus (1937). Though the patient died, he and his medical collaborators defined the ethical position for risk taking and experimental surgery. This standard has been widely followed.

Swan, Henry, MD

Denver, Colorado

1. Performed early resection of aneurysms with aortic homograft replacement (1949), and performed the first peripheral arterial replacement with homografts.
2. Performed the first series of open heart operations under hypothermia. (Lewis preceded with atrial septal defect closure, and Varco with open correction of pulmonic stenosis without hypothermia.)

Swann, HJC, MD

Los Angeles, California

1. The cardiologist and physiologist who developed the pulmonary artery catheter that bears his name and his co-worker's, 'Swann–Ganz'.

Taussig, Helen B, MD

Baltimore, Maryland

1. Recognised that cyanotic children often died when the ductus closed.
2. Inspired by Gross's closure of patent ductus arteriosus, she sought a surgeon to 'build a ductus'. Persuaded Blalock to try it in the laboratory, then in humans.
3. Her cyanotic patients for the Blalock–Taussig operation were the first to be palliated by surgery.

Trusler, George, MD

Toronto, Canada

1. Pre-eminent Canadian paediatric surgeon at the Hospital for Sick Children, Toronto.
2. Developed the aortic valve repair technique for patients with ventricular septal defect and prolapsed cusps.

Turina, Marko, MD

Zurich, Switzerland

1. Pioneer in thoracic aortic surgery.
2. Collaborator with Senning in many paediatric advances.
3. Outstanding Editor of *The European Journal of Cardiothoracic Surgery*.

Tubbs, Oswald, FRCS

London, England

1. Developed an improved dilator for closed mitral valvotomy.
2. Performed the first ligation of ductus arteriosus for endocarditis.

Urschel, Harold C, MD

Dallas, Texas

1. Innovator and extender of revascularisation procedures.
2. Past President of American College of Chest Physicians.

Varco, Richard, MD

Minneapolis, Minnesota

1. Collaborated in early open heart surgery with Dennis (1951).
2. Collaborated with Lillehei in cross-circulation (1954).
3. Actively pursued ileal bypass as a metabolic prophylaxis against atherosclerosis.

Vineberg, Arthur, MD

Montreal, Canada

1. Creator of Vineberg mammary artery implantation for coronary artery disease (1946).
2. His work was based on extensive experimental laboratory research until graft patency was proved by Sones.

Wada, Juro J, MD

Tokyo, Japan

1. Bubbled and debubbled venous blood to oxygenate (1953), and developed a pump oxygenator.
2. Pioneered tilting disc hingeless Wada–Cutter Heart Valve (1966).
3. Used a hyper basic oxygenation chamber for severe cyanotic heart disease (1967).
4. Performed total aortic arch replacement with immersion hypothermia (1960).
5. Performed first ascending aortic aneurysm resection in Japan (1959).
6. Performed the only heart transplantation in Japan (1968), and was severely criticised because there was no definition of brain death.

Wallace, Robert, MD

Washington DC

1. Developed surgical techniques in congenital heart disease with McGoon and Kirklin at the Mayo Clinic.
2. Past President of the American Association for Thoracic Surgery.

Waterston, David J, FRCS

London, England

1. Devised aortopulmonary anastomosis.
2. Outstanding surgeon and teacher.

Wiggers, Carl J, MD

Cleveland, Ohio

1. A cardiac physiologist who linked laboratory experiments to clinical findings in medicine and surgery.

Wolner, Hans, MD

Vienna, Austria

1. Pioneer of artificial heart technology
2. Pre-eminent Austrian Professor of cardiac surgery and proponent of thoracic aortic surgical technique.
3. President of the European Society of Cardiothoracic Surgery.

Wooler, Geoffrey, FRCS

Leeds, England

1. Pioneer of mitral valve repair techniques.
2. Developer of tissue valve prostheses with Marion Ionescu.

Yacoub, Sir Magdi, FRCS

London, England

1. World-renowned surgical technician and pioneer of operative techniques for congenital and acquired heart disease.
2. Most prolific heart and lung transplanter in the world.
3. Proponent of new scientific methods in cardiac surgery, particularly in the field of molecular biology.

Zerbini, Euriclides DeJesus, MD

São Paulo, Brazil

1. Brilliant innovator of surgical techniques and instruments.
2. Performed a multitude of regional first operations and led Brazilian manufacturers to create equipment not otherwise available from the outside world.
3. Innovator of biological valves (dura mater).
4. Modest and creative teacher, clinician, and founder of Brazilian Heart Institute.

Zoll, Paul M, MD

Boston, Massachusetts

1. Pioneer of external, then implantable cardiac pacemakers.
2. Made precise anatomical studies of coronary arteries in health and disease with Blumgart and Schlessinger.
3. Collaborated with Harken as the cardiologist in World War II foreign body work.

Zuhdi, Nazih, MD

Oklahoma City, Oklahoma

1. Developed a rotating screen oxygenator with Clarence Dennis and Karl Karlson (1953); and collaborated in the first mechanical pump support for chronic heart failure (1955).
2. Combined efforts in developing plastic sheet oxygenator (bubble type) with Gott, DeWall and others (1956).
3. Developed several heat exchange systems and the double helical reservoir heart–lung machine.
4. First used glutaraldehyde fixed porcine valves in the aortic and mitral positions in humans (with Warren Hancock, 1970).
5. Used the first total haemodilution prime of a heart–lung machine (with 5% dextrose in water), combined with moderate hypothermia (experimentally and clinically, 1960).

Names Index

Biographies are in **bold** type

Subject Index

Page numbers in *italic* indicate illustrations